P9-BBQ-509

RESEARCH IN
OCCUPATIONAL
THERAPY

Methods of Inquiry
for Enhancing Practice

Gary Kielhofner, DrPH, OTR/L, FAOTA

Professor and Wade-Meyer Chair
Department of Occupational Therapy
College of Applied Health Sciences
University of Illinois at Chicago

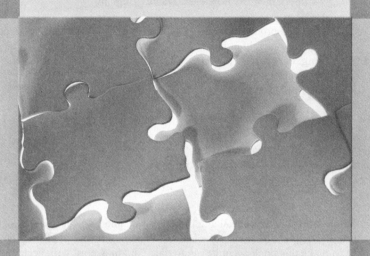

Research in Occupational Therapy

Methods of Inquiry for Enhancing Practice

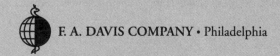

F. A. DAVIS COMPANY • Philadelphia

F. A. Davis Company
1915 Arch Street
Philadelphia, PA 19103
www.fadavis.com

Printed in the United States of America

Last digit indicates print number: 10 9 8 7 6 5 4 3

Acquisitions Editor: Christa A. Fratantoro
Manager of Content Development: Deborah J. Thorp
Developmental Editor: Peg Waltner
Design Manager: Carolyn O'Brien

As new scientific information becomes available through basic and clinical research, recommended treatments and drug therapies undergo changes. The authors and publisher have done everything possible to make this book accurate, up to date, and in accord with accepted standards at the time of publication. The authors, editors, and publisher are not responsible for errors or omissions or for consequences from application of the book, and make no warranty, expressed or implied, in regard to the contents of the book. Any practice described in this book should be applied by the reader in accordance with professional standards of care used in regard to the unique circumstances that may apply in each situation. The reader is advised always to check product information (package inserts) for changes and new information regarding dose and contraindications before administering any drug. Caution is especially urged when using new or infrequently ordered drugs.

Library of Congress Cataloging-in-Publication Data

Kielhofner, Gary
  Research in occupational therapy : methods of inquiry for enhancing practice /
Gary Kielhofner.
     p. cm.
  Includes bibliographical references and index.
  ISBN-13: 978-0-8036-1525-0
  ISBN 10: 0-8036-1525-6
  1. Occupational therapy—Research. I. Title.
  RM735.K54 2006
  615.8′515—dc22

                                                                    2006041013

This book is dedicated to:

A. Jean Ayres,
for role-modeling the vocation of a scientist in
the field

Mary Reilly,
for providing timeless insights into the nature
of knowledge and discovery in occupational
therapy

Noomi Katz,
for demonstrating open and persistent inquiry
into a complex clinical problem

Anne Mosey,
for logically critiquing how scholarship should
advance the practice of occupational therapy

Elizabeth Yerxa,
for demonstrating how to love the questions
posed by our field

And to all others who have passed on to a
current generation of scholars the passion,
persistance, and perspectives necessary to
scholarship in occupational therapy

CONTRIBUTORS

Beatriz C. Abreu, PhD, OTR, FAOTA
Clinical Professor
Department of Occupational Therapy
School of Allied Health Sciences
University of Texas Medical Branch;
Director of Occupational Therapy
Transitional Learning Center at Galveston
Galveston, Texas

Marian Arbesman, PhD, OTR/L
Clinical Assistant Professor
Department of Rehabilitation Science
University at Buffalo; President, ArbesIdeas, Inc.
Consultant, AOTA Evidence-Based Literature
    Review Project
Buffalo, New York

Nancy A. Baker, ScD, OTR/L
Assistant Professor
School of Health and Rehabilitation Sciences
University of Pittsburgh
Pittsburgh, Pennsylvania

Brent Braveman, PhD, OTR/L, FAOTA
Clinical Associate Professor
Director of Professional Education
Department of Occupational Therapy
College of Applied Health Sciences
University of Illinois at Chicago
Chicago, Illinois

Lisa Castle, MBA, OTR/L
Director of Occupational Therapy
University of Illinois Medical Center at Chicago
Chicago, Illinois

Sherrilene Classen, PhD, MPH, OTR/L
Assistant Professor
University of Florida
College of Public Health and Health Professions
Gainesville, Florida

Mary A. Corcoran, PhD, OTR, FAOTA
Research Professor
The George Washington University
Department of Health Care Sciences
School of Medicine and Health Sciences
Washington, DC;
Professor
Department of Occupational Therapy
Shenandoah University
Winchester VA

Susan Corr, DipCOT, MPhil, DIPMed ED, PhD
Reader in Occupational Science
School of Health
The University of Northampton
Park Campus,
Northampton, England

Wendy J. Coster, PhD, OTR/L, FAOTA
Associate Professor and Chair
Department of Occupational Therapy and
    Rehabilitation Counseling
Sargent College of Health & Rehabilitation
    Sciences
Boston University
Boston, Massachusetts

Anne Cusick, BAppSc(OT), MA, PhD
College of Science and Health
University of Western Sydney
Penrith South, Australia

Jean Crosetto Deitz, PhD, OTR/L, FAOTA
Professor & Graduate Program Coordinator
Department of Rehabilitation Medicine
University of Washington
Seattle, Washington

Anne E. Dickerson, PhD, OTR/L, FAOTA
Professor and Chair
Department of Occupational Therapy
East Carolina University; Co-Director of
    Research for Older Adult Driver Initiative
    (ROADI)
Editor of Occupational Therapy in Health Care
Greenville, North Carolina

M. G. Dieter, MLIS, MBA
Clinical Assistant Professor, Health Informatics
Department of Biomedical and Health
    Information Sciences
University of Illinois at Chicago
Chicago, Illinois

Heather Dillaway, PhD
Assistant Professor, Sociology
Wayne State University
Detroit, Michigan

Claire-Jehanne Dubouloz, OT(c), PhD
Associate Professor
Associate Dean of the Faculty of Health Sciences
Director of the School of Rehabilitation Sciences
University of Ottawa
Ontario, Canada

**Edward A. S. Duncan, PhD, BSc(Hons),
    Dip.CBT, SROT**
Postdoctoral Research Fellow
Nursing, Midwifery and Allied Health
    Professions Research Unit
The University of Stirling
Stirling, Scotland
Clinical Specialist Occupational Therapist
Occupational Therapy Department
The State Hospital
Carstairs, Scotland

Mary Egan, PhD, OT(C)
Associate Professor
School of Rehabilitation Sciences
University of Ottawa
Ontario, Canada

Marcia Finlayson, PhD, OT(C), OTR/L
Associate Professor
Department of Occupational Therapy
College of Applied Health Sciences
University of Illinois at Chicago
Chicago, Illinois

Gail Fisher, MPA, OTR/L
Associate Department Head for Administration
Clinical Associate Professor
Department of Occupational Therapy
University of Illinois at Chicago
Chicago, Illinois

Kirsty Forsyth, PhD, OTR
Senior Lecturer
Occupational Therapy Department
Queen Margaret University College
Edinburgh, Scotland

Ellie Fossey, DipCOT (UK), MSC
Senior Lecturer - Postgraduate Courses
    Coordinator
School of Occupational Therapy
La Trobe University;
PhD Candidate
School of Social Work
The University of Melbourne
Victoria, Australia

Patricia Heyn, PhD
Senior Research Instructor
Division of Geriatric Medicine/School of
    Medicine
University of Colorado Health Sciences Center
Denver, Colorado

Frederick J. Kviz, PhD
Professor
Community Health Sciences
School of Public Health
University of Illinois at Chicago
Chicago, Illinois

Mark R. Luborsky, PhD
Professor of Anthropology and Gerontology
Director of Aging and Health Disparities Research
Institute of Gerontology
Wayne State University
Detroit, Michigan

Cathy Lysack, PhD, OT(C)
Associate Professor, Occupational Therapy and
    Gerontology
Wayne State University
Detroit, Michigan

Annie McCluskey, PhD, MA, DipCOT
Senior Lecturer in Occupational Therapy
School of Exercise & Health Sciences
University of Western Sydney
Penrith South, Australia

Jane Melton, MSc, DipCOT (UK)
Lead Occupational Therapist for Practice
    Development & Research
Gloucestershire Partnership NHS Trust
The Charlton Lane Centre
Cheltenham, England

Jaime Phillip Muñoz, PhD, OTR, FAOTA
Assistant Professor
Department of Occupational Therapy
Duquesne University
Pittsburgh, Pennsylvania

David L. Nelson, PhD, OTR, FAOTA
Professor of Occupational Therapy
College of Health Sciences
Medical University of Ohio at Toledo
Toledo, Ohio

Kenneth J. Ottenbacher, PhD, OTR/L
Professor and Director
Division of Rehabilitation Sciences
University of Texas Medical Branch
Galveston, Texas

Sue Parkinson, BA, DipCOT
Practice Development Advisor for OTs
Derbyshire Mental Health Services NHS Trust
Derby, England

Amy Paul-Ward, PhD
Assistant Professor
Department of Occupational Therapy
Florida International University
Miami, Florida

Nadine Peacock, PhD
Associate Professor
Community Health Sciences
School of Public Health
Adjunct Associate Professor
Department of Anthropology
University of Illinois at Chicago
Chicago, Illinois

Geneviève Pépin, PhD, OTR
Adjunct Professor
Occupational Therapy Program
Rehabilitation Department
Laval University
Quebec, Canada

Mick Robson, DipCOT
Formerly a Senior Research Practitioner within
    the Central and North West
        London Mental Health NHS Trust
        (CNWL)/UK Centre of Outcomes Research
        and Education (UKCORE) Partnership
London, England

Yolanda Suarez-Balcazar, PhD
Associate Professor
Department of Occupational Therapy
Associate Director, Center for Capacity Building
    for Minorities with Disabilities Research
University of Illinois at Chicago
Chicago, Illinois

Pimjai Sudsawad, ScD, OTR
Assistant Professor
Occupational Therapy Program
Department of Kinesiology
University of Wisconsin-Madison
Madison, Wisconsin

Lynn Summerfield-Mann, DipCOT, SROT, MSc
Doctoral Student
Principal Lecturer in Occupational Therapy
Department of Allied Health Professions
Faculty of Health & Social Care
London South Bank University
London, England

Renée R. Taylor, PhD
Associate Professor
Department of Occupational Therapy
University of Illinois at Chicago
Chicago, Illinois

Machiko R. Tomita, PhD
Clinical Associate Professor
Department of Rehabilitation Science
Director, Aging and Technology Projects
School of Public Health and Health Professions
University at Buffalo
Buffalo, New York

Hector W. H. Tsang, PhD, OTR
Associate Professor
Department of Rehabilitation Sciences
The Hong Kong Polytechnic University
Hong Kong

Toni Van Denend, MS, OTR/L
RehabWorks
Staff Therapist
Hunt Valley
Maryland

Craig A. Velozo, PhD, OTR
Associate Professor and Associate Chair
Department of Occupational Therapy
College of Public Health and Health Professions;
Research Health Scientist
North Florida\South Georgia Veterans Health
    System
University of Florida
Gainesville, Florida

Elizabeth White, PhD, DipCOT
Head of Research and Development
College of Occupational Therapists
London, England

Suzie Willis, DipCOT, SROT, MSC, MA
Head Research Practitioner
Central and Northwest London Mental Health
    Trust
Tamarind Centre
Park Royal Centre for Mental Health
London, England

Don E. Workman, PhD
Executive Director
Office for the Protection of Research Subjects
Northwestern University
Chicago, Illinois

Yow-Wu B. Wu, PhD
Associate Professor
School of Nursing
University at Buffalo
Buffalo, New York

REVIEWERS

Catherine Emery MS, OTR/L, BCN
Assistant Professor
Occupational Therapy Program
Alvernia College
Lancaster, Pennsylvania

Karen Funk, OTD, OTR
Assistant Professor
University of Texas, El Paso
El Paso, Texas

Heather A. Gallew, OTD, OTR/L
Assistant Professor of Occupational Therapy
Xavier University
Cincinnati, Ohio

Robert W. Gibson, MSOTR/L
Research Associate
University of Florida
Gainesville, Florida

Stacie Lynn Iken, PhD, MS, OTR/L
Occupational Therapy Program Director &
   Associate Professor
University of Mary
Bismarck, North Dakota

Panelpha L. Kyler, MA, OT, FAOTA
Public Health Analyst & Adjunct Faculty Genetic
   Services Branch
Maternal & Child Health Bureau
Health Resources & Services Administration
Department of Health & Human Services
Towson University
Bethesda, Maryland

Jennie Q. Lou, M.D., M.Sc., OTR
Associate Professor of Public Health & Associate
   Professor of Occupational Therapy
Nova Southeastern University
Ft. Lauderdale, Florida

Ferol Menks Ludwig, PhD, OTR, FAOTA, GCG
Professor & Director of Doctoral Program
Nova Southeastern University
Ft. Lauderdale, Florida

Rosemary M. Lysaght, PhD, OTR/L
Assistant Professor
University of Utah
Salt Lake City, Utah

Maralynne D. Mitcham, PhD, OTR/L, FAOTA
Professor & Director
Occupational Therapy Educational Program
College of Health Professions
Medical University of South Carolina
Charleston, South Carolina

Carol Reed, EdD, OTR, FAOTA
Professor & Chair
Occupational Therapy Department
Nova Southeastern University
Plantation, Florida

Pat Sample, PhD
Associate Professor
Occupational Therapy
Colorado State University
Fort Collins, Colorado

Barbara A. Boyt Schell, PhD, OTR/L, FAOTA
Professor & Chair
Occupational Therapy
Brenau University
Athens, Georgia

Karen Sladyk, PhD, OTR, FAOTA
Professor & Chair
Bay Path College
Longmeadow, Massachusetts

Janet H. Watts, PhD, OTR, CRC
Associate Professor & Director of Post-
   Professional Graduate Studies
Virginia Commonwealth University
Richmond, Virginia

Shirley A. Wells, MPH, OTR, FAOTA
Assistant Professor
University of Texas
Brownsville, Texas

Those who enter the profession of occupational therapy come with a desire to enable people to participate more fully in everyday life. The profession's mission is practical and humanistic. Not surprisingly, the mention of research in occupational therapy can engender expectations of an uninteresting and technical topic of limited relevance. This is not surprising. Research is often written about as though it were mysterious and quite apart from practical therapeutic work. As a consequence, discussions of research can sometimes make it appear inaccessible and remote from occupational therapy practice.

Investigators, such as those who have contributed to this book, do research because they find the process of discovery exhilarating and because they see how it enhances occupational therapy practice. Thus, in this text, we have sought to underscore two themes. First, we have sought to illustrate how research is a creative process of discovering and sharing new information. We have aimed to demonstrate that research is not only comprehensible but also engaging. Second, we have made specific efforts to demonstrate how research is both essential to and can support and improve occupational therapy practice. We sought to accomplish this not only through constant use of occupational therapy research examples, but also through addressing issues of how research contributes to professional knowledge and how research can be used by members of the profession.

> Investigators, such as those who have contributed to this book, do research because they find the process of discovery exhilarating and because they see how it enhances occupational therapy practice.

DEFINITIONS OF RESEARCH

One can readily find a number of definitions of research as it pertains to the field of health care. For instance, research has been defined as:

> " a systematic and principled way of obtaining evidence (data, information) for solving heath care problems" Polgar and Thomas, S.A. (2000, p 3)

> "a systematic search for and validation of knowledge about issues of importance..." Polit and Hungler (1999, p 3)

> "a structured process of investigating facts and theories and exploring connections" Portney and Watkins (2000, p 4)

> "Multiple, systematic strategies to generate knowledge about human behavior, human experience and human environments in which the thought and action processes of the researcher are clearly specified so that they are logical, understandable, confirmable, and useful". Depoy and Gitlin (1998, p 6)

Taken together, these definitions emphasize a number of important points. First, research is systematic, principled, structured, and logical. Second, it involves a process of investigation or obtaining evidence in order to generate knowledge, and test theories Third, research aims to study issues of importance and solve practical problems. These characteristics of research have been our point of departure and are emphasized throughout the text.

SCOPE, CONTENT, AND ORGANIZATION OF THE BOOK

This book discusses contemporary research methods and tools. It aims to comprehensively cover the range research relevant to occupational therapy. The book is designed to build an appreciation of the kinds of perspectives, strategies and specific tools that are used by researchers. It should also allow the reader to become a competent consumer of most types of research. Finally, it includes the necessary information to prepare one for being a competent collaborator in research.

Because the book is broad in scope, many topics are covered at the most basic level. Therefore, many chapters will provide the reader with many additional resources for understanding research reports and for participating in research.

Deciding how to organize and sequence the chapters in a text such as this is no small challenge; everyone consulted offered up differing opinions. Our strategy has been to organize the book into nine fairly small sections. Each section is designed to stand alone; however, some sections do rely on material discussed in other sections and the reader will profit from referring to those other chapters. Within each section, the chapters are generally best read in sequence.

Importantly, the sequence of the sections and the chapters within the sections is not intended to convey anything about importance. To a large extent, sequence was driven by how we felt the underlying logical with which we sought to explain research would best unfold.

Reading this book can be approached in a variety of ways. Most readers will find it helpful to complete section one first, since it discusses some of the broadest and most basic topics related to research in occupational therapy. Beyond this first section, the sequence can depend on the reader's interest or the organization for a course or coursework for which to book is being used. Below each section is described to give a sense of its purpose and contents.

The first section introduces the reader to the nature and scope of research and its place in occupational therapy. Chapters address why research is needed, philosophical underpinnings of research, the range of research methods, the basic process common to all forms of research, and the various roles and responsibilities that members of the profession should and can take on related to research. By the end of the section, the reader should have a very broad idea of aims of research, the assumptions, principles and concerns that guide research, and the different ways that research can be conducted. Additionally, the reader should appreciate what the results of research have to do with the profession and what members of the profession should have to do with research.

The second section covers major forms of quantitative research designs (i.e., exploratory, group comparison, survey, retrospective, longitudinal, and single subject) These chapters aim to provide an overview of both the logic and methods that belong to each design. Readers should glean a substantial understanding of what types of research questions quantitative designs can address and how such designs answer these questions.

Section three addresses a specific issue underlying quantitative research, namely; how investigators quantify or measure the phenomena they study. The rigor of all quantitative investigation rests on how adequately the researcher has operationalized the variables of interest. Thus, the quantification of research variables must be carefully approached. Three chapters address this issue from the different perspectives of classical test theory, contemporary item response theory, and a critical reflection on the aims, value, and limits of quantification.

The fourth section completes coverage of quantitative research by discussing the major statistical methods used in such research. In addition to the overview of statistics provided by the chapters, this section includes tables that provide, at a glance: summaries of the questions various statistics answer, requirements for appropriate application of the statistic, and how the numbers generated by the statistic should be interpreted.

Section five covers qualitative research methods. These chapters provide an overview of the logic and methods of qualitative research, and discuss how qualitative data are collected, managed and analyzed. This section aims to provide the reader with an understanding of the logic and range of qualitative methods, the various purposes to which qualitative research is put, and the major methodological procedures involved in doing qualitative research.

The sixth section covers research designs that do not neatly fit into either the broad quantitative or qualitative categories. Two chapters cover research approaches that achieve insights through systematically eliciting opinions or perspectives. A third chapter discusses how qualitative and quantitative research methods can be combined in a rigorous way.

Section seven covers in detail the various steps and procedures the investigators complete when they conduct research. The first chapter provides an overview of the main steps of research which are discussed in more detail in subsequent chapters. These include: searching the literature; identifying research questions; designing the study; assuring the research is ethically sound; obtaining funding for the research; securing samples; collecting, managing and analyzing data; disseminating findings; and writing a research report. This section aims to discuss the research process in such a way that the reader appreciates all the elements that go into research and so that a first-time researcher can systematically anticipate and plan for what is involved in a study.

Section eight discusses how research methods can specifically be used to enhance occupational therapy practice. It includes illustrations of how research methods can be applied to needs assessment and to program development and evaluation. Additionally this section features three chapters that address participatory research approaches. These approaches represent a promising way to conduct research that is grounded in and addresses the issues and perspectives of occupational therapy practitioners and consumers.

> We hope the book conveys the deep commitment that all who contributed feel toward the research process.

best suited their discussion. Because of its classic use certain key concepts still use the term, subject, in the phraseology (e.g., between-subjects variance or single-subject design). In such instances authors have retained classical terminology to avoid confusion. Other authors preferred use of the contemporary terms, such as participants, stakeholders or partners for their discussion.

Section nine discusses evidence based practice. The chapters in this section cover the definition, history and purpose and implementation of evidence-based practice. This section also addresses how practice can effectively be changed in response to evidence and how evidence can be generated in ways that are more relevant to practice.

A NOTE ON TERMINOLOGY

Convention about how to refer to persons who are being studied in an investigation has changed over the years. The classical term, subject, connoted that individuals were objects of inquiry and/or were subjected to experimental procedures. Contemporary researchers generally prefer the term, participant. This terminology stresses the extent to which people who are studied freely contribute time, personal information, and effort to a study. Still other researchers, who emphasize the importance of involving people who are being studied as partners in the research enterprise, use terms such as partners or stakeholders to refer to individuals whose circumstances are being investigated.

Throughout this text the authors of chapters were given freedom to use the terminology which

CONCLUSION

Writing this book was a challenging enterprise for all involved and reading it will be no less challenging. Nonetheless, the reader will find that the chapter authors are not only knowledgeable and passionate about their topic, but made substantial effort to help the reader comprehend the topic. We hope the book conveys the deep commitment that all who contributed feel toward the research process. Most of all, we hope that the reader will share some of that commitment after having digested this volume.

Gary Kielhofner

REFERENCES

DePoy, E. & Gitlin, L. (1998) *Introduction to Research: Understanding and Applying Multiple Strategies*. St. Louis: C.V. Mosby.

Polgar, S. & Thomas, S.A. (2000). *Introduction to Research in the Health Sciences*. Edinburgh: Churchill Livingston.

Polit, D.F. & Hungler, B.P. (1999). *Nursing Research: Principles and Methods*. Philadelphia: Lippincott.

Portney, L.G. & Watkins, M.P. (2000). *Foundations of Clinical Research: Applications to Practice*. (2nd Ed) Upper Saddle River, New Jersey: Prentice-Hall.

ACKNOWLEDGMENTS
Scholarship of Practice

No book of this size and scope comes into existence without the contributions of many people. First of all, I am grateful for the privilege of working as editor with the esteemed colleagues from throughout the world who contributed chapters to this text. Each brought unique qualities to the chapters they created, writing from the informed perspectives of experience and expertise. In the course of editing their work, I learned a great deal.

I owe a debt of gratitude for the commitment and the many hours of careful work that my team at UIC put into this project. Research assistants and graduate students, Jenny Fox-Manaster, Annie Ploszaj, and Jessica Kramer provided outstanding leadership that helped guide this manuscript to fruition at various stages. They had able editorial help of their peers: Mona Youngblood, Stefanie Conaway, Sun-Wook Lee, and Kathleen Kramer. My assistant, Felicia Walters, ably oversaw the process of acquiring photographs, while post-doctoral fellow Patty Bowyer gave helpful feedback throughout the process.

We relied heavily on external reviewers to improve the clarity and content of the book. Their guidance and feedback were instrumental to improving the final quality of this text. I am grateful to the following persons who reviewed the book at its various stages of development:

Julie Bass-Haugen, Bette R. Bonder, Barbara A. Boyt Schell, Jane Case-Smith, Sherrilene Classen, Susan Doble, Regina Doherty, Edward Duncan, Catherine Emery, John Fleming, Ellie Fossey, Linnea Franits, Karen Funk, Linda Gabriel, Heather A. Gallew, Kilian Garvey, Robert W. Gibson, Stacie Lynn Iken, Panelpha L. Kyler, Lori Letts, Jennie Q. Lou, Ferol Menks Ludwig, Rosemary M. Lysaght, Nancy MacRae, Maralynne Mitcham, Maggie Nicol, Jane O'Brien, Genèvieve Pépin, Carol Reed, Pat Sample, Dianne F. Simons, Karen Sladyk, Roger Smith, Barry Trentham, Kerryellen Vroman, Janet H. Watts, Shirley A. Wells, Don Workman, and Hon Yuen. Thanks are also owing to Marcia Ciol, who created many graphs for figures in *Chapter 11, Single Subject Research*.

This book would not have come into existence but for the friendship and persistent badgering of Christa Fratantoro and Margaret Biblis. Margaret convinced me that the book was a good idea and artfully talked me into taking it on, despite my initial hesitations. Christa was there at every stage and willing to do whatever it took to make this a great book. Deborah Thorp provided able editorial guidance and the final look and layout of the text is a reflection of her hard work.

Over the years, F.A. Davis has supported projects that began as ideas without much precedent, including my very first text. I am grateful for their ongoing faith in and support of me.

TABLE OF CONTENTS

SECTION 9

Evidence-Based Practice

C H A P T E R   1

The Necessity of Research in a Profession

Gary Kielhofner

A. Jean Ayres provided occupational therapy to children with learning disabilities (Figure 1.1). She observed that some of these children had difficulty processing sensory information from their bodies and from the environment. She also noted that these sensory processing problems appeared related to problems in motor and academic learning. Spurred by her observations, Ayres began developing a conceptualization of how the brain organizes and interprets sensory information (Ayres, 1979). She used this theory, referred to as Sensory Integration, to understand the functional difficulties found in some children with learning disabilities.

Ayres went on to conduct research on large samples of children to describe the different types of sensory problems that certain children exhibited. As part of this research, she constructed tests to study the behavioral manifestations of sensory processing problems. Findings from a series of nation-wide studies comparing normal children and children with problems processing sensory information eventually identified patterns of sensory integrative impairment (Bundy, Lane, &

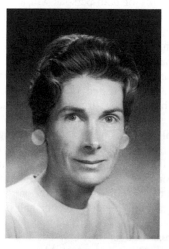

Figure 1.1 Dr. A. Jean Ayres. (Reprinted with permission from Kielhofner, G. Conceptual foundations of occupational therapy, 3rd ed. Philadelphia: FA Davis, 2004, p. 47.)

Murray, 2002). Armed with empirical support for the existence of certain patterns of sensory processing problems and with a conceptualization of those problems, she refined strategies of intervention. Her own research and hundreds of studies by others over several decades have served to improve understanding of sensory integration problems, to develop and refine a battery of tests designed to help therapists identify and understand sensory integrative impairments, and to test the effectiveness of interventions designed to remediate them (Walker, 2004).

Lucy Jane Miller began research developing norm-referenced standardized scales for preschool children after working as an occupational therapist in the Head Start program (Figure 1.2). During that time she realized that most of the children who later demonstrated problems were "missed" by traditional screening tests. She was awarded federal funding to standardize the Miller Assessment for Preschoolers and to develop the FirstSTEP, a shorter screening tool (Miller, 1982, 1988, 1993). Dr. Miller later developed and standardized the Toddler and Infant Motor Evaluation and made a large step forward in intelligence testing when she co-authored the Leiter International Performance Scale, which provides a nonmotor, nonverbal alternative to traditional IQ scales (Miller, 1988, 1982; Roid & Miller, 1997).

Dr. Miller used tests as a way to identify and evaluate children with sensory processing problems and developmental delays. Since 1995, Dr. Miller and her team have run a full-time program of research investigating the underlying mechanisms of sensory dysfunction and evaluating the effectiveness of occupational therapy for children with these disorders (McIntosh, Miller, Shyu, & Hagerman, 1999; Miller et al., 1999). This research has included diverse investigations such as quantitative studies of the sympathetic nervous system based on descriptions of children's "fight or flight" responses and qualitative studies of parental hopes for therapy outcomes.

Dr. Laura Gitlin, an applied research sociologist, has a long-standing passion for developing

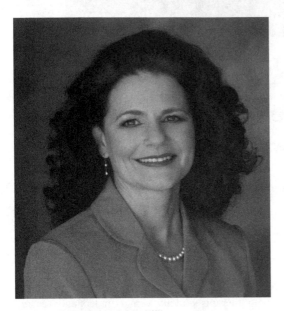

Figure 1.2 Dr. Lucy Jane Miller.

and testing innovative health and human services that can make a difference in the lives of persons with disabilities and their families (Figure 1.3). Working out of the traditions of Kurt Lewin's field theory and M. Powell Lawton's competence-environmental press framework in aging research, her collaboration with occupational therapy has

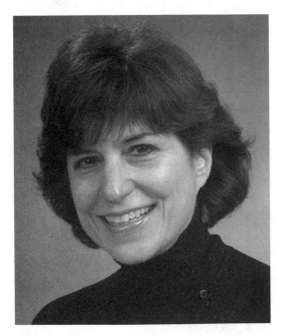

Figure 1.3 Dr. Laura N. Gitlin.

been a natural fit. Since 1988, in partnership with her occupational therapy colleagues, Dr. Gitlin has received federal and foundation funding to study the adaptive processes of older adults, the role and benefits of adaptive equipment and home environmental modification for older people with functional impairments, the quality of life of persons with dementia living at home, and interventions to enable older adults with functional difficulties to age in place at home (Gitlin & Corcoran, in press; Gitlin, Luborsky, & Schemm, 1998; Gitlin, Swenson Miller, & Boyce, 1999). Her recent study on physical frailty has demonstrated the effectiveness of a combined occupational therapy and physical therapy intervention in reducing difficulties with activities of daily living.

In addition, Dr. Gitlin and her team have been investigating the most effective approaches to supporting families to manage dementia-related care challenges (Gitlin, Schinfeld, Winter, Corcoran, & Hauck, 2002). This research has involved developing various measures such as a standardized assessment of the physical features of home environments that support or hinder functionality (Home Environmental Assessment Protocol [HEAP]), a tool to measure the type and range of care strategies families use (Task Management Strategy Index [TMSI]), and a tool to evaluate the strength of the therapeutic engagement process with families (Therapeutic Engagement Index [TEI]) (Gitlin et al. 2002).

This program of research has yielded an effective intervention with families, the Environmental Skill-building Program (ESP). It has also generated other related approaches that enhance the quality of life of both persons with dementia and their families (Gitlin, et al., 2003). Currently, Dr. Gitlin and her team are working on ways of translating these evidence-based interventions into reimbursable services.

Kerstin Tham, a Swedish occupational therapist, became interested in a particular problem some of her clients with a cerebrovascular accident (CVA) experienced (Figure 1.4). This problem, unilateral neglect, meant that, following a CVA, people no longer recognized half of their own bodies nor did they perceive half of the world. As a consequence, they neglected these regions of the self and the world, washing only one side of the body, eating only the food on one half of the plate, and so on.

A great deal of research has been published about the problem of neglect. Moreover, a number of training approaches have been developed to help people with neglect overcome the problem.

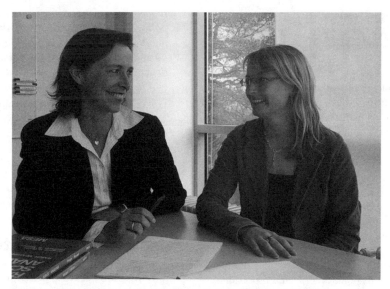

Figure 1.4 Dr. Kerstin Tham (left) and student Ann-Helen Patomella.

However, these approaches have not been shown to be very successful in improving function.

Dr. Tham became convinced that the research that had described unilateral neglect had one large flaw. It always examined how neglect appeared from the outside—that is, how it appeared to clinicians and researchers. It never asked the person with CVA how it was to experience neglect. So, she decided to undertake research that would describe neglect phenomenologically (i.e., from the point of view of the person who had it), with the aim of better providing services for it.

In a qualitative study in which she observed and interviewed four women over an extended period of time, she and her colleagues came to provide some startling insights into the nature of unilateral neglect (Tham, Borell, & Gustavsson, 2000). For instance, they found that people with neglect believed that the neglected body parts were not their own or not attached to their bodies. Their research described a natural course of discovery in which persons with neglect came to understand that they had neglect and were able to make sense of their strange and chaotic experiences of the self and the world.

> Without the development of a research base to refine and provide evidence about the value of its practice, occupational therapy simply will not survive, much less thrive, as a health profession.

In a subsequent investigation, Dr. Tham and a colleague went on to examine how behaviors of other people influenced the experiences and behavior of the person with neglect (Tham & Kielhofner, 2003). She continues this line of research, which offers a new approach to understanding and providing services to persons with unilateral neglect. She and her doctoral students are now also examining the experience of persons having other types of perceptual cognitive impairments after acquired brain damage (Erikson, Karlsson, Söderström, & Tham, 2004; Lampinen, & Tham, 2003).

Each of these four researchers has engaged in widely different programs of occupational therapy research. They used different methods on very different populations and sample sizes. Nonetheless, the work of each of these investigators stands as an example of why research is important to the field overall. That is, their research has provided:

• Knowledge and know-how that guides therapists in their everyday work, and
• Evidence that assures others about the impact of occupational therapy services.

The Profession's Research Obligation

Every health profession asks its clients and the public to have a level of confidence in the worth of its services. To justify that confidence, the profession must enable its members to offer high-quality services which will benefit the client. Thus, when healthcare professionals provide service to clients, the knowledge and skills they use should be "justified in terms of a systematic and shared body of professional knowledge" (Polgar & Thomas, 2000, p. 3). This knowledge includes the theory that informs practice and the tools and procedures that are used in practice. Research is the means by which the profession generates evidence to test and validate its theories and to examine and demonstrate the utility of its practice tools and procedures. Therefore, every profession has an ongoing obligation to undertake systematic and sustained research (Portney & Watkins, 2000).

The Necessity of Research for Professional Recognition and Support

The existence of occupational therapy depends on societal support. This support ranges from subsidizing educational programs that prepare occupational therapists to reimbursing occupational therapists for their services. Societal support for healthcare professions cannot be assumed. For instance, those who make public policy and decide what healthcare services are needed increasingly rely on scientific evidence to decide where limited public and private resources should be directed. As a result, research is increasingly necessary to ensure that resources will be available to support the profession. Along these lines Christiansen (1983) notes:

> "The goal of research in an applied discipline such as occupational therapy is to enhance and refine the knowledge base relevant to practice so that consumers receive the best available treatment." (Ottenbacher, 1987, p. 4)
> "It is incumbent upon a developing profession to insure that its steadily growing body of knowledge be verified through research…" (West, 1981, p. 9)

It seems clear that as administrators and policymakers render decision about how health care providers are used and reimbursed, those disciplines with objective evidence of their effectiveness and efficiency will have a competitive advantage. (p.197)

He concludes, quite correctly, that research is an economic imperative for the profession:

Without the development of a research base to refine and provide evidence about the value of its practice, occupational therapy simply will not survive, much less thrive, as a health profession (Christiansen, 1983)

Evidence-Based Practice

The obligation of the profession to conduct research that refines and validates its knowledge base is paralleled by an obligation of individual therapists to engage in evidence-based practice (Taylor, 2000). Accordingly, whenever possible, practitioners should select intervention strategies and tools that have been empirically demonstrated to be effective (Eakin, 1997). Evidence-based practitioners integrate their own expertise with the best available research evidence. The next section briefly examines some of the ways that research provides evidence for practice.

How Research Supports Practice

Research supports practice in many different ways including:

- Generating foundational knowledge used by therapists,
- Providing evidence about the need for occupational therapy services,
- Developing and testing theory that underlies practice, and
- Generating findings about the process and outcomes of therapy.

In the section below we examine each of these ways that research generates knowledge to support and advance practice

Generating Foundational Knowledge

Much of the background information that occupational therapists use on a daily basis would not exist without research. Often, a long history of investigation is behind what has become taken-for-granted knowledge. Knowledge of musculoskeletal anatomy, neuronal transmission, the milestones the characterize child development, the nature of personality, and the etiology and prognosis of diseases have resulted from thousands of studies.

Over decades, investigators examined these phenomena, providing accounts that were subsequently verified or corrected by others. In time, this knowledge was accumulated and refined until it became part of the repository of knowledge that informs occupational therapy practice. This knowledge is ordinarily generated by persons who are not occupational therapists, but their research is, nonetheless, important to occupational therapy practice.

Providing Evidence of the Need for Occupational Therapy Services

Without clear identification of need, one can neither decide what services to provide nor accurately evaluate the value of any service. Needs assessment research determines what clients require to achieve some basic standard of health or to improve their situation (Witkin & Altschuld, 1995). It focuses on identifying gaps between clients' desires and their situations (Altschuld & Witkin, 2000).

Needs assessment is particularly important in identifying the nature and consequences of new types of disabilities or new circumstances affecting persons with disabilities, and in identifying problems not previously recognized or understood. For example, studies recently indicated that human immunodeficiency virus/acquired immunodeficiency syndrome (HIV/AIDS) increasingly affects individuals from disadvantaged minority populations, and individuals with histories of mental illness, substance abuse, poverty, limited education, and limited work experience (Centers for Disease Control and Prevention [CDC], 2000; Karon, Felming, Steketee, & De Cock, 2001; Kates, Sorian, Crowley, & Summers, 2002). Research has also shown that while newer drug therapies have lowered AIDS mortality, the chronic disabling aspects of the disease and numerous associated conditions continue to pose challenges for those affected (CDC, 2000). Many people with HIV/AIDS struggle to overcome personal, financial, and social challenges that impact their desire to live independently and return to the workforce (McReynolds & Garske, 2001). Moreover, despite these general characteristics of the AIDS population, a needs assessment study also demonstrated that individuals' perceptions of needs differed by race, ethnicity, and gender (Sankar & Luborsky, 2003).

Together these studies indicated that persons with HIV/AIDS would potentially benefit from an individualized intervention designed to help them achieve independent living and employment as they envisioned it. These studies provided a foundation on which to propose a study of such an occupational therapy intervention which is in process as the book goes to press (Paul-Ward, Braveman, Kielhofner, & Levin, 2005).

Developing and Testing Occupational Therapy Theory that Explains Practice

Every profession makes use of theories that underlie and explain its practice. By definition, the explanations offered by a theory are always tentative. By testing these explanations, research allows theory to be corrected and refined so that it provides increasingly useful explanations for practice. As will be discussed in the next chapter, ideas about how research refines and tests theory have evolved over the centuries, but research remains the primary tool by which a theory can be improved.

In professions, theories are ordinarily organized into frameworks or models that are used to guide practice. These theories explain problems that therapists address and to justify approaches to solving them that are used in therapy. Consequently, the testing and refinement of such theories through research contributes to advancing practice. Therapists should always judge and place their confidence in the explanations provided by any theory in relation to the extent to which that theory has been tested and developed by research.

A wide range of research can be used to test and develop theory. No single study can ever test all aspects of a theory. The following kinds of studies are ordinarily used to examine and develop theory:

- Studies that aim to verify the accuracy of the concepts. These types of studies ask whether there is evidence to support the way the concept describes and/or explains some phenomena.
- Studies that ask whether there are relationships between phenomena as specified by the theory.
- Studies that compare different groups of participants on concepts that the theory offers to explain the differences between those groups.
- Studies that examine the potential of the theory to predict what will happen.

Over time, as the evidence accumulates across such studies, informed judgments can be made about the accuracy and completeness of a theory. Findings from such research ordinarily lead to alterations in the theory that allow it to offer more accurate explanations. Since the theories used in occupational therapy typically seek to explain problems that therapists encounter in practice and to explain how therapists go about solving those problems, these types of studies directly inform practice.

The following is an example of research that tests theory with implications for practice. Occupational therapy practice with persons who have central nervous system damage has been guided by a theory of how people control movement, the motor control model. Toward the end of the 20th century, this model, which previously saw the control of movement as being directed exclusively by the brain, began to change. A new conceptualization (Mathiowetz & Bass-Haugen, 1994, 2002) argued that movement is a result of the interaction of the human nervous system, the musculoskeletal system, and the environment. This theory emphasized the importance of the task being done and of the environment (e.g., the objects used) in influencing how a person moves. The implication of this theory was that the tasks chosen and the objects used in therapy would have an impact on recovery of coordinated movement. Occupational therapists conducted research that illustrated clearly that the nature of the task being done and the environment do affect the quality of movement (Lin, Wu, & Trombly, 1998; Mathiowetz & Bass- Haugen, 1994; Wu, Trombly, & Lin, 1994). These and other studies (Ma and Trombly, 2002; Trombly & Ma, 2002) now provide evidence that tasks involving meaningful objects and goal-oriented activities positively influence performance and motor learning.

Providing Evidence About the Nature and Outcomes of Therapy

Many types of studies examine aspects of occupational therapy practice and its outcomes. The most typical of these studies are those that:

- Are undertaken to develop and test assessments that are used in practice,
- Examine the clinical reasoning of therapists when they are making decisions about therapy,
- Determine the kinds of outcomes that result from therapy,
- Examine the process of therapy, asking what goes on in therapy, or
- Use participatory methods to investigate and improve services in a specific context.

Below we examine each of these kinds of studies in more detail.

Studies that Test Assessments Used in Therapy

A number of interrelated forms of inquiry are used to develop and test assessments used in the field; the aim of such research is to ensure the dependability of those methods (Benson & Schell, 1997). Dependable assessments are reliable—that is, they yield consistent information in different circumstances, at different times, with different clients, and when different therapists administer them. A dependable information-gathering method must also be valid—that is, it must provide the information it is intended to provide. Typical of studies examining whether an assessment is valid are those that:

- Ask experts whether the content of an assessment is coherent and representative of what is intended to be gathered (i.e., content validity).
- Analyze the items that make up an assessment to determine whether they coalesce to capture the trait they aim to measure.
- Ask whether the assessment correlates with measures of concepts that are expected to concur and whether it diverges from those with which no relationship is expected.
- Determine whether they can differentiate between different groups of people.

In addition to studies that examine reliability and validity of assessments, there are studies that examine the clinical utility of assessments. Such studies may ask therapists and/or clients whether they find the assessments informative and useful for identifying problems and making decisions about theory. The development of any assessment ordinarily involves a series of studies that contribute to the ongoing improvement of the assessment over time.

Studies of Clinical Reasoning

Occupational therapists work with clients to identify their clients' problems and choose a course of action to do something about them. This process is referred to as clinical reasoning (Rogers, 1983; Schon, 1983). An important area of research in occupational therapy has been investigations that examine clinical reasoning.

One of the most influential studies of clinical reasoning by Mattingly and Flemming (1994) identified different types of reasoning that characterized occupational therapy practice. Their research has served as a framework for understanding how occupational therapists make sense of and take action with reference to their clients' problems and challenges in therapy.

Outcomes Research

Outcomes research is concerned with the results of occupational therapy. Investigations that examine the outcomes of occupational therapy services include:

- Investigations of a specific intervention strategy or technique,
- Studies of comprehensive occupational therapy programs, and
- Inquiries that examine the contribution of occupational therapy to an interdisciplinary program of services (Kielhofner, Hammel, Helfrich, Finlayson, & Taylor, 2004).

The study of occupational therapy techniques and approaches helps refine understanding of these discrete elements of practice. This type of research examines outcomes specific to an intended intervention. Such studies may also seek to determine the relative impact of different techniques or approaches (e.g., comparisons between individual versus group interventions).

Studies of comprehensive occupational therapy programs ask whether an entire package of services produces a desired outcome. Such studies typically examine the impact of services on such outcomes as independent living, employment, or enhanced school performance. A well-known example of this type of research is a study by Clark et al. (1997), which documented the positive outcomes of an occupational therapy program for well elderly persons. Finally, studies that examine the impact of interdisciplinary services can also document the impact of the occupational therapy component of such services.

Inquiry Into the Processes of Therapy

It is important not only to understand whether interventions work, but also to know why they work or do not work. Studies that examine the impact of interventions increasingly focus on identifying the underlying mechanism of change (Gitlin et al., 2000). Often an important prelude to designing intervention outcome studies is to examine what goes in therapy in order to improve upon services before they are more formally tested.

An example is a study by Helfrich and Kielhofner (1994) that examined how client occupational narratives influenced the meaning clients

assigned to occupational therapy. This study showed how the meanings of therapy intended by therapists were often not received by or in concert with the client's meaning. The study findings underscored the importance of therapists having knowledge of the client's narrative and organizing therapy as a series of events that enter into that narrative. Such studies of the process of therapy provide important information about how therapy can be improved to better meet client needs.

Participatory Research

A new and rapidly growing approach to investigation is participatory research. This approach involves researchers, therapists, and clients doing research together to develop and test occupational therapy services. Participatory research embraces the idea of partnership in which all the constituents work together and share power and responsibility to investigate, improve, and determine the outcomes of service. It also involves innovation in which new services are created to respond to problems that are mutually identified by researchers and therapists/clients.

This type of research is especially useful for contributing knowledge that practitioners can readily use and that consumers will find relevant to their needs. A recent example of this kind of study involved developing and evaluating a consumer-driven program for individuals with chronic fatigue syndrome. This program provided clients with an opportunity to learn self-advocacy skills; improve quality of life, functional capacity, and coping skills; acquire resources; and achieve increased quality of life (Taylor, 2004).

Conclusion

This chapter introduced the necessity of research for occupational therapy. We saw that research gives clients and the public reason to have confidence in occupational therapy. We also saw that it provides the rationale for administrators and policymakers to support the occupational therapy services.

The chapter also examined how research creates the knowledge and know-how that therapists use in practice by testing theory and practice. Figure 1.5 summarizes the dynamic relationship between theory, research, and practice. As it illustrates, each of these key elements of the profession has an influence on the other. Theory and research evidence guides practice. Practice raises problems

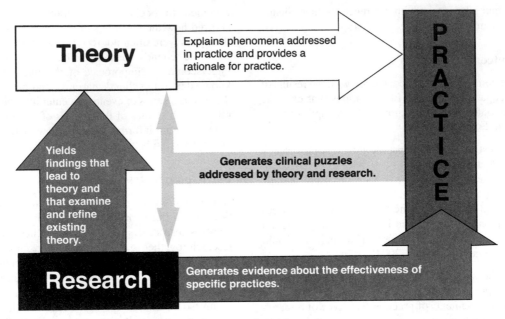

Figure 1.5 The relationship of theory, research, and practice.

and questions to be addressed in theory and research. Research tests theory and practice, providing information about their validity and utility, respectively.

The remainder of this text explains the nature, scope, design, methods, and processes that make up research. It also illustrates the wide range of tools that researchers use for their inquiries. Throughout the text, as one encounters multiple discussions of how research is done, it is important not to lose sight of why it is done. One would do well to remember Yerxa's (1987, p. 415) observation that "Research is essential to achieving our aspirations for our patients and our hopes and dreams for our profession."

REFERENCES

Altschuld, J. W., & Witkin, B. R. (2000). *From needs assessment to action: Transforming needs into solution strategies*. Thousands Oak, CA: SAGE Publications.

Ayres, A. J. (1979). *Sensory integration and the child*. Los Angeles: Western Psychological Services.

Benson J., & Schell, B. A. (1997). *Measurement theory: Application to occupational and physical therapy*. In J. Van Deusen, & D. Brunt (Eds.), Assessment in Occupational Therapy and Physical Therapy. Philadelphia: W. B. Saunders.

Bundy, A. C., Lane, S. J., & Murray, E. A. (2002). (Eds.), *Sensory integration: Theory and practice* (2nd ed., pp. 169–198). Philadelphia: F. A. Davis.

Centers for Disease Control and Prevention (CDC). (2000). *HIV/AIDS Surveillance Supplemental Report, 7* (1). Atlanta: U.S. Department of Health and Human Services, Centers for Disease Control and Prevention.

Christiansen, C. (1983). An economic imperative. *The Occupational Therapy Journal of Research, 3* (4), 195–198.

Clark, F., Azen, S. P., Zemke, R., Jackson, J., Carlson, M., Mandel, D., et al. (1997). Occupational therapy for independent-living older adults: A randomized controlled trial. *Journal of the American Medical Association, 278*, 1321–1326.

Eakin, P. (1997). The Casson Memorial Lecture 1997: Shifting the balance—Evidence based practice. *The British Journal of Occupational Therapy, 60* (7), 290–294.

Erikson, A., Karlsson, G., Söderström, M., & Tham, K. (2004). A training apartment with electronic aids to daily living: Lived experiences of persons with brain damage. *American Journal of Occupational Therapy, 58*, 261–271.

Gitlin, L. N. & Corcoran, M. (in press). *An occupational therapy guide to helping caregivers of persons with dementia: The home environment skill-building program*. American Occupational Therapy Association.

Gitlin, L. N., Corcoran, M., Martindale-Adams, J., Malone, M. A., Stevens, A., & Winter, L. (2000). Identifying mechanisms of action: Why and how does intervention work? In R. Schulz (Ed.). *Handbook of dementia care giving: Evidence-based interventions for family caregivers*. New York: Springer.

Gitlin, L. N., Luborsky, M., & Schemm, R. L. (1998). Emerging concerns of older stroke patients about assistive device use. *The Gerontologist, 3* (2), 169–180.

Gitlin, L. N., Schinfeld, S., Winter, L., Corcoran, M., & Hauck, W. (2002). Evaluating home environments of person with dementia: Interrater reliability and validity of the home environmental assessment protocol (HEAP). *Disability and Rehabilitation, 24*, 59–71.

Gitlin, L. N., Swenson Miller, K., & Boyce, A. (1999). Bathroom modifications for frail elderly renters: outcomes of a community-based program. *Technology and Disability, 10,* 141–149.

Gitlin, L. N., Winter, L., Corcoran, M., Dennis, M., Schinfeld, S., & Hauck, W. (2003). Effects of the Home Environmental Skill-building Program on the caregiver-care recipient dyad: Six-month outcomes from the Philadelphia REACH initiative. *The Gerontologist, 43* (4), 532–546.

Gitlin, L. N., Winter, L., Dennis, M., Corcoran, M., Schinfeld, S., & Hauck, W. (2002). Strategies used by families to simplify tasks for individuals with Alzheimer's disease and related disorders: Psychometric analysis of the task management strategy index (TMSI). *The Gerontologist, 42,* 61–69.

Helfrich, C. & Kielhofner, G. (1994). Volitional narratives and the meaning of therapy. *The American Journal of Occupational Therapy, 48,* 319–326.

Karon, J. M., Fleming, P. L., Steketee, R. W., & De Cock, K. M. (2001). HIV in the United States at the turn of the century: An epidemic in transition. *American Journal of Public Health, 91* (7), 1060–1068.

Kates, J. R., Sorian, J. S., Crowley, T. A., & Summers, T. A. (2002). Critical policy challenges in the third decade of the HIV/AIDS epidemic. *American Journal of Public Health, 92* (7), 1060–1063.

Kielhofner, G., Hammel, J., Helfrich, C., Finlayson, M., & Taylor, R. R. (2004). Studying practice and its outcomes: A conceptual approach. *American Journal of Occupational Therapy, 58,* 15–23.

Lampinen, J., & Tham, K. (2003). Interaction with the physical environment in everyday occupation after stroke: A phenomenological study of visuospatial agnosia. *Scandinavian Journal of Occupational Therapy, 10,* 147–156.

Lin, K. C., Wu, C. Y., & Trombly, C. A. (1998). Effects of task goal on movement kinematics and line bisection performance in adults without disabilities. *American Journal of Occupational Therapy, 52,* 179–187.

Ma, H., & Trombly, C. A. (2002). A synthesis of the effects of occupational therapy for persons with stroke, part II: Remediation of impairments. *American Journal of Occupational Therapy, 56,* 260–274.

Mathiowetz, V., & Bass-Haugen, J. (1994). Motor behavior research: Implications for therapeutic approaches to central nervous system dysfunction. *American Journal of Occupational Therapy, 48,* 733–745.

Mathiowetz, V., & Bass-Haugen, J. (2002). Assessing abilities and capacities: Motor behavior. In C. A. Trombly & M. V. Radomski (Eds.), *Occupational therapy for physical dysfunction* (5th ed., pp. 137–158). Baltimore: Lippincott Williams & Wilkins.

Mattingly, C., & Flemming, M. (1994). *Clinical reasoning: Forms of inquiry in a therapeutic practice.* Philadelphia: F. A. Davis.

McIntosh, D. N., Miller, L. J., Shyu, V., & Hagerman, R. (1999). Sensory-modulation disruption, electrodermal responses, and functional behaviors. *Developmental Medicine and Child Neurology, 41,* 608–615. The Psychological Corporation.

McReynolds, C. J., & Garske, G. G. (2001). Current issues in HIV disease and AIDS: Implications for health and rehabilitation professionals. *Work, 17,* 117–124.

Miller, L. J. (1988, 1982). *Miller assessment for preschoolers.* San Antonio, TX:The Psychological Corporation.

Miller, L. J. (1993). *FirstSTEP (screening test for evaluating preschoolers): Manual.* San Antonio, TX: The Psychological Corporation.

Miller, L. J., McIntosh, D. N., McGrath, J., Shyu, V., Lampe, M., Taylor, A. K., et al. (1999). Electrodermal responses to sensory stimuli in individuals with fragile X syndrome: A preliminary report. *American Journal of Medical Genetics, 83* (4), 268–279.

Ottenbacher, K. J. (1987). A scholarly rite of passage. *Occupational Therapy Journal of Research, 7* (1), 3–5.

Paul-Ward, A., Braveman, B., Kielhofner, G., & Levin, M. (2005). Developing employment services for individuals with HIV/AIDS: Participatory action strategies at work. *Journal of Vocational Rehabilitation, 22,* 85–93.

Polgar, S., & Thomas, S. A. (2000). *Introduction to research in the health sciences.* Edinburgh: Churchill Livingston.

Portney, L. G., & Watkins, M. P. (2000). *Foundations of clinical research: Application to practice* (2nd ed.). Upper Saddle River, NJ: Prentice-Hall.

Rogers, J. C. (1983). Eleanor Clarke Slagle Lectureship—1983; Clinical reasoning: The ethics, science, and art. *American Journal of Occupational Therapy, 37* (9), 601–616.

Roid, G. H., & Miller, L. J. (1997). *Leiter International Performance Scale Revised.* Wood Dale, IL: Stoelting Co.

Sankar, A., & Luborsky, M. (2003). Developing a community-based definition of needs for persons living with chronic HIV. *Human Organization, 62* (2), 153–165.

Schon, D. (1983). *The reflective practitioner: How professionals think in action.* New York: Basic Books.

Taylor, M. C. (2000). *Evidence-based practice for occupational therapists.* Oxford, UK: Blackwell Science.

Taylor, R. (2004). Quality of life and symptom severity in individuals with chronic fatigue syndrome; findings form a randomized clinical trial. *American Journal of Occupational Therapy 58* (1), 35–43.

Tham, K., Borell, L., & Gustavsson, A. (2000). The discovery of disability: A phenomenological study of unilateral neglect. *American Journal of Occupational Therapy, 54,* 398–406.

Tham, K., & Kielhofner, G. (2003). Impact of the social environment on occupational experience and performance among persons with unilateral neglect. *American Journal of Occupational Therapy, 57* (4), 403–412.

Trombly, C. A., & Ma, H. (2002). A synthesis of the effects of occupational therapy for persons with stroke, part I: Restoration of roles, tasks, and activities. *American Journal of Occupational Therapy, 56,* 250–259.

Walker, K. F. (2004). A. Jean Ayres. In K. F. Walker & F. M. Ludwig (Eds.), *Perspectives on theory for the practice of occupational therapy* (3rd ed., pp. 145–236). Austin, TX: Pro-ed.

West, W. (1981). A journal of research in occupational therapy: The response, the responsibility. *Occupational Therapy Journal of Research, 1* (1), 7–12.

Witkin, B. R., & Altschuld, J. W. (1995). *Planning and conducting needs assessments: A practical guide.* Thousand Oaks, CA: SAGE Publications.

Wu, C. Y., & Trombly, C. A., & Lin, K. C. (1994). The relationship between occupational form and occupational performance: A kinematic perspective. *American Journal of Occupational Therapy, 48,* 679–687.

Yerxa, E. J. (1987). Research: The key to the development of occupational therapy as an academic discipline. *American Journal of Occupational Therapy, 41* (7), 415–419

CHAPTER 2

The Aim of Research: Philosophical Foundations of Scientific Inquiry

Gary Kielhofner

Although the philosophical underpinnings of studies are rarely discussed in research publications, they are always lurking in the background. Consider, for instance, the following contrasts. Some researchers will take pains to demonstrate how subjectivity and personal bias were eliminated from their studies, while others will detail how their personal histories and subjective experiences shaped and informed their investigation. Some researchers will be concerned with what their findings tell us about the nature of reality, while others focus instead on helping the reader understand how reality was experienced by those who where studied. Some investigators carefully distance themselves from subjects, while other investigators immerse themselves in the lives of those they study. Still other investigators invite those they study to be equal partners in the research enterprise.

Such differences in the conduct of research are not simply incidental to the methods used. They reflect fundamentally different philosophical stances on reality, objectivity, and human knowing. Anyone who participates in research or wishes to be a consumer of research should appreciate the philosophic underpinnings that shape the fundamental attitudes and beliefs of those who conducted the research. In the end, these may be as important and consequential as the researcher's adherence to accepted methods and protocols (Kaplan, 1964).

This chapter examines the philosophical foundations of scientific inquiry and illustrates how ideas about inquiry and the knowledge it creates have evolved. This historical account will examine four periods of the philosophy of science:

- Classicism,
- Modernism,
- Critical Modernism, and
- Postmodernism.

As will be seen, each of these periods offers a different understanding of the aims and consequences of conducting inquiry.

There is no attempt here to provide a comprehensive discussion of the philosophy of science. Rather, the aims are to capture some key ideas and highlight the epistemological stances that are likely to be implied in the range of research found in occupational therapy.

Classicism: Origins of the Scientific Method

Aristotle is generally considered the first philosopher of science in the Western world inasmuch as he formulated the foundations of empiricism. He proposed that the world could be understood by detailed observation combined with a systematizing of those observations. To this end, Aristotle outlined research as a process of going from observations of the natural world (i.e., the objects and events that we perceive through the senses) to explanation, and then back to observations (Losee, 1993). The first part of this process, induction, involves creating explanations (i.e., theory) from specific observations. In the second phase, deduction, one derives from the theory specific statements or predictions that could be examined to see if they bear up under observation of the natural world. When statements deduced from a theory were shown to correspond to what was observed, one had proof of the veracity of the theory. This induction–deduction process (Figure 2.1) is still at the core of all research, though different types of research view it differently, emphasize one or another of the phases, and have different ideas about the role of the investigator in the process.

> Although the philosophical underpinnings of studies are rarely discussed in research publications, they are always lurking in the background.

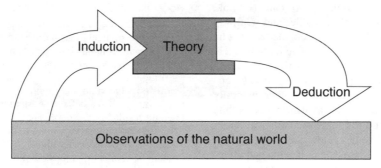

Figure 2.1 Aristotle's inductive–deductive method.

The Search for Truth

Aristotle and other early philosophers of science were fundamentally concerned with separating scientific knowing from the fallibility of ordinary knowing. Thus, they focused on how to ensure the truthfulness of knowledge generated through the inductive–deductive cycle (Klee, 1997; Losee, 1993). This truth, they believed, depended on logic. They reasoned that if pure logic was used to connect the natural world to scientific knowledge, the latter could be demonstrated to be true. Thus, they critically examined how logic was used in both the inductive and deductive phases of research.

For Aristotle and many who followed, the deductive stage readily conformed to rigorous logic—that is, the specific statements that were tested through research could be deduced from the

Theory and Its Components

Theory is a network of explanations; it provides concepts that label and describe phenomena and postulates that specify relationships between concepts. Concepts describe, define, and provide a specific way of seeing and thinking about some entity, quality, or process. For example, the concept of "strength" refers to a characteristic of muscles (i.e., their ability to produce tension for maintaining postural control and for moving body parts). Exercise is a concept that refers to a process (i.e., the use of muscles to produce force against resistance).

Postulates posit relationships between concepts, asserting how the characteristics or processes to which concepts refer are organized or put together. An example of such a postulate is: exercise increases the ability of muscles to produce force. When several concepts and postulates are linked together, they constitute a whole network of explanations that make up a given theory

larger theory following strict logical principles. However, the inductive phase was problematic. It required something more than logic. Induction involved an intuitive leap. In arriving at explanations, a scholar had to invent first principles that were the foundation of the explanation that any theory provided. These first principles could only be assumed to be true, since they could not be proved. Confronted with this problem, Aristotle opted for a faith in their truth. He justified this faith by arguing that the natural world presented itself in a fashion that explicated its most basic laws. In other words, the first principles were self-evident.

In the late 15th and early 16th centuries, Galileo criticized Aristotle's self-evident first principles as being too metaphysical and therefore unscientific. Galileo sought, instead, to ground scientific explanations in the "obvious truth" of mathematical descriptions that perfectly fit the natural world (Klee, 1997; Losee, 1993). He and his contemporaries reasoned that the correspondence between mathematical concepts and the natural world could not be coincidental, and therefore represented an obvious truth.

Nonetheless, like Aristotle, Galileo was ultimately confronted with the fact that the process of induction involved intuition. He made extensive use of imagining phenomena that he could not observe (e.g., free fall in a vacuum) to arrive at explanations. In the end this imaginative process also required him to use certain unavoidable nonmathematical assumptions to construct his explanations. Thus, a complete logical connection between the natural world and theory was still not achieved for the inductive process.

Descartes, a contemporary of Galileo, was not convinced that mathematical correspondence was sufficient to constitute the truth of theoretical first principles. He sought to resolve the problem by doubting all potential first principles in search for those that were beyond doubt (Watson, 2002). His search for principles beyond all doubt resulted in the famous dictum: *Cogito, ergo sum.* (I think, therefore I am.) Like Aristotle and Galileo, Descartes also was unable to avoid the fact that he made intuitive leaps in his inductive reasoning. He referred to these intuitive leaps as using analogies (e.g., inferring planetary movement had to be circular based on observations of other naturally occurring phenomena such as whirlpools). While he sought to defend the logic of analogical thinking, like those before him, Descartes was unable to reduce induction to pure logic. It remained a creative act that went beyond logical thought.

In the end, philosophers of science were unable to avoid the conclusion that induction involved more than pure logic. Even today, it is understood that induction is an intuitive and creative process. Moreover, they were also unable to resolve the problem that the first principles that were generated through induction could not be proven. Early philosophers attempted to justify the first principles that resulted from induction on the grounds of self-evidence, mathematical correspondence, and truth beyond doubt. No matter how well argued these justifications, the bottom line was that they each demanded some type of belief that went beyond logic. That intuition and faith remained unavoidable parts of induction eventually led philosophers to search for truth in the deductive phase.

Modernism: From Absolute Truth to Positivistic Science

A critical turning point in the philosophy of science was ushered in by Newton and his contemporaries in the 17th century (Cohen, 1958; Klee, 1997; Losee, 1993). These early researchers replaced the concern for absolute truth with concern for how to correct errors in knowledge. They envisioned science as a process of testing and verification of the theory created through inductive reasoning. Newton accepted the idea of intuition and creativity in generating theory as a necessary process, since he made extensive use of such thinking in his own theorizing. Thus, in order to establish confidence in his theories, Newton focused on the deductive phase.

To specify how error could be identified in theory through testing, he outlined an axiomatic method (Cohen & Smith, 2002). It contained three steps:

- Identifying within the theory those first principles that could not be deduced from any others that were, therefore, ultimately not provable (these first principles were labeled axioms and

Modernism and Progressive Science

> The philosophical ideas referred to as "logical positivism" contained an important idea of progress that is also a cornerstone of modernism. Born out of 18th century Enlightenment, modernism included not only faith in science as a method but also a belief that true human progress would result from science. That is, science was expected to continually improve the human condition as knowledge accumulated and was used to the betterment of society and its institutions. Thus, modernism optimistically sought "universal human emancipation through mobilization of the powers of technology, science, and reason (Harvey, 1990, p. 41).

the other theoretical principles that could be deduced from the first principles were labeled theorems),
- Specifying how the theorems were correlated with the empirical world so that they could be systematically tested, and
- Testing the theorems through observation of the natural world.

Although this approach admitted that the first principles could not be proved, they had to yield theorems that did not contradict the natural world. Hence, first principles that yielded incorrect theorems would ultimately be understood to be false and, therefore, could be eliminated (Cohen, 1958).

Logical Positivism

This approach to research meant that theories had to be contingent and subject to revision as the evidence generated in research required it. Thus, the approach of Newton and his contemporaries did not seek to claim that their theories were true. Rather, they asserted that any theory was a possible, but not necessarily infallible, explanation. A theory's plausibility depended on whether statements that could be logically deduced from it held up in the natural world. If observations of the natural world did not bear out what was logically deduced from a theory (i.e., were disproved), then the theory would ultimately be rejected. Within this framework, while truth was not immediately at hand, scientists could make progress toward it. Research could systematically identify what was false through empirical testing. What survived the test of time and evidence would be increasingly closer to the truth. This view that research allowed theory to progress toward truth came to be known as logical positivism.

Subsequent philosophers of science in the logical positivist tradition focused on improving the logical rigor of methods through which researchers induced theory from observation and then went about testing the fit of theoretical explanations with the empirical world. The work of these philosophers of science represents a complex and often subtly nuanced discussion of how empiricism was possible. Below we examine only a few highlights of the kinds of contributions that major philosophers made to refine the understanding of how knowledge was generated and refined.

In the 18th century, two of the most important philosophers refining ideas about the logical processes that linked the theoretical explanation to the observable world were David Hume and Immanuel Kant (Klee, 1997; Losee, 1993). They represent two distinct schools of thought. Thus, each emphasized different aspects of the empirical method.

Hume believed that all human understanding began with sensations of the world and that all human knowledge comes from experience (Jenkins, 1992). Thus, for him, research was the systematic means of building up knowledge from experience of the world. Kant disagreed with Hume's assertion that all human knowledge was built up incrementally through experience (Kant, 1996). Rather, his thesis of "Transcendental Idealism" argued that the human mind played an active role in how humans experience and make sense of the world. Nonetheless, he emphasized, along with Hume, that objective knowledge of the natural world was possible.

Hume refined the logic by which one could explain the experienced world and test the veracity of those explanations (Jenkins, 1992). He differentiated between two types of scientific statements: (1) relational statements that derived their truth from their internally consistent logic, irrespective of any relationship to the empirical world and (2) matter-of-fact statements whose truth could be claimed only by reference to empirical data. Hume was primarily concerned with how matter-of-fact statements could be tested and disproved if they were inaccurate and he helped to refine the logic of this process.

Because Kant focused on how the human mind ordered understanding of the world, his primary contributions are in the area of theory construction. He argued that logic provided the ultimate rules according to which theories could be constructed. He argued for the importance of any new theory being able to be incorporated logically into older empirically established ones. In his view, the dependability of theories relied on their logical interconnectedness.

In the 19th century, John Stuart Mill continued the search to identify rigorously logical procedures for arriving at theoretical explanations (Skorupski, 1998). His greatest contributions were the further systemization of the logical process of induction. He developed four laws that governed theorizing about causation:

• Agreement,
• Concomitant variation,
• Residues, and
• Difference (Skorupski, 1998).

According to the method of agreement, when a researcher observed that a certain variable preceded another variable under a number of circumstances, it was reasonable to assert the probability that the first variable caused the second. In concomitant variation, causation could be asserted based on the observation that two variables are noted to vary together and in the same direction (e.g., more of one is accompanied with more of another). In the method of residues, a causal relationship between one variable and another could be made when the causal relationships among other variables are removed and the relationship of one variable preceding another variable remains.

Mill considered the method of difference to be the most important. In this instance, causation is asserted when the presence of the first variable is followed by the second and when, in the first variable's absence, the second does not occur. The method of difference led to the use of experiments in which presence of a presumed causable variable is systematically manipulated.

In the 20th century, philosophers of science continued to construct a logical framework of science. Two important philosophers, Hempel and Oppenheim, exemplify the efforts of this period (Klee, 1997; Losee, 1993). They underscored the importance of theory being able to predict phenomena. For one to have confidence in an explanation, it had to be capable of generating predictions that could be investigated through research. Their work focused on how one logically derived observable predictive statements from theoretical explanations.

Nagel (1949) built on their work by specifying the difference between theoretical and observational statements. Observational statements, he argued, did not go beyond what was actually observed, and were therefore not "contaminated" by theory. This was an important point since, if the actual test of a theory is to be objective, then the statement that is being tested cannot be "biased" by the theory. It has to stand apart from the theory and merely link the theory logically to something that can be observed in order to determine whether or not the theory accurately predicts the phenomena under question.

The Critique of Positivism

Logical positivism underscored the importance of deriving hypotheses logically from theory so that they could be tested by research and, when incorrect, shown to be false. However, a major problem that arose was whether a hypothesis, much less a theory, could actually be demonstrated to be false. The whole foundation of logical positivism was based on the falsifiabilty of hypotheses that allowed research to correct theories.

The popular notion was that a crucial experiment could be designed for each hypothesis that would, once and for all, decide whether it was false. However, the idea of the crucial experiment came to be strongly criticized. For instance, Grunbaum (1970) argued that no hypothesis derived from a theory could be as sufficiently isolated from the theory as to provide an absolute test of the theory. This was, in part, because the meaning of any hypothesis was not contained solely in the statement of that hypothesis but also in the entire matrix of concepts from which the hypothesis was deduced. This means that the understanding of the hypothesis, including what evidence could constitute its falsity, also depends on the theory from which it is derived.

Therefore, evidence that contradicts a particular hypothesis can easily be explained away. A convenient shift in the sense of the hypothesis will suffice to protect the theory from which the hypothesis was derived. Grunbaum's argument led to the conclusion that there could be no logic of proof and disproof external to any theory. Rather, any proposed test of a theory depends on the theory for its sensibility. For instance, Hesse (1970) pointed out that all observational terms contained in hypotheses are theory-dependent. That is, their meaning cannot stand apart from the theory. Therefore, any attempt to capture the empirical world in the language of a hypothesis irrevocably commits the researcher to the theory that makes sense of the hypothesis in the first place.

These were not small problems for logical positivism. If the very observational terms necessary to generate evidence about a theory are themselves reliant on the theory for their meaning, then:

• A theory can never truly be shown to be false.
• Evidence cannot be used to show that one theory is better than another (Hesse, 1970; Scriven, 1970).

These two conclusions basically undermine the whole idea of a progressive, self-correcting science that incrementally eliminates error and thereby moves toward truth. Instead, these arguments point out that a theory, at best, represents one possible explanation of the events it addresses (Hesse, 1970; Scriven, 1970).

Critical Modernism: Rethinking the Role of Empiricism

Criticisms of logical positivism ushered in an important new direction in the understanding of science. This perspective has been labeled critical modernism (Midgely, 2003). As already noted, an earlier shift had redirected the ideal of science as achieving necessary truth toward a conception of science as progressing toward truth through self-correcting empiricism. Despite their differences, both of these views ultimately sought to identify logical principles and procedures that would emancipate science from the fallibility of ordinary human thinking and knowing.

However, the more philosophers attempted to isolate the logic of science from other psychological processes (e.g., intuition and creativity), the more apparent it became that this was not possible. The logical principles that were once considered to specify the very nature of science came to be understood as only one property of science. While logic is necessary, it is not sufficient for doing research. Within this new framework the role of intuition in induction, the nonprovability of first principles, and the embeddedness of observations within their theoretical contexts were looked at anew.

Take for instance, what White has to say about the problem of intuition in the process of induction. He notes that the process of "reducing concrete experience to artificial abstractions, or to put it more precisely, the act of substituting concepts, 'free inventions of the human intellect'....for concrete experiences of the senses...is the very essence of sciencing" (White, 1938, p. 372).

Moreover, philosophers of science came to see the incorrigibility of the first principles upon which all theories must be based, not as a fundamental problem, but as an important clue about the nature of science. That is, if the most abstract components of a theory cannot be shown to be grounded in the empirical world, it is because theory imparts meaning on, rather than extracts meaning from, the natural world. Theory is a creation of the human mind that makes sense of the world. The creative process by which researchers originate ideas to make sense of their observations of the natural world is as much a part of the research process as the logic by which researchers link the theoretical with the observed (Bronowski, 1978).

These critics of logical positivism identified flaws in its assertion that research would advance theory toward truth. Moreover, they were able to give creative and meaning-making processes a place in the research process. However, if research does not advance knowledge toward truth, what then is its purpose? Exactly how does research advance knowledge? The answers to these questions have been greatly influenced by Thomas Kuhn's (1962) historical analyses of how research was conducted in physical sciences. His work refined understanding of what researchers do when they empirically test theory. Along with other critics of positivism, Kuhn (1977) argues that when investigators collect data they do not directly test that theory, since "the scientist must premise current theory as the rules of his game" (p. 270). He further notes that all theories "can be modified by a variety of ad hoc adjustments without ceasing to be, in their main lines, the same theories" (Kuhn, 1977, p. 281). So, instead of testing theory, evidence generated in research allows the theory to be adjusted to better fit whatever phenomena it is designed to explain.

Kuhn's insights point out that research does not prove or disprove the theory. However, it does improve the theory. Research serves as the basis for generating theories and, thereafter, can be used to enhance the fit of that theory to the natural world. Said another way, research allows investigators to advance the particular understanding of the phenomena that a given theory offers. As noted earlier, theory serves as a way to impart meaning on observations made in research. Once in place, theory serves as a schema for guiding the systematic observation of the world. Finally, because theory explains the world in a particular way, it leads to investigations that refine that explanation. All of these processes result in the accumulation of knowledge. Studies thus add to the stockpile of information related to any theoretical system.

Over time the knowledge accumulated through research does appear somewhat like the progression of knowledge envisioned by the logical positivists—with one important difference. Instead of progressing toward truth, theories progress by becoming better at the particular way they make sense of the world.

How Theories Change

Kuhn also provided an account of how theories were eventually rejected and replaced with newer theories. It was not, as supposed in the logical positivist tradition, the result of critical experiments that proved the theory wrong. Instead, theories were replaced when they were no longer fruitful for generating insights, yielding new problems for analysis and/or when they no longer were effective in making sense of new observations. In essence, theories were abandoned not because they were shown to be untrue, but because they simply ran out of steam. They were replaced with newer theories that were more effective in generating insights and problems to investigate and that made sense of things the old theory could not decipher.

Kuhn also underscored the importance of the scientific community sharing a common theoretical perspective (what he refers to as the paradigm). This common understanding refers not only to the explanations that are given by the theory but also to:

- What problems are considered most important to investigate and
- What techniques or approaches to collecting and analyzing data are considered acceptable or preferable.

Toulmin (1961) agrees with Kuhn, noting that theories both select what the researcher will see as problems to be investigated and also impart particular meanings to the phenomena that are studied. These problems are not the only possible problems and the meanings are not the only meanings that might be brought to bear on the world. However, they are the ones that make sense to the community of researchers at the time. Without them, the research process could not take place.

The perspectives, norms, rules, and so forth that guide how research is done in a particular arena are not absolute. Rather they constitute the "culture" of the research community. They are binding because:

- They represent a world view that is shared by all those doing research in a particular area. This allows them to makes sense of what they are studying and to make sense of the very process by which they go about studying it.
- Anyone wanting to be taken seriously as a researcher in the area must conform to them.

Kuhn's work underscores, then, that the scientific community needs theories or paradigms as contexts for doing research. They give the community of researchers a shared way of making sense of empirical objects and events so that they can be pondered in a particular way. As White (1938) notes, theories are arbitrary points of view from which scientists examine and consider reality. Theories are inescapable intellectual spaces within which researchers conduct their research.

Postmodernism

Postmodernism represents the most recent set of ideas in the philosophy of science. It is not a coherent single argument, but rather a set of loosely related themes. Postmodernists are particularly critical of the logical positivist perspective in more extreme ways than the critical modernists (Harvey, 1990). The critique of modernism discussed earlier pointed out how it is impossible to disentangle the language of a hypothesis from the theoretical system in which it is embedded. The philosopher, Wittgenstein (1953) went even further, asserting that language constructs reality. His argument leads to the conclusion that, since language determines what humans perceive, science cannot escape its own linguistic blinders. In other words, the very language of science determines what the scientist can come to know.

> Theories give the community of researchers a shared way of making sense of empirical objects and events so that they can be pondered in a particular way.

Wittgenstein is generally attributed with beginning what has come to be known as "social constructivism," a standpoint that pervades postmodern thought. It asserts, in essence, that all knowledge, including scientific knowledge, is socially constructed and, therefore, relative. In this postmodern framework scientific knowledge is no more privileged than any other source of knowledge. It is the particular perspective of a particular group of people who have a particular purpose in mind.

Lyotard's (1979) critique of the state of scientific knowledge directly assaults the positivist approach of modernism. He argues that science is a form of metanarrative. According to Lyotard, the scientific metanarrative claims that science is a project of human enlightenment based on logic and empiricism and that promises to create a unified understanding of the word, work for the good of all, and improve the human condition. Lyotard and other postmodernists point out the many failures of science in this regard (e.g., contributions of science to the atrocities of modern warfare and ecological problems and the failure of modern science to address the needs of oppressed groups, women, ethnic minorities, and members of third world countries).

Lyotard further argues that scientific disciplines are like games with their own rules, boundaries, and permissible moves. Importantly, what is permissible in the game is determined by power structure of any particular branch of science. Foucault (1970), in particular, emphasizes this relation between power and knowledge, arguing that the production of knowledge is closely tied to social control and domination. His work provides a basis for many postmodern critiques of how science serves to perpetuate oppression.

As a result of Lyotard's and Foucault's work, postmodernists are particularly critical of any broad theories that they see as forms of metanarrative. They argue that these metanarratives privilege certain groups and certain perspectives, while they have no more validity than any other "story" that might be narrated. Postmodernists emphasize the right of groups to have their own voice and speak for their own reality (Harvey, 1990). For this reason, postmodern thinking has been used by scholars whose work has championed disenfranchised groups (e.g., women's studies [Weedon, 1987] and disability studies [Rioux, 1997]).

In the end, most postmodernists paint a negative view of science. They not only discount the methodological claims made by the logical positivists, but also call into question the value of much of the information science has created. The ultimate conclusion of postmodernism is that "there can be no universals, that absolute truth is an illusion" (Midgley, 2003, p. 48). Moreover, postmodernists have critiqued science as being ideologically biased, tied to power structures, and ultimately contributing to oppression by replacing local knowledge with falsely claimed universal knowledge. Consequently, postmodernists seek to "promote variety, undermine certainty, and promote local, critical thought" (Midgley, 2003, p. 55).

Critiques of Postmodernism

A number of severe critiques of postmodernism exist (Harvey, 1990; Midgley, 2003). Some of these are directed at apparent self-contradictory arguments within postmodernism. For example, the most frequently cited contradiction within postmodernism is that, while it disparages grand theories (metanarratives), it proposes a grand theory that is supposed to supersede all previous theories. Or conversely, if one accepts the proposition that no universal claims about knowledge are true, then one has to reject the postmodernist claim that all knowledge is socially constructed. Postmodernists typically admit that there are ironic and self-contradictory elements of the postmodern argument, but they dismiss criticisms of this aspect of postmodernism as a misplaced concern for logic and coherence.

The most salient criticism of postmodernism, however, is that while it has successfully pointed out some of the limitations and failures of modernism, it has not offered any alternative (Midgley, 2003). In fact, extreme postmodernists argue that any attempt at creating universal knowledge is essentially pointless.

Conclusion

This chapter documented the history of thought in the philosophy of science. It illustrated how research was classically conceived as a means of attaining truth based on self-evident principles and proof. This perspective was replaced by the logical positivist view of science as a self-correcting

process that would progress toward truth. Later, critical modernists challenged this view and argued that theories cannot be corrected by research but only improved as explanatory systems. Finally, postmodernists called into question all of science as a privileged form of knowing, suggesting that no universal knowledge can be achieved. Table 2.1 illustrates these four periods in the philosophy of science and their major arguments concerning theory, empiricism, and scientific knowledge. It represents not only the evolution of ideas about research, but also a continuum of perspectives, some of which are embraced, either implicitly or explicitly, by researchers today.

For instance, most quantitative research employs logical methods developed in the logical positivist tradition. Many qualitative researchers embrace ideas represented in critical modernism and postmodernism. Every study draws in some way upon the kinds of ideas that have been developed in the philosophy of science.

What, then, are the lessons that researchers can take from the continuum of philosophical perspectives discussed in this chapter? First of all, few today would embrace the classic idea that science produces truth. However, with the exception of extreme postmodernists, most would agree that science produces potentially useful knowledge. Representing the view of critical modernists, Kuhn (1977) ultimately concluded that scientific efforts should be judged on their utility—that is, "the con-

Table 2.1 A Continuum of Ideas in the Philosophy of Science

	Classicism	Modernism	Critical Modernism	Postmodernism
The nature of theory	Theory is built on first principles that are self-evident (i.e., revealed by the world).	Theory is a logical system that explains and can predict events in the world.	Theory is a product of creative imagination that enables scientists to appreciate the world in a particular way.	Theory is a meta-narrative that falsely claims privileged status over other possible narratives.
The role of empiricism	Theory can be proved by deducing empirically demonstrable statements.	Theory can be disproved through empirical tests of logically derived hypotheses.	Theory can be improved by empirical testing.	Empirical testing proves nothing; it only reinforces claims to power/legitimacy.
View of scientific knowledge	Scientific knowledge represents truth.	Scientific knowledge is tentative but can be made increasingly true over time.	Scientific knowledge is one possible version of the world, which must be critically judged for its consequences.	All knowledge, including scientific knowledge, is socially constructed/relative.

crete technical results achievable by those who practice within each theory" (p. 339). Kuhn's comments suggest that scientific efforts in occupational therapy should be judged on their ability to help therapists effectively solve the kinds of problems their clients face.

Postmodernism is generally not useful as a philosophical premise for doing research. Nonetheless, postmodernism can be useful as a critical stance from which to judge scientific efforts. In particular, it is useful in calling attention to how science can be shaped by ideology, power, and interest.

One of the most relevant examples for occupational therapy are disability studies that use the postmodern social constructivist argument as a basis for critiquing much existing research on disability. As Rioux (1997) points out, the various research efforts to classify, count, and study relationships among variables associated with disability appear to be objective and scientific. However, this science is informed by an ideology about the nature of disability that focuses on disability as an individual deviation from norms. Importantly, the understanding of disability that has resulted from this approach is at variance with how people with disabilities experience their situation. Thus, the dominant modern understanding of disability is a social construction, not a fact. Scholars in disability studies have called for the voices of disabled persons to be added to the scientific discourse about disability in order correct this prevailing misunderstanding of disability (Scotch, 2001).

A second important lesson to be taken from postmodernism is the need to contextualize knowledge in the circumstances of its production—that is, to place any claims to knowledge in the context within which the knowledge was generated. A number of investigators, especially those involved in qualitative research, where the investigator's interpretation is a major analytic tool, do carefully context their research efforts in their personal and other relevant histories. By doing so, the investigator gives the reader an additional perspective from which to understand and judge the research findings.

While the ideas about the nature of research in the philosophy of science have changed dramatically over the centuries, each era has offered certain principles, ideas, and understandings that are useful to keep in mind regarding research. While they might be formulated in a number of ways, this chapter concludes with the following key insights and guidelines.

Regarding Theory

- Theories are human creations that seek to impart meaning on the world.
- First principles or underlying assumptions are unavoidable and untestable parts of any theory.
- Theories always represent one way of explaining or making sense of things.
- While theories cannot be disproved, their ability to explain the natural world can be improved through research.
- The ultimate worth of any theory is its ability to generate solutions to practical problems.
- It is not possible to undertake research, no matter how open-ended and free of presuppositions, without some underlying theory and first principles, even if they are not made explicit. Thus, whether a researcher is using only a handful of loosely connected assumptions and concepts or a complex theory, some conceptual context is necessary to any research.

Regarding the Research Process

- Research is part of an inductive–deductive process in which theory is derived from and tied back to the world through empiricism.
- Logic is necessary to connect the concepts and propositions that make up a theory with each other and to connect them with the things in the world to which they refer.
- All research is embedded in theory (whether or not it is made explicit). The theory is what makes sense of the phenomena examined, the scientific problems addressed, and the way those problems are solved.
- Research does not advance theory toward truth, but instead improves the way that any theory makes sense of the world.

Regarding Researchers

- Researchers always impart meaning on what they observed by creating theories.
- Investigators bring to bear all their characteristics (including personal history, training, theoretical understandings, and assumptions) on the research process.
- Researchers are part of a social community that shares a perspective that makes sense of what is studied as well as related norms and rules that set out what should be studied and how.

Regarding the Impact of Research

- Research is not inherently value-free or benign.
- Research can be tied to particular ideologies and used to reinforce power structures and to disenfranchise or oppress groups.
- Research can be used for positive ends and by advancing understanding and prediction of certain phenomena, it can inform practical action.

REFERENCES

Bronowski, J. (1978). *The origins of knowledge and imagination.* New Haven: Yale University Press.

Cohen, I. B. (Ed.). (1958). *Isaac Newton's papers & letters on natural philosophy.* Cambridge, MA: Harvard University Press.

Cohen I. B., & Smith, G. (Eds.). (2002). *The Cambridge companion to Newton.* Cambridge, UK: Cambridge University Press.

Foucault, M. (1970). *The order of things: An archeology of the human sciences.* New York: Pantheon.

Grunbaum, A. (1970). Can we ascertain the falsity of a scientific hypothesis? In E. Nagel, S. Bromberger, & A. Grunbaum (Eds.), *Observations and theory in science* Baltimore: John Hopkins University Press.

Harvey, D. (1990). *The condition of postmodernity.* Cambridge, MA: Blackwell.

Hesse, M. (1970). Is there an independent observation language? In R. G. Colodny (Ed.). *The nature and function of scientific theories.* Pittsburgh: University of Pittsburgh Press.

Jenkins, J. (1992). *Understanding Hume.* Edinburgh: Edinburgh University Press.

Kant, I. (1996). *Critique of pure reason* (W. S. Pluhar, Trans.). Indianapolis: Hackett.

Kaplan, A. (1964). *The conduct of inquiry: Methodology for behavioral science.* San Francisco: Chandler.

Klee, R. (1997). *Introduction to the philosophy of science: Cutting nature at its seams.* New York: Oxford University Press.

Kuhn, T. (1962). *The structure of scientific revolutions.* Chicago: University of Chicago Press.

Kuhn, T. (1977). *The essential tension.* Chicago: University of Chicago Press.

Losee, J. (1993). *A historical introduction to the philosophy of science* (3rd ed.). New York: Oxford University Press.

Lyotard, J. (1979). *The postmodern condition: A report on knowledge.* Minneapolis: University of Minnesota Press.

Midgley, G. (2003). Five sketches of post-modernism: implications for systems thinking and operational research. *International Journal of Organizational Transformation and Social Change. 1,* 47–62.

Nagel, E. (1949). The meaning of reduction in the natural sciences. In R. C. Stauffer (Ed.), *Science & civilization* (pp. 327–338). Madison: University of Wisconsin Press.

Rioux, M. H. (1997). Disability: The place of judgment in a world of fact. *Journal of Intellectual Disability Research, 41,* 102–111.

Robson, J. M. (1996) *Collected works of John Stuart Mill.* New York: Routledge.

Scotch, R. K. (2001). *From good will to civil rights: Transforming federal disability policy* (2nd ed.). Philadelphia: Temple University Press.

Scriven, M. (1970). Explanations, predictions and laws. In H. Feigl & G. Maxwell (Eds.), *Minnesota studies in the philosophy of science.* Minneapolis: University of Minnesota Press.

Skorupski, J. (Ed.). (1998). *The Cambridge companion to John Stuart Mill.* Cambridge, UK: Cambridge University Press.

Toulmin, S. (1961). *Foresight and understanding: An inquiry into the aims of science.* Bloomington, IN: University of Indiana Press.

Watson, R. (2002). *Cogito ergo sum: The life of Rene Decartes.* Boston: Godine Press.

Weedon, C. (1987). *Feminist practice and poststructuralist theory.* Cambridge, MA: Blackwell.

White, L. (1938). Science is sciencing. *Philosophy of Science, 5,* 369–389.

Wittgenstein, L. (1953). *Philosophical investigations.* Oxford: Basil Blackwell.

CHAPTER 3

The Range of Research

Gary Kielhofner • Ellie Fossey

Research studies are almost as varied as they are numerous. Even within a specific field such as occupational therapy, there is considerable diversity of investigations. For example, studies may differ along such dimensions as:

- The sample size, or number of study participants (from one to hundreds or thousands),
- What participants are asked to do (being observed versus undergoing complex interventions),
- How information is gathered (following participants in their ordinary activities and context versus taking measurements in a laboratory setting), and
- How the data are analyzed (identifying underlying narrative themes versus computing statistical analyses).

One way to appreciate this diversity of research is to examine different ways it is classified. In this chapter, we consider three ways that research is differentiated: by method, by design, and by purpose (Table 3.1). Since all the approaches to research that we discuss here are detailed in this book, the aim of this chapter is to give the reader a broad appreciation of the range of research that will be discussed later.

Research Methods: Qualitative and Quantitative

One of the most common distinctions is that between qualitative and quantitative research methods. Terminology suggests these methods differ by the presence or absence of quantification. However, it is important to note that these two broad categories of research are also distinguished by important philosophical differences (Crotty, 1998). Hence, we describe the origins of qualitative or quantitative research and their differing assumptions, approaches to rigor, and research focus, as well as examining how they gather, analyze, and interpret data.

Quantitative Methods

Quantitative research originated in the physical sciences. Fields such as astronomy and physics were the first to develop sophisticated research methods; they were followed by the biological sciences. As a result, approaches to doing research were first developed in the context of studying the physical world (Johnson, 1975). Later, fields that studied human behavior (e.g., psychology and sociology) emulated perspectives and methods that were already flourishing in the physical and life sciences.

Assumptions About the Phenomena Under Inquiry

Fundamental to any inquiry are its assumptions about the nature of the phenomena being studied (Neuman, 1994). The quantitative tradition is grounded in the assumption that there is one, objective reality that is stable over time and across situations. So, for example, the laws of gravity are presumed to remain the same over the centuries and to apply equally throughout the universe. Similarly, in the biological domain, it is assumed that the laws of kinematics that govern how the body produces movement apply equally when one is an adolescent and when one is older and that they are the same across people. Therefore, the aim of quantitative methods is to discover the rules or laws underlying the objective world as a basis for scientific prediction and control (Guba & Lincoln, 1994).

Table 3.1 Typical Ways of Categorizing Research

Research methods	Qualitative methods
	Quantitative methods
Research designs	Experimental and quasi-experimental studies
	Single subject designs
	Field studies and naturalistic observation
	Surveys
	Psychometric studies
Research purposes	Basic
	Applied
	Transformative

Research in occupational therapy began to develop in earnest in the mid-20th century. At that time occupational therapy practice was dominated by an approach that emulated medicine's emphasis on scientific methods developed in the physical and life sciences, such as chemistry and biology (Kielhofner, 2004). Not surprisingly, the research that began to appear around this time was quantitative. The following two examples of research, reported in the *American Journal of Occupational Therapy*, are characteristic of the period.

Drussell (1959) reported a descriptive study that asked whether the industrial work performance of adults with cerebral palsy was related to their manual dexterity, as measured by the Minnesota Rate of Manipulation Test (MRM). The MRM is a standardized measure of manual dexterity originally used for testing workers' ability to perform semiskilled factory operations. Work performance was measured with a widely used industrial measure, the Service Descriptive Rating Scale. In this study both tests were administered to 32 adults with cerebral palsy who were enrolled in an adult vocational training program. The results of the study indicated that the two measures were positively correlated. This finding was interpreted as indicating that the MRM could be a valuable tool in assessing vocational potential for this population.

Cooke (1958) reported results of an experimental study that investigated whether adding a weight to the dominant upper extremity of patients with multiple sclerosis would improve their coordination. The rationale was that the addition of weight would mitigate patients' intention tremors and thus increase coordination. In this study of 39 patients in a physical rehabilitation program, the subjects were tested with and without a weighted cuff using the MRM Test (used in this study as the measure of coordination). The results of the study failed to support the hypothesis that the addition of a weight would improve coordination. In fact, the opposite was observed; subject scored significantly lower when wearing the weighted cuffs. This author concluded, then, that the addition of the cuff slowed the speed of movement, negatively affecting coordination.

The characteristics of these two studies, quantification of the variables under study through use of standardized measures, use of experimental conditions in the second study, and statistical analyses (descriptive in the first study; inferential in the second study) are hallmarks of quantitative research. Since these studies were conducted, the use of more complex experimental designs, including pre- and post- intervention testing, randomization of study participants, and test development, has developed in occupational therapy. Nevertheless, the underlying logic of the research designs used in these two studies is similar to that of contemporary quantitative research in occupational therapy.

This assumption of a stable world governed by timeless laws is also applied to the study of human behavior. For example, early in the field of psychological research, behaviorism sought to discover the laws that governed how positive or negative consequences influenced behavior. It was expected that these laws would allow the articulation of causal models to predict behavior across people and across the course of development. Thus this tradition of psychological research was predicated on a view of human behavior as observable, measurable, and predictable (Rice & Ezzy, 1999).

> ...the aim of quantitative methods is to discover the rules or laws underlying the objective world as a basis for scientific prediction and control.

Rigor: An Emphasis on Objectivity

Quantitative methods place importance on the scientist maintaining an objective stance. The quantitative researcher must take great care to see the outside world as it is by avoiding the influence of subjective error or bias. This concern for scientific objectivity permeates quantitative research and its methodological procedures. Thus, in quantitative research the investigator ordinarily employs standardized and predetermined designs and procedures (Seltiz, Wrightsman, & Cook, 1976). Because quantitative researchers aim to discover invariant laws that apply across situations, they are also concerned with being able to generalize from the sample studied in the particular investigation to a larger population that the samples represent. Thus, the use of standard sampling procedures aims to ensure the generalizability of the findings.

A Focus on Theory Testing

Because of how they view the world, quantitative researchers tend to focus on:

- Creating theory that explains the laws governing the phenomena under study, and
- Testing that theory to verify and refine it through research (Filstead, 1979).

Thus, translating abstract theory into specific answerable questions and concrete observable hypotheses (statements of expected observations based on the theory) is key to quantitative research (Filstead, 1979).

Data Representation and Analysis: Quantification and Statistics

Quantification involves transforming observations into numerical data for manipulation using statistics. The researcher assigns numbers in a systematic, objective way to capture some essential characteristic of the variables under study. Quantification can include enumeration based on assignment to differential categories, determination of degree (ranking or rating), or determination of amount (measurement). There are many different procedures and tools for analyzing data statistically, dependent on the type of data and the nature of the research question and design. However, in general, statistical analyses are used to:

- Characterize or describe aggregated data (e.g., to indicate frequency, variability, averages), and
- To draw inferences about the data collected (e.g., to determine whether the average value of a characteristic differs across two groups).

Findings are presented in the form of statistics that characterize the sample and the population it represents, answer questions, and/or test hypotheses.

Qualitative Methods

Qualitative methods are typically used in research that aims to describe and explain persons' experiences, actions and interactions, and social contexts. Qualitative research is an umbrella term for a range of methodologies originating from the fields of anthropology, sociology, philosophy, and psychology. Today, they are widely used in the health sciences. Many researchers in occupational therapy have embraced these methodologies to study occupation and practice issues, viewing them as congruent with the profession's philosophical orientation (Hammell, 2002).

The perspectives and methods of qualitative research originally grew out of the challenges of studying groups of people who were dramatically different from the investigator. Because qualitative researchers encountered foreign languages, perspectives, and practices, they recognized that behavior reflected rules specific to the social and cultural context (Denzin, 1971; Edgerton & Langess, 1974; Johnson, 1975; Pelto & Pelto, 1978; Schutz, 1954). Qualitative methods developed in response to the recognition that the everyday world that people experience is a valid focus of inquiry (Crotty, 1998; Neuman, 1994). Thus, qualitative research traditions generated a unique set of assumptions about, and approaches to studying, the phenomena they investigated.

Qualitative research is generally divided into ethnographic, phenomenological, and narrative inquiry approaches, each of which represents a somewhat different standpoint. Ethnography emphasizes the societal and cultural context that shapes meaning and behavior. Phenomenology focuses on how people experience and make sense of their immediate worlds, and narrative inquiry seeks to understand how people construct storied accounts of their and others' lives and of shared events (Rice & Ezzy, 1999).

Assumptions About the Phenomena Under Study

Early qualitative researchers justified their approach by emphasizing the differences between the phenomena they studied and the approach of the traditional physical scientists. For instance, Schutz (1954) argues:

The world of nature, as explored by the natural scientist, does not "mean" anything to the molecules, atoms and electrons therein. The observational field of the social scientist, however, namely the social reality, has a specific meaning and relevance structure for the human beings living, acting, and thinking, therein. (p. 266)

Qualitative researchers asserted that human behavior was guided by meaning, not objective laws (Blumer, 1969; Lofland, 1976; Pelto & Pelto, 1978). Moreover, qualitative researchers recognize not one single human reality but, instead, multiple realities reflected in the different meaning structures of different groups.

Qualitative researchers have also stressed that individual and collective actions require those involved to assess and interpret the ongoing and typical situations that confront them (Blumer, 1969; Lincoln & Guba, 1985; Rice & Ezzy, 1999). Thus, unlike the phenomena studied by the physical and life sciences that are governed by invariant and timeless laws, the phenomena studied in qual-

Qualitative research began to appear in occupational therapy literature during the 1980s. At that time, there was a resurgence of interest in ideas about occupation, its meanings and significance for health, on which occupational therapy practice was founded (Kielhofner, 2004). This led occupational therapists to seek relevant research designs for exploring the meanings and contexts of people's everyday lives, occupations, and experiences of illness, disability, or therapy, and to argue for the use of qualitative designs in occupational therapy (Kielhofner, 1982a, 1982b; Krefting, 1989; Yerxa, 1991). Early examples of qualitative research published in occupational therapy most commonly used ethnographic designs, originating in anthropological fieldwork methods, of which the following is an example.

This study examined the daily life experiences of 69 adults with developmental delay who were discharged from state hospitals to residential facilities as part of the deinstitutionalization movement. In this study, the project team (anthropologists, sociologists and clinicians followed the study participants over a 3-year period, participating with them in their daily life events in the five residential facilities where they lived. Researchers recorded observational data in field notes, conducted ongoing open-ended interviews with the residents, and videotaped them. Analysis of the data form this field study resulted in several publications (Bercovici, 1983; Goode, 1983; Kielhofner, 1979, 1981). Kielhofner (1979) reported how the participants experienced and organized their behavior in time. He described how the participants did not progress through the usual life events that tend to demark maturation (e.g., graduating high school, marriage, parenthood). Rather, their lives were largely unchanged over time with the result that the participants tended not to be future oriented; they did not expect things to be change, nor did they make plans for achieving change in their lives. Hence, he argues among other things that the participants:

> ...have ceased to become in the sense of the dominant culture, and from their own point of view, they are off the career time track. They are, in a sense, "frozen in time." (Kielhofner, 1979, p. 163)

Another feature of how these study participants experienced their lives uniquely was that unlike many other members of American culture, they had a surplus of time and a deficiency of things to do that would fill up their time. As a result, they did not experience long periods waiting for events to occur with the impatience or frustration that characterized the investigators' reactions. Rather, waiting was something that helped to fill time. These and other findings pointed out that these adults approached the organization of their daily activities and their lives in a radically different way from mainstream American culture (Kielhofner, 1981).

This study highlights the emphasis of ethnographic research on illuminating the social and cultural context of human action and its meaning. It also illustrates the use of this type of research in examining how changes in health policy and services may impact persons. Since this study was conducted, qualitative research in occupational therapy has diversified, using phenomenological, narrative, and, more recently, participatory approaches. It has also expanded in focus to explore occupational therapists' clinical reasoning and practice issues in many settings, as well as the everyday lives and occupations of clients of occupational therapy services.

itative research are seen as dynamic, relational, and embedded in a particular context.

Rigor: An Emphasis on Understanding and Representing Subjective Reality

Since qualitative researchers seek to understand the actions of people, they must know the everyday meaning and contexts that inform and shape those actions (Strauss & Corbin, 1990). Qualitative researchers are concerned with accurately capturing research participants' subjective meanings, actions, and perceptions of their social contexts (Popay, Rogers, & Williams, 1998). Consequently, qualitative researchers use methods to actively engage their study participants in dialogue, and participate with them in the activities under study, in order to achieve an insider (or emic) understanding.

Unlike quantitative researchers who sought to maintain an objective stance on the phenomena they studied, qualitative researchers aim to immerse themselves in the subjective reality of the persons whom they study (DePoy & Gitlin, 1998; Pelto & Pelto, 1978; Rice & Ezzy, 1999). Qualitative researchers also reflect on their own personal reactions in the research setting to gain better access to how study participants experience their reality (Denzin, 1971). The greatest threat to rigor in qualitative research is that researchers may erroneously substitute their own meaning for the meanings of those they are studying, creating fictitious, and thus invalid, findings.

A Focus on Authenticity and Groundedness

Qualitative research aims to "illuminate the subjective meaning, actions and context of those being researched" (Popay, Rogers, & Williams, 1998, p. 345). Thus, central to the quality of qualitative research is:

- "Whether participants' perspectives have been genuinely represented in the research (authenticity), and
- Whether the findings are coherent in the sense that they 'fit' the data and social context from which they were derived" (Fossey, Harvey, McDermott, & Davidson, 2002, p. 723).

Qualitative researchers ordinarily begin their inquiry, like quantitative researchers, with guiding theoretical concepts and questions. However, they formulate broad questions, rather than narrowly defined questions or specific hypotheses. As data are gathered and inform these broad questions, they are refined, leading to more focused sampling and information-gathering. Thus, qualitative research is flexible, emergent, and responsive to the study setting, data, and its analysis. The participants and their social context shape the kinds of information gathered, and the themes and explanations that emerge in the study.

This means that, in qualitative research, the resulting abstractions, or theory developed, are grounded in the participants' experiences and social contexts. Valid representation centers on the transformation of the meanings, perspectives, and behaviors of those studied into theoretical abstractions. These abstractions must authentically represent how those studied experience and organize their world (Rice & Ezzy, 1999).

Data Representation and Analysis: Textual Description and Theory Grounded in Data

Data collection in qualitative research focuses on gaining understanding of the phenomena under study as they are experienced by the participants. This means that researchers strive to preserve the ways in which participants characterize their experiences and actions. Audiotaped interviews that allow extensive quotation of participants' own words, detailed notes that describe events and actions, written and visual documents, and recordings are typical data. These data provide a rich source for the qualitative investigator, but they also pose a challenge to coherently and concisely present findings.

Qualitative findings are represented as textual descriptions or narratives. Consequently analysis involves translating a wealth of detailed qualitative information to a textual account. Importantly, this account or narrative must authentically describe the phenomena being studied. That is, it must preserve for the reader the same essence of what was studied.

Qualitative data analysis requires the researcher to explore the meanings, patterns, or connections among data. This process involves the researcher's own thought, reflection, and intuition. There are many different qualitative procedures and tools for analyzing qualitative data. They share the common feature of progressively exploring the data, and comparing and contrasting different parts of the data in order to evolve a more sophisticated understanding (Tesch, 1990).

Often data gathering and data analysis occur iteratively, with each influencing the other. Since the researcher seeks to generate findings that are clearly grounded in participants' viewpoints, various safeguards are built into the analytic process. For example, qualitative research requires adequate sampling of information sources (i.e., people, places, events, types of data) so as to develop a full description of the phenomenon being studied (Rice & Ezzy, 1999). In addition, qualitative researchers typically return to the participants to seek their feedback as to whether the findings generated truly characterize their experiences.

Presentations of findings must enable the reader to appreciate the phenomena studied, and to gain insights into how they are experienced by the participants. One way of accomplishing this is through "thick description" (Geertz, 1973). Thick description refers to a sufficiently detailed depiction, drawn from the raw data, of people's experiences, actions, and situations to convey the layers of personal and contextual meanings that inform them (Denzin, 1971). For this reason, qualitative findings are generally presented with substantial

> ...in qualitative research, the resulting abstractions, or theory developed, are grounded in the participants experience and social context.

quotes, verbatim field notes, and other data that help point to the essence of the phenomena that the researcher is attempting to characterize.

The Qualitative–Quantitative Distinction

Table 3.2 illustrates how quantitative and qualitative methods differ across the dimensions discussed above. One way of thinking about these two methods is that quantitative research tends to emphasize the deductive logical phase, focusing on the testing of theory, whereas the qualitative tradition tends to emphasize the inductive phase, generating theory out of the careful observation of the nature situation (DePoy & Gitlin, 1998). These two modes of inquiry are also distinguished by different assumptions and approaches to achieving scientific rigor (Crotty, 1998; Fossey, Harvey, McDermott, & Davidson, 2002).

Despite their differences, these research methods have long been integrated in the social sciences. More recently, they are used together in health and human and services research (DePoy & Gitlin, 1998). Increasingly, occupational therapy researchers understand and draw upon both methods. As noted earlier, quantitative methods have their origins in the study of physical phenomena. In occupational therapy, whenever the object of inquiry is the structure and function of the human body, quantitative methods are the appropriate research approach to use. Quantitative methods are also used to study such things as cognitive functioning, sense of mastery, life satisfaction, adaptation, playfulness, and coping. When the aim of research is to compare different groups on these variables, study their relationships, or to determine whether intervention changes them, then quantitative research is the method of choice.

Qualitative research is better suited to the study of subjective experience, meaning, and the subjective and contextual aspects of human action and interaction (Guba & Lincoln, 1994; Neuman, 1994). Qualitative methods are especially appropriate for studies that seek to understand individuals' and groups' subjective experiences of impairment, occupation, and daily life, as well as to explore social and cultural factors that influence these experiences. Consequently, there are many issues about which occupational therapy researchers are interested to learn (e.g., how clients experience therapy, the thinking process behind therapists' decisions about their clients, what it is like to experience a particular disability) for which qualitative research is the method of choice.

Research Designs: An Overview of Common Basic Designs

Research can also differ by its basic design. Design refers to the fundamental strategy or plan of how the research will be structured. Research designs each have their own inherent logic. While the intention here is not to exhaustively list all research designs, we will cover the most common designs found in occupational therapy investigations. They include:

• Experimental and quasi-experimental studies,
• Single subject studies,
• Field studies and naturalistic observation,
• Survey studies, and
• Psychometric studies.

Experimental and Quasi-experimental Studies

Experimentation grew out of research in the life sciences and uses quantitative research methods. The basic characteristic of all experimental research is that the investigator manipulates an independent variable, the antecedent variable that is expected to produce an effect on a dependent variable. These designs aim to provide evidence that the independent variable is the cause of changes or differences in the dependent variable.

Experimental and quasi-experimental designs are specific blueprints for how to conduct an experiment (Campbell & Stanley, 1963). The fundamental aim of experimentation is to control, as much as possible, extraneous influences that might lead to an incorrect conclusion about the influence of the independent variable on the dependent variable. In a true experiment, two or more groups of participants are subjected to different independent variables. A fundamental characteristic of these research designs is the inclusion of a control group as a basis for comparison with the experimental group, which undergoes the condition of primary interest (such as an occupational therapy intervention) in the study.

A simple example of an experiment in occupational therapy is a study in which one group of persons receives therapy and a second group does not. In such a study, the researcher measures some characteristic (dependent variable), such as the independent self-care performance. The aim of the experiment would be to attribute any differences in self-care independence (dependent variable)

Table 3.2 **Key Differences Between Qualitative and Quantitative Research Methods**

Characteristic	Quantitative Research Tradition	Qualitative Research Tradition
Origin	Physical and life sciences	Study of people different from the investigator (anthropology, philosophy, sociology)
Assumptions	Objective reality contains stable preexisting patterns or order that can be discovered	Social reality is dynamic, contexted, and governed by local meanings.
Aims	To discover natural laws that enable prediction or control of events	To understand social life and describe how people construct social meaning
Approach to rigor	Maintain objectivity	Authentically represent the viewpoints of those studied.
Data presentation	Numbers (statistics)	Textual, "thick" descriptions in language of participants
Data analysis	Describes variables and their relationships and tests hypotheses in order to test theory	Identifies meaning, patterns, and connections among data; describes experience/social scene; produces theory "grounded" in the data.

between the two groups to the independent variable (receipt of occupational therapy services). However, in this case, the dependent variable might be influenced by the initial level of functioning of participants. If one group were generally better functioning than the other group at the beginning of the experiment, then this difference in functioning could account for differences in self-care independence. We might find this difference between the two groups whether or not they received occupational therapy services. Thus, in experimental studies subjects are randomly assigned to the two different conditions to achieve equivalent groups.

Quasi-experimental designs follow the same logic as experimental designs; they typically include a control group, or one or more comparison groups, and experimental manipulation of the independent variable of interest, but lack the degree of rigor found in true experiments (Cook & Campbell, 1979). For example, a study in which participants are not randomly assigned to groups would be considered quasi-experimental.

Occupational therapy researchers sometimes undertake less rigorous quasi-experimental research because true experiments research can be difficult to undertake in real-life contexts. For example, one of the authors is involved of an investigation of the effects of occupational therapy services, compared to a less intensive standard educational intervention, on independent living and employment (dependent variables). In this study, services are delivered to residents in the facilities where they live. Random assignment was not feasible because delivering different types of

services to persons living in the same house was likely to create other situations that would bias the results. For example, if a person in one group shared information and resources he or she received from services with a roommate who was not receiving those services, it would contaminate the findings. Consequently, for this study, a quasi-experimental design was chosen. All residents in one setting receive the same services and are compared with residents of another setting who receive different services. This type of design opens the experiment to alternative explanations for any differences in independence or employment found other than the services received, such as group personality, types of people in each house, and house staff. However, it was the most rigorous design practicable in this context. Thus, despite their limitations, quasi-experimental designs are valuable when the constraints in health or human service environments mean random assignment is not appropriate, ethical, or feasible (De Poy & Gitlin, 1998).

Single-Subject Studies

Experimental designs rely on comparisons of averages in groups. Individual variation in response to an intervention is not a focus of such studies. For that reason, practitioners sometimes find large group experiments to have limited relevance to decision-making about what services or strategies would be best for an individual client. Single-subject designs follow the logic of experimentation, but examine the impact of interventions on single subjects who serve as their own controls.

Examples of Experimental and Quasi-experimental Designs

A study examining the value of combined sensory integration and perceptual–motor treatment for children with developmental coordination disorder (DCD) provides an example of a quasi-experimental design. Davidson and Williams (2000) assessed 37 children with DCD, using the Movement ABC and the Beery-Buktenica Developmental Test of Visual–Motor Integration, before and after they had received combined sensory integration and perceptual–motor treatment for 10 weeks. The children were also reassessed with the same measures at 1-year follow-up. The authors reported results that indicated these children made statistically significant but relatively small gains in fine motor skills and visual–motor integration. They concluded that 10 weeks o therapy may be ineffective to achieve improvements in motor skills and motor integration for children with developmental coordination disorder.

In contrast, an experimental design was used in a study to determine whether occupational therapist home visits targeted at environmental hazards reduce the risk of falls in community-based frail older adults in Sydney, Australia (Cumming et al., 1999). The sample comprised 530 older adults (mean age 77 years), recruited from a hospital prior to discharge and randomly assigned to a control group or to occupational therapy intervention (experimental group). The latter group received a post-discharge home visit by an experienced occupational therapist, who assessed the home for environmental hazards, made home safety recommendations, and facilitated minor home modifications. A monthly falls calendar was used to ascertain falls over a 12-month follow-up period. The intervention was effective among those ($n = 206$) who reported one or more falls in the year prior to the study: at 12 months the risk of falling and of recurrent falls and the likelihood of being admitted to hospital were all significantly lower in the occupational therapy intervention group than in the control group. The authors concluded that home visits by occupational therapists can prevent falls among older people at increased risk of falling. Further, this effect may not be caused by home modifications alone, given only about 50% of recommended home modifications were in place at a 12-month follow-up visit.

Both these studies were designed to examine the effectiveness of an occupational therapy intervention. They each involved taking measurements for the outcome variables of interest pre- and post-intervention, both also included a 1-year follow-up. The principal differences between them lie in the inclusion of a control group, and random assignment of participants to this and the experimental group. This allowed the researchers (Cumming et al., 1999) to determine whether those who received occupational therapy intervention benefited compared to those others who receive no intervention (control group), and to have greater confidence that detected benefits are attributable to the intervention. As can be seen, it was also a substantially more ambitious undertaking to conduct an experimental study of this type.

These designs permit a controlled experimental approach within which to observe single subjects under ongoing treatment conditions in clinical settings (Portney, & Watkins, 2000).

Single-subject designs generally involve two major strategies that allow the subject to represent both a control and an experimental condition(s):

- Gathering baseline data over time during which the experimental condition is absent and then gathering data over time during which the experimental condition is present, and
- Gathering data during alternating periods in which the experimental condition is present or withdrawn.

Quantitative data are gathered on the dependent variable during the different experimental and control phases, and are analyzed both visually and using statistics designed for single-subject experimentation.

As noted above, single-subject designs follow an experimental logic and thus are not to be confused with qualitative studies that may involve a single participant. Both types of studies are characterized by a sample of one, but their underlying logic is different. Qualitative research that includes only one study participant follows the logic of qualitative methodology. In this instance, the judgment is made that one participant is of sufficient interest or adequately characterizes the phenomena under question. Thus, additional participants are not necessary to inform the intent of the study.

Field Studies and Naturalistic Observation

Field studies and naturalistic observation are forms of research that take place in the actual settings. Investigators study events as they happen and persons in their natural context. Both qualitative and qualitative research methods make use of this type of design.

Example of a Single-Subject Experimental Design

To investigate the effectiveness of a new somatosensory retraining program to improve tactile and proprioceptive discrimination in adults with sensory loss due to stroke, Carey, Matyas, and Oke (1993) designed a study involving two series of four single-subject experiments. In the first series involving four medically stable adults with stroke, data were gathered using the Tactile Discrimination Test on 10 occasions within each phase: the baseline (prior to training) and intervention (somatosensory retraining), and then a follow-up at an interval similar to the time taken to complete the baseline and intervention phases. The second series involved another four stroke participants in a similar procedure, except that both the Tactile Discrimination Test and the Proprioceptive Discrimination Test were administered in this series. Graphic and statistical interrupted time-series analyses show clearly the changes between the phases in each case. Improvements were clinically significant, with all participants reporting improved performance comparable to that of their other hand. These effects were maintained in follow-up tests.

Sensory training was a relatively new area of investigation and the population of adults with sensory loss post-stroke potentially diverse. Given these factors, the authors chose a single subject experimental design to allow individual responses to this intervention to be systematically examined. Often papers reporting single-subject experiments will report results on several subjects, as Carey et al. (1993) did. These are considered replications since the results from each single subject's experiment are analyzed separately.

In qualitative field studies, investigators seek to gain an insider's view of the phenomena under study through intensive and extended immersion. Investigators ordinarily collect data in multiple ways (e.g., gathering documents and artifacts, informal interviewing and observation) over some extended period of time. Researchers also use their growing appreciation of the phenomena under study to continuously evolve the kinds of data collected, the methods for acquiring data, and who is sought out as a source of data.

Naturalistic observation refers to quantitative research that takes place in natural settings. Such research aims to study the phenomena "undisturbed" by laboratory conditions or experimental procedures. For example, naturalistic observation can be used to study specific behaviors as they occur in classrooms, hospitals, or nursing homes. In naturalistic observation studies the observer seeks to make "unbiased" observations of how events or behaviors actually take place. The investigator does not participate in the events under study, but rather seeks to be as unobtrusive as possible.

Naturalistic observations generally seek to determine the kinds of behaviors that occur, their frequency, the conditions under which they occur, and so forth. For instance, the investigator may use a time sampling approach in which observations are recorded at specific time intervals, those intervals being chosen randomly or according to some logical schema. Data are ordinarily collected using some kind of coding procedure, determined prior to beginning the research, which enables the behavioral observations to be recorded in a manner that can be enumerated.

Survey Studies

Survey studies are nonexperimental designs undertaken to investigate the characteristics of a defined population (Depoy, & Gitlin, 1998; Portney, & Watkins, 2000). They are often conducted with large samples. Survey studies are used to investigate such things as conditions or needs within a defined community, or the extent of disease or disability in a population. Generally, survey research aims to randomly select the sample so that the findings can be generalized to the population from which the sample was chosen.

The most common form of survey research is implemented through the use of mailed questionnaires. More recently, the Internet has been used as a method of questionnaire distribution. Also, surveys can be conducted through Web-based survey sites, to which selected subjects are directed. Questionnaires are usually designed to gather quantitative data, although open-ended questions may be asked to elicit qualitative responses that are used to supplement quantitative findings.

Other survey research methods include telephone and face-to-face interviews. When surveys follow the logic of quantitative methods research, the investigator uses a structured interview protocol so that all the participants respond to the same standardized questions. In qualitative surveys, the investigator is more likely to use an interview guide that allows participants to influence the direction of the interview, but also emphasizes strategies for probing, which seek to elicit the respondents' perspective.

Examples of Naturalistic Field Studies

Field studies are conducted in the natural context and thus are particularly suited to examining how some behavior or natural process occurs, such as how mothers facilitate their children's play at home, or how persons discover what they are able to do in daily life when their capacities have been altered by trauma or disease. The following two studies exemplify qualitative field studies in occupational therapy.

The study by Pierce (2000) was designed to develop a theoretical description of the developmental progressions in how 1- to 18-month-old infants play within the home, using intensive longitudinal observation and grounded theory methods of analysis (Glaser & Strauss, 1967). Pierce (2000) gathered extensive monthly data in the homes of 18 American mothers and infants over a period of 18 months, including written play observations, multiple interviews with the mothers, and many hours of videotapes of the infants at play with the usual objects and spaces in their home environments. One reported aspect of this study focused on how mothers manage the spaces and objects in their homes to create and support their infants' play (Pierce, 2000; Pierce & Marshall, 2004). These findings describe the everyday tasks of mothers in selecting playthings for their infants (e.g., household implements, clothing, commercial toys), as well as organizing their spatial arrangement to support and control the infants' play in the home. Pierce (2000) concluded that this study makes visible the behind-the-scenes work of mothers in supporting infant play.

In a naturalistic study of a different kind, Tham, Borell, and Gustavsson (2000) designed a phenomenological study to investigate how adults with unilateral neglect experienced their disabilities in the context of their everyday lives. The study participants were four Swedish women with left hemiparesis and unilateral neglect following stroke. To explore their experiences of unilateral neglect, Tham and colleagues interviewed these women five to seven times over a 16-week period during their rehabilitation, including 4 weeks of an occupational therapy intervention that utilized meaningful everyday occupations as means to improve awareness of disabilities (Tham, Ginsburg, Fisher, & Tegner, 2001). A phenomenological method was used to create a description of how these women learned to live with unilateral neglect. The findings describe a discovery process in which the participants moved from experiencing their disabilities as new and unfamiliar, to beginning to discover and understand the consequences of unilateral neglect during performance of everyday activities, and then learning to handle the experience of neglect in everyday life situations. The authors suggest increased understanding was a prerequisite to being able to use strategies to compensate for disability. They concluded therefore that through participating in meaningful occupational situations, the participants gradually discovered their disabilities and began to recapture the left half of their worlds.

The research designs used in these two field studies illustrate different traditions of qualitative research. Nevertheless, several of their characteristics typify much qualitative research: extended engagement with participants in a natural setting; data collection that involves extensive interaction between the researchers and study participants; and the presentation of findings as a textual description.

Psychometric Studies

Psychometric studies are specifically designed to investigate the properties of clinical assessment tools, or data collection instruments, intended for use in research. Strictly speaking, this type of research is aimed at determining the validity and reliability of these instruments. Following quantitative logic, instruments with known validity and reliability provide objective measurement of the variables under study. Research with the primary purpose of the development and evaluation of clinical assessment tools may also include research questions that address their practical significance in clinical contexts. Psychometric research is largely quantitative, although qualitative methods are sometimes used to determine the kinds of content that should go into an assessment before it is developed, as well as to examine its clinical utility.

Validity refers to whether an instrument measures what it is intended to measure. Because instruments are designed to operationalize an underlying concept or construct, this aspect is often referred to as construct validity. There are many methods of determining validity. These include, for instance, concurrent validity and predictive validity. Concurrent validity follows the logic that an instrument designed to capture a variable should show an association with another variable that is theoretically expected to be related to it. Predictive validity asks whether a measure of some characteristic (e.g., ability to perform activities of daily living) is able to predict some future outcome, such as whether a person is able to perform those activities with or without assistance. Thus studies designed

A Survey Study Example

Survey research designs have frequently been in used in occupational therapy to investigate professional attitudes, knowledge, and practices. In this study, Dysart and Tomlin (2002) aimed to estimate the prevalence of evidence-based practice among occupational therapists in the United States. They designed a questionnaire to obtain demographics, information about current evidence-based practice use, and factors related to its use. The questionnaire was mailed to 400 randomly selected clinically practicing American Occupational Therapy Association members, and 209 completed the questionnaire for a 58% response rate. The authors analyzed the survey data using descriptive and inferential statistics to respectively describe the distribution of opinions and associations between demographic and evidence-based practice variables. Their findings suggested that therapists were engaging in a modest amount of evidence-based practice: they occasionally accessed research information through from various sources, with the majority (57%) implementing one to five new research-based treatment plans in the past year. However, less experienced respondents more frequently believed that research conclusions translated into treatment plans for individual clients than those with 15 or more years of clinical experience. Time available at work to access research information, high continuing education costs, weak research analysis skills, and placing higher value on clinical experience than on research were reported barriers to research utilization. The authors suggested mitigating these barriers may increase evidence-based practice use among clinically practicing occupational therapists.

to test expected associations, or predictions, provide evidence on behalf of the validity of an assessment tool or data collection instrument.

Reliability refers to whether a given instrument provides stable information across different circumstances. Thus studies designed to test reliability might examine whether a given instrument is reliable, for instance, when multiple raters use the instrument to gather data and when data are gathered on more than one occasion (referred to as inter-rater and test–retest reliability, respectively).

Psychometric studies in occupational therapy have used a range of research designs. Examples include the development of observation-based performance measures, such as the Assessment of Motor and Process Skills (Fisher, 1997; see also http://www.ampsintl.com/) and interview-based tools, such as the Canadian Occupational Performance Measure (COPM) (Carswell et al., 2004) and the Occupational Performance History Interview-II (Kielhofner et al., 2004), the development of which is summarized in the feature box titled Instrument Development in Occupational Therapy.

Research Purposes: Applied, Basic, and Transformative

Research can be differentiated according to its underlying purpose: basic, applied, or transformative. Basic, applied, and transformative types of research each have different stances on how information generated from research informs practice, so we also draw attention to these differences in relation to occupational therapy.

Basic Research

Basic research includes investigations undertaken for the purposes of generating evidence about some phenomena or testing theory about some phenomena (Depoy & Gitlin, 1998; Portney & Watkins, 2000). Basic research is undertaken for the sake of generating new knowledge without direct concern for its applicability or practical significance. The full range of research methods and designs previously described may be used in basic research, although traditionally, basic research emphasized the importance of value-free science that was disinterested in questions of application in order to avoid undue bias. It was thought that basic science would inform practice by identifying the underlying laws that governed phenomena and thus providing the logic for professions that applied that knowledge (Schon, 1983). This approach has been criticized by some scholars who argue that basic science knowledge does not translate readily into practice (Peloquin, 2002; Thompson, 2001).

Throughout much of its history, occupational therapy has relied on basic research conducted by other disciplines to inform practice. For instance, research that identified the anatomy of the musculoskeletal system and the physiology of nerve conduction are two examples of information generated from basic research in the fields of anatomy and physiology that form part of the foundation of occupational therapy knowledge. More recently, some occupational therapists have argued for the development of a basic science concerned with the study of occupation, referred to as occupational science. Its proposed purpose was to generate

Instrument Development in Occupational Therapy

Psychometric research is an ongoing process that usually represents a series of studies leading to progressive refinement of an assessment or measure (Benson & Schell, 1997). The following is a description of some of the early studies that examined the reliability, validity, and clinical utility of the Occupational Performance History Interview II (OPHI-II) (Kielhofner et al., 2004), an occupational therapy interview with an accompanying rating scale.

The OPHI was originally studied with a sample of 154 occupational therapy clients from psychiatry, physical disabilities, and gerontology practice in the United States and Canada (Kielhofner & Henry, 1988). This investigation found that the raw total score obtained from the rating scale had only marginally acceptable inter-rater reliability and test–retest reliability. A second study (Kielhofner, Henry, Walens, & Rogers, 1991) sought to improve the reliability of the OPHI rating scale by developing more specific guidelines for conducting the interview and completing the rating scale. The scale was found to be acceptably stable in this study.

Lynch and Bridle (1993) examined the concurrent validity of the OPHI, finding moderate correlations between OPHI raw scores and measures of depression and pain in persons with traumatic spinal cord injury. This was an expected relationship since other studies had shown that function in everyday life is associated with pain and depression. Following the logic that one's occupational life history represents strengths and weaknesses for future adaptation, Henry, Tohen, Coster, and Tickle-Degnen (1994) found that the OPHI (administered with young adults during hospitalization for a first psychotic episode) predicted psychosocial functioning and symptomatic recovery 6 months after discharge, thus providing evidence of its predictive validity. Fossey's (1996) and Neistadt's (1995) studies provided evidence that therapists perceived the OPHI to be a useful assessment in a range of contexts. Studies such as these provide cumulative evidence about an instrument's reliability, validity, and clinical utility.

Beyond the studies reported above, subsequent studies lead to further revision of the interview itself to improve the kind of data collected and creation of new rating scales to accompany it (Kielhofner & Mallinson, 1995; Mallinson, Kielhofner, & Mattingly, 1996; Mallinson, Mahaffey, & Kielhofner, 1998). The OPHI-II rating scales were eventually shown to be more reliable and valid than the previous scale (Kielhofner, Mallinson, Forsyth & Lai, 2001), and several recent studies have illustrated the kind of information about people's occupational lives gained using the OPHI-II interview and its clinical usefulness (Bravemann & Helfrich, 2001; Chaffey & Fossey, 2004; Goldstein, Kielhofner & Paul-Ward, 2004; Gray & Fossey, 2003).

---

explanations of humans as occupational beings (Yerxa et al., 1989). Like that of other basic research, the role of occupational science was envisioned as describing, explaining, and predicting events as part of the search for knowledge and truth (Primeau, Clark, & Pierce, 1989). Mosey (1992a, 1993) questioned the legitimacy of a basic science in occupational therapy on the grounds that the allocation of human and other resources to basic inquiry would detract from badly needed applied inquiry. Its proponents, nevertheless, argue that occupational science will likely influence how occupational therapists perceive and approach their work (Zemke & Clark, 1996).

Basic research may vary in how closely it relates to practical problems and practice issues, on which applied research focuses. To illustrate, Pierce's (2000) study (see related feature box) offers insights into the occupation-related tasks and routines of American mothers facilitating play with very young children at home. This study's purpose is consistent with basic research: to generate a theory of infant play development within the home. Consequently, the study did not address questions concerning occupational therapy practice for mothers or the children with identified occupational dysfunction, ill health, or disability. However, it provides information about the kinds of questions that occupational therapists could ask about facilitating play at home, both in practice and future applied research with mothers of very young children with identified occupational dysfunction, ill health, or disability.

Applied Research

Investigations that seek to solve some practical problem, or to generate information specifically to inform practice, are referred to as applied research (Depoy & Gitlin, 1998; Portney, & Watkins, 2000). Historically, applied research was most often undertaken by professions to address their practical concerns and held less status in academic circles where basic science was considered to be most rigorous because it was deemed to be value-free and thereby not biased by the practical concerns or less rigorous conditions under which applied research was conducted. This viewpoint has changed; most scientists now recognize the importance of applied research.

Many important research problems or questions generated in health and human service environments are applied in nature. Applied research generally seeks to investigate the merits of practice strategies (e.g., assessments and interventions). In occupational therapy, applied research address issues such as:

• Whether an assessment used in practice provides dependable and useful information to guide practice,
• How therapists reason in the context of practice, and
• What outcomes are achieved by providing particular services as part of therapy.

Applied research is often viewed as particularly important for achieving external credibility (i.e., influencing those who make policy and economic decisions that impact on the delivery of occupational therapy services). Indeed, Mosey (1992b) argued that this type of research is critical to occupational therapy since it provides information about the value of what the profession does. However, practitioners have critiqued applied research for testing practice strategies under ideal conditions that cannot be reproduced in practice (Dubouloz, Egan, Vallerand, & Von Zweck, 1999; Dysart & Tomlin, 2002). Applied research in occupational therapy ranges from psychometric studies, to qualitative investigations of the therapy process, to controlled experiments that compare different therapeutic approaches (see examples in feature boxes in this chapter).

Transformative Research

Transformative research refers to inquiry that is designed specifically to bring about change in some practical situation, or a specific context. Its emphasis is on transforming social realities so that people's lives are improved. Transformative research aims to foster self-reflection, mutual learning, participation, and empowerment (Letts, 2003; Reason 1994; Wadsworth & Epstein, 1998). Hence, this type of research has been used to enable groups of people who are in some way marginalized, deprived, or oppressed to bring about change in their lives and communities (Rice & Ezzy, 1999).

Examples of transformative research are relatively new in occupational therapy (Letts, 2003). The most common form of research with a transformative purpose in health care and in occupational therapy is participatory research. Some common features of participatory types of research are that it:

• Is always grounded in a practical context,
• Involves people not simply as data sources but as partners in the research process,
• Emphasizes power sharing between the researchers and local stakeholders (e.g., therapists and clients), and
• Is action-oriented, focusing on making change in the practice setting and on examining the impact of that change from the perspectives of those who are most influenced by it.

Transformative research is newer than either basic or applied research. Transformative research calls for embedding the research process in the practice setting and giving stakeholders (e.g., practitioners and clients) a voice in shaping the research process. It aims to alter and empirically examine services, while empowering the stakeholders and embedding change processes within the context to which they are relevant. In this way, it attempts to combine research, education, and action or to link theory (knowing) and practice (doing) (Rice & Ezzy, 1999).

On the face of it, such research has special relevance to practitioners and clients in fields such as occupational therapy since it is much more directly driven by their agendas and aimed at having a positive impact on their circumstances (Crist & Kielhofner, 2005). Proponents argue that research grounded in and directly helping to evaluate practice in natural contexts should be given high priority in the field.

Conclusion

This chapter provided an overview of the range of research that one is likely to encounter in occupational therapy. It examined three different ways of differentiating research: method, design, and purpose. The aim was to be illustrative rather than exhaustive in examining variation in research. It should be obvious from the discussion that

> Research can take on many different forms, each with its own aims, approach to generating knowledge, and strategies for achieving rigor.

research can take on many different forms, each with its own aims, approach to generating knowledge, and strategies for achieving rigor

In this discussion, we also mentioned some of the debates about the relative merits of differing types of research. Such debates are ongoing, and rightfully so. It is important to also recognize that, while researchers of particular traditions have previously been more divided in their allegiance to and use of one or another approach to research, it is not uncommon for contemporary research to use multiple methods and to incorporate more than one purpose in a single study.

REFERENCES

Benson, J., & Schell, B. A. (1997). Measurement theory: Application to occupational and physical therapy. In J. Van Deusen, & D. Brunt (Eds.), *Assessment in occupational therapy and physical therapy* (pp. 3–24). Philadelphia: W. B. Saunders.

Bercovici, S. (1983). *Barriers to normalization*. Baltimore: University Park Press.

Blumer, H. (1969). *Symbolic interactionism*. Englewood Cliffs, NJ: Prentice-Hall.

Braveman, B., & Helfrich, C. A. (2001). Occupational identity: Exploring the narratives of three men living with AIDS. *Journal of Occupational Science, 8*, 25–31.

Campbell, D. T., & Stanley, J. C. (1963). *Experimental and quasi-experimental designs for research*. Chicago: McNally & Co.

Carey, L. M., Matyas, T. A., & Oke, L. E. (1993). Sensory loss in stroke patients: effective training of tactile and proprioceptive discrimination. *Archives of Physical Medicine and Rehabilitation, 74*, 602–611.

Carswell, A., McColl, M. A., Baptiste, S., Law, M., Polatajko, H., & Pollock, N. (2004). The Canadian Occupational Performance Measure: A research and clinical literature review. *Canadian Journal of Occupational Therapy, 71*(4), 210–222.

Chaffey, L., & Fossey, E. (2004). Caring and daily life: Occupational experiences of women living with sons diagnosed with schizophrenia. *Australian Occupational Therapy Journal, 51*(4), 199–207.

Cook, T. D., & Campbell, D. T. (1979). *Quasi-experimentation: Design and analysis issues for field settings*. Boston: Houghton Mifflin.

Cooke, D. M. C. (1958). The effect of resistance on multiple sclerosis patients with intention tremor. *American Journal of Occupational Therapy, 12*(2), 89–92.

Crist, P., & Kielhofner, G. (2005). *The scholarship of practice: Academic and practice collaborations for promoting occupational therapy*. Binghamton, NY: Hayworth Press.

Crotty, M. (1998). *The foundations of social research: Meaning and perspective in the research process*. Crows Nest, Australia: Allen & Unwin.

Cumming, R. G., Thomas, M., Szonyi, G., Salkeld, G., O'Neill, E., Westbury, C., et al. (1999). Home visits by an occupational therapist for assessment and modification of environmental hazards: A randomized trial of falls prevention. *Journal of the American Geriatrics Society, 47*, 1397–1402.

Davidson, T., & Williams, B. (2000). Occupational therapy for children with developmental coordination disorder: A study of the effectiveness of a combined sensory integration and perceptual-motor intervention. *British Journal of Occupational Therapy, 63*, 495–499.

Denzin, N. (1971). The logic of naturalistic inquiry. *Social Forces, 50*, 166–182.

DePoy, E., & Gitlin, L. N. (1998). *Introduction to research: Understanding and applying multiple strategies* (2nd ed.). St. Louis: C. V. Mosby.

Drussell, R. D. (1959). Relationship of Minnesota rate of manipulation test with the industrial work performance of the adult cerebral palsied. *American Journal of Occupational Therapy, 13*, 93–105.

Dubouloz, C., Egan, M., Vallerand, J., & VonZweck, C. (1999). Occupational therapists' perceptions of evidence based practice. *American Journal of Occupational Therapy, 53*, 445–453.

Dysart, A. M., & Tomlin, G. S. (2002). Factors related to evidence-based practice among US occupational therapy clinicians. *American Journal of Occupational Therapy, 56*, 275–284.

Edgerton, R., & Langess, L. (1974). *Methods and styles in the study of culture*. San Francisco: Chandler and Sharp.

Filstead, W. J. (1979). Qualitative methods: A needed perspective in evaluation research. In T. Cook, D. Campbell, & C. Reichart (Eds.), *Qualitative and quantitative methods in evaluation research* (pp. 33–48). Beverly Hills: SAGE Publications.

Fisher, A. G. (1997). Multifaceted measurement of daily life task performance: Conceptualizing a test of instrumental ADL and validating the addition of personal ADL tasks. *Physical Medicine and Rehabilitation: State of the Art Reviews, 11*, 289–303.

Fossey, E. (1996). Using the Occupational Performance History Interview (OPHI): Therapists' reflections. *British Journal of Occupational Therapy, 59*(5), 223–228.

Fossey, E., Harvey, C. A., McDermott, F., & Davidson, L. (2002). Understanding and evaluating qualitative research. *Australian & New Zealand Journal of Psychiatry, 36*, 717–732.

Geertz, C. (1973). Thick description: Toward an interpretive theory of cultures. In C. Geetrz (Ed.), *The interpretation of culture: Selected essays* (pp. 3–30). New York: Basic Books.

Glaser, B., & Strauss, A. (1967). *The discovery of grounded theory*. New York: Aldine.

Goldstein, K., Kielhofner, G., & Paul-Ward, A. (2004). Occupational narratives and the therapeutic process. *Australian Occupational Therapy Journal, 51*, 119–124.

Goode, D. (1983). Who is Bobby? Idealogy and method in the discovery of a Down's syndrome person's competence. In G. Kielhofner (Ed.), *Health through occupation: Theory & practice in occupational therapy* (pp. 237–255). Philadelphia: F. A. Davis.

Gray, M., & Fossey, E. (2003). The illness experiences and occupations of people with chronic fatigue syndrome. *Australian Occupational Therapy Journal, 50*, 127–136.

Guba, E. G., & Lincoln, Y. S. (1994). Competing paradigms in qualitative research. In N. K. Denzin & Lincoln, Y. S. (Eds.), *Handbook of qualitative research* (pp. 105–117). Thousand Oaks, CA: SAGE Publications.

Hammell, K. W. (2002). Informing client-centered practice through qualitative inquiry: Evaluating the quality of qualitative research. *British Journal of Occupational Therapy, 65*, 175–184.

Henry, A., Tohen, M., Coster, W., & Tickle-Degnen, L. (1994). *Predicting psychosocial functioning and symptomatic recovery of adolescents and young adults following a first psychotic episode.* Paper presented at the Joint Annual Conference of the American Occupational Therapy Association and the Canadian Association of Occupational Therapists, Boston.

Johnson, J. (1975). *Doing field-research.* New York: Free Press.

Kielhofner, G. (1979). The temporal dimension in the lives of retarded adults: A problem of interaction and intervention. *American Journal of Occupational Therapy, 33,* 161–168.

Kielhofner, G. (1981). An ethnographic study of deinstitutionalized adults: Their community settings and daily life experiences. *Occupational Therapy Journal of Research, 1,* 125–142.

Kielhofner, G. (1982a). Qualitative research: Part One—Paradigmatic grounds and issues of reliability and validity. *Occupational Therapy Journal of Research, 2(2),* 67–79.

Kielhofner, G. (1982b). Qualitative research: Part Two—Methodological approaches and relevance to occupational therapy. *Occupational Therapy Journal of Research, 2(2),* 67–79.

Kielhofner, G. (2004). *Conceptual foundations of occupational therapy* (3rd ed.). Philadelphia: F. A. Davis.

Kielhofner, G. & Henry, A. (1988). Development and investigation of the Occupational Performance History Interview. *American Journal of Occupational Therapy, 42,* 489–498.

Kielhofner, G., Henry, A., Walens, D., & Rogers, S. (1991). A generalizability study of the Occupational Performance History Interview. *Occupational Therapy Journal of Research, 11,* 292–306.

Kielhofner, G., & Mallinson, T. (1995). Gathering narrative data through interviews: Empirical observations and suggested guidelines. *Scandinavian Journal of Occupational Therapy, 2,* 63–68.

Kielhofner, G., Mallinson, T., Crawford, C., Nowak, M., Rigby, M., Henry, A., & Walens, D. (2004). *Occupational Performance History Interview II (OPHI-II)* (Version 2.1). Model of Human Occupation Clearinghouse, Department of Occupational Therapy, College of Applied Health Sciences, University of Illinois at Chicago, Chicago, IL.

Kielhofner, G., Mallinson, T., Forsyth, K., & Lai, J. S. (2001). Psychometric properties of the second version of the Occupational Performance History Interview. *American Journal of Occupational Therapy, 55,* 260–267.

Krefting, L. (1989). Disability ethnography: A methodological approach for occupational therapy research. *Canadian Journal of Occupational Therapy, 56,* 61–66.

Letts, L. (2003). Occupational therapy and participatory research: A partnership worth pursuing. *American Journal of Occupational Therapy, 57(1),* 77–87.

Lincoln, Y. S., Guba, E. G. (1985). *Naturalistic inquiry.* Thousand Oaks, CA: SAGE Publications.

Lofland, J. (1976). *Doing social life.* New York: John Wiley & Sons.

Lynch, K., & Bridle, M. (1993). Construct validity of the Occupational Performance History Interview. *Occupational Therapy Journal of Research, 13,* 231–240.

Mallinson, T., Kielhofner, G., & Mattingly, C. (1996). Metaphor and meaning in a clinical interview. *American Journal of Occupational Therapy, 50,* 338–346.

Mallinson, T., Mahaffey, L., & Kielhofner, G. (1998). The Occupational Performance History Interview: Evidence for three underlying constructs of occupational adaptation (rev.). *Canadian Journal of Occupational Therapy, 65,* 219–228.

Mosey, A. C. (1992a). *Applied scientific inquiry in the health professions: An epistemological orientation.* Rockville, MD: American Occupational Therapy Association.

Mosey, A. C. (1992b). The issue is—Partition of occupational science and occupational therapy. *American Journal of Occupational Therapy, 46,* 851–853.

Mosey, A. C. (1993). The issue is—Partition of occupational science and occupational therapy: Sorting out some issues. *American Journal of Occupational Therapy, 47,* 751–754.

Neistadt, M. (1995). Methods of assessing client's priorities: A survey of adult physical dysfunction settings. *American Journal of Occupational Therapy, 49,* 420–436.

Neuman, W. L. (1994). *Social research methods: Qualitative and quantitative approaches.* Needham Heights, MA: Allyn and Bacon.

Peloquin, S. M. (2002). Confluence: Moving forward with affective strength. *American Journal of Occupational Therapy, 56,* 69–77.

Pelto, P., & Pelto, G. (1978). *Anthropological research: The structure of inquiry.* New York: Cambridge University Press.

Pierce, D. (2000). Maternal management of the home as a developmental play space for infants and toddlers. *American Journal of Occupational Therapy, 54,* 290–299.

Pierce, D., & Marshall, A. (2004). Maternal management of the home space and time to facilitate infant/toddler play and development. In S. Esdaile & J. Olson (Eds.), *Mothering occupations: Challenge, agency and participation* (pp. 73–94). Philadelphia: F. A. Davis.

Popay, J., Rogers, A., & Williams, G. (1998). Rationale and standards for the systematic review of qualitative literature in health services research. *Qualitative Health Research, 81,* 341–351.

Portney, L. G., & Watkins, M. P. (2000). *Foundations of clinical research: Applications to practice* (2nd ed.). Upper Saddle River, NJ: Prentice-Hall.

Primeau, L. A., Clark, F., & Pierce, D. (1989). Occupational therapy alone has looked upon occupation: Future applications of occupational science to pediatric occupational therapy. *Occupational Therapy in Health Care, 6,* 19–32.

Reason, P. (1994). Three approaches to participatory inquiry. In N. K. Denzin & Lin Y. S. Lincoln. (Eds.), *Handbook of qualitative research* (pp. 324–339). Thousand Oaks, CA: SAGE Publications.

Rice, P. L. & Ezzy, D. (1999). *Qualitative research methods, a health focus.* Melbourne: Oxford University Press.

Schutz, A. (1954). Concept and theory formation in the social sciences. *Journal of Philosophy, 51,* 266–267.

Schon, D. (1983). *The reflective practitioner.* New York: Basic Books.

Seltiz, C., Wrightsman, L., & Cook, S. (1976). *Research methods in social relations.* New York: Holt, Rinehart & Winston.

Strauss, A., & Corbin, J. (1990). *Basics of qualitative research.* Thousand Oaks, CA: SAGE Publications.

Tesch, R. (1990). *Qualitative research: analysis types and software tools.* New York: Palmer Press.

Tham, K., Borell, L., & Gustavsson, A. (2000). The discovery of disability: a phenomenological study of unilateral neglect. *American Journal of Occupational Therapy. 54,* 398–406.

Tham, K., Ginsburg, E., Fisher, A. G., & Tegner, R. (2001). Training to improve awareness of disabilities in clients with unilateral neglect. *American Journal of Occupational Therapy, 55,* 46–54.

Thompson, N. (2001). *Theory and practice in human services.* Maidenhead: Open University Press.

Wadsworth, Y., & Epstein, M. (1998). Building in dialogue between consumers and staff in acute mental health services. *Systemic Practice and Action Research, 11,* 353–379.

Yerxa, E. J. (1991). National speaking: Seeking a relevant, ethical, and realistic way of knowledge for occupational therapy. *American Journal of Occupational Therapy, 45,* 199–204.

Yerxa, E. J., Clark, F., Frank, G., Jackson, J., Parham, D., Pierce, D., et al. (1989). An introduction to occupational science: A foundation for occupational therapy in the 21st century. *Occupational Therapy in Health Care, 6,* 1–17.

Zemke, R., & Clark, F (1996). *Occupational Science: The evolving discipline.* Philadelphia: F. A. Davis.

CHAPTER 4

Characteristics of Sound Inquiry and the Research Process

Gary Kielhofner

Despite their varying methods, designs, and purposes, all research studies share some common features and procedures. The aim of this chapter is to overview those elements that characterize all research. First, accepted characteristics of good research are identified and examined. Second, the activities that ordinarily make up the research process from the time it is planned until its completion are identified.

Characteristics of Research

The following characteristics are hallmarks of all research (Crotty, 1998; DePoy & Gitlin, 1998; Polgar & Thomas, 2000; Polit & Hungler, 1999; Portney & Watkins, 2000; Stein & Cutler, 1996):

- Rigor,
- A scientific/scholarly attitude of skepticism and empiricism,
- Logic, and
- Communality.

Each of these is interrelated with the others. Moreover, quality research exhibits all of these characteristics.

Rigor in Research

Research is distinguished from ordinary searching for knowledge by its degree of rigor. The concept of rigor means that investigators carefully follow rules, procedures, and techniques that have been developed and agreed upon by the scientific community as providing confidence in the information generated by research (Neuman, 1994; Thompson, 2001).

These rules, procedures, and techniques that make up rigorous research are quite varied and specific to the research questions, the methods and design of the research, and the topic or phenomena under investigation. The following are three examples of how investigators achieve rigor in research:

- In experimental research, investigators use standardized research designs that provide control over factors that could bias or confound the results. In a classic text, Campbell and Stanley (1963) outlined the threats to validity in experimental research and detailed a series of experimental and quasi-experimental designs that to various extents controlled for these threats. Today, when investigators use one of these experimental or quasi-experimental designs, members of the research community readily recognize the logic of their design and the extent of rigor it provided in the experiment. The confidence that is placed in the findings corresponds to the rigor of the design used.

- In survey research, investigators are concerned that the sample accurately represents the population of interest (Rea & Parker, 1997). To ensure representativeness, investigators must identify the population and sample from it so as to ensure that those asked to participate in the study characterize the total population. Then, the investigator must engage in a series of steps to ensure that as many of those asked to participate actually do. Finally, the investigator must ask whether there is any evidence that those who respond to the survey are systematically different from those who did not respond.

- In qualitative research investigators follow procedures to ensure that they have penetrated and comprehended how the people they are studying think about, choose, and experience their actions (Rice & Ezzy, 1999; Strauss & Corbin, 1990). Since these procedures cannot be pre-standardized as in experimental or survey research, investigators maintain a record of the natural history of the study that documents how insights and new questions arose from the data, how decisions were made to gather new information, how the participants in the study were selected, how the data were coded, and what procedures were used to extract themes and meaning from the data. When researchers have formulated their findings, they return to those they have studied and share these findings to verify that they have authentically captured their experience.

These are but a sampling of the many approaches and procedures that investigators use to ensure rigor in research. In each of these instances, the rules and procedures that the investigators follow have been worked out over time by communities of investigators who sought to improve the soundness of their research. These rules and procedures have been shared, scrutinized, discussed, and debated in the scientific community. Eventually, through consensus, they have become prevailing standards by which investigators do research and by which completed research is judged (Crotty, 1998).

As the previous examples illustrate, rigor requires investigators to be thoroughly aware of the accepted rules and procedures for the type of research they plan to undertake. Investigators must also be cognizant of unique approaches that are typically used by other researchers who conduct research on the specific topic of the investigation. This second type of information is often critical for knowing how to effectively apply rules and procedures in a given context or with the uniquely challenging characteristics of the study topic and/or subjects. While the formal rules and procedures for rigorous research can be found in methodological texts, the specific processes that are used in a given area of investigation are often shared through various forms of communication including published reports of research, scientific presentations, and direct communication among investigators in a particular area.

With this kind of procedural knowledge as background, investigators must form sound judgments about what rules, procedures, and techniques (referred to as research design and methods) will be used in their studies to generate knowledge in which the scientific community can have the most confidence (Seltiz, Wrightsman, & Cook, 1976). When implementing their research, investigators are further responsible to ensure adherence to these chosen methods and, in some stances, to make additional informed decisions about methods as the research unfolds (Lincoln & Guba, 1985).

As can be seen, research is meticulous, detailed, and reflective. Investigators strive to achieve the highest degree of rigor possible in a given study so as to optimize the confidence that can be placed in the information generated. Finally, researchers are obligated to honestly let others know what their procedures were, any problems that were encountered, and what limitations of rigor are inherent in the study. With this information, research consumers know how much confidence to place in the findings.

The Scientific/Scholarly Attitude: Skepticism and Empiricism

All research is characterized by a scientific or scholarly attitude that incorporates two elements:

• Skepticism and
• Empiricism (Polit & Hungler, 1999; Portney & Watkins, 2000).

Skepticism is the idea that any assertion of knowledge should be open to doubt, further analysis, and criticism. Skepticism is important because it prevents prematurely accepting something as accurate. Continual questioning of proposed knowledge allows the scientific community to ensure that claims to knowledge are not taken as accurate unless they survive constant scrutiny over time (Thompson, 2001).

The scientific or scholarly attitude also demands proof rather than opinion. Empiricism means that scientific knowledge emerges from and is tested by observation and experience (Portney, & Watkins, 2000). Thus, all research involves generating data. Data are information about the world gathered through observation, listening, asking, and other forms of acquiring or extracting information from a situation, event, or person.

Data are valued over opinion because the latter is prone to error and personal bias. However, data are gathered systematically so that the influence of error and bias are minimized (Benson & Schell, 1997). Moreover, it is common that more than a single opinion will be held about any topic. Consequently, the most systematic way of deciding between or among differing perspectives is by asking how well they bear up under scrutiny. Empiricism, then, includes the notion that scientists can refine what they know by consistently checking it against the world.

Logical Reasoning

Another cornerstone of research is logic. Importantly, logic is used to systematically link knowledge to what the knowledge is supposed to explain. This occurs through the process of inductive and deductive reasoning (DePoy & Gitlin, 1998). As pointed out in Chapter 2, the logic of inductive and deductive reasoning has been a topic of constant dialogue, debate, and refinement in the scientific community.

Inductive reasoning, or induction, involves making generalizations from specific observations. For instance, suppose over the course of a week, an occupational therapy investigator observes on several occasions clients who suddenly become aware of another client or a therapist observing them. The researcher also notices that on these occasions, clients appear to increase their efforts. From these observations, the investigator might arrive at the general assertion that clients feel socially obligated to make the most of therapy and that there sense of obligation is strengthened when clients feel socially visible. Creating such a generalization is an example of the process of induction.

As the example illustrates, induction involves synthesizing information to generate a theory or an explanation about observed patterns. Induction makes sense of observations by identifying them as belonging to a larger class of phenomena that exhibit an underlying pattern or meaning.

Such a generalization is plausible, but, of course, it is not yet tested or verified. To test it, an investigator would have to use deductive reasoning—that is, to logically derive from this generalization statements that reference observable phenomena. The following are some examples:

- If asked whether they feel clients in therapy should put forth all the effort they can, clients will respond affirmatively.
- If observed doing therapy alone and in the presence of other clients, clients would demonstrate more effort when in the presence of others.
- While engaged in a therapy session, clients' efforts would increase or decrease according to whether the therapist was paying attention to them or not.

Each of these statements could be used as a test of the veracity of the larger generalization created through induction. This is because these observational statements were logically derived. That is, it was deduced that, if persons feel social pressure to put forth effort in therapy, and if being observed increases social pressure, then each of these statements should be true. If they are shown not to be true, then the investigator would have to abandon or revise the general statement from which they were derived.

Induction and deduction allow the investigator to go back and forth between explanations and observations. As shown in Figure 4.1, observations are the basis on which scientists induce generalizations and test statements deduced from those generalizations. The cycle of creating

general propositions or theory by induction from data, followed by deduction of specific statements that can be verified or dismissed by data, is the most basic process by which scientific knowledge is advanced.

Different research approaches emphasize either the inductive or the deductive phase. For example, in experimental research, hypotheses deduced from theories are tested. This deductive–empirical approach is typical of quantitative research. On the other hand, qualitative research tends to emphasize the inductive phase. Rich data gathered from participation, observation, and interviews with people are used to generate new insights, concepts, or theories. While different research traditions may emphasize one or another aspect of the data–induction–generalization–deduction–data cycle, all research ultimately makes use of both elements.

Communality

Research occurs within a community of scientists who consider how research in a given area should be conducted, who scrutinize individual studies, and who collectively arrive at judgments about what conclusions should be drawn about a body of research findings (Crotty, 1998; DePoy & Gitlin, 1998; Polgar & Thomas, 2000; Polit & Hungler, 1999; Portney & Watkins, 2000; Stein & Cutler, 1996). Every study is submitted to a public process in which both the knowledge acquired and the means of acquiring that knowledge are laid bare for others to scrutinize, criticize, and replicate. Research is most typically made public through scientific presentations or posters at conferences or meetings and through publication in scientific journals. A review process (typically done by anonymous peers) ensures that the study to be presented or published meets a basic threshold of rigor.

Once a study has been presented and/or published, others in the scientific community have the opportunity to scrutinize and criticize it. Criticism of existing studies is also a public process that occurs in presentations or publications. In fact, a very typical prelude to presenting the findings of any study is to point out both the findings and limitations of previous investigations, arguing how the current study both builds and improves upon them.

> Every study is submitted to a public process in which both the knowledge acquired and the means of acquiring that knowledge are laid bare for others to scrutinize, criticize, and replicate.

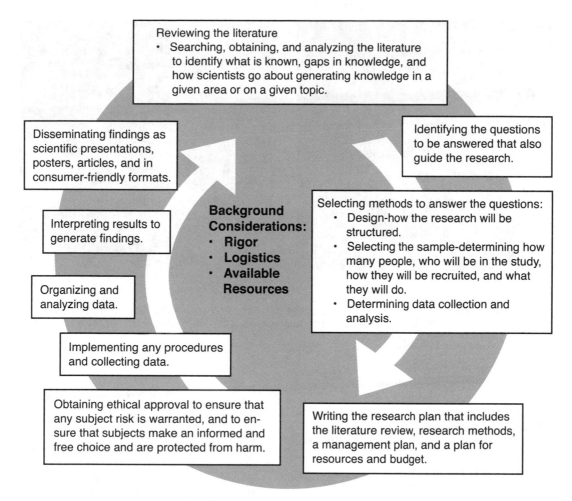

Figure 4.1 The research process.

Finally, it is common practice for scientists to replicate a published study (often improving on some aspect of it or doing it under different conditions) to determine whether they achieve the same results. For this reason, when a study is offered to the scientific community, it is important that it is explained sufficiently so that others can understand exactly what was done and how the conclusions of the study were generated (verifiability) and so that others can repeat the study to see if the same results are obtained (replicability).

Researchers build upon and place new knowledge in the context of existing knowledge generated by the scientific community. All research is informed by what has gone before. This is why the report of a study always begins with a review of existing literature. The literature review serves to situate the study in the context of what the scientific community already knows. Importantly,

researchers not only learn from each other the findings generated by research, they also learn from others' mistakes and inventions. Innovations in research methods generated by one investigator are routinely used by other investigators to improve their own research. In this way, the scientific community tends to advance together, with each investigator learning from the experiences of others.

Research as a Set of Interrelated Activities

As illustrated in Figure 4.1, all research involves the following key activities (DePoy & Gitlin, 1998; Polgar, & Thomas, 2000; Polit & Hungler, 1999; Portney & Watkins, 2000; Stein & Cutler, 1996):

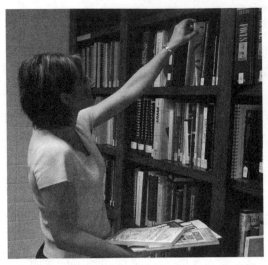

A

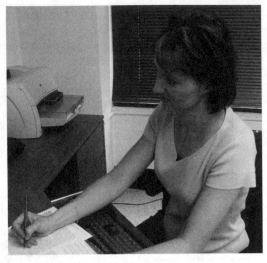

B

Figure 4.2 (A, B) Kim Eberhardt, MS, OTR/L, a research coordinator with the Spinal Cord Injury Program at the Rehabilitation Institute of Chicago conducts a literature review to identify a research question.

- Reviewing the literature,
- Identifying the research questions,
- Selecting the research methods,
- Writing a research plan,
- Obtaining ethical review,
- Implementing research procedures and collecting data,
- Organizing and analyzing data,
- Interpreting results to generate findings, and
- Disseminating findings.

These activities are listed in the sequence that investigators generally follow when planning and implementing a study. However, it is often the case that an investigator moves back and forth between these activities. For example, all research begins with a review of the literature. Nonetheless, at the end of the study when the findings are being prepared for dissemination, an investigator would be remiss without going back to the literature to see if anything new has been published in the interim.

In the following sections, each of these activities are discussed. They are briefly examined to provide a general orientation to the research process. Later chapters will significantly expand each of these topics.

Reviewing the Literature

The aim of reviewing the literature is to identify, evaluate, and understand the existing published theory and research on a given topic. By doing a thorough literature review, investigators learn:

- What kind of information has been generated on the topic, and
- What kind of research methods investigators have used to generate that information.

Thus, the literature review serves to justify or provide a rationale for the research since it allows the investigator to decide what knowledge is lacking and how to best go about generating it.

Reviewing the literature first requires a systematic literature search. This search is ordinarily accomplished through a variety of means. Today the most common method is using Web-based searching and search engines that retrieve publications based on key words. Another common method is a manual search that involves examining the references of existing publications to see what publications previous investigators have considered important.

Once one has exhaustively identified and obtained the relevant literature, it is necessary to analyze it. When analyzing the literature, an investigator asks the following kinds of questions:

- What is known about this topic?
- What theories are used to explain it?
- What methods are used to generate this knowledge?
- What are the strengths and weaknesses of these methods?
- What gaps exist in knowledge about this topic?

By applying these kinds of questions to the existing literature as a whole, the investigator arrives at judgments that allow one to identify the research questions and select the methods. A well done literature review makes it clear why the study is important and needed, and provides important information concerning how it should be undertaken.

Identifying Research Questions

A key step in any study is deciding what question the research will seek to answer. Researchers often begin with broad questions and then narrow them. Creating the research question is closely tied to the literature review, as it requires the investigator to identify what is not currently known that the investigation will address. In addition to reviewing the literature, investigators generally consult with other researchers in the area to make sure the question they are developing is warranted and useful.

Identifying the research question also involves selecting a theoretical approach that frames the question. For example, an investigator wants to examine the broad area of what factors increased motivation of clients to participate in therapy. To formulate a question, the investigator has to begin with some kind of theoretical idea about what constitutes motivation. This process can be fairly straightforward if there is a single well-formulated theory that characterizes a particular research topic. In some other cases, there may be competing theories, so that one has to select from among them. In still other instances there may not be a clear theoretical approach, so that one has to identify a theoretical approach that might be appropriate to the topic. Even if an investigator does not specify a theory, certain assumptions and concepts will be implicit in how any question is posed. Thus, research is more logical and transparent when the theory is made explicit.

How the research question is formulated determines much of the rest of the study. In particular, the question asked shapes the selection of the research methodology. For example, if an investigator formulates a question about motivation that asks what factors influence motivation, then the design of the study will be largely descriptive and could involve either qualitative or quantitative approaches. On the other hand, if an investigator wants to know whether an intervention improves motivation, then a quantitative design such as a control group study or a single subject study will be required. If an investigator wants to know unique factors that motivate individuals in a particular context, a qualitative field study is likely to be the design of choice. Finally, if an investigator

wanted to know whether different factors motivate persons of different ages, then a quantitative survey is needed.

Deciding the Research Methodology

Deciding the methodology of any study involves making decisions about the research design, sample, data collection, and analysis. In approaching these decisions the investigator must first determine whether to draw from one or both of the quantitative and qualitative traditions of research. Each tradition will be suited to answer certain types of research questions and not others.

Deciding the design of the research involves several interrelated decisions. First, the investigator has to decide the overall approach of the study. This involves such broad considerations as whether the investigation will be:

- A field study in which the investigator becomes immersed in the phenomena under question,
- An experimental study in which the investigator will control different conditions in which subjects will be examined, or
- A survey study in which participants will respond to a written questionnaire.

As noted earlier, when making such decisions, the investigator is deciding on the best overall approach to answer the type of question the study is seeking to answer.

Once the broad decision about research design is made, other types of decisions must also be made to refine the study design. For example, in an experimental study, the investigator will need to decide whether random assignment is feasible and what will constitute the different conditions to be compared. In a survey study, the investigator will have to decide whether subjects will participate in the study only once, or whether they will be contacted multiple times over a longer period. In a qualitative study, the investigator will need to decide, for instance, whether it will be an extended participant observation or a brief series of key informant interviews. In designing any given study, investigators will often consider a number of possibilities. It is not uncommon to redesign a study several times while planning. All of these design decisions affect the rigor of the study as well as the resources that will be needed to carry out the study.

The investigator must also decide who will participate in the study. This decision involves what characteristics the subjects will have (e.g., age, how they will be recruited and chosen, and how many will be included and what they will be asked to do in the study). This aspect is referred to as sampling.

The final aspect of deciding the research methods is determining how data will be collected and analyzed. The answers to the study questions depend on the quality of data collected and how they are analyzed. Once again the choices may range widely. For example, data may be collected with open-ended methods that evolve over the course of the research or they may be collected through the use of highly standardized procedures and are stable from subject to subject and over time. No matter what type of data are collected, investigators are concerned with their dependability.

The approach of data analysis also depends on whether the study is qualitative and/or quantitative. Qualitative data are ordinarily coded and classified and then thematically analyzed. Qualitative data analysis tends to unfold as the research unfolds (Hammell, Carpenter, & Dyck, 2000). Often data analysis is both shaped by and shapes the kind of data that gets collected. Quantitative data analysis involves the use of statistics. Statistics may be used to describe what was found or to draw inferences about it (e.g., to decide whether two groups differ on a characteristic or whether one variable predicts another).

How an investigator goes about making decisions about study design and methods also depends on the overall type of research being done. In most quantitative research, most if not all of the decisions will be made before the research commences. However, in qualitative research, some of the decisions may be made before the research begins but others will depend on and respond to how the research unfolds.

Writing the Research Proposal

In most instances, investigators will write up a plan of the research in order to organize the planning process and to communicate the plan to others. A research proposal is a document that details the need and rationale for the study question, describes the anticipated methods that will be used to address the question, and provides the anticipated logistics and necessary resources for conducting the research.

The proposal serves first to organize the research plan in the investigator's mind and as a kind of blueprint for later implementing the research. A proposal is also typically used to secure approval (e.g., administrative approval or supervisory approval when the investigator is in training). In other instances, the proposal is used to request funding for the research. When the proposal is used to request funding, it is referred to as a grant proposal.

The research plan includes the elements already discussed (i.e., the literature review and the research methods). Another component of the research proposal is a management plan. It includes a description of the major tasks necessary to complete the project, who will do them, and when they will be done. Along with the management plan, larger studies include an organizational plan that includes all the personnel involved in the study, what their responsibilities will be, and how they will relate to each other.

A final component of a research plan is consideration of the necessary resources for conducting the research. These include, for instance, space and equipment, personnel, and supplies. A budget is also typically prepared for a research plan and is always required for a grant proposal, since it forms the rationale for the funds that are being requested. The budget covers necessary costs of the research for such things as personnel to help carry out the research, supplies necessary for the research, and so on.

Obtaining Ethical Review

Studies involving human beings as subjects undergo ethical review, which is a process designed to:

• Protect subjects from any harm,
• Ensure that subjects' effort and any risk involved is warranted by the study's importance, and
• Ensure subjects freely give informed consent to participate.

Persons who are not directly involved in the research conduct a review of the proposed study to make sure it meets these ethical standards. Institutions in which research is routinely conducted maintain ethics boards (sometimes called Institutional Review Boards), whose purpose is to review and approve research. Obtaining ethical approval is ordinarily the last step before beginning implementation of a study.

Implementing Research Procedures and Collecting Data

Implementation of a study can vary dramatically with the nature of the research. For example, implementing a qualitative field study may involve months of participation with subjects in their natural context, during which time the investigator takes field notes, records interviews, and collects documents. On the other hand, implementing a controlled study comparing groups receiving different therapy approaches may involve assigning subjects randomly to the two intervention conditions, collecting baseline data, providing the interventions, documenting their conformity to the intervention protocol, and collecting post-intervention data. Implementing a survey study may require obtaining a random sample of subjects with addresses, mailing the survey instrument, and doing follow up mailings to ensure the highest possible response rate.

Research designed to develop assessments may involve a series of sequential steps (Benson & Schell, 1997). For example, the investigator may begin with collecting qualitative information from clients and/or therapists to ascertain what kind of information should be included in the assessment. Then, once a prototype is designed, a pilot study may be conducted to obtain systematic feedback from those who used or experienced the assessment. Following this, the assessment may be revised and then data will be collected and analyzed to examine whether they have the properties of a sound assessment. Next, revision of the assessment may be followed by further data collection and analysis to determine whether it has improved psychometrically.

Depending on the type of research being conducted, the implementation may be either emergent or highly structured. For instance, qualitative field studies generally begin with an overall question and plan, but the investigation will be guided by what happens and what is found in the field. The selection of what to observe, whom to interview, and what types of data to collect will be shaped by the unfolding understanding of the topic under investigation. In this case, rigor depends on the investigator's careful attention to the situation under study and strategic development of research strategies to faithfully create an understanding of the situation that reflects how those in the situation experience it (Lincoln & Guba, 1985).

In contrast, a controlled experimental study requires strict adherence to protocols defined before the implementation begins. In this case, the investigator will seek to avoid the interference of natural conditions on the study process and will carefully document any aberration from the plan of the research. Here, rigor is achieved through strict adherence to protocol.

A pivotal aspect of implementing any study is recruiting and retaining the participants or subjects necessary for the study. Subjects can be recruited for studies using a variety of approaches such as presentations that invite participation, fliers or brochures, and mailings. Once subjects have indicated an interest, the investigator must adequately inform the potential participants about the study and obtain and document informed consent (a process in which potential subjects learn about the purpose of the study and what is being asked of them as participants and subsequently decide whether or not to participate).

When the research involves a single point of contact with subjects, as in a survey, consent and data collection may occur at the same time. However, many studies require participants to be involved over a period of time and thus require careful attention to subject retention. Once again, a number of strategies, such as subject reimbursement, ongoing contact, and messages to thank and remind, are used to maintain interest and involvement with the study.

An important consideration in all research is to make sure that the necessary data are collected. Once again, concerns about data collection will depend on the design of the research. In qualitative research, the investigator is concerned that each topic has been saturated (i.e., that enough data have been collected from enough different circumstances to ensure that a particular topic is fully informed). In survey research, as noted above, the researcher will be concerned with getting responses from as many persons as possible from the sample chosen. In experimental research, the investigator will be careful to avoid missing data from the pre- and post-group conditions.

No matter what the type of research, the investigator must always be vigilant during the research implementation to make sure that the research unfolds in ways that optimize confidence in the findings. Understanding the logic behind the research design allows the investigator to determine how to respond to the inevitable unexpected circumstances that occur in implementing research.

Managing and Analyzing Data

After data are collected, managing, storing, and analyzing the data is the next important step. During this step, it is important to monitor data collection to make sure it is being carried out as planned and that the accumulated data are comprehensive. Thus, data are routinely monitored and logged in as they are collected. Next, data must be prepared for the analytic process—that is, transformed into a format appropriate to either qualitative and/or quantitative analysis. For qualitative analysis, most data are typically in the form of text or narrative and are usually entered into a qualitative software package. Quantitative data are transferred to an electronic database appropriate to the software that will be used for statistical analysis. Another important aspect of data management is to ensure that data are secured so that they will not be accidentally destroyed and to ensure that only members of the research team have access to the data in order to protect the confidentiality of the study subjects.

Data analysis involves manipulating the data in order to answer the research question. As noted earlier, qualitative data analysis typically involves coding and sorting the data in order to identify key themes that will make up the findings, whereas quantitative data analysis involves computing descriptive and inferential statistics. Data analysis is a complex process and there are a large number of qualitative and quantitative approaches to analyzing data as will be discussed in detail later in this text.

Interpreting Results and Generating Findings

Perhaps the most critical and exciting aspect of any research is the process of making sense of patterns in the data and transforming them into a coherent set of findings to be shared with other members of the scientific community. As with other aspects of the research process, how one

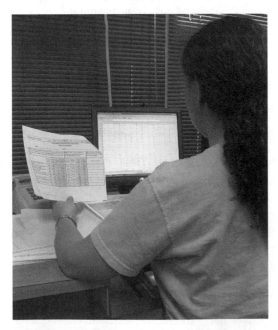

Figure 4.3 A graduate student checks research data entered into the database to prepare for analysis.

goes about interpreting the data collected in research and generating the findings is quite variable depending on the type of research and the topic of inquiry.

In some research, the process is quite formal. For instance, in an experiment where hypotheses (statements of expected results) have been postulated, the major task will be to decide whether the data analysis supports or requires one to reject the veracity of the hypothesis. In qualitative research, the investigator must ponder the themes and patterns in the data to generate insights into their meaning (Hammell, Carpenter, & Dyck, 2000). This can be a highly creative process in which the investigator's theoretical background as well as knowledge of the subjects and their life contexts comes into play.

In addition to the major work of generating an understanding or assigning meaning to the patterns in the data, the process of interpreting results also requires the investigator to skeptically examine the data for alternative explanations to the ones being pursued, and to make sure there are not problems in the data set (e.g., missing or incomplete data, or an unexpected pattern in the data that affects how it can be statistically analyzed) that need to be considered or corrected in the analysis. Finally, the investigator has to carefully consider the degree of confidence that should be assigned to the findings. This aspect involves several considerations including such things as how persuasive the data patterns are in supporting the conclusions being drawn, and the limitations of the research methods used to generate the findings.

Increasingly, investigators conduct this aspect of the research in public. For example, they may present preliminary findings and seek feedback from peers. They may ask consultants with specialized expertise in the analytical methods (e.g., statistics) to give their opinions about the data and their meaning. They may share their findings with other persons doing research in the same area to gain their insights.

Dissemination

No study is complete until it has been formally shared with other members of the scientific community and other interested constituencies. As noted earlier, investigators typically disseminate their findings through refereed presentations, posters, and published papers. In some instances, the investigator may write a book to disseminate findings.

The purpose of disseminating research findings in the scientific/scholarly community is twofold.

First, one is sharing the information generated through the research with others, thus contributing to what is known about the phenomena under study. A second and equally important element is that by making the research public, other scientists/scholars can examine the work to determine its rigor and, therefore, form opinions about how dependable the findings are.

> No study is complete until it has been formally shared with other members of the scientific community and other interested constituencies.

Understanding research and, in particular, being able to conduct research, requires detailed knowledge of all the elements that were only touched on in this chapter. Subsequent sections of this book will offer this kind of specific information.

It has become increasingly important to share research results with nonscientific groups who are affected by the research (e.g., persons whose situations or conditions were studied in the research). In the current information age, consumers are increasingly desirous of accessing information generated by research themselves in order to make informed judgments. For this reason, many investigators also seek to disseminate their findings in formats that are more user-friendly to those outside of the scientific/scholarly community. Such formats include nonscientific articles, books, Web sites, videos, and brochures.

The Full Circle of Research

At the point research findings are disseminated, the research process has come full circle. Each investigation began as an examination of the literature to find out what was known about a topic and how such knowledge was generated. Once published, the research becomes part of that body of literature. By culminating the research process with publication, investigators link their work back to the community of scientists/scholars working in a particular area. Without publication, the research, for all practical purposes, does not exist.

Conclusion

This chapter discussed the elements that characterize all forms of research. It examined characteristic hallmarks of good research and overviewed the ordinary activities that make up the research process. This chapter aimed to give the reader a broad sense of what research involves.

REFERENCES

Benson J., & Schell, B. A. (1997). Measurement Theory: Application to occupational and physical therapy. In J. Van Deusen & D. Brunt (Eds.), *Assessment in occupational therapy and physical therapy*. Philadelphia: W. B. Saunders.

Campbell, D. T., & Stanley, J. C. (1963). *Experimental and quasi-experimental designs for research*. Chicago: McNally & Co.

Crotty, M. (1998). *The foundations of social research: Meaning and perspective in the research process*. Crows Nest, Australia: Allen & Unwin.

DePoy, E. ,& Gitlin, L. (1998). *Introduction to research: Understanding and applying multiple strategies*. St. Louis: C. V. Mosby.

Hammell, K. W., Carpenter, C., & Dyck, I. (2000). *Using qualitative research: A practical introduction for occupational and physical therapists*. Edinburgh: Churchill Livingston.

Lincoln, Y. S., & Guba, E. G. (1985). *Naturalistic inquiry*. Thousand Oaks, CA: SAGE Publications.

Neuman, W. L. (1994). *Social research methods: Qualitative and quantitative approaches*. Needham Heights, MA: Allyn and Bacon.

Polgar, S. & Thomas, S. A. (2000). *Introduction to research in the health sciences*. Edinburgh: Churchill Livingston.

Polit, D. F., & Hungler, B. P. (1999). *Nursing research: Principles and methods*. Philadelphia: Lippincott.

Portney, L. G., & Watkins, M. P. (2000). *Foundations of clinical research: Applications to practice* (2nd ed.) Upper Saddle River, NJ: Prentice-Hall.

Rea, L., & Parker, R. (1997). *Designing and conducting survey research: A comprehensive guide*. San Francisco: Jossey-Bass.

Rice, P. L., & Ezzy, D. (1999). *Qualitative research methods, a health focus*. Melbourne: Oxford University Press.

Seltiz, C., Wrightsman, L., & Cook, S. (1976). *Research methods in social relations*. New York: Holt, Rinehart & Winston.

Stein, F., & Cutler, S. (1996). *Clinical research in allied health and special education*. San Diego: Singular Press.

Strauss, A., & Corbin, J. (1990). *Basics of qualitative research*. Thousand Oaks, CA: SAGE Publications.

Thompson, N. (2001). *Theory and practice in human services*. Maidenhead: Open University Press.

CHAPTER 5

Professional Responsibility and Roles in Research

Anne Cusick • Gary Kielhofner

Mary smiles to the audience as she accepts the award for her contribution to occupational therapy research. Over a 40-year career, her achievements include published books and papers reflecting studies funded by large competitive grants.

Lingson rushes from his part-time clinical job to college to teach a class, across town to pick up his children, and then back to the university ceremonial hall. He wonders if he will ever see a day when he does not feel tired. Donning unfamiliar clothes, he proceeds into the hall to receive his doctorate and postdoctoral fellowship.

Hannah completes the final editing of her project investigating an aspect of practice: "I'll never do that again: I'll just read other folk's research and concentrate on putting that into practice" she thinks.

Ellamal goes to work early as she has done for 20 years. She approaches some new clients, inviting them to participate in a study, fills out screening forms, and administers informed consent before sending their information on to the Principal Investigator. Then she starts her day's work.

Carlos and Maria meet at a café and spread out their papers. Going through piles of data and background articles, they spend hours working on a critical review of research papers, preparing a presentation for therapist peers in which they will recommend changes to practice.

Christa tells the student she is supervising that she's never felt the need to read research articles since her on-the-job experience has taught her all she needs to know about what works.

The occupational therapists in these scenarios each hold a personal view about the importance of research in their profession. They have made choices about whether and how to support, use, or produce research to enhance occupational therapy practice. These choices and judgments have an impact on their professional and personal lives. Moreover, their decisions about creating and consuming research evidence affect the profession as a whole.

This chapter explores professional responsibility and roles in conducting and consuming inquiry. It examines ways in which occupational therapists might view research and make choices about research roles in professional life. The chapter describes knowledge and skills central to various research roles, and it illustrates some strategies that can be used to develop them.

Responsibility, Uncertainty, and Research

Being a professional brings with it responsibilities, and ethical practice is one of them. Evidence from research can be used to inform practice decisions, guide therapeutic processes, and provide relevant information about how to interpret outcomes of service (Cusick, 2001a). When therapists use research evidence in their clinical decisions, they can better know what to do, with whom, when, why, and how best to do it. They can also be more accountable as they are aware of potential and actual outcomes of their service (Barlow, Hayes, & Nelson, 1984; Cusick, 2001b). Occupational therapists, thus, have an ethical responsibility to be aware of research and to engage with it.

Occupational therapists also have a professional responsibility to use research to help enhance the quality of their clinical decisions. If problems addressed by therapists in practice were straightforward, and if issues and answers were certain, solutions could be provided by unthinking

> Evidence from research can be used to inform practice decisions, guide therapeutic processes, and provide relevant information about how to interpret outcomes of service.

implementation of protocol. There would be no need at all for the training, responsibility, discretion, expertise, and autonomy of professionals. Professionals operate within uncertainty in the many complex and high-impact decisions they make every day. Professionals must therefore find ways to negotiate the uncertainty that comes with practice (Charles, 2001; Dew, Dowell, McLeod, Collings, & Bushnell, 2005; Mullavey-O'Byrne & West, 2001). In the past, professional authority or expertise was considered sufficient (Basmajian, 1975). However, in the 21st century, decision-making in professional practice needs to be backed by rigorous and transparent evidence. In recognition of this demand for evidence, occupational therapy research productivity has steadily increased (Majnemer et al., 2001; Paul, Liu, & Ottenbacher, 2002). Developments in evidence-based practice have provided further opportunities for scientific knowledge to be integrated with expert opinion in professional judgments. When used intelligently, evidence-based approaches systematically use a variety of forms of information including research, therapist, and client opinion to make meaningful and relevant decisions (Bury & Mead, 1998; Dawes et al., 1999; Taylor, 2000). This approach means therapists can responsibly exercise professional discretion in practice within known limits of their information base.

Therapists need to be discerning about practice priorities, and research information can help them do this. When resources are scarce, difficult decisions must be made about how best to use them. A research orientation to practice helps therapists deal with the inter-professional competition, budget cuts, insurance denials, and other challenges that can emanate from limited resources. Further, when professionals have a research orientation, they can respond to challenges about one's knowledge or service values as opportunities to rationally examine evidence rather than interpreting criticism as personal affronts.

Research Roles

Individual therapists can engage with research in a variety of ways. For instance, they can do original research, collaborate in studies, or engage in reading and critiquing research with peers. Therapists can take on one or more of the following roles (summarized in Table 5-1) (American Occupational Therapy Foundation, 1983; Barlow et al., 1984; Cusick, 1994, 2000, 2001b, 2001c; Cusick, Franklin, & Rotem, 1999; Murray & Lawrence, 2000):

- Research producer,
- Research collaborator,
- Research consumer, or
- Research advocate.

Research Producers

Research producers can be academics, practitioner-researchers, and students who actively engage in research in university, clinical, and community settings (Barlow et al., 1984; Cusick, 2000, 2001c; Hinojosa, 2003; Murray & Lawrence, 2000; Polatajko & MacKinnon, 1987). Research producers develop high levels of research expertise. They design and lead investigations, develop teams of dedicated staff, and bring together research resources to produce new knowledge. Research producers generate published papers, conference presentations, books, and sometimes multimedia or creative works. These resource products are widely disseminated and critically reviewed prior to and after release.

Some research producers choose this role early in their careers; others take a different route. Occupational therapists who select research producer roles must commit themselves to the highest level of precision and rigor. For this, they must complete specialized research training at the doctoral and postdoctoral levels (Paul, 2001). Doctoral training emphasizes advanced knowledge and skills in both theoretical and methodological domains. It culminates in the production of a dissertation that requires conception, implementation, and documentation of a major study or study series.

Dissertation research is completed under the supervision of a committee of seasoned researchers who guide doctoral candidates in their research and who ultimately judge whether or not the research is sufficiently rigorous and important. Often, the doctoral dissertation process culminates with a "defense," in which the doctoral candidate presents their work, answers critical questions, and responds to probing comments about the research from supervisory committees and sometimes a public audience. The defense reflects the very public nature of the research enterprise and serves as a way to evaluate the individual's readiness to engage in the public process of science as discussed in Chapter 34.

While the doctoral degree is increasingly common in occupational therapy, postdoctoral training is still rare. In mature research fields, postdoctoral training is required before one enters into a fully independent research role. Postdoctoral trainees work alongside accomplished researchers and/or within a research team/laboratory. They are advanced "apprentices" who learn more sophisticated analytical techniques, and develop specific expertise in an area of study, a theoretical domain, or a specialized kind of inquiry. They also typically gain experience in grant writing and publication during postdoctoral training.

Research Collaborators

Collaboration can occur in a range of ways and, although a working knowledge of research is always required, not all collaboration needs to be at the level of a research producer. Examples of collaborative activity that do not involve leading research include:

- Being subjects/participants in a study by answering surveys or participating in focus groups,
- Referring and screening clients for studies,
- Collecting data for an investigation,
- Implementing services that are being tested in an intervention study,
- Serving on the advisory board of a funded research grant,
- Helping investigators negotiate the politics and administrative processes of research in a clinical site, and
- Identifying a research question and helping interpret the results of a study of practice.

Collaboration is the most common research involvement by therapists in clinical settings (Majnemer et al., 2001). Without therapists who are willing to train for study requirements, to implement protocols, to volunteer time, and to maintain quality records, many clinical studies could not be completed. Research collaboration is critical for the field.

Collaboration needs careful negotiation, planning, good communication, and relationships of trust (Brown, 1994; Cusick, 1994). Chapter 40 discusses challenges and opportunities that arise in collaboration between practitioners. Among other things, expectations relating to requirements, authorship, and intellectual property need to be negotiated and clear. Depending on the intellectual contribution made to the design, interpretation, and writing up of the study, collaborators may or may not be considered "co-investigators" or "co-authors." (See Chapter 29 for a discussion of authorship guidelines.)

Preparation and expertise required for research collaboration vary widely depending on the nature of the research endeavor. In many instances, the professional education and experience of occupational therapists are all that is needed to be a valuable collaborator. In other instances, therapists may bring skills they learned in a thesis project or research courses taken as part of professional or post-professional education. Sometimes therapists will receive specialized training that enables them to implement an intervention being studied or collect data in a reliable and valid manner. Often this training is provided in preparation for or as part of therapists' involvement in a particular study. Thus, therapists who collaborate learn important skills and knowledge through the research process itself.

Research Consumers

All therapists should use research to inform their practice. Applying research information in practice has been called "consuming research" (AOTF, 1983), "research utilization" (Brown & Rodger, 1999; Craik & Rappolt, 2003), and being "research sensitive" (Cusick, 2001a). It is part of being a "reflective practitioner" (Fleming & Mattingly, 1994; Parham, 1987). More recently, therapists have been encouraged to become evidence-based practitioners, routinely consuming and using research in practice (Cusick & McCluskey, 2000; Taylor, 2000).

The preparation for research consumer roles varies depending on how one goes about it. Most professional programs in occupational therapy provide at least the basic knowledge required to intelligently read a research report. Critical appraisal (such as that discussed in Chapter 42) requires more advanced skills to formulate a question, identify appropriate literature, and even calculate some basic statistics that summarize the information available in research literature. Critical appraisal skills are taught in some occupational therapy programs and are often available through continuing education. These skills are likely to become a requirement of professional competency in the future.

While all therapists should consume, use, and apply research evidence to inform practice, some will take their role as critical consumers one step further. They will publicize knowledge gaps in practice as well as the information they find that fills those gaps. They do this through conference papers, letters to editors, discussion papers, and critically appraised topics. This form of critical consumerism is important both because it stimulates debate and further investigation, and because it contributes knowledge to others. The proliferation of occupational therapy resources such as critically appraised topics in journals, Internet sites, and discussion boards are examples of the growing

Postdoctoral Training

Dr. Patricia Bowyer is an occupational therapist who recently earned a doctoral degree. Dr. Bowyer's goal is to do clinically relevant research related to the Model of Human Occupation using a range of research methodologies. She came to the University of Illinois at Chicago, where she is completing a postdoctoral fellowship in the occupational therapy department.

In addition to taking two advanced courses in theory and statistics, she is working on a number of research projects that will give her experience in developing assessments and studying service outcomes. For instance, she is currently working on developing a pediatric assessment. In this project, she has sought input from a national pool of clinicians and she will go on to collect data internationally that will be used to examine the psychometrics of this tool.

Dr. Bowyer is also collaborating to complete a qualitative study on the impact of Enabling Self Determination, an occupational therapy service program for persons with HIV/AIDS. The focus of this inquiry is to understand how staff in transitional living facilities viewed the impact of these new occupational therapy services on the clients and the facility.

During her postdoctoral training, Dr. Bowyer will also gain experience reviewing grants and developing grant-writing expertise through participating in grant submissions. She also has opportunities to write and submit papers for publication. By working full time on a range of research projects and processes, she is developing advanced skills for the role of a research producer.

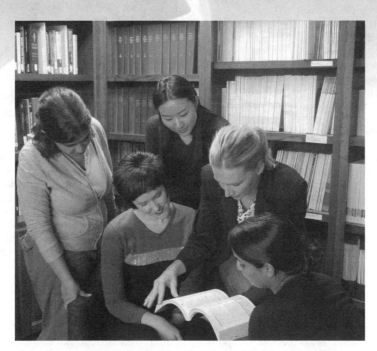

Postdoctoral fellow, Dr. Bowyer (center) discusses concepts related to her research with several graduate students.

importance of this type of research consumer role and contribution.

Research Advocates

Some therapists support research by finding knowledge gaps, generating relevant questions, identifying research priorities, and lobbying professional leaders to "do something" to help therapists working on practice problems. They work as research advocates by providing the momentum and support for research even though they do not produce it themselves. The following are some examples of research advocacy:

Research Collaborator

Heidi Waldinger Fischer is a research occupational therapist working at the Rehabilitation Institute of Chicago (RIC). When Heidi graduated from the University of Illinois at Chicago, she went to work at RIC as a staff therapist providing services on inpatient and outpatient units to individuals with spinal cord injury, traumatic brain injury, stroke, and orthopedic conditions. During that time, Heidi became more and more aware that the need for evidence-based practice was growing. She was also concerned about the lack of evidence to guide many aspects of her practice.

After 3 years of working as a staff therapist, she was offered the opportunity to assist engineers in the Sensory Motor Performance Program to explore the potential of rehabilitation robotics for the upper extremity following stroke. Heidi saw this as an opportunity to contribute toward the building of a more substantial evidence base. For the past 2 years, she has assisted in the Neuromuscular Hand Rehabilitation and Arm Guide Laboratories of the Sensory Motor Performance Program at RIC. Her current research experience focuses on stroke rehabilitation. She works on projects aimed at understanding underlying mechanisms of impairment, developing individualized treatment protocols, and development and use of robotic devices to improve upper extremity function. Her responsibilities include participation in the collection and analysis of data related to muscle activity, muscle stimulation, brain imaging, and kinematics. Most recently, she also has experience working at RIC's Center for Rehabilitation Outcomes Research assisting in the development and implementation of a physical activity promotion program for persons with arthritis. As an occupational therapist, Heidi is able to offer a clinical perspective to motor control and robotics research. She is able provide her interdis-

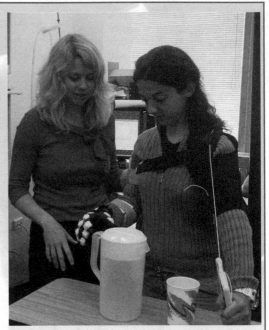

Heidi Waldinger Fischer (left), a research occupational therapist working at the Rehabilitation Institute of Chicago (RIC), works with a participant in a study of upper extremities utilizing rehabilitation robotics.

ciplinary colleagues with a unique understanding of a person's occupational performance. This knowledge directly impacts the way robotic devices are developed and guides her fellow researchers in maintaining a client-centered focus to their work. Heidi hopes her work will not only serve to supplement the much needed evidence to inform practice, but also will ultimately improve the quality of life of those individuals she serves.

• Being involved in a local or national professional association that funds or otherwise supports research,
• Lobbying policymakers/legislators to improve access to research databases, funds, and professional development for occupational therapists,
• Asking employers to provide Internet access to therapists at work so they can consult easily accessible databases for "just in time" information,
• Donating money to various causes and projects or to organizations that fund occupational therapy research,
• Encouraging colleagues involved in research

through emotional support, praise, and recognition to create research supportive cultures, and
• Responding to agency invitations to comment on research priorities or goals.

Often persons who advocate research have no specialized training or background in research. Their primary qualification is that they appreciate the importance of research to the vitality of the profession.

Research Role Contributions

Every research role makes valuable contributions to the profession. Without research producers,

Practitioner-Researcher

Natasha Lannin has been an occupational therapist for just over 10 years; she has mostly worked in the area of neurological rehabilitation. As a new graduate working in rural and remote settings, she sought out research information on the Internet to inform her practice decisions and support her choice of clinical evaluations. She attended and later presented at regional and national conferences. She did this to ensure that she stayed up to date with practice trends and received feedback on her practice through peer review. Natasha also made regular personal contacts with leading practitioners and researchers at conferences and developed a lively e-mail network that helped overcome her geographical isolation. As part of her post-professional development, Natasha completed a postgraduate diploma in case management by distance education. This diploma helped broaden her practice skill base at the same time as focusing her interest on research methods that might be used to solve clinical problems.

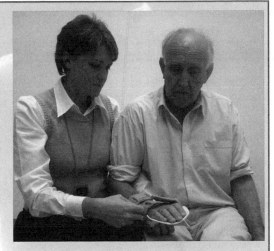

Natasha Lannin (left), practicing therapist and doctoral student at the University of Western Sydney, as part of her doctoral studies applies a splint to a client in a clinical setting.

Following a challenge by hospital colleagues to her use of splinting intervention for people who had had a stroke, she critically appraised the literature and identified a significant knowledge gap. Identifying this knowledge gap was a turning point in her career. She decided to address it by becoming involved in research. She identified clinical experts and researchers who were willing to assist "long-distance" in the design of a study. She engaged in individual study to learn more about research methods. She sought out supportive interdisciplinary networks in the hospital and across the region by phone.

With these resources, she began the long process of study design, ethical approval, and implementation of a small randomized controlled trial. After the study was published in the *Archives of Physical Medicine*, queries from her occupational therapy colleagues made it clear that there were further questions in need of answers.

Next, Natasha decided to pursue a research degree. It had become increasingly apparent to her

that she needed the kind of expertise and resources that could only be obtained through a graduate degree program. By this time, Natasha had moved to the city, and had a supervisory team and wide network of hospital clinicians ready and willing to support her work by acting as recruiters. Natasha obtained a scholarship for her research work, but continued in a part time practice role, which permitted time for research and family responsibilities. Natasha Lannin has now completed her research degree, received a national award for her research work, and published several clinical studies that address questions and issues she faced as a therapist. These include instrument studies, outcome studies, critical appraisals, and systematic reviews. Practitioner-researchers like Natasha Lannin keep occupational therapy research focused on the difficult, complex, and urgent questions of day-to-day practice.

there is no original knowledge base. Without collaborators, clinical studies could not be implemented. Without supporters, resources needed for research or research dissemination and uptake are not available. Without therapists to advocate for research and guide research questions and priorities, research will not be relevant. Without therapists to use or consume research in their service for the public, the quality of practice suffers. All therapists can help support inquiry-based practice in some way. Not everyone will conduct research;

however, everyone can contribute to the profession becoming evidence-based (Cusick, 2003; Rodger, Mickan, Tooth & Strong, 2003).

Taking on Research Roles

Choosing and developing a research role unfolds much as any other life role (Cusick, 2001c) (Table 5.1). Role development is part of the "social self" (Blumer, 1969), and developing a "researching

Collaboration between academics and practitioners is commonplace in clinical research. Each person brings different role skills, knowledge, resources, and attributes to the inquiry process. Iona Novak (left) is an occupational therapist with specialist practice expertise in cerebral palsy. She has worked for many years in a specialist cerebral palsy service with her professional roles ranging from direct care therapist, to institution-wide roles facilitating professional development. Most recently, she has become manager of research and innovation activities in her institution. This role involves participation and leadership in national and international cerebral palsy forums.

Anne Cusick (right) is an occupational therapy academic who has worked for more than 20 years in a university doing research, teaching, and administration following her years as a clinician. Anne's inquiry has focused primarily on issues related to practitioner research. More recently, she has become involved in clinical outcome studies, particularly randomized controlled trials.

Iona and Anne have been working together on research projects for more than 5 years, and their plans extend well into the next 5 years. They knew each other by reputation prior to meeting at a conference where they discussed issues relating to outcome evaluation. From that conversation, a series of research questions emerged, and a long-term research relationship was born. Their collaborative projects have included evaluations of occupational therapy home program interventions, instrumentation studies, and multidisciplinary intervention outcome trials. Iona's clinical contacts resulted in ongoing research collaborations involving physicians, other therapists, people with cerebral palsy, and families. Anne's research contacts resulted in collaborations with statisticians, research therapists, students, research assistants, and administrators. Iona has completed her first research postgraduate qualification with Anne (a Master of Science Honors Degree) and is now an industry sponsored PhD candidate working with Anne on a randomized controlled trial investigating occupational therapy intervention efficacy with children who have cerebral palsy. This clinical trial involves research leadership of a multidisciplinary team, working with industry sponsorship, international trial registration, and management of project staff. The scope and logistics of this study are made possible by Iona's and Anne's collaboration. Their partnership has involved not only administrative negotiation, transparency, and accountability, but also a genuine relationship of trust and respect driven by a shared vision of the research project benefits for people with cerebral palsy.

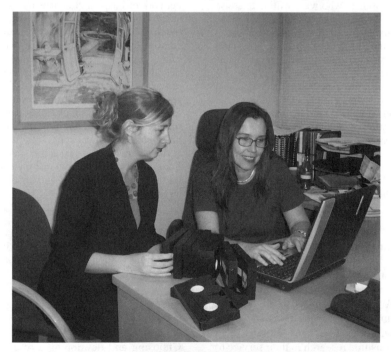

Occupational therapy academic, Dr. Anne Cusick (right) collaborates with practitioner-researcher Iona Novak (PhD candidate).

Research-Resistant Practitioners

Despite the widely acknowledged importance of research to the profession, there are individuals in the field who are "research resistant." These therapists adopt fearful, hostile, or neglectful positions toward information generated by research. Such therapists have clinical skills based on experience, but they have no way to ensure that their practice is not limited or based on outdated information. They may also be guided primarily by personal frames of reference and world views outside professional approaches (Cusick, 2001d). Therapists may be research resistant because they actively devalue research or, by default, because they have chosen to do nothing. Research resistance is not consistent with professional responsibility.

Therapists who are research-resistant may be concerned that their experience and expertise is being de-valued by the increasing attention being given to research information. However, scientific knowledge is viewed as complementary to knowledge gained through experience and the latter is valued in the context of evidence-based practice (Richardson, 2001; Titchen & Ersser, 2001).

Ironically, therapists who resist using research information place themselves at risk of having their hard-earned expertise dismissed by interdisciplinary colleagues, administrators, and others.

Sometimes therapists feel intimidated by research since their own professional training did not include research or treated it in a cursory manner. However, even those who have limited research training or understanding have choices. For example:

- They can choose to use research-based clinical guidelines that are presented in practical user-friendly ways,
- They can adopt service recommendations of managers or supervisors who use research information, or
- They can be open to new ideas that students or colleagues bring that might be founded in research and ask questions.

In the future, being research-resistant may not be a role choice available. There are likely to be credentialing or employment conditions that require therapists to have skills for and to use research information for practice.

self" is an intensely social process (Magoon & Holland, 1984). One must be socialized to research just as with other professional roles (Lewis & Robinson, 2003). The process of identifying, reflecting on, and constructing a research role is called "role taking" (Turner, 1956, 1990). Role taking occurs as one observes and comes to value different roles, tries out role behaviors, gets feedback, and eventually finds a good fit between the self and a role (Biddle, 1979).

Most investigation and discussion of research role development has occurred in relation to research producers (Cusick, 2000, 2001c, 2001d), but the processes of role development can be equally applied to other research roles. It starts with the particular stance a therapist takes toward research. That stance is predisposed by personal biography and context (Cusick, 2000, 2001c, 2001d).

An occupational therapist's research standpoint may be:

- Sparked by an event such as meeting someone or experiencing a difficult situation, (e.g., deciding to become more involved in research because of funding cuts or insurance denials that referenced a lack of evidence about occupational therapy),
- Incidental to daily obligations, (e.g., when

charged to develop and justify new services, a therapist becomes engaged with evidence about service outcomes),
- Inspired by meeting an investigator (e.g., at a conference or at a university),
- Fueled by personal desires (e.g., enriching one's work experience, becoming more credible and able to justify decisions with good quality information, or achieving the autonomy and flexibility that research roles can bring with them),
- Based on a drive to achieve enhanced status and participate in higher status groups where one can have an influence on important issues in occupational therapy (e.g., gaining national research grants that provide resources to study therapy, influencing policy decisions, developing advanced educational opportunities for occupational therapists, and creating new services for an underserved population),
- Based on a sense of obligation to contribute to research as part of professional identity,
- Fueled by a sense of generosity and gratitude toward the profession coupled with a desire to "give something back," or
- A strategic response to opportunities.

Most therapists in research-related roles will identify that a combination of these factors

Table 5.1 **Research Roles and Related Training, Education, Expertise, and Activities**

Role	Typical Education/Training	Expertise	Activities
Research producer	• Doctorate • Postdoctoral training	• Advanced knowledge of theoretical and research methods	• Identify original research questions and design/methods for answering them. • Secure funding for research. • Supervise/oversee the implementation of research. • Work with interdisciplinary collaborators, statistical consultants and others with specific research expertise. • Prepare research reports for presentation or publication.
Research collaborator	• Professional training • Specialized training related to study involvement	• Practice • Knowledge • Specialized knowledge/ skills • For particular studies	• Serve as subjects/ participants. • Refer and screen potential subjects. • Collect data. • Implement services that are being tested. • Provide clinical advise/expertise. • Help negotiate the politics and administrative processes. • Help identify a research question and interpret results.
Research consumers	• Professional training • Training in critical appraisal skills	• Practice expertise to appraise relevance of findings • Skills in evidence-based practice/ critical appraisal of research	• Read research and use findings to guide practice. • Identify practice knowledge gaps. • Complete and present/publish critical appraisals.
Research advocates	• Appreciation of the value of research that can accrue from training and/or experience	• Administrative/ Organizational expertise • Personal commitment to supporting research	• Serve in professional associations that fund/ support research. • Lobby policymakers & legislators. • Ask employers for resources. • Donate money encouraging/supporting colleagues involved in research. • Comment on research priorities or goals.

sparked their interest and then influenced their own research role taking.

Strategies for Research Roles

A research standpoint is only the beginning. Therapists need to then identify, reflect on, and construct research roles that suit them and their life/work context. Building one's own research role requires:

• Exposure to role models and role alternatives,
• Opportunities to reflect on and try out role behaviors,

• Opportunities to get feedback, and
• Opportunities to evaluate new standpoints and experiences.

Exposure provides opportunities to identify what particular research roles look like. It can happen through encounters in occupational therapy education programs, at conferences, on the job, and socially. Strategies for enhancing one's first-hand role exposure include:

• Attending colloquia by visiting speakers,
• Joining journal clubs,
• Attending professional association meetings,
• Seeking supervision or field work placements where research is taking place,
• Volunteering to participate in a research project, and
• Being employed as a research assistant.

One can also gain exposure through written profiles, biographies, seminars, and other media that describe not only the technical aspects of research roles, but also its social dimensions and personal processes. This type of information is useful to consider the kinds of attributes required for various research roles and for learning how people balance home and work responsibilities and negotiate the obligations, demands, and politics of research involvement. It is also important to learn about the impact one can have through research involvement and the personal satisfaction that can accrue from it.

Taking on a research role is an important and conscious decision. Consequently, opportunities to figuratively try on potential research roles are useful. Therapists need to be able to not only think about a particular research role "out there," but also think about themselves in relation to the role. Conversations with trusted mentors, supervisors, managers, friends, and colleagues permit thinking out loud and provide different views of what is required for various roles. Such conversations can offer realistic feedback on one's capacity, encourage different scenario planning, identify practical constraints and implications of particular role choices, and provide a "reality check."

Once particular research roles are selected, occupational therapists need opportunities to try out different research role behaviors, and to acquire knowledge and technical skills for their preferred role. Depending on the role, technical knowledge and skills may range from reading research in an informed way, to developing research questions, preparing designs and protocols, to collecting and analyzing data, to deciding how to apply published findings to practice.

Depending on the role one chooses, the necessary skills may be readily learned or they may take years of training. For example, many of the technical research skills required for research consumer roles such as evidence-based practice are taught in professional entry level courses or continuing education. On the other hand, as noted earlier, learning to be a research producer requires earning a doctoral degree and gaining postdoctoral training and/or experience.

In addition to research-specific skills, successful researchers in occupational therapy must also:

• Accept responsibility and maximize their own autonomy,
• Clearly articulate the values that underpin their work,
• Engage in forward planning by setting priorities, deadlines, and goals,
• Integrate and carefully schedule various activities, and
• Understand the system in which they work and manage colleagues, gatekeepers, and people of influence to get resources (Cusick, 2000, 2001c, 2001d).

Research-specific and the above mentioned general inquiry skills are facilitated through training opportunities that provide realistic and respectful feedback, and that couple clear expectations for performance with high degrees of autonomy (AOTF, 1983; Bland & Ruffin, 1992; Cusick, 2000; Magoon & Holland, 1984; Murray & Lawrence, 2000; Paul, Stein, Ottenbacher, & Liu, 2002; Pelz & Andrews, 1976). This type of training and feedback often begins with the student role wherein students learn whether or not their literature review, critically appraised topic, or research methods assignment met standards and expectations. It will assuredly continue for the developing researcher when submitting conference papers, journal articles, grants, or requests for release time to be involved in research. Over time, these repeated experiences are opportunities for learning, role feedback, and, if positive, research role validation. Therapists therefore don't just "do" research' they "become" research producers, consumers, advocates, or collaborators through a reflective process and social process (Cusick, 2001c, 2001d; Young, 2004). They think about desired roles, select and try on research role behaviors, get feedback on their relative role attainment, and consider whether or not the role feels worthwhile. This self-reflective process involves a continual internal dialogue with oneself about the emerging and changing research role. That dialogue is more meaningful when conversations with trusted friends, mentors, or colleagues can provide opportunities to "think out loud" and, in doing so, further refine one's research standpoint, role taking choices, and views about the worth of the research enterprise in one's life.

Conclusion

In this chapter, we have stressed that research involvement is a professional responsibility. We indicated that occupational therapists make conscious choices about research roles, which include those of advocate, consumer, collaborator, or producer of research. Strategies of research role development were also discussed.

While this chapter focused on individual research role development, no one can be successful in a research role when functioning only as an individual. Research roles emerge only in relation to others. Research involvement of any form is an intensely social process. Whether involvement is as a leader or member of a research team, joining a journal club, serving on a editorial board, having one's grant reviewed by a panel, or presenting a paper at a conference, one is always engaged with others. Even the process of publishing a research paper, which can take weeks of private writing time, ends up in a highly public process.

At one time, research was viewed as a solo enterprise. The ideal of the independent investigator was viewed as the epitome of science. Today, however, it is recognized that the best research is created by teams that include diverse members who can bring their different expertise and perspectives to the research enterprise. Participatory methods (such as those described in Chapters 38, 39, and 40) typically bring researchers together with practitioners, consumers, and community members, all of whom function as integral partners in the research process. Research is also becoming increasingly interdisciplinary in nature. This means that occupational therapists must be prepared to extend their research involvement to those beyond the profession.

Research roles and responsibility are key features of professional life. They underpin ethical practice and provide ways to enhance practice quality and to be accountable in addition to the broader endeavor of contributing to the development of the profession. Research involvement is part of a community of effort in which people collaborate together to advocate for, create, critique, and make use of research evidence for the betterment of the profession and the people we service

in practice. Each of the therapists at the beginning of this chapter had a particular approach to his or her practice and a demonstrable impact on the profession. Each had a different research standpoint and each had his or her own story concerning his or her research role. What will your story be?

REFERENCES

American Occupational Therapy Foundation (1983). Research competencies for clinicians and educators. *American Journal of Occupational Therapy, 37*, 44–46.

Barlow, D. H., Hayes, S. C., & Nelson, R. O. (1984). *The scientist-practitioner: Research and accountability in clinical and educational settings.* New York: Pergamon Press.

Basmajian, J. V. (1975). Research or retrench: The rehabilitation professions challenged. *Physical Therapy, 55*, 607–610.

Biddle, B. J. (1979). *Role theory: Expectations, identities and behaviors.* New York: Academic Press.

Bland, C. J., & Ruffin, M. T. (1992). Characteristics of a productive research environment: Literature review. *Academic Medicine, 67*, 385–397.

Blumer, H. (1969). *Symbolic interactionism: Perspective and method.* Englewood Cliffs, NJ: Prentice-Hall.

Brown, G. T. (1994). Collaborative research between clinicians and academics: Necessary conditions, advantages and potential difficulties. *Australian Occupational Therapy Journal, 41*, 19–26.

Brown, G. T., & Rodger, S. (1999). Research utilization models: Frameworks for implementing evidence-based occupational therapy practice. *Occupational Therapy International, 6*, 1–23.

Bury, T., & Mead, J. (Eds.). (1998). *Evidence-based health care: A practical guide for therapists.* Oxford: Butterworth-Heinemann.

Charles, C. (2001). The meaning(s) of uncertainty in treatment decision-making. In J. Higgs & A. Titchen (Eds.), *Professional practice in health, education and the creative arts.* Oxford, UK: Blackwell Science, pp. 62–71.

Craik, J., & Rappolt, S. (2003). Theory of research utilization enhancement: A model for occupational therapy. *Canadian Journal of Occupational Therapy, 70*, 266–275.

Cusick, A. (1994). Collaborative research: Rhetoric or reality? *Australian Occupational Therapy Journal, 41*, 49–54.

Cusick, A. (2000). Practitioner-researchers in occupational therapy. *Australian Occupational Therapy Journal, 47*, 11–27.

Cusick, A. (2001a). The research sensitive practitioner. In J. Higgs & A. Titchen (Eds.), *Professional practice in health, education and the creative arts.* Oxford: Blackwell Science, pp. 125–135.

Cusick, A. (2001b). 2001 Sylvia Docker Lecture: OZ OT EBP 21C: Australian occupational therapy, evidence-based practice and the 21st century. *Australian Occupational Therapy Journal, 48*, 102–117.

Cusick, A. (2001c). The experience of practitioner-researchers in occupational therapy. *American Journal of Occupational Therapy 55*, 9–18.

Cusick, A. (2001d). Personal frames of reference in professional practice. In J. Higgs & A. Titchen (Eds.), *Practice knowledge and expertise in the health professions.* Oxford: Butterworth-Heineman, pp. 91–95.

Cusick, A. (2003). Clinical research: A room of one's own. *Australian Occupational Therapy Journal, 50*(1), 44–47.

Cusick, A., Franklin, A., & Rotem, A. (1999). Meanings of 'research' and 'researcher'—the clinician perspective. *Occupational Therapy Journal of Research, 19*, 101–125.

Cusick, A., & McCluskey, A. (2000). Becoming an evidence-based practitioner through professional development. *Australian Occupational Therapy Journal, 47*, 159–170.

Dawes, M., Davies, P., Gray, A., Mant, K., Seers, K., & Snowball, R. (1999). *Evidence-based practice: A primer for health care professionals*. Edinburgh: Churchill Livingstone.

Dew, K., Dowell, A., McLeod, D., Collings, S., & Bushnell, J. (2005). This glorious twilight zone of uncertainty: Mental health consultancies in general practice in New Zealand. *Social Science in Medicine* (online March 2005, Science Direct).

Fleming, M., & Mattingly, C. (1994). Action and inquiry: Reasoned action and active reasoning. In C. Mattingly and M. H. Fleming (Eds.), *Clinical reasoning: Forms of inquiry in a therapeutic practice*. Philadelphia: F. A. Davis, pp. 316–342.

Hinojosa, J. (2003). Therapist or scientist—How do these roles differ? *American Journal of Occupational Therapy, 57*, 225–226.

Lewis, S. J., & Robinson, J. W. (2003). Role model identification by medical radiation science practitioners: A pilot study. *Radiography, 9*, 13–21.

Magoon, T. M., & Holland, J. L. (1984). Research training and supervision. In S. D. Brown & R. W. Lent (Eds.), *Handbook of counselling psychology*. New York: John Wiley & Sons.

Majnemer, A., Desrosiers, J., Gauthier, J., Dutil, E., Robichaud, L., Rousseau, J., & Herbert, L. (2001). Involvement of occupational therapy departments in research: A provincial survey. *Canadian Journal of Occupational Therapy, 68*, 272–279.

Mullavey-O'Byrne, C., & West, S. (2001). Practising without uncertainty: Providing health care in an uncertain world. In J. Higgs & A. Titchen (Eds.), *Professional practice in health, education and the creative arts*. Oxford, UK: Blackwell Science, pp. 49–61.

Murray, L., & Lawrence, B. (2000). *Practitioner-based enquiry: Principles for post-graduate research*. London: Falmer Press.

Parham, D. (1987). Toward professionalism: The reflective therapist. *American Journal of Occupational Therapy, 41*, 555–561.

Paul, S. (2001). Postdoctoral training for new doctoral graduates: Taking a step beyond a doctorate. *American Journal of Occupational Therapy, 55*, 227–229.

Paul, S., Liu, Y., & Ottenbacher, K. J. (2002). Research productivity among occupational therapy faculty members in the United States. *American Journal of Occupational Therapy, 56*, 331–334.

Paul, S., Stein, F., Ottenbacher, K. J., & Liu, Y. (2002). The role of mentoring on research productivity among occupational therapy faculty. *Occupational Therapy International, 9*, 24–40.

Pelz, D. C., & Andrews, F. M. (1976). *Scientists in organizations productive climates for research and development* (rev. ed.). Ann Arbor, MI: Institute for Social Research, University of Michigan.

Polatajko, H., & MacKinnon, J. (1987). Occupational therapy graduate education: The scientist practitioner model. *Canadian Journal of Occupational Therapy, 54*, 119–138.

Richardson, B. (2001). Professionalisation and professional craft knowledge. In J. Higgs & A. Titchen (Eds.), *Practice knowledge and expertise in the health professions*. Oxford: Butterworth-Heineman, pp. 42–47.

Rodger, S., Mickan, S., Tooth, L., & Strong, J. (2003). Clinical research: Room for all? *Australian Occupational Therapy Journal, 50*, 40–43.

Taylor, M. C. (2000). *Evidence-based practice for occupational therapists*. Oxford: Blackwell Science.

Titchen, A., & Ersser, S. J. (2001). The nature of professional craft knowledge. In J. Higgs & A. Titchen (Eds.), *Practice knowledge and expertise in the health professions*. Oxford: Butterworth-Heineman, pp. 35–41.

Turner, R. H. (1956). Role taking, role standpoint, and reference group behaviour. Abridged from *American Journal of Sociology, 61*, 316–328. In B. J. Biddle & E. J. Thomas (Eds.), *Role theory: Concepts and research*. New York: John Wiley & Sons, pp. 151–158.

Turner, R. H. (1990). Role change. *Annual Review of Sociology, 16*, 87-110.

Young, A. F. (2004). Becoming a practitioner-researcher: A personal journey. *British Journal of Occupational Therapy, 67*, 369–371.

CHAPTER 6

Descriptive Quantitative Designs

Gary Kielhofner

Descriptive research depicts naturally occurring events or characteristics of research participants (e.g., behaviors, attitudes, and other attributes) (DePoy & Gitlin, 1998; Polit & Hungler, 1999; Portney & Watkins, 2000). Descriptive research is common in occupational therapy and serves a number of purposes. It should also be noted that descriptive research is often the aim, or one of the aims, of retrospective designs that use existing databases, as discussed in Chapter 9 or survey research, as discussed in Chapter 8. Strictly speaking, descriptive research also includes studies that compare groups when there is not experimenter manipulation of an independent variable. However, since the logic of group comparisons is similar across a range of experimental and descriptive designs, descriptive group comparison studies are discussed in Chapter 7. The aim of this chapter is to address other forms of descriptive research.

In many situations, too little is known to undertake studies in which independent variables are manipulated and their effects on dependent variables are observed. Descriptive research often takes advantage of naturally occurring events or available information in order to generate new insights through inductive processes. Consequently, descriptive investigations often serve an exploratory purpose. Such studies typically lead to greater understanding of phenomena, and the resulting conceptualizations are then later tested through more rigorous research designs.

Sometimes basic descriptive information is needed in order to indicate norms, trends, needs, and circumstances that inform and guide practice. Finally, descriptive research is a component of all research studies, since it is used to characterize subjects and other relevant circumstances that surround the research.

There are two types of descriptive research:

- Univariate research in which data are collected on a single variable or a series of single variables and then characterized with descriptive statistics, and
- Correlational research in which relationships between two or more variables are examined.

These two types of descriptive studies and their uses in occupational therapy research are presented in this chapter

Univariate Descriptive Studies

Univariate investigations are typically used to:

- Characterize the sample or circumstances that make up any study,
- Characterize a problem or phenomena,
- Document incidence and prevalence of health related conditions,
- Establish norms,
- Document developmental phenomena, and
- Document case studies.

Chapter 15 provides an overview of descriptive univariate statistics that are used for these types of investigations. These univariate descriptions are ordinarily in the form of frequencies, central tendencies (e.g., mean) and dispersion (e.g., range or standard deviation). Below, the nature and purposes of these types of descriptive research are discussed.

> Descriptive research often takes advantage of naturally occurring events or available information in order to generate new insights through inductive processes.

Characterizing a Study Sample and Characteristics

No matter how complex the design of a study, all investigations include components of basic descriptive design through which the participants and other relevant circumstances in the study are characterized. Basic descriptive data are always collected, analyzed, and reported in any research. This is true for qualitative research as well, in which basic quantitative information is typically used along with qualitative information to characterize the study participants.

Essential to any study report is information about the subjects of a study on key demographic variables (e.g., age, sex, race or ethnicity, diagnosis, type of impairment). In addition to characterizing research participants, it is also important to characterize other conditions that make up a study. For example, in a study of intervention outcomes, the investigator would describe the types of services provided, the length of time over which the service was provided, the frequency of service provision, and how much service in total was provided.

Characterizing a Phenomenon or Problem

Descriptive studies in occupational therapy often serve the purpose of illuminating some phenomena or circumstance that is of interest to the field. For instance, Bar-Shalita, Goldstand, Hahn-Markowitz, and Parush (2005) studied the response patterns of typical 3- and 4-year-old Israeli children to tactile and vestibular stimulation. This study was undertaken to generate basic knowledge about the response patterns of typically developing children to sensory stimuli. The investigators sought to describe sensory response patterns and to determine whether they changed from age 3 to age 4.

The study results indicated that these children were neither hypo- nor hyper-responsive to tactile and vestibular stimuli. By providing evidence that typically developing children do not swing between hyper- and hypo-responsivity, this study provided a framework for identifying children whose sensory responsiveness is atypical. The investigators also found no evidence of change in responsiveness from the 3- to 4-year-olds. This finding suggested that children's patterns of response to tactile and vestibular stimulation have stabilized by age 3. As this investigation illustrates, descriptive research that characterizes typical phenomena, such as sensory responsiveness, can be very useful in occupational therapy.

In addition, descriptive studies are often used in occupational therapy to characterize functional aspects of a disability. Such investigations are helpful in understanding what types of occupational challenges are faced by certain popula-

tions. When such studies describe ways that individuals with disabilities adapt, they are helpful as guidelines for practitioners. The first feature box that follows contains an example of such a study.

Incidence and Prevalence Studies

Another important purpose of descriptive studies is to document the incidence and prevalence of health-related conditions. Studies that address this purpose are referred to as epidemiological studies. Although incidence and prevalence studies are usually conducted by public health and medical researchers, their results are widely used in occupational therapy. In addition, occupational therapy researchers are increasingly contributing to and conducting incidence and prevalence studies that focus on functional aspects of impairment.

Prevalence is a proportion of a total population who have a particular health-related condition (Polit & Hungler, 1999; Portney & Watkins, 2000). Prevalence (P) is calculated as:

$$P = \frac{\text{Number of observed cases of a condition at a given time point or during a given interval}}{\text{Total population at risk}}$$

When prevalence is examined at a specific time point, it is referred to as point prevalence. When it is calculated based on observed cases during a time period (e.g., over a year), it is referred to as period prevalence (Portney & Watkins, 2000). Prevalence is calculated without reference to the onset of the condition; thus, it aims to characterize what proportion of a population has a condition at a point or period of time without consideration of when the condition began. The feature box on prevalence rates for chronic fatigue syndrome presents an example of a prevalence study.

Incidence is concerned with how many persons have onset of a condition during a given span of time. Incidence refers to the number of new cases of a disease or disability in a population during the specified time period. It can be calculated as either cumulative incidence or incidence rate (MacMahon & Trichopoulos, 1996).

Cumulative incidence is calculated as:

$$CI = \frac{\text{Number of observed new cases during a specified period}}{\text{Total population at risk}}$$

Liedberg, Hesselstrand, and Henriksson (2004) used a diary method to collect data on the time use and activity patterns of women with long-term pain (diagnosed with fibromyalgia). The women were asked to fill in a diary for 7 consecutive days and again 3 months later over 4 consecutive days. In the diary they noted what they were doing during each time period, where they were, with whom they were doing the activity, whether they had physical problems, and their mood. The investigators then coded the diary entries in a number of ways. For example, they coded activities as belonging to one of seven spheres of activity (care of self, care of others, household care, recreation, travel, food procurement or preparation, and gainful employment). Within these general categories the activities were further sorted into more detailed activity categories (e.g., sweep, vacuum, scrub, and dust as categories of household care). This study yielded data that could be compared with existing Swedish population data. For example, the authors found that the women in this study spent more time in self-care than women in the general population. The study also included an intervention component for all women (i.e., they were supported to examine the results of the analysis of their initial diary entries and to identify goals for changing their daily activity patterns). More than half of the women were successful in achieving some of their long-term, comprehensive goals by the second period of data collection.

This descriptive study provided a detailed portrayal of these women's daily lives. Such descriptive findings are helpful for understanding how persons with chronic pain often organize and experience activities in their lives. The findings also point to the value of this kind of data collection and analysis as a tool for educating clients in rehabilitation, and as a framework for helping clients think about how they will accommodate and cope with their condition.

Prevalence Rates for Chronic Fatigue Syndrome

Chronic fatigue syndrome (CFS) is an ambiguous and debilitating condition. Initially, it was considered a rare syndrome and it was believed to occur only among Caucasian, affluent persons who were "overachievers." Early attempts to estimate the prevalence of CFS utilized physician referrals as a means by which to count individuals with the diagnosis. The problem with this approach was that many physicians either did not believe in the existence of CFS or were unfamiliar with the diagnostic criteria. In addition, prior studies neglected to account for the large proportion of people within the United States that do not have access to medical care and do not have the opportunity to receive an evaluation and diagnosis.

Jason et al. (1999) conducted a study to estimate the prevalence of CFS in a randomly selected, community-based sample that was free of biases imposed by access to medical care and attitudes about CFS held by referring physicians. To estimate the CFS prevalence, researchers made telephone contact with a sample of 18,675 adults residing in Chicago. These individuals completed a brief telephone interview about fatigue. Those who reported symptoms that matched CFS diagnostic criteria (screened positives) and a non-fatigued control group (screened negatives) received a complete medical and psychiatric evaluation. The purpose of the evaluation was to rule out other medical and psychiatric conditions that might explain a participant's symptoms. Descriptive statistics that included univariate and multivariate approaches were used to estimate the overall prevalence of CFS and the prevalence of CFS according to sex, ethnicity, age, and socioeconomic status. Results produced an estimate of CFS as occurring in approximately 0.42% of the sample. This translates to a prevalence estimate that CFS occurs in 4.2 per thousand persons. Moreover, when the prevalence was broken down according to sociodemographic categories, CFS was found to be highest in women, in members of numerical minority groups, and in individuals of lower socioeconomic status.

Findings from this study challenged prior perceptions of CFS as a rare disorder that affected only Caucasian upper-class women. This study exemplifies the potential that descriptive epidemiological studies have in changing existing knowledge and attitudes about health conditions and the people who experience them. When the results of this study were replicated by a similar methodology, the Centers for Disease Control and Prevention revised their official estimates of prevalence rates. Moreover, the official recognition that this was not a rare disease led to increased federal funding to address the needs of this population and increased awareness of health providers that it was a prevalent disorder and that it occurred among minority populations

Incidence rate (*IR*) is calculated as:

$$IR = \frac{\text{Number of observed new cases during a specified period}}{\text{Total person-time}}$$

In the formula for *IR*, the denominator is calculated as person-periods. For example, if a condition was studied over a 10-year period and 100 persons were enrolled, the total possible person-years are 1,000 (100 persons observed over 10 years). However, if two persons died and were no longer in the sample after 5 years, they would contribute only 10 person-years (5 years x 2 persons) to the formula, reducing the denominator by 10 person-years. Unlike cumulative incidence, which assumes all subjects are at risk during the entire period studied, incidence rate characterizes the number of new cases as a proportion of persons who were actually at risk during each of identified segments of the total period studied (e.g., for each year of a 10-year period).

Prevalence and incidence rates are important to providing both an understanding of the magnitude of a health-related condition (i.e., how common or prevalent it is) and risk (i.e., what are the chances of someone incurring a given health-related condition). For example, in 2003, the Centers for Disease Control and Prevention (CDC) estimated that there were between 800,000 and 900,000 people living with human immunodeficiency virus (HIV) in the United States. Calculated as a proportion of the population, these existing cases would represent prevalence of HIV in the United States. At that time, the CDC also estimated that approximately 40,000 new (HIV) infections occur annually in the United States (CDC, 2004). When calculated as a proportion of the total U.S. population, these cases would represent the cumulative incidence of HIV infection. The prevalence of HIV infection provides researchers and healthcare providers an understanding of the magnitude of the problem of HIV infection in the United States, since it provides information about both the absolute number of cases and the proportion of the total population affected by the condition. The incidence estimate provides an understanding of risk.

Incidence and prevalence are ordinarily calculated for subpopulations as well (e.g., different ages, males versus females), since the occurrence of new and existing cases of conditions is not evenly distributed across the population. For example, early studies of HIV in the United States indicated that males who engaged in homosexual activity were at highest risk. However, over the past 20 years, the incidence of the disease has changed. That is, HIV increasingly affects women, individuals from minority populations, and individuals with histories of mental illness and substance abuse (CDC, 2000; Karon, Fleming, Steketee, & DeCock, 2001; Kates, Sorian, Crowley, & Summers, 2002; Orenstein 2002). Findings on the incidence of new cases thus help identify which populations are at greatest risk.

Normative Research

Investigators undertake normative research in order to establish usual or average values for specific variables. This type of research is helpful for identifying and characterizing performance problems (i.e., knowing how extreme a person's deviation from a norm is) and doing treatment planning. As Portney and Watkins (2000, p. 171) note, norms are "often used as a basis for prescribing corrective intervention or predicting future performance." For example, research that led to the description of what is normal strength for different populations is used routinely in occupational therapy practice. These types of norms serve as a basis for evaluating performance of a given individual by comparing that individual with what is typical for someone with the same characteristics (e.g., age and sex). Research that aims to establish norms must be particularly careful to avoid sampling bias. For this reason, normative studies use random samples and ordinarily rely on large sample sizes.

Developmental Research

Developmental research seeks to describe "patterns of growth or change over time within selected segments of a population" (Portney & Watkins, 2000, p. 14). Such studies may describe patterns of change that characterize typical growth and development. Developmental research has been important in documenting the course of acquiring functional abilities in childhood (e.g., crawling, walking, talking, grasping) as well as the functional changes associated with aging.

Other developmental investigations seek to characterize the course of disease or disability over time (e.g., the course of functional recovery from a traumatic event or the course of functional decline in degenerative conditions).

Developmental research usually involves a cohort design in which a sample of participants is followed over time and repeated measures are taken at certain intervals in order to describe how the variable(s) under study have changed (Stein & Cutler, 1996). Sometimes developmental research is accomplished through a cross-sectional design in which the investigator collects data a one time point from a sample that is stratified into different age groups (e.g., children who are 6, 12, 18, and 24 months of age or older adults who are 60–64, 65–69, 70–74, 75–79, etc.). Observed differences between the sample in each age strata are then attributed to the process of development or aging. Cohort studies have the advantage of eliminating effects of sample bias on observed changes, but they are subject to the influence of historical events that are unrelated to the course of development. Cross-sectional designs avoid the latter problem but are prone to cohort effects (i.e., effects that are unrelated to age and are due to some circumstance unique to a particular age cohort). In both cases, random sampling is critical in order to generalize from the sample to the population the study is intended to characterize.

Descriptive Case Studies

Descriptive case studies are in-depth descriptions of the experiences or behaviors of a particular individual or a series of individuals. Case studies are most typically undertaken to describe some new phenomena or to document a client's response to a new intervention. While many case studies in occupational therapy are qualitative in nature, quantitative case studies can also be useful in characterizing how an individual has responded following a traumatic event and/or intervention.

Descriptive case studies differ from the single-subject designs described in Chapter 11 in that there is no experimental manipulation of an independent variable. Rather, the investigator documents variables as they naturally occur or documents an intervention and what happens following it (but without the comparison to the absence of the intervention or to another intervention). Case studies are most valuable when the information reported is comprehensive. Thus, investigators undertaking a case study will either attempt to provide data on several variables of interest or provide repeated measures of some variable over time.

While such case studies are readily related to practice, they are one of the least rigorous forms of research since they lack control and generalizability (Portney & Watkins, 2000). For this reason, a series of, or several, case studies are often used as the basis from which to generalize concepts which then lead to more controlled studies.

Case studies can be particularly useful for investigating new interventions or interventions that require substantial individualization or trial and error. For example, Gillen (2002) reported a case in which occupational therapy services based on concepts of motor control were used to improve mobility and community access in an adult with ataxia. The study reported baseline information from the Functional Index Measure (FIM™) and then reported occupational therapy techniques of "adapted positioning, orthotic prescription, adapted movement patterns, and assistive technology" that were used to address client-centered functional goals (Gillen, 2002, p. 465). The study reported positive changes in the client's FIM score following the intervention.

Correlational Research

Correlational research aims to demonstrate relationships between variables under study (Portney & Watkins, 2000). Correlation refers to an interrelationship or association between two variables (i.e., the tendency for variation in one variable to be either directly or inversely related to variation in another variable). This type of research is sometimes referred to as exploratory, since it is frequently undertaken to identify whether specified variables are related or to determine which variables are related in a multivariable study.

Correlational studies also can provide evidence that is consistent or inconsistent with causal assertions and thus they can provide important evidence for developing theoretical propositions that assert causal relationships between variables (see the following feature box). An important limitation of correlational studies with reference to making causal assertions is that, without experimental control, there is no way to rule out the possibility that two variables might be related by virtue of their association with a third, unobserved variable. Correlational studies can serve as helpful first steps in sorting out causal relationships (i.e., if two variables are not correlated, then there is no reason to anticipate or test for a causal relationship between them). Many correlational studies serve as precursors to experimental studies that exert experimental control over independent and dependent variables in order to draw inferences about causation.

While many correlational studies are concerned with relationships between pairs of variables, investigators are often interested to know the relationship between several variables that are hypothesized or presumed to have a causal relationship with a dependent variable. For example, many studies have examined factors that influence return to work following an injury. In this case, whether or not a person returns to work is the dependent

Correlational studies are often useful for testing hypothesized relationships derived from theory. For example, the Model of Human Occupation (Kielhofner, 2002) argues that volition leads to choices about occupational participation. Based on this theoretical argument, it can be hypothesized that volitional traits should be associated with observed patterns of occupational participation. Correlational studies have been implemented to test this proposed relationship.

For example, Neville-Jan (1994) examined the correlation between volition and patterns of occupation among 100 individuals with varying degrees of depression. Her study found, as hypothesized, a relationship between the adaptiveness of the subjects' routines and a measure of their personal cau-

sation, independent of the level of depression. Another example is a study by Peterson et al. (1999) that examined the relationship between personal causation (feelings of efficacy related to falling) and the pattern of occupational engagement in 270 older adults. They found, as expected, that lower personal causation (i.e., lower falls self-efficacy) was related to reduced participation in leisure and social occupations. These two studies thus provided evidence in support of the proposition that volitional traits (in this case, personal causation) influence the choices persons make about engaging in occupations. As noted in this chapter, however, these correlations are consistent with but cannot be taken as proof of causation.

variable of interest and a study may examine the influence of number of supposed causal or predictive variables (e.g., age, education, extent of impairment, personality, worker identity, and previous work history) on return to work. This type of study ordinarily uses regression analysis (discussed in Chapter 17). The aim of such studies is to identify the amount of variance in the dependent variable that is explained by a set of predictor variables.

In correlational research, there may or may not be a temporal sequence between the hypothesized predictor variables and the dependent variable of interest. Sometimes correlational studies are retrospective and the information on all variables is collected simultaneously. However, in prospective studies data on the predictor variables are collected first and the dependent variable is observed at a later time or at several later time points. Obviously, when there is temporal sequence, inferences about causal relationships have greater weight.

Conclusion

Descriptive research is common in occupational therapy. As noted in this chapter, it serves a number of important purposes, not the least of which is leading to more sophisticated research designs such as those discussed in the following chapters. This chapter focused on descriptive research in which investigators obtained observational data directly from subjects. Other types of studies, including retrospective studies that examine existing data sets and survey research, also sometimes employ designs whose purpose is descriptive. When that is the case, the underlying logic of these studies is the same as described in this chapter.

REFERENCES

Bar-Shalita, T., Goldstand, S., Hahn-Markowitz, J., & Parush, S. (2005). Typical children's repsonsivity patterns of the tactile and vestibular systems. *American Journal of Occupational Therapy, 59,* 148–156.

Centers for Disease Control and Prevention. (CDC). (2000). *HIV/AIDS Surveillance Supplemental Report* (Vol. 7). Atlanta: U.S. Department of Health and Human Services, Centers for Disease Control and Prevention.

Centers for Disease Control and Prevention (CDC). (2004). *HIV/AIDS Surveillance Report, 2003* (Vol. 15). Atlanta: U.S. Department of Health and Human Services, Centers for Disease Control and Prevention.

DePoy, E., & Gitlin, L. N. (1998). *Introduction to research: Understanding and applying multiple strategies* (2nd ed.). St. Louis: C. V. Mosby.

Gillen, G. (2002). Improving mobility and community access in an adult with ataxia. *American Journal of Occupational Therapy, 56,* 462–465.

Jason, L. A., Richman, J. A., Rademaker, A. W., Jordan, K. M., Plioplys, A. V., Taylor, R. R., et al. (1999). A community-based study of chronic fatigue syndrome. *Archives of Internal Medicine, 159,* 2129–2137.

Karon, J. M., Fleming, P. L., Steketee, R. W., & DeCock, K. M. (2001). HIV in the United States at the turn of the century: An epidemic in transition. *American Journal of Public Health, 91*(7), 1060–1068.

Kates, J., Sorian, R., Crowley, J. S., & Summers, T. A. (2002). Critical policy challenges in the third decade of the HIV/AIDS epidemic. *American Journal of Public Health, 92*(7), 1060–1063.

Kielhofner, G. (2002). *A model of human occupation: Theory and application* (3rd ed.). Baltimore: Williams & Wilkins.

Liedberg, G., Hesselstrand, M., & Henriksson, C. M. (2004). Time use and activity patterns in women with long-term pain. *Scandinavian Journal of Occupational Therapy, 11,* 26–35.

MacMahon, B., & Trichopoulos, D. (1996). *Epidemiology: Principles & methods* (2nd ed.). Boston: Little, Brown.

Neville-Jan, A. (1994). The relationship of volition to adaptive occupational behavior among individuals with varying degrees of depression. *Occupational Therapy in Mental Health, 12*(4), 1–18.

Orenstein, R. (2002). Presenting syndromes of human immunodeficiency virus. *Mayo Clinic Proceedings, 77*(10), 1097–1102.

Peterson, E., Howland, J., Kielhofner, G., Lachman, M. E., Assmann, S., Cote, J., & Jette, A. (1999). Falls self-efficacy and occupational adaptation among elders. *Physical & Occupational Therapy in Geriatrics, 16*(1/2), 1–16.

Polit, D. F., & Hungler, B. P. (1999). *Nursing research: Principles and methods.* Philadelphia: Lippincott.

Portney, L. G., & Watkins, M. P. (2000). *Foundations of clinical research: Applications to practice* (2nd ed.). Upper Saddle River, NJ: Prentice-Hall.

Stein, F., & Cutler, S. (1996). *Clinical research in allied health and special education.* San Diego: Singular Press.

CHAPTER 7

Group Comparison Studies: Quantitative Research Designs

David L. Nelson

Designs that compare groups are among the most common in quantitative research. Group comparison designs range from true experiments to comparisons between naturally occurring groups, and from elegantly simple designs to complex combinations of different kinds of interventions, outcomes, and controls. Interestingly, although some of the simplest designs have the best claim to validity and utility, relatively complex designs are appropriate for certain research questions.

Experimental designs provide evidence about *probable causality*. An experiment tests the probability that an intervention has an effect on an outcome, or the probability that one intervention has a different effect on an outcome than another intervention. Geniuses such as Thorndike and Woodward (1901); Fisher (1935); and Amberson, McMahon, and Pinner (1931) integrated concepts such as randomization and controls with probabilistic statistics, and the result is a rational and logical basis for if–then statements. When if–then statements are drawn from theory or from clinical observations and transformed into testable hypotheses, science advances. Embedded in this chapter are procedures to enhance validity as well as practical discussions about the assumptions that must be made in quantitative research.

Nonexperimental group comparison designs (sometimes called quasi-experimental designs) lack the degree of control achieved by experimental designs. In some cases, these kinds of designs can lay the groundwork for subsequent experimental investigations. In other cases, where the researcher needs to know about the differences between different kinds of people, true experimentation is impossible. The researcher must build other kinds of controls into these designs.

This chapter begins with a discussion of experimental designs and proceeds through other types of group comparison designs. A basic premise is that no design is best for all research questions; each has its advantages and disadvantages.

Basic Experiments

Basic experimental design is the most rigorous type of group comparison study (Campbell & Stanley, 1963; Kerlinger, 1986). This type of design will be examined by starting with a definition of and then explaining each part of the definition using examples.

Definition of a Basic Experiment

- There is one sample that is drawn representatively from one population.
- There is one categorical independent variable.
- Study participants are randomly assigned to as many groups as there are conditions to the independent variable.
- The independent variable is administered as planned.
- Potentially confounding variables are minimized, and otherwise uncontrollable events are equally likely across the groups.
- There is one dependent variable on which all subjects are measured or categorized.
- The experimental hypothesis tested is the probability of a causal effect of the independent variable on the dependent variable within the population.

> Writing about group designs is a humbling experience. The methodological literature concerning group research designs is so broad and so deep that every statement in this chapter could be followed by 20 reference citations. As an alternative, this chapter cites only key references thought to be of the most direct benefit to the reader. Those interested in more in-depth treatments of group research designs are referred the list of publications in the "Additional Resources" section at the end of the chapter. Both the primary references and this additional bibliography are sources from which I have learned and continue to learn, and collectively they support the statements made in the chapter.

In the following sections, each element is examined in detail.

Explaining the Definition

There Is One Sample that Is Drawn Representatively from One Population.

A population is any set of people (or in some cases, animals) who share common features. "Americans 70 years of age or older residing in extended care facilities (ECFs)" is a population. Similarly, "persons with Parkinson's disease (stage II through IV)" is another population, and "6-year-old children with autism (but not mental retardation) attending special education classes" also makes up a population.

A sample consists of the persons (participants or subjects) who are in the study. The sample is a subset of some population. A study sample could consist of 120 persons 70 years of age or older, residing in extended care facilities (ECFs) in the United States. This subset of 120 persons is drawn from the entire population (hundreds of thousands of people) who are older than 70 years of age and reside in American ECFs. It is critical that the persons who make up the sample in an experiment are representative of the population from which they are drawn. Research procedures for making sure that the sample is representative of the population are described in Chapter 31.

There Is One Categorical Independent Variable.

There are two kinds of variables: categorical and continuous. The conditions of a categorical variable are qualitatively different from each other, whereas the conditions of a continuous variable are quantitatively different from each other. Type of intervention is an example of a categorical variable. Neurodevelopmental therapy is one type of intervention, and biomechanically based therapy is a different kind of intervention. Each of these interventions could be a condition of a categorical variable; in this case the categorical variable would have two, qualitatively different conditions. Another example of a categorical variable could have three conditions: authoritarian group structure, laissez-faire group structure, and democratic group structure.

In contrast, continuous variables involve quantitative, ordered relationships. Measured height is a continuous variable. The score on a sensory integration test is also a continuous variable.

A categorical variable is an independent vari-able when the researcher examines its probable effects on an outcome (called a dependent variable). The independent variable is the possible cause, and the dependent variable is the possible effect. In an occupational therapy study, designed to test whether an occupationally embedded exercise protocol produces a different outcome from a rote exercise protocol, one condition of the categorical independent variable might be stirring cookie batter and another condition might be the same kind of stirring but with no batter. The dependent variable could be the number of times that the circular motion is completed.

Study Participants Are Randomly Assigned to as Many Groups as There Are Conditions to the Independent Variable.

Study participants are assigned by the researcher into groups, each of which receives one condition of the independent variable. For example, if there are 120 study participants and if there are two conditions of the independent variable, 60 persons could be assigned to one condition and 60 to the other condition. For an experiment with four conditions to the independent variable and with N (overall sample size) = 120, 30 persons could be assigned to each group.

As in the previous examples, a one-to-one ratio is usually used in assigning participants to groups, but not always. For example, a researcher might have a good reason for assigning more participants to one group than to another. Regardless of ratio, randomization is absolutely essential. In a one-to-one ratio, randomization means that every participant in the sample will have an equal chance of being in each of the groups. Procedures for randomization are presented in Chapter 31. Randomization ensures that there is no bias that favors one group over the other. If randomization is done properly, then the rules of chance make it probable that the groups are equivalent to each other at the beginning of the experiment.

Each of the conditions of the independent variable might consist of alternative, previously untested interventions or stimuli (e.g., comparing a parallel group task to a project group task). A sec-

> A common error is to say "independent variables" when referring to the multiple conditions of a single independent variable. Remember: a variable must vary.

In her 2000 Eleanor Clarke Slagle lecture, Dr. Margo Holm reasoned that embedding exercise within everyday tasks (what I term *occupationally embedded exercise*) is one of the few ideas in occupational therapy that has been supported by a systematic review of multiple experiments. Dr. Holm (2000) cites this area of inquiry as an example of the highest level of research evidence.

ond option is to compare an intervention to a control condition (i.e., the absence of any research-induced intervention or stimulus). For example, the control group in a study of an occupation-based wellness program for middle-aged, overweight male professors could be given no special intervention, as a way of finding out if the wellness program is effective.

A third option is to compare an intervention or stimulus to an attention-placebo condition. A placebo condition in drug studies involves administration of a nonactive substance (e.g., a pill) that looks, smells, and tastes the same as the active drug in the study. An attention-placebo condition involves administration of human contact that mimics the intervention under study, without involving the essence of what is under study. For example, in a study of neurodevelopmental therapy (NDT), the children in the attention-placebo condition receive the same amount of touching and time with an adult as the children receiving NDT. A technique to ensure equality of attention is yoking, whereby each person in the attention-placebo group receives the same amount of attention as a specific person in the intervention group. With reference to the previous NDT study example, this technique would mean that each child in the attention-placebo condition would receive the same amount of touching and time as a specific child in the NDT group. Fourth, a common type of comparison condition involves usual care or standard care, which is compared to some new type of intervention. For ethical reasons, subjects in any of these different types of comparison conditions often receive the intervention condition (if found effective) after the experiment is completed.

The Independent Variable Is Administered as Planned.

A study is said to have fidelity if there is documentation that the independent variable is administered just as planned (Moncher & Prinz, 1991). Using the earlier example of a study of occupationally embedded exercise, a problem of fidelity occurs if the research assistant by mistake tells a

participant in the rote exercise condition to "make cookies." Also, a subject in the image-based condition might become distracted, fail to think about stirring cookies, and just do the stirring as a rote exercise. Both of these situations exemplify bleeding: a participant assigned to one condition actually experiences some or all of the comparison condition.

In addition to bleeding, there are other problems of fidelity. Consider an experiment whereby each participant is supposed to attend four specially designed family education sessions (versus a usual-care condition) and some subjects arrive late and miss part of the sessions. Here the problem is that some of the subjects simply are not experiencing what they are supposed to be experiencing. A problem of delivery occurs, for instance, when the interventionist fails to spend the required time with the participant, or forgets to administer all of the protocol (e.g., leaving out a component of one of the family education sessions). A problem of receipt is a failure of the participant to pay attention to the therapist's instructions (e.g., a subject is present at the educational session but is distracted because of a problem at work). A problem of enactment is a failure of participants to do something they are supposed to do (e.g., following the advice given in the educational session). Documentation of fidelity is especially important in studies that involve complex interventions administered over long periods of time, and in studies involving the participant's generalization of learning from one context to application in another.

Potentially Confounding Variables Are Minimized, and Otherwise Uncontrollable Events Are Equally Likely Across the Groups.

In an ideal experimental world, the independent variable is the only thing affecting the participants while they are in the experiment. But in the real

I (your chapter author) first learned about intervention fidelity from Dr. Laura Gitlin (please see selected references under her name), at a meeting of the Center for Research Outcomes and Education (CORE) on a sunny day in Chicago. As attested by the smiles of the participants, learning about experimental research can be fun. Dr. Virgil Mathiowetz, who was also in attendance that day, and I later wrote about fidelity (Nelson & Mathiowetz, 2004). Virgil wrote the better parts of the paper.

world, there are many potentially confounding variables (things that could affect the participants in addition to the conditions of the independent variable). Potentially confounding variables are also sometimes called confounds, extraneous variables, nuisance variables, and sources of error. For example, in a study comparing occupationally embedded exercise to rote exercise in older nursing home residents, a nursing aide could interrupt the participant while stirring the cookie dough or the older person could lose attentiveness because of poor sleep the night before. Therefore, one's experimental design incorporates practical strategies for minimizing the chances of potentially confounding variables. For example, the researcher can explain the need for privacy to the staff; select a quiet, out-of-the-way room for the study; and put up a do-not-disturb sign.

Despite any researcher's best efforts, there are always events that cannot be controlled. This is especially true of intervention studies taking place over many months. For example, a study of the effects of a multisite, school-year-long, occupation-based fitness program for overweight children (versus an attention-placebo control condition) involves potentially confounding variables such as differing school-based practices, differing levels of family participation, family and community events (positive as well as negative), differing exposures to mass media, differing opportunities for sports participation, changes resulting from growing older, and illnesses that may occur. Experimental design cannot eliminate all these potentially confounding variables, and there are practical limitations even on monitoring them. The researcher's goal is that these potentially confounding variables are equally likely to occur in each of the comparison groups. In other words, the researcher tries to ensure that bias does not occur (where one of the conditions is systematically favored). Other terms used to refer to a biasing confounding variable are artifact and sources of systematic error.

To eliminate certain artifacts, researchers frequently use masking (also called blinding). In a "double-blind" study, neither the participants (one blind) nor the researcher (the other blind) is aware of which groups receive which condition of the independent variable. This is usually done through use of a placebo. However, total double-blinds are impossible in most occupational therapy studies, because the participant is usually aware of what is happening and the administrators of the independent variable (often occupational therapists) are professionally responsible for being aware of the service they are providing. In occupational therapy

research, other types of blinding may sometimes be used:

- The person conducting the randomization can be masked from the subsequent randomization sequence,
- The person measuring the dependent variable (see below) can be masked from knowing who has received which condition, and
- The statistician can be masked from knowing who has received which condition.

There Is One Dependent Variable on Which All subjects Are Measured or Categorized.

The dependent variable is the criterion used to compare the conditions of the independent variable to each other. All participants are measured or categorized on the dependent variable. For example, for an independent variable involving a comparison between occupationally embedded exercise and rote exercise, the dependent variable might be the number of exercise repetitions (a continuous variable that can be measured). Alternatively, the dependent variable in a special skin protection program for wheelchair users (compared to a usual-care condition) might be the presence or absence of skin breakdown (a categorical variable).

The method used to collect data on the dependent variable must be valid and reliable. Experimenters often try to improve reliability and validity through a variety of strategies:

- Measuring each participant several times so that the dependent variable is the mean,
- Providing training that exceeds the minimum specified in the measurement protocol,
- Using multiple, simultaneous raters or judges in measuring or judging the dependent variable, and
- Masking (see above) the measurers/judges.

In selecting a dependent variable for a study, the researcher has to be especially concerned about its responsiveness. Responsiveness (also called sensitivity in the nonmedical literature) is the capacity of the dependent variable to show small but meaningful increments of change over time. For example, a nonresponsive measure might be a three-point scale for measuring self-care: independent, partly dependent, and dependent. A research participant can make much meaningful progress in taking care of oneself, but the person's progress does not show up in the measure. For example, if a female participant starts out with the ability to do very little self-care and ends with the ability to take care of herself except for one or two

The term *sensitivity* is a good example of a research term meaning two totally different things. In the medical literature, *sensitivity* refers to predictive validity of a diagnostic test. In the literature of psychology, sensitivity often refers to the capacity of a measurement to reflect change in participants over time (what is called *responsiveness* in the medical literature).

things, her rating would not change since she is still partly dependent.

Another kind of nonresponsive measure is one that has ceiling or floor effects. A ceiling effect occurs where the sample's scores are already so high on the scale that little improvement is possible. A floor effect occurs when the opposite is the case. For example, adolescents with conduct disorders are unlikely to demonstrate a reduction in aggressive episodes in a one-day study if the typical participant engages in only a few aggressive incidents per week.

Ideally, the experimenter–researcher uses a method of capturing the dependent variable that is recognized as the criterion standard (sometimes called the gold standard) in the field. Thus in selecting a data collection procedure for the dependent variable, the investigator asks if there is a consensus in the field concerning the best way to measure or categorize that variable. For example, 5-year survival rate is a criterion standard for interventions addressing certain types of cancers. However, occupational therapy researchers frequently address research questions that have not been studied adequately in the past. An excellent way to address this problem is for the designer of an experiment to ask experts in the field to confirm the validity of a dependent variable. At the same time, the investigator can ask the experts to identify how much of a difference between comparison groups at the end of the study is required to be meaningful. For example, the investigator might ask whether a 10% reduction in rehospitalization rates is a meaningful difference in a study of interventions for participants with chronic schizophrenia.

Knowing how much change one can expect to see in the dependent variable can be factored into a decision about the number of subjects needed in the study. There is a calculation called power analysis that allows one to make this determination. It is discussed in detail in Chapter 17.

The Experimental Hypothesis Tested Is the Probability of a Causal Effect of the Independent Variable on the Dependent Variable Within the Population.

The first thing about this definition to notice is the word prediction. It is a hallmark of quantitative research that all the variables under study and their possible relationships, one way or the other, are determined in advance. A hypothesis is a prediction about the relationship between variables within a population. The end result of an experiment can have only two possibilities: support for this hypothesis, or a lack of support. Consider the following experimental hypothesis: Occupationally embedded exercise elicits more exercise repetitions than rote exercise in nursing home residents aged 65 years or more. Even though the present tense (elicits, not will elicit) is used, a prediction is implied, because the hypothesis is stated before the research starts. The independent variable has two conditions: occupationally embedded exercise versus a control condition. The dependent variable consists of exercise repetitions. And the sample is drawn from the population of nursing home residents 65 years of age or older. The type of relationship between the variables under study is the hypothesized effect of the independent variable on the dependent variable. Probable causality is involved: the independent variable is the hypothesized cause, and the dependent variable is the hypothesized effect. Quantitative research deals with probability, not with certainty or truth. See Chapter 17 on statistics to find out how probability is used to assess research outcomes.

> Type I error involves reporting a relationship when there really is no relationship.

The logic of the basic experiment is as follows:

* If groups assigned to conditions of the independent variable are probably equal at the start of the experiment (the chance processes of randomization ensure probable equivalence),
* If groups are treated the same except for the independent variable, and
* If there are differences between groups at the end of the experiment, then the differences were probably caused by the independent variable acting on the dependent variable. This is the basis for experimental design's claim to study probable causality.

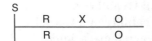

S = Start
R = Randomization
X = Condition of independent variable
O = Observation (measurement or categorization used
    for dependent variable)

Figure 7.1 Basic experimental design, with true control group, one intervention, and no pretest. After the sample is randomized (*R*) into two groups, one group receives an intervention (*X*) while the control group does not. Both groups are measured or categorized (*O*) in the same way. *The symbolic format for these figures is adapted from Campbell and Stanley (1963).

The following is another experimental hypothesis: In nursing home residents 65 years of age or older, there are differences among occupationally embedded exercise, imagery-based exercise, and rote exercise in terms of exercise repetitions. Here, the independent variable has three conditions that are compared with each other. This is also an example of a nondirectional hypothesis. A nondirectional hypothesis does not predict which condition will end up with the superior outcome; it simply predicts that one of the conditions will be superior. Still implied is probable causality. In contrast, a directional hypothesis is clear as to which group is predicted to have higher scores (or higher proportions in the case of categorical variables). Figures 7.1 to 7.3 illustrate three basic experimental designs.

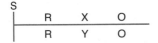

S = Start
R = Randomization
X = Condition of independent variable
Y = A different intervention, usual care, or attention-placebo
O = Observation (measurement or categorization used
    for dependent variable)

Figure 7.2 Basic experimental design comparing two conditions of the independent variable, and no pretest. After the sample is randomized (*R*) into two groups, one group receives an intervention (*X*) while the other group receives (a) a different intervention, (b) usual care, or (c) an attention-placebo (*Y*). Both groups are measured or categorized (*O*) in the same way.

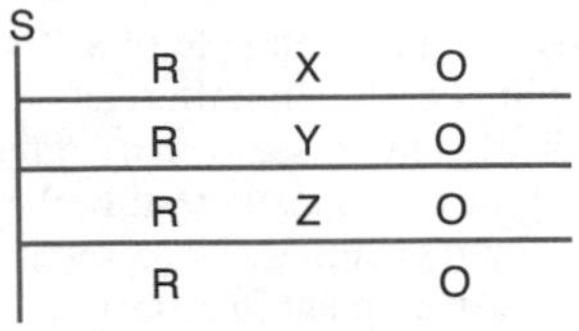

S = Start
R = Randomization
X = An intervention
Y = A different intervention or usual care
Z = A different intervention, usual care, or attention-placebo
O = Observation (measurement or categorization used
    for dependent variable)

Figure 7.3 Basic experimental design (pretest–posttest) comparing three conditions of the independent variable to each other and to a control group. After the sample is randomized (*R*) into four groups, three groups receive *X, Y, Z* respectively while the fourth receives nothing. All groups are measured or categorized (*O*) in the same way.

Evaluating the Validity of Group Comparison Designs

Type I Error

Type I error involves reporting a relationship when there really is no relationship (Rosenthal & Rosnow, 1991). The reader of the research report can never be absolutely certain that a type I error has been made. However, the reader of the research report may reason that weaknesses in the research design make the chances of a type I error unacceptably large.

To understand this point, consider the following nonexperimental research design that is highly prone to type I error: the pretest–posttest no-control group design (Figure 7.4). In this design, a single group of participants receive a test, an intervention, and another test after the intervention. Consider the statement: Manipulation of the spine

Campbell, D. T., & Stanley, J. C. (1963). *Experimental and quasi-experimental designs for research*. Chicago: Rand McNally is the classic reference concerning type I error and how to prevent it. It is a remarkably brief book filled with an intense logic that many a graduate student has practically memorized. It is highly recommended by this author as a resource for understanding group comparison designs.

decreases pain in adult males with acute lumbar pain secondary to lifting-related injuries.

The researcher following this design simply:

- Selects persons with acute lumbar pain secondary to lifting-related injuries,
- Measures the level of pain (a pretest),
- Administers a series of manipulation interventions,
- Measures the level of pain once again (a posttest), and
- Compares the pretest to the posttest.

If pain decreases significantly from the pretest to the posttest, the researcher concludes that the spinal manipulation is effective. The problem with this researcher's logic is that the design does not protect against type I error: it is quite likely (no one knows exactly how likely) that the manipulation has nothing to do with the improvement in pain levels. The following potentially confounding variables unrelated to manipulation may have caused the improvement:

- Acutely ill persons might recover without any intervention through natural healing.
- The research participants might have received other interventions between the pretest and the posttest.
- There might have been something about being tested twice on the pain scale that resulted in lower scores the second time around.

There are many possible explanations for the observed change, and so the bottom line is that we do not know anything more than we knew before the research study. Possible sources of type I error are not controlled in this study design.

Another nonexperimental research design often highly at risk for a type I error is the nonrandomized control group design (Figure 7.5). Consider the following hypothesis: Splinting technique A is superior to splinting technique B in improving

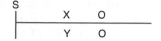

S = Start
X = An intervention
Y = A different intervention, usual care, or attention-placebo
O = Observation (measurement or categorization used for dependent variable)

Figure 7.5 Nonrandomized comparison group design (no pretest). The subjects in one naturally occurring group receive one intervention (*X*), and the subjects in a different naturally occurring group receive a different intervention. A measurement or categorization is then done (*O*). It is important to note that this design is not recommended except for pilot testing in advance of future research.

wrist range of motion for persons with carpal tunnel syndrome. Instead of randomly assigning participants to groups, the researcher assigns one naturally occurring group (e.g., patients at one hand clinic) to receive technique A and assigns another naturally occurring group (e.g., patients in a different hand clinic) to receive technique B. At the end of 2 weeks of being splinted, the patients in the first clinic who received technique A actually have greater wrist range of motion than the patients in the other clinic who received technique B. Consequently, the researcher reports the superiority of splinting technique A.

However, the chances of a type I error are unacceptably high. The problem is that the patients at the first clinic might have been different from, or nonequivalent to, the patients in the second clinic (even before splinting, they might have been less severely disabled). Also, they might have had special opportunities for progress, based on the quality of the clinic's staff or on demographic factors, or they might have had less risk for re-injury. Even if the researcher uses a pretest–posttest nonrandomized control group design and finds that the two groups do not differ on the baseline, there is still a high chance of a type I error. Patients at the first clinic might have a greater potential for change than the patients at the second clinic. For example, it is possible that the range- of-motion scores are equal at pretest even though the patients at the first clinic have relatively recent, acute injuries whereas the patients at the second clinic have chronic injuries unlikely to change in a short period of time.

The basic experiment was invented to reduce the chances of a type I error to some small, controllable amount. Randomization ensures that the

S
| O   X   O

S = Start
X = An intervention
O = Observation (measurement or categorization used for dependent variable)

Figure 7.4 Pretest–posttest design with no control or comparison group. After a pretest, an intervention is given, to be followed by a posttest. It is important to note that this design is not recommended except for pilot testing in advance of future research.

comparison groups are probably equivalent at the outset of the study. A comparison condition balances potentially confounding variables (thereby preventing systematic bias). For example, both groups in a basic experiment are equally likely to be exposed to the same processes of healing, maturation, extraneous interventions, repeated testing, and other factors. The basic experiment was developed within the tradition of scientific skepticism: the biggest danger to scientific development is to report a relationship when one does not exist.

Type II Error

Type II error is the failure to find and report a relationship when the relationship actually exists (Rosenthal & Rosnow, 1991). Like type I error, the reader of a research report can never be certain that a type II error has occurred. But certain research designs and situations are prone to increasing the risks of type II error to unacceptable levels. Recommendations by Ottenbacher (1995) and Ottenbacher and Maas (1998) for identifying risks of type II error and for how to avoid type II error are particularly recommended for those who wish to understand more about this issue.

Sources of type II error include:

- A small sample size,
- A subtle (yet real) independent variable,
- Much dispersion on the dependent variable within groups:
  - Dispersion due to individual differences among subjects, or
  - Dispersion due to measurement error, and
- A stringent or nonrobust statistical test of the hypothesis.

Although the basic experiment provides the best protection against type I error, it sometimes provides poor protection against type II error. Consider a study with the following hypothesis: an occupational therapy program will increase the organizational skills of clients with traumatic brain injury (vs. an attention-control condition). The occupational therapy program takes place once a week for 4 weeks, and the measurement of organizational ability involves a nonstandardized rating system whereby a therapist makes judgments concerning the client's organizational ability while shopping from a list in the supermarket. The researcher has ensured a lack of bias by:

- Selecting 20 clients for the study,
- Randomizing them to groups,
- Making sure of high fidelity within groups and no bleeding between groups,
- Ensuring that the measurer remains masked (i.e., unaware of the intervention condition of the participants), and
- Following the plan for statistical analysis.

Following the logic discussed earlier, this design allows little chance of a type I error, because neither group is favored by biasing variables. However, the chances of a type II error are so great that it is very unlikely that a difference will be found between groups even if the type of intervention under study is actually effective. This is because:

- The intervention is not intensive enough to produce a large effect,
- The number of subjects in each group is small, and
- The quality of the measure of the dependent variable is unknown and may not be reliable or sensitive.

To decrease the chances of a type II error, the researcher can:

- Increase the sample size by extending the study over time or by finding additional sites for the research,
- Increase the effect of the independent variable by providing therapy more often per week and over a longer period of time, and
- Decrease dispersion due to measurement error by using a test of organizational ability that has been demonstrated to be accurate (reliable) yet sensitive to change (responsive) in past studies.

In fact, all three strategies are warranted in this case to avoid type II error.

There are several strategies to decrease dispersion on the dependent variable that is due to individual differences. The most straightforward way to decrease dispersion is to select participants who are homogeneous (similar to each other, as opposed to heterogeneous). In our example of persons with brain injury, the researcher could decide in advance that research participants are included only if at a similar stage of recovery.

Another way to decrease dispersion is to use a pretest–posttest experimental design, as opposed to a posttest-only experimental design. Figures 7.6

> Type II error is the failure to find and report a relationship when the relationship actually exists.

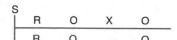

S = Start
R = Randomization
X = Condition of independent variable
O = Observation (measurement or categorization used
for dependent variable)

Figure 7.6 Basic experimental design (pretest–posttest), with true control group and one intervention. After the sample is randomized (*R*) into two groups, both groups are pretested (*O* to left) in the same way. Next, one group receives an intervention (*X*) while the control group does not. Finally both groups are posttested (*O* to right).

and 7.7 illustrate two such designs. To use the same example again, a pretest of organization ability administered before the independent variable would permit statistical procedures that control for individual differences in the final analysis. The dependent variable is adjusted, correcting for the individual differences. This is done in an unbiased way, so that neither group being compared to each other receives a special advantage. Several different statistical procedures are capable of making this adjustment.

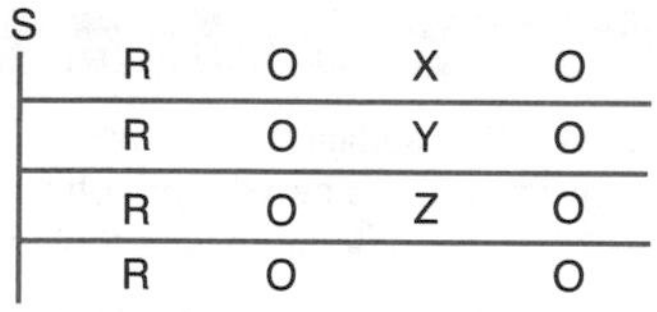

S

R	O	X	O
R	O	Y	O
R	O	Z	O
R	O		O

S = Start
R = Randomization
X = An intervention
Y = A different intervention, usual care, or attention-placebo
Z = A different intervention, usual care, or attention-placebo
O = Observation (measurement or categorization used for dependent variable)

Figure 7.7 Basic experimental design (pretest–posttest) comparing three conditions of the independent variable to each other and to a control group. After the sample is randomized (*R*) into four groups, groups are pretested (*O* to left) in the same way. Next, three groups receive *X, Y, Z* respectively while the fourth receives nothing. Finally, all groups are measured or categorized (*O* to right) in the same way.

Sometimes it is impossible to do a pretest. For example, in a study of occupationally embedded exercise, it is impossible to do a pretest of repetitions because the repetitions can be counted only in the simultaneous context of the independent variable (e.g., while actually stirring). In this case, some other variable can be measured in advance that is probably associated with the dependent variable. This kind of variable is called a covariate. For example, in a study in which the dependent variable involves stirring repetitions, a likely covariate is grip strength. Individual differences reflecting grip strength can be controlled through analysis of covariance. The point here is that a covariate, properly chosen in advance of the study, can reduce individual differences and thereby reduce dispersion on the dependent variable. The result is less of a chance of a type II error, making it possible to demonstrate that the independent variable probably makes a real difference. Figures 7.8 and 7.9 (on p. 74) illustrate two such designs.

Yet another strategy to decrease individual differences is to use a randomized matched subjects design (Figure 7.10 on p. 74); it is called a randomized matched pairs design where there are two conditions of the independent variable. This design is also referred to as a type of randomized block design. In this instance, participants are matched to each other in advance on some relevant variable, and then they are randomly assigned to groups (each of which receives a different condition of the independent variable). Consider the hypothesis: community-dwelling persons with dementia who receive added home-based occupational therapy are less likely to enter extended care facilities than community-dwelling persons with dementia

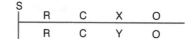

S = Start
R = Randomization
C = Covariate(s) reflecting variable(s) associated with the dependent variable
X = Condition of independent variable
Y = A different intervention, usual care, or attention-placebo
O = Observation (measurement or categorization used for dependent variable)

Figure 7.8 Experimental design comparing two conditions of the independent variable, with planned covariate(s). After the sample is randomized (*R*) into two groups, the covariate (*C*) is measured. Next, each group receives interventions *X* or *Y*. Both groups are measured or categorized (*O*) in the same way.

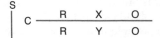

S = Start
R = Randomization
C = Covariate reflecting variable associated with the
    dependent variable
X = An intervention
Y = A different intervention, usual care, or attention-
    placebo
O = Observation (measurement or categorization
    used for dependent variable)

Figure 7.9 Experimental design comparing two conditions of the independent variable, with a planned covariate available prior to randomization. After the sample is randomized (*R*), each group receives *X* or *Y*. Both groups are measured or categorized (*O*) in the same way.

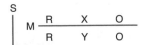

S = Start
M = Matching
R = Randomization
X = Condition of independent variable
Y = A different intervention, usual care, or attention-
    placebo
O = Observation (measurement or categorization used
    for dependent variable)

Figure 7.10 Matched subjects (matched pairs) experimental design comparing two conditions of the independent variable. First, subjects are paired based on some relevant similarity. Randomization (*R*) is done in blocks of two (randomized block design). Next, one group receives *X* or *Y*. Both groups are measured or categorized (*O*) in the same way.

receiving usual care. Participants can be paired to each other in terms of level of dementia, and then randomly assigned to either the occupational therapy condition or to usual care. The statistical analysis for this design involves comparisons of persons who are similar to each other, thereby reducing unsystematic error due to individual differences.

In summary of our discussion of type I and type II error, the basic experiment is a great means of preventing type I error. But special adjustments must often be made to prevent type II error. Table 7.1 is a way of depicting how likely a type II error is in occupational therapy research in comparison to research in some other fields. But we are not alone. Researchers in psychotherapy, special education, and many branches of medicine must overcome the same disadvantages. Statistical presentations in Chapter 17 discuss the importance of

Table 7.1 Inherent Dangers of Type II Error in Occupational Therapy Research

Common Causes of Type II Error	Laboratory Animal Studies	Occupational Therapy Studies
Small sample size	Animals are readily available at reasonable cost.	Persons with disabilities are small minorities of the population, often with major health and financial problems.
Dispersion due to individual differences	Healthy animals are highly homogeneous (often genetically matched).	Persons with disabilities vary from each other more than the general population; all persons respond somewhat differently to occupational forms.
Dispersion due to measurement error	Measurement systems in most animal research is highly precise.	Most measurement systems in occupational therapy generate high levels of error.
Dispersion due to random events	Highly controlled environments are typical.	People's lives are full of chance events that cannot be eliminated in multisession studies.
Robustness of the independent variable	Biological interventions are often powerful; subtle effects can be investigated after robust effects are demonstrated.	A single short-term occupation usually has little long-term effects; ethical considerations preclude risky interventions.
Powerful statistical procedures	Biostatisticians are familiar with techniques to reduce unsystematic error.	Much occupational therapy research in the past has not employed sophisticated procedures to reduce unsystematic error.

reporting the effect size of a comparison, not just the *p* value. What is important to note here is that an experiment reporting a substantial but statistically nonsignificant difference must be interpreted with great caution: the chances of a type II error might be high.

External Validity

External validity has to do with generalizability, whether the results of a research project can be applied to the nonresearch environment (the real world out there) (Campbell & Stanley, 1963). Unfortunately, it is possible that an experiment can avoid making type I and type II errors (i.e., it could have internal validity) and yet have no external validity. For example, a laboratory study of how people interact under experimental conditions might have excellent internal validity but might not reflect how people interact when not under close examination.

External validity can be threatened by two main factors:

- Artificiality in the experimental environment (things are so different that subjects behave differently from how they do in everyday life), and
- Unrepresentative samples (a mismatch exists between the intended population and the actual sample that is studied).

Artificiality can apply to the independent variable or the dependent variable. Lab coats, unusual settings, excessively complex informed consent procedures, and unusual equipment can threaten external validity. For example, in studies of perception, participants asked to discriminate among carefully projected images might make discriminations that they cannot make in the blooming and buzzing confusion of everyday life, where they focus on individually meaningful things. An example of artificiality in measuring the dependent variable can be seen in an electrogoniometer strapped onto the participant's arm, to measure elbow flexion. The participant might reach differently when wearing this bulky contraption (e.g., he or she might lean forward more than usual, thereby decreasing elbow flexion artificially).

To decrease artificiality, the researcher can strive to design the independent variable so that it takes place (as much as possible) under everyday conditions. Instead of studying perception in a controlled lab, it can be studied in the participant's home. The problem in this instance is that naturalistic settings involve potentially confounding variables (the ring of the telephone or the voices of others in the home) that threaten to cause problems of internal validity. For this reason, careful investigators may gather preliminary evidence under controlled laboratory conditions, and later in subsequent experiments show that the effect also can be demonstrated in the everyday world. As for artificiality of the dependent variable, unobtrusive measurements can sometimes be used. For example, there are motion detection systems that do not involve strapping objects to participants' arms.

Unrepresentativeness of the sample can be addressed in two ways: subject selection procedures and dealing with study dropouts. The basic idea of this strategy is to ensure that the participants in the study do not represent some special subpopulation that responds differently to the independent variable from the population that is supposedly under study. Examples of unrepresentative samples are studies supposedly of U.S. nursing home residents where the sample is 80% male, or studies of children with autism where the sample is 80% female. A proper experimental write-up details the relevant demographic characteristics of the sample so that the reader can decide to whom the study can be generalized. There is nothing wrong with a study of male nursing home residents as long as the researcher does not say that the results can be generalized to all nursing home residents.

Dropouts are particularly likely in long-term experiments: participants might lose interest over time, become ill in ways that are not relevant to the experiment, or move away. The danger to external validity is that the participants who drop out might be different from the participants who remain in the study (e.g., dropping out might be a way of avoiding unpleasant side effects of the intervention under study, or dropping out might reflect special frailty). Strategies to prevent dropouts include careful explanation of the study in advance, frequent positive communications over the course of the study, and due consideration for the inconveniences participants experience (e.g., lost time, transportation, etc.). The experimental

> External validity has to do with generalizability, whether the results of a research project can be applied to the nonresearch environment (the real world out there).

plan should include procedures for recording and reporting any dropouts; ideally dropouts can be compared to non-dropouts to see if differences exist.

Variations on Randomized Designs

We have already discussed three variations on basic posttest-only experimental design:

- Pretest–posttest experimental design,
- Use of a covariate to adjust for individual differences, and
- Randomized matched subjects design.

There are other variations that can be helpful, given particular research problems. They are discussed below.

Interim Repeated Measures, Post–Post Tests, and Long-Term Follow-up Tests

Sometimes it is desirable to measure the outcome repeatedly over the course of an experiment (Fleiss, 1986). For example, in a study in which sensory integrative therapy is administered to children with learning disabilities over a full year (compared to a true control group), the researcher might measure school achievement each quarter. In this way, the researcher can gain insight as to quarter-by-quarter rates of change. It is possible that there might be little difference between groups at the end of the first quarter, but a large difference at the end of the second quarter. This provides important information concerning the duration required for this intervention to have an effect. The researcher using repeated measures should be clear in advance as to the primary (most important) endpoint, the measurement that will be used to test the main hypothesis of the study. For example, in the study of sensory integration, the primary endpoint might be the final quarter's measurement of school performance, at the end of the school year. In this case, the earlier quarter-by-quarter measures are interim measures. However, if the researcher designates the second-quarter measurement of school performance as the primary endpoint, then the third- and fourth-quarter measurements are called post–posttests. Figure 7.11 illustrates a repeated measures design.

Sometimes the organizations responsible for the protection of human subjects require interim measurements (Friedman, Furberg, & DeMets, 1998). For example, in a study of a daily-walking

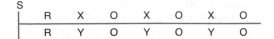

S = Start
R = Randomization
X = An intervention
Y = A different intervention, usual care, or attention-placebo
O = Observation (measurement or categorization used for dependent variable)

Figure 7.11 Experimental design (no pretest) comparing two conditions of the independent variable with repeated observations (repeated measures). After the sample is randomized (*R*) into two groups, each group receives *X* or *Y*. Both groups are observed (*O*) in the same way. Observations (*O*) occurring before the designated primary end point are called interim measures. Observations (*O*) occurring after the primary endpoint are called post–posttests.

intervention to reduce falls in community-dwelling older persons (versus an attention-control condition), the Institutional Review Board wants to rule out the possibility that the daily walking might actually increase the rate of falling. These are unique statistical procedures for analyzing the dependent variable when there are repeated measures. The more statistical tests that are done, the more likely it is that some of those tests appear to be statistically significant by chance alone.

The difference between post-posttests and long-term follow-up tests is that long-term follow-up test occurs after a period of no intervention. To take the example of the year-long program of sensory integration, a long-term follow-up test can take place a year after the conclusion of intervention and the posttest. The long-term follow-up test sheds light as to whether the effects of the intervention are still detectable a year after the withdrawal of the intervention. Figure 7.12 illustrates an experimental design with long-term follow ups.

Multiple Dependent Variables Tested in Reference to the Same Independent Variable

Researchers frequently want to know whether an intervention affects several dependent variables (Stevens, 1986). For example, in a study of the effects of added levels of occupational therapy in comparison to usual care in subacute rehabilitation patients, the researcher might want to know if the added sessions affect three separate outcomes: objectively measured self-care, discharge out-

S
R	O	X	O	O	O
R	O	Y	O	O	O
R	O	Y	O	O	O

S = Start
R = Randomization
X = Condition of independent variable
Y = A different intervention, usual care, or attention-placebo
Z = A different intervention, usual care, or attention-placebo
O = Observation (measurement or categorization used for dependent variable)

Figure 7.12 Experimental design (pretest–posttest) comparing three conditions of the independent variable with repeated observations (repeated measures) and two long-term follow-ups. After the sample is randomized (*R*) into three groups, each group is pretested. Next, each group receives *X, Y,* or *Z*. Groups are observed (*O*) in the same way immediately after the intervention and at two additional points in time.

S
R	X	OPQ
R		OPQ

S = Start
R = Randomization
X = An intervention
O = Observation (a dependent variable)
P = Observation (another dependent variable)
Q = Observation (yet another dependent variable)

Figure 7.13 Experimental design (posttest-only), with three dependent variables (*O, P, Q*) and a true control group. After the sample is randomized (*R*) into two groups, one group receives an intervention (*X*) while the control group does not. Both groups are measured or categorized (*O, P, Q*) in the same way.

come, and patients' self-reports of goal achievement. There is a statistically testable hypothesis for each of the dependent variables, and there is also a way to do a single test of the effectiveness of the intervention across all three dependent variables (multivariate analysis of variance). Figure 7.13 illustrates an experimental design with three dependent variables.

The advantage of having multiple dependent variables is obvious. It is great to know about all three outcomes without having to do three studies. A possible problem, however, is that measurement of the first dependent variable has an effect on the second dependent variable. A person could have fatigue after the first measurement, or the first measurement might sensitize the person to the second measurement (a measurement of vestibular ability might artificially inflate a subsequent measure of alertness). A design strategy to deal with this problem is counterbalancing of the dependent variables (Figure 7.14 on p. 78), where the different variables are experienced in different sequences, so each dependent variable sometimes occurs early in the testing protocol and sometimes late. Note that this counterbalancing of the dependent variables should not be confused with counterbalancing of

the independent variables, to be discussed later in the section on crossover designs.

Another problem encountered by having several outcomes is multiplicity: the increase in type I error due to multiple statistical tests on the same participants. The more tests that are done, by chance alone it is likely that some of those tests will appear to be statistically significant. Unless special care is taken, the chances of a type I error increase for multiple statistical tests, especially if these tests are done on the same participants. For instance one might have 20 dependent variables, if one wishes to look at each aspect of self-care (tooth-brushing, hair-combing, buttoning, etc.) If each of these 20 variables is tested independently at the .05 level, the chances are that at least 1 of the 20 tests will be found significant even if the independent variable had no effect at all (a type I error). Therefore investigators use special corrective procedures discussed in Chapter 17. It is also good practice that a researcher interested in multiple outcomes clearly identify and justify a primary dependent variable and discriminate in statistical procedures between analysis of the primary dependent variable and secondary dependent variables.

> The more statistical tests that are done, the more likely it is that some of those tests appear to be statistically significant by chance alone.

Mechanisms of Change

A special argument in favor of multiple dependent variables occurs when the researcher theorizes that the intervention under study works in a chain reac-

S
	R	X		OPQ
	R			OPQ
	R	X		PQO
	R			PQO
	R	X		QOP
	R			QOP

S = Start
R = Randomization
X = An intervention
O = Observation (a dependent variable)
P = Observation (another dependent variable)
Q = Observation (yet another dependent variable)

Figure 7.14 Experimental design (posttest-only), with true control group and three dependent variables (*O*, *P*, *Q*) that are counterbalanced according to a Latin Square. After the sample is randomized (*R*) into six groups, three groups receives an intervention (*X*) while three groups serve as controls. All groups are measured or categorized on *O*, *P*, and *Q*, but in different sequences, so that two groups receive *O* first, two receive *P* first, and two receive *Q* first. The alternative is to assign subjects to all possible sequences of the three measurements (which would result in 12 groups).

tion style, in which first one aspect of the person is affected, which in turn influences some other aspect (Gitlin et al., 2000). For example, consider a comparison between a client-centered approach to occupational therapy and an impairment-reduction approach, in which the primary dependent variable is functional outcome. The researcher may theorize that the reason the former approach is superior is that it increases the patient's sense of volition. Therefore, the researcher not only measures functional outcome but also measures volition. Depending on the researcher's theory, volition might be measured at the midpoint of the study, at the end of the study when functional outcome is measured, or at multiple points. The measurement of hypothesized mechanisms of change strengthens the interpretation of the results and contributes to theory confirmation. Figure 7.15 illustrates such a design.

Tests of Fidelity

A desirable feature of research design is to conduct quantitative tests for intervention fidelity (Lichstein, Riedel, & Grieve, 1994). Figure 7.16 illustrates this type of design. In the comparison between the client-centered and impairment-reduction approaches to therapy (discussed above),

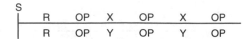

S
	R	OP	X	OP	X	OP
	R	OP	Y	OP	Y	OP

S = Start
R = Randomization
X = Condition of independent variable
Y = A different intervention, usual care, or attention-placebo
O = Observation (primary dependent variable)
P = Observation (measurement indicating theory-based mechanism of change)

Figure 7.15 Experimental design comparing two interventions, with pretest and interim repeated measure on primary dependent variable (*O*) as well as on a measure indicating a theory-based mechanism of change (*P*).

the researcher could document that the therapists administering the two types of intervention actually follow the intended protocol, with no bleeding from condition to condition and with adherence to "doses" (i.e., amount of intervention) called for in the protocol. Another example is to compare statistically the amount of time spent with subjects in an attention-control group to the amount of time spent with intervention subjects. The researcher in this instance generates a methodological hypothesis (a test of the validity of the research procedures).

Completely Randomized Factorial Designs

Completely randomized factorial designs have more than one independent variable; otherwise they resemble basic experiments. For example, a researcher may want to test the effects of a home safety program on falls prevention in older, community-dwelling persons, while also testing

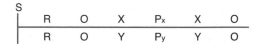

S
	R	O	X	P_x	X	O
	R	O	Y	P_y	Y	O

S = Start
R = Randomization
X = An intervention
Y = A different intervention
O = Observation (primary dependent variable)
P_x = Measure of fidelity of intervention X
P_y = Measure of fidelity of intervention Y

Figure 7.16 Experimental design (pretest–posttest) comparing two interventions, with an interim measure of the degree to which the conditions of the independent variable were administered as called for by the research protocol (P_x and P_y).

the effects of a lower extremity strengthening program on falls prevention in the same population. In a completely randomized factorial design, the researcher randomly assigns participants to one of four groups:

- A group that receives the lower extremity strengthening program only,
- A group that receives the home safety program only,
- A group that receives both interventions, and
- A group that receives attention-control only.

In factorial design, both interventions can be tested, and a special bonus is that the interaction of the two interventions can be studied. An interaction occurs when the effects of one intervention depend on (i.e., augment or decrease) the effects of the other intervention. For example, one kind of interaction is that the home safety program is effective only when combined with the lower extremity strengthening program, such that the two interventions together are more effective than the lower extremity strengthening program alone.

When two independent variables each have two conditions (as in our falls prevention example), we call it a 2 × 2 factorial design. If one of the independent variables has three conditions (e.g., lower extremity weight training versus Tai Chi training vs. attention-placebo) and the other has two conditions, then we call it a 2 × 3 factorial design (Figure 7.17). In this case, subjects are randomly assigned to six groups. If there are three independent variables (let us say that we are adding a vision-training program to the 2 × 3 design, then we call it a 2 × 2 × 3 factorial design. Here participants are randomly assigned to 12 groups. Some interesting interactions can be studied in such an instance. Still another factorial design (2 × 2 × 2) is shown in Figure 7.18 on p. 80. Another advantage of factorial designs is that statistical analysis (through analysis of variance) often reduces error, thus tending to prevent type II error. The main problems with factorial design are that many more subjects are needed to fill up all those groups, and there are many more things that can go wrong in a complex factorial design than in a relatively straightforward basic experiment.

Randomized Treatments by Levels Design

A different kind of factorial design involves a randomized independent variable along with another independent variable that reflects two or more types of persons (Figure 7.19 on p. 80). This kind of independent variable is sometimes called an

S

R	O	XY₁	O
R	O	XY₂	O
R	O	X	O
R	O	Y₁	O
R	O	Y₂	O
R	O		O

S = Start
R = Randomization
X = An intervention (one of two conditions of an independent variable-the other condition is control)
Y₁ = An intervention of type Y (one of three conditions of an independent variable- the other conditions are Y₂ and control)
Y₂ = An intervention of type Y (one of three conditions of an independent variable- the other conditions are Y₁ and control)
O = Observation (a dependent variable)

Figure 7.17 Completely randomized 2 × 3 factorial design (pretest–posttest), with true control condition. After randomization (R) and the pretest (O), one group receives a combination of two interventions (X and Y_1); the next group receives a combination of X and Y_2; three groups receive a single intervention (respectively X, Y_1, or Y_2); and one group serves as a true control. The posttest follows.

organismic variable, a nonmanipulated variable, or a variable consisting of preexisting conditions. Basically, this kind of variable cannot be randomly assigned (e.g., you cannot randomly assign some people to the older group and others to the younger group). Sex is a commonly studied organismic variable. Consider a study or men and women wherein the randomized independent variable is a parallel group (in which each person completes a task in the presence of others) versus a project group (in which each person works together on a shared, common project). The dependent variable in this study is a measure of nonverbal socialization (e.g., the frequency that participants make eye contact). The researcher recruits an equal number of men and women. A positive design feature is to ensure that the men and women match up well to each other on potentially confounding variables, such as age and socioeconomic status. Next, the researcher assigns half the men to the parallel condition and half to the project condition, and proceeds to assign half the women to the parallel condition and half to the project condition. This design permits the study of the interaction of sex and parallel/ project group status. For example, it could be found that women interact nonverbally

S

R	C	$X_1Y_1Z_1$	O
R	C	$X_2Y_1Z_1$	O
R	C	$X_1Y_2Z_1$	O
R	C	$X_2Y_2Z_1$	O
R	C	$X_1Y_1Z_2$	O
R	C	$X_2Y_1Z_2$	O
R	C	$X_1Y_2Z_2$	O
R	C	$X_2Y_2Z_2$	O

S = Start
R = Randomization
C = Covariate (a variable associated with the dependent variable)
X_1 = An intervention of type X (one of two conditions of an independent variable- the other condition is X_2)
X_2 = An intervention of type X (one of two conditions of an independent variable- the other condition is X_1)
Y_1 = An intervention of type Y (one of two conditions of an independent variable- the other condition is Y_2)
Y_2 = An intervention of type Y (one of two conditions of an independent variable- the other condition is Y_1)
Z_1 = An intervention of type Z (one of two conditions of an independent variable- the other condition is Z_2)
Z_2 = An intervention of type Z (one of two conditions of an independent variable- the other condition is Z_1)
O = Observation (a dependent variable)

Figure 7.18 Completely randomized $2 \times 2 \times 2$ factorial design (posttest-only with covariate). After randomization (R) and measurement of the covariate (C), the eight groups receive all possible combinations of the three types of interventions, each of which has two conditions. The posttest follows.

more when working in a parallel situation, whereas men interact nonverbally more in a project situation.

The following are other examples of randomized treatments by levels design:

• Studying the effects of an intervention (vs. usual care) in persons with left hemiparesis in comparison to persons with right hemiparesis,
• Comparing the effectiveness of an educational strategy (vs. typical classroom strategy) in first-year versus second-year occupational therapy students, and
• Studying the effects of an intervention (vs. a usual care condition) at multiple sites, where by subjects are randomly assigned within each site.

S

		R	O	X	O
T_1	M	R	O	Y	O
T_2	M	R	O	X	O
		R	O	Y	O

T_1 = One type of person (e.g., persons with a specific health problem, or persons of one gender)
T_2 = A different type of person (e.g., persons with a different health problem/persons with no health problem, or persons of the other gender)
S = Start
M = Matching of the two types of persons on potentially confounding variables
R = Randomization
X = An intervention
Y = A different intervention
O = Observation (a dependent variable)

Figure 7.19 Randomized treatments by levels design (2×2) (pretest–posttest with matching on potentially confounding variables). There are two types of people before the start of the research (T_1 and T_2). The two types of people are matched (M) in relevant ways. The first type of persons are then randomly assigned to one of two interventions, and the second type of persons are also assigned to one of the two interventions.

Randomized Controlled Trials (RCTs)

A randomized controlled trial (sometimes called a clinical trial) is an experiment wherein an important health outcome is the dependent variable, a clinical intervention is part of the independent variable, and research participants are recruited and randomly assigned over time as they become available (Friedman, Furberg, & DeMets, 1998). Many of the examples used already in this chapter reflect hypotheses that could be studied by RCTs (e.g., falls prevention studies, the effects of various occupational therapy interventions on functional outcomes). However, not all the examples discussed in this chapter dealt with outcomes; several dealt with short-term effects of theoretical interest to occupational therapy (e.g., the effects of occupationally embedded exercise on exercise repetitions, or the comparison of parallel versus project groups in terms of nonverbal socialization). These theory-based studies of short-term effects are experiments but not RCTs. These non-RCT experiments add to the theoretical base of occupational therapy and occupational therapy models of practice, but they do not directly test whether occupational therapy produces health outcomes or not.

Randomized controlled trials reflect a tradition of experimentation that developed in medicine and pharmacology. A major problem faced in drug outcome studies that is not so much of a problem in short-term, non-RCT experimentation is the fact that dropouts can threaten the validity of results. Another problem in studying long-term outcomes is that bias can easily be introduced if there are not special procedures for masking randomization codes. For example, if a research assistant is screening a particularly weak patient who nevertheless meets the criteria for inclusion, and if the research assistant knows that the randomization code indicates that the next person accepted into the study is assigned to the research assistant's preferred intervention, the temptation (conscious or unconscious) is for the research assistant to reject the patient from the study. Another feature of RCTs is that outcomes are often categorical (e.g., life or death) rather than measurable; therefore, biostatisticians have paid particular attention to branches of statistics dealing with categorical outcomes (e.g., survival rates).

Authors within the RCT tradition often use different terms from other experimenters (e.g., in psychology, agriculture, or sociology). Instead of saying independent variable, they often say interventions. Instead of saying that participants are randomly assigned to conditions of the independent variable, they often say that subjects are randomly assigned to arms. Instead of saying dependent variable, they often say outcome. In the RCT literature, a distinction has been made between studies of efficacy and studies of effectiveness. Efficacy deals with the study of an intervention under nearly ideal conditions (where random error is highly controlled, where interventionists have special training, and where costs are not considered). On the other hand, studies of effectiveness test whether the intervention works in typical clinical conditions.

A special issue related to dropouts involves a choice between intention-to-treat analysis and per-protocol analysis (Hollis & Campbell, 1999). In intention-to-treat analysis, dropouts are sought out for outcomes testing even if they discontinued the intervention to which they were assigned, and even if they ended up experiencing the opposing intervention (the other condition of the independent variable). Part of the rationale for intention-to-treat analysis is that participants who drop out or choose the opposite intervention might do so because of adverse side effects brought about by the intervention to which they were originally assigned. Advocates of intention-to-treat analysis argue that the clinician and the patient need to know the likelihood that a particular intervention will be effective in advance of a prescription. In contrast, per-protocol analysis excludes dropouts, with the rationale that inclusion of dropouts only causes random error and increases the chances of a type II error. Currently, intention-to-treat analysis tends to be the favored methodology, with the possibility of a secondary test on a per-protocol basis after the primary test.

Much effort has been devoted to the improvement of RCT design and RCT reporting. A result of this effort is the CONSORT (Consolidated Standards of Reporting Trials) Statement. The current version of CONSORT provides a checklist of essential items that should be included in an RCT (Table 7.2), and a diagram for documenting the flow of participants through a trial (Figure 7.20 on p. 83) (Moher, Shulz, & Altman, 2001).

Table 7.2 **CONSORT Criteria for Randomized Control Trials**

Paper section topic	Item	Description
Title and abstract	1	How participants were allocated to interventions (e.g., "random allocation," "randomized," or "randomly assigned").
Introduction	2	Scientific background and explanation of rationale.
Method		
Participants	3	Eligibility criteria for participants and the settings and locations where the data were collected.
Interventions	4	Precise details of the interventions intended for each group and how and when they were actually administered.
Objectives	5	Specific objectives and hypotheses.
Outcomes	6	Clearly defined primary and secondary outcome measures and, when applicable, any methods used to enhance the quality of measurements (e.g., multiple observations, training of assessors).

(continued)

Table 7.2 **CONSORT Criteria for Randomized Control Trials** (continued)

Paper section topic	Item	Description
Sample size	7	How sample size was determined and, when applicable, explanation of any interim analyses and stopping rules.
Randomization: Sequence generation	8	Method used to generate the random allocation sequence, including details of any restriction (e.g., blocking, stratification).
Randomization: Allocation concealment	9	Method used to implement the random allocation sequence (e.g., numbered containers or central telephone), clarifying whether the sequence was concealed until interventions were assigned.
Randomization: Implementation	10	Who generated the allocation sequence, who enrolled participants, and who assigned participants to their groups.
Blinding (masking)	11	Whether or not participants, those administering the interventions, and those assessing the outcomes were blinded to group assignment. When relevant, how the success of blinding was evaluated.
Statistical methods	12	Statistical methods used to compare groups for primary outcome(s); Methods for additional analyses, such as subgroup analyses and adjusted analyses.
Results		
Participant flow	13	Flow of participants through each stage (a diagram is strongly recommended). Specifically, for each group report the numbers of participants randomly assigned, receiving intended treatment, completing the study protocol, and analyzed for the primary outcome. Describe protocol deviations from study as planned, together with reasons.
Recruitment	14	Dates defining the periods of recruitment and follow-up.
Baseline data	15	Baseline demographic and clinical characteristics of each group.
Numbers analyzed	16	Number of participants (denominator) in each group included in each analysis and whether the analysis was by "intention-to-treat." State the results in absolute numbers when feasible (e.g., 10/20, not 50%).
Outcomes and estimation	17	For each primary and secondary outcome, a summary of results for each group, and the estimated effect size and its precision (e.g., 95% confidence interval).
Ancillary analyses	18	Address multiplicity by reporting any other analyses performed, including subgroup analyses and adjusted analyses, indicating those prespecified and those exploratory.
Adverse events	19	All important adverse events or side effects in each intervention group.
Discussion		
Interpretation	20	Interpretation of the results, taking into account study hypotheses, sources of potential bias or imprecision, and the dangers associated with multiplicity of analyses and outcomes.
Generalizability	21	Generalizability (external validity) of the trial findings.
Overall evidence	22	General interpretation of the results in the context of current evidence.

Cluster Randomized Controlled Trials

A cluster randomized controlled trial (Figure 7.21 on p. 84) is a special kind of RCT, in which clinical sites are randomly assigned to arms (conditions of the independent variable), as opposed to randomly assigning individual participants (Friedman, Furberg, & DeMets, 1998). For example, in a study of the effects of intensive, repeated home evalua-tions on acute rehabilitation patients with hip fracture (vs. usual care), 20 rehabilitation hospitals can be involved. Ten are randomly assigned to the special home evaluation condition, with the other 10 assigned to usual care. Perhaps each hospital can supply 15 patients, and all patients at a given site are treated the same because they are in the same experimental condition. Sometimes this is called a *nested design* (participants are "nested" together

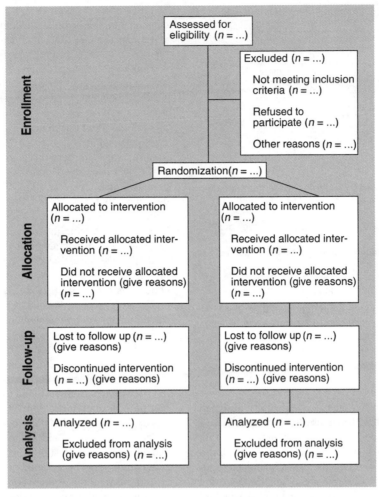

Figure 7.20 CONSORT flow diagram for reporting randomized controlled trials.

within each site). One advantage of this design is the prevention of bleeding from one condition to the other (e.g., when patients see their roommates getting special treatment). Another advantage is that differing skill levels and possible biases of those administering the interventions can be assumed to be more balanced across conditions than is the case when interventionists observe each other in close quarters. The main disadvantages are complexity, expanded training, fidelity issues, and ethical compliance within the rules and cultures of many different organizations (Spilker, 1991). Another disadvantage is a loss of power in the statistical analysis, caused by within-site similarity. It is important to distinguish this design from the multisite design discussed above in the section on randomized treatments by levels design, in which participants at each site are randomized (as opposed to being nested, as in this design).

Crossover Design (Also Called Counterbalanced Design)

A crossover design starts off like a basic experiment, in which participants are randomly assigned to as many groups as there are conditions of the independent variable. But each group then goes on to experience both conditions of the independent variable (Chow & Lui, 1998). In the case of two conditions of the independent variable, one randomly assigned group receives condition X first, is measured on the dependent variable, then receives condition Y, and then is measured again. The other randomly assigned group receives condition Y first, then X. If Y consistently leads to different effects of the dependent variable, regardless of order, it is concluded that the independent variable is probably responsible for the difference.

S

	Rs	O	X	O
	Rs	O	X	O
	Rs	O	X	O
Eight Sites	Rs	O	X	O
	Rs	O	Y	O
	Rs	O	Y	O
	Rs	O	Y	O
	Rs	O	Y	O

S = Start

Rs = Randomization by site (each site and all persons at that site have an equal chance of being assigned to X or Y

X = An intervention administered to each subject at the site

Y = A different intervention administered to each subject at the site

O = Observation of each person (measurement or categorization used for dependent variable)

Figure 7.21 Randomized cluster design, comparing two interventions at eight research sites. Four research sites are randomly assigned (R_s) to one condition (X) , and the other four sites are assigned to the other condition (Y).

Consider the hypothesis: A specially designed wheelchair seat will increase work productivity in adults with cerebral palsy and mental retardation (in comparison to an off-the-shelf, standard sling-seat wheelchair). Half the participants are randomly assigned to experiencing the special seating system first, and then experiencing the standard seating system. The other half are randomly assigned to the standard system first, and then to the special system. If productivity is greater for both groups when seated in the special system, the directional hypothesis is supported.

This design controls against type I error through counterbalancing the conditions of the independent variable. A faulty design not controlling for type I error is the administration of one condition of the independent variable to all participants first, and then the administration of the other condition second. The difference on the dependent variable might be due to many factors other than the independent variable. For example, participants might have scored high on the second condition because they were warmed up on the first, or because they learned what they have to do to score well on the dependent variable. On the other hand, participants might have scored low on the second condition because of fatigue or boredom. These are potentially biasing confounding variables. In contrast to this faulty design, the counterbalancing

of order in a crossover design addresses all these causes of type I error. If participants score higher when experiencing one intervention than another, regardless of order of presentation, factors such as warming up, learning, fatigue, and boredom probably cannot account for the results.

The advantage of crossover design is the reduction of the chances of a type II error. Dispersion due to individual differences is controlled because each participant is compared to oneself. In addition, two measurements per person increase statistical power in comparison to designs in which each person is measured once. The disadvantage of this design is that a sequence effect or a carryover effect can prevent a clear interpretation that one intervention is superior, regardless of order. For example, the researcher must be hesitant to conclude that the special seating system is superior if productivity was approximately equal between conditions for the group that experienced the special seating system second. Crossover design is therefore not recommended for studies of interventions that are hypothesized to lead to enduring changes within the person. Crossover designs are also not recommended for studies in which the dependent variable involves certain kinds of learning (in which participants tend to do better the second time through a problem). On the other hand, this design is particularly appropriate for studies of assistive technology and compensatory methods, and for the study of stimuli that have short-term effects (e.g., effects on mood or arousal).

If there are three or more conditions to the independent variable, counterbalanced design offers two options: the Latin Square (Figure 7.22) or random assignment to all possible sequences (Figure 7.23). Consider the hypothesis of comparing occupationally embedded exercise (coded O), imagery-based exercise (coded I), and rote exercise (coded R). One third of the sample is randomly assigned

S

	R	X	O	Y	O	Z	O
	R	Y	O	Z	O	X	O
	R	Z	O	X	O	Y	O

S = Start

R = Randomization

X = An intervention

Y = A different intervention

Z = Another different intervention

O = Observation (primary dependent variable)

Figure 7.22 Randomized counterbalanced design (Latin Square), with an independent variable consisting of three conditions (X, Y, Z).

S							
	R	X	O	Y	O	Z	O
	R	Y	O	Z	O	X	O
	R	Z	O	X	O	Y	O
	R	X	O	Z	O	Y	O
	R	Y	O	X	O	Z	O
	R	Z	O	Y	O	X	O

S = Start
R = Randomization
X = An intervention
Y = A different intervention
Z = Another different intervention
O = Observation (primary dependent variable)

Figure 7.23 Randomized counterbalanced design (fully randomized), with an independent variable consisting of three conditions (*X, Y, Z*).

S			
	O	X	O
	O		O

S = Start
X = Intervention
O = Observation (measurement or categorization used for dependent variable)

Figure 7.24 Nonrandomized comparison group design (pretest–posttest, with true control group). After a pretest and before the posttest (*O*), the subjects in one naturally occurring group receive an intervention (*X*), and the subjects in a different naturally occurring group receive nothing. It is important to note that this design is not recommended except for pilot testing in advance of future research.

to an *O–I–R* sequence; another one third is assigned to *I–R–O*, and the rest of the sample is assigned to *R-O-I*. This is a Latin Square. Note that each of the interventions occurs first once, second once, and third once. The Latin square uses three of the six possible sequences; other possible sequences are *I–O–R*, *O–R–I*, and *R–I–O*. The alternative counterbalancing strategy is to randomly assign the sample into six groups, each of which experiences one of the six possible sequences.

Group Designs Not Involving Randomization

Nonrandomized Comparison Group Design

The nonrandomized comparison group design (Figure 7.24) is also called a nonrandomized trial when the dependent variable is a valued health outcome. When type I error was discussed earlier, nonrandomized comparison group designs were described as similar to experiments, but using convenient preexisting groupings as the method of assigning participants to conditions of the independent variable, as opposed to randomization. For example, classrooms of children make up convenient preexisting groups, so that all the children in two classrooms can be assigned to one condition and all the children in two different classrooms can be assigned to the other condition. The problem is that the children in two sets of classrooms might be systematically different from each other (e.g., due to class placement procedures, such as grouping the academically talented children in one class-

room). Confounding variables might account for any difference found on the dependent variable. Hence this design is often called the nonequivalent group design.

A variation on this kind of design is the waiting list control group design, in which those at the top of a waiting list for an intervention are assigned to an intervention and those at the bottom of the list serve as the control group. After the completion of the study, those at the bottom of the list receive the intervention, so this design is favored for humanitarian reasons. Another advantage of this design is that it permits the study of expensive interventions (e.g., home modifications) without the researcher having to fund the intervention because all the persons on the waiting list will ultimately receive the intervention. However, as with other nonrandomized designs, it is possible that the people at the bottom of the list are systematically different from those at the top (e.g., those at the top might be more knowledgeable on how to work the system, more resourceful, and/or more assertive).

An important design strategy when conducting nonrandomized designs is to match the groups at the outset on potentially confounding variables as illustrated in Figure 7.25 on p. 86. Consider the hypothesis that an occupational therapy handwriting program increases legibility in first-grade children identified as educationally at-risk because of poverty. The school principal and teachers welcome the research and offer four classrooms of children, but only if classes are not disrupted by randomization. The researcher gathers data on exact age and standardized educational scores. Then the researcher makes sure that the children in the two classrooms to receive the intervention are matched to the children in the other two class-

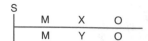

S = Start
M = Matching on the dependent variable or some
    variable associated with the dependent variable
X = Intervention
Y = A different intervention
O = Observation (measurement or categorization used
    for dependent variable)

Figure 7.25 Nonrandomized comparison group design, with matching. The subjects in one naturally occurring group are matched to the subjects in another group, either on the dependent variable (O) or on a variable associated with the dependent variable. Each group then receives X or Y. Although the matching procedure improves the design somewhat over other nonrandomized designs, it is always possible that some relevant variable has not been matched. It is important to note that this design is not recommended except for pilot testing in advance of future research.

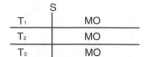

T_1 = One type of person (e.g., persons with a specific
    health problem)
T_2 = A different type of person (e.g., persons with a
    different health problem)
T_3 = Another different type of person (e.g., persons
    with a different health problem, or persons with no
    health problem)
S = Start
M = Matching of the two types of persons on
    potentially confounding variables
O = Observation (a dependent variable)

Figure 7.26 Cross-sectional design (three conditions), with matching. The nonmanipulated independent variable (three types of persons to be compared) preexists the research. The three types of persons are matched (M) on potentially confounding variables, and immediately observed (O) for possible differences.

rooms. Means and dispersions of age and standardized educational scores as well as proportions of sex are approximately equal between children receiving the intervention and those not receiving it. This process of matching necessarily involves the exclusion of some children at the extremes of the ranges who are preventing an overall match. Ideally, the matching and exclusion are done by someone masked to the hypothesis and to knowledge of which group will receive which condition of the independent variable (dealing only with numbers). Despite all this, it is still possible that the two groups are systematically different from each other in some way that the researcher did not or could not measure. For example, one of the classroom teachers might emphasize penmanship in ways that the other classroom teachers do not.

An alternative strategy to matching is the use of special statistical procedures designed to correct for initial differences between groups. Here, potentially confounding variables must be identified, measured, and entered into statistical calculations. These procedures are controversial (Huitema, 1980). On the one hand, it can be argued that appropriate statistical control permits a researcher to make an end-of-study claim that an independent variable probably affected the dependent variable. However, others place little confidence in the results of nonrandomized comparison designs and claim that the write-ups of these designs should not infer probable causality. Perhaps the best use of this design is in the collec-

tion of pilot data to justify a much more expensive randomized controlled trial.

Cross-Sectional Design (Immediate Ex Post Facto Comparisons)

The purpose of this design (Figure 7.26) is to compare different types of persons in terms of some immediately measurable dependent variable. For example, the researcher might want to compare children with cerebral palsy to children without a known disorder in terms of spatial perception. The researcher wants to know if children with cerebral palsy have a special problem with spatial perception. Another example is the cross-sectional developmental study, where children of different age groups (let us say 36-month-olds, 42-month-olds, and 48-month-olds) are compared in terms of attention to task. A third example is to compare persons with left hemiplegia to persons with right hemiplegia in terms of standing balance.

In this design, the researcher does not manipulate the assignment of subjects to groups, as in experiments. This kind of independent variable is sometimes called an organismic variable or a variable consisting of preexisting conditions. Because the independent variable took place in the past before the researcher came along, the Latin phrase ex post facto is also used to describe this design.

Cross-sectional designs are needed to answer questions concerning the special characteristics of disability groups. The problem, of course, is that a difference on the dependent variable might well be due to some confounding variable (a type I error). For example, a difference in spatial perception between children with cerebral palsy and non-disabled children might be due to factors that have nothing to do with cerebral palsy (e.g., parental skill, access to older siblings, etc.). As with other nonrandomized designs, cross-sectional designs require careful matching on potentially confounding variables (i.e., matching means, dispersions, and proportions). Usually a sample from the relatively rare population (e.g., the disability group) is selected in some representative way, and then members of the comparison group (e.g., matched nondisabled controls) are assembled. Once again, masking the matcher is a positive strategy. The other strategy employed with this and all other nonrandomized designs is to use statistical methods to make adjustments on the dependent variable when comparison groups differ in relevant ways. It is important to remind ourselves that this strategy has vigorous adherents as well as vigorous critics.

In the field of human development, aspects of cross-sectional designs are frequently combined with longitudinal approaches (in which the same sample is repeatedly measured at planned intervals over time) (Rosenthal & Rosnow, 1991). The general idea is that the researcher can have a relatively high degree of confidence if the cross-sectional and the longitudinal approaches confirm each other. The longitudinal approach eliminates the possible bias likely in comparing different populations, and the cross-sectional approach eliminates the possible bias of repeated testing. The same logic could be applied to studies of the progression of specific disabilities.

Case-Control Design (Case-Referent Design or Case Comparison Design)

This design (Figure 7.27) was developed in the field of epidemiology. The purpose of the design to find out if some specific variable from the past discriminates between people who today have a disease (or disability) and people who do not. The classic example is to investigate past levels of smoking habits of persons with lung cancer and matched controls who do not have lung cancer. An example that is more relevant to occupational therapy is to compare newly admitted patients with hip fracture to matched controls in terms of past injurious falls requiring medical care. Because the data collected refers to past events, case-control designs are termed retrospective studies.

The advantage of this design is the relative ease with which possible causal or risk factors can be explored, without waiting for years to see how

		S		
E or no E	T_1		M	O_E
E or no E	T_2		M	O_E

E = An event hypothesized to be a risk factor
T_1 = A type of person with a specific health problem
T_2 = A type of person without the health problem
S = Start
M = Matching of the two types of persons on potentially confounding variables
O_E = Observation (dependent variable) of the hypothesized risk factor through retrospective documentation

Figure 7.27 Case-control design investigating a single risk factor in a single health condition (in comparison to a matched group of persons without the health condition). A group with a health problem (T_1) is identified and matched (M) to a group without the health problem (T_2). The researcher documents (O_E) whether or not each group experienced a specific risk factor event (E) prior to the development of the health problem in T_1.

events unfold. As with many other kinds of nonrandomized designs, research questions can be studied in humans that are unethical or impossible to study through random assignment. However, in addition to the possibility that the comparison groups might be different from each other in other ways beside the dependent variable, retrospective studies frequently depend on unreliable data. For example, one common way to collect data concerning past events is to interview the participant. As a general rule, self-reports become less accurate as distance in time increases. In addition, the interviewer may be biased, consciously or unconsciously, in the way that questions are asked to the participant. Another type of measurement error occurs when using archival information (e.g., medical records). In prospective studies (involving measurement of future events), a plan can be formulated to collect data that includes special training for raters and tests of inter-rater independent agreement. This is impossible in retrospective studies. Another common problem with case-control studies involves multiplicity, in which the researcher investigates a host of past events, some of which might discriminate between currently assembled groups by pure chance. Special statistical procedures are needed to deal with specificity as well as the possibility of complex interactions.

Multigroup Cohort Design (Cohort Analytic Study)

In this design (Figure 7.28 on p. 88), the researcher matches a sample that has a hypothesized risk fac-

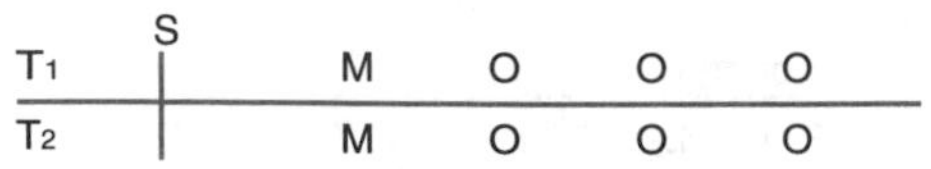

```
          S
T₁        |        M    O    O    O
                                        ——————
T₂        |        M    O    O    O
```

T₁ = Persons with a specific risk factor
T₂ = Perspns without the risk factor
S = Start
M = Matching of the two types of persons on poten-
    tially confounding variables
O = Observation (a dependent variable)

Figure 7.28 Multigroup cohort design (two conditions), with matching and longitudinal follow-ups.
Persons with (T_1) and without (T_2) a possible
risk factor are matched on potentially confounding variables. Repeated observations (O) over
time indicate whether or not the hypothesized
risk factor leads to the health problem.

tor to a sample that does not. Then the researcher
picks a future point in time (or a series of points if
using repeated measures) to see if the hypothesized risk factor truly predicts the disease or disability. A classic example in epidemiology is to see
if high levels of cholesterol in middle age predict
heart disease in old age. An example more relevant
to occupational therapy is to investigate if mild left
hemiplegia predicts automobile accidents in comparison to matched cohorts of (a) persons with
mild right hemiplegia and (b) healthy controls.

This design is similar to nonrandomized comparison group design. Indeed, some authors use the
term cohort design for what we earlier defined as
nonrandomized comparison group design. A difference between designs is that multigroup cohort
design deals with the study of risk factors not
under the researcher's control and resulting in poor
outcomes, whereas nonrandomized comparison
group design deals with interventions under the
control of the researcher and hypothesized to have
positive outcomes. Given this logic, a study of
whether brain injury predicts psychiatric disorders
(at higher rates than controls) is a multigroup
cohort design, whereas a study of a special intervention designed to prevent psychiatric disorders
in persons with brain injury is a nonrandomized
comparison group design if participants are
assigned to conditions in some way other than randomization.

Prospective multigroup cohort studies generally have stronger claims to validity than retrospective studies because measurements can be
planned and possible confounding variables can be
monitored. Multigroup cohort studies are stronger
than single cohort studies because the presence of
a matched control group makes it possible to estimate not only the rate of the outcome but also the
differential rate in comparison to a control group.
This controls for the possibility that the outcome
will develop whether or not the risk factor is present. Another weak alternative to the multigroup
cohort study is the use of previously collected
demographic data on the healthy population as a
control condition, as opposed to using matched
controls. Problems with previously collected
demographic data are: (a) the data were collected
under different circumstances by different data
collectors and (b) the life experiences of a prospective cohort are different from archival information
collected at a different point in time.

Conclusion

In summary, choice of a research design depends
on five factors: prevention of type I error; prevention of type II error; external validity; the resources
available to the researcher; and the theoretical or
clinical importance of the research question. If the
researcher wishes to study the effects of a powerful independent variable (i.e., one that produces a
large effect in the dependent variable) and if generous resources are available, the basic posttest-
only experimental design (perhaps configured as a
randomized controlled trial) provides the strongest
evidence. However, the researcher is often
unaware of how powerful the independent variable
is until years of study have passed. Therefore, the
desire for protection against type II error (which is
almost always more likely in the best of designs
than type I error) enhances the attractiveness of
alternative randomized research designs. Each of
these has its advantages and disadvantages,
depending on the research question and resources
available. Though questionable in terms of type I
error, nonrandomized designs are important as
cost-efficient pilot studies. Nonrandomized
designs can also address research questions of special importance to the field of occupational therapy
and to the understanding of persons with disability.

> The introduction to group comparison designs in
> this chapter encourages occupational therapy stu-
> dents and practitioners to learn more about spe-
> cific designs for specific research questions. The
> author's intent will be served if this chapter
> results in some eager young colleague doing
> experimental research that advances occupa-
> tional therapy knowledge and helps the profes-
> sion to better serve our clients and students.

No single design is best for all circumstances. Hopefully this chapter provides an introduction to the advantages and disadvantages of the main group comparison designs.

REFERENCES

Amberson, J. B., McMahon, B. T., & Pinner, M. (1931). A clinical trial of sanocrysin in pulmonary tuberculosis. *American Review of Tuberculosis, 24*, 401–435.

Campbell, D. T., & Stanley, J. C. (1963). *Experimental and quasi-experimental designs for research.* Chicago: Rand McNally.

Chow, S. C., & Lui, J. (1998). *Design and analysis of clinical trials.* New York: John Wiley & Sons.

Fisher, R. A. (1935). *The design of experiments. London: Oliver and Boyd.*

Fleiss, J. L. (1986). *The design and analysis of clinical experiments.* New York: John Wiley & Sons.

Friedman, L. M., Furberg, C. D., & DeMets, D. L. (1998). *Fundamentals of clinical trials* (3rd ed.). New York: Springer-Verlag.

Gitlin, L. N., Corcoran, M., Martindale-Adams, J., Malone, C., Stevens, A., & Winter, L. (2000). Identifying mechanisms of action: Why and how does intervention work? In R. Schulz (Ed.), *Handbook on dementia caregiving: Evidence-based interventions for family caregivers.* New York: Springer.

Hollis, S., & Campbell, F. (1999). What is meant by intention to treat analysis? Survey of published randomised controlled trials. *British Medical Journal, 319*, 670–674.

Holm, M. B. (2000). Our mandate for the new millennium: Evidence-based practice, 2000 Eleanor Clark Slagle Lecture. *American Journal of Occupational Therapy, 54*, 575–585.

Huitema, B. E. (1980). *The analysis of covariance and alternatives.* New York: John Wiley & Sons.

Kerlinger, F. N. (1986). *Foundations of behavioral research* (3rd ed.). New York: Harcourt Brace.

Lichstein, K. L., Riedel, B. W., & Grieve, R. (1994). Fair tests of clinical trials: A treatment implementation model. *Advances in Behaviour Research and Therapy, 16*, 1–29.

Moher, D., Schulz, K. F., & Altman, D. G. (2001). The CONSORT statement: Revised recommendations for improving the quality of reports of parallel-group randomized trials. *Annals of Internal Medicine, 134*, 657–662.

Moncher, F. J., & Prinz, R. J. (1991). Treatment fidelity in outcome studies. *Clinical Psychology Review, 11*, 247–266.

Nelson, D. L., & Mathiowetz, V. (2004). Randomized controlled trials to investigate occupational therapy research questions. *American Journal of Occupational Therapy, 58*, 24–34.

Ottenbacher, K. J. (1995). Why rehabilitation research does not work (as well as we think it should). *Archives of Physical Medicine and Rehabilitation, 76*, 123–129.

Ottenbacher, K. J., & Maas, F. (1998). How to detect effects: Statistical power and evidence-based practice in occupational therapy research. *American Journal of Occupational Therapy, 53*(2), 181–188.

Rosenthal, R., & Rosnow, R. L. (1991). *Essentials of behavioral research: Methods and data analysis* (2nd ed.). New York: McGraw-Hill.

Spilker, B. (1991). *Guide to clinical trials.* Philadelphia: Lippincott Williams & Wilkins.

Stevens, J. (1986). *Applied multivariate statistics for the social sciences.* Hillsdale, NJ: Lawrence Erlbaum.

Thorndike, E. L., & Woodworth, R. S. (1901). The influence of improvement in one mental function upon the efficiency of other functions. *Psychological Review, 8*, 247–261, 384–395, 553–564.

RESOURCES

http://consort-statement.org/

OTseeker.com

Altman, D. G., Schulz, K. F., Moher, D., Egger, M., Davidoff, F., Elbourne, D., et al. (2001). *The revised CONSORT statement for reporting randomized trials: Explanation and elaboration.* Retrieved September 7, 2002, from http:/consort-statement.org/newene.html

Begg, C., Cho, M., Eastwood, S., Horton, R., Moher, D., Olkin, I., et al. (1996). Improving the quality of reporting of randomized controlled trials: The CONSORT statement. *Journal of the American Medical Association, 276*, 637–639.

Berk, P. D., & Sacks, H. S. (1999). Assessing the quality of randomized control trials: Quality of design is not the only relevant variable. *Hepatology, 30*, 1332–1334.

Bork, C. E. (1993). *Research in physical therapy.* Philadelphia: Lippincott.

Cadman, D., Law, M., DeMatteo, C., Walter, S., Rosenbaum, P., & Russell, D. (1989). Evaluation of treatment in occupational therapy: Part 2. Practical issues in conducting clinical trials. *Canadian Journal of Occupational Therapy, 56*, 243–247.

Cohen, J. (1988). *Statistical power analysis for the behavioral sciences* (2nd ed.). Hillsdale, NJ: Lawrence Erlbaum.

Cooper, H., & Hedges, L. V. (Eds.). (1994). *The handbook of research synthesis.* New York: Russell Sage Foundation.

Dhingra, V., Chittock, D. R., & Ronco, J. J. (2002). Assessing methodological quality of clinical trials in sepsis: Searching for the right tool. *Critical Care Medicine, 30*, 487–488.

Donner, A., & Klar, N. (2000). *Design and analysis of cluster randomization trials in health research.* London: Arnold.

Egger, M., Juni, P., & Bartlett, C. (2001). Value of flow diagrams in reports of randomized controlled trials. *Journal of the American Medical Association, 285*, 1996–1999.

Everitt, B. S., & Pickles, A. (1999). *Statistical aspects of the design and analysis of clinical trials.* Singapore: Regal Press.

Hennekens, C. H. (1999). *Clinical trials in cardiovascular disease: A companion to Braunwald's heart disease.* Philadelphia: W. B. Saunders.

Hinkle, D. E., Wiersma, W., & Jurs, S. G. (1998). *Applied statistics for the behavioral sciences* (4th ed.). Boston: Houghton Mifflin.

Huwiler-Muntener, K., Juni, P., Junker, C., & Egger, M. (2002). Quality of reporting of randomized trials as a measure of methodological quality. *Journal of the American Medical Association, 287*, 2801–2804.

Kazdin, A. E. (2003). *Research design in clinical psychology* (3rd ed.). Boston: Allyn & Bacon.

Law, M., Cadman, D., Rosenbaum, P., Russell, D., DeMatteo, C., & Walter, S. (1989). Evaluation of treatment in occupational therapy. Part 1. Methodology issues in conducting clinical trials. *Canadian Journal of Occupational Therapy, 56*, 236–242.

McFadden, E. (1998). *Management of data in clinical trials*. New York: John Wiley & Sons.

Moher, D., Jones, A. J., & Lepage, L. (2001). Use of CONSORT statement and quality of reports of randomized trials: A comparative before-and after evaluation. *Journal of the American Medical Association, 285*, 1992–1995.

Montori, V. M., & Guyatt, G. (2001). Intention-to-treat principle. *Canadian Medical Association Journal, 165*, 1339–1341.

Neter, J., Wasserman, W., & Kutner, M. H. (1985). *Applied linear statistical models* (2nd ed.). Homewood, IL: Richard D. Irwin.

Olkin, I. (1995). Meta-analysis: Reconciling the results of independent studies. *Statistics in Medicine, 14*, 457–472.

Ottenbacher, K. J. (1998). A quantitative evaluation of multiplicity in epidemiology and public health research. *American Journal of Epidemiology, 147*, 615–619.

Portney, L. G., & Watkins, M. P. (2000). *Foundations of clinical research: Applications to practice* (2nd ed.). Upper Saddle Rive, NJ: Prentice-Hall Health.

Prien, R. F., & Robinson, D. S. (Eds.). (1994). *Clinical evaluation of psychotropic drugs: Principles and guidelines*. New York: Raven Press.

Reisch, J. S., Tyson, J. E., & Mize, S. G. (1989). Aid to the evaluation of therapeutic studies. *Pediatrics, 84*, 815–827.

Rennie, D. (2001). CONSORT revised: Improving the reporting of randomized trials. *Journal of the American Medical Association, 285*, 2006–2007.

Schulz, K. F., Chambers, I., Hayes, R. J., & Altman, D. G. (1995). Empirical evidence of bias. Dimensions of methodological quality associated with estimates of treatment effects in controlled trials. *Journal of the American Medical Association, 273*, 408–412.

Schwartz, D., Flamant, R., & Lellouch, J. (1980). *Clinical Trials*. London: Academic Press.

Yeaton, W. H., & Sechrest, L. (1981). Critical dimensions in the choice and maintenance of successful treatments: Strength, integrity, and effectiveness. *Journal of Consulting and Clinical Psychology, 49*, 156–167.

CHAPTER 8

Survey Research Design

Kirsty Forsyth • Frederick J. Kviz

Survey research is a method of inquiry characterized by collecting data using structured questions to elicit self-reported information from a sample of people (Aday, 1996; DePoy & Gitlin, 1998). Surveys are characterized by these key dimensions:

- Identifying the population of interest and appropriately sampling that population,
- Identifying the research aims and question and generating survey questions to systematically gather the necessary information, and
- Developing statistical estimates that can be generalized to the population under study.

The main advantages of survey research are that investigators can:

- Reach a large number of respondents[1] with relatively minimal expenditure,
- Collect data on numerous variables, and
- Perform statistical manipulation during data analysis that permits multiple uses of the data set (Rea & Parker, 1997).

There are two main factors that can influence the rigor of survey research (Fowler, 2002). The first is potential nonresponse bias (i.e., respondents selected for the sample who elect not to respond). These second is potential response bias, which may result from factors such as:

> Survey research is a method of inquiry characterized by collecting data using structured questions to elicit self-reported information from a sample of people.

- Respondents being unable to recall information accurately,
- Respondents interpreting the meaning of a question differently than the meaning intended by the researcher, or
- Response choices that do not accurately express respondents' experiences or opinions.

When designing survey research, investigators must take care to reduce these two forms of bias as much as possible, as discussed throughout the chapter.[2]

Surveys collect data using self-administered questionnaires, telephone interviews, or face-to-face interviews. Self-administered questionnaires may be mailed, administered online, or distributed and collected at convenient points of contact such as in schools, workplaces, clinics, or hospitals. This chapter focuses on:

- How to choose the specific survey data gathering method,
- How to build the questionnaire/interview,
- How to administer the survey (including sampling), and
- Preparation for data analysis.

Choosing Data Gathering Methods

As noted in the preceding section, survey research uses questionnaires, (administered directly, by mail, and online), and interviews (telephone and face-to-face) to collect data. Quantitative survey interviews are quite distinct from interviews used in qualitative studies. In a survey, the interview questions are fixed, and the interviewer seeks to administer the interview in an objective manner following the interview protocol.

---

[1]The term "respondent" refers to people responding to the survey.

[2]Another important consideration in survey research is governmental regulations affecting the privacy of patients. This varies, of course, by country. In the United States the Health Insurance Portability and Accountability Act (HIPAA) privacy rule has requirements which must be followed in medical research. Medical research that falls under HIPAA regulations conform to these rules. While these rules govern all forms of research involving patients, they can have particular implications for survey research. A useful source of information on how HIPAA regulations affect research is the National Institutes of Health Web site.

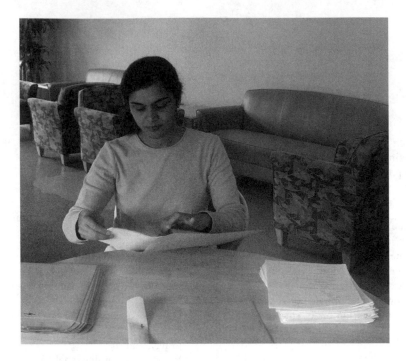

Figure 8.1 A research assistant stuffs envelopes in preparation for a mailed survey.

When choosing a survey data gathering method, the advantages and disadvantages of each method need to be considered. These are discussed below and illustrated in Table 8.1.

Mailed Questionnaires

Traditionally, the most common method of collecting survey data has involved the dissemination of printed questionnaires through the mail to a sample of respondents. Respondents are asked to complete the questionnaire on their own and return it to the researchers. One advantage of the mailed questionnaire is its relatively low cost (Abramson & Abramson, 1999). Another advantage over interviews is that the questionnaire can be completed at the respondent's convenience with no time constraint. Finally, since there is no personal contact with an interviewer, respondent anonymity may be better preserved and potential interviewer bias is not a factor (Rea & Parker, 1997).

A potential disadvantage of all questionnaires is that they require literacy skills. When studying certain disadvantaged or intellectually impaired populations, researchers may have to deal with a lack of or limited literacy. Moreover, the lack of interaction with the respondent means that any parts of the questionnaire that are misunderstood for any reason cannot be clarified by the data collector.

A specific disadvantage of mailed questionnaires is that the response rate tends to be lower than that for interview methods. Moreover, many follow-ups may be required to obtain an acceptable response rate. In addition, mailing and return of questionnaires, along with any necessary follow-ups to secure sufficient respondents, can be time consuming (Abramson & Abramson, 1999). Mail surveys usually take 3 to 4 months for respondents to complete and return the questionnaires in response to the three mailings (initial plus two follow-ups) that are typically required. Later in the chapter, strategies for follow-up are discussed in more detail.

Directly Administered Questionnaires

Directly administered questionnaires have the same advantages as mailed questionnaires, with the exception that the investigator may ask for the questionnaire to be completed within a given time frame. Direct administration of questionnaires has the additional advantage that it does not take the long period of time required for mailed surveys. Finally, it is the least costly survey method.

The major disadvantage of direct administration is sampling. Since direct administration requires a clustering of respondents in a specific physical setting, the usual strategies for obtaining

Table 8.1 Advantages and Disadvantages of Different Methods of Data Collection in Survey Research

	Questionnaires	Interviews
Advantages	• Relatively low cost • Respondent anonymity may be better preserved • Interviewer bias is not a factor	• Greater flexibility to probe for more detail, and administer more complex questionnaires • Ensure the integrity of the questionnaire
Disadvantages	• Response rate tends to be lower • Any confusion about the questions cannot be clarified • Requires literacy skills	• Expensive (personnel and training costs)

	Mail	Direct	Online	Telephone	Face-to-face
Advantages	• Can be completed at the respondent's convenience • No time constraint	• Take less time • No mailing cost	• Fast • Web-based • Administration can incorporate features that paper questionnaires cannot • Data can be directly imported for analysis	• Potentially short data collection period • Usually cost less • Afford more perceived anonymity • Easier to sample a large geographical area	• Ideal for contacting hard-to-reach populations • Reduces/eliminates missing data
Disadvantages	• Can be time consuming • Many follow-ups may be required	• Limits sampling strategies • Less flexibility in time frame	• Only people with computers or computer skill can be contacted • Raises concerns over privacy and anonymity	• Less interviewer control • Limited ability to support questionnaires with visual aids • Only people with telephones can be contacted • Opportunity to establish credibility is more limited	• Cost of travel • Longer data collection period • Interviewer can be a source of bias • Concerns about personal safety of the interviewers and lack of respondent anonymity

a representative sample are not possible. Thus, directly administered questionnaires are most useful when the setting where the data are collected is the focus of the study and/or the persons in that setting are the population of interest. However, this is often not the case. Consequently, surveys done through direct administration are limited in their generalizability. Direct administration of questionnaires is most often used to pilot (and thus refine) the questionnaire, or to collect pilot data for a larger study that will use appropriate sampling strategies.

Online Questionnaires

While online methods of administering questionnaires are relatively new, they are increasingly used. There are two main methods of online administration (Bowers, 1999; Bradley, 1999; Ramos, Sedivi, & Sweet 1998; Sheehan & Hoy, 1999). The first is an e-mail survey. In this method, the questionnaire is contained in the body of the e-mail or in a document that is sent with the e-mail as an attachment. The respondent is requested to complete the survey and return it (as an e-mail or an attached completed document depending on how the survey was sent). The second method of online administration is posted on the World Wide Web. Respondents are sent a request to complete the survey by e-mail with a link to the URL for the survey.

The advantages of both means of online administration are that they are fast. The Web-based administration has the potential to incorporate features not available on a printed questionnaire such as pull-down menus and check-boxes. An additional benefit of the Web-based survey is that data can typically be exported directly to a statistical analysis package, bypassing the need to do manual data entry.

The main disadvantage of this method of questionnaire administration is that it requires minimally access and knowledge of computer use on the part of the respondent. In the case of Web-based administration, somewhat more skill on the part of the respondent and substantial technological skill on the part of the researcher is required. For these reasons, there can be particular problems of sampling or nonresponse bias. There can also be substantial concerns about privacy and anonymity of the respondent.

Telephone Interviews

Some surveys collect data through interviews conducted via telephone by trained interviewers. All interviews have the advantage of greater flexibility as interviewers can probe for more detail and administer more complex questionnaires. Interviewers can also maintain the integrity of the ordering of the questions (whereas someone completing a questionnaire may not complete it in sequence resulting in bias) (Aday, 1996).

A unique advantage of telephone interviews is a potentially short data collection period. In some situations; data can be gathered and processed within several days. While they are more expensive than mailed questionnaires (i.e., they involve personnel and training costs), telephone interviews usually cost less and afford more perceived anonymity than face-to-face interviews. In particular, telephone interviews (along with mailed questionnaires) offer an advantage over face-to-face interviews when the sample is distributed over a large geographical area (Rea & Parker, 1997).

A disadvantage of phone interviews is that the interviewer has less control than in a face-to-face interview. The interviewer's opportunity to establish credibility is more limited over the phone. Moreover, respondents can put down the phone at anytime. A disadvantage that affects sampling is that only people with telephones can be contacted. Thus, in some studies, constituents of the population of interest may be missed. Finally, there is limited ability to support questionnaires with visual aids that can clarify questions in the interview (Abramson & Abramson, 1999).

Face-to-Face Interviews

Survey data can be collected in person by trained interviewers. These interviews are typically conducted at the respondent's residence. However, other sites such as schools, workplaces, or clinics may also be used. This method has many of the same strengths as phone interviews. Face-to-face interviews are ideal for contacting hard-to-reach populations, for example, homeless or incarcerated criminal offenders and they are usually completed with little or no missing data.

Some disadvantages of face-to-face interviews are the high costs (for travel as well as personnel and training), and the time involved in traveling for and doing the data collection period. Despite the potential advantages of face-to-face interviews, the interviewer can also be a source of bias. For example, the face-to-face encounter may influence the respondent to seek approval from the interviewer. Moreover, sex, age, or cultural differences may bias the respondent. Finally, face-to-face interviews can raise concerns about personal safety of the interviewers and lack of anonymity for the respondent (Abramson & Abramson, 1999).

Selecting and Combining Data Collection Methods in Surveys

In making a decision about which data collection method to use in survey research, there are multiple considerations. In the end, the investigator must select the method that best suits the research question, the population under study, and the available resources and constraints for the study. In some studies, a combination of methods may be used to lower costs and improve data quality. For example, telephone interviews may be conducted with persons who do not respond to a mailed questionnaire. Or, a respondent to a face-to-face interview may be asked to complete and return by mail a self-administered questionnaire that requires consulting household records or other household/family members (Hoyle, Harris, & Judd, 2002; Siemiatycki, 1979).

Building the Questionnaire/Interview

At the heart of the survey process is development of the questionnaire or interview schedule (i.e., the written form or guide to be used by the interviewer). Many of the principles for constructing the survey data collection method are the same whether it is a questionnaire or an interview. Therefore the following discussion pertains to both unless specific points are made about one or the other. The usual steps in building an interview or questionnaire are:

- Defining and clarifying the survey variables,
- Formulating the questions,
- Formatting the questionnaire or interview schedule, and
- Piloting and revising the questionnaire/interview schedule.

These steps are discussed below.

Defining and Clarifying Survey Variables

The first step in building the survey is to identify key variables to be measured. This can be done through a review of the literature and/or interacting (e.g., via focus groups or unstructured interviews) with the target population to gain a full understanding of the issues to be studied. There is not an ideal number of variables for a survey study. The rule, "as many as necessary and as few as possible," is sound advice so as to minimize respondent burden and survey costs (Abramson & Abramson, 1999).

The variables chosen for a survey study depend on the aim and research question(s) of the study. Some survey research aims primarily to describe particular phenomena. For example, the periodic survey conducted by the National Board for the Certification of Occupational Therapists (NBCOT) in the United States (National Board for Certification in Occupational Therapy, 2004) aims to characterize the practice of entry-level occupational therapists in order to guide the development of the certification exam. This survey is guided by questions concerning what theory or models therapists use, what assessments they use, the types of interventions they do, and so on. In this survey, the variables of interest were those that characterized entry-level practice.

Other surveys aim to determine whether relationships exist between variables. In this case, the study questions will ask whether and how variables under study covary (i.e., correlate), or whether a number of variables can be shown to account for variability in a selected variable.

Each of the variables should be clearly defined both conceptually and operationally. Part of the process of clarifying each variable is identifying the appropriate level of data desired, (i.e., nominal, ordinal, ratio, interval, as discussed in Chapter 13) and corresponding format for collecting that level of data. For example, in the NBCOT survey, most of the variables were nominal, such as which model of practice or which assessment was used. The survey asked for this information by asking therapist to name the models they used. The same type of information might also have been asked in order to obtain ordinal data. For instance:

How frequently do you use the biomechanical model in your practice?
Rarely 1
Often 2
Always 3

Deciding the variables under study and the level of data to be collected is a critical step. It not only affects the overall quality of the study but also determines the type of analysis that can be carried out with the data. Hence, when doing this step, investigators should anticipate the statistical analyses they plan to undertake.

Formulating Questions

Once the variables have been identified, questions are formulated to elicit data on those variables. For a complex variable, it may be necessary to develop

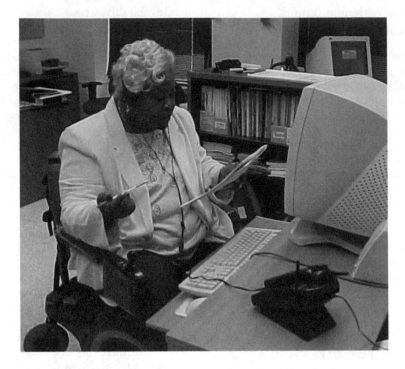

Figure 8.2 Phone interviews are a frequently used method of data collection in research.

several questions. Moreover, when several questions are asked about a variable in order to form a scale, the variable can be captured with greater reliability and validity (see Chapters 12 and 13). Questions should:

- Have face validity, that is, they should reflect what the investigator wants to know and be obvious in meaning for the respondents,
- Ask about things for which the respondent can be expected to know the answer, and
- Be clear and unambiguous, user friendly, and not be offensive (Bradburn, Sudman, & Wansik, 2004).

Questions must not contain assumptions that might confuse a respondent or introduce potential bias. For example, the question, "What was your experience of occupational therapy during your last hospital admission?" assumes that the respondent recalls which of the services received during the hospitalization were occupational therapy.

Complex and lengthy sentences are particularly likely to be misunderstood by respondents. Thus, questions should be short and simple (Converse & Presser, 1986). Questions that have two components should be avoided; the following is an example of such a question: "Recalling how many times you came to occupational therapy, do you think it was adequate?" Breaking these double-barreled questions into separate questions would be more straightforward. For instance: "How many times did you come to occupational therapy?" followed by, "Do you think that was adequate?"

Sometimes a filter question is employed to find out if the respondent has knowledge/experience of an issue before asking him or her to answer more specific questions about the issue (Hoyle et al., 2002). For example, "Do you remember receiving occupational therapy during your hospitalization?" If the respondent answers "yes" to this question, then it would be appropriate to ask about the experience of occupational therapy. If not, then there is no point in asking further about occupational therapy.

Questions may be asked in two general forms: closed questions or open questions. A closed question provides specific response choices and therefore allows for more uniformity in response and simplifies the analysis. The following is an example of a closed question:

Which of the following factors is the most important in your documentation?
Identification of clients occupational needs . . .1
Communication to the interdisciplinary team . .2
Capturing the client's narrative 3

Also, by presenting response choices, the researcher is providing the same frame of reference to all respondents. Closed questions provide options to be considered and therefore can act as a memory prompt (Hoyle et al., 2002). There is, however, concern that they may force people to choose among alternatives that are predetermined by the researcher instead of answering in their own words (Converse & Presser, 1986).

> The design of the questionnaire needs to allow for making the task of reading questions, following instructions, and recording answers as easy as possible.

The following is an example of an open question:

> What factors influence the content
> of your documentation?

Open-ended questions, such as this one, are useful for eliciting a more detailed narrative response. While answers to this type of open-ended question may provide rich information, they may also be challenging to categorize for analysis (Converse & Presser, 1986).

Investigators sometimes use open-ended questions initially with a small pilot study sample of the population to generate the closed questions for the main survey (Schuman & Presser, 1981). This approach helps to generate closed questions with options that are understandable to the respondents.

Often researchers use both types of questions in a survey. A common approach is to give some response choices and then provide an "other (please specify)" category. For example:

> Which of the following do you use to assess a
> client's occupational participation?
> Formal outcome measure 1
> Informal interview with the client 2
> Informal observation of the client 3
> Other 4
> Please specify_____

Formatting the Questionnaire

The design of the questionnaire needs to allow for making the task of reading questions, following instructions, and recording answers as easy as possible. This section should be read with Figures 8.3 and 8.4 in mind. Mailed questionnaires must be clear and attractive to complete. They require formatting that ensures ease of use and accuracy of response. With telephone and face-to-face interviews, more weight is given to formatting the written questionnaire for interviewer convenience and to allow the interviewer to easily record the responses. Sometimes for telephone interviews, the interviewer may use a computer-based questionnaire that allows the data to be entered directly to the computer. This method avoids the extra step of data entry that occurs when responses are recorded by the interviewer on paper.

Formatting Principles

There are a number of overall formatting principles that should guide questionnaire construction (Table 8.2). The first is to develop a clear, attractive front cover. It should contain:

- The title of the study,
- Directions for completion of the survey, and
- The name of the financial sponsor and/or institution of the principle investigator (Dillman, 1978).

Respondents are more likely to trust a known institution rather than a named individual whom they do not know. Adding a picture or illustration can be informative and add interest. The back cover of the questionnaire should not have any questions on it. It should contain only an invitation for further comments, a statement of thanks, instructions for returning the completed questionnaire, and a mailing address for the survey.

Having an uncluttered appearance to the survey is paramount. Using extra paper is preferable to condensing the questionnaire into fewer pages, which can lead to confusion and errors (Salant & Dillman, 1994). For clarity of reading, 12-point type in a standard font (e.g., Arial or Times New Roman) is preferable. For a questionnaire that will be mailed to respondents who may have lowered vision, such as elderly persons, a larger type size, such as 14-point, should be used.

Thorough instructions must be provided so that it is clear how the interviewer or respondent should indicate their response to a question (e.g., "circle the number of your answer"), directions for completing the questionnaire should be distinguished from the questions by using special typographic formatting for emphasis, such as italics, bold, parentheses, or brackets. Caution is urged when using all capital letters; this format is difficult to

```
                                              SPN_____{Private}
                                              Interviewer ID_____


        ROYAL INFIRMARY OCCUPATIONAL THERAPY PROGRAM FOLLOW-UP
                         (Telephone interview)


        Hello, my name is _____ and I'm calling from the Royal Infirmary
        occupational therapy department. May I please speak with _____? We
        are interviewing previous clients of the Royal Infirmary occupational therapy
        service to learn more about how occupational therapy can help people to get
        back to doing everyday activities following discharge from the Royal Infirmary.
        We are calling you because the occupational therapy records show that you
        have difficulty doing everyday activities, and we would like to ask you some
        questions about your clinic experiences, health, and everyday activities.

        Time interview began:        :              (use 24-hour clock)
                                _____ _____


        1.   In general, how would you describe your health at this time? Would you
             say it is. . .

                              Very poor, ....................................................... 1
                              Poor, ............................................................. 2
                              Good, or.......................................................... 3
                              Very good ...................................................... 4
                              Don't know ...................................................... 8


        2.   Compared to other people about your age, how would you describe your
             health in general? Would you say it is . . .

                              Worse than average, ...................................... 1
                              About average, or .......................................... 2
                              Better than average ...................................... 3
                              Don't know..................................................... 8


        3.   If 1 is not important and 5 is very important, how important is it for some-
             one your age to be able to do everyday activities independently?

             Not                                    Very
             Important                              Important           DK

               1          2          3          4       5               8
```

Figure 8.3 Format of a telephone survey.

read when applied to more than a few words. There need to be very clear instructions about negotiating "skip patterns," in situations in which a certain subset of questions may not apply to some respondents (e.g., because they apply only to one sex or a particular age group). Figure 8.4, question 4 illustrates how a skip pattern can be indicated in a questionnaire.

Each question should be assigned a number sequentially throughout the questionnaire. The questions should be written out in full rather than using a one-word variable label, for example,

"What is your age?" rather than, "Age?" The questions should all start at the left margin. All response choices should be indented and all start at the same place. Leader dots can be helpful for visually linking the response choices with the numerical codes. All the parts of the same question and its response choices should be on the same page, never split between two pages. Response categories should be presented in a vertical list format rather than a horizontal format (Bradburn et al., 2004). Each response choice should be assigned a numerical code that will be circled by

SPN_____{Private}

**ROYAL INFIRMARY OCCUPATIONAL THERAPY SERVICE
SURVEY OF HEALTH AND EVERYDAY ACTIVITY BEHAVIOR**

*Please circle one response code number according to your answer
except where instructed otherwise.*

1.   In general, how would you describe your health at this time?

Very poor, ... 1
Poor, ... 2
Good, or.. 3
Very good 4

2.   Compared to other people <u>about your age</u>, how would you describe your
health in general?

Worse than average, ... 1
About average, or 2
Better than average 3

3.   What was your <u>main</u> reason for attending occupational therapy?

Difficulty doing self care 1
Difficulty doing work tasks 2
Difficulty doing leisure activities 3
Other *(Please specify)* 4

_____

4.   Do you feel satisfied with your occupational therapy experience?

Yes...............................1   *(SKIP to Q.30)*
No.................................2

Figure 8.4 Format of a mailed survey.

the respondent or interviewer to record each response. These numerical codes are likely to yield fewer mistakes than using check boxes when coding and processing the completed questionnaire for data entry (Dillman, 1978).

Creating a vertical flow by aligning response codes along the right-hand margin helps to reduce the number of errors. Vertical flow and a generous use of spacing and indentation give the survey an uncluttered, user-friendly appearance. For a series of items that share the same root question and the same response choices, an efficient format is illustrated by Figure 8.5, question 19.

Sequencing Questions

The sequence of questions is also important. Every questionnaire should start with a few easy

questions that have obvious relevance to the topic of the survey (Dillman, 1978). Following these few introductory questions, the main study questions are presented. Usually issues related to a respondent's beliefs, behaviors, and attitudes are explored related to the study topic. Topically related subjects should be clustered together.

Some respondents regard questions about their demographic background as invasive, and the relevance of such questions to the study topic is often not apparent if they are asked early in a questionnaire. Therefore, questions about the respondent's demographic background are often placed at the end of the questionnaire, except where it is necessary to screen a respondent's eligibility to answer a particular group of subsequent questions (e.g., only questions about recent therapy outcomes

Table 8.2 **General Principles of Survey Formatting**

- The front cover should be clear and attractive.
- The back cover of the questionnaire should not have any questions.
- The survey should have an uncluttered appearance.
- A 12-point type font is preferable.
- Questions need an assigned number sequentially.
- Clear instructions need to be provided.
- Questions need to be written out in full rather than one word.
- The questions should all start at the left margin.
- All the parts of a question should be on the same page.
- Response categories should have a vertical response format.
- Response choices should have a numerical code to be circled.
- Space generously to avoid a cluttered look.

would be asked of respondents who have received therapy recently).

It is helpful to have smooth transitions between topics. This may be achieved by presenting questions in a chronological order when appropriate, by using section headings, or by inserting a brief statement introducing a group of questions about a new topic. This is especially important for sensitive questions that may provoke embarrassment, be viewed as private or personal, or ask about illegal behaviors. Respondents will be more likely to respond to such questions if there is an appropriate context given for the questions and the respondent can see the relevance of the questions to the study purpose.

Within a topical area of the survey, one should structure the questions in a logical sequence. The "funnel" principle, which is used frequently, starts with general questions followed by ones that become increasingly more specific (Hoyle et al., 2002). It is also important to avoid a potential question sequence effect (Tourangeau & Rasinski, 1988). That is, one should avoid asking a question sequence in which a previous question will likely bias the response to the next question.

Formatting Questions for Different Scales

By their nature, nominal and ordinal scales have finite categories. For example, a question using a nominal scale is:

What is your sex?
Male 1
Female 2

The respondent can respond only by choosing one of the two finite categories.

Nominal categories may be randomly listed to eliminate the possibility of any sequencing effect. Other alternatives for nominal categories are to list them in descending order, starting with the ones that are likely to be chosen most frequently, or to list them alphabetically.

An ordinal scale asks the respondent to choose one of a number of finite categories. The following is an example of an ordinal scale that asks the respondent to choose one of three ratings on an ordinal scale of importance.

How important is your relationship with your client to the outcomes of therapy?
Not so important 1
Important 2
Extremely important 3

19. What kind of occupational therapist support would you find helpful?

	Very helpful	Somewhat helpful	Not at all helpful	Don't know
a. Self-help materials	1	2	3	8
b. A lifestyle class	1	2	3	8
c. An activity support group	1	2	3	8
d. One-to-one activity coaching	1	2	3	8
e. Something else (*specify*)	1	2	3	8

Figure 8.5 A sample question from an occupational therapy survey.

12. The following are some statements about how occupational therapists (OT) might deal with clients who are having difficulty doing everyday activities. For each statement, please indicate if you strongly disagree, disagree, agree, or strongly agree.

	Strongly Disagree	Disagree	Agree	Strongly Agree
a. My OT should <u>advise</u> me how to engage in daily activity.........	1	2	3	4
b. My OT should <u>teach</u> me how to engage in daily activity.........	1	2	3	4

Figure 8.6 An example of Likert scales from a survey of occupational therapy practice.

Ordinal responses should be listed in logical order. Listing ordinal responses from lowest to highest (as in the example above) not only makes them clearer, but also avoids the need to reverse the coding scheme for the analysis.

Responses to an interval scale may be assigned to an infinite number of possible points or to specified ranges. Deciding on categories for interval scales involves judgment. For example, if asking respondents about their age, it is generally fine to ask how many years old one is, since people can easily retrieve their age from memory. However, if the question is about income, people may have more difficulty recalling the exact amount and thus the use of ranges such as $30,000 to $35,000 may be preferable. The decision about using actual amounts versus ranges depends on consideration of this factor along with how important it is to have exact information versus information characterized by a range. When using ranges, one should use boundaries that conform to traditional rounded breaking points. For example in asking for years of experience it is better to ask: "0–4 years, 5–9 years" rather than "0–4.5 years, 4.6–9.5 years."

Scaled response mechanisms, such as Likert scales, have response choices to elicit opinions. Likert scales are bipolar, ranging from the most negative point at one end of a continuum to the most positive point at the opposite end, for example, using an "agree/disagree" continuum. The questions should be focused on one issue or domain. The response choices should be balanced, with an equal number of similar points ranging from low to high, for example, "strongly agree," "agree," "disagree," and "strongly disagree" (e.g., Figure 8.6, question 12).

Piloting the Questionnaire

Piloting of the questionnaire is essential before the main study. By doing a pilot study, an investigator can find out if respondents can understand the questions and if they can reasonably understand

and respond to the questions. Piloting can also determine in an interview-based survey whether the interviewers will be able to convey the questioning format as it is written.

Within a pilot study, investigators can gather data to evaluate the intended survey instrument. Three of the most common ways of gathering such data are focus groups, field pretesting, and individual interviews (Presser et al., 2004). They are discussed below.

Focus Groups

Every researcher's views can be widened by systematic discussions within a focus group (Stewart & Shamdasani, 1990). Focus groups ordinarily involve a small group of persons who represent the range of characteristics expected in the study sample. The investigator guides the group through a discussion that aims to elicit every member's opinion.

Focus groups can be used during the initial planning of the investigation to help define the key study. They can also be used to evaluate the questions once they have been developed into the questionnaire. Focus groups can provide information about the complexity of what is being asked and how people understand the terms in the questionnaire. In some instances, focus groups can involve a question-by-question review of the questionnaire.

Field Pretesting

For telephone or face-to-face interviews, investigators ordinarily will conduct a small number of interviews (usually about 15 to 30), with people who are similar to those who will be respondents in the planned survey. For mailed questionnaires, respondents who are from the study population are asked to complete the questionnaire. There can be some debriefing questions at the end of the questionnaire asking for feedback on such factors as what was unclear or confusing. Field pretests also provide critical information on the practical aspects of administering the survey tool that allows unforeseen problems to be addressed before doing the larger study (Fowler, 1995). A valuable tool for assessing these aspects is to conduct a debriefing interview with pretest interviewers.

Debriefing Interview

A debriefing interview with respondents about their understanding of questions can be helpful (Lessler & Tourangeau, 1989). The focus of the interview is to find out the respondent's reactions to the questions. The debriefing interview involves three steps:

1. Asking the questions or providing the questionnaire,
2. Allowing the respondent to answer the questionnaire or interview, and
3. Asking the respondent what was going though his/her mind during the process.

An investigator may also ask respondents to:

• Paraphrase their understanding of the questions,
• Define the terms used in the interview, and/or
• Identify any confusion or concern.

Debriefing interviews are very helpful in identifying how the respondent experiences the questionnaire or interview process and whether anything needs to be changed to improve the accuracy of the data they yield.

> A hallmark of a well designed survey study is that the respondents are selected randomly from the target population.

Implementing a Survey Study

The procedures used in implementing a survey study will have a large impact on the rigor of the investigation (Fowler, 2002). Three key factors that influence study rigor are:

• Sampling,
• Response rates, and
• How the survey is carried out.

Each is discussed in the following sections.

Sampling Strategies

As noted at the beginning of this chapter, most survey data are collected from a sample of a relatively small number of members of a target population. These sample data are used to make estimates of the target population's characteristics (parameters). A census is a special case, in which survey methods are used to collect data from or about every member of a population, that is, a 100% sample.

The main reason for collecting data from a sample instead of from an entire population is that it is much less expensive. Also, when available funding is fixed, resources can be allocated to collect information about more variables than would be possible in a survey of the entire population. Another important reason for sampling is that it usually reduces the data collection period, making the study findings available for dissemination and application much sooner. Finally, in cases in which gaining access to population members requires special strategies (e.g., negotiating access to worksites, or screening randomly composed numbers for a telephone interview survey), the strategy can be done more effectively and efficiently with a sample than with the entire population.

Some survey samples are selected by nonprobability methods (e.g., selecting respondents who are convenient or who have volunteered). Selecting a sample using such procedures, which depend on subjective judgments (by the respondents or by the researcher) about who should be included, may result in a sample that constitutes an unrepresentative (biased) population subgroup. Although such a sample may be useful for an exploratory or pilot study about a new topic or new population, great caution must be exercised in generalizing from a nonprobability sample to a target population. There are no systematic methods to account for possible selection bias. Also, standard statistical methods (e.g., confidence intervals) that are based on a random sampling theoretical model cannot be applied appropriately to data from a nonprobability sample.

Consequently, a hallmark of a well designed survey study is that the respondents are selected randomly from the target population. Random (probability) sampling, in conjunction with good questionnaire design and data collection procedures, provides the foundation on which reliable estimates of population characteristics may be derived from sample data.

In random sampling, the selection of each respondent is independent of the selection of any and all others. Thus, for example, a person would not be included automatically in a sample because someone else in his or her household (e.g., spouse) is selected. Each population member has a unique, independent chance of being selected. That chance must be greater than zero, and it must be known or it must be possible to calculate it. Although it often is desirable that the probability of selection is the same for each population member, this is not an essential aspect of random sampling. In cases in which the probability of selection varies (e.g., in a disproportionate stratified sampling design), the researcher must calculate weights to adjust for this in the analysis.

The basic model underlying sampling theory and inferential statistics is simple random sampling with replacement (i.e., returning the respondent selected to the population after sampling so that he or she has an equal change of being selected subsequently) (Cochran & Williams, 1973). In common survey practice, however, it is not practical or desirable to collect data from the same population members more than once. Therefore, virtually all survey samples are selected without replacement. The first step in selecting any random sample is to obtain or compile a list of all (or as near as possible) of the members of the target population (e.g., all the members of the British College of Occupational Therapists). This list is called the sampling frame. In simple random sampling without replacement, every element (population member) on the frame is assigned a unique

number from 1 to N (N = the number of elements). Then n (n = the desired sample size) elements are identified to be in the sample by referring to a random number source (such as a random number table, or a random number generator on a calculator or computer), from which the researcher selects n unique numbers corresponding to elements on the sampling frame. When sampling without replacement, once an element's number is selected, it is set aside and not used again, that is, it is ignored if it is derived more than once from the random number source.

In many cases, the sampling process is greatly simplified by using systematic random selection, which is used commonly in survey research (Levy & Lemeshow, 2003). Again, every element on the frame is assigned a unique number from 1 to N. Next, a selection interval (k) is calculated by dividing the population size by the sample size: $k = N/n$. For example, to select a sample of 200 elements from a population of 1600, $k = 1600/200 = 8$. Then, after selecting a random starting point in the interval from 1 to k (1 to 8 in this example), the researcher selects that first element from the sampling frame and every k element thereafter. Thus, if the random starting point is 4, using a selection interval = 8, the sample will consist of elements on the sampling frame that previously were assigned the numbers 4, 12, 20, 28 …1596 (Figure 8.7).

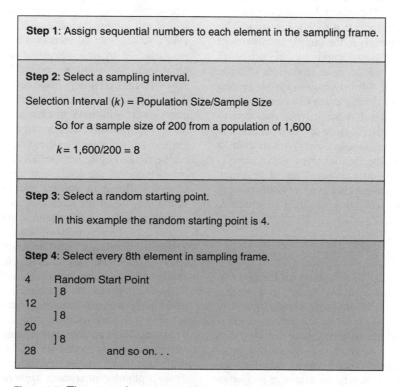

Figure 8.7 The steps for systematic random selection.

Before using systematic random selection, however, the sampling frame must be assessed for any preexisting periodic arrangement of elements that might coincide with the selection interval. This is because a random procedure is used only once, when the first selection point is identified. Thereafter, all the other elements selected in the sample are identified by their relative position on the sampling frame. For example, if for some reason every eighth person listed on the sampling frame in our example (starting with person number 4) happens to be a certain sex or in a certain occupational category, the sample may be biased. Fortunately, in most studies potential periodicity bias may be avoided effectively by first arranging the sampling frame in a random or near random order, usually alphabetically by surname.

A stratified random sample may be selected using information that is already available about the population members to divide them into subgroups (strata) that are of special interest for the study purpose. For example, a sample of occupational therapists might be stratified according to length of employment, which would be available from employee records. Then a separate random sample would be selected from within each of the length of employment strata. For example, three samples might be selected, one each from among those employed less than 1 year, 1 to 4 years, and 5 years or longer. The main advantages of stratification is that it ensures that each subgroup will be included appropriately in the sample and there will be more stability (less sampling error) across all possible samples of the same size. Both of these aspects contribute toward obtaining more precise estimates of population parameters from the sample statistics. Several strategies may be used to decide how to construct strata and to determine the number of elements to select from each stratum. In some cases, stratification involves giving population members unequal probabilities of selection. Accordingly, the researcher must adjust for this in the analysis by weighting the data (Cochran & Williams, 1973).

Response Rate

An important aspect of the quality of the data collected from a representative sample is how successful a survey is in obtaining cooperation from the persons selected into the sample. As noted at the beginning of the chapter, failure to collect data from a high percentage of the sample is a major source of potential survey error, called nonresponse bias. In addition to the degree of nonpartic-

ipation, nonresponse bias depends on the extent to which nonrespondents differ systematically from respondents in terms of their characteristics on key variables under study (Fowler, 2002; Groves, 1989; Kviz, 1998). In such cases, the absence of nonrespondents from the analysis may cause survey estimates of population parameters to be lower or higher than their true value. For example, if persons who engage in risky behaviors are less willing than others to participate in a survey about health risks, then the estimates of the prevalence of those behaviors based on data from the survey sample will be too low (Tourangeau & Smith, 1996).

Availability is another source of nonresponse, especially in telephone and face-to-face interview surveys. If the data collection times are within working times then it will be challenging to gather data on a working population. Less educated people and those older than 65 years of age are less willing to be interviewed in a random-digit telephone procedure (Groves & Couper, 1998). Even with a relatively high response rate, there still is a potential for nonresponse bias if the reason for nonresponse is related strongly to the survey topic. Therefore, it is important that efforts are put into reducing nonresponse and/or comparing any systematic difference between respondents and nonrespondents.

Reducing nonresponse rates in telephone and face-to-face interview surveys involves ensuring access and gaining cooperation (Groves & Couper, 1998). Access can be increased by making multiple calls and by ensuring these happen at varied times including evenings and weekends. An average of 10 calls is usually made before deciding that the person being called is a nonrespondent. Having interviewers who have flexible schedules and can make appointments at the respondents' convenience enhances access to the sample. Cooperation can be elicited by an advanced letter clearly stating the purpose of the study and the content of the interview. Being clear at the start of the interview of the purpose of the questions and reassuring the respondents their information is important to the outcome of the research will support cooperation. Training interviewers who understand the importance of good response rates and who can handle challenging questions with sensitivity is essential. Reducing nonresponse in a mailed survey involves developing a well presented questionnaire and sending multiple mailings to nonrespondents. Three mailings of the questionnaire and a cover letter are recommended about one month apart (Dillman, 2000). If questionnaires are mailed to a general population without appropriate follow-up techniques, the response rate is likely to be less than 50% (Edwards et al., 2002; Heberlein & Baumgartner, 1978).

The response rate is an important mechanism for assessing the potential for nonresponse bias. In general, the response rate is calculated as the number of sample members from whom a completed questionnaire is collected, divided by the number of sample members who are eligible to participate in a particular survey, expressed as a percentage (Kviz, 1977). However, special considerations often must be taken into account depending on various aspects of any particular survey. Although there still is no generally accepted standard for computing response rates, many survey professionals have adapted the guidelines set forth by the American Association for Public Opinion Research (2004), which are available from the organization's Web site along with a response rate calculator that may be downloaded free at http://www.aapor.org.

Response rates vary widely across the various survey data collection modes, and even across studies using the same mode. In general, response rates are highest and quite similar for the two interview survey methods, with response rates tending to be about 5 percent higher for face-to-face interviews than for telephone interviews. Response rates generally are lower for mailed questionnaires (Aday, 1996). A review by Goyder (1985) found that response rates for mailed questionnaires using the strategies we recommend here range from about 30 percent to as high as 80 percent or higher, with the 60 to 70 percent range being regarded by some survey experts as a realistic average expectation for a well implemented mail survey. Response rates for "typical" face-to-face interview surveys range from about 70 to 90 percent or higher (Goyder, 1985). Czaja and Blair (2004) suggest the following response rates may be expected for most typical surveys: 65% to 95% for face-to-face interviews, 60% to 90% for telephone interviews, and 45% to 75% for mailed questionnaires.

There is no agreed-upon standard minimum for an acceptable response rate. Some have suggested 50% to 60% as adequate (Rea & Parker, 1997) while others have suggested above 70% is acceptable (Fowler, 2002). Of course, as discussed earlier, in addition to the response rate, any assessment of potential nonresponse bias must consider whether and to what extent nonrespondents are likely to differ from respondents in terms of key variables under study. However, even with a 90% response rate there may be some nonresponse bias.

Carrying Out the Survey

Face-to-face interviews afford the opportunity for an advance letter that informs the potential respondent of the details of the study. Telephone random digit dialing is always a cold contact. However, other telephone surveys may afford the opportunity to send a letter prior to the call to increase response rates. Mail surveys can send an advance letter that explains a questionnaire will be mailed to respondents shortly. Cover letters are critical to response rates of mailed survey (Salant & Dillman, 1994). It is the only opportunity the researcher has to anticipate and deal with the respondents' questions and concerns about participating in the survey. The cover letter should be printed on letterhead stationery, and have the mailing date and the name and address of the anticipated respondent. It should include at a minimum why the study is important, why the respondent's answers are important, assurance of confidentiality of their answers, and whom to contact if they have questions about the survey. The letter should conclude with a thank you and be signed with an original signature whenever possible.

Telephone and face-to-face interviews obtain higher cooperation rates in the evenings and weekends, which is when most respondents are likely to be available for interview (Weeks, Kulka, & Pierson, 1987). Interview schedules need to be developed to reflect when the sample can be accessed. Interviewers generally are instructed to allow a phone to ring up to 10 rings to allow respondents sufficient time to pick up the phone. Leaving a message on an answering machine or voice-mail system usually is not advised unless this will be the last attempt to contact a respondent. It is best for the interviewer to make direct contact. Few respondents return a call in response to a message left by an interviewer.

All forms of survey need appropriate follow-up procedures to maximize response rates. The majority of face-to-face interviews are carried out within six contact attempts (Kalsbeek, Botman, Massey, & Lui, 1994). The number of follow-ups is dependent on cost. A careful cost–benefit analysis should be completed before deciding how many repeat calls the interviewers make before assigning a nonresponse status to a sample unit.

It is more cost effective to complete contacts to nonrespondents in telephone interview surveys. If there is a busy signal, for example, it has been recommended to call back a maximum of three times, 3 minutes apart (Survey Research Laboratory, 1987). When the sample is selected from a list, a minimum of 10 call backs at different times on dif-

Table 8.3 **Procedure for Administration of Mailed Surveys**

Timeframe	Action
Before survey is sent	Mail a personalized, advanced letter to everyone in the sample.
Round 1	Mail personalized cover letter with more detail of the study, a questionnaire and a stamped, addressed return envelope.
4–8 days later	Send a follow-up postcard or letter to thank everyone who has responded and ask those who have not done so to respond.
Round 2 4 weeks after first questionnaire was sent	To nonrespondents send a new personalized cover letter, replacement questionnaire, and stamped self-addressed envelope.
Round 3: 8 weeks after first questionnaire was sent out	To nonrespondents send a new personalized cover letter, replacement questionnaire and stamped address envelope.
End data collection 12 weeks after first questionnaire was sent out	

ferent days is usually completed to nonrespondents. When working with a random digit dialing sample, where there is a chance for more nonresidential telephone numbers to be included in the sample, most survey research organizations attempt a minimum of about 15 calls.

Mailed surveys require a systematic approach to administration to ensure acceptable response rates (Table 8.3). Follow-up mailings to everyone in the sample (even those who have responded) are not efficient and may confuse or irritate those who have already responded. Targeted repeated administrations can be achieved if there is a way of identifying those who have not responded. This can be achieved if a sample point number (SPN) is placed at the top right hand corner of the questionnaire. This number corresponds to the respondent's entry in the sampling frame, which should be kept in a locked physical file and/or in a password-protected computer file to protect respondent confidentiality. It is good practice to tell people what the number is for in the covering letter. If it is important that the respondent not be identifiable even to the researcher then a postcard procedure can be employed (Fowler, 2002), whereby a postcard bearing the respondent's SPN is enclosed with the questionnaire along with a request for the respondent to mail it separately when he or she mails back the completed questionnaire. The text of the postcard states: "Dear researcher, I am sending this postcard at the same time that I am sending my completed questionnaire. Since the questionnaire is completely anonymous (the SPN is not recorded on the questionnaire in this case) this will let you know I have returned my questionnaire." This procedure maintains anonymity while enabling the researcher to track who has responded to the survey. Whatever procedure is used, it must be

approved by an ethical board (see Chapter 29) that judges the procedure to be warranted in light of the potential respondents' rights to consent and to confidentiality.

Preparing for Data Analysis

The formal process of gathering survey data has been outlined earlier. The data this process generates must now be presented in an understandable format. During the planning stage of the research, the researcher should know how the data will be analyzed to meet the objectives of the study. This process of thinking forward to the analysis phase early on can often identify and allow correction of gaps in the data that will be obtained through the questionnaire.

Survey data are usually entered into a computer data file for statistical analysis. Each statistical program has different criteria in how the data should be formatted. To facilitate computer processing and analysis, codes must be assigned to all responses on a completed questionnaire. There should be clear rules as to which numbers are assigned to which answers on the survey. A code book should be developed that clearly indicates which codes are reflective of which questionnaire answers and which column the questionnaire can be found in the electronic dataset (Figure 8.8).

If the coding is complex, detailed coding instructions will need to be developed. These need to be clear in order to ensure coding reliability. Codes need to be assigned to missing data to identify if the respondent refused to answer a question, left a response blank inadvertently, a question was not applicable to the respondent, or the respondent did not know the information requested by a ques-

Variables in Export Sequence

Column Location	Content of Column
1-3:	subject identifier (001-999) (3 numeric code)
4-6:	repeat code (001-999) (3 numeric code)
7-8:	translation used (1 character code/1 numeric code) missing data: 09
9-11:	country in which data was collected code (3 character code) missing data: 009
12-13:	age (2 numeric code) missing data:99
14:	gender (M or F) missing data: 9
15-17:	nationality (3 character code) missing data: 009
18:	ethnicity (single numeric code) missing data: 9
19:	years of education (single numeric code) missing data: 9
20-21:	degree earned (2 character code) missing data: 09
22-23:	employment status (2 character code) missing data: 09
24-25:	living situation (2 character code) missing data: 09
26:	independence in occupational behavior (1 character code) missing data: 9
27-28:	major disabling condition category (2 character code) missing data: 09
29-32:	specific major disabling condition (4 numeric code) missing data: 0009

Figure 8.8 An example of the demographic information section of a code book.

tion. Codes need to be generated for open questions, or for "other" choices, where the responses were not predictable. The researcher identifies categories that emerge as themes in the answers to the open question.

Quality control procedures include having trained coders, independently checking each coder's work, and coders should write notes about codes of which they are not sure so that they can be checked by the supervisor. Other quality control methods include using a well developed interface between the computer and the data entry personnel. Computer programs (e.g., ACCESS, SPSS, SAS, Epi-Info) now can develop data entry screens to ease the process of entering data. These programs can be set to accept only a certain range of codes in a particular field, thereby reducing error codes in a field. The data can be entered twice in two different files and then the files can be correlated to identify potential errors in data entry. This can be expensive and therefore a 10% random sample can be entered in twice to check accuracy. The rate of error from data entry should be less than 1% (Fowler, 2002).

Precoded forms that can be scanned electronically are becoming used more often. This option may not be financially viable at present for smaller surveys; however, this may become an option in the future with the reduction in cost of the equipment. Current options are discussed in Bloom and Lyberg (1998). Also, as noted earlier, survey researchers are increasingly exploring effective ways of collecting survey data using the Internet (Couper, 2000; Dillman, 2000)

Conclusion

Surveys allow for the systematic collection of information from a sample of people to generate an understanding of the population from which the sample was drawn. Completing a rigorous survey study requires careful attention to building the survey, administering the survey, and processing the data. If these procedures are followed, the summary statistics can be generalized to the population under study, which is the aim of survey research.

REFERENCES

Abramson, J., & Abramson, Z. (1999). *Survey methods in community medicine* (5th ed.). New York: Churchill Livingstone.

Aday, L. (1996). *Designing and conducting health surveys.* San Francisco: Jossey-Bass.

American Association for Public Opinion Research (2004). *Standard definitions: Final dispositions of case codes and outcome rates for surveys.* Retrieved in March 2005, from http://www.aapor.org.

Bloom, E., & Lyberg, L. (1998). Scanning and optical character recognition in survey organizations. In M. Couper, R.P. Baker, J Bethlehem, C.Z.F. Clark, J. Martin, W. Nicholls, & J.M. O'Reilly (Eds.), *Computer assisted information collection* (pp. 449–520). New York: John Wiley & Sons.

Bowers, D. K. (1999). FAQs on online research. *Marketing Research, 10*(1), 45–48.

Bradburn, N. M., Sudman, S., & Wansik, B. (2004). *Asking questions.* San Francisco: Jossey-Bass.

Bradley, N. (1999). Sampling for Internet Surveys: An examination of respondent selection for Internet research. *Journal of the Market Research Society, 41*(4), 387–395.

Cochran, W.G., & Williams, G. (1973). *Sampling techniques.* New York: John Wiley & Sons.

Converse, J., & Presser, S. (1986). *Survey questions: Handcrafting the standardized questionnaire* (2nd ed.). Beverly Hills, CA: Sage.

Couper, M. P. (2000) Web Surveys: A review of issues and approaches. *Public Opinion Quarterly, 64,* 464–494.

Czaja, R., & Blair, J. (2004). *Designing surveys: A guide to decisions and procedures.* Thousand Oaks, CA: Pine Forge Press.

DePoy, E., & Gitlin, L. (1998). *Introduction to research: Understanding and applying multiple strategies.* St. Louis: Mosby.

Dillman, D. A. (1978). *Mail and telephone surveys: The total design method.* New York: John Wiley & Sons.

Dillman, D. A. (2000) *Mail and Internet surveys: The tailored design method.* New York: John Wiley & Sons.

Edwards, P., Roberts, I., Clarke, M., DiGuiseppi, C., Pratap, S., Wentz, R., et al. (2002). Increasing response rates to postal questionnaires: Systematic review. *British Medical Journal, 324*(7347), 1183–1191.

Fowler, F. (1995). *Improving survey questions. Applied social research methods series* (Vol. 38). Thousand Oaks, CA: Sage.

Fowler, F. (2002). *Survey research methods. Applied social research methods series* (Vol. 1). Thousand Oaks, CA: Sage.

Goyder, J. (1985). Face-to-face interviews and mailed questionnaires: The net difference in response rate. *Public Opinion Quarterly, 49,* (2, summer), 234–252.

Groves, R., & Couper, M. (1998). *Nonresponse in household interview surveys.* New York: John Wiley & Sons.

Groves, R. M. (1989). *Survey errors and survey costs.* New York: John Wiley & Sons.

Heberlein, T., & Baumgartner, R. (1978). Factors affecting response rates to mailed questionnaires: A quantitative analysis of the published literature. *American Sociological Review, 43,* 447–462.

Hoyle, R. H., Harris, M. J., & Judd, C. M. (2002). *Research methods in social relations* (7th ed.). Pacific Grove, CA: Wadsworth.

Kalsbeek, W., Botman, S., Massey, J., & Lui, P. (1994). Cost efficiency and the number of allowable call attempts in the National Health Interview Survey. *Journal of Official Statistics, 10,* 133–152.

Kviz, F. J. (1977). Toward a standard definition of response rate. *Public Opinion Quarterly, 41,* 265–267.

Kviz, F. J. (1998). Nonresponse in sample surveys. In T. Cotton & P. Armitage (Eds.), *Encyclopedia of biostatistics.* Chichester, UK: John Wiley & Sons.

Lessler, J.,Tourangeau, R., & Salter W. (1989, May). Questionnaire design research in the cognitive research laboratory. *Vital and Health Statistics* Series 6, No.1; DHHS Publication No. PHS-89-1076. Washington, DC: US Government Printing Office.

Levy, P. S., & Lemeshow, S. (2003). *Sampling of populations: Methods and applications.* New York: John Wiley & Sons.

National Board for Certification in Occupational Therapy. (2004). A practice analysis study of entry-level occupational therapist registered and certified occupational therapy assistant practice. *OTJR, Occupation, Participation and Health, Spring, Volume 24, Suppl. 1.*

Presser, S., Couper, M. P., Lessler, J. T., Martin, E., Martin, J., Rothgeb, J. M., et al. (2004). Methods for testing and evaluating survey questions. *Public Opinion Quarterly, 68* (Spring), 109–130.

Ramos, M., Sedivi, B. M., & Sweet, E. M. (1998). Computerized self-administered questionnaires. In M. P. Couper, R. P. Baker, J. Bethlehem, C. Z. E. Clark, J. Martin, W. L. Nichols, & J. M. O'Reilly (Eds.), *Computer assisted survey information collection* (pp. 389–408). New York: John Wiley & Sons.

Rea, L., & Parker, R. (1997). *Designing and conducting survey research: A comprehensive guide.* San Francisco: Jossey-Bass.

Salant, P., & Dillman, D. (1994). *How to conduct your own survey.* New York: John Wiley & Sons.

Schuman, H., & Presser, S. (1981). *Questions and answers in attitudes surveys*. New York: Academic Press.

Sheehan, K. B., & Hoy, M. G. (1999). Using e-mail to survey Internet users in the United States: Methodology and Assessment. *Journal of Computer Mediated Communication, 4* (3). Available: http://www.ascusc.org/jcmc/vol4/issue3/sheehan.html.

Siemiatycki, J. (1979). A comparison of mail, telephone, and home interview strategies for Household Health Surveys. *American Journal of Public Health, 69* (3), 238–245.

Stewart, D., & Shamdasani, P. (1990). *Focus groups*. Newbury Park, CA: Sage.

Survey Research Laboratory, University of Illinois. (1987). *Chicago area general population survey on AIDS* (SRL No. 606), Interviewer Manual. Chicago: Author.

Tourangeau, R., & Rasinski, K. (1988). Cognitive processes underlying context effects in attitude measurement. *Psychological Bulletin, 103*, 299–314.

Tourangeau, R., & Smith, T. W. (1996). Asking sensitive questions: The impact of data collection mode, question format, and question content. *Public Opinion Quarterly, 60*, 275–304.

Weeks, M., Kulka, R., & Pierson, S. (1987). Optimal call scheduling for a telephone survey. *Public Opinion Quarterly, 51*, 540–549.

RESOURCES

Web Sites

American Association for Public Opinion Research (AAPOR). *Best practices for survey and public opinion research*. 2002. Available at AAPOR Web site: http://www.aapor.org/default.asp?page=survey_methods/standards_and_best_practices.

American Association for Public Opinion Research (AAPOR). *Code of professional ethics and practices*. 2002. Available at AAPOR Web site: http://www.aapor.org/default.asp?page=survey_methods/standards_and_best_practices/code_for_professional_ethics_and_practices

American Association for Public Opinion Research (AAPOR). *Response rate calculator*, available at: http://www.aapor.org/default.asp?page=survey_methods/response_rate_calculator. A free copy of an Excel spreadsheet (AAPOR Outcome Rate Calculator Version 2.1) may be downloaded to facilitate computing rates according to the methods described in AAPOR's document, "Standard Definitions: Final Dispositions of Case Codes and Outcome Rates for Surveys."

American Statistical Association, Survey Research Methods Section. Proceedings. Online proceedings of the American Statistical Association Survey Research Methods Section from 1978 to present. Also includes papers from the Joint Statistical Meetings and some papers from the American Association of Public Opinion Research meetings. More than 3000 papers in all. http://www.amstat.org/sections/srms/proceedings/

Sage Publications. *The survey kit*. A collection of brief, applied books by various authors, about survey research methods. Information is available at http://www.sagepub.com. NOTE: Search for "survey kit."

U.S. Office of Management and Budget. *Revisions to the Standards for the Classification of Federal Data on Race and Ethnicity*, (October 30, 1997). Available online at http://www.whitehouse.gov/omb/fedreg/omb-dir15.html.

Articles

Couper, M. P., Traugott, M. W., & Lamias, M. J. (2001). Web survey design and administration. *Public Opinion Quarterly, 65*, 230–253.

Schaeffer, N. C., & Presser, S. (2003). The science of asking questions. *Annual Review of Sociology, 29*, 65–88.

Schwarz, N. (1999). Self-reports: How the questions shape the answers. *American Psychologist, 54*(2), 93–105.

Books

Couper, M. P., & Nicholls, II, W. L. (1998). The history and development of computer assisted survey information collection methods. In M. P. Couper, R. P. Baker, J. Bethlehem, C. Z. F. Clark, J. Martin, W. L. Nicholls II, et al. (Eds.), *Computer assisted survey information collection* (pp. 1–21). New York: John Wiley & Sons.

DeVellis, R. F. (2003). *Scale development: Theory and applications*. Newbury Park, CA: SAGE Publications.

Fink, A. (1995). *How to ask survey questions*. Thousand Oaks, CA: Sage.

Fowler, F. J., Jr. (1998). Design and evaluation of survey questions. In L.Bickman & D. J. Rog (Eds.), *Handbook of applied social research methods* (pp. 343--374). Thousand Oaks, CA: SAGE Publications.

Harkness, J. A., van de Vijver, F.J. R., & Mohler, P. P. (2002). *Cross-cultural survey methods*. San Francisco: Jossey-Bass.

Presser, S., Rothgeb, J. M., Couper, M. P., Lessler, J. T., Martin, E., Martin, J., et al. (Eds.) (2004). *Methods for testing and evaluating survey questionnaires*. New York: John Wiley & Sons.

Schwarz, N., & Sudman, S. (Eds.) (1996). *Answering questions: Methodology for determining cognitive and communicative processes in survey research*. San Francisco: Jossey-Bass.

Sudman, S., Bradburn, N. M., & Schwarz, N. (1996). *Thinking about answers: The application of cognitive processes to survey methodology*. San Francisco: Jossey-Bass.

Tourangeau, R., Rips, L. J., & Rasinski, K. (2000) *The psychology of survey response*. New York: Cambridge University Press.

Willis, G. B. (2005). *Cognitive interviewing: A tool for improving questionnaire design*. Thousand Oaks, CA: SAGE Publications.

*Note: Many universities have expertise in survey design and can be consulted when creating a survey.

CHAPTER 9

Study Designs for Secondary Analysis of Existing Data

Sherrilene Classen

Secondary analysis involves the use of data that were gathered for previous research studies or other primary purposes (e.g., medical records, databases from surveys). The main purpose of using this type of research is to describe or explore phenomena that may lead the researcher to ask more specific questions, to generate hypotheses, or to engage in prospective research (gathering of data at some point in the future).

For example, consider a researcher who wants to determine if there is a relationship between medication use and functional status of older adults. Such a researcher could begin to answer this question by exploring the medication and functional status data from existing records in a nursing home or rehabilitation facility. If the researcher found negative associations between sedatives and cognitive functioning, it would be possible to ask more specific questions (e.g., why is there a negative relationship between sedatives and cognitive functioning, or what is the relationship between sedatives and instrumental activities of daily living [ADL] functioning in older adults?). The researcher may then choose to engage prospectively in a follow-up study to answer these questions.

Secondary analysis is a valid mode of inquiry, widely used in such fields as public health and nursing. It is also beginning to be used in occupational therapy. This method holds many advantages. For example, it is cost effective, decreases subject burden, and is useful for exploring new areas of research. Nonetheless, many pitfalls exist and investigators must plan for managing and acknowledging those.

This chapter defines secondary analysis and describes how retrospective analysis and the use of existing databases fit within this type of design. The definitions, advantages, limitations, and application of this type of research are outlined. The chapter also describes different datasets, how they can be accessed, their purposes, and how to manage their limitations.

Definition of Secondary Analysis

Secondary analysis involves using available information. As noted earlier, this information may be available in existing records that were generated for purposes of documenting health care. Another important source of data for secondary analysis is existing databases (i.e., data that were originally collected for another study and are now available for further analysis). When using records for secondary analysis, the investigator observes, records, classifies, counts, and analyzes this existing information. In the case of existing databases, data are already organized into a format for analysis, so the investigator chooses what data to access and how to analyze those.

Designs for Secondary Analysis

Although the data already exist in both circumstances, it is important that the researcher considers the design that will be used to guide how data are extracted from existing records or databases and how they will be analyzed. Secondary analysis includes both descriptive and analytical designs. Descriptive designs depict the distribution and frequency of health conditions. Their purpose is to identify populations at high risk for developing a condition and to formulate hypotheses for further investigation. For example, using data from a health survey, an investigator may wish to describe the health status of people in a community. After analyzing the data, the researcher may identify high-risk groups and plan to examine the risks further in follow-up studies.

Analytical designs are concerned with identifying or measuring the effects of risk factors or health conditions, and with testing hypotheses. The com-

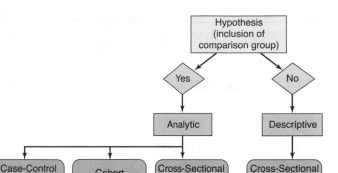

Figure 9.1 Decision tree for retrospective study designs.

mon types of analytical studies are cross-sectional, case control, and cohort. Figure 9.1 presents a decision tree for designs that involve secondary analysis of existing data. If the researcher wants to test a hypothesis, the analytical path will be followed, resulting in a choice among case control, cohort, or analytical cross-sectional studies. If no hypothesis is involved and the researcher wants to describe the population, a descriptive cross-sectional design is appropriate.

Cross-Sectional Design

Cross-sectional studies are also sometimes referred to as prevalence studies, when the aim is to examine the extent to which a health behavior or condition exists among some group (e.g., the prevalence of exercise behavior among physically disabled persons or the prevalence of acquired immunodeficiency syndrome [AIDS] among intravenous drug users).

In cross-sectional studies, investigators usually examine the relationship between a health outcome and some other variables. All the variables under study were captured at the same point in time and thus provide a "snapshot" of the subjects under study. In this type of study, the most common measure of association used is called the odds ratio (OR) as explained in the feature box below.

The odds ratio indicates the direction (positive or negative) and the size of the effect of those exposed to birth anoxias who were likely to show sensory integrative disorder. To interpret the odds ratio adequately one needs to calculate a confidence interval. One may say that this proposed exposure acts as a significant risk to disease if the odds ratio is greater than one (as it is in this case), and the lower bound of the confidence interval does not go below 1. This chapter does not address the actual way of calculating odds ratios, as this procedure is described in any statistics textbook, or

The Odds Ratio

The odds ratio is the ratio of two odds, which is an estimate of risk. For example, consider the following notation for the distribution of a binary exposure (exposed or not exposed) and a binary health outcome (sensory integrative disorder/no sensory disintegrative disorder) in a population.

		Outcome: Sensory integrative disorder	
		Yes	No
Exposure: Birth anoxia	Yes	a	b
	No	c	d

The odds ratio in the example above is $(a \times d) / (b \times c)$

If such a study involved 100 subjects it might result in the following data:

		Outcome: Sensory integrative disorder	
		Yes	No
Exposure: Birth anoxia	Yes	43	7
	No	2	48

In this case the odds ratio is $43 \times 48/ 7 \times 2 = 2,064/14 = 147.43$. The odds ratio indicates that someone who has been exposed to birth anoxia is 147 times more likely to have sensory integrative disorder, than someone not exposed to birth anoxia.

may be obtained by using a statistical software program such as SPSS or SAS.

The major advantages of the cross-sectional design are that it:

• Is relatively easy to do,
• Does not require a long time to execute,
• Is usually less expensive than other secondary analyses, and
• Provides a snapshot of the population.

The limitations of this type of study are that it:

• Is not appropriate for studying rare health conditions or those with a short duration,
• Cannot distinguish the temporal sequence of cause and effect,
• May falsely classify a person with a health problem in remission as not having the problem (because the design only provides a snapshot of a person's status at a point in time), and
• Is not suitable to examine rare outcomes, or outcomes of short duration (Mausner & Kramer, 1985).

The following is an example of a cross-sectional study. An occupational therapy researcher wants to determine the relationship between medications in the senior adult population and their activities of daily living status. To answer this question, the investigator analyzes an existing dataset containing information on medication management and on the functional status of a cohort of older adults. After analysis, the descriptive statistics will provide information about the associations between the explanatory variable (types of medication taken) and the outcome variable (independence in activities of daily living). The researcher may formulate a hypothesis from these associations that will facilitate further investigation.

Case-Control Design

Also called a case-history study, case control designs represent a true retrospective study and are described in detail in Chapter 7. The researcher compares cases with controls and determines the outcome of interest by looking backwards in time to determine which factors may lead to a particular outcome. The risk estimate is also expressed as an odds ratio. The major advantages of this design are:

• It is quick and inexpensive compared to other designs,
• It is appropriate for evaluating rare health outcomes or those with long latency periods (i.e., a long time between a precipitating factor and the outcome of interest), and

• Multiple factors can be evaluated for a single disease.

Limitations of this design are:

• Various forms of bias are inherent in the study design,
• Information on risk factors and confounding variables may be difficult to identify,
• Difficult to assess whether health condition causes exposure to a factor or the factor causes the health condition, and
• Difficult to identify and assemble case group representatives and identify a control group (Mausner & Kramer, 1985).

The following is an example of a case control study. An occupational therapy researcher wants to know what activity risk factors are associated with repetitive motion injuries in the upper extremity. From clinics serving such persons in a given state, the researcher obtains reports on subjects who have been diagnosed with repetitive motion injuries (cases). In addition, the researcher solicits records of people without repetitive motion injuries (controls) from general practitioner clinics in the same state. To determine the most important risk factors associated with upper extremity pain, the researcher identifies the different activity exposures associated with these cases and controls.

Cohort Design

Cohort studies may be prospective or retrospective. The prospective cohort is described in Chapter 7. The retrospective cohort, which is the version of this design used in secondary analysis, is also called a longitudinal, incidence, follow-up, or historical cohort study. The incidence of health outcomes is determined in persons who were exposed versus those who were not exposed to a certain factor or factors. The major advantages of this design are that:

• The study factor (independent variable) is observed on each subject before the health outcome is observed,
• Bias, for example, recall bias, is excluded in the exposure as the researcher observes the development of an outcome based not on the memory of the subjects, but on the exposure, and
• One can study additional associations with the outcome.

Limitations of this study design include:

• The attrition or drop-out of subjects, and
• Changes in criteria, practice standards, or methods occurring over time (Mausner & Kramer,

1985). (For example, a researcher studies the association between multiple medication use and functional limitations in a group of older adults, using a 10-year-old database and realizes that many of the older subjects died or "dropped out," which greatly affects the sample size at the end of the 10-year period. In addition, some of the medications that were used as standard practice 10 years ago are not being used today.)

The following is an example of a retrospective cohort study. From an existing dataset, an occupational therapy researcher examines the association between medications (exposure) used by senior adults and safe driving (outcome). The researcher identifies age, race, sex, and comorbidities as explanatory variables. She targets senior adults, age 65 and older, and examines their historical records retrospectively for 5 years. Annually and at the end of the 5-year period she determines the association between medication use and safe driving.

Summary

This section discussed secondary analysis designs consisting of descriptive and analytical designs.

The three major retrospective studies—cross-sectional, case-control, and cohort—were described with examples pertaining to occupational therapy practice. Table 9.1 summarizes the strengths and weaknesses of these designs.

Managing Bias and Confounding

In retrospective analysis, the researcher does not have control over the data because they were generated in the past. Consequently, the researcher must be aware of two existing sources of error that may distort findings of the study:

• Bias and
• Confounding (Mausner & Kramer, 1985).

Bias

Bias, which is systematic rather than random error, may occur during any stage of the study: during the design and conduct, in the analysis, and in the

Table 9.1 **Summary of Advantages and Disadvantages of Retrospective Studies**

Type of Study	Advantages	Disadvantages
Cross-sectional	• Is relatively easy to do. • Can be done quickly. • Provides a snapshot of the population. • Is usually less expensive than other designs for secondary analyses.	• Not appropriate for rare health conditions or those with a short duration. • Cannot determine temporal sequence of cause and effect. • Because the design only provides a snapshot of a person's status, a person with a health problem in remission may be falsely classified as not having the problem.
Case-control	• Quick and inexpensive compared to other designs. • Appropriate for evaluating rare health outcomes or those with long latency periods. • Multiple factors can be evaluated for a single disease.	• Various forms of bias are inherent in the study design. • Information on risk factors and confounding variables may be difficult to identify. • Difficult to assess whether health condition causes exposure to a factor or the factor causes the health condition. • Difficult to identify and assemble case group representatives and identify control group.
Cohort (historical)	• The study factor is observed on each subject before the outcome is observed. • Lack of bias in exposure. • Yields relative risk and incidence rates, which are measures of absolute risk. • Can study additional health outcome associations.	• Problems of attrition. • Changes over time in criteria and methods.

interpretation of the study results (Sackett, 1979). Two major sources of bias are:

- Selection bias and
- Information bias.

The following is an example of a selection bias in retrospective analysis. Consider a study in which an investigator wants to do retrospective analysis of nursing home records to examine assistive device and adaptive equipment utilization. In such a study clients who did not give consent to have their records accessed may differ systematically from those who did give consent (e.g., they may have more involved impairments). If this were so, the researcher may potentially not capture the information of "more involved clients" and underestimate the extent to which assistive devices and adaptive equipment are used by nursing home residents.

This same example can be used to illustrate information bias. Nursing home records may contain information about assistive devices and adaptive equipment that clients were provided. However, this information may not be an accurate estimate of utilization if more devices and equipment were provided to residents than were used by residents. Table 9.2 presents sources of selection

Table 9.2 Bias: Explanation, Impact, and Ways to Avoid or Manage in Retrospective Studies

Bias	Explanation	Impact	Ways to Avoid or Manage
Selection bias			
Prevalence/incidence bias (Neyman's bias)	Results from inclusion of prevalent or existing cases rather than incident or new cases.	The use of prevalent cases can lead to an overrepresentation of cases of long duration, because those who have rapidly cured, or died, have a lower probability of being included.	Use incident cases, or prevalent cases with a short interval between the diagnosis and onset of disease/disability.
Self-selection or membership bias	Refers to the characteristics of an individual that may consciously or unconsciously affect membership in a group.	May increase or decrease the risk estimate.	Can be minimized in selecting groups that are closely related in terms of activity, occupations, environment, etc.
Loss to follow-up or withdrawal bias	Most relevant in cohort studies and refers to the completeness of follow-up or rate of withdrawal, which may be different in the exposed vs. nonexposed.	May increase or decrease the risk estimate depending on whether or not the outcome experience is different among those lost.	Compare loss group to follow-up group on baseline data to determine important differences.
Berkson's bias	Relevant in case-control studies, refers to selective factors that lead hospital cases and controls to be different from what is seen in the general population.	May increase or decrease the risk estimate.	Use controls, without the outcome under investigation, that are equal to the cases. For example, if hospital cases are used, then choose hospital controls (not healthy controls) as a comparison group.
Information bias			
Recall bias	Differences, generally among cases and controls, in accuracy or completeness of recall to memory of prior events or experiences.	Increase the risk estimate.	Validate exposure information from independent source; use hospital controls and/or more than one control group.

(continued)

Table 9.2 **Bias: Explanation, Impact, and Ways to Avoid or Manage in Retrospective Studies** (continued)

Bias	Explanation	Impact	Ways to Avoid or Manage
Interviewer bias	The interviewer is subconsciously or consciously gathering selective information. For example, an interviewer may probe for more information about exposure among cases, because of the expectation of exposure.	Increase the risk estimate.	Theoretically by blinding the interviewer to the case/control status; use of trained interviewers and standardized interview form; re-interview a sample of study subjects.
Family information bias	Most relevant in case-control studies. Cases may be more aware of family history of disease or risk factors because the occurrence of disease has stimulated discussion of past history.	Increase the risk estimate.	Validate disease and exposure status; use controls with another disease state.

and information bias, their impact, and ways to manage these biases in retrospective designs.

Confounding

Confounding is the mixing of the effects of extraneous variables with the variables under study. An extraneous variable may fully or partially account for the apparent association between variables under study. Alternatively, it may mask or hide an underlying true association. A variable must meet two criteria for being considered a confounding variable:

• It must be a risk factor for the outcome under study, or associated with the outcome, but not necessary causal, and
• It must be associated with the exposure under study, but not a consequence of the exposure.

Confounding can be controlled in the design through restriction or matching. It can be controlled in the study analysis through stratification, or multivariate analysis, or both.

Restriction allows one to narrow the ranges of values of potential confounders. For example, when sex, age, and race are expected to be confounding factors, an investigator might restrict a study sample to white men, ages 35 to 40. While such subject restriction would control for age, race, and sex, the results would be restricted to a narrow sample. Matching by pairs occurs where one or more controls are chosen for each case based on specific characteristics or range of variables. For example, consider a retrospective study that aims to determine factors that account for difficulty remaining employed among persons with mental

illness. Each individual who was not employed for the last 5 years might be matched on the basis of sex, age, and education level if these were not variables of interest and are likely to be confounding variables.

Matching by frequency occurs by first knowing or estimating the expected number of cases within each level of the confounding variable or variables, such as white females aged 20 to 24, white females aged 25 to 29, white females 30 to 34, and so forth. The appropriate number of controls for each stratum is then selected from the pool of potential controls until the number needed in each stratum is achieved (Kelsey, Whittemore, Evans, & Thompson, 1996).

Stratification involves partitioning the data according to the levels of the confounder. For example, consider a study of physically disabled persons in which the study focus is the relationship between extent of physical impairment and employment. If a comorbid condition (e.g., affective disorder) is a confounder of employment outcomes, then one may stratify the information according to whether or not the subjects had a diagnosis of depression, bipolar disorder, or no affective disorder. Controlling for more than two or three confounding variables is usually not recommended.

Finally, multivariate analysis is the construction of mathematical models to simultaneously describe the effect of exposure and other factors that may be confounding. Chapter 17 covers multivariate analyses and how they are used. The following is an example of using multivariate analysis to control for a confounding factor. Using an existing workman's compensation database, a researcher wants to examine the incidence of carpal tunnel syndrome in computer operators. The researcher identifies possible confounding factors (e.g., certain kinds of leisure time activities) that may contribute to the carpal tunnel condition and decides to control for leisure time activities in the analysis.

Existing Databases: Advantages and Disadvantages to Occupational Therapy Researchers

An existing health database is a set of information collected at some point in the past for the purpose of shedding light on health conditions (Miller, 1982). Secondary analysis of existing data is receiving increased attention in health care. Shrinking grant dollars, pressure to produce replicable findings, and a growing interest in outcomes investigation have all contributed to an increasing use of existing data for multiple research purposes. Secondary data analysis may offer the practitioner and researcher ready access to large datasets with multiple variables.

Types of Secondary Data

Two types of secondary data exist:

* Aggregate and
* Individual.

Aggregate data are summary-level data, the result of applying statistical analyses to micro-level datasets. Analysis may entail summing the number of each type of response for a given variable, then applying additional calculations such as weighting and estimation of sampling error. These procedures are meant to provide reliable inferences about an entire population based on data collected from the sample, or set of samples, surveyed (Disability Statistics Center, 2005). Aggregate data provide:

* Estimates of selected characteristics of the entire population surveyed (e.g., how many people in the United States have a disability), or
* A specific subset of the population (e.g., the proportion of working-age men with disabilities who have college degrees).

Aggregate data are frequently used to describe trends over specific time periods (e.g., how the unemployment rate for people with AIDS has changed from year to year since 1995). One limitation of these prepared aggregate data is that they might not use all the variables of interest to the user. Examples of aggregate data sources include:

* Census tract statistics,
* Centers for Disease Control and Prevention (CDC) records of reportable diseases by geographic areas, and
* Hospital data reported by diagnosis-related group (DRG) or conditions.

Individual level data are those for which separate information is available for each person or member of a list of individuals. The most common sources of individual level data include:

* Administrative (e.g., claims data),
* Operational (e.g., rehabilitation or discharge reports),
* Analytic (e.g., cost reports),
* Patient medical records, and
* Primary data collected in previous studies.

Existing databases can be obtained from a variety of population-based (e.g., National Center for Health Statistics), state (e.g., State Health Department), regional (e.g., County Health Department), and local resources (e.g., a local rehabilitation facility) (Freburger & Konrad, 2002). Routinely collected data, for example, National Center for Health Statistics data, are often used to provide descriptive statistics underlying the health condition and an indication of the frequency of the occurrence of a health condition. Such data also serve to provide leads concerning the etiology (causes) of outcomes or conditions, and to generate hypotheses (Mainous & Hueston, 1997).

> Shrinking grant dollars, pressure to produce replicable findings, and a growing interest in outcomes investigation have all contributed to an increasing use of existing data for multiple research purposes.

The following example illustrates the use of an existing database. An occupational therapy researcher wishes to study the relationship between travel patterns (e.g., night vs. day driving, distances driven, frequency of trips taken, and destinations of trips) of older adult drivers and crashes. Using data from the National Travel Household Survey, the researcher examines the association between exposure variables (age, race, sex, and geographic region) and explanatory variables (type of car, medical status, use of medications, comorbidities, socioeconomic status) on the outcome variable, crashes. The researcher identifies descriptive information and associations that will help explain the relationship between risk factors and crashes.

Some data are readily available, in that they are routinely abstracted, tabulated, and published, or can easily be obtained in nonpublished forms upon request. Included in this category are:

- Surveys from the National Centers for Health Statistics, and
- Data from the Centers for Disease Control and

Prevention (CDC); and data on a variety of health conditions reported in the CDC's *Morbidity and Mortality Weekly Report (MMWR)*.

Researchers may also obtain data by abstracting and tabulating information from records that have been kept primarily for other purposes, such as hospital records, occupational therapy records, industrial records, insurance records, university student health records, and Armed Forces and Veterans Administration records. Prior to spending time on abstracting and tabulating information from records, researchers should enquire if these records are available in computerized form (Pabst, 2001). Table 9.3 presents a summary of data types useful for determining some aspects of health conditions.

Use of existing databases may produce a cost–benefit advantage (Castle, 2003). Although the researcher will have to invest time in defining, collaborating with the dataset owners, or abstracting and tabulating the data, dollars in collecting the data will be saved. Researchers, who oftentimes

Table 9.3 Summary of Data Sets Useful for Determining Aspects of Health Status

Category of Data	Importance	Examples of Variables
Community health data	Provide a profile of the community health necessary for development of goals and objectives.	Mortality rates, disability rates; incidence and prevalence; morbidity rates; unemployment rates.
Health system data	Has limited impact on health status. Data for utilizing process evaluation and cost benefit analysis.	Utilization data (admissions, discharges, client demographics, accessibility); facility data (institutional and human resources); cost data (primary care, indirect, clinic maintenance, personnel, and insurance costs).
Lifestyle data	National data, e.g., the Behavior Risk Factor Surveillance System (BRFSS) provides useful data for identifying risk factors and risk groups.	Lifestyle components defined as behavioral habits, or risk-taking behavior, e.g., smoking, obesity, exercise, substance use and marital patterns.
Human biology data	Provide identification of target groups or subgroups at risk, or for promotion, prevention, or intervention activities.	All demographic characteristics (age, sex, racial/ethnic groups, occupation); genetic risk information.
Environmental data	Provide identification of risk factors, confounders or the identification of subgroups.	Air, water, soil conditions; climate, general environmental quality; housing data; occupational data.
Socioeconomic data	Provide data for identification of "at risk" groups and to examine subgroups of the community.	Income, distribution of wealth, employment status, poverty levels; living environment; level of education; social order; physical and mental health; social status; recreation and leisure.

work with limited funding, may benefit from using existing datasets.

For example, an occupational therapy researcher is ultimately interested in developing an occupation-based health promotion program to curtail or prevent depression in senior adults. To begin, the investigator wants to examine, in persons with chronic illnesses, the association between activity restriction (exposures) and depression (outcome). Confounding variables are age, sex, race, and geographic area. The researcher decides to use the National Health Interview Survey, a U.S. survey with respondent data from approximately 130,000 people from 50,000 households. In this survey, individuals are asked to report conditions that resulted in activity restrictions occurring close to the time of the interview and they also report depressive symptoms. This database, while it has certain limitations in the quality of the data, can provide important findings about the relationship of activity restriction and depression across a large and diverse sample. The researcher would be able to formulate a hypothesis from the findings of this exploratory data analysis to further examine inactivity and depression in the senior adult population.

Purposes, Nature, and Sources of Existing Data

Existing data may be used to examine estimates of such variables as:

• Hospitalizations,
• Frequency of visits to rehabilitation settings,
• Impairment and disability,
• Measures of cost,
• Risk factors,
• Socioeconomic indicators, and
• Occupational indicators.

Such data can be found in national surveys, surveillance programs, and vital statistics from a variety of Web-based resources. In addition, such information may be obtained from organizations (e.g., hospitals, insurance companies and state health departments). Table 9.4 presents data sources, URL addresses, and a description of a range of data sources.

Modern databases may incorporate linked databases, which provide population-based, statewide, computerized, and probabilistic data. For example, The National Highway Traffic Safety Administra-

Table 9.4 Sources of Existing Data: Access to National Databases

Data Source and URL Address	Description
Centers for Disease Control and Prevention http://www.cdc.gov	The Centers for Disease Control and Prevention (CDC) is the lead federal agency for protecting the health and safety of people, providing credible information to enhance health decisions, and promoting health. Many datasets for developing and applying disease prevention and control, environmental health, and health promotion and education activities are available from the CDC. Some are discussed below.
National Center for Health Statistics (NCHS) http://www.cdc.gov/nchs/express.htm	Some NCHS data systems and surveys are ongoing annual systems while others are conducted periodically. NCHS has two major types of data systems: • Systems based on populations, containing data collected through personal interviews or examinations and • Systems based on records, containing data collected from vital and medical records.
Healthy Women: State trends in health and mortality http://www.cdc.gov/nchs/healthywomen.htm	This site contains tables that describe the health of people in each state by sex, race, and age. Currently, mortality tables and health behavior and risk factor tables can be accessed by downloading a free data dissemination software called Beyond 20/20®.
WISQARS: Web-based Injury Statistics Query and Reporting System http://www.cdc.gov/ncipc/wisqars/	WISQARS™ (Web-based Injury Statistics Query and Reporting System) is an interactive database system that provides customized reports of injury-related data. These include fatal and non-fatal injury reports, leading causes of nonfatal injuries and years of potential life lost

(continued)

Table 9.4 Sources of Existing Data: Access to National Databases (continued)

Data Source and URL Address	Description
National Center for Chronic Disease Prevention and Health Promotion http://www.cdc.gov/nccdphp	CDC's National Center for Chronic Disease Prevention and Health Promotion's mission is to prevent and control chronic diseases. The center conducts studies to better understand the causes of these diseases, supports programs to promote healthy behaviors, and monitors the health of the nation through surveys.
CDC: Behavioral Risk Factor Surveillance System (BRFSS) http://www.cdc.gov/brfss/	The BRFSS, the world's largest telephone survey, tracks health risks in the United States. Information from the survey is used to improve the health of the American people. The following subsets of data are available: Prevalence Data: Information on health risks in your state and in the nation; Trends Data: Data of selected risk factors in a state or in the nation; SMART Selected Metropolitan/Metropolitan Area Risk Trends: Information on health risks for selected local areas; BRFSS maps illustrating health risks at national, state, and local levels. Historical Questions: The historical record of BRFSS Survey Questions by category.
CDC WONDER http://wonder.cdc.gov/	WONDER provides a single point of access to a wide variety of reports and numeric public health data. These include data on health practice and prevention, injury prevention, and environmental and occupational health.
National Health Information Center (NHIC) http://www.health.gov/nhic/	The National Health Information Center (NHIC) is a health information referral service. NHIC puts health professionals and consumers who have health questions in touch with those organizations that are best able to provide answers. NHIC was established in 1979 by the Office of Disease Prevention and Health Promotion (ODPHP), Office of Public Health and Science, and the Office of the Secretary, U.S. Department of Health and Human Services.
U.S. Census Bureau http://www.census.gov/	The Census Bureau has extensive data at the U.S. level and substantial data for states and counties, somewhat less for cities. At present they release data for the very smallest areas (census tracts, block groups, and blocks) only once a decade after tabulating the results of the Population and Housing Census. The home page has key links (People, Business, Geography) to help you. Subjects A to Z gives you a large list of topics through which to search. You can find the population of a state, county, or city in FedStats.
National Health Examination Survey http://webapp.icpsr.umich.edu/cocoon/NACDA-SERIES/00197.xml	Reports on data collected through direct examination, testing and measurement of a national sample of the civilian noninstitutionalized U.S. population
National Survey of Family Growth http://www.nichd.nih.gov/about/cpr/dbs/res_national5.htm	Reports based on data collected in periodic surveys of a nationwide probability sample of women 15–44 years of age.
National Hospital Discharge Survey http://www.cdc.gov/nchs/about/major/hdasd/nhdsdes.htm	Data are obtained from sampling records of short-term general and specialty hospitals in the United States Within each sampled hospital, discharges are randomly sampled from daily listing sheets and information on diagnoses, surgical procedures, and length of stay are abstracted.
The National Ambulatory Medical Survey http://www.cdc.gov/nchs/about/major/ahcd/namcsdes.htm	This survey includes nonfederally employed physicians sampled from the American Medical Association and the American Osteopathic Association, in office-based patient care practices. During a random week in a year, the physician-patient visit is recorded in terms of the diagnosis, treatment, disposition and length of visit.

(continued)

Table 9.4 Sources of Existing Data: Access to National Databases (continued)

Data Source and URL Address	Description
National Health Care Survey http://www.cdc.gov/nchs/ nhcs.htm	Data collection from healthcare settings such as hospitals, outpatient clinics, emergency rooms, ambulatory care facilities, outpatient and free standing surgical units, health agencies, hospitals, and community-based long-term care facilities. A Patient Follow-up Component is included, providing information on outcomes of patient care and subsequent use of care through periodic contacts with patients or patient's families.
The National Health and Nutrition Examination Survey I http://www.cdc.gov/nchs/ nhanes.htm	Provides data from physical examinations, clinical and laboratory tests, and questionnaires on a sample of non-institutionalized civilian population of the U.S. NHANES I was a prevalence study undertaken during 1971–1975, and included about 20,000 individuals in the age range 1–74 years. It was designed to measure overall health status, with emphasis on nutritional status, dental health, skin problems, and eye conditions. Detailed information from a subset of individuals is available on chronic lung disease; disabling arthritis, cardiovascular disease; hearing level; health-care needs; and general well-being.
The National Health and Nutrition Examination Survey II http://www.cdc.gov/nchs/nhanes.htm	Provides data from 20,000 individuals age 6 months to 74 years, carried out during 1976–1980. This prevalence study was designed to permit some assessment of changes in the population's nutritional status, and certain other variables over time. Health and nutritional status of three Hispanic groups were included in the Hispanic Health and Nutritional Survey (HHANES) carried out in 1982–1984.
The National Health and Nutrition Examination Survey III http://www.cdc.gov/nchs/nhanes.htm	Carried out in 1988–1994, this survey includes data on persons 2 months of age and older with no upper age limit. All participants undergo physical examination, body measurements, and a dietary interview.
The Longitudinal Study of Aging http://www.cdc.gov/nchs/ products/elec_prods/subject/ lsoa.htm	Group of surveys based on the Supplement on Aging to the 1984 National Health Interview Survey. Data were obtained on the family structure, frequency of contacts with children, housing, community and social support, occupation and retirement, ability to perform work-related functions, conditions and impairment, functional limitations, and providers of help for those activities. Information was obtained from 160,000 people aged 55 years and older. Sub samples of participants have been interviewed in subsequent years, mainly in order to measure changes in various social and health-related variables over time.
National Highway Traffic Safety Administration: Crash Outcome Data Evaluation System (CODES) http://www.nhtsa.dot. gov/people/perform/trafrecords/ pages/codes/codes.htm	Statewide, population-based, computerized data related to motor vehicle crashes for two calendar years These include crash data collected by police on the scene, EMS collected by ENTs who provide treatment en route and Emergency department/hospital data collected by hospital and outpatient medical staff. Probabilistic linkage of the crash, hospital and either EMS or emergency department data are possible so that persons involved and injured in a motor vehicle crash can be tracked from the scene through the healthcare system. Linkage also makes it possible to evaluate the medical and financial outcome for specific event, vehicle and person characteristics.
National Highway Traffic Safety Administration: Fatality Analysis Reporting System (FARS) http://www-nrd.nhtsa. dot.gov/departments/nrd-30/ ncsa/fars.html	Fatality information derived from FARS includes motor vehicle traffic crashes that result in the death of an occupant of a vehicle or a non-motorist within 30 days of the crash. FARS contains data on all fatal traffic crashes within the 50 states, the District of Columbia, and Puerto Rico. The data system was conceived, designed, and developed by the National Center for Statistical Analysis (NCSA) to assist the traffic safety community in identifying traffic safety problems, developing and implementing vehicle and driver countermeasures, and evaluating motor vehicle safety standards and highway safety initiatives.

tion's (NHTSA, 2004) CODES (Crash Outcome Data Evaluation System) database provides crash data (collected by police at the scene), Emergency Management System (EMS) data (collected by emergency medical technicians [EMTs] who provide treatment at the scene), and en route-emergency department (ED) and hospital data (collected by physicians, nurses, and others who provide treatment in the ED, hospital, or outpatient setting). Probabilistic linkage exists among the crash, hospital, and EMS or ED data so that persons involved and injured in a motor vehicle crash can be tracked from the scene of the accident through the healthcare system. Linkage makes it possible to evaluate a variety of variables such as the following:

- Demographic variables associated with increased risk for injury,
- Vehicle registration, driver license, and citation data,
- Roadway, vehicle, or human behavior characteristics,
- Medical insurance, medical conditions, mental health, and substance abuse data,
- Injury patterns by type of roadway and geographic location, and
- Safety needs at the community level.

The availability of large datasets, the potential of accessing existing data through collaboration with organizations, and capabilities that modern databases afford provide substantial opportunities for the occupational therapist to engage in research.

Examples of Using Existing Databases to Shed Light on Practice, Service Needs, and Outcomes

Existing data may be used to shed light on practice, service needs, and outcomes. This section discusses some existing databases and provides examples of how these databases could be used by occupational therapy researchers and practitioners.

Computerized data systems used in hospitals, rehabilitation clinics, outpatient, and home health settings make it readily possible to obtain clinical and health information from a patient. These data include administrative information, laboratory and diagnostic tests, medications and blood products received, admitting and discharge diagnoses, procedures performed, and treatment received (Iezzoni, 2002). Within a few minutes the user can identify patients with various combinations of attributes, and display or download the associated information. For example, a researcher could use computerized data from a rehabilitation clinic to

determine the type, duration, and frequency of services needed and delivered over a period of time, and to track the rehabilitation outcomes, including discharge destinations and follow-up status. Such information may be used to develop staffing models, marketing plans, and budgets for the following fiscal year.

Other computerized information may reveal information from subpopulations of hospitalized patients and produce comparisons of characteristics of subpopulations. Statistical applications, assisting the user to analyze the data, are often integrated into such a system. For example, based on a description of the subpopulation's distribution, stratified by age, days of therapy required, and people power required, an occupational therapy researcher could determine the most important service needs and intervention areas for this subpopulation.

Studies using industrial records, can examine whether the environment is contributing to an occupational health condition. For example, an occupational therapy researcher could use industry data to determine the incidence and prevalence of work-related injuries, and the most common risk factors associated with them. Such information may be foundational for developing an injury prevention and education program.

People enrolled in health insurance groups have a financial incentive to obtain all of their care through the plan. Thus data from such groups can provide opportunity for researchers to link records of earlier health conditions, treatment, and medications, to records of later health conditions. Often computerized records are available over time, making them potentially very useful for longitudinal analysis. For example, an occupational therapy researcher could determine, in the senior adult population, the psychogeriatric medications most associated with falls leading to injuries, and the subsequent cost of rehabilitation services. After operationalizing each variable of importance, the researcher could request these data from the health insurance group. The insurance company could provide de-identified data (data stripped of any personal identifiers) to the researcher who may now perform the analysis and obtain the results.

Two major sources of mental health data exist on the prevalence of psychiatric disorders in the general U.S. population. The National Institute of Mental Health Epidemiologic Catchment Area (ECA) Program provides data on the incidence, prevalence, and other characteristics of several psychiatric disorders in about 18,000 community residents. The Division of Biometry, National Institute of Mental Health, collects hospital admission statistics throughout the country and issues reports

(Kelsey et al., 1996). Using this type of data, an occupational therapy researcher could conduct a study of the incidence, prevalence, and type of psychiatric disorders in this community, as background to developing a community-based program. The therapist could also learn about other important characteristics of the population, including risk factors, needs, and likely insurance availability to reimbursement for occupational therapy services.

The National Institute of Occupational Safety and Health (NIOSH, 2005) publishes documents on frequency of diseases of presumed occupational etiology in a variety of industries and on a variety of etiologic agents found in the occupational environment. An occupational therapy researcher could use data from NIOSH to determine areas of potential intervention for prevention of occupational injuries. Identified risk factors could be used for the development of a workplace health education and promotional program.

Utilizing an Existing Database

Utilizing an existing database requires an investigator to know how to access the database, what its protocols are, how to sort through the database, and what challenges to expect. This section overviews these issues.

Accessing and Retrieving Data

In many cases a researcher may access data from national organizations via the Internet. The researcher must follow the published guidelines for data access and data manipulation; these may vary considerably with each dataset. Some datasets can be downloaded or installed to the researcher's own personal computer and used with an appropriate software package. To load the data and translate them into a form that can be read by the software, executable files are often included with the data. Other public domain files can be accessed through the Internet only by using specific query language that is available on the Web site where the data are housed.

For example, the National Center of Health Statistics (NCHS) provides public information on health status by compiling statistical information from medical records, by conducting medical examinations, examining birth and death registries, and conducting various health surveys. NCHS releases this information in a variety of datasets. An occupational therapy researcher uses the National Health Interview Survey (NHIS) to

develop a clinical assessment tool for activities of daily function. He or she downloads the NHIS dataset, a text file, from the NCHS Web site and uses Statistical Package for the Social Sciences (SPSS) software input statements to convert the downloaded text file into a SPSS file. He then selects the variables of interest based on ability to perform various daily living tasks. The missing data, and subsequent reduction in sample size, is the biggest problem for this analysis. However, by using existing data, he or she could retrieve and start developing an assessment tool ready for psychometric evaluation.

Accessing person level data from known sources (e.g., obtaining existing data from a research organization or another researcher) ordinarily involves a number of steps including:

- Negotiating administrative approval for access,
- Undergoing an Institutional Review Board (IRB) protocol (i.e., human subjects ethical review), and
- Assuring compliance with any privacy regulations (e.g., in the United States complying with Health Information Portability and Privacy Act [HIPAA]).

Another point of access may be achieved by contacting private organizations, such as a rehabilitation hospital or insurance company. In this case the researcher will also have to complete the steps noted earlier. Moreover, the investigator would need to learn and follow the policies of the organization, often having to pay a fee for obtaining the abstracted strip data.

Accessing and retrieving the data can present a number of challenges. Becoming familiar with retrieval policies and procedures can sometimes pose technical problems. To address these challenges, a researcher may:

- Seek formal training provided by the dataset keeper,
- Rely on the resources of the primary data analyst,
- Seek assistance from a computer information specialist,
- Obtain abstracted data (data ready for use based on specific variables that the researcher require), or
- Utilize a statistical analyst to help with data retrieval and analyses.

Compliance with Privacy and Ethical Protocols

The use of patient-identifiable data in research is subject to increasingly complex regulation. Moreover, it may vary by country and by organization.

While this section briefly overviews some of the steps required to comply with privacy and ethical protocols, investigators will need to become familiar with what is required in each setting.

Ordinarily, when analyzing existing data, an investigator may apply for exempt IRB approval since no new data are collected. When using data from another researcher, approval must be obtained by submitting a letter to the review committee outlining the proposed secondary analysis study and the keeper of the original data. The investigator doing the secondary analysis is bound by the same confidentiality and privacy restrictions as the primary investigator. Ordinarily, the primary principal investigator and secondary researcher sign a document of agreement. This document outlines the rights, responsibilities, and obligations of the primary principal investigator and secondary researcher. This document usually describes the data that were accessed (e.g., interviews, demographic data), method of access (i.e., via computer software), and provisions for reference citations in publications and presentations. The primary principal investigator and secondary researcher also sign a Certificate of Confidentiality as assurance that the primary principal investigator will protect the confidentiality and privacy of the subjects.

When patient-identifiable information is needed to link data from two sources for analysis, the process is increasingly more complex (Malfroy, Llewelyn, Johnson, & Williamson, 2004). The process of establishing a study may involve obtaining ethical research and development and data protection approval, including application to the Patient Information Advisory Group, set up under Section 60 of the Health and Social Care Act, 2001.

Obtaining Data

Once the important data approval issues have been decided, the researcher can consider how the data will be obtained and moved to the selected data storage medium. Steps need to be taken to ensure that data are handled (i.e., retrieved and stored) a minimum number of times. Ideally, data should be handled only once (Pollack, 1999).

Each additional time data are accessed before they are put into the storage medium, there is a chance that they can be damaged or changed. Software packages, such as BrainMaker (2004), may enable the researcher to combine data that had been previously stored in smaller files and put into a large data set for analysis.

When data are being obtained from a medium that requires data conversion into study variables, a protocol for this process must be developed. Personnel who will obtain data must be trained and periodically checked for accuracy. For example, if a study is using medical records, personnel may need to review individual records to locate and code data, and enter the data into a computer program for analysis. A procedure for how data will be located, coded, and entered will need to be developed and personnel will need to be trained and checked for accuracy.

The Challenges of Using Existing Databases

There are a number of limitations associated with using existing databases (Brown & Semradek, 1992; Clarke & Cossette, 2000; Pollack, 1999). The following are some key limitations or problems:

- It is often difficult to know all the details about the secondary data. Information on the source data (i.e., the original dataset, its purpose, function and use), instruments, and procedures used for data collection are often limited, missing, or not easily found.
- Secondary analysis does not afford the investigator complete control over operationalizing variables. Consequently, there may not be congruence between the investigator's conceptual definition of a variable and what is available in the dataset. There may be a lack of congruence between the conceptual definition in the secondary study and the operational definition used in an original study. It is also possible that the unit of analysis may not be the same (e.g., data collected from people cannot be translated to family-level data).
- The original study may lack a theoretical framework, challenging the secondary investigator's use of a conceptual framework for the secondary analysis.
- There may be threats to reliability including problems with the instruments (e.g., unknown psychometric properties), poor training and supervision of the data collectors, and inconsistent data collection procedures.
- There may be threats to validity such as the instruments not fitting the concepts, large amount of data being missing, confusion about coding missing data, or inaccuracy in data entry.
- There may be selection and information bias in the data that are difficult to detect or manage.
- The secondary researcher has no choice in the selection of the instruments. Instruments used in the study may not be the best matches for

measuring the variables under study, yielding measurement concerns (Strickland, 1997).

- Data may be out of date owing to changes in case definitions, classifications of diagnoses, and changes in clinical practice. For example, the CDC has revised the case definition of AIDS three times. Similarly, what was called a cerebral hemorrhage at the beginning of the decade was tending to be called cerebral thrombosis at the end of the decade (Kelsey et al., 1996).
- The investigator lacks control in conceiving, generating, and recording the dataset.
- Data may be incomplete, erroneous, or misleading. For example, U.S. hospitals are usually reimbursed according to the Diagnostic Related Group System (DRG); thus, the diagnosis may be influenced by reimbursement considerations.

These limitations illustrate the potential pitfalls associated with using existing databases. The next section describes necessary strategies to limit or eliminate these pitfalls.

Dealing with the Challenges of Existing Databases

This section discusses nine general strategies for managing some pitfalls associated with use of existing databases (Brown & Semradek, 1992; Clarke & Cosette, 2000; Pollack, 1999).

Consider the Research Question

The variables contained within each dataset are a function of the original purpose for the compilation of the data. In using data for a secondary analysis, the issues of variable conceptualization, operation, and availability become paramount. Before working with a dataset, the researcher needs to generate:

- Carefully conceptualized research problem and question, and
- Identified variables required for the investigation.

Then the investigator must ask how well the problem, question, and variables match the way existing data were defined and collected. Delving into an existing dataset without first constructing the conceptual foundation and methodological approach for the inquiry increases the potential of introducing threats to both reliability and validity.

> Retrospective research and analysis offer many uses and much promise for occupational therapy practice, service, and research.

Consider the Database, the Study Methodology, and the Study Conclusions

Motheral and colleagues (2003) developed a retrospective research checklist of 27 questions to guide consideration of the database, the study methodology, and the study conclusions. This checklist covers a wide range of issues, including relevance, reliability and validity, data linkages, eligibility determination, research design, treatment effects, sample selection, censoring, variable definitions, resource valuation, statistical analysis, generalizability, and data interpretation. Use of this checklist can be very helpful in evaluating and using a database for retrospective analysis.

Select the Most Appropriate Database to Answer the Research Questions

The properties of the database can either facilitate or hinder addressing the intended research questions. For example, in considering a database to examine the determinants of unsafe driving among senior adults, the most desirable database would be routinely collected, up-to-date, and linked; it would provide population-based, statewide computerized and probabilistic data pertaining to motor vehicle crashes. The CODES database is an example of such data. Figure 9.2 represents a flow diagram of CODES linked data. From this diagram one can easily see how environmental information (e.g., description of the injury event) is linked to medical (e.g., inpatient rehab) and claims (e.g., HMO) information, affording the researcher with opportunities to follow the client from the scene of the accident through discharge from the medical or rehabilitation setting.

Obtain a Thorough Description of the Data

Many archives provide a codebook, or data dictionary, for each dataset. The codebook contains the list of variables as well as information on the sampling design, instruments, and procedures. Some archives of single datasets offered by individual researchers may not provide all this information. In this case, the secondary investigator should contact the primary researcher to request the codebook, copies of instruments and instrument

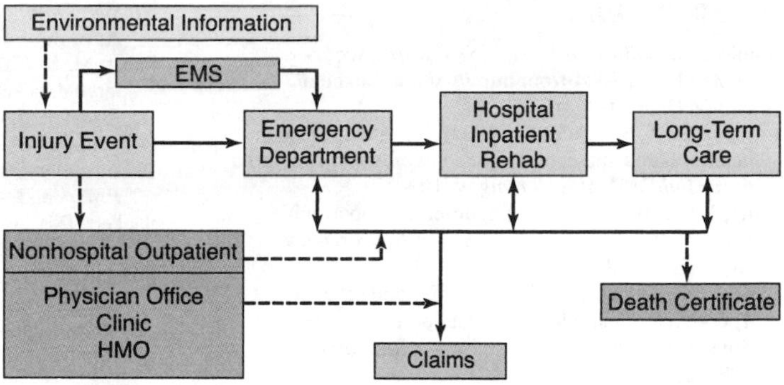

Figure 9.2 Flow diagram explaining the CODES linked data. (Reprinted with permission from National Highway Transportation Safety Administration [NHTSA]).

descriptions, written protocols, and instructions to data collectors. In some cases, the secondary researcher may wish to speak with the data collector(s) to better understand the context of the study and to elicit any problems that arose during data collection.

Choose a Timely Data Source

Timeliness can be an issue when there is a long time interval between the original study and the secondary study. It may be necessary for the secondary researcher to choose another dataset that has less time-sensitive data or that was collected more recently.

Talk to Program Staff

Program staff may help in abstracting the data. Although most national organizations, for example, the Census Bureau, provide data for free on the Internet, investigators sometimes need to access the data in a format not available over the Internet. In those cases, they may be able to get the data with help of the program staff (and, perhaps, at some additional cost).

Training

Some organizations provide extensive on-site training in use of the dataset. While such training can be very valuable, the researcher may have to incur travel and training costs to become educated in the use of the dataset.

Use a Computer Information Specialist

With continued advancements in technology, researchers may want to work with a computer scientist or analyst to optimize effectiveness and efficiency in data retrieval, storage, management, and analysis. These professionals have skills and knowledge that may ease the task of analysis, and

save time and money. They can provide database construction; database management, data monitoring, data cleaning, and reduction; data dictionary development; and data table construction.

Manage Missing Data

If missing data are nonrandom, steps should be taken to determine whether the data could be recovered, as might happen if a certain set of files did not link during a data merge (Kneipp & McIntosch, 2001). The most commonly used methods are to:

* Delete those subjects for whom there are missing data (listwise deletion),
* Delete those subjects only when the variable with missing data is used in an analysis (pairwise deletion), and
* Impute some value to replace the missing data, or by using regression (McCleary, 2002).

Conclusion

Retrospective research and analysis offer many uses and much promise for occupational therapy practice, service, and research. By carefully evaluating datasets before choosing one, researchers can capitalize on the benefits, and at the same time, minimize the potential pitfalls of secondary analyses. Any inquiry using existing data must be carefully designed to optimize integrity, reliability, and validity of the study. The research question, database, study methodology, data description, timeliness, use of support, managing data entry errors, and missing data are all important concepts in ensuring scientific rigor. Once practitioners and researchers fully recognize the challenges inherent in a secondary analysis, rich opportunities exist for studying health-related questions of relevance to occupational therapy.

REFERENCES

BrainMaker. *California Scientific software*. Accessed September 5, 2004 from http://www.calsci.com/tsLargeDataSets.html.

Brown, J. S., & Semradek, J. (1992). Secondary data on health-related subjects: Major sources, uses, and limitations. *Public Health Nursing, 9,* 162–171.

Castle, J. E. (2003). Maximizing research opportunities: Secondary data analysis. *Journal of Neuroscience Nursing, 35,* 287–290.

Clarke, S. P., & Cossette, S. (2000). Secondary analysis: Theoretical, methodological, and practical considerations. *Canadian Journal of Nursing Research, 32,* 109–129.

Disability Statistics Center. Finding disability data on the web. Retrieved May 5, 2005 from http://dsc.ucsf.edu/main.php?name=finding_data

Freburger, J. K., & Konrad, T. R. (2002). The use of federal and state databases to conduct health services research related to physical and occupational therapy. *Archives of Physical Medicine and Rehabilitation, 83,* 837–845.

Iezzoni, L. I. (2002). Using administrative data to study persons with disabilities. *The Milbank Quarterly, 80,* 347–379.

Kelsey, J. L., Whittemore, A. S., Evans, A. S., & Thompson, W. D. (1996). *Methods in observational epidemiology* (2nd ed.). New York: Oxford University Press.

Kneipp, S. M., & McIntosh, M. (2001). Handling missing data in nursing research with multiple imputation. *Nursing Research, 50,* 384–389.

Mainous, A. G., III, & Hueston, W. J. (1997). Using other people's data: The ins and outs of secondary data analysis. *Family Medicine, 29,* 568–571.

Malfroy, M., Llewelyn, C. A., Johnson, T., & Williamson, L. M. (2004). Using patient-identifiable data for epidemiological research. *Transfusion Medicine, 14,* 275–279.

Mausner J. S., & Kramer, S. (1985). *Epidemiology: An introductory text*. Philadelphia: W. B. Saunders.

McCleary, L. (2002). Using multiple imputation for analysis of incomplete data in clinical research. *Nursing Research, 51,* 339–343.

Miller, J. D. (1982). Secondary analysis and science education research. *Journal of Research in Science Teaching, 19,* 719–725.

Moriarty, H. J., Deatrick, J. A., Mahon M. M., Feetham, S. L., Carroll, R. M., Shepard, M. P., & Orsi, A. J. (1999). Issues to consider when choosing and using large national databases for research of families. *Western Journal of Nursing Research, 21,* 143–153.

Motheral, B., Brooks, J., Clark, M. A., Crown, W. H., Davey, P., Hutchins, D., Martin, B. C., & Stang, P. (2003). A checklist for retrospective database studies—report of the ISPOR Task Force on Retrospective Databases. *Value Health, 6,* 90–97.

National Highway Traffic Safety Administration (NHTSA). *Crash Outcome Data Evaluation System (CODES)*. Retrieved September 10, 2004 from http://www-nrd.nhtsa.dot.gov/departments/nrd30/ncsa/CODES.html

NIOSH: Databases and information resources. Retrieved April 2005 from http://www.cdc.gov/niosh/about.html.

Pabst, M. K. (2001). Methodological considerations: Using large data sets. *Outcomes Management in Nursing Practice, 5,* 6–10.

Pollack, C. D. (1999). Methodological considerations with secondary analyses. *Outcomes Management Nursing Practice, 3,* 47–52.

Sackett, D. L. (1979). Bias in analytical research. *Journal of Chronic Disability, 32,* 51–63.

Strickland, O. L. (1997). Measurement concerns when using existing databases. *Journal of Nursing Measurement, 5,* 115–117.

RESOURCES

Best, A .E. (1999). Secondary databases and their use in outcomes research: A review of the area resource file and the Healthcare Cost and Utilization Project. *Journal of Medical Systems, 23,* 175–181.

Byar, P. B. (1980). Why databases should not replace randomized clinical trials. *Biometrics, 36,* 337–342.

Estabrooks, C. A., & Romyn, D. M. (1995). Data sharing in nursing research: Advantages and challenges. *Canadian Journal of Nursing Research, 27,* 77–88.

Feinstein, A. R. (1984). Current problems and future challenges in randomized clinical trials. *Circulation, 70,* 767–774.

Greenland, S., & Finkle, W. D. (1995). A critical look at methods for handling missing covariates in epidemiological regression analyses. *American Journal of Epidemiology, 142,* 1255–1264.

Jacobson, A. F., Hamilton, P., & Galloway, J. (1993). Obtaining and evaluating data sets for secondary analysis in nursing research. *Western Journal of Nursing Research, 15,* 483–494.

Kashner, T. M. (1998). Agreement between administrative files and written medical records: A case of the Department of Veterans Affairs. *Medical Care, 6,* 1324–1336.

Kneipp, S. M., & Yarandi, H. N. (2002). Complex sampling designs and statistical issues in secondary analysis. *Western Journal of Nursing Research, 24,* 552–566.

Kraft, M. R. (2003). Database research. *Science of Nursing, 20,* 43–44.

Landerman, L. R., Land, K. C., & Pieper, C. F. (1997). An empirical evaluation of the predictive mean matching method of imputing missing values. *Sociological Methods & Research, 26,* 3–33.

Last, M. (2001). *A dictionary of epidemiology* (4th ed.). New York: Oxford University Press.

Rotnitzky, A., & Wypij, D. (1994). A note on the bias of estimators with missing data. *Biometrics, 50,* 1163–1170.

Szabo, V., & Strang, V. R. (1997). Secondary analysis of qualitative data. *Advances in Nursing Science, 20,* 66–74.

Victora, C. G., Habicht, J., & Bryce, J. (2004). Evidence-based public health: Moving beyond randomized trials. *American Journal of Public Health, 94,* 400–405.

Longitudinal Research: Design and Analysis

Yow-Wu B. Wu • Kirsty Forsyth • Gary Kielhofner

Longitudinal research is useful for investigators who want to gain a detailed understanding of patterns of stability and change in occupational participation over time. It is also valuable for developing a coherent explanation of how and why the occupational change has occurred.

Longitudinal research involves collecting data over time using repeated measures and completing a longitudinal analysis of the data. Longitudinal research has focused on understanding people's engagement in activities of daily living and is, therefore, relevant to occupational therapists (Sonn, Grimby, & Svanborg, 1996; Spector & Takada, 1991).

The purpose of this chapter is to provide a basic understanding of the longitudinal study methodology (design and analysis), and opportunities for applying this approach in occupational therapy research. The chapter covers:

- What constitutes longitudinal research,
- Longitudinal research designs, and
- Selected techniques in analyzing longitudinal data.

This should be viewed as an introductory discussion of longitudinal research; only the basic concepts of designs and selected number of analytical techniques are discussed. Readers who are interested in more detailed discussions should consult materials in the Resources list.

> Spector and Takada (1991) describe an analysis based on 2,500 residents in 80 nursing homes in Rhode Island. Multivariate models were used to estimate which aspects of care were associated with resident outcomes after controlling for resident characteristics. Outcomes, measured over a 6-month period, included death, functional decline, and functional improvement. Results suggest that higher staff levels and lower staff turnover were related to functional improvement. Facilities with high catheter use, low rates of skin care, and low participation in organized activities were associated with negative outcomes. Facilities with few private-pay residents were also associated with negative outcomes.

are referred to as dependent variables. In some longitudinal designs, investigators make inferences about causal links between intervention variables and dependent variables related to time.

Since this type of research includes different designs and analytical methods, it is difficult to give a definition that applies to all situations. The aim of longitudinal research is to study the phenomena in terms of time-related constancy and change. For example, longitudinal research would be the method of choice if one wanted to know what happens to older persons' engagement in everyday activities over time after they enter a nursing home. An appropriate longitudinal design to answer this question could involve measuring the numbers of residents' everyday activity at admission, and at 1, 3, 6, 9, and 12 months after admission. The analysis of these data would focus on identifying change or stability of these everyday activity measures, and if data were collected on other variables, the study might also aim to identify what causes this change or stability.

> The defining characteristic of longitudinal research is that data are collected at multiple time points.

The Nature of Longitudinal Research

The defining characteristic of longitudinal research is that data are collected at multiple time points.

In longitudinal studies, the variables that are examined as to their stability or change over time

Intra-individual and Inter-individual Variability

Baltes and Nesselroade (1979) point out that longitudinal research is focused on studying both:

- Intra-individual differences (i.e., differences within each participant over time), and
- Inter-individual patterns (i.e., differences in the pattern of change or stability across participants in the study).

For example, consider a study in which the investigator collected information on the number of life roles a person reports every 6 months for 5 years starting from the age of 65 to 70. In such a study, the researcher would be interested in finding out whether there is a change in number of life roles across the 5 (65 to 70) years. This would be intra-individual change. The investigator would also want to know whether the patterns of these changes vary from person to person. This would be inter-individual change.

In the study just mentioned, the investigator would also likely want to know the reasons for any differences in the pattern of change between individuals. Keeves (1988) identified three major systems that affect the change and stability in human development:

- Biological factors,
- Environmental factors, and
- Planned learning or interventions.

With regard to the example, the pattern of life role change may vary from person to person because of biological factors such as whether or not the person had a chronic illness. Similarly, the pattern of life role change may differ because of different opportunities in participants' families and neighborhoods (environmental factors). Finally, differences in number of life roles may be due to whether the older adults participated in a lifestyle and wellness program offered by an occupational therapist (planned learning and intervention factors).

Types of Longitudinal Questions

According to Singer and Willett (2003), there are two types of questions that can be asked about change over time:

- Descriptive questions, and
- Questions that examine relationships between predictors and patterns of change.

Descriptive questions aim to characterize each individual's pattern of change over time. They might ask:

- What is the direction of the change? (e.g., increase or decrease in number of life roles over time?)
- Is the change linear or nonlinear? (e.g., do life roles decrease for a period and then plateau?)
- Is the change consistent or does it fluctuate from time to time? (e.g., are the number of life roles highly variable across time according to the health status of the person at the time of measurement?)

The following are examples of questions about the relationship between predictors and the pattern of change:

- Is the pattern of life role change predicted by the health status of the person?
- Do men and women show different patterns of change in life roles over time?

To answer this type of question, investigators would test hypotheses about the variables that account for differences in patterns of change over time.

Longitudinal Research Designs

All longitudinal research designs are characterized by the following two features:

- They must have a measure of time (i.e., observed change or stability in variables must be associated with time), and
- Observations must be made at more than two time points to identify the impact of time on trajectories.

Longitudinal research designs can vary as to whether the time intervals at which data are collected are fixed (i.e., every participant must be observed or interviewed at a fixed time point such as 3, 6, and 9 months) or flexible (i.e., data can be gathered at flexible time points). The advantage of flexible time points is, for example, that if a participant was supposed to be interviewed at 3 months and was quite ill at that time, the data can be gathered at either 3.5 or 4 months. Whether data are collected at fixed or flexible time points has implications for how the data can be analyzed (i.e., using fixed models vs. more flexible random or mixed models for analyzing data). Finally, an important consideration in all longitudinal designs is that in longitudinal research, missing data are inevitable.

Five Longitudinal Research Designs

Kessler and Greenberg (1981) identify five different types of longitudinal research designs:

- Simultaneous cross-sectional studies,
- Trend studies,
- Time series studies,
- Intervention studies, and
- Panel studies.

Each of these designs has its special focus in answering different types of questions. In this section, we briefly introduce these designs and discuss their strengths and weaknesses. We also address the questions that are associated with these designs.

Simultaneous Cross-Sectional Studies

In a simultaneous cross-sectional study, investigators collect data at one time point using samples of participants representing different age groups. The purpose of this design is to investigate whether there is an age group difference on certain variables. Notably, time in these studies is a function of the different ages of participants in each sample. Consequently, this design is unique among longitudinal designs in the way the investigator operationalizes the metric of time. Rather than collecting data across time, it collects data from samples that represent a span of time.

A researcher who plans to use this design needs to consider:

- How many participants are required in each group for the analysis, and
- How samples can be selected to represent a defined population.

In addition, there are also typical considerations about how to best sample in order to answer the substantive question. For example, consider an occupational therapy researcher who wishes to know if the amount of time spent in self-care activities is a function of age in persons 60 to 80 years old. There are two major factors to consider in this type of longitudinal study design. The first is how to determine the age group. For instance, should the investigator select the age groups by consecutive years, by every other year, or every 5 years? This is a substantive issue that must be determined by theory, previous research, or clinical evidence.

An investigator may decide to gather information every other year. Table 10.1 illustrates such a design. It is a typical simultaneous cross-sectional longitudinal design, in that all data are collected simultaneously from different samples, each of

Table 10.1 Simultaneous Cross-Sectional Study Layout

Different Age groups	Samples*	Data Collection Time
60	1	01/04
62	2	01/04
64	3	01/04
66	4	01/04
68	5	01/04
70	6	01/04
72	7	01/04
74	8	01/04
76	9	01/04
78	10	01/04
80	11	01/04

*Each different number represents a different sample set

which represents a different time point. The second factor is how to select representative samples from the specified age groups. This requires identification of the population from which the sample will be drawn. If the target population is all persons older than 65 years of age in the United Kingdom, then one might generate the sample from the government register of retired people.

If the intent of the study was to examine the impact of other variables, such as sex and race on time spent in self-care activities, then the sampling strategy might stratify the sample according to these variables. See Chapter 31 for a more in-depth discussion of stratification.

This type of design is based on the assumption that the chronological age is related to the dependent variable. The advantages of the simultaneous cross-sectional design are:

- It is easy and economical to execute because data are collected at one time point, and
- Environmental confounding factors are reduced because they are all measured at the same time.

The following are requirements of this type of design (Keeves, 1988):

- The age samples must be drawn from the same common population, and
- The influencing factors and their effects must remain constant across the time span during which the different age samples have been exposed to the factors.

If these requirements are not met, the findings will be confounded by other factors unrelated to age. For example, if the samples selected in 60-year-old group are predominantly African males, the 62-year-old group are predominantly white females and the 64-year-old group are predominantly Asian males and females, then the first assumption would not be met. If all the samples were drawn randomly from the same common population, one would expect sex and race to be equalized across the groups. With the kind of sample described above, the factors that influence the time spent in self-care activities could very well differ by race and sex. Therefore, any conclusion about the effect of aging on self-care activities would be misleading, since it is confounded by race and sex.

The primary weakness of this design is that it does not provide data on the change pattern of individual participants, since it does not follow individuals over time. If individual pattern of change is a major concern of the study question, this is not an appropriate design to use (Singer and Willett, 2003). Another weakness is that each time period is represented by a different sample; these samples may differ on characteristics other than age. Taking the preceding example, one would expect that not all those in the 60-year-old group are likely to live until 80. Thus, the sample of those who are 80 may differ from those in the 60-year-old age group who will not survive to 80 because of significant biological or other differences. Nonetheless, these potential differences are unknown.

A further weakness in this type of study is that the factors that impact the dependent variable may not be the same across different samples. Since we do not use the same participants at different times, caution must be taken if we assume the variable that has influenced the self-care activities will be the same across different times.

Trend Studies

In trend study designs, investigators collect data from samples of participants representing the same age group at different time points. Therefore, the pool of participants selected to represent each time point are different, although they are from the same age group. The purpose of this type of study is to examine trends in certain phenomenon as time progresses. For example, consider an investigator who wants to know whether the amount of time spent in leisure and in school work has changed in the decade from 1994 to 2003 for children ages 10 to 14 years old. In this case, the investigator would

Table 10.2 Trend Studies Layout

Age Group	Sample*	Data Collection Times
10–14	1	1994
10–14	2	1995
10–14	3	1996
10–14	4	1997
10–14	5	1998
10–14	6	1999
10–14	7	2000
10–14	8	2001
10–14	9	2002
10–14	10	2003

*Each different number represents a different sample set.

have to collect data spanning a 10-year period, selecting a sample of 10- to 14-year-olds that represent the target population for each time period. Thus, the participants would be different each time but their mean age would be the similar. Table 10.2 provides a layout of this design.

Investigators can use this type of design not only to describe the trend, but also to explain observed trends. For example, adolescents in public versus private schools could be sampled and the effects of type of school enrollment on leisure and schoolwork could be examined. Such a study might find, for instance, that in one of these groups study time increased while it remained constant in the other. In addition, this type of study can be used to examine the impact of historical variables on the trend. For example, the introduction of school testing during the 10-year period could be examined to see if it had an effect on the dependent variables.

The strength of this approach is that data for this type of study can be obtained either retrospectively (which is economical) or prospectively. A retrospective application of this design would require the investigator to sample persons who were 10 to 14 years of age during the targeted years. An obvious limitation of this type of design is that it asks subject to recall their leisure and school work involvement. Notably, the period since the behavior occurred will differ across the different year samples (e.g., the 2003 group would be asked to recall behavior of a year ago, while the 1995 group would be asked to recall what they did a decade earlier. A prospective application of this design would require the investigator to conduct the study over a 10-year period, sampling 10- to

14-year-olds each year. An obvious limitation of this design is the amount of time required.

A requirement of this design is that the environmental factors (with the exception of any that are measured) are the same across all different times. Otherwise, if there are unknown environmental factors, they might be confounded with the effect of time.

In addition to the limitations noted in the preceding paragraphs, the major limitation of the trend study design is that this type of design does not allow the investigator to explain any trends based on biological, environmental, or intervention variables (Keeves, 1988). One possible exception is the natural occurrence of an event in a prospective study that can be examined for its effect on the dependent variable.

Time Series and Intervention Studies

In time series studies, investigators collect data from the same participants at different time points. The purpose of this type of study is to observe the pattern of changes within (intra-individual) and across (inter-individual) individuals. Time series designs can be used both for nonexperimental situations and experimental purposes. The latter are intervention studies. A researcher who uses a time series design selects one or more sample(s) of participants and follows these participants, gathering data from time to time. Table 10.3 illustrates a time series study in which data are first collected from the subjects when they are age 45 and each year thereafter for a total of 10 years.

Table 10.3 **Time Series Study Layout**

Different Age Group	Sample*	Data Collection Times
45	1	1995
46	1	1996
47	1	1997
48	1	1998
49	1	1999
50	1	2000
51	1	2001
52	1	2002
53	1	2003
54	1	2004

*Numbers representing the sample are the same since data are collected from the same subjects each year.

The following are advantages of time series studies:

• This design can directly identify intra-individual constancy and change through time.
• It is possible to examine whether or not patterns over time (trends) are homogeneous across individuals.
• It is possible to examine relationship of change patterns to demographic and other variables (including experimental/intervention variables).
• It is possible to use advanced statistical techniques to make causal inferences (von Eye, 1985).

An example of a time series design that examines relationships between change patterns and demographic variables is a study of whether patterns of recovery following a stroke differ between sexes or between persons of different initial health status.

In time series studies, a researcher can also add intervention at a selected time point (Keeves, 1988). This can be used as a one group design, in which the researcher is interested in comparing the changes on the dependent variable before and after the intervention. The design can also be used with two or more groups. For example, both a one-group and a two-group time series design could be used to examine the impact of occupational therapy on people who have had a stroke. In a one-group time series design, persons with stroke could be measured for functional ability every month beginning in the 6th month post-stroke. An occupational therapy intervention could be offered to all the participants in a study following the 8th month observation and three more observations could be completed. This type of time series design follows the same logic as single-subject designs as discussed in Chapter 11. A two-group design might involve an occupational therapy intervention immediately following the stroke for one group that would be compared to a control group that did not receive the intervention or that received a control intervention. In this case, data might be collected on both groups at 6, 12, 18, and 24 months post-intervention. In this instance, the logic of the design is the same as control group designs, which are discussed in Chapter 7.

An important design consideration in time series studies is whether the sequence of observations is adequate to examine the process of change. In designing a study, one needs to consider both how long and how frequently it is necessary to gather data in order to capture the relevant trends in the dependent variable.

There are three shortcomings to using time series studies:

1. Repeated measurement can introduce a measurement effect (i.e., the act of collecting data once may influence the participant's score on the subsequent occasion of data collection.) For example, when the dependent variable is measured with a performance test, there may be practice effect (i.e., taking the test improves the ability being tested).
2. There is a greater tendency for missing data because of participant attrition.
3. Time series studies are costly.

Panel Studies

The term "panel" refers to a sample of participants involved in the context of a longitudinal study. Keeves (1998) described a panel study design as a series of different samples (panels) that are initiated at different times; data are collected from each sample at the same time intervals. The longitudinal panel study is often referred to as a multiple cohort design, since it investigates multiple cohorts on multiple occasions (Bijleveld et al., 1998). Figure 10.1 illustrates a panel study in which data are collected from six sets (panels) of subjects beginning at age 1 and every other year thereafter until age 9. As illustrated in the figure, the first cohort of participants begins in 1991 when children are age 1, and data are collected from this cohort every 2 years until 1999 when they are age 9. The second cohort starts from 1993 when they are 1 year of age and follows the same pattern of data collection until 2001. A total of six cohorts are included following this pattern. Close examination of Figure 10.1 shows that the diagonals under chronological age correspond to a trend design, each row corresponds to time series design, and each column corresponds to a cross-sectional design.

Panel studies ordinarily yield more information than trend and cross-sectional studies because the same groups of participants are measured repeatedly. In a time series study, observations are usually taken on a single entity at a relatively large number of time points. In a panel study, data are collected from many participants, but ordinarily at relatively fewer points in time than in a time series study (Markus, 1979).

In a panel study, investigators can examine the simultaneous influence of time, cohort (C), time of measurement (T), and age (A) (Schaie, 1965); these are noted on Figure 10.1. Consequently, a strength of this design is that researchers can explore many different factors that may influence the observed patterns in dependent variables. For example, a researcher is able to examine the interaction effects of A × C, A × T, and C × T. For example, A × C is used to examine if the pattern of change differs among six different dates of birth cohorts. It will answer the question of whether the growth pattern of 1990 is the same as the growth patterns of 1992, 1994....... and 2000. The A × T is used to examine if there is any difference among different age groups. For example, we can compare to see if year 1 versus year 3 makes any difference. The C × T is used to examine the differences among the same ages across different years of birth. The challenge of this design is that it is very time consuming, costly, and subject to high attrition rates. Unless there is a strong financial support, this design is not easy to implement. For example, one challenge of this design is to extend the length of the study sufficiently to differentiate cohort and age (Keeves, 1988).

Date of Birth (C)	Chronological age at time of measurement (A)									
1990	1	3	5	7	9					
1992		1	3	5	7	9				
1994			1	3	5	7	9			
1996				1	3	5	7	9		
1998					1	3	5	7	9	
2000						1	3	5	7	9
Time of Measurement (T)	'91	'93	'95	'97	'99	'01	'03	'05	'07	'09

Figure 10.1 Panel design showing ages of 5-year cohorts measured at 2-year intervals.

Summary

The previous sections discussed major longitudinal study designs. Each of these designs combines different approaches to sampling and to operationalizing time. Each has its own strengths and weaknesses. Table 10.4 summarizes these designs and their strengths and weaknesses.

Table 10.4. A Comparison of Longitudinal Study Designs

Design	Description	Strengths	Weaknesses
Simultaneous cross-sectional	Data are collected at one time point, using different samples of participants representing different age groups.	• Easy and economical to execute because there is only one time of data collection. • Environmental confounding factors are reduced since they are all measured at the same time.	• Does not provide data on the change pattern of individual subjects. • Each time period is represented by a different sample; samples may differ on characteristics other than age. • Factors that impact the dependent variable may not be the same across different cohorts.
Trend studies	Data are collected on samples of participants representing the same age group at different time points.	• Can be implemented either retrospectively (which is very economical), or prospectively.	• Does not allow explanation of trends based on biological, environmental, or intervention variables. • Prospective: requires substantial time. • Retrospective: can introduce bias due to differential recall requirements.
Time series studies	Data are collected from the same participants at different time points.	• Can directly identify intra-individual constancy and change through time and individuals serve as their own controls. • Can examine whether or not patterns over time (trends) are homogeneous across individuals. • Can examine relationship of change patterns to demographic and other variables (including experimental/intervention variables). • Can use advanced statistical techniques to make causal inferences.	• Repeated measurement can introduce a measurement effect. • There is a greater tendency for missing data due to participant attrition. • Time series studies are costly.
Panel studies	A series of different samples (panels) are initiated at different times; data are collected from each sample at the same time intervals.	• Can explore many different factors that may influence the observed patterns in dependent variables.	• Panel studies are very time consuming, costly, and subject to high attrition rates leading to missing data.

Statistical Analysis of Longitudinal Studies

Two primary functions in analyzing longitudinal data are:

- Descriptive and
- Explanatory.

Descriptive analysis is used to characterize the dependent variable at different time points and to identify patterns of the dependent variable over time. Explanatory analysis is used to explore the relationship of observed patterns with other variables. This section introduces selected analytical approaches for analyzing longitudinal data. For purposes of illustration, we use previously mentioned designs as examples for introducing different analytical techniques. Our discussion focuses only on continuous dependent variables, since those who are interested in analyzing dichotomous, categorical, or count-dependent variables in longitudinal data are referred to readings in the Resources list.

Analysis for Simultaneous Cross-sectional Studies

Consider the example of a researcher who wishes to know if the amount of time spent in self-care activities is a function of age in people 60 to 80 years old. In the study example provided in Table 10.1, the investigator collected data at one time point with 11 samples each of different age groups, each 2 years apart (60, 62, 64,...78, 80).

For descriptive analysis, this researcher would calculate the means and standard deviations for each of these 11 groups. The investigator could also make a line chart to examine if the amount of time spent in self-care activities has changed from age 60 to age 80. These analyses describe the data, but do not test whether the means are significantly different from each other.

The investigator can ask not only if there is any difference among these age groups in time spent in self-care, but also which age groups make the differences. Answers to these questions can be found by using a one-way analysis of variance (ANOVA) (as described in Chapter 17 with post hoc tests because in this design, independent samples represent each age group).

Analysis of Trend Studies

For trend analysis, the question to be answered by the analysis is whether time has any impact on the outcome for a specific age group.

Both descriptive statistics and explanatory statistics can be used to answer the research question of this design. Descriptive statistics present the means and standard deviations of each time measure and plot the findings. This visual presentation will demonstrate the impact of time on the outcome variable. Both ANOVA and regression analyses can be used to study the relationship between other variables and the trend.

Since this is not a within-subject design, there is no guarantee that the participants for the sample representing each year will be homogeneous. Therefore, the more heterogeneous participants' demographic characteristics are across samples, the more caution one must exercise in interpreting trends as due to time. Table 10.2 presents an example of a trend study in which children ages 10 to 14 years were sampled across a 10-year period to examine changes in time spent in leisure and schoolwork. If, in such a study, there was a substantially different composition of participants according to sex or race across the samples for each year represented, these differences might account for observed changes or be confounded with the influence of time.

Statistical Analysis for Time Series Studies

Time series studies are within subject designs, which mean that data are collected on each participant at more than one time point. In these designs, data from each time point are interrelated to data collected at other time points. For instance, a person's score on a functional measure at one time point in a time series study is likely to be correlated with subsequent scores and so on. Therefore, multilevel data analysis (sometimes called hierarchical linear models or mixed models) can be used for data analysis.

In multilevel data analysis for longitudinal data, each individual person will be used as a unit of analysis at the first level. Time is treated as a predictor to model the growth pattern of the dependent variable. Thus each individual will have an intercept and regression coefficient(s). The researcher can then study if these intercepts and regression coefficients vary among different individuals. If they do, the next step is to model these intercepts and regression coefficients to find out what factors contribute to these variations. We will demonstrate how to use this multilevel data analysis technique in the "Analytic Examples" section.

Statistical Analysis for Panel Studies

Panel data studies include both within and between designs, each participant is measured at at least more than two time points, and each participant belongs to one cohort. Usually, panel data studies have fewer numbers of time points than time series studies. In our example, each cohort has five time points in the panel study and there are ten time points in the time series study.

In panel studies, we can use either ANOVA with repeated measures, fixed model ANOVA, or multilevel data analysis. The choice depends on the researcher's focus of interests as well as how the data were collected. If the researcher is interested in comparing the differences among time points within the same cohort, ANOVA with repeated measures can be used to achieve the goal. If the interest is focusing on the pattern of changes among persons or groups, multilevel data analysis would be a better choice. Multilevel analysis is more flexible in terms of using random time intervals. For example, in ANOVA with repeated measures, the time intervals are fixed to all individuals; however, there is no such limitation for multilevel data analysis.

Analytical Example

The following example is based on a fictitious data set. We assumed that 20 participants were randomly assigned to an experimental group and 20 to a control group. The participants in the experimental group received an intervention treatment that is designed to enhance clients' communication and interaction skills. Each participant's skills were measured four times by observation using the Assessment of Communication and Interaction Skills (ACIS) (Forsyth, Lai, & Kielhofner, 1999; Forsyth, Salamy, Simon, & Kielhofner, 1998), before intervention (initial) and 3 months, 6.5 months, and 12 months after intervention. The

One example of a study that utilized a repeated-measures design is a follow-up study of long-term quality of life outcomes for individuals with chronic fatigue syndrome (Taylor, Thanawala, Shiraishi, & Schoeny, in press). Researchers used a within-subjects, repeated-measures cohort design to evaluate the long-term effects of an integrative rehabilitation program. Twenty-three participants with chronic fatigue syndrome attended eight sessions of an illness-management group followed by 7 months of individualized peer counseling that took place once per week for 30 minutes. Quality of life was measured five times (i.e., at baseline, following the group phase, following the one-on-one phase, and 4 and 12 months following program completion). A within-subjects repeated measures ANOVA revealed significant increases in overall quality of life for up to 1 year following program completion ($F (4, 21) = 23.5, p < 0.001$). Although definitive conclusions about program efficacy were limited by the lack of follow-up data on a control group (necessitating a within-subjects design), findings suggested that the program may have led to improvement in quality of life for up to 1 year following program completion.

patterns of changes are presented in Figures 10.2 and 10.3.

Figure 10.2 presents the ACIS measures of 20 participants in the experimental group. The majority of participants have lower measures on the initial ACIS, and they have a significant improvement 3 months later, except two participants whose measures drop from initial to 3 months. Almost all (except one) subjects had a small drop from 3 to 6.5 months and later on. Communication and interaction skills stabilized between 6.5 and 12 months,

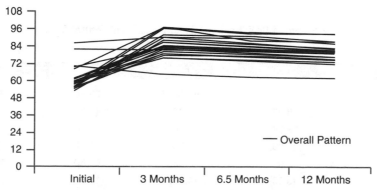

Figure 10.2 Communication and interaction skill scores for the experimental group.

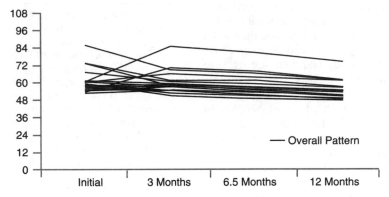

Figure 10.3 Communication and interaction skill scores for the control group.

as there are no obvious changes between these two time points.

In the control group (see Figure 10.3), four participants significantly dropped from initial to 3 months. Three participants showed major improvements from initial to 3 months. Other participants stayed about the same from baseline to 12 months. Approximately four to five participants in each group had very different initial ACIS measures when compared to the remaining group members. These people also showed a different pattern of change compared to the remaining members of the group. Descriptive statistics for these two groups are presented in Table 10.5.

ANOVA with Repeated Measures

We will demonstrate the ANOVA with repeated measures approach because it is a frequently used method in analyzing longitudinal data. Basic concepts of ANOVA are covered in Chapter 17, so we will not repeat them here. In our interaction and communication intervention example, the dependent variable is collected at four different timepoints. Since time is a factor nested within each individual, it is called a *within*-subject factor. Whether or not the participants received the occupational therapy intervention is called a *between*-subjects factor. Consequently, this is a one within-factor and one between-factor ANOVA with repeated measures design. Three major questions can be asked by this analysis:

1. Is there a time effect on participants' ACIS measures? This question asks whether there is a difference on the ACIS measure at the four different time points, regardless of whether the participant received the intervention.
2. Is there a group mean difference (average of four time points) on ACIS measures between experimental and control groups?
3. Is there an interaction effect between time and intervention?

Usually, the second question is not important to a researcher in a longitudinal study because the investigator is more interested in the time effect and interaction effect between time and intervention. It is more useful to know if the intervention

Table 10.5 ACIS Means and Standard Deviations for Experimental and Control Group at Four Different Times

	Initial	3 Months	6.5 Months	12 Months
Experimental	60.06	81.84	79.20	76.80
	(8.88)	(7.92)	(7.32)	(7.20)
Control	59.94	58.26	55.80	52.98
	(7.86)	(7.56)	(7.32)	(6.12)
Overall	60.00	70.08	67.50	64.86
	(8.28)	(14.16)	(13.86)	(13.74)

Numbers in parentheses are standard deviations.

resulted in a difference of communication skills over time. If the interaction effect is significant, it means we cannot conclude (as would be stated in the null hypothesis) that the pattern of change is the same between experimental and control groups.

Results of this hypothetical study show that the time factor and intervention factor have an interaction effect on the ACIS measures because the patterns of change between intervention and control groups are different (see Figure 10.2). The experimental group showed an increase in communication skills after receiving the intervention and then declined slightly before stabilizing. In contrast, the control group (see Figure 10.3) that did not receive the intervention showed an overall decline in communication skills over time.

As shown in Table 10.5, before the intervention, the ACIS measures do not differ significantly between experimental and control groups. Three months after the intervention, the ACIS measures of the experimental group are significantly improved; however, the control group decreases slightly compared to its initial ACIS measure. Both groups have shown a similar stable rate of decreasing from 3 months on.

ANOVA results shown in Table 10.6 indicated that both a time effect (initial to 3 months, 3 months to 6.5 months, and 6.5 months to 12 months, $p < .001$), and a time and intervention interaction effect (initial to 3 months, $p < .01$) exist. The interaction effect exists only at the initial and 3-month data collection points and is not significant for the remaining data collection points.

Multilevel Data Analysis

Multilevel data analysis uses a different approach to analyzing longitudinal data from that of the traditional ANOVA with repeated measures. The multilevel analysis approach focuses on the changes of the trajectories instead of comparing the mean differences across time points. Multilevel longitudinal data analysis is based on the concept that there is a relationship between the time factor and the outcome variable and that this relationship can be either linear or nonlinear. This relationship is reflected by a rate of change that indicates the relationship between the outcome variable and time. The rate of change may differ from person to person, and multilevel analysis uses this rate of change as a dependent variable, and further explores what factors have a relationship with this rate of change.

The researcher can examine variations within and between individuals. There are three advantages of using this approach:

1. This approach has less stringent restrictions concerning the characteristics of data being analyzed, compared to univariate ANOVA with repeated measures. For example, the time interval is not required to be fixed, which means that a subject does not have to be measured at certain fixed time points.
2. The parameter estimations are more precise because of using more advanced estimating methods.
3. Missing data in first level are not an obstacle of using this approach.

By examining the four time points in the ACIS data example, we find a trend that the relationship between time and the ACIS score for experimental group is not merely a straight line (linear model), but the trend of ACIS has one bend. This is the reason why we add a quadratic component in the regression model and treat it as a nonlinear model. In the experimental group, the improvement is dramatic from initial to 3 months, then it drops slowly

Table 10.6 Findings on ANOVA with Repeated Measures Testing Within-Subjects' Contrasts

		SS	df	MS	F	p
Time	Initial–3 months	4,052.16	1		34.3	<.001
	3 months–6.5 months	261.90	1		129.4	<.001
	6.5 months–12 months	280.44	1		157.4	<.001
Time × Group	Initial–3 months	5,498.09	1		46.5	<.001
	3 months–6.5 months	.40	1		.2	.657
	6.5 months–12 months	1.90	1		1.1	.309
Error	Initial–3 months	4,490.64	38	118.17		
	3 months–6.5 months	76.68	38	2.02		
	6.5 months–12 months	67.68	38	1.78		

Table 10.7 **Final Estimation of Fixed Effects and Variance Components**

Fixed Effect	Coefficient	Standard Error	t-ratio	Approximate df	p-value
Final estimation of fixed effects:					
Status around 6 month					
Control	56.64	1.72	32.95	38	<.001
Exp−Control	25.54	2.49	10.24	38	<.001
Linear slope					
Control	−.60	.17	−3.45	38	0.002
Exp−Control	2.21	.30	7.45	38	<.001
Quadratic slope					
Control	.006	.04	0.16	38	0.871
Exp−Control	−.39	.06	−6.86	38	<.001

Final estimation of variance components:

Random Effect	Standard Deviation	Variance Component	df	Chi-square	p-value
Status around 6 months	7.45	55.57	38	182.28	<.001
Linear slope	.80	.64	38	110.42	<.001
Quadratic slope	.16	.02	38	62.43	0.008
Level 1	4.62	21.31			

from 3 months to 12 months. In the control group, several people dropped very fast from initial to 3 months; other ACIS scores were stable from initial to 3 months, and then dropped at a minimal but consistent rate. Based on this information, it is more appropriate to model the growth trajectories in a nonlinear fashion.

This involves estimating each person's communication status at around 6 months after beginning this study (referred to as the intercept), linear term of growth (expressed as positive or negative regression coefficient), and quadratic term of growth (expressed as an accelerating or deaccelerating regression coefficient). These estimated values of the intercept, regression coefficient for the linear term, and regression coefficient for the quadratic term are then used as dependent variables to compare the difference between experimental and control groups on second-level data analysis.[1]

In multilevel longitudinal data analysis, one first models the growth trajectories in the first-level

data analysis. The estimated components in this level data analysis include:

• The intercept, and
• The regression coefficients related to linear and nonlinear (quadratic, cubic, or other types) components.

Each participant will have an intercept, a regression coefficient for the linear part, and a quadratic part in our example. If the pattern of change is a straight line, then we do not need to model the quadratic component. The second step of analysis is to treat these three estimated variables (intercept, regression coefficients for linear and quadratic components) as three dependent variables in the second-level analysis. We then use coded variables to indicate if the participant belongs to the experimental or control group as a predictor.

Based on the aforementioned logic, we will be able to obtain the following information in Table 10.7. The communication skill measure, around 6 months of the study, for the control group is 56.64 and for the experimental group is 25.54 higher than for the control group. The linear growth trajectories for the control group is decreasing by .60 per month; however, for the experimental group it increases 1.61 (2.21−.60) per month. The differ-

[1]Multilevel data analysis is also known as mixed effects models. There are different software programs that can be used to analyze such data, among them, the most frequently used are Hierarchical Linear Models (HLM), ML-Win (Multi-level and SAS for Windows). This example is based on the results of HLM.

ence between the control and experimental groups is significantly different ($p < .001$). For the control group, the quadratic slope is .006, which is not significantly different from 0. This means that for the control group the communication skill decreasing rate is kept consistent from month to month. For the experimental group, the communication skill measure improves at beginning. However, when time progresses, this growth rate slows down by $-.38$ ($-.39 + .006$) per month. The differences of quadratic slopes between experimental and control groups are also statistically significant ($p < .001$).

By examining the lower part of Table 10.7, we found that the residual variances of the second level three variables (intercept, regression coefficients for linear and quadratic components) are still significantly different from 0 after we model the intervention variable. This means that the researcher can still explore other predictors in addition to the intervention to explain the variations among individuals, such as if sex or age make a difference or not.

Conclusion

This chapter introduced longitudinal methods. We noted that longitudinal research involves different designs and analytical techniques. Since each design has its purpose, strengths, and weaknesses, researchers need to know specifically what they want to study to determine the most appropriate design and analytical technique to use.

REFERENCES

Baltes, P. B., & Nesselroade, J. R. (1979). History and rationale of longitudinal research. In J. R. Nesselroade, & P.B. Baltes (Eds.), *Longitudinal research in the study of behavior and development*. New York: Academic Press.

Bijleveld, C. C. J. H., van der Kamp, L. J. Th., Mooijaart, A., van der Kloot, W. A., van der Leeden, R., & van der Burg, E. (1998). *Longitudinal data analysis: Designs, models and methods*. London: SAGE Publications.

Forsyth, K., Lai, J., & Kielhofner, G. (1999). The assessment of communication and interaction skills (ACIS): Measurement properties. *British Journal of Occupational Therapy, 62*(2), 69–74.

Forsyth, K., Salamy, M., Simon, S., Kielhofner, G. (1998). *A user's guide to the assessment of communication and interaction skills (ACIS)*. Bethesda: The American Occupational Therapy Association.

Keeves, J. P. (1988). Longitudinal research methods. In J. P. Keeves (Ed.), *Educational research, methodology, and measurement: An international handbook*. Oxford: Pergamon Press.

Kessler, R. C., & Greenberg, D. F. (1981). *Linear panel analysis: Models of quantitative change*. New York: Academic Press.

Markus, G. B. (1979). *Analyzing panel data*. London: Sage.

Schaie, K. W. (1965). A general model for the study of developmental problems. *Psychological Bulletin, 64*, 92–107.

Singer, J. D., & Willett, J. B. (2003). *Applied longitudinal data analysis: Modeling change and event occurrence*. New York: Oxford University Press.

Sonn, U., Grimby, G., & Svanborg, A. (1996). Activities of daily living studies longitudinally between 70 and 76 years of age. *Disability and Rehabilitation, 18*(2), 91–100.

Spector, W. D., & Takada, H. A. (1991). Characteristics of nursing homes that affect resident outcomes. *Journal of Aging and Health, 3*(4), 427–454.

Taylor, R. R., Thanawala, S. G., Shiraishi, Y., & Schoeny, M. E. (In press). Long-term outcomes of an integrative rehabilitation program on quality of life: A follow-up. *Journal of Psychosomatic Research*.

von Eye, A. (1985). Longitudinal research methods. In T. Huaén & T. N. Postlethwaite, (Eds.), *The international encyclopedia of education* (Vol. 5, pp. 3140–3152). Oxford and New York: Pergamon.

RESOURCES

For Longitudinal Designs
Menard, S. (2002). *Longitudinal research*. Thousand Oaks, CA: SAGE Publications.

Ruspini, E. (2002). *Introduction to longitudinal research*. London: Routledge.

Schulsinger, F., Mednick, S. A., & Knop, J. (1981) (Ed). *Longitudinal research: Methods and uses in behavioral science*. Boston: Martinus Nijhoff.

For Longitudinal Analysis
Lindsey, J. K. (1993). *Models for repeated measurements*. Oxford and New York: Oxford University Press..

Little, T. D., Schnabel, K. U., & Baumert, J. (2000). *Modeling longitudinal and multilevel data: Practical issues, applied approaches, and specific examples*. Mahwah, NJ: Lawrence Erlbaum.

For Web sites of longitudinal studies: Ruspini (2002).

Panel design
Hsiao, C. (1986). *Analysis of panel data*. New York: Cambridge University Press.

CHAPTER 11

Single-Subject Research

Jean Crosetto Deitz

A therapist working in a technology center wanted to know if her client, an individual with a high-level spinal cord injury, would be more successful in terms of text entry using system A as opposed to system B. A second therapist, working with four individuals who were institutionalized with chronic depression, wanted to know if these individuals would initiate conversation more in their group therapy session if it followed a pet therapy session. These are the types of questions that therapists continually ask, and both of these questions can be addressed using single-subject research methods. According to Backman, Harris, Chisholm, and Monette (1997), these methods "can inform and illuminate clinical practice" and "provide concrete data to validate existing theories in rehabilitation as well as formulate new ones" (p. 1143).

> Single-subject research methods are useful for answering questions regarding the effectiveness of specific interventions for specific individuals by providing experimental control and by contributing to clear and precise clinical documentation.

Single-subject research, sometimes referred to as single-system research, is based on within-subject performance, with the unit of study being one person or a single group that is considered collectively. Each participant serves as his or her own control and there are repeated measurements over time of the same dependent variable or variables. Also, while other factors are held constant, there is systematic application, withdrawal, and sometimes variation of the intervention (independent variable).

Single-subject research methods are useful for answering questions regarding the effectiveness of specific interventions for specific individuals by providing experimental control and by contributing to clear and precise clinical documentation. They are especially suited to occupational therapy research because groups of persons with similar characteristics are not required, and thus these methods are appropriate for use when the therapist has one, or at most, a few clients with whom a particular intervention is employed, or in situations in which the therapist is working with an individual with a low-incidence diagnosis or impairment. A further advantage of single-subject research is that it does not require the withholding of treatment from a no-treatment control group. Because each participant serves as his or her own control, the treatment typically is withheld from the participant for one or more periods of time and then it is instituted or reinstituted. Also, because only one or a small number of individuals are studied, the financial and time demands are realistic for practice settings. Even though only one or a small number of individuals are studied, the findings from single-subject research can be used to inform practice and to justify and inform larger scale investigations (Ottenbacher, 1990). Information learned in the process of single-subject research can be used in designing more costly group experimental studies involving numerous participants and multiple sites.

Common Single-Subject Research Designs

A simple notation system is used for single-subject research designs where *A* represents baseline; *B* represents the intervention phase; and *C* and all other letters represent additional interventions or conditions.

The *A–B* Design and Variations

The design upon which all others are built is the *A–B* design, where *A* indicates a baseline phase and *B* indicates a treatment (or intervention) phase. This can be exemplified by looking at both the first baseline phase (*A*) and the treatment phase (*B*) in Figure 11.2 in the feature box for the therapy ball study. This displays the data for Emily for percentage of intervals seated. The vertical axis of the graph indicates the percentage of intervals seated and the horizontal axis indicates the days. During the first baseline phase (*A*), Emily experienced 12 days of sitting on classroom chairs as usual and data were systematically kept on percentage of intervals seated. Note that Emily's percentages of intervals seated were consistently below 60%. Following the novelty week, phase *B* (intervention) was started and Emily used the therapy ball

for seating during language arts. Note that the percentage of intervals seated increased substantially during the treatment phase. If the study had stopped after data were collected for only a baseline phase and an intervention phase, this would have been an *A–B* design.

A common variation of the *A–B* design is the *A–B–C* successive intervention design. With this design, a second intervention is introduced in the *C* phase. For example, the therapist studying the

The Therapy Ball Study

Example of a Single-Subject Research Study Designed to Answer a Practice Question

An interdisciplinary group wanted to know if the use of therapy balls as classroom seating devices affected the behavior of students with attention deficit hyperactivity disorder (ADHD) (Schilling, Washington, Billingsley, & Deitz, 2003). Their first research question was, "What effect does using therapy balls as chairs have on in-seat behavior?" (Schilling et al., 2003, p. 535). The convenience sample for the study consisted of three children (two males and one female) with ADHD and average intelligence. The three children were from the same fourth-grade public school classroom and, during language arts, all demonstrated out-of-seat behavior requiring repeated teacher verbal and/or physical prompts.

The dependent variable, "in-seat behavior," was measured whereby following each 10-second observation a rater scored the participant's behavior as either "out-of-seat" or "in-seat" (Schilling et al., 2003). Each participant was observed for five 2-minute periods during language arts, for a total of 60 observations per session. Data systematically were collected for "in-seat behavior" for each of the participants individually. During language arts, the three participants and all other class members experienced (1) a series of days during which chairs were used for seating (first baseline phase); (2) a 1-week novelty period during which balls were used for seating; (3) a series of days during which balls were used for seating (first intervention phase); (4) a series of days during which chairs were used for seating (second baseline phase); and (5) last, a series of days during which balls were used for seating (second intervention phase). Throughout the study, efforts were made to hold all factors constant that could potentially have influenced the results of the study. For example, the teacher was the same each day, data were collected at the same time each day, and, throughout the duration of the study, each

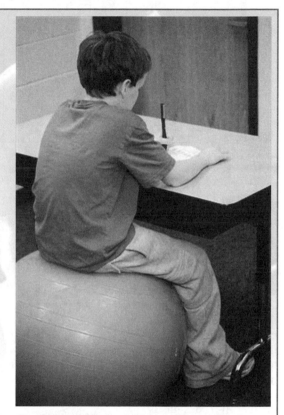

Figure 11.1 A study participant is observed working while using a therapy ball as a chair.

participant's medication for ADHD was held constant in terms of type and dosage.

Throughout all baseline and intervention phases, even though all of the children in the classroom participated in the intervention, data were collected only for the three children with ADHD. Data were graphed and examined for each of the three participants individually. Refer to Figure 11.2 for an example of graphed data for percentage of intervals seated for Emily (pseudonym).

(continued)

The Therapy Ball Study (continued)

The data indicates that Emily was "in-seat" a higher percentage of intervals when using the therapy ball for seating during language arts than when using a chair for seating. For Emily, confidence in the effect of the intervention is supported since her "in-seat behavior" increased immediately following institution of the intervention, dropped markedly when the intervention was removed, and again increased when the intervention was reinstituted. The graphs for the other two participants were similar to the graph depicted in Figure 11.2, thus providing additional support for the use of therapy balls for classroom seating for fourth-grade students with ADHD. Studies such as the one just described support evidence-based practice.

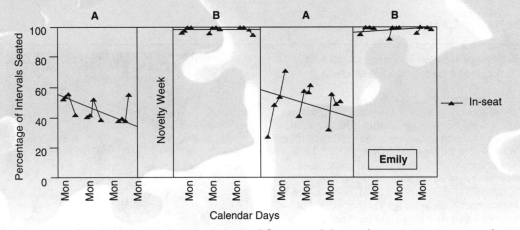

Figure 11.2 Graph of Emily's "in-seat behavior." Connected data points represent consecutive days within the same week. Variability in the number of data points was the result of a non-school day or absence from class. (Copyright 2003 by the American Occupational Therapy Association, Inc., Reprinted with permission.)

effects of the alternative seating devices might have chosen to introduce the ball for seating in the B phase and an air cushion for seating in the C phase in an attempt to see if one device was more effective than the other. Another variation of the A–B design is the A–B–C changing-criterion design, which is characterized by having three or more phases with the criterion for success changing sequentially from one intervention phase to the next. This design is suited to interventions that are modified in a stepwise manner since the criterion for success is changed incrementally with each successive intervention phase (Hartmann & Hall, 1976). It is appropriate for situations

> Multiple-baseline designs require repeated measures of at least three baseline conditions that typically are implemented concurrently with each successive baseline being longer than the previous one. Multiple-baseline designs can be (a) across behaviors; (b) across participants; or (c) across settings.

in which the goal is stepwise increases in accuracy (e.g., quality of letters written), frequency (e.g., number of repetitions completed), duration (e.g., length of exercise session), latency (e.g., time it takes to begin to respond after a question is asked), and magnitude (e.g., pounds of weight lifted) (Hartmann & Hall, 1976). Consider a client who seldom or never exercises and is enrolled in a health promotion program because of health concerns. The baseline phase (A) might involve recording the number of continuous minutes the individual walks on a treadmill at 1.5 miles per hour. During the first intervention phase (B) the criterion for success might be 30 continuous minutes of treadmill walking at 1.5 miles per hour; during the second intervention phase (*C*) the criterion for success might be 30 continuous minutes of treadmill walking at 2.0 miles per hour; and during the third intervention phase (*D*) the criterion for success might be 30 continuous minutes of treadmill walking at 2.5 miles per hour. This could continue until the desired rate of walking was achieved. The changing criterion design also is useful in situations in which stepwise decreases in specific behaviors are desired.

With both the *A–B* and *A–B–C* designs, no causal statements can be made. In the therapy ball study, if data had been collected only for an initial baseline phase and a treatment phase (see Figure 11.2 located in the feature box on the therapy ball study), the therapist would not have known if some factor other than the introduction of the therapy ball for classroom seating resulted in Emily's increase in "in-seat behavior." For example, at the beginning of the intervention phase, the language arts assignments might have changed to a topic of greater interest to Emily and that change, rather than the therapy ball, might have influenced Emily's "in-seat behavior." Therefore, this design is subject to threats to internal validity.

Withdrawal Designs

The *A–B–A* or withdrawal design has stronger internal validity than the *A–B* and *A–B–C* designs. This design consists of a minimum of three phases: baseline (*A*), intervention (*B*), and baseline (*A*) or conversely *B–A–B*. However, it can extend to include more phases, with the *A–B–A–B* being one of the most common. The latter has ethical appeal in situations in which the intervention is effective since you do not end by withdrawing the intervention. Withdrawal designs are exemplified by the therapy ball study in which the therapy ball for seating was removed after the intervention phase and data were again collected under baseline conditions and then the intervention was reinstituted (see Figure 11.2 in the therapy ball study featured earlier in this chapter). Because this design involves a return to baseline, it is most appropriate for behaviors that are reversible (likely to return to the original baseline levels when intervention is withdrawn). This is a true experimental design in the sense that causal inferences can be made related to the participant or participants studied. For example, in the therapy ball study, because the percentage of "in-seat behavior" increased during the intervention phase and then returned to the original baseline levels during the second baseline phase and then increased when the intervention was reinstituted, it is possible to say that the use of

the therapy ball likely resulted in an increase in "in-seat behavior" for Emily during language arts.

Multiple-Baseline Designs

Multiple-baseline designs, the next category of designs, require repeated measures of at least three baseline conditions that typically are implemented concurrently with each successive baseline being longer than the previous one. Multiple-baseline designs can be (a) across behaviors; (b) across participants; or (c) across settings.

Multiple-Baseline Design Across Behaviors

In a multiple-baseline design across behaviors, the same treatment variable is applied sequentially to separate behaviors in a single participant. Consider the hypothetical example of an adult with dementia who frequently displays three antisocial behaviors: swearing, door slamming, and screaming. The therapist is interested in knowing whether or not her intervention is successful in reducing or eliminating the frequency of occurrence of these behaviors. For 5 days, during a 2-hour socialization group the researcher collects baseline data on these behaviors, making no change in intervention (Figure 11.3 on p. 144). On the sixth day, the researcher introduces the intervention, thus starting the treatment phase (*B*) for the first behavior (swearing). The researcher makes no change in the treatment program for door slamming and screaming. These two behaviors remain in baseline (*A*). After 10 days the researcher initiates the same intervention for door slamming, and, after 15 days, she initiates this same intervention for screaming. If the researcher can demonstrate a change across all three behaviors following the institution of the intervention, this provides support for the effectiveness of the intervention in decreasing antisocial behaviors in the adult studied. This exemplifies a multiple-baseline design across behaviors.

Multiple-Baseline Design Across Participants

With a multiple-baseline design across participants, one behavior is treated sequentially across matched participants. For example, if you had three men with limited grip strength, you might institute a specific intervention for the first on the 8th day, for the second on the 16th day, and for the third on the 26th day. Figure 11.4 on p. 145 displays hypothetical data for such a study.

A variation of the multiple-baseline design across participants is the nonconcurrent multiple-

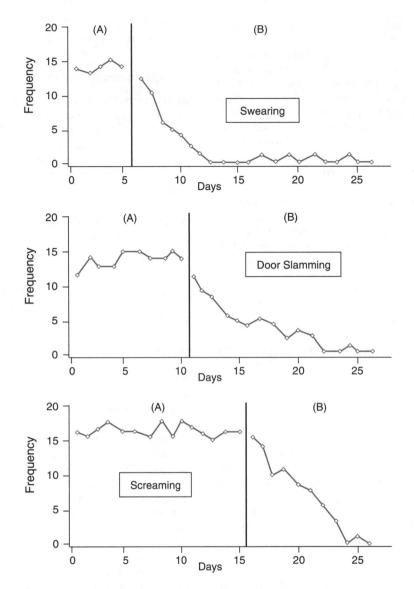

Figure 11.3 Multiple-baseline design across behaviors—example of graphed data.

baseline design across individuals (Watson & Workman, 1981), whereby different individuals are studied at different times, a feature that makes it ideal for clinical settings where it often is impractical to start multiple clients in a study simultaneously. With this design, the researcher predetermines baseline lengths and randomly assigns these to participants as they become available. For example, in a nonconcurrent multiple baseline design across three individuals, the researcher might choose baseline lengths of 6 days, 10 days, and 13 days. The first participant might start the study on April 1st, the second might start on April 13th, and the last might start on April 26th. For

each of the three participants, the researcher would randomly select without replacement one of the baseline lengths. See Figure 11.5 on p. 146 for a graphic display of hypothetical data. Since baseline data collection typically is continued until a stable pattern emerges, Watson and Workman (1981) recommend dropping a participant if his or her baseline data do not achieve stability within the predetermined time for the participant's baseline. Because each of the participants in a nonconcurrent multiple baseline study starts the intervention at a different randomly determined time, some control is provided for other variables that could result in desired changes in the target behavior.

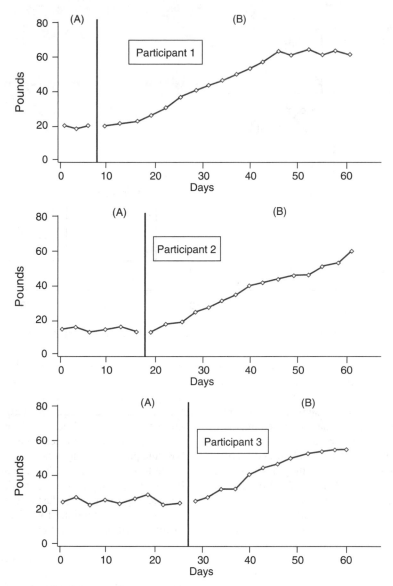

Figure 11.4 Multiple-baseline design across participants—example of graphed data.

Multiple-Baseline Design Across Settings

With a multiple-baseline design across settings, the same behavior or behaviors are studied in several independent settings. Consider the child with an autism spectrum disorder who is in an inclusive school setting. This child repeatedly interrupts. He does this in the classroom, in the cafeteria, and on the playground. The therapist collects baseline data in all three settings for 5 days. Then, she tries an intervention in the classroom (the first setting), while simultaneously continuing to collect base-line data in the other two settings. After 3 more days, she introduces the intervention in the second setting (the cafeteria), while continuing to collect baseline data in the third setting. Last, after 3 more days, she introduces the intervention in the third setting (the playground). Refer to Figure 11.6 on p. 147 for a graph of hypothetical data.

With multiple-baseline designs, intervention effectiveness is demonstrated if a desired change in level, trend, or variability occurs only when the intervention is introduced. In addition, the change in performance should be maintained throughout the intervention phase.

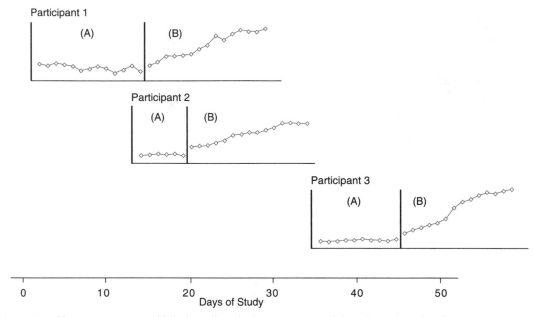

Figure 11.5 Nonconcurrent multiple-baseline design across participants—example of graphed data.

Multiple-baseline designs have three major strengths. The first relates to internal validity. Because the intervention is started at a different time for each individual, behavior, or setting, these designs help to rule out the internal validity threat of history as described by Campbell and Stanley (1963). For more detail regarding internal and external validity, refer to Chapter 7. Also, because results of research using these designs can show that change is effected in multiple individuals, behaviors, or settings, support is provided for the demonstration of causal relationships. The second strength of multiple-baseline designs is that they require no reversal or withdrawal of the intervention, a characteristic that makes them appealing and practical for research when discontinuing therapy is contraindicated. The third strength of multiple-baseline designs is that they are useful when behaviors are not likely to be reversible. Often, therapists expect that an intervention will cause a difference that will be maintained even when the intervention is withdrawn. For example, once a therapist has taught a client who has had a spinal cord injury to dress independently, the therapist expects the client will be able to dress independently, even when therapy is withdrawn. This makes it inappropriate to use the withdrawal design discussed earlier, because with this design, intervention effectiveness is demonstrated when the behavior returns to the original baseline level following withdrawal of the intervention.

The primary weakness of multiple-baseline designs is that they require more data collection time because of the staggered starting times for the intervention phases. Because of this, some behaviors or participants are required to remain in the baseline phase for long periods of time, which may prove to be problematic. For example, in the first hypothetical study involving an adult with dementia (see Figure 11.3), the last behavior (screaming) was allowed to continue for 15 days prior to the institution of the intervention.

Alternating-Treatments Design

The alternating-treatments design and/or minor variations of it also have been termed the multi-element baseline design, the randomization design, and the multiple schedule design (Barlow & Hayes, 1979). These designs can be used to compare the effects of intervention and no intervention, or they can be used to compare the effects of two or more distinct interventions. This can extend to comparing the effectiveness of two or more different therapists or the effectiveness of providing a specific intervention at one time of day versus another. In all cases, these designs involve the fast alternation of two or more different interventions or conditions. Though they typically have a baseline phase, it is not essential. These designs are not appropriate when behavior is expected to take time to change, when effects are expected to

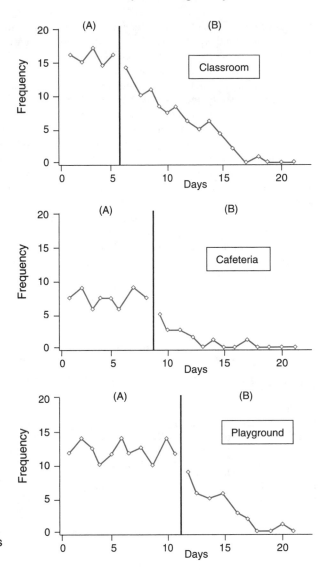

Figure 11.6 Multiple-baseline design across settings—example of graphed data.

be cumulative, or when multiple treatment inter-ference (described in Chapter 7) is anticipated.

Alternating-treatments designs are useful in sit-uations when change is expected in the dependent variable over time because of factors such as a dis-ease process (e.g., rheumatoid arthritis) or a natu-ral recovery process (e.g., strokes, burns). With other designs, such factors could result in changes in the dependent variable that could compromise interpretation of study results. However, with the alternating-treatments design, effects from these changes largely are controlled because each inter-vention is instituted within a short period of time, typically 1 or 2 days. See the feature box titled Example (Hypothetical) Study Using an Alternating-Treatments Design to further illustrate the use of this design.

Because alternating-treatments designs require interventions that will produce immediate and dis-tinct changes in behavior, they are suited to inde-pendent variables that can be instituted and removed quickly and whose effects typically are immediate. Thus, they are suited to studying the effects of independent variables such as splints, orthoses, positioning devices, and assistive tech-nology. This design also has been used when studying the effects of interventions on dependent variables such as self-report measures, overt behavior exhibited during specific interventions, and exercise repetitions. For example, Melchert-McKearnan, Deitz, Engel, and White (2000) stud-ied the effects of play activities versus rote exercise for children during the acute phase fol-lowing burn injuries. Outcome measures were number of repetitions of therapeutic exercise completed, number and type of overt distress behaviors displayed, scores on self-report scales of pain intensity, and self-report of overall enjoyment of the activity. The alternating-treatments design was chosen for this study because it was expected that there would be changes in the children as a result of the recovery process and it was expected that the effect of the intervention on each of the outcome variables would be immediate.

The alternating-treatments design has three primary strengths. First, it does not require a lengthy withdrawal of the intervention, which may result in a reversal of therapeutic gain. Second, it often requires less time for a comparison to be made because a second baseline is not required. Third, with this design, it is possible to proceed without a formal baseline phase. This is useful in situations where there is no practical or meaningful baseline

condition or where ethically it is difficult to justify baseline data collection.

The primary weakness of the alternating-treatments design stems from its vulnerability to a validity threat relating to the influence of an intervention on an adjacent intervention (multiple treatment interference). As a partial control for this threat, all variables that could potentially influence the results of the study should be counterbalanced. For example, if a therapist was trying to determine which of two electric feeders was best for his client relative to time to complete a meal, and feeder A always was used at lunch and feeder B always was used at dinner, it might be that the client did more poorly with feeder B because he strained his neck when using feeder A at lunch and this influenced his use of feeder B. Randomizing the order of use of the feeders, though it would not eliminate order effects, would allow for order

Example (Hypothetical) Study Using an Alternating-Treatments Design

A woman's productivity on an assembly line is compromised because of arthritis. The therapist wants to know if use of a specific splint will result in an increase in productivity. The independent variable is the splint and the dependent variable is the number of assembly units completed per hour. See Figure 11.7 for a graph of hypothetical data, noting that data for both the intervention and non-intervention conditions are plotted on the same graph.

During the first phase of the study, baseline data on the number of assembly units completed

per hour were collected for five sessions. The woman did not wear the splint during this phase. Phase 2 began after the woman wore the splint for a 1-week accommodation period. During the 16 days of phase 2, the order of the two conditions (with and without splint) was counterbalanced by random assignment without replacement. Therefore, for 8 of the 16 days in phase 2, the woman wore the splint at work; for the other 8 days she did not use the splint. In both conditions, data were systematically collected on number of assembly units completed per hour. As depicted in the graph, the woman's work productivity improved, thereby providing support for the use of the splint in the work setting for this woman.

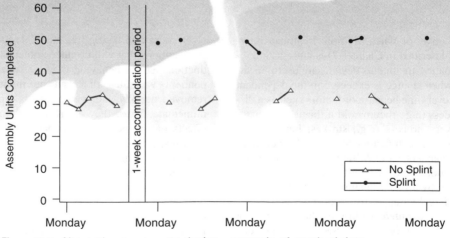

Figure 11.7 Alternating-treatments design—example of graphed data.

effects to be identified if they did exist (Hains & Baer, 1989).

Variations

The research designs described are only a sample of the possibilities. The literature is replete with creative examples of design variations. For example, Wacker and colleagues (1990) advocated for the sequential alternating-treatments design, a combination of the alternating-treatments and multiple-baseline designs, and others have suggested extending the withdrawal design to include more phases and multiple intervention conditions (e.g., *A–B–A–C–A–D–A–C–A–D–A–B–A*).

Definition of Variables and Collection of Data

Similar to group research, dependent variables have to be operationally defined and data collection methods that are replicable and reliable must be used. In addition to using physiologic measures (e.g., oxygen saturation), strength or endurance measures (e.g., pounds of grip strength, time spent exercising at a given level), frequency measures (e.g., number of bites of food taken without spilling during a meal), and self-report measures (e.g., level of pain, level of satisfaction), interval-recording techniques often are used. There are three common interval-recording techniques: momentary time sampling, partial interval recording, and whole interval recording (Harrop & Daniels, 1986; Richards, Taylor, Ramasamy, & Richards, 1999). With momentary time sampling, a response is recorded if it occurs precisely at a predetermined moment. For example, consider a study in which "in seat behavior" was the dependent variable. Using momentary time sampling, a data collector, listening to a tape of beeps recorded at 5-second intervals, would record whether or not the child was "in seat" at the moment of each beep. By contrast, with partial-interval recording, a response is scored if it occurs in any part of the interval. For example, in the previous example, the child would be scored as "in seat" if she was in her seat during the first 2 seconds of the 5-second interval and out of her seat during the last 3 seconds of that interval. With whole-interval recording, the child would have to be in her seat during the full 5-second interval in order to be scored as "in seat."

Typically, with interval-recording techniques, either the data collector uses headphones to hear a tape of beeps recorded at regular intervals,

such as every 5 or 10 seconds, or uses videotapes of recorded sessions with beeps superimposed on the tapes. The data collector typically records responses on a recording sheet such as the one presented in Figure 11.8 on p. 150, which was designed for use for 10 minutes of data collection with 5-second intervals. For each interval, the researcher circles either an "I" for "in-seat" or an "O" for "out of seat." This approach of making the same mark (a circle) regardless of whether "in seat" or "out of seat" is scored, is important in situations where two data collectors, in close proximity, must collect data simultaneously for reliability checks. Otherwise, the subtle sounds of making an "I" or an "O" might inadvertently provide a cue to the other data collector, possibly biasing results.

Data Reporting and Analysis

Data Graphs

Typically, with single-subject research, data for each variable for each participant or system are graphed with the dependent variable on the *y*-axis and time (e.g., days, weeks) on the *x*-axis. Vertical lines indicate phase changes, and lines connect data points reflecting consecutive days. See Figure 11.2 for an example. When graphing data for one variable for more than one participant, the scale for each graph should be the same to facilitate comparisons across graphs. For example, if one participant's data ranged from 3 to 29, and another's ranged from 20 to 58, both graphs should start at 0 and extend to at least 60. This facilitates visual comparison across participants. Carr and Burkholder (1998) described the process for creating graphs for single-subject research using Microsoft Excel ™.

Researchers graph data on either equal interval graph paper or the standard behavior chart (sometimes referred to as six-cycle graph paper). The primary benefit of the former is that it is easily understood. Benefits of the standard behavior chart are that behaviors with extremely high or low rates can be recorded on the chart and the graph progresses in semilog units thus facilitating the estimation of linear trends in the data (Carr & Williams, 1982).

Phase Lengths

Though the researcher estimates phase lengths prior to implementation of the study, typically the

Data Recording Sheet for In-Seat/Out-of-Seat Study

Instructions: For each interval, circle either "I" for "in-seat" or "O" for "out of seat."

min. 1	I O	I O	I O	I O	I O	I O	I O	I O	I O	I O	I O	I O
min. 2	I O	I O	I O	I O	I O	I O	I O	I O	I O	I O	I O	I O
min. 3	I O	I O	I O	I O	I O	I O	I O	I O	I O	I O	I O	I O
min. 4	I O	I O	I O	I O	I O	I O	I O	I O	I O	I O	I O	I O
min. 5	I O	I O	I O	I O	I O	I O	I O	I O	I O	I O	I O	I O
min. 6	I O	I O	I O	I O	I O	I O	I O	I O	I O	I O	I O	I O
min. 7	I O	I O	I O	I O	I O	I O	I O	I O	I O	I O	I O	I O
min. 8	I O	I O	I O	I O	I O	I O	I O	I O	I O	I O	I O	I O
min. 9	I O	I O	I O	I O	I O	I O	I O	I O	I O	I O	I O	I O
min. 10	I O	I O	I O	I O	I O	I O	I O	I O	I O	I O	I O	I O

```
KEY
I = In seat
O = Out of seat
```

Figure 11.8 Sample recording sheet for interval recording (momentary time sampling, whole-interval recording, or partial-interval recording).

actual length of each phase is determined during the course of the study with data collection within a phase continuing until a clear pattern emerges. In determining estimates for phase lengths prior to study implementation, several factors should be taken into account. First, the researcher should decide whether or not he or she intends to use statistical analyses because these often necessitate a specified minimum number of data points in each condition in order to meet the required assumptions for their use. Second, in situations where change is expected due to factors such as development or a disease process, the researcher should consider making the lengths of baseline and intervention phases comparable. This facilitates the visual analyses of the resulting data. Third, the researcher should consider the variability in the expected data and the magnitude of the expected change. In cases where high variability and/or small (but important) changes are expected, longer phases are advised.

Visual Analysis

Visual analysis of graphically presented data to infer conclusions about cause and effect involves looking for a change in level, trend, or variability between phases when treatment is instituted or withdrawn (Ottenbacher & York, 1984; Wolery & Harris, 1982). See Figure 11.9 for potential patterns of data reflecting no change and change.

In some cases, incorporating additional descriptive information into graphs can be used to augment visual data analyses. For example, the split-middle technique can be used to describe data and predict outcomes given the rate of change. The accuracy of these predictions depends on the number of data points on which the prediction is based and on how far into the future a prediction is being made. The split-middle technique also can be used to facilitate the examination and comparison of trends in two or more phases.

Using the split-middle technique, once data for a phase are plotted on a graph, a celeration line reflecting the direction and rate of change is determined. For details concerning the process for using the split-middle technique and creating celeration lines refer to Kazdin (1982), Barlow and Hersen (1984), or Ottenbacher (1986). Though these strategies typically are used to facilitate visual analyses, statistical change can be evaluated

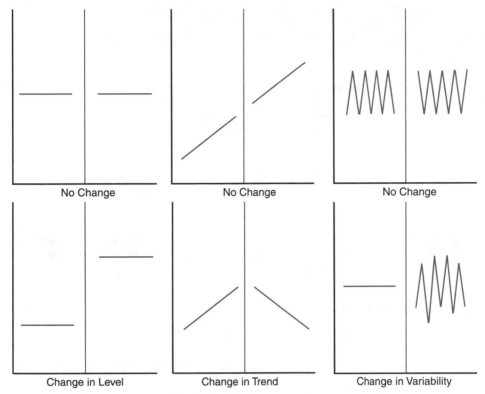

Figure 11.9 Patterns of data reflecting no change and change.

by applying a binomial test to determine whether or not a significant proportion of data points in an intervention phase fall above or below the celeration line projected from baseline. For computational details refer to the writings of White (1972), Barlow and Hersen (1984), or Ottenbacher (1986).

Another example of descriptive information that can be incorporated into graphs to augment visual analyses is the use of a dashed line across each phase demarcating the mean for that phase. Though useful in some situations, this approach can contribute to misinterpretations of the data when the data reflect either an upward or downward trend, when there are few data points within a phase, and when data points within a phase are highly variable. For example, relative to the former, it is possible to have similar means in adjacent A and B phases, thus suggesting no effect from the intervention. However, if there was a steady increase in an undesirable behavior (upward trend) in the A phase and a steady decrease in the undesirable behavior (downward trend) in the B phase, comparison of the means could lead to the erroneous conclusion of no difference between the two phases. See Figure 11.10 on p. 152 for a hypothetical example.

Statistical Significance

If the researcher using single-subject methods plans to determine statistical significance for a study to supplement visual analysis, the researcher needs to design the study to meet the necessary assumptions. One of the best and most underutilized statistical tests appropriate for use in single-subject research is the randomization test (Edgington, 1980, 1995; Onghena & Edgington, 1994; Todman & Dugard, 2001; Wampold & Worsham, 1986). It is a conservative way to evaluate shifts in time-series data and is ideal because it is robust to serial dependency (i.e., correlation among successive responses in one individual) and systematic trends in the data and it does not require a normal distribution. It focuses exclusively on the data available, evaluating the probability of the actual outcome when compared to the set of all possible outcomes. If a researcher plans to use randomization tests to analyze data from single-subject research, it is important that the researcher randomly assign experimental conditions (Edgington, 1980, 1995). In doing this, the researcher should consider the need to control for systematic trends over the course of the study that may be attributable to developmental or recovery processes.

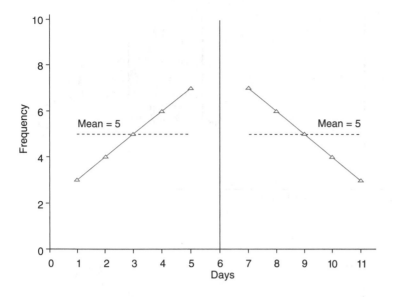

Figure 11.10 Example of misleading use of comparison of means across phases.

Incorporation of Social Validation Procedures into the Design

According to Schwartz and Baer (1991), the purpose of assessing social validity is to evaluate the acceptability or viability of an intervention. Typically this is accomplished through use of one or more questionnaires directed to the research participants and others in their environments (e.g., family members, teachers). Social validation is important since it is possible for an intervention to result in desirable changes in the dependent variable, but still be identified by research participants or other stakeholders as being unacceptable. For example, results from a research study may indicate that use of a specific type of splint decreases daily reports of pain and increases range of motion. However, in a social validation questionnaire, the research participant may indicate that the splint limits function and is cosmetically unacceptable and therefore would not be chosen for use.

Social validation procedures were used in the therapy ball study described in the feature box that appeared earlier in this chapter (Schilling et al., 2003). This involved three steps. First, the target children and all other children in the class and the teacher filled out social validity questionnaires. Second, at the conclusion of the study, all were instructed to write about what they "liked" and "didn't like" about using balls for classroom seating. Last, evidence of social validity was obtained by observing the teacher's choices following the completion of the study. She continued to use therapy balls for seating for the children with ADHD and she ordered additional balls for other students, thus supporting the social validity of the intervention.

The Issue of Generality

Though a well-designed and implemented single-subject study completed with one individual has strong internal validity, it is weak relative to external validity (discussed in Chapter 7). Thus, though we may have confidence in the findings for the individual studied, we do not know the extent to which these findings generalize to other comparable individuals. Generality in single-subject research is achieved only through replication with other individuals, in other settings, and with other therapists. For example, in the therapy ball study

> Social validation is important since it is possible for an intervention to result in desirable changes in the dependent variable, but still be identified by research participants or other stakeholders as being unacceptable.

Questions to Answer When Designing a Single-Subject Research Study

(Though the following questions are listed in an order, in practice, the process is iterative and may vary in sequence.)

- What is the purpose of my study and why is it important?
- What is my research question?
- What literature do I need to review in order to understand the topic, the measurement issues, the research design, etc.?
- Who are my participants and how will I select them?
- What is the independent variable (intervention strategy)?
- How will I ensure that the intervention implemented in my study is consistently exact and true

to the intervention as intended and described (intervention fidelity)?

- What is (are) the dependent variable(s)?
- How will I ensure that my measurements are reliable?
- What is the design of my study and what is my rationale for selecting that design? (Do I plan to use a test for statistical significance, and if so, how will that influence the design of my study?)
- How will I graph and analyze my data?
- How will I assess social validity?
- What are the strengths and limitations of my proposed study?
- What ethical factors should I address and what are the Institutional Review Board requirements?

described previously, two other children, in addition to Emily, were studied. Because results for all three children were similar, some support is provided for the generality of the findings. Additional replications by other researchers, in other settings, and with different children would further increase generality if comparable outcomes continued to be achieved.

> Both the process of single-subject research and the products of single-subject research support evidence-based practice.

Kazdin (1982) distinguished between direct replication that involves systematically applying the same procedures across different, but similar, individuals and systematic replication that involves repeating the study with systematic variations. An example of the latter would be to design and conduct a replication study using different types of participants (e.g., children with autism instead of children with attention deficit hyperactivity disorder [ADHD]). Ideally, in a systematic replication study, only one variable is changed at a time. Systematic replications expand understanding regarding with whom and under what conditions the intervention is effective.

Conclusion

Single-subject research methods are useful in addressing many important questions related to the extent to which different intervention strategies are

successful with different clients. These methods are congruent with responsible occupational therapy practice in that they emphasize clearly articulating desired outcomes, defining intervention and measurement strategies, and collecting data reliability over time. Both the process of single-subject research and the products of single-subject research support evidence-based practice. Questions for the clinician/researcher to answer when designing a single subject research study appear in the following feature box.

REFERENCES

Backman, C., Harris, S. R., Chisholm, J., & Monette, A. D. (1997). Single-subject research in rehabilitation: A review of studies using AB, withdrawal, multiple baseline, and alternating treatments designs. *Archives of Physical Medicine and Rehabilitation, 78,* 1145–1153.

Barlow, D. H., & Hayes, S. C. (1979). Alternating treatments design: One strategy for comparing the effects of two treatments in a single subject. *Journal of Applied Behavior Analysis, 12,* 199–210.

Barlow, D. H., & Hersen, M. (1984). Single case experimental designs strategies for studying behavior change (2nd ed.). New York: Pergamon Press.

Campbell, D., & Stanley, J. (1963). *Experimental and quasi-experimental designs for research.* Chicago: Rand McNally.

Carr, J. E., & Burkholder, E. O. (1998). Creating single-subject design graphs with Microsoft Excel™. *Journal of Applied Behavior Analysis, 31,* 245–251.

Carr, B. S., & Williams, M. (1982). Analysis of therapeutic techniques through use of the standard behavior chart. *Physical Therapy, 52,* 177–183.

Edgington, E. S. (1980). Random assignment and statistical tests for one-subject experiments. *Behavioral Assessment, 2,* 19–28.

Edgington E.S. (1995). Single subject randomization tests. In E. S. Edgington (Ed.), *Randomization tests* (3rd ed., pp. 263–301). New York: Marcel Dekker.

Hains, H., & Baer, D. M. (1989). Interaction effects in multielement designs: Inevitable, desirable, and ignorable. *Journal of Applied Behavior Analysis, 22,* 57–69.

Harrop, A., & Daniels, M. (1986). Methods of time sampling: A reappraisal of momentary time sampling and interval recording. *Journal of Applied Behavior Anlaysis, 19,* 73–77.

Hartmann, D. P., & Hall, R. V. (1976). The changing criterion design. *Journal of Applied Behavior Analysis, 9,* 527–532.

Kazdin, A. E. (1982). *Single-case research designs: Methods for clinical and applied settings.* New York: Oxford University Press.

Melchert-McKearnan, K., Deitz, J., Engel, J., & White, O. (2000). Children with burn injuries; Purposeful activity versus rote exercise. *The American Journal of Occupational Therapy, 54,* 381–390.

Onghena, P., & Edgington, E. S. (1994). Randomization tests for restricted alternating treatments designs. *Behaviour Research & Therapy, 32,* 783–786.

Ottenbacher, K. (1986). *Evaluating clinical change: Strategies for occupational and physical therapists.* Baltimore: Williams & Wilkins.

Ottenbacher, K. (1990). Clinically relevant designs for rehabilitation research: The idiographic model. *American Journal of Physical Medicine & Rehabilitation, 69,* 286–292.

Ottenbacher, K., & York, J. (1984). Strategies for evaluating clinical change: Implications for practice and research. *The American Journal of Occupational Therapy, 38,* 647–659.

Richards, S. B., Taylor, R. L., Ramasamy, R., & Richards, R. Y. (1999). *Single subject research applications in educational and clinical settings.* San Diego: Singular.

Schilling, D. L., Washington, K., Billingsley, F., & Deitz, J. (2003). Classroom seating for children with attention deficit hyperactivity disorder: Therapy balls versus chairs. *The American Journal of Occupational Therapy, 57,* 534–541.

Schwartz, I. S., & Baer, D. M. (1991). Social validity assessments: Is current practice state of the art? *Journal of Applied Behavior Analysis, 24,* 189–204.

Todman, J. B., & Dugard, P. (2001). *Single-case and small-n experimental designs a practical guide to randomization tests.* Mahwah, NJ: Lawrence Erlbaum Associates.

Wacker, D., McMahon, C., Steege, M., Berg, W., Sasso, G., & Melloy, K. (1990). Applications of a sequential alternating treatments design. *Journal of Applied Behavior Analysis, 23,* 333–339.

Wampold, B. E., & Worsham, N. L. (1986). Randomization tests for multiple-baseline designs. *Behavioral Assessment, 8,* 135–143.

Watson, P. J., & Workman, E. A. (1981). The non-concurrent multiple baseline across-individuals design: An extension of the traditional multiple baseline design. *Journal of Behavior Therapy and Experimental Psychiatry, 12,* 257–259.

White, O. R. (1972). *A manual for the calculation and use of the median slope – a technique of progress estimation and prediction in the single case.* Eugene, OR: University of Oregon, Regional Resource Center for Handicapped Children.

Wolery, M., & Harris, S. (1982). Interpreting results of single-subject research designs. *Physical Therapy, 62,* 445–452.

RESOURCES

Selecting Target Behaviors

Kazdin, A. E. (1985). Selection of target behaviors: The relationship of the treatment focus to clinical dysfunction. *Behavioral Assessment, 7,* 33–47.

CHAPTER 12

Developing and Evaluating Quantitative Data Collection Instruments

Gary Kielhofner

Both everyday practice and research in occupational therapy require the use of sound quantitative data collection instruments. These instruments can include such things as:

• Self-report forms,
• Interviews with rating scales,
• Observational checklists or rating scales,
• Calibrated measurement devices, and
• Tests.

Chapter 32 includes a more detailed discussion of the various type of data collection procedures and instruments. The purpose of this chapter is to examine the concepts and methods that underlie the development of assessments and the criteria that may be applied to examine the quality of a data collection assessment.

This chapter mainly discusses an approach to quantitative instrument development and analysis referred to as classical test theory (CTT) (Hambleton, & Jones, 1993; Nunally, 1978). Chapter 13 discusses a more recent and complementary approach, item response theory (IRT). Further, Chapter 14 discusses an additional set of considerations for choosing or developing an instrument.

> This process of measurement is classically defined as a rule-bound procedure by which one assigns numbers to variables in order to quantify some characteristic.

Quantifying Information

Many of the things that occupational therapists seek to measure can be directly observed and judged in a commonsense way. For example, one can readily recognize strength and coordination (i.e., some persons are obviously stronger or more coordinated than others). However, everyday powers of observation are not very precise or reliable. For example, when two persons have similar strength, it may be difficult to say who is stronger. Moreover, if two different people are asked to judge who of a small group of individuals is the most coordinated, they are likely to arrive at different judgments. This kind of imprecision and inaccuracy of judgment is unacceptable in research and clinical practice. Both situations require that occupational therapists make much more precise judgments than are possible through everyday powers of observation.

Quantitative instruments seek to achieve accuracy and consistency by translating information about some aspect of a person into numbers (Cronbach, 1990; Guilford, 1979). This process of measurement is classically defined as a rule-bound procedure by which one assigns numbers to variables in order to quantify some characteristic.[1]

All measurement requires a specific procedure and instrumentation that allows quantification of the characteristic of interest. For example, therapists measure muscle strength using instruments that quantify strength as an amount of pressure generated or an amount of weight lifted. Similarly, coordination can be quantified by transforming the observed speed and accuracy of standardized task performance into a score.

---

[1]As discussed in Chapter 13, item response theory approaches use a more restrictive definition of measurement, but this chapter follows the more classic definition. The IRT definition is referred to as objective measurement to differentiate these two approaches.

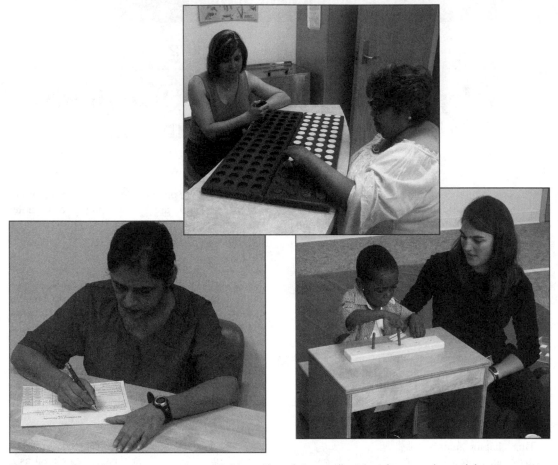

Figure 12.1 Sound measures are essential to gather data on clients and research participants.

Two Key Elements of Measurement

Returning to the earlier example, the problems that occur in everyday judgments about who is stronger or more coordinated are linked to the fact that:

- Strength or coordination might mean different things to different persons, and
- Each person may have a different procedure or criteria for arriving at judgments about strength or coordination.

For example, one person may think of strength as an observable muscle mass. Another person may think of strength in terms of some performance (e.g., winning an arm wrestling contest). In each instance, the person who seeks to make a judgment about strength is working with an idea

of what strength is (e.g., muscularity or ability to demonstrate strength in performance) and has some way to observe that idea (e.g., looking at who appears more muscular or watching to see who lifts more, or wins an arm wrestling contest).

These two elements tend to be implicit in everyday judgments leading to the kinds of inaccuracy or disagreement noted earlier. Consequently, they are made explicit in measurement. That is, underlying all measurement are two essential steps:

- Definition of the construct to be measured, and
- Operationalizaiton of the construct through formal instrumentation.

Constructs and Their Operationalization

All variables that are measured must first be abstractly conceptualized as constructs. For example, consider the phenomena "movement." If one wishes to measure some aspect of movement, one must first conceptualize or define the specific characteristic of movement that one wishes to measure. For example, the measurement of movement could involve such things as:

• Freedom of movement,
• Speed of movement, and
• Efficiency of movement.

Once one has chosen an element of movement for measurement (e.g., freedom of movement) then one must clearly define or conceptualize what will be measured. The most common measure of the freedom of movement is joint range of motion, which is defined as the movement about the axis of a joint. Joint range is further specified as active and passive. Active range of motion refers to the range of movement about the axis of a joint that a person can produce using his or her own strength.

Once a very specific definition of a construct is developed, then a procedure and/or instrument for operationalizing that construct can be developed. In the case of active range of motion, the procedure involves asking a client or research participant to move the part of the body of interest and then to apply an instrument that operationalizes the movement and represents it in terms of numbers. In the case of a goniometer, movement about the axis of a joint is operationalized as degrees of a circle (i.e., 0 to 360 degrees).

If one wished to measure another aspect of movement, such as efficiency of movement, then a specific construct would need to be defined and an appropriate method of operationalizing that construct developed. Consequently, all measurement begins with identifying the construct that one intends to measure and proceeds to a specific method of operationalizing that construct.

The Rule-Bound Nature of Measurement

Measurement is rule bound in that there are specific rules or laws that govern how numbers can be used to stand for some quality of the construct that is being measured. Physical measurements of human traits (e.g., height, weight, strength, and range of motion) build upon physical measures that have been developed for characterizing a whole range of objects. Other human traits (e.g., abilities, attitudes, aspects of the personality, and

so on) rely upon the development of unique new forms of measurement. For the most part it is these latter forms of measurement that are discussed in this chapter.

Scales of Measurement

The rules of measurement reflect the basic scales of measurement. That is, numbers may be used to:

• Differentiate one characteristic from another,
• Indicate order from less to more of a characteristic,
• Indicate an amount of a characteristic on a continuum from less to more, and
• Indicate an absolute amount of a characteristic.

These purposes correspond to the nominal, ordinal, interval, and ratio level scales. Each of these scales of measurement has a specific purpose, meaning of the number, and rules that govern how numbers are assigned and how they can be mathematically manipulated as summarized in Table 12.1.

Nominal Scales

Nominal scales are used to classify characteristics such as sex. In this case numbers are used to identify a specific category (e.g., 1 = female; 2 = male). In nominal scales numbers have no other meaning than identifying the category or characteristic to which a person belongs. The basic rule underlying nominal scales is that each category must be exclusive of the other categories. The only mathematical operation that is allowed with nominal scales is that they can be counted. Thus, research variables based on nominal characteristics are usually represented as frequency counts and proportions derived from those counts (e.g., 20 males and 80 females = 1/5 male).

Ordinal Scales

Ordinal scales are used to classify ranked categories. A typical example of ranking in occupational therapy is degree of dependence and independence (e.g., 1 = totally independent, 2 = needs minimal assistance, 3 = needs moderate assistance, 4 = needs maximal assistance, 5 = totally dependent). In ordinal scales, the number refers to a rank order. Using the example above, 2 is the second most independent rating.

Importantly, in ordinal scales the intervals between ranks are not necessarily the same. That is, the difference between "totally independent" and "needs minimal assistance" may not be the

Table 12.1 **Scales of Measurement**

Type of Scale	Purpose of Scale	Meaning of Numbers	Requirement	Possible Mathematical Manipulation	Examples
Nominal	Classification	Identify a category	Mutual exclusivity	Counting (i.e., compilation of frequencies)	Sex, ethnicity/race, religion, diagnosis
Ordinal	Ranking (i.e., position within a distribution categories)	Indicate rank order	Mutual exclusivity/Ordinality	Strictly speaking, same as nominal. In practice, often used as if they are interval	Degree of independence, grade of muscle strength (i.e., good, fair, poor)
Interval	Represents continuum of a characteristic using equal-interval units	Indicate position on a continuum partitioned into equal unit intervals	Mutual exclusivity, ordinality, and equivalency of units	Can be added and subtracted	Pounds of pressure generated as a measure of strength
Ratio	Indicates amount	Indicate absolute amount (zero equals total absence of characteristic measured)	Mutual exclusivity, ordinality, equivalency of units, and absolute zero point	All mathematical and statistical operations	Height, weight

same as the distance between "needs moderate assistance" and "needs maximal assistance." This means that the numbers used in ordinal scales do not represent an amount. Rather they are categorical labels that indicate ranking within a distribution of categories.

Strictly speaking, then, ordinal scales are descriptive scales like categorical scales and the numbers used are not true quantities. Thus, mathematical operations to which they can be subjected in the strictest sense are the same as nominal variables. While it is common to calculate such numbers as an average rank or a change score that involves mathematical operations (i.e., addition, subtraction, multiplication, and division), the resulting numbers are not "meaningful as true quantities" (Portney & Watkins, 2000, p. 55). Thus, when ordinal scores are subjected to these mathematical operations they are treated "as if" they had the properties of interval scales. This common practice is considered controversial by some researchers for reasons discussed in Chapter 13. To an extent the widespread treatment of ordinal data as if it were interval data reflects the fact that in occupational therapy, like other disciplines that seek to measure a range of human

traits, ordinal scales are the most commonly used scales.

Interval Scales

Interval scales demonstrate equal distances (i.e., intervals) between the units of measurement. Interval scales represent the continuum of a characteristic (from less to more) using equal interval units. They allow the investigator or practitioners to determine relative difference. For example, on an interval score the difference between 2 and 3 is the same as the difference between 3 and 4, 4 and 5, and so on.

Interval scales do not indicate absolute amount or magnitude of a characteristic because they do not have a true zero point indicating the absence of any of the characteristics. It should be noted that while some interval scales do have a zero point (along with plus and minus values), these are arbitrarily zero points without meaning. A true zero point must represent the absence of the characteristic being measured.

Importantly, interval scales are additive since the intervals between numbers are the same. Thus, total scores (addition) and change scores (subtraction) can be calculated. Because interval scales can be subjected to a number of mathematical operations without violating the underlying rules, they are preferable to ordinal scales. This is why there is increasing interest in the IRT methods discussed in Chapter 13 that convert ordinal scale data into interval scales.

Ratio Scales

Ratio scales demonstrate equal distances between units of measure and they also have an absolute zero point. Therefore, they indicate absolute amounts of the characteristics measured. Unlike interval scales, numbers from ratio level scales can be interpreted as ratios; for example, someone who is 6 feet tall can be said to be twice as tall as someone who is 3 feet tall. Moreover, all forms of mathematical and statistical operations are permissible with ratio scales. An example of ratio scales used in occupational therapy is strength measures (e.g., a dynamometer) where the zero point represents a total lack of strength (i.e., inability to generate any pressure).

Measurement Error

Returning again to the example of estimating strength and coordination, the underlying problem was inaccuracy of judgment. The aim of measurement is to achieve the most accurate judgment possible. Theoretically, there is always some error present in measurement, but measurement seeks to minimize the amount of measurement error. To think about and minimize error, classical test theory uses two concepts. The first concept is true score, which refers to the actual quality or amount of the underlying characteristic measured that a person has. The second concept is the observed score, which refers to the number that the observer assigns to the individual using an instrument.

In classical test theory, the observed score is considered to be a function of two factors:

• The true score, and
• The error of measurement (Hambleton & Jones, 1993).

This relationship is represented by the equation:

$$X = T + E$$

where X = bserved score; T = true score; E = error.

When the error term is known, the true score is defined as the observed score minus the error score or:

$$T = X - E$$

Thus T is the score that will be assigned to an individual or that an individual would achieve on an instrument if the instrument were error-free.

Types of Measurement Error

There are two types of errors that can occur when applying instruments:

• Systematic error, and
• Random error.

Systematic errors are consistent or predictable errors; they occur when an instrument misestimates the true score by a consistent amount and in the same direction (too low or too high).[2] Random error occurs by chance and is, thus, unpredictable.

Typical sources of error on a measurement instrument include:

• The instrument itself,
• The individual who is administering the instrument (i.e., rater or tester error), and
• Fluctuations in the characteristic measured.

A variety of instrument factors contribute to measurement error. These include such things as:

• Problems in the conceptualization of the construct being measured and how it is translated into an instrument,
• Lack of precision that requires the person administering or taking the instrument to estimate or guess,
• Complexity or lack of clarity in how the instrument is to be used, and
• Ambiguity that leads to differential interpretation of items or tests that are part of the instrument.

Strategies for Reducing Measurement Error

There are a number of ways that developers and users of instruments seek to reduce measurement error. The most common are:

• Standardization of the instrument,

[2]Classical test theory ordinarily conceptualizes systematic error as a problem of validity (Portney & Watkins, 2000). However, one of the most common sources of systematic error is inter-rater disagreement due to differences in severity/leniency. This form of systematic error has been largely overlooked because the statistical methods used to examine reliability do not account for systematic covariation coupled with differences in severity/leniency.

- Methods of informing, training, and ensuring accuracy of raters, and
- Taking repeated measures.

Standardization

One of the most important and effective ways to reduce the measurement error of an instrument is to standardize it. Standardization refers to specifying a process or protocol for administering the assessment. Instruments may involve varying degrees of standardization, depending on the nature of the instrument. The following are examples. Tests such as the Minnesota Rate of Manipulation Test (Lafayette Instruments, 1969) or the Sensory Integration and Praxis Tests (Ayres, 1989) require a specific administration protocol along with a standard test kit. Observational instruments such as the Assessment of Motor and Process Skills (Fisher, 1993) may require standardized situations while allowing a certain amount of discretion on the part of the administrator. Semistructured clinical interviews such as the Occupational Circumstances Interview and Rating Scales (Forsyth et al., 2005) may allow substantial flexibility in how the interview is conducted but require the therapist to complete a standardized rating scale. Self-administered instruments such as the Child Occupational Self Assessment (Keller, Kafkes, Basu, Federico, & Kielhofner, 2005) rely on the structure of the paper-and-pencil form and clear instructions and guidance on the part of the therapist administering the assessment.

In each of these instances, the developer of the instrument considered and often completed many trials to determine what procedures would optimize gathering comprehensive and stable information. In the case of testing sensory–motor abilities, a set of specific highly structured motor tasks was considered optimal. In the case of doing an interview, flexibility to respond to clients and make them feel comfortable was considered optimal for gathering the personal information for which the interview asks.

Reducing Rater or Tester Error

Rater or tester error is ordinarily caused by such factors as mistakes, guessing, or variability in test administration or circumstances. This source of error is minimized by ensuring that the person using the instrument:

- Understands the construct the instrument is designed to measure,

- Knows the administration protocol, and
- Understands the content of the instrument.

Standardization of instruments helps to reduce variability in how raters administer a test. Other approaches to minimizing rater or tester error are:

- Providing detailed instrument instructions or an administration manual,
- Training, and
- Credentialing those who will administer an instrument (credentialing ordinarily involves both formal training and some kind of practical test or other demonstration that the person is competent to administer the instrument).

Repeated Measurement

In instances in which the characteristic that the instrument seeks to measure tends to fluctuate, testers typically take multiple measurements in order to note the range and central tendency of the variability. In this way the practitioner or investigator can avoid using only an extreme or unusual score and thus misestimating the true or more usual value of the characteristic being measured. Regression toward the mean (the tendency for extreme scores to be followed with scores that are more average) makes taking repeated measures a good strategy for reducing error. Use of this strategy depends, of course, on how feasible it is to take multiple measures and on how much the fluctuation affects the precision of the measure.

Instrument Reliability

Reliability refers to the property of consistency in a measure. Implied in the definition of reliability is that any difference in the score obtained (e.g., from time to time or from different individuals) should be due to true differences in the underlying characteristic and not due to error. Reliability, then, reflects the extent to which an instrument is free from sources of error (Cronbach, 1990)

The Reliability Coefficient

Reliability is expressed as a ratio of the variance of the true score to the total variance observed on an instrument, or:

$$\frac{T}{T + E}$$

where T = true score variance and E = error variance.

The value of this ratio is referred to as the reliability coefficient. It ranges from 0.0 to 1.0; 1.0, which indicates there is no error. The larger the error, the more the reliability coefficient will deviate from a perfect coefficient of 1.0.

The reliability coefficient is interpreted as the "proportion of observed variance that is attributed to true score variance" (Bensen & Schell, 1997, p. 5). Thus, for example, a reliability coefficient of .90 is considered to be an estimate that 90% of the variance observed can be attributed to variance in the characteristic measured (true score) as opposed to error variance. When the reliability of assessments is being investigated, reliability coefficients are calculated as correlation coefficients, which are discussed in the following sections and explained in detail in Chapter 17.

Empirical Evaluation of Instrument Reliability

When instruments are being developed or evaluated for particular use, their reliability is empirically investigated. In the context of classical test theory, reliability of an instrument is empirically assessed using the following methods:

- Test–retest or stability,
- Split-half reliability,
- Alternate forms reliability, and
- Internal consistency.

Test–Retest or Stability

One of the most common ways of determining whether an instrument provides consistent results is to administer the same instrument on two different occasions. When readministering an instrument to assess reliability, there is no empirical way to separate differences that are due to:

- Changes in the underlying trait, and
- Changes that are due to error.

Therefore, consideration has to be given to how likely it is that the underlying trait will change or has changed in the period between administrations. This is a consideration in both choosing the period of time between administrations and in interpreting the statistical results.

Choosing the period for readministration also requires consideration of possible effects of the first administration on subsequent administration. For example, memory can inflate agreement if the subject recalls and repeats the responses given on an instrument when taking the instrument a second time. In tests of ability, the practice effect of taking the test the first time may inflate the score the indi-

vidual receives on the second administration. For this reason, investigators generally want to include a period that is:

- Long enough to erase the effects of memory or practice, yet
- Not so long as to result in a genuine change in the underlying characteristic that will be confounded with error.

Moreover, when reporting findings on test–retest reliability, investigators should indicate both the time interval between administrations and any rationale for whether the underlying trait is expected to change during that period.

Test–retest reliability correlations are calculated based on the two administrations of the instrument; the time 1 score is the first variable and the time 2 score is the second variable. The Pearson Product Moment correlation is typically used for test–retest reliability. Generally, correlations (r-values) above .60 for longer time intervals, and higher values for shorter intervals, are considered evidence of reliability. In the end, interpretation of the statistic should be based on theoretical expectations. If there is no reason to suspect that the underlying characteristic changed, then a higher correlation will be expected.

The following is an example of test–retest reliability. Doble, Fisk, Lewis, and Rockwood (1999) examined the test–retest reliability of the Assessment of Motor and Process Skills (AMPS) (Fisher, 1993). They administered the AMPS to a sample of 55 elderly adults and then reassessed them within 1 to 10 days, calculating Pearson Product Moment Correlations. The two administrations of the AMPS were highly correlated (i.e., Motor $r = .88$ and Process $r = .86$), providing evidence of good test–retest reliability.

Split-half Reliability

Split-half reliability is a technique most often used when testing reliability of questionnaires. It is preferred since the alternative way to test reliability is to readminister the entire questionnaire. If it is readministered too soon, reliability may be overestimated because of memory (i.e., the respondents fill it out based on how they recall having filled it out before). If it is readministered too far apart, then the underlying characteristic may have changed, leading to an underestimation of reliability since true score change is confounded with error.

To avoid these problems, investigators divide the items into two smaller questionnaires (usually by dividing it into odd and even items, or first half–last half) and then correlating the scores obtained from the two halves of the instrument. In this case, the Spearman–Brown prophecy statistic is typically used. The correlation (r) should be .80 or higher.

Alternate Forms or Equivalency Reliability

For some instruments, it is important to be able to administer different versions of the instrument. For example, national certification tests or aptitude tests use different combinations of items to avoid cheating and also to ensure that the item pool reflects contemporary material (Benson & Schell, 1997). In other cases, investigators are concerned with different administration formats of an instrument (e.g., an instrument that can be administered as a paper-and-pencil checklist or a card sort procedure). In these instances, it is important that different versions, or forms, of an instrument provide consistent results.

Alternate forms reliability involves administration of the alternative forms to subjects at the same time. In order to avoid the effects of sequence (e.g., fatigue), the order in which the forms are administered may be counterbalanced (i.e., half the subjects take one instrument first and the other half take the other instrument first), or the items that make up the two forms may be integrated randomly or in alternating sequence in a single test. Alternate forms reliability is assessed using the Pearson Product Moment Correlation. It is generally accepted that the correlation (r) should be .80 or higher.

Internal Consistency

Investigators often examine whether the items that make up an instrument covary or correlate with each other. This property is often referred to as homogeneity.[3] This is tested by asking whether the items covary. For example, if the items on a scale of cognition all reliably measure cognition, then a person with low cognition would tend to score lower on all the items and a person with high cognition would tend to score higher on the items. If this is the case across a sample, then the items will demonstrate consistent variance.

[3]Although internal consistency is generally discussed as a measure of reliability, it overlaps with validity. That is, the homogeneity of items indicates the items converge or work together to measure the same underlying construct. In item response theory, this property is known as unidimensionality (see Chapter 13). In contrast to simply asking whether the items covary, this method asks instead whether the observed scores of items fit with expectations based on the item's placement on the continuum of the characteristic being measured.

It should be noted that internal consistency and construct validity, which is discussed later, are closely related. However, internal consistency is considered an issue of reliability because if many items measure the underlying construct and some do not, the latter will be adding error to the instrument. Consequently, internal consistency is generally taken as evidence of both reliability and validity.

Internal consistency is typically assessed using Cronbach's coefficient alpha (α) (Cronbach, 1951). Alpha is the average of all split-half reliabilities for the items that make up the instrument. It can be used with both dichotomous and ordinal scales. Like other correlations, alpha ranges from 0.0 to 1.0 and the larger the alpha coefficient, the stronger the inter-correlation among items and, therefore, homogeneity of the scale as a whole. Generally, alpha values that approach .90 are indications of high homogeneity. Since alpha is affected by the number of items, longer scales will tend to generate higher coefficients. While alpha gives an indication of overall consistency, it does not provide information about which items may be inconsistent and, thereby, contributing error to the instrument.

Another approach to examining internal consistency or homogeneity is item-to-total correlations. In this method, each item is correlated to the total test score. Pearson Product Moment correlations are used unless items are dichotomous in which case a point-biserial correlation coefficient is used. Generally, authors suggest that item-total correlations should yield correlations between .70 and .90 (Streiner & Normal, 1995). The advantage of item-total correlations over alpha is that they allow an instrument developer to identify individual items that may be inconsistent with the total score and, thereby, contributing error to the instrument.

Evaluating Instrument Reliability

The choice of which approach(s) to use for evaluating reliability depends on what sources of measurement error are relevant to the measurement instrument. For example, if an instrument targets a characteristic that is somewhat variable from time to time (e.g., mood state or fatigue), test-retest is not a very good estimate of stability since there is no way to empirically sort out what variability is due to error versus fluctuation in the underlying trait. In this case, split-half reliability is a more relevant approach. On the other hand, if an instrument measures a characteristic that is relatively stable, then test–retest is a relevant form of reliability to examine.

In cases in which different items or administration formats are used in versions of an instrument (e.g., the national certification examination taken by occupational therapists) the approach of choice is equivalency or parallel forms. Thus, in developing or assessing evidence about reliability of an instrument, consideration needs to be given to what the instrument measures and how the instrument is intended to be used.

It is important to recognize that reliability assessment based on classical test theory is sample dependent (Hambleton & Jones, 1993). This means that the obtained reliability coefficient will differ from sample to sample, largely because of differences in the variability of different samples drawn from the same population. For this reason, Benson and Schell (1997) recommend that whenever an instrument is used within a study, reliability evidence should be reported for that sample. In practice, it is often the case that, if an instrument is used with a group for which there has previously been reported reliability data, investigators will make reference to this previous research, but not reevaluate reliability in the context of the study. However, it is common practice and highly desirable to report reliability findings when an investigation uses an instrument with a population that differs from previous research or when some aspect of the administration varies from previously reported studies.

Rater/Observer Effects on Reliability

In occupational therapy many types of instruments require the administrator to complete a checklist, form, or rating scale based on information gathered about a client based on observation, testing, or interview. As noted earlier, the rater or observer can be a source of error and certain strategies can be used to reduce rater error. Rater or observer error is also assessed empirically. For this purpose, there are two sources of observer/rater error that are typically examined:

• The biasing effects of observer presence or observer characteristics, and
• Rater bias.

Observer Presence or Characteristics

In many instances of observation, interview, or testing, the rater's presence (and characteristics) may have an impact on the behavior or information provided by the client. For instance, clients who are aware of being observed may alter their behavior to influence the observer's conclusion. In addition, the characteristics of an observer (e.g., sex,

race, age) may impact how a person behaves. For example, in responding to an interview, clients who perceive the interviewer to be more able to understand their situation may give more complete information or note problems that would be withheld from another interviewer who is not perceived to be as capable of understanding. Moreover, a client may seek to create a particular impression on the part of the interviewer based on perceived characteristics of the interviewer.

Rater Bias

Rater bias may occur when the rater translates the information obtained into a classification or rating. In this situation, any number of characteristics of the rater may introduce error. Rater characteristics that might result in error include demographic characteristics, experience, training, or theoretical orientation of the rater. Rater demographics might result in error, for example, when the rater shares characteristics with the person rated and overempathizes or judges the person too harshly or with too much leniency because of personal experience. Differences in experience, training, and theoretical orientation may result in raters bringing different perspectives or understandings to the instrument, thereby introducing error.

Assessing Inter-rater Reliability

The extent of rater bias is assessed through investigations of inter-rater reliability. Inter-rater reliability is typically studied by having two or more raters observe the same clients, either directly or through videotape or audiotape. The inter-rater reliability coefficient that is used depends on the nature of rating that is done.

For example, when raters classify clients on characteristics, investigators sometimes calculate percent agreement. While percent agreement can provide some information about rater agreement, it tends to inflate agreement when fewer categories are used. For example, when there are only two categories, raters will agree 50% of the time just by chance. Thus, 75% agreement represents only a 25% agreement above chance. For this reason, a more accurate estimate of agreement takes chance agreement into consideration. Thus investigators use the kappa statistic (Cohen, 1960), which corrects for chance. When there is concern about magnitude of disagreement a weighted kappa statistic is used, since kappa assumes all disagreements are of equal weight or importance. For example, if raters were classifying client mood states as depressed, anxious, happy, or tranquil, there would be more concern about two raters who judged a client to be happy and depressed, respectively than if they rated the client depressed and anxious, respectively. The latter is a smaller amount of disagreement than the former. In this instance a weighted kappa (Cohen, 1968) can be used to consider the extent of disagreements; it would distinguish between the two types of disagreements given in the example above.

The kappa statistic is influenced by sample size, subject variability, and the number of categories used, so it must be interpreted with care. Fleiss (1981) provides the following guidelines for interpretation of kappa values:

* > 0.75 = excellent agreement,
* 0.40 to 0.75 = fair to good agreement, and
* <0.40 = poor agreement.

The following is an example of the use of the kappa statistic. Clemson, Fitzgerald, Heard, and Cumming (1999) examined the inter-rater reliability of the Westmead Home Safety Assessment (WeHSA), a checklist of categories of potential fall hazards. Since this is a dichotomous assessment (i.e., items are assessed as to whether or not they present a potential falls hazard), kappa is an appropriate statistic for assessing inter-rater reliability.

A previous study had shown inadequate reliability for a third of the items. Therefore the instrument was revised to clarify items and a manual and a training program was developed. In this study, pairs of therapists, who were trained in the use of the assessment, completed normally scheduled home visits during which one therapist administered, the other observed, and both independently scored the WeHSA. Based on evaluations of 21 homes of clients who were referred for home modification assessment, falls risk management and other functional reasons, kappa statistics were calculated. The investigator reported that:

* 52 of the items received kappa values greater than 0.75,
* 48 of the items received kappa values between 0.40 and 0.75, and
* None of the items received kappa values lower than 0.40.

The results of this study indicated that the instrument's inter-rater reliability had improved and met recommended criteria for reliability.

When ordinal scales are used, the most appropriate measure of agreement is a nonparametric correlation coefficient, the Spearman rho. For interval and ratio scales the parametric, Pearson Product Moment Correlation is typically used.

An important limitation of correlation coefficients in estimating rater agreement is systematic disagreement, which occurs when there are differences in rater severity or leniency. For example, on a 10-point rating scale, two raters may consistently give different ratings that covary as shown in Table 12.2. While the two raters are always in disagreement about the appropriate rating, their disagreement is systematic (i.e., rater 2 always gives a higher score that is 3 points higher than rater 1's score). For this reason, investigators increasingly estimate inter-rater reliability with more powerful statistics than these traditional correlations.

Generalizabilty Theory and Intraclass Correlations

Alternatives to traditional correlational approaches to estimating inter-rater reliability include Item Response Theory (discussed in Chapter 13) and the variance components approach of generalizability theory (Benson & Schell, 1997). The latter approach allows for the estimation of multiple sources of error in addition to the random error considered in classical test theory. Moreover, classical approaches to assessing reliability estimate reliability only by examining one source of error at a time, whereas the variance components approach estimates reliability while accounting for several different sources of error simultaneously. Thus, this method can be used to calculate the reliability of an observed score in estimating the true score by partitioning error due to several factors (referred to as facets) such as variations in the raters and testing conditions, alternate forms, and administration at different times. This approach uses Analysis of Variance (ANOVA) (discussed in Chapter 17) to estimate sources of variation and their interactions. A reliability coefficient, called the intraclass correlation coefficient (ICC), can be computed. Unlike

Table 12.2 A Hypothetical Illustration of Systematic Disagreement Due to Differences in Rater Severity/Leniency

Observation	Rater 1	Rater 2
1	2	5
2	3	6
3	5	8
4	1	4
5	6	9
6	4	7

other reliability estimates it is not sample dependent; therefore the components approach is also referred to as generalizability theory. Another important value of this statistic is that it reflects the extent of agreement between raters including systematic disagreement which is not reflected in other estimates of reliability (Ottenbacher & Tomchek, 1993).

Validity

Validity means that measure derived from an instrument represents the underlying construct that the instrument is designed to measure. Strictly speaking, an instrument is never validated. Rather, investigators seek to validate an interpretation of the scores the instrument yields (Benson & Schell, 1997; Cronbach, 1971; Nunally, 1978). This distinction underscores the fact that all measurement instruments are used to make inferences about a specific characteristic of a person (or group in the case of community or group assessments). It is the validity of that inference that is ultimately of concern. Thus, when an instrument is said to have validity, it means that the interpretation of the measurement that is made with the instrument is correct in its meaning.

As noted earlier, all instruments are designed to measure some abstract characteristic or construct. A construct is a theoretical creation and so it is important to demonstrate the usefulness of the construct for explanation and for practice (e.g., making sense of a client's behavior, identifying a client's problems or strengths, predicting future functioning). Inevitably, concerns for validity also interrelate with the intended use and demonstrated utility of the results obtained from an instrument.

Validity is not an all-or-nothing property of an instrument, but rather a matter of degree (Benson & Schell, 1997). The validity of an instrument is demonstrated by the accumulation of several types of evidence produced over many studies. An instrument should be judged by a body of evidence that provides or fails to provide support for its validity. Moreover, ongoing research should continue to provide evidence about the validity of an instrument long after it is published and in use.

> The validity of an instrument is demonstrated by the accumulation of several types of evidence produced over many studies.

How one goes about generating or assessing the evidence of validity depends on both the underlying trait is seeks to measure and the intended use of the assessment. Generally, the following are indices that are used to develop and assess validity of an instrument:

- Face validity,
- Content validity,
- Criterion validity, and
- Construct validity.

Each is discussed and illustrated below.

Face Validity

Face validity means that an instrument has the appearance of measuring an underlying construct. For example, if an assessment is designed to measure an attitude about leisure (i.e., how important leisure is), and the items all are made up of statements about leisure, the instrument can be said to have face validity. Face validity is, however, the weakest evidence of validity. For example, consider the following statements about leisure:

- I always try to make time for leisure activities.
- I often feel there is not enough time to do the things I enjoy.
- Doing leisure activities helps one achieve relaxation and refreshment.
- Engaging in leisure always enhances my mood.

On the face of it, the items all ask about leisure and, arguably, reflect how much a person values leisure. However, the second item may reflect more about how much a person works or fulfills other non-leisure obligations than how much leisure is important to that person. Similarly, the last item may reflect whether a person is depressed instead of how much leisure is valued.

Consequently, face validity alone is insufficient to demonstrate the validity of an instrument. However, it is often a good place to start when one is trying to generate or create items to make up an instrument. Moreover, face validity can be helpful in deciding whether or not to use an instrument. If the items that make up an instrument are not, on the face of it, relevant or meaningful to what one aims to measure or to the intended audience, then the instrument is not likely to be valid for that purpose. Finally, in the absence of any other evidence about the validity of an instrument, face validity is the minimum criterion that one should apply when deciding whether to use an instrument. However, since there is no formal way of evaluating face validity, it is ultimately an informal process. Consequently, two experts may review the same instrument and one might say it has face validity and the other may not.

Content Validity

Content validity refers to the adequacy with which an instrument captures the domain or universe of the construct it aims to measure (Nunally, 1978). The constructs that instruments are intended to measure inevitably include a range of content. For example, self-care includes such content as brushing teeth, bathing, and dressing. When developing or judging an instrument, one must ask whether the universe of content represented by the underlying construct is adequately reflected in the instrument.

In addition to the concern about whether all the relevant content is included in an instrument, content validity is also concerned that irrelevant content be excluded from the instrument. So, for example, an assessment of self-care should not have items that reflect socializing with friends or performance at work, since these occupations are not part of the occupation of self-care.

Content validation requires one to conceptually define the domain that is being measured and specify how this domain is to be operationally defined (i.e., making concrete the elements of the conceptual definition) (Benson & Schell, 1997). Only then can one determine that the items that make up an instrument adequately represent the universe of the construct.

Assessing content validity often begins with developing a set of specifications about what domains make up the construct of interest. This can be done by:

- Reviewing relevant literature,
- Reviewing existing instruments that target the construct to see what content is included, and
- Seeking the opinions of an expert panel (i.e., a group of individuals who have in-depth knowledge or expertise concerning the domain of interest).

Sometimes expert panels are consulted in several rounds as an instrument is being developed. For example, in the first round members of the panel may be asked to brainstorm content that should be included. In the second round they may be asked to examine a list of content for its comprehensiveness and focus. In a third round they may be asked to generate or evaluate specific items that reflect the content.

The following is an example of how one group of instrument developers approached the issue of content validity. In developing the Volitional Questionnaire (de las Heras, Geist, Kielhofner, & Li, 2003), investigators first identified the broad construct of volition that includes a person's thoughts and feelings about personal causation (effectiveness and capacity), interests, and values. Moreover, included in the definition of the construct was that volition was manifested across a continuum of exploratory, competency, and achievement motivation. This instrument was designed to capture volition as it is manifested in behavior. Thus, to operationalize the construct of volition the authors had to specify ways that a person demonstrated a sense of capacity and efficacy, interest, and value or meaningfulness in action across the continuum from exploration to competency to achievement. Items were generated based on clinical experience and using feedback from a panel of experts who used the concept of volition in practice (Chern, Kielhofner, de las Heras, & Magalhaes, 1996).

The resulting items that were designed to capture the universe of volition are shown in Table 12.3. Later research, using Item Response Theory, identified that the items all belonged to the construct of volition and represented a continuum from exploration to competency (Li & Kielhofner, 2004).

One important consideration in identifying the universe or domain of a construct is how broadly it is defined since it affects the degree of inference that someone using the instrument must make. Borg and Gall (1983) note that a low-inference construct is one that is readily or easily observed and that requires only limited judgment on the part of the observer. In contrast, a high-inference item may involve a series of events or behaviors and/or one that requires the observer to assemble different aspects of a client's behavior into a judgment. High-inference items tend to produce less reliable observation. Therefore, low- inference items have the virtue of making observational scales more reliable. This is often the case when the trait of interest is relatively concrete.

However, in occupational therapy there are variables of interest that are more difficult to translate into low-inference items. The Volitional Questionnaire, which was described earlier, is an example of this situation. The developers of this instrument wanted to measure volition from observing the behavior of individuals who could

Table 12.3 Items that Make Up the Volitional Questionnaire

ACHIEVEMENT

Seeks challenges.
Seeks additional
    responsibilities.
Invests additional
    energy/emotion/attention.
Pursues an activity
    to completion/
    accomplishment.

COMPETENCY

Tries to solve problems.
Shows pride.
Tries to correct
    mistakes/failures.
Indicates goals.
Stays engaged.

EXPLORATION

Shows that an activity is special
    or significant.
Tries new things.
Initiates actions/tasks.
Shows curiosity.
Shows preferences.

not self-report their volitional thoughts and feelings. Making inferences about motivation based on behavior requires a level of abstraction and judgment. Consequently, the instrument's developers had to create a detailed manual with definitions and examples of each item. Moreover, it is important that the person using the Volitional Questionnaire have a theoretical understanding of volition, the construct that the instrument seeks to measure.

As this example illustrates, it is important in high-inference instruments that the observer/rater have adequate background and understanding of the intended construct and how it is operationalized. Sometimes, this need can be addressed though a detailed user's manual. Moreover, in some instances, training in how to use the instrument is also desirable or necessary (Benson & Schell, 1997). It also seems that in these types of instruments, the user must have both a solid theoretical background and commitment to applying theory in practice.

Assessing content validity is inherently a subjective and conceptual process that involves consideration of the various domains that make up a construct. Sometimes these domains are specified by consensus, as in the case of self-care. Other times, the domains must be identified from a particular theoretical perspective, as in the earlier examples of the Volitional Questionnaire

Finally, when developing a questionnaire or self-report, it is often important to identify the domain from the perspective of persons who will be responding to the instrument. For example, if the intention of a self-report assessment is to capture environmental barriers to disabled persons' independent living, content validity would require that it include all the things that persons with disabilities encounter as barriers. In this case, using focus groups of persons with disabilities to generate ideas about and to evaluate the content of such an instrument would be advisable.

Criterion Validity

Unlike face and content validity, criterion validity involves collecting objective evidence about the validity of an assessment. Criterion validity refers to the ability of an instrument to produce results that concur with or predict a known criterion instrument or known variable. As the definition implies, criterion validity includes two types of evidence:

• Concurrent validity, and
• Predictive validity.

When assessing criterion validity, it is important to select a criterion instrument that is recognized and demonstrated to have good reliability and validity. Often such an instrument is referred to as the "gold standard" instrument (i.e., an instrument that is widely recognized and empirically demonstrated to be a reliable and valid measure of the intended construct). Benson and Schell (1997) also recommend and provide a formula for estimating the upper bound (highest possible value) of a validity coefficient. If it is too low, then they recommend improving one of the two measures or selecting a different criterion measure. They also provide a related formula for estimating how high a validity coefficient would be if the two measures were perfectly correlated; if the value of this estimate is too low, then they recommend choosing a different criterion measure.

Concurrent Validity

Concurrent validity refers to evidence that the instrument under development or investigation concurs or covaries with the result of another instrument that is known to measure the intended construct or with another criterion. Concurrent validity is often the method of choice when there is an existing "gold standard" instrument. One may ask, if such an instrument exists, why develop a new assessment? There may be a variety of reasons. For example, the existing instrument(s) may be too lengthy or costly to administer regularly. Moreover, the existing assessments may demand capabilities for participation that the intended clients do not possess. Finally, the existing instruments may simply not be practical for use in the situation for which the new instrument is intended.

Concurrent validity is assessed by administering the new assessment that is under development or investigation at the same time as the criterion instrument or variable and then calculating a correlation. If the two instruments are found to be highly correlated then there is evidence of concurrent validity. For example, Sudsawad, Trombly, Henderson, and Tickle-Degnen (2000) studied the relationship between the Evaluation Tool of Children's Handwriting (ETCH) and teachers' perceptions of handwriting legibility (the criterion variable) using a questionnaire that asked about the student's handwriting performance in the classroom. Contrary to expectations, there was no significant relationship between the ETCH and teacher questionnaire scores in legibility or task-specific legibility. The findings of this study brought into question whether the ETCH validly measures handwriting legibility.

Predictive Validity

Predictive validity involves evidence that a measure is a predictor of a future criterion. Assessment of predictive validity is achieved by administering the instrument under question first and then collecting data on the criterion variable at a later time. For example, if an assessment is designed to capture a client's ability for independent living or return to work, then the appropriate criteria would be whether the person is living independently or employed at a future date.

Predictive validity is often challenging to demonstrate because it requires a longitudinal study. All other forms of validity and reliability testing can essentially be done through simultaneous data collection. Nonetheless, it can be powerful evidence of validity.

Construct Validity

Construct validity refers to the capacity of an instrument to measure the intended underlying construct. In reality, construct validity is the ultimate objective of all forms empirically assessing validity, but the process of empirically assessing construct validity involves a series of studies that provide cumulative evidence. Construct validity is ultimately concerned with the underlying construct that the instrument targets. Construct validity is crucial when the "interpretation to be made of the scores implies an explanation of the behavior or trait" (Bensen & Schell, 1997, p. 11).

As noted earlier, the idea of a construct is a theoretical conceptualization. As such, it is tied to a network of explanatory ideas that make sense of the trait. This network of explanation is foundational to how construct validation is accomplished. It includes not only a clear definition of the construct but also how it is related to other constructs. A well articulated theory that explains a construct and its relationship to other constructs allows for a stronger approach to validation.

> A well articulated theory that explains a construct and its relationship to other constructs allows for a stronger approach to validation.

Construct validity testing is sometimes referred to as hypothesis driven, since studies that provide evidence of construct validity test hypotheses that are based on theoretical assertions about the construct and its relationship to other variables.

There are several approaches to demonstrating construct validity; the most common include:

- Known groups method,
- Convergent and divergent methods, and
- Factor analytic methods.

Each is discussed below.

Known Groups Method

The known groups method involves identifying subjects who are demonstrated to differ on the characteristic the instrument aims to measure. So, for example, if an instrument is designed to measure capacity of independent living, it might be administered to people who are living in nursing homes and those living independently in the community. In this instance, the instrument should produce different scores for the two groups of persons (i.e., document differences known to exist in the two different groups).

With the known groups method, it is also common to perform a discriminant analysis (see Chapter 17) to evaluate the ability of the measure(s) derived from the instrument to correctly classify the subjects into their known groups. Discriminant analysis is a form of regression analysis in which independent variables (in this case, test scores) and categorical dependent variables (group membership) are analyzed. Based on an equation generated by the discriminant analysis, individuals are assigned to groups in the analysis. If the measure accurately discriminates subjects into known groups, there is evidence of validity.

Convergent and Divergent Methods

Assessment of convergent and divergent validity involves theoretically derived comparisons. Convergence is the principle that two measures intended to capture the same underlying trait should be highly correlated. Convergence obviously overlaps with the concept of concurrent validity. Implied in the concept of concurrent validity is that the association between two measures of the same construct should be demonstrated across different circumstances of place, sample, and time.

Divergence (or discriminant validity) is the principle that tests designed to measure different traits should show patterns of association that discriminate between the traits. Thus, for example two measures of unrelated traits such as attitudes toward leisure and motor capacity should be unrelated. Similarly, measures of associated but not identical constructs should be moderately related. Thus, in using convergent and divergent methods, investigators examine how closely the results of an instrument correlate with measures of characteris-

tics that are closer and more distant conceptually from the intended construct and asking whether the strength of association is related.

Campbell and Fiske (1959) proposed a combination of convergent and divergent validity for assessing validity; it is referred to as the multitrait–multimethod approach. According to this approach an investigator would examine two or more traits using two or more instruments (methods) for measuring each trait. For example, if one is developing an instrument to measure problem-solving, it should correlate strongly with another test of problem-solving and moderately with a test of attention. Similarly, two tests of attention should correlate more strongly than tests of different traits such as a test of attention and a test of problem solving. The logic is that the two tests designed to measure the same thing should be more correlated than two tests designed to measure concepts whose functions overlap as illustrated in Figure 12.2.

Factor Analytic Method

When investigators believe that a construct is or may be multidimensional, factor analysis (see Chapter 17) is sometimes used to empirically demonstrate the dimensions of the construct. Factor analysis examines a set of items that make up an instrument and determines whether there are one or more clusters of items.

Sachs and Josman (2003) used factor analysis to study the Activity Card Sort (ACS), a standardized assessment that aims to measure the amount and level of involvement in various activities. The ACS requires persons to sort cards depicting peo-

Figure 12.2 An illustration of the multitrait–multimethod matrix: Expected pattern of concurrence–divergence based on theoretical associations of problem-solving and attention.

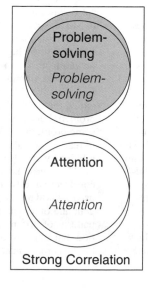

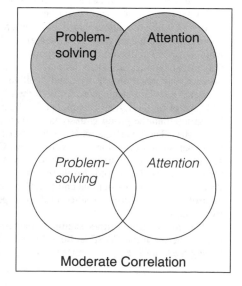

ple engaged in real-life activities into categories. The investigators administered the ACS to 184 participants (53 students and 131 elderly persons). Factor analysis revealed five factors (i.e., demanding leisure, instrumental activities of daily living, maintenance, leisure, and social recreation) for students and four factors (i.e., instrumental activities of daily living, leisure, demanding leisure, and maintenance) for older persons based on 60 pictures. The results of this study indicate an important feature of factor analysis (i.e., its sample dependency). Factors from an instrument identified for one group cannot be assumed to be the same for another group. Moreover, factors should be previously hypothesized based on the underlying theory. Exploratory factor analysis that looks for patterns after the fact does not provide evidence of validity.

Summary

As noted earlier, evidence about construct validity is ordinarily reflected in a number of the types of construct validity just discussed. The feature box below includes an example of an investigation designed to provide evidence about construct validity. The study reported in this feature box is one of a series of studies that ultimately contribute to the construct validity of the instrument in question.

Interrelationship of Reliability and Validity

The reliability and validity of instruments are interrelated. If an instrument is unreliable because of random measurement error, it cannot be valid.

A Study of Construct Validity

Koning and Magill-Evans (2001) studied the construct validity of the Child and Adolescent Social Perception Measure (CASP) (Magill-Evans, Koning, Cameron-Sadava, & Manyk, 1995), an instrument that measures the ability to use nonverbal cues to identify the emotions of others. This instrument involves 10 videotaped scenes that depict situations that children and adolescents frequently encounter (with verbal content removed). After viewing each scene, the persons being tested are asked to identify the emotions portrayed by each of the characters and to note which cues they used to identify the emotions. The instrument generates two scores: an emotion score (ES) that reflects the ability to correctly identify emotions and a nonverbal cues score (ESC) that reflects the ability to correctly identify the cues that were present in the scene for inferring emotions.

In this study, the authors used a known groups approach. Participants were 32 adolescent males who had social skills deficits consistent with the diagnosis of Asperger's Disorder and 29 controls who were matched on sex, age, and intelligence quotient (IQ). The mean score for both the ES and ESC scores on the CASP was higher for the control group than the group with social skills deficits ($p < .001$). The investigators also used discriminant analysis to determine how well the two CASP scores together could discriminate the subjects into the two groups. The found that 96.9% of the children with social skills deficits and 86.2% of the controls were correctly classified in their respective groups.

The investigators further examined the correlation between the CASP and the Social Skills Rating System (SSRS), a standardized assessment of general social skills (which does not measure social perception). This instrument can be used by a parent, a teacher, or completed via self-report. Because it measures a construct (general social skills) that is related to (but not identical to) the construct of social perception measured by the CASP, moderate correlations were predicted. Correlations between the ES and ESC and the parent, child, and teacher ratings on the SSRS ranged from .34 to .63, as expected. The pattern of correlations (stronger association for parent and teacher than for students) was as expected, since children with social skills problems tend to have difficulty admitting their problems with peers. Similarly, moderate correlations were predicted with IQ (i.e., 59 for both the ES and ESC).

Correlations with three scores from the Clinical Evaluation of Language Fundamentals-Revised (CELF-R), a standardized evaluation of expressive and receptive language skills (a construct not expected to be highly related to social perception), ranged from .29 to .40. Correlations of the CASP with scores obtained from the Child Behavior Checklist (CBCL), a standardized questionnaire in which the teacher or parent report the frequency of problem behaviors, ranged from .38 to .57. Since some problem behaviors are related to difficulties in reading social cues, these somewhat higher correlations were also consistent with expectations.

This study illustrates a systematic approach to construct validity for the CASP. The investigators used a known groups method, along with convergent and divergent methods. They demonstrated patterns of difference/discrimination and association that fit based on theoretical arguments about the construct under study.

However, a reliable instrument is not, de facto, valid. That is, an instrument might produce consistent results but the items may not be targeted to the intended variable; in this instance the items would consistently measure something other than the intended construct.

In the end, a desirable instrument achieves consistent results that clearly target the underlying construct the instrument is designed to measure. Factors that make for a weak instrument generally affect both reliability and validity. For example, if an instrument includes several items that are ambiguous, the instrument will have high error (unreliability) and will fail to consistently target the underlying characteristic of interest (invalidity). Efforts to enhance any instrument ordinarily target both reliability and validity simultaneously.

Creating and Evaluating Evidence of Reliability and Validity

As noted earlier, validity is always a matter of degree that is reflected in the extent of accumulated evidence about an instrument. Moreover, the more variability in evidence (e.g., across types of validity, populations, and situations), the more confidence one can have in the validity of a measure.

Deciding how to go about validating an instrument or judging the evidence on behalf of an instrument depends in part on the intended use of the instrument. For example, Law (1987) argues that different approaches are relevant depending on whether the purpose of an instrument is descriptive, predictive, or evaluative. If the purpose is descriptive, then evidence of content and construct validation is most relevant. If the purpose is predictive, then content and criterion-related validity are important to assess. If the purpose is evaluative, content and construct validity is most important.

In the end, each instrument developer must pursue a logic and strategy that provides evidence connected to:

• The nature of intended construct,
• The purpose to which the instrument will be put,
• The population(s) with whom the instrument is intended to be used, and
• The types of circumstances in which the instrument will be applied.

When all these factors are reflected in the evidence of validity, one can have a degree of confidence in the validity of the instrument.

Other Psychometric Properties

Reliability and validity are fundamental to any good instrument. However, since instruments are used in practice and research to measure traits in ways that influence clinical and research decisions, a good instrument must have other properties that include:

• Precision,
• Sensitivity and specificity,
• Criterion or norm referencing, and
• Standardized scores and standard error of measurement.

Each of these psychometric properties is discussed below.

Precision

Precision refers to the exactness of a measure (i.e., the extent of its ability to discriminate differing amounts of a variable). The more precise a measure is, the finer its ability to discriminate between different amounts. For example, a ruler that is calibrated only to 1/8 of an inch cannot accurately discriminate smaller amounts. A ruler that is calibrated to 1/16th of an inch is more sensitive in measuring distance and, thus, has more precision. Similarly, a scale that measures only pounds is less precise than a scale that measures pounds and ounces. The precision of physical measures is determined by the fineness of the calibration they use.

All other things being equal, the precision of measures of psychological or behavioral traits (e.g., measures that are based on self-reports or rating scales) is generally related to the number of items on the scale. If each item is conceptualized as an "estimate" of the underlying trait, precision increases with each estimate. Of, course other factors affect precision including the error associated with each item and how well the items are targeted to the person being measured (see Chapter 13 for a discussion of this issue).

Because more items increase precision, it would seem logical to compose instruments of as many items as possible. However, lengthy instruments are often not feasible in either practice or research. Moreover, when instruments are too lengthy, error can be increased because of such factors as fatigue. Thus, in constructing an assessment a balance must be struck between enhancing precision through increased items and practical issues of instrumentation (e.g., time, cost demands on the client or subject).

Precision is closely linked to the ability of an instrument to measure change (sometimes referred to as responsiveness to change) as well as to power and effect size (discussed in Chapter 16). For instance, if a scale is calibrated to the nearest pound only and a child grows by gaining 7 ounces, no change will be detected. In choosing or developing an instrument for research or practice, one will need to consider how much change is relevant or important to detect and select an instrument with the appropriate level of sensitivity. For example, if one were studying the influence of an intervention on the growth rates of premature infants, a scale calibrated to ounces might be very important. On the other hand, a study of weight loss among obese adults would not require the same level of sensitivity.

There is no standard way to assess the precision of an instrument since desired precision is always a function of the purpose to which an instrument is being applied. One common approach is to readminister an assessment following a time interval or circumstance that is expected to produce a change and determine through statistical testing whether a change in the mean score is detected. Another solution is to calculate an effect size (see Chapter 16) in the same circumstances.

Sensitivity and Specificity

When instruments are used to determine the existence of a problem or the need for therapy, sensitivity and specificity are concerns. Sensitivity refers to the ability of an instrument to detect the presence of a problem or condition when it is present. Specificity is the ability of an instrument to produce negative results when the problem or condition is not present.

Most occupational therapy instruments do not result in simple dichotomous decisions about the presence or absence of a problem. Rather, they typically produce continuous data that illustrate where the individual falls on a continuum of less to more of the trait measured. Instruments require a cutoff score when they are used to make a clinical decision about whether a problem is present (or sufficiently present to warrant intervention or some other decisions such as discharge placement).

A cutoff score is the point beyond which a person is determined to have a problem, or to be unable to perform an activity or achieve a level of independence. In establishing a cutoff score, one has to take into consideration the sensitivity and specificity of the cutoff. That is, one does not want

to detect the presence of a problem when it does not exist, nor does one want to incorrectly decide a problem is not present.

In establishing the cutoff, increasing sensitivity will also likely reduce specificity. In other words, if a higher score means a problem is present and the cutoff is set at a lower level, then sensitivity is increased (persons with the problem will likely be detected) but at the same time specificity is probably reduced (some persons without the condition will be judged to have it). If the cutoff is set higher specificity can be increased (fewer or no persons will be incorrectly judged to have the problem), but sensitivity will be decreased (some persons with the problem may not be detected). The extent to which this is an issue depends on how precise an assessment is, but since all instruments have limited precision and some error, one has to decide in which direction it is better to err.

Norm Referencing and Criterion Referencing

The aim of any instrument is to allow the user to make judgments. Two typical ways that judgments are formed are through norm referencing or criterion referencing. Criterion referencing refers to making judgments or interpretations of a score with reference to what is considered adequate or acceptable performance (Portney & Watkins, 2000). In occupational therapy, criterion may be typically linked to such factors as performance (i.e., adequacy for completing a task), participation (i.e., ability to partake in a occupation such as work or leisure or live independently in the community), and quality of life or well being (e.g., adequate feelings of efficacy).

Sometimes a criterion is clearly linked to the content of a scale (e.g., if a scale includes all the abilities that are necessary to drive safely, then passing all the items may be the criterion). In other cases criteria are tied to a level of knowledge or ability such as passing a certain percentage of items on a test. Criterion referencing works best when it is clearly linked to a relevant outcome. In some instances it will be necessary to gather empirical data on the measure and compare it to the criterion in order to determine the logic for the criterion.

Norms are summarized data from the sample on which an instrument is developed (Benson & Schell, 1997). Norms are created by administering an instrument in a standardized way and then combining and summarizing the scores obtained from all those on whom data were collected. Norms should be created by testing a large sample that meets a profile (e.g., that proportionally represents all those with whom the instrument is intended to be used).

Norms are usually reported in terms of means, standard deviations, percentiles, and standard scores. It is important to recognize that norms are sample dependent, so that it is important that the sample on which norms are based is thoroughly described (Benson & Schell, 1997). When considering the usefulness of norms one should consider whether the sample on which norms are based is sufficiently similar to the intended population. For instance, one might ask whether the ages, cultural background, and sex of the sample are the same as in the target population.

Considerable misunderstanding and controversy exists over the use of norm-versus criterion-referenced tests. Proponents of norm-referencing argue that norms provide important points of reference from which to judge whether or not a person's performance or characteristic is of concern or warrants intervention. Critics of norm-referencing point out that norms often fail to take into consideration variability in development and performance and they argue that use of norms unfairly devalues or stigmatizes persons who are different from the average. Proponents of criterion-referencing point out that criteria are more "objective" in that they link judgments to something that is rational and not biased by a preference for the typical. Critics of criterion referencing point out that a criterion can sometimes be arbitrarily imposed. In the end, the use of both norm and criterion referencing should be done with clear attention to the purposes for which they are being used and the consequences of making judgments.

In clinical practice, these considerations must be individualized for a client. For example, identifying a child's deviation from developmental motor or cognitive norms may be important to determining the need for early intervention services for one child with developmental disability. On the other hand, some developmental norms may be much less relevant than criteria for making judgments about treatment intervention with a child who is severely developmentally delayed.

Standardized Scores and Standard Error of Measurement

Standardized scores (i.e., *t*-scores) are sometimes developed for instrument scores to facilitate comparison of an individual's score to that of others on

whom norms have been developed for the instrument. The *t*-scores are computed by setting the mean at 50 and the standard deviation at 10. They allow a person's raw score to be converted to a percentile for comparison to normative data.

If any instrument was applied to an individual an infinite number of times, it is reasonable to assume that the scores obtained would vary somewhat each time. Theoretically, the distribution of these scores would resemble a normal curve (see Chapter 15 for discussion of the normal curve). Moreover, the mean of all these measures would be equal to the person's true score (i.e., the actual amount of the variable or characteristics in the person being measured) and the scores would be evenly distributed on either side of this mean with fewer and fewer obtained scores the more extreme the deviation from the mean. The more accurate or error free a measure, the more closely the obtained scores will be distributed around the mean.

The standard deviation of all the measurement errors is referred to as the standard error of measurement (SEM). The SEM for a given instrument is estimated from a sample of subjects using the following formula:

$$SEM = s_x \sqrt{1 - r_{xx}}$$

where s_x = the standard deviation of the observed scores and r_{xx} = the reliability coefficient for the instrument (e.g., test–retest or inter-rater reliability) (Portney & Watkins, 2000).

The SEM can be interpreted according to the characteristics of the normal curve. That is, there is a 68% chance that an individual's true score falls within ± 1 SEM of the obtained score and a 95% chance that the true score falls within ± 2 SEM of the obtained score. An important limitation of the SEM is that its interpretation is dependent on the type of reliability coefficient that is used to compute it. So, for example if it is based on test–retest reliability the SEM reflects the error expected based on readministration; it will not take into consideration error due to rater bias.

Conclusion

This chapter provided an overview of the main issues of concern in the development and evaluation of measurement instruments from the perspective of classical test theory. Entire books are devoted to detailed discussions of the concepts and methods of measurement and instrument construction. Therefore, this chapter is best taken as an orientation to these issues and as a guide for examining literature that reports the development and empirical study of measurement instruments. Moreover, the next two chapters will add additional considerations for evaluating and developing measures.

The Process of Instrument Development

Instrument development is an ongoing process that, arguably, has no clear endpoint. Basically, an instrument should be developed and judged following a stream of evidence about its reliability and validity. Different authors have recommended the sequence of steps that should go into the construction and investigation of instruments (Benson & Clark, 1982; Benson & Hagtvet, 1996).

Nonetheless, there is no standard process for developing assessments. The following is a recommendation of steps that can be followed based on the literature and the experience of this author in developing a number of instruments. Since this chapter focuses on classical test theory, these steps will mainly refer to the methods that belong to that approach. Other approaches to instrument development are discussed in Chapter 13 and are followed by many instrument developers. It should be noted that the steps of instrument development noted below are not strictly linear. Often, instrument developers will move back and forth between steps as an instrument is being refined.

- **Identify the need for the instrument.** A large number of instruments both within and relevant to occupational therapy exist. Thus, before embarking on the development of an instrument, one should first identify the need for the assessment. Typical reasons for developing an assessment are the lack of adequate assessments for the intended construct and the inapplicability of existing assessments for the intended population or context of administration. This step obviously requires that one comprehensively review the literature to identify existing instruments and their properties.
- **Identify the purpose and the intended population.** Measurement instruments are tools for accomplishing particular aims with a particular group of clients or subjects. One should clearly outline the purpose of the instrument, including what type of information it is intended to generate and for what ends the information will be used. In addition, one needs to consider the intended population in terms of such factors as age, cultural background, and what types of impairment may be present. This information is important to determining both the content and the format of the instrument.

For the investigator who is seeking to develop an assessment, the references cited in this chapter and the resources listed below are a good beginning. In addition, the feature box includes a discussion of the general steps involved in developing and empirically assessing instruments.

- **Specify the underlying construct.** Good measurement begins with a clear articulation of the underlying construct an instrument is designed to measure. Instrument developers focus not only on clearly articulating the trait or variable the instrument targets, but also on whether this trait is homogeneous or multifaceted.
- **Create a plan of how the construct will be operationalized.** This step involves identifying the range or universe of content that will be included. If a multidimensional construct is intended, each subconstruct needs to be clearly defined and its content identified. If the instrument targets a single homogeneous construct, the content within this domain needs to be identified. During this stage, it is also helpful to think about what represents the continuum of the construct. Particular attention should be paid to the upper and lower ends of the characteristics to be measured to ensure that the content covers the whole range of variation in the characteristic (construct) to be measured.

During this stage it is often useful to consult with experts (i.e., with persons who have knowledge and experience relevant to the intended construct, purpose, and population of the instrument). Focus groups with such experts (including clients for whom the instrument is intended) can be helpful in brainstorming appropriate content.
- **Decide the format of the instrument.** This step is linked to identifying the purpose of the instrument. It involves deciding the actual mechanism by which information will be gathered and translated into numbers. Some typical choices are self-report forms or card sorts that will be scored, observational instruments that use categorical or ordinal rating forms, interviews accompanied by rating forms, tests of various capacities, and so on. This step should also give consideration to the population for which the instrument is intended to make sure the format of the instrument is suited to their age, capacity, and so forth.

An important consideration at this stage is how the instrument will be administered and by whom. If it is intended to be a self-administered instrument, then consideration has to be given to the persons who will be taking it (e.g., their

(continued)

reading level and their perspective). If it is to be administered by a tester or observer, consideration needs to be given to how much knowledge and skill will be assumed.

During this stage, developers consider details of the instrument. For example, if the instrument is a rating form one needs to consider whether the items will be rated as dichotomous (yes/no) or on an ordinal scale. If an ordinal rating is used, then developers must consider how many rating points should be included. This decision is influenced by considering conceptually how many values or points are important to identify. For example, in creating a rating of self-care independence, investigators have generally sought to discriminate between levels of assistance that are needed so that a three-point scale (e.g., independent, needs assistance, dependent) is considered insufficient to discriminate the levels of independence that are of clinical relevance.

Another consideration is variability. Scales generally provide more variability when there are more rating points. One exception, however, is that, sometimes, scales with middle points (e.g., a five-point scale) provide less variability than scales without a neutral rating (e.g., a four-point scale) since the latter forces persons who other-wise would overuse the neutral rating to make discriminations. A final consideration is how fine a discrimination the respondent or user can make. Providing a seven-point scale to clients who do not make such fine discriminations in their judg-ments will only add error to the instrument.

• **Develop items.** Once the target construct and format for the instrument are clearly defined and operationalized, the developer will go about cre-ating the actual items that make up the question-naire, test, and rating scale. This process is critical since an instrument will only be as good as the items of which it is constructed. Develop-ment of items often involves:

• Asking for feedback from a panel of experts on initial items. This helps to ensure that the con-tent targets the intended variable (when experts are knowledgeable about the variable of inter-est) and that the content is relevant to practi-cal/clinical considerations (when experts are experienced practitioners). This can be done in a focus group format or through a survey. Often it is helpful to create a survey of intended items and ask experts to provide feedback on several dimensions of each intended item (e.g., clarity, relevance, importance).

• Doing focus groups with persons with whom the instrument will be used and/or with practi-tioners who will use the assessment. This is often done to ensure the relevance of the items to those for whom it is intended. Relevance may mean that the items are:

• At the right level of difficulty,
• Understandable,
• Applicable to the circumstance of the respondent, and
• Reflect what they consider important about the thing being measured.

When focus groups are not feasible, it may be useful to approach a series of individuals for their opinions on these issues.

• **Develop supporting materials.** This step involves clearly delineating and writing out instructions, procedures, meanings of items, and so on. Usually, at this stage one will create an administration guide or manual to accompany the instrument.

• **Pilot the instrument.** During this stage, a first version of the intended instrument should be applied as it is intended to be used and with the administrators and/or population for which it is intended. Pilot testing almost inevitably results in the identification of one or more of the following:

• Unforeseen difficulties in administration,
• Problems with content (e.g., too difficult or irrelevant),
• Ambiguity in items,
• Difficulty with test instructions or proce-dures, and
• Difficulties in using the categories or rating scale.

• **Revise the instrument and develop supporting materials.** Feedback from the pilot testing typi-cally results in identification of items that need to be clarified or revised and the need to more clearly spell out instructions, procedures, and meanings of items, and so on. Usually the pilot will result in revision of the administration guide or manual. Depending on the extent of revision needed, one may repeat the pilot phase and once again revise. Some instrument developers who use a participatory research process (see Chapters 38, 39, and 40) use an iterative process in which the instrument is successively piloted and revised with therapists and/or consumers acting as peers in the instrument development process.

• **Empirically assess reliability and validity in successive stages.** This step is actually a series of steps or studies that progressively assess the instrument. As noted in this chapter, how one goes about this depends on the nature of the instrument being developed. One should develop a plan of the sequence of questions that are to be asked about reliability and validity. Generally, it is useful to start with smaller samples that are necessary for the statistics to be performed, since early studies often result in further revision of the instrument. Once the instrument is finalized, larger samples necessary for creating norms or identifying criterion (cutoffs) can be studied.

REFERENCES

Ayres, A. J. (1989). *Sensory integration and praxis texts (manual)*. Los Angeles: Western Psychological Services.

Benson, J., & Cark, F. (1982). A guide for instrument development and validation. *American Journal of Occupational Therapy, 36*, 789–800.

Benson, J., & Hagtvet, K. (1996). The interplay between design and data analysis in the measurement of coping. In M. Zeidner & N. Endler (Eds.), *Handbook of coping* (pp. 83–106). New York: John Wiley & Sons.

Benson J., & Schell, B. A. (1997). Measurement theory: Application to occupational and physical therapy. In J. Van Deusen & D. Brunt (Eds.), *Assessment in occupational therapy and physical therapy* (pp. 3–24). Philadelphia: W. B. Saunders.

Borg, W., & Gall, M. (1983). *Educational research: An introduction* (4th ed.). New York: Longman.

Campbell, D. T., & Fiske, D. W. (1959). Convergent and discriminant validation for the multitrait-multimethod matrix. *Psychological Bulletin, 56*, 81–105.

Chern, J., Kielhofner, G., de las Heras, C., & Magalhaes, L. (1996). The volitional questionnaire: Psychometric development and practical use. *American Journal of Occupational Therapy, 50*, 516–525.

Clemson, L., Fitzgerald, M. H., Heard, R., & Cumming, R. G. (1999) Inter-rater reliability of a home fall hazards assessment tool. *Occupational Therapy Journal of Research, 19*, 83–100

Cohen, J. (1960) Coefficient of agreement for nominal scales. *Educational and Psychological Measurement, 20*, 37–46.

Cohen, J. (1968). Weighted kappa: nominal scale agreement with provision for scaled disagreement or partial credit. *Psychological Bulletin, 70*, 213–220.

Cronbach, L. J. (1951). Coefficient alpha and the internal structure of tests. *Psychometrika, 16*, 297–334.

Cronbach, L. J. (1971). Test validation. In R. L. Thorndike (Ed.), *Educational measurement* (2nd ed., pp. 443–507). Washington, DC: American Council on Education.

Cronbach, L. J. (1990). *Essentials of psychological testing* (5th ed.). New York: Harper and Row.

de las Heras, C. G., Geist, R., Kielhofner, G., & Li, Y. (2003). *The Volitional Questionnaire* (version 4.0). Model of Human Occupation Clearinghouse, Department of Occupational Therapy, College of Applied Health Sciences, University of Illinois at Chicago, Chicago, IL.

Doble, S., Fisk, J. D., Lewis, N., & Rockwood, K. (1999). Test–retest reliability of the assessment of motor and process skills in elderly adults. *Occupational Therapy Journal of Research, 19*, 203–219.

Fisher, A. G. (1993). The assessment if IADL motor skills: An application of many faceted Rasch analysis. *American Journal of Occupational Therapy, 47*, 319–329.

Fleiss, J. L. (1981). *Statistical methods for rates and proportions*. New York: John Wiley & Sons.

Forsyth, K., Deshpande, S., Kielhofner, G., Henriksson, C., Haglund, L., Olson, L., Skinner, S., & Kulkarni, S. (2005). *The Occupational Circumstances Assessment Interview and Rating Scale* (version 4.0). Model of Human Occupation Clearinghouse, Department of Occupational Therapy, College of Applied Health Sciences, University of Illinois at Chicago, Chicago, IL.

Guilford, J. (1979). *Psychometric methods* (2nd ed.). New York: McGraw-Hill.

Hambleton, R. K., & Jones, R. W. (1993). Comparison of classical test theory and item response theory and their applications to test development. *Educational Measurement: Issues and Practice, 12*, 38–47.

Keller, J., Kafkes, A., Basu, S., Federico, J., & Kielhofner, G. (2005) *The Child Occupational Self-Assessment (COSA)* (version 2.1). Model of Human Occupation Clearinghouse, Department of Occupational Therapy, College of Applied Health Sciences, University of Illinois at Chicago, Chicago, IL.

Koning, C., & Magill-Evans, J. (2001). Validation of the child and adolescent social perception. *Occupational Therapy Journal of Research, 21*, 41–67.

Lafayette Instruments (1969). *The Complete Minnesota Dexterity Test*. Examiner's manual. Lafayette Instruments, Lafayette Instrument Co., Lafayette, IN.

Law, M. (1987). Measurement in occupational therapy: Scientific criteria for evaluation. *Canadian Journal of Occupational Therapy, 54*(3), 133–138.

Li, Y., & Kielhofner, G. (2004). Psychometric properties of the Volitional Questionnaire. *Israeli Journal of Occupational Therapy, 13*, 85–98.

Magill-Evans, J., Koning, C., Cameron-Sadava, A, & Manyk, K. (1995). The child and adolescent social perception measure. *Journal of Nonverbal Behavior, 19*, 151–169.

Nunally, J. C. (1978). *Psychometric theory* (2nd ed.). New York: McGraw-Hill.

Ottenbacher, K. J., & Tomchek, S. D. (1993). Measurement in rehabilitation research: Consistency versus consensus. In C. V. Granger & G. E. Gresham (Eds.), *Physical medicine and rehabilitation clinics of North America: New developments in functional assessment* (pp. 463–473). Philadelphia: W. B. Saunders.

Portney, L. G., & Watkins, M. P. (2000). *Foundations of clinical research: Applications to practice* (2nd ed.). Upper Saddle River, NJ: Prentice-Hall.

Sachs, D., & Josman, N. (2003). The activity card sort: A factor analysis. *OTJR: Occupation, Participation and Health, 23*, 165–174.

Streiner, D. L., & Normal, G. R. (1995). *Health measurement scales: A practical guide to their development and use* (2nd ed.). New York: Oxford University Press.

Sudsawad, P., Trombly, C. A., Henderson, A., & Tickle-Degnen, L. (2000). The relationship between the evaluation tool of children's handwriting and teachers' perceptions of handwriting legibility. *American Journal of Occupational Therapy, 55*, 518–523.

RESOURCES

Benson, J., & Cark, F. (1982). A guide for instrument development and validation. *American Journal of Occupational Therapy, 36*, 789–800.

Cronbach, L. J. (1990). *Essentials of psychological testing* (5th ed.). New York: Harper and Row.

Nunally, J., & Bernstein I. H. (1994). *Psychometric theory* (3rd ed.). New York: McGraw-Hill.

Thorndike, R. L., & Hagen, E. (1990). *Measurement and evaluation in psychology and education* (5th ed.). New York: John Wiley & Sons.

Van Deusen J., & Brunt D. (Eds.) (1997). *Assessment in occupational therapy and physical therapy*. Philadelphia: W. B. Saunders.

CHAPTER 13

Objective Measurement: The Influence of Item Response Theory on Research and Practice

Craig A. Velozo • Kirsty Forsyth • Gary Kielhofner

As presented in Chapter 12, standardization, reliability, and validity are the cornerstone of developing sound instruments in occupational therapy and health care. Standardization in administering and scoring instruments is critical to ensure that scores obtained from different raters or administrations of an instrument are comparable. The consistency of results, as established by reliability testing, provides researchers and therapists with the confidence that the scores from assessments will be consistent at different times and across different raters. Furthermore, studies of validity, especially construct validity, provide evidence that instruments measure what they intend to measure.

Standardization, reliability, and validity of instruments are important since the correctness of judgments depends on them. Decisions of whether a client needs a given service, has improved, or should be discharged are typical judgments therapists make in everyday practice. Occupational therapy researchers make judgments about whether a tested intervention works, or whether one group differs from another on variables of interest. For such judgments to be sound, they must depend upon standardized, reliable, and valid assessment instrumentation.

In spite of the well-established psychometric procedures upon which occupational therapy and healthcare measures have been built, these assessments have always lacked the degree of accuracy found in measurement in the basic sciences. Obviously, many of the constructs assessed in occupational therapy (e.g., functional ability, burden of care, volition) are intrinsically more global or abstract than those found in the physical sciences (e.g., distance, temperature, and weight). Nonetheless, examining occupational therapy constructs from an objective measurement perspective

> Accurate, consistent, and meaningful measurement is possible only with standardized, reliable, and valid instruments.

reveals that many present and future instruments can emulate the precision of measures used in the physical sciences.

Accurate, consistent, and meaningful measurement is possible only with standardized, reliable, and valid instruments. The purpose of this chapter is to build upon and go beyond the traditional psychometric analyses that are discussed in Chapter 12. The chapter introduces concepts and examples of objective measurement. It also discuss methodologies that can provide additional value to existing instruments and provide a framework for developing new measures with features not attainable via traditional psychometrics. For reasons that will become apparent later in this chapter, the numbers attached to the majority of occupational therapy and healthcare assessments are referred to here as scores. Only those numbers that have the attributes of objective measurement are referred to as measures.

Comparison of Measures to Scores

One way to clarify the differences between objective measures and the present-day "scores" used in occupational therapy is to compare how basic-science measures distance with how occupational therapy attempts to rate or score self-care. Table 13.1 on p. 178 presents a summary of this comparison.

Equal Intervals

On all measures of distance, markings indicating increments of distance have equal intervals. For instance, markings of inches or centimeters have

Table 13.1 **Comparison of Measures to Scores**

Ruler (Measure)	ADL (Score)
Equal intervals—Markings on ruler represent equal intervals.	Unequal intervals—Ratings do not necessarily represent equal intervals.
Efficiency—Use only the aspect of the ruler that is most relevant to the object being measured.	Inefficiency—All items of the assessment are administered, independent of the ability of the individual.
Precision—Once the distance of an object is estimated, attention is paid to the finer markings of the ruler to gain precision.	Imprecision—No logical method to achieve precision.
Transparency—Distance can be translated across numerous instruments and converted across different scales.	Nontransparency—No convenient, reliable ways to translate scores between assessments.

equal distances along the entire length of the measurement instrument (e.g., the distance between 3 and 4 inches is the same as the distance between 1 and 2 inches, 5 and 6 inches, and so on). In contrast, the markings for scores on activities of daily living (ADL) assessments do not have this characteristic of equal intervals. The ratings of the items (or questions) of an assessment may appear to be equidistant since one often rates them with numbers (e.g., 1 = total dependence assist, 2 = needs maximal assist, 3 = moderate assist, 4 = minimal assist, and 5 = independent). Nonetheless, on this type of rating it cannot be guaranteed that the intervals between numbers are all the same. For example, is the interval between total dependence and maximum assistance equivalent to the interval between minimum assistance and independence? When studies have examined this type of question, answer is almost invariably, no. Even when rating scales are labeled with percentages (e.g., 25%, 50%, 75% independent) there is no guarantee that the distances between these ratings are equivalent.

Efficiency

The application of the ruler[1] (e.g., a 12-inch ruler, a yardstick, or a tape measure) to the task of measurement is easily learned and thus can be done with acceptable efficiency by virtually everyone. To measure the width of a small object, we do not have to use the entire ruler, just the part of the ruler that is relevant to the object that is being measur-

ing. That is, when measuring an object that is $8\frac{1}{2}$ inches wide, one uses only the markings close to $8\frac{1}{2}$ inches. One does not have to test the object against the markings at 2, 3, 4, 5 inches and so on. In contrast to using a ruler, the generating a score for ADL is not particularly efficient. The great majority of ADL instruments require that the client be scored on all items of the instrument. That is, even if an individual is capable of walking up stairs, according to standardized procedures, the assessor is required to evaluate whether or not that individual is capable of transferring to a toilet seat or in or out of a tub. Deriving a score from the instrument requires that all of the items of the instrument be rated so that they can be totaled.

Precision

Not only is a ruler efficient, but even the crudest of rulers is quite precise and can be used according to the level of precision desired. A quick observation may give an estimated width of the object (e.g., $8\frac{1}{2}$ inches) that may be adequate for many purposes. However, if desired, one can more closely observe with the ruler to more precisely measure the width of an object. By lining the finer markings on the ruler to the edge of the object one might arrive at the conclusion that 8 and $\frac{7}{16}$th inches is the more accurate measurement of its width.

Unfortunately, with traditional ADL instruments, there is no analogous method of achieving greater precision in measuring ADL status. Independent of the ability level of an individual, all items of the instrument must be used to obtain a score. This means that many items that provide little information on the person's ADL ability (i.e., items well below and/or well above the persons' ability level) are used to measure ADL ability. This approach sacrifices both efficiency and precision.

---

[1]This example of measurement is taken from continued American use of the English system of measurement. We are aware that in many other parts of the world the metric system is used for everyday measurement. The example we give can be easily extrapolated to this form of measurement.

Transparency

Measures of distance are "transparent" (Fisher, 1997). That is, the measures exist independently of the instruments used to generate them. When provided with a particular measure of distance (e.g., inch, centimeter, yard, meter, or mile), there is no need to indicate the instrument used to attain that measurement in order to understand what the measure means. Furthermore, translating scores across scales (e.g., inches to centimeters) is commonplace and easily accomplished by placing both scales on the same ruler or with simple conversion formulas.

The assessment of ADL is not so transparent. The meaning of scores is tied to the instrument used to generate the scores. Scores from one scale, such as the Functional Independence Measure (FIM™) are not easily translated into other ADL scales such as the Barthel Index. This limitation prevents monitoring clients across settings that use different ADL instruments (e.g., inpatient rehabilitation and skilled nursing facilities) and similarly makes it difficult to compare findings across studies that use different instruments.

Limitation of Scores Versus Measures

The terms measure and measurement are widely used to refer to occupational therapy and healthcare assessments that yield numerical values. However, such usage is not entirely accurate. Although all measures are numbers, all numbers are not measures (Wright, 1997b). It is common to assign numbers to information gathered in practice and research, especially when therapists or clients are asked to rate or judge information. In doing so, it is also common to ignore that one has made a major conceptual jump when attaching numbers to the qualitative statements used to characterize observations.

Because of its familiarity to many occupational therapists, the FIM is used throughout this chapter to demonstrate the limitations of using scores instead of measures in occupational therapy and health care. This is not intended to be an indictment of the FIM. The FIM shows sound psychometric qualities and efforts have been made to convert scores produced by the FIM to true meas-

ures using Rasch and IRT methodologies (Linacre, Heinemann, Wright, Granger, & Hamilton, 1994; Marino & Graves, 2004).

Scores Are Not Measures

Scores from most occupational therapy and healthcare instruments produce frequency counts, not measures. Total values obtained from these types of instruments represent the number of items the client passed (i.e., in yes/no or pass/fail instruments) or a total of the number of items with a rating of 1, 2, 3, 4, etc. Scores or frequency counts produced from most assessments used by occupational therapists fail to reflect the qualities of objective measurement and they fail to adequately capture the underlying construct that the instruments intend to represent.

> While all measures are numbers, all numbers are not measures.

Ordinal ratings produced by scores are not the same as interval ratings produced by measures. A measure is a number with which arithmetic and linear statistics can be accomplished (Wright & Linacre, 1989). That is, even the simplest form of mathematics requires interval values in which distances between consecutive ratings are equal (Merbitz, Morris, & Grip, 1989; Wright & Linacre, 1989). Scores fail to achieve interval-based measurement.

For example, on the FIM, item ratings indicating that total dependence is 0%, maximum assistance is 25%, moderate assistance is 50%, and so forth suggest that the adjacent ratings are equidistance from each other. However, these labels do not ensure that the distances between ratings are equal as is the case on an interval scale. Figure 13.1 on p. 180 shows a true interval scale and the typical type of ordinal scale used for rating ADL; as shown the latter usually has unequal intervals across the ratings. On such a scale, there is no mathematical guarantee that an improvement from total dependence to maximum assistance equals an improvement from modified independence to total independence. Without the guarantee that the distances between the numbers produced by instruments are interval, analyses from scores can lead to misinterpretations. For example, if improvement from total dependence to maximum assistance actually represents a larger change than an improvement from moderate assistance to minimum assistance, ordinal scores would underestimate improvements made by more severely impaired clients.

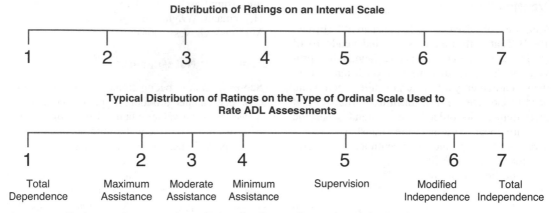

Figure 13.1 Rating scale comparison: Interval rating scale versus ordinal ratings.

There are other problems in how scores represent characteristics of clients or subjects. For example, on the FIM, the lowest score, 18, represents getting a 1 (total dependence) on all 18 items and the highest score, 126, reflects getting a 7 (independence without equipment) on all 18 items. A score of 18 on the FIM implies the lowest possible functional ability and score of 126 implies the highest possible functional ability.

These implications are incorrect. The lowest score of 18 does not differentiate a range of abilities (e.g., the individual who responds to only pinprick and the individual who only has the ability to bring a face cloth to his/her face). These two individuals would both would get the same, lowest score on the FIM while they actually have different ability levels. Similarly, a score of 126 does not reflect highest possible functional ability. This score would be assigned only to a certain range of individuals: those individuals with only minor physical and cognitive abilities, to individuals who are fully functional in all their life roles. Thus, the FIM would fail to differentiate these individuals. As with the FIM, scores produced by most instruments used by occupational therapists fail to adequately represent the true range of ADL abilities. These are ways in which the FIM and other assessments fail to achieve the requirements of objective measurement.

Scores Are Test Dependent

Inherent in producing scores instead of measures is test dependency. That is, instruments with different items, number of items, and/or rating scales generate different total scores. Test dependency leads to the almost endless development of assessments that are intended to measure the same construct. At

present, there are more than 85 assessments of ADL (McHorney, 2003). Ironically, while the items included in these assessments overlap considerably (e.g., almost all assessments include items that represent eating, dressing, grooming/hygiene, etc.), instrument developers and users seem to have incessant debates on which assessment is the best and there have been few efforts to create methods to translate scores between the different instruments.

Test dependency leads to an almost total lack of communication in healthcare research and outcomes. Researchers often explain their failure to reproduce findings from previous studies as a result of the inability to compare findings from different assessments. Furthermore, test dependency prevents the monitoring of patients across healthcare settings that use different instruments. For example, it is difficult, if not impossible, to empirically determine if a patient who is transferred from a rehabilitation inpatient facility (which uses the FIM as an outcome measure) deteriorates, maintains, or improves after transferring to a skilled nursing facility (which use the Minimum Data Set [MDS] as an outcome measure).

Scores May Lack Unidimensionality

An essential characteristic of measurement is the quality of unidimensionality. That is, a measure should define a single, unidimensional variable (Wright & Linacre, 1989). For example, speed, weight, and length are all unidimensional constructs; a score that reflected both weight and length would be confusing. How such confusion arises from multidimensional instruments in occupational therapy can be exemplified with the FIM. While it is common practice to use a total score on the FIM, studies suggest that the FIM total score reflects both a motor and cognition-communication component (Linacre et al., 1994). Without separating these two constructs, improvement in an FIM score could reflect several combinations of events (e.g., improvement in both motor and cognition, improvement in motor but not in cognition, or improvement in cognition but not motor abilities). Since a score does not reflect which of these or other combinations of factors it is based on, it is difficult to interpret a score.

Wright and Linacre (1989) note that no assessment can ever achieve perfect unidimensionality. This is even true for the physical sciences. Nonetheless, Wright and Linacre (1989) argue that the ideal of unidimensionality must be approximated in a measure.

Objective Measurement in Occupational Therapy and Health Care

The Institute of Objective Measurement (2004) defines objective measurement as follows:

> *Objective measurement is the repetition of a unit amount that maintains its size, within an allowable range of error, no matter which instrument is used to measure the variable of interest and no matter who or what relevant person or thing is measured. (http://www.rasch.org/define.htm)*

This definition points out several characteristics of measurement to which occupational therapy instruments should aspire. The phrase *repetition of a unit amount that maintains its size* refers to equality of intervals between units on the instrument. It underscores the importance of having interval-based, not ordinal-based values as discussed earlier. As stated in the definition, the unit of measure should be independent of the instrument is used to measure the variable of interest. This means that measures must be test free (i.e., that different instruments should be able to generate comparable measures). Finally, the phrase *no matter who or what relevant person or thing is measured* refers to measures being "sample free," or independent from the person or object being measured.

Creating measures in occupational therapy and health care requires a different conceptual framework than that which has been used to develop tra-

ditional assessments. Below some of the key concepts to this framework are noted.

The Measure Is Separate From the Instrument That Generates the Measure

First, it must be recognized that the measure is separate from the instrument used to generate the measure. Wright (1997b) describes the measure as a theoretical construct and the unit of measurement as a perfect idea. For example, in the physical sciences, distance is a theoretical construct. Measuring with rulers is so commonplace in daily life that we often do not recognize that our instrument, the ruler, only estimates the perfect idea of distance.

While there are many distances that are practical and measured on a daily basis, measured distances can range from the fraction of a micron that separates two electrons to the span between solar systems that are light years apart. Moreover, there are literally thousands devices for measuring distance ranging from micrometers that measure very small distances to astronomical instruments that capture distances in terms of the speed of light. Despite the almost infinite ways of measuring distance, it is relatively easy to compare or transpose the units produced by all of these instruments. This is true even when the unit of measurement is based on a different scale. Often, measurement instruments place different units of measurement on the same instrument (e.g., inches and centimeters on a ruler). Otherwise, simple formulas or tables can be readily used to translate measures across different scales.

Once one recognizes that instruments and the measures they represent are not one in the same, one can take advantage of the pragmatic features of objective measurement. For example, ADL, like distance, can be thought to be a theoretical construct, a perfect idea. While the FIM represents possible ADL activities, these activities are limited. ADL can theoretically range from the ability of lifting a facecloth to one's face to fulfilling a daily life role, such as being a worker. As there are different rulers to measure the theoretical construct of distance, different ADL instruments also should be able measure ADL. Some ADL measures could measure low levels of ADL ability while others could measure higher levels of ADL ability.

Furthermore, the theoretical construct of ADL connects the different ADL instruments. This opens up the possibility of translating measures generated by different ADL instruments and scales. Theoretically, like the measurement of distance, someday the ADL construct could become transparent. That is, it would be possible to refer to an amount of ADL ability independent of the measurement instrument used to generate the ADL ability measure.

Items Represent Differing Amounts of the Intended Construct

When using occupational therapy and healthcare measures, it is important to recognize that the questions or items on instruments do not represent the same amount of the construct being measured. When measuring distance, different parts of the ruler represent different amounts of distance. For example, objects that reach the 12-inch mark on a ruler are obviously longer than objects that reach the 2-, 3-, or 4-inch mark. Measures in occupational therapy and health care can similarly be conceptualized as representing more or less of the construct being measured. For example, ADL tasks represent different levels of complexity and demand. That is, bathing and dressing arguably involve more motor activity and more steps than brushing teeth or combing hair. If this is so, it should be easier to achieve a rating of "minimal

assist" on combing hair than achieving a "minimal assist" rating on bathing. Said another way, bathing requires more ADL ability than hair brushing. Figure 13.2 illustrates what the ADL assessment likely appears like when compared to the theoretical continuum of ADL independence.

Viewing an instrument's items in a hierarchical arrangement, representing more or less of a construct, offers tremendous advantages in measuring constructs in occupational therapy and health care. First, if a person is capable of challenging tasks, there is a high probability that he or she will be successful at accomplishing less challenging tasks. In our example (Figure 13.2), if an individual is capable of bathing or dressing, there is a high probability that he or she will be successful at brushing teeth or combing hair. For the technical purpose of measuring ADL, it would be unnecessary to assess lower amounts of the construct (e.g., brushing teeth and combing) if the individual is capable of performing items that represent greater amounts of the construct (e.g., dressing or bathing). It should be noted, that this is in no way to suggest that practitioners should limit their evaluation of relevant ADL activities. Nonetheless, for purposes of measurement, it should be unneces-

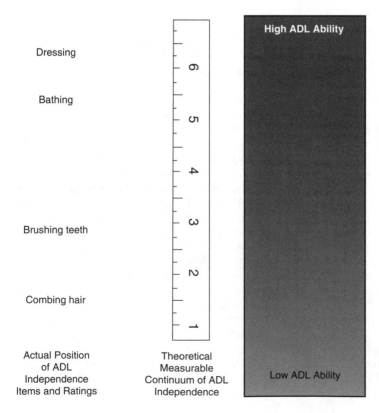

Figure 13.2 Items on a hypothetical ADL independence instrument compared to the theoretical continuum of ADL independence.

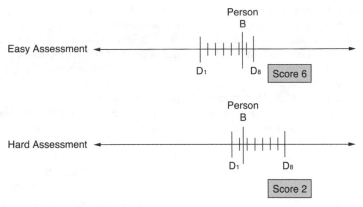

Figure 13.3 Demonstration of scores for an individual (B) when taking an easy assessment versus a hard assessment using CTT. $D_1 - D_8$ represents items of different difficulty. One point is achieved for every item that B gets correct. While the individual's ability does not change across tests, his/her score is dependent on the test taken.

sary to assess all possible ADL activities in order to measure a client's ADL ability.

As described earlier, precision in measuring distance typically proceeds first with an estimate of the length of an object followed by a focus on the finer markings of the ruler to increase precision. Once items from occupational therapy and healthcare instruments are identified as representing more or less of the construct they intend to measure, a process analogous to measuring distance can take place. For example, in measuring ADL, once it is determined that an individual has the ability to accomplish activities such as bathing, items of similar difficulty (e.g., dressing) or items representing finer levels of the item (e.g., amount of assistance, amount of time, etc.) can be asked to more finely discriminate the ADL abilities of this individual. This procedure, in addition to being efficient (e.g., avoiding questions far above or far below the ADL ability of the individual), has the potential of achieving precision by focusing more detailed questions at the ability level of the individual.

Classical Test Theory

Many of the limitations faced in achieving objective measurement in occupational therapy and health care is a function of the mathematical theories that traditionally underlie instrument development and psychometrics. Test development in education and health care has been based on classical test theory (CTT). The classical test model is a simple linear relationship that links the observed score (X) to the sum of the true score (T) and error score (E), $X = T + E$ (Hambleton & Jones, 1993).

When error is defined,[2] the true score (T) is defined as the observed score (X) minus the error score.

Test Dependency

The serious limitation of this model is that scores obtained with CTT are test dependent. That is, a respondent's true score is dependent on the questions or tasks of particular assessment on which they are tested (Hambleton & Jones, 1993). On more challenging assessments, respondents will get lower observed scores and on easier assessments they will get higher observed scores (Figure 13.3). Test dependency leads to challenges in translating scores across similar assessments.

Reliability

While internal consistency, test–retest, and inter-rater reliability are necessary they are not sufficient for objective measurement. All reliability statistics are sample dependent and instrument dependent. For example, internal consistency, as determined by Cronbach alpha levels, is not only dependent on the inter-correlations among items but by the number of items (i.e., more items produce higher alpha levels) (Streiner & Norman, 1989).

Reliability statistics also have other limitations. Inter-rater reliability at times can mask the qualities of a measure. For instance, instruments with ceiling or floor effects can show high test–retest reliability despite the instruments' failure to differentiate clients in the ceiling or floor. Reliability

[2]Three assumptions are necessary: (1) true scores and error scores are uncorrelated, (2) average error score for a population is zero, and (3) error scores on parallel tests are uncorrelated.

statistics also are limited in their ability to reveal covariance in rater agreement. For example, raters may show high correlations across their ratings and therefore have high inter-rater agreement, but they may systematically differ in the severity of their ratings (e.g., one rater consistently rate patients two points higher than another rater). Systematic difference in ratings can have serious implications in the scoring of individuals, that is, more lenient raters providing consistently higher ratings than more severe raters.

Validity

Similar critiques can be levied on evaluating instruments on the basis of validity criterion. While predictive validity is commonly used as a means to evaluate the measurement qualities of instruments in occupational therapy and health care, this methodology would be highly suspect in evaluating measures in the physical sciences. For example, to validate measures of distance (e.g., length of an object) as to whether or not they would predict a single event, for example, whether an object would fit through a doorway, would seem absurd. Measures of distance have a myriad of uses beyond this simple objective.

Furthermore, the prediction of any event is never simply a function of the instrument under study. For example, using the FIM to predict length of stay (LOS) at first glance may seem logical (reflecting the importance of ADL function to return home), but in reality, there are many factors that influence LOS and there can be complex inter-relationships between these factors (e.g., secondary conditions, exacerbation of a medical condition, medical capitation for inpatient services, etc.). In summary, validity, like reliability, is not sufficient for determining measurement quality. The exclusive focus on concurrent, discriminant, and predictive validity (all which follow the same logic) may actually obscure more fundamental qualities of objective measurement such as efficiency and precision.

Norms

One of the psychometric characteristics often considered critical for the acceptance of a healthcare instrument is the availability of norms. That is, the quality of an instrument is considered to depend on whether or not its values are connected to averages of a particular population (e.g., children of a given age, males or females, individuals with a particular impairment, and so on). While normative samples can be extremely useful in occupational therapy

and health care, they are not required for objective measurement. For example, in the physical sciences the quality of the measurement of distance is not dependent on norms. In fact, one can readily see the absurdity of having to generate norms for heights or widths for all objects that could be potentially measured.

Thurstone (1928) notes that a measurement instrument must not be seriously affected in its measuring function by the object (or person) it is measuring. Once an instrument has established measurement qualities, such as precision, it can be used to produce norms if they are desired and useful for some purpose. Although norms have pragmatic utility (e.g., to determine if an item or person being measured is within normal limits or if a child has reached a milestone) they are not an essential feature of objective measurement.

Rasch Measurement and Item Response Theory

The solution to object measurement lies in item response theory (IRT) models and methodologies.[3] In contrast to CTT, IRT focuses on the item rather than the test. Three IRT models are prevalent in the literature and are described as the one-, two-, and three-parameter models. All models relate person ability to one or more parameters. The one-parameter model, often referred to as the Rasch model, includes item difficulty. The two-parameter includes both item difficulty and item discrimination. Finally, the three-parameter model includes item difficulty, item discrimination, and guessing. The focus of the remainder of this chapter is on the one-parameter, or Rasch model. In addition to this being the most basic of the IRT models, from a technical perspective, it most closely reflects the tenants of objective measurement as outlined above.

Rasch Model

In 1953, the Danish mathematician George Rasch (1960) generated solutions to Thurstone's measurement requirements with the simple relationship of person ability (B), item difficulty (D), and the probability of a correct solution (P). The most basic version of the Rasch formula is presented below (Velozo, Kielhofner, & Lai, 1999).

[3]Fredrick Lord is often credited as the father of IRT, with his observation that ability scores, in contrast to true scores, are more fundamental to measurement since they are test independent (Hambleton & Jones, 1993; Lord, 1953).

Fundamental Objective Measurement

Wright (1997a,b) notes that much of the critical literature on fundamental, objective measurement has been ignored by classic test theory. Nonetheless, its beginnings can be traced to Normal Campbell's (1920) deduction that fundamental measurement requires the possibility of physical "concatenation," like the joining of sticks to concatenate length or piling of bricks to concatenate weight (Campbell, 1920; Wright, 1997a). Louis Thurstone, in the late 1920s and early 1930s outlined the following requirements of useful measurement:

- Unidimensionality—the universal characteristic of all measurement is that it describes only one attribute of the object measured (Thurstone, 1931).
- Linearity—measurement implies a linear continuum, for example, the qualitative variations of scholastic achievement must be forced into a linear scale (Thurstone & Chave, 1929).
- Abstraction—the linear continuum implied in all measurement is an abstraction, not the measuring device (Thurstone, 1931).
- Invariance—the unit of measurement can be repeated without modification in the different parts of the measurement continuum (Thurstone, 1931).

- Sample free calibration—a measuring instrument must not be seriously affected in its measuring function by the object being measured (Thurstone, 1928).
- Test-free measurement—it should not be required to submit every subject to the whole range of the scale (Thurstone, 1926).

In addition to Thustone's requirements for measurement, another critical development was Guttman's (1950) concept of "conjoint transitivity." That is, the concept of a total raw score can be clarified only by specifying the response to every item or question in a test or assessment. He proposed that if a person endorses or passes a challenging (hard) item, he/she should endorse all less challenging (easy) items. While this concept is critical to objective measurement, Rasch (1960) replaced the Guttman's deterministic model (i.e., the requirement that *all* less challenging items must be "passed" and *all* more challenging items must be "failed") with a probabilistic model of passing and failing (i.e., very easy items have a high probability of being passed, items at the persons ability level have a 50% probability of being passed, and very challenging items have a high probability of being failed).

$$\text{Log } [P_{ni}/1 - P_{ni}] = B_n - D_i$$

where

P_{ni} = probability of person n passing item i,

$1 - P_{ni}$ = probability of person n failing item i,

B_n = ability of person n, and

D_i = difficulty of item i.

The left side of the formula represents the linear transformation of the probability of passing a particular item divided by the probability of failing a particular item. The logarithmic transformation is critical in the creation of linear, interval-based measures.

The core of the Rasch formula is the relationship of person ability (B_n) to item difficulty (D_i). The attractiveness of this simple formula is that it captures the fundamental element of all testing, the relationship of a person to the assessment item. That is, the most basic description of any assessment situation is whether or not the person is successful in passing the item that he or she is attempting. Consider for instance, the ADL item "brushing hair." If an individual's ADL ability is high relative to "brushing hair," he or she will have a high probability of passing that item. If the indi-

vidual's ADL ability is low relative to "brushing hair," he or she will have a high probability of failing that item. When an individual's ability matches item difficulty, there is a 50% probability of passing the item.

The relation of person ability to item difficulty is an accurate representation of the process of measuring, even in the basic sciences. For example, if we consider parts of the ruler as "items" of different difficulty, we can replicate the operation of the Rasch formula. When measuring an object approximately $3\frac{1}{2}$ inches in width, the object has a "high probability of passing" (i.e., exceeding) a marking of 1 inch, 2 inches, and 3 inches. That object also has a "high probability of failing" (i.e., falling short of) markings of 6 inches, 5 inches, and 4 inches. As one attempts to determine the *exact width* of an object, one must have less confidence in the correctness of our measurement. That is, one can be confident that the object is at least 1, 2, or 3 inches in width, and not 4, 5, or 6 inches. However, one cannot be as confident that the object is exactly $3\frac{1}{2}$ inches. It could be 3 and $^{15}/_{32}$ inches or 3 and $^{17}/_{32}$ inches. Ironically, as one approaches the calibrations closer to the true width of the object, one has a 50% probability of being exactly correct.

It is interesting to note that the above measurement process typifies the strategy a therapist may use when interviewing new clients about their functional ability. First questions may be off target. That is one may ask about ADL tasks that are far above or far below the person's ADL ability level. If one receives affirmative answers to the questions asked about ADL independence, then one moves on to more difficult ADL tasks and ask about them. If one receives negative answers, one moves to easier ADL tasks. Eventually, as when one is asking about ADL tasks that are nearer the actual abilities of the individual, one starts getting less clear answers, such as "I think I can do that." Once the ADL tasks one asks about are at the ability level of the individual, there is a 50% probability of the individual answering similar ADL questions in either the affirmative or negative.

Slightly more advanced Rasch formulas can take into account more complicated assessment situations. For example, instead of the dichotomous situations described above, rating scales can be analyzed. Rasch rating scale models allow consideration of more detailed information about the level of independence (i.e., 1 = unable to do, 2 = needs maximal assistance, 3 = needs minimal assistance, 4 = independent). To analyze this situation, as an alternative to investigating the probabilities of a person passing or failing an item, the formula determines for individuals of different abilities the probability of passing or failing an item at a particular rating (e.g., whether or not the individual with low ability passes combing hair at the level of needing minimal assistance).

Similarly, many-faceted Rasch formulas can take into account rater severity. That is, while raters may be consistent in their ratings, there is a high likelihood that some raters have a tendency to be more severe or more lenient than other raters. With CTT scoring methods, clients that are rated by more severe raters will get lower scores while clients rated by less severe raters will get higher scores, independent of their true ability levels. By comparing the probabilities of ratings across raters, multifaceted Rasch analysis can determine the relative severity of raters and correct for this severity in determining a person's true measure.

Rasch Measurement Model Statistics

Rasch measurement statistics, while having some analogs in traditional psychometrics, differ owing to their focus on analysis at the person and item level versus the test level (Table 13.2). In contrast to traditional psychometrics, Rasch provides detailed information on rating scales, items, persons, and other factors (called facets) such as rater severity. These statistics provide an analysis of critical objective measurement features of assessments.

Rasch analysis first converts ordinal data generated by dichotomous or rating scale data into interval measures called log equivalent units (logits) (Merbitz, Morris, & Grip, 1989; Wright & Linacre, 1989). Logits are based on the natural log of getting a correct response and have the characteristic of interval data by retaining the same mathematical length throughout the continuum of the variable (Linacre & Wright 1989; Smith, 1992). The logit scale is usually set at the average difficulty level of the items of the particular assessment. Person ability, item difficulty, and facets such as rater severity are all expressed in the same unit of measurement, the logit.

Person measures, or calibrations, are generated by estimating the position of each person assessed on the continuum from less to more of the underlying construct. Persons with higher measures are those persons with more of the construct being measured and vice versa. In the case of an ADL scale, a person's calibration is the measure of how much ADL ability the person has.

Item measures, or calibrations, indicate how much of the underlying construct an item represents. The order in which items of a scale are calibrated is also important for assessing the validity of a scale. Items with higher calibrations should be those that are expected to represent more of the construct measured. Similarly, items calibrated lower should be those expected to represent less of the characteristic. For example, on an ADL scale

> The core of the Rasch formula is the relationship of person ability (B_n) to item difficulty (D_i). The attractiveness of this simple formula is that it captures the fundamental element of all testing, the relationship of a person to the assessment item.

Table 13.2 Rasch Statistics*

Statistic Name	Comparable Traditional Statistic	Explanation of Rasch Statistic	Desired Values
Person Measure	Person total raw score	Logistic transformation of the person's raw score (logit)—represents person ability	Can range from $-\infty$ to $+\infty$. No particular desired values though the distribution of person measures should overlap the distribution of item measures (see person–item match below)
Item Measure	p-value—proportion of the sample that passed the item	Logistic transformation of the p-value (logit)	Can range from $-\infty$ to $+\infty$. No particular desired values though the distribution of item measures should overlap the distribution of person measures
Item Discrimination	Item discrimination index—difference between the proportion of high and low scores passing an item	Proportional to the slope of the function of the probability of passing an item relative to person ability. The Rasch model holds this constant for all items while two- and three-parameter models calculate a value for each item	Rasch model holds item discrimination constant at 1.0 Two- and three-parameter models—high positive values (low positive and negative values should be of concern) (Hambleton & Jones, 1993, p. 45)
Item or Person Fit - Infit–inlier-sensitive or information-weighted fit - Outfit–outlier-sensitive fit	For item fit—point biserial correlation—correlation of the item to rest of the test No analog for person fit.	Mean square residual (MnSq)—ratio of observed scores to expected scores—amount of distortion of the measurement system Standardized mean square (ZSTD) —conversion of MnSq to α normally distributed standardized score	MnSq—ideal is 1.0. Values > 1.0 indicate unpredictability (unmodeled noise, data underfitting the measurement model) Values < 1.0 indicate over predictability (Redundancy, data overfitting the measurement model) Recommended ranges for surveys is 0.6–1.4 and for clinical assessments is 0.5–1.7 (Wright & Linacre,1994) ZSTD—ideal value is 0.0. Less than 0 indicates too predictable; greater than 0.0 indicates to erratic. Acceptable ranges are between –2.0 and 2.0. Note high n-sizes result in inflated ZSTD
Reliability	Cronbach alpha or Kuder-Richardson 20 (K-R 20)—an indication of internal consistency analogous to doing multiple split-half reliability tests	Separation reliability—ratio of unbiased sample standard deviation to average standard error of the test (Fisher, 1993)	Similar in estimate to Cronbach alpha or K-R 20— satisfactory values are between 7.0 and 8.0 (Bland & Altman, 1997)

(continued)

Table 13.2 **Rasch Statistics*** (continued)

Statistic Name	Comparable Traditional Statistic	Explanation of Rasch Statistic	Desired Values
Person Separation and Person Strata	Standard deviation of distribution of raw scores	Person separation—person spread divided by error Person strata—number of statistically distinct strata = $(4Gp + 1)/3$, where Gp = person separation (Wright & Masters, 1982, p. 106)	In general, person separation over 2. Technically, person strata over 2 means the instrument divides the sample into at least two statistically distinct strata
Person-Item Match	Proportion of individuals passing or failing items	Comparison of person measure distribution to item measure distribution	Typical distribution comparisons (e.g., visual comparison of distributions, person and item means within 2 standard deviations)

*Adapted from Fisher (1993).

we would expect dressing to be calibrated higher than combing hair.

Since items and persons are calibrated on the same continuum, one can determine whether items are appropriately targeted to the levels of the trait represented by the client under study. In general, an instrument should have items whose mean is near the mean of the clients. Furthermore, the items should spread out so that they cover the range of variation represented by the clients, and thus avoid ceiling and floor effects. A scale without higher-level items to measure higher-level persons and lower level items to measure lower level persons will have ceiling and/or floor effects (i.e., everyone above or below a certain level will get the same score despite differences between them in the construct being measured).

Rater measures, or calibrations, indicate how severe or lenient a rater is when assigning scores on the scale. A rater with a higher calibration is more severe in assigning ratings and a rater with a lower calibration is more lenient in assigning ratings. Ideally, differences in raters' severity should be small, so that the measure a person receives is not greatly impacted by who did the rating. When this is not the case, rater calibrations can be used to correct person measures for rater severity (Fisher, 1993; Forsyth, Lai, & Kielhofner, 1999; Lai, Velozo, & Linacre, 1997).

The most critical statistic in Rasch analysis is the fit statistic (Haley, McHorney, & Ware, 1994; Wright & Stone, 1979). Fit statistics are generated for persons, items, and raters. Rasch analytic programs usually separate fit statistics into infit and outfit. Infit, or inlier-sensitive/information-weighted fit, is more sensitive to the pattern of responses targeted on the items or persons. For example, persons showing high infit are demonstrating an unexpected pattern of responses on items that are most reflective of their ability level. Outfit, or outlier-sensitive fit, is more sensitive to responses far from the persons or items. For example, a person showing high outfit is demonstrating an unexpected pattern on items that are easy or hard for the individual.

Fit mean-square (MnSq) values represent the observed variance from the data divided by the expected variance estimated by the Rasch mathematical model. The ideal MnSq ratio is 1.0, whereby the observed variance from the data equals the expected variance from the Rasch model. MnSq illustrates the extent to which the item, person, or rater fit the expectations of the model. MnSq above 1.0 indicates the item, person, or rater is increasingly erratic (i.e., observed variance is higher than expected variance) while MnSq below 1.0 represents data that is overly predictable. High MnSq are taken to indicate misfit (i.e., that an item was not a valid indicator of a construct, that a client was not validly measured, or that a rater was not using the scale in a valid manner).

Low MnSq below 0.5–0.6 indicates that the item, person, or rater shows too little variability or that the scoring pattern is too deterministic. Wright and Linacre (1994), recommend MnSq ranges for surveys to be 0.6–1.4 and for clinical observations to be 0.5–1.7. High-fit statistics are generally of more concern because they represent a greater threat to the validity of the assessment.

Fit statistics can be useful in identifying a variety of aberrations in the assessment process. High person fit may indicate a survey respondent who is providing false information. It also can be diagnostic; for example, a person performing unexpectedly poorly on an ADL item which for most persons is easy (e.g., eating) may be indicative of a particular problem (e.g., difficulty with swallowing). Item misfit can be an indication of a poorly worded item or can be an indication of multidimensionality in an assessment.[4] Individual erratic items can be removed from an assessment. A rater showing high fit statistics may be an indication that he or she is misinterpreting the scoring criterion. This could lead to removing that rater's data from a dataset. It also can mean that the rater requires further training to use the assessment correctly.

Rasch statistical programs also produce statistics that are analogous to those used in traditional psychometrics. Person separation reliability is analogous to Cronbach's alpha (Bland & Altman, 1997) and similarly serves as a measure of internal consistency. Person separation represents the number of levels into which subjects and raters are classified by their calibrations. When persons are well separated, the scale effectively discriminates different levels of the trait being measured. When applied to persons, the separation statistic represents the sensitivity of the scale to detect differences in subjects. On the other hand, rater separation represents the extent of rater bias due to severity/leniency.

Applications of Item Response Theory in Health Care

IRT and the associated methodologies provide a revolutionary framework for the investigation of existing instruments and development of new instruments. This capability emerges from the ability to analyze at the item level instead of the test level. While CTT methodologies provide general indications of problems or limitations of existing instruments, IRT methodologies provide more detailed information on the potential cause of the limitation. In combination with clinical experience, analysis of instruments at the item level can

lead to pragmatic solutions to measurement challenges in health care.

Analyzing Existing Healthcare Instruments

Many researchers have begun to use IRT methodologies to reexamine instruments that were originally developed following CTT. For instance, IRT methodologies have been used to investigate the item-level characteristics of existing instruments. Rasch analyses of the FIM (Linacre et al., 1994), Patient Evaluation Conference System (PECS; Silverstein, Fisher, Kilgore, Harley, & Harvey, 1991) and the Level of Rehabilitation Scale (LORS-III; Velozo, Magalhaes, Pan, & Leiter, 1995) have produced parallel results that provide new insights into these assessments.

Rasch analysis item fit statistics indicate that the items of these instruments are multidimensional. That is, the items of global functional status instruments appear to represent more than one underlying latent trait. For example, Velozo and colleagues (1995) showed that when all the items of LORS are analyzed together, items representing ADL (e.g., eating, grooming, dressing, etc.) show good fit statistics while items representing the cognition/communication (e.g., memory, expression, problem solving, etc.) showed unacceptably high fit statistics. When the items representing each of these constructs are analyzed separately, they show acceptable fit statistics. These findings and findings similarly found in the Rasch analysis of the FIM (Linacre et al., 1994) led both research groups to conclude that these global functional status instruments measure two unique constructs. The above findings have now led to the practice of scoring FIM ADL and cognition/communication separately when reporting clinical outcomes (e.g., Bates & Stineman, 2000).

Item calibrations produced from the analysis also provided insights on how well these instruments were measuring the samples under study. As noted earler, in addition to producing both item difficulty measures and person ability measures, Rasch analysis places these measures on the same linear continuum. This item person relationship reveals not only the presence of ceiling or floor effects, but also the relationship of instrument items to these effects. This is illustrated on Figure 13.4, which shows both items and person measures on the same graph for the LORS. Velozo and colleagues (1995) used this methodology to investigate the effectiveness of the ADL items of the LORS in measuring patients at admission and discharge. An analysis of 3,056 rehabilitation inpa-

---

[4]Fit statistics alone are not adequate in identifying multidimensionality. Even when all items fit the Rasch model, factor analysis can reveal multiple constructs (Linacre, 1998; Smith, 2002).

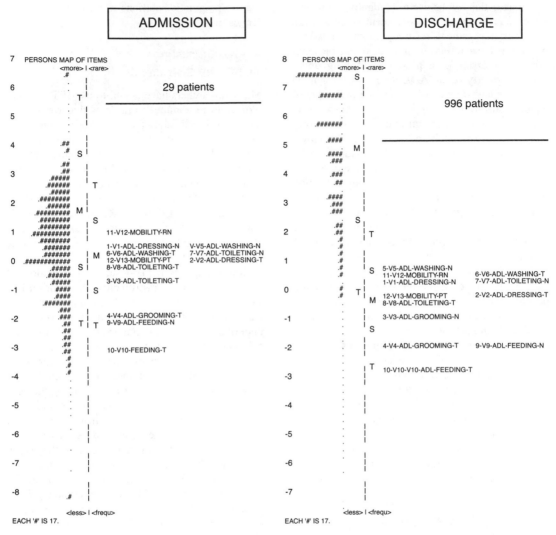

Figure 13.4 Person ability–item difficulty match at admission and discharge for the Level of Rehabilitation Scale–III. (Adapted from Velozo et al., 1995.)

tients with admission and discharge measures revealed that while there was no ceiling effect at admission (see left-hand side of Figure 13.4), 32% of the inpatients were in the ceiling (i.e., above the highest calibrated items) at discharge (see right-hand side of Figure 13.4). That is, 32% of the inpatients received the maximum measure on the instrument. Even more dramatic were the ceiling effects for the cognition/communication scales of the LORS demonstrating 35.5% of the patients in the ceiling at admission and 49.9% of the patients in the ceiling at discharge.

Further, item-based analyses of the LORS provided insights on how to eliminate these effects. The ADL item difficulty hierarchy for the LORS

showed a distinct pattern. Items representing feeding and grooming, were easy and items representing washing (bathing) and mobility (locomotion) were the most difficult. Therefore, elimination of the ceiling effect at discharge could likely be achieved by including more challenging ADL items such as carrying items while walking or climbing several flights of stairs.

The comparisons of item difficulties to person abilities also provide some evidence why global functional measures would not be effective in measuring outcomes for outpatient rehabilitation. Individuals discharged from inpatient rehabilitation are likely to be competent with basic ADLs. This does not suggest that these individuals are fully rehabilitated. More challenging items, such as more strenuous locomotor tasks or instrumental activities of daily living would more likely differentiate persons discharged from inpatient services. Furthermore, these findings would suggest the need for further rehabilitation.

Development of New Instruments

While IRT models are useful in analyzing existing healthcare instruments, their true value may be in the development of new instruments. Well-known assessments used by occupational therapists that have been developed though Rasch analysis include the: Assessment of Motor and Process Skills (Fisher, 1993), Assessment of Communication and Interaction Skills (Forsyth, Salamy, Simon, & Kielhofner, 1998), Pediatric Evaluation of Disability Inventory (Haley, Coster, Ludlow, Haltiwanger & Andrellos, 1992), Occupational Performance History Interview (OPHI) (Kielhofner et al., 2004), and Worker Role Interview (Braveman et al., 2005).

In contrast to instruments that have been developed using CTT models, instruments developed using IRT models are more likely to incorporate item difficulty when measuring individuals. By doing this, researchers are able to test the underlying theory or logic of the item hierarchy, thus critically examining the validity of the instrument in measuring the underlying construct. Instruments developed to systematically reflect an item hierarchy are less likely to demonstrate ceiling and floor effects and are more likely to be sensitive in detecting differences between those being assessed. Most important of all, Rasch analysis provides detailed information that can provide insights into how to improve the instruments under development.

For example, Velozo and Peterson (2001) used Rasch measurement as a basis to develop the University of Illinois (UIC) Fear of Falling Measure. The purpose of this measure was to identify and differentiate fear of falling among community dwelling elderly. Velozo and Peterson (2001) used Stone's (1997) method of item development, whereby fear of falling was expressed as a variable representing a range of items that would elicit fear in the most fearful individuals (e.g., "getting out of bed," "getting on/off a toilet") to items that would elicit fear only in the least fearful individuals (e.g., "using an escalator" and "walking outside when it was icy"). Furthermore, middle-difficulty items were developed such as "walking on a crowded street" and "climbing stairs." More subtle degrees of item difficulty were generated by incorporating

environmental challenge to the items, for example, "climbing well-lit stairs," "climbing poorly lit stairs," carrying bundles up well-lit stairs," carrying bundles up poorly lit stairs."

Rasch analysis of 106 community dwelling respondents revealed only 1% of the sample in the floor of the instrument, and 7.5% in the ceiling. In general, the resultant item calibrations verified the construct validity of the instrument. The easiest items in the instrument were "getting in/out of bed," "get on/off toilet," and "get dressed" while the most challenging items were "walk outside when it was icy," "carry bundles up poorly lit stairs," and "use a step stool to reach in kitchen cabinet." Furthermore, as hypothesized, common items with differing environmental challenges calibrated in the expected hierarchy (e.g., carrying bundles up poorly lit stairs was more difficult than carrying bundles up well-lit stairs).

In addition to providing evidence of construct validity, the ability to place person measures and item calibrations on the same linear continuum provides a critical link between the qualitative content of the instrument and the measures produced by the instrument. Following Rasch analysis, each person ability measure becomes connected with an item calibration. Velozo and Peterson (2001) demonstrated this connection between person measures and the qualitative content of the UIC Fear of Falling Measure. For example, the average measure of the sample they studied was associated with being moderately worried about standing on a moving bus and carrying objects up well-lit stairs. These investigators postulated that this connection between the quantitative values could be used to determine clinical significance, i.e., an individual showing adequate improvement on the fear of falling scale so that they were "not fearful about walking on a crowded street" could be a criterion for an individual living in an urban setting.

Innovative Measurement Methodologies Based on Item Response Theory

In addition to its utility as a means of developing assessments, the use of the Rasch measurement model has also opened up other possibilities for advancing measurement methodologies. Below we discuss three of these advances:

- The development of keyforms for instantaneous measurement and quality control,
- Computer adapted testing, and
- Linking existing measures.

Development of Keyforms for Instantaneous Measurement and Quality Control

Despite the advantages of Rasch-based measures in generating interval measures versus ordinal scores, use of the former in everyday occupational therapy practice is still limited. One obvious barrier is that raw data must be converted into Rasch-based interval measures. With few exceptions (e.g., the Assessment of Motor and Process Skills, Fisher, 1993), methods of generating interval measures via computer scoring are not readily available to practitioners. Therefore, even when using assessments that were originally developed using the Rasch measurement model, practitioners ordinarily do not have available means to generate Rasch-based interval measures.

Linacre (1997) first proposed an alternative to using computers to obtain interval measures. He introduced the idea of a keyform, that is, a paper-and-pencil method that "combine into one graphi-cal presentation the essential steps of data collection and measurement construction" (Linacre, 1997, p. 316). While the keyform does require Rasch analysis (commonly done by the instrument developer), once the keyform is created, Rasch-based interval measures can be generated directly from the form without further computer analysis. The first example of keyforms for an occupational therapy instrument was developed for the second version of the Occupational Performance History Interview (OPHI-II) (Kielhofner et al., 2004). Prior to developing the keyforms, research using the Rasch measurement model supported the conclusion that the three OPHI-II scales were reliable and valid measures. The OPHI-II keyforms allow generation of instantaneous measures from raw rating scale data, while also exercising intuitive quality control of the data obtained (Kielhofner, Dobria, Forsyth, & Basu, 2005; Kielhofner, Mallinson, Forsyth, & Lai, 2001).

The basis of a keyform is that there is a relationship between raw scores and interval measures.

Completing the OPHI-II Keyforms

Below are the instructions for completing the OPHI-II Keyforms. The reader should refer to the keyform for the Occupational Identity Scale (Figure 13.5). The process for completing all three OPHI-II keyforms is identical.

When All Items Are Rated:

1. Turn the OPHI Key on its side (landscape format).
2. Record the ratings in the leftmost column marked "rate client here."
3. Calculate the sum of the ratings and record on the total score line.
4. Turn the form back upright (portrait format).
5. Locate the total score you obtained in the first (left) column of the box at the right, marked total score.
6. Now, look at the corresponding numbers in the two following columns. The first number (middle column) is the client measure—it is based on a 100-point scale where 0 is the least amount of occupational identity and 100 is the most occupational identity that can be captured with this rating scale. The second number is the standard error of that the measure.
7. Record the client measure and standard error numbers in this box onto the lines titled client measurement and standard error.

Examining the Pattern of Scores

In addition to adding up the scores and obtaining the client measure from the raw total score, it is also useful to circle the numbers in order to inspect what the pattern reveals. There are two things that can be readily discovered. First, if someone's pattern of ratings are all or mostly at the extreme (i.e., all or mostly 1's or 4's), then the person has likely demonstrated a ceiling or floor effect—that is, he or she has either more or less identity then this scale could measure.

Obtaining a Measure With Missing Data

1. If you have not scored all the items, then the procedure is as follows:
2. Turn the OPHI Key on its side (landscape format).
3. Circle all the items you DID rate.
4. Draw a line across the body of the key form, by eye, through the average of the ratings.
5. The line will intersect a client measure and corresponding standard error, as shown in example 2, in the box immediately below the key.
6. Turn the form back upright (portrait format).
7. Look at the numbers intersected by your line in the left box, immediately below the key. The left column represents client measure, and the right column standard error.
8. Record the numbers intersected by the line you drew onto the lines titled client measurement and standard error.

Raw scores can be used to estimate interval measure in two ways. When all items are rated, the sum of the raw scores estimates the measure. At first blush, this statement may seem to contradict the challenges identified with adding up raw scores. However, if a person measured fits the expectations of the Rasch model, in a Rasch-based instrument such as the OPHI-II, raw scores reflect the position of items on the unidimensional continuum. Increasingly higher sums of the raw scores are achieved through higher ratings on increasingly higher-level items. Thus, when the person's ratings conform to that expected pattern, the sum of the raw score ratings can be readily converted to linear measures via a keyform table.

An important step in completing the keyforms is to visually determine whether the pattern of ratings conforms to these expectations. Referring to Figure 13.5 on p. 194, the OPHI Identity Scale keyform, the expectation is that there is a higher probability in getting higher ratings on the lower-level items (e.g., "Made occupational choices (past)") and lower ratings on the higher-level items ("Has personal goals and projects"). If the ratings violate these expectations (e.g., unexpectedly low ratings on a lower-level items or unexpectedly high ratings on a higher-level item), a judgment must be made about whether the anomalous pattern means the assessment was valid for the client in question. If the judgment is that the pattern is not valid, all of the client's data can be disregarded or just the anomalous rating could be treated as missing data in deriving a measure. When the ratings are as expected, they can be summed to derive a total raw score for which the keyform will provide a corresponding person measure along with its standard error. When some items are not rated a total raw score cannot be calculated. However, the remaining items can be used to estimate the person measure. In this case, a visual representation of the relationship between raw scores and measures is used (see Figure 13.5). The keyforms combine both these features together.

Keyforms, therefore, allow therapists to combine the steps of data collection, quality control, and measurement into a single process. By eliminating the necessity to computer score every assessment, keyforms provide the therapist with Rasch-based interval measures and provide a means of deriving measures when there is missing data. While keyforms are available only for two occupational therapy assessments as of this writing (keyforms are also available for the Occupational Self-Assessment, Baron et al., 2006), their availability and use is likely to grow because of their ease in deriving interval measures.

Computerized Adaptive Testing (CAT)

One of the most dramatic advances in modern measurement is the combination of IRT with computer technology to develop computerized adaptive tests (CAT). As proposed by Thurstone (1926) and described earlier in this chapter, a distinct characteristic of measurement is that it eliminates the need to use all the items of an instrument to derive a measure. The relevance of this feature of measurement in health care is demonstrated in Figure 13.6 on p. 195. Portrayed is a continuum of physical function represented by "easy" items such as "sitting balance," "grooming," and "upper extremity dressing" on the left of the continuum, and "difficult" items such as "jogging," "biking 10 miles," and "running 10 miles" to the far right. Logically, individuals of different abilities should be tested with different items along the continuum. For example, an individual with severe multiple sclerosis would be likely be tested with less challenging items such as "sitting balance," and an individual with a moderate level cerebrovascular accident tested with more challenging items such as "toilet transfers" and "ambulation. An individual with mild osteoarthritis would likely be tested with even more challenging items such as "jogging" and "biking 10 miles."

While IRT statistics can provide the item calibrations to identify the items that are most appropriate for an individual of a particular ability, paper-and-pencil instruments are not a practical means of administering these items. Personal computers, on the other hand, readily provide the technology to selectively administer items to an individual depending on the answers or performance on items previously administered to the individual. An algorithm for the administration of items via a computerized adaptive test (CAT) is presented in Figure 13.7 on p. 195. The algorithm starts with setting an initial estimated person measure and then items are directed to an individual that are close in calibration to the last calibrated person measure. The stopping rule can be based on a confidence interval or amount of precision set by the administrator. Once the desired confidence interval is achieved, the respondent receives a measure for the construct and the algorithm gets initiated for the next construct to be measured. The program stops when all constructs have been measured.

Extensive development of CATs took place in the 1980s (Martin, McBride, & Weiss, 1983; Olsen, Maynes, Slawson, & Ho, 1986; Weiss, 1985), and by 1994 a variety of CATs were being administered in the field of education. In spite of

Occupational Identity Key

Measure client here. Circle ratings and draw line ⟶

	Rate Client Here	1		2			3		4	Client Measure	Standard Error
Has personal goals and projects	3	1·········1		2			③		4········4		
Identifies a desired occupational lifestyle	3	1·········1		2			③		4········4		
Expects success	2	1·········1		②			3		4········4		
Accepts responsibility	3	1·········1		2			③		4········4		
Appraises abilities and limitations	3	1·········1		2			③		4········4		
Has commitments and values	3	1·········1		2			③		4········4		
Recognizes identity and obligations	?	1·········1		2			3		4········4		
Has interests	3	1·········1		2			③		4········4		
Felt effective (past)	1	(1·········1)		2			3		4········4		
Found meaning and satisfaction in lifestyle (past)	1	(1·········1)		2			3		4········4		
Made occupational choices (past)	1	(1·········1)		2			3		4········4		
Total Score _____ ?											

Client Measure scale (center column):

```
— 100    13
 -98
 -96
 -94
 -92
— 90     8
 -88
 -86
 -84     6
 -82     5
— 80     5
 -78     5
 -76     4
 -74     4
 -72     4
— 70     4
 -68     4
 -66     4
 -64     5
 -62     5
— 60     5
 -58     5
 -56     5
 -54     5
 -52     4
— 50     4
 -48     4
 -46     4
 -44     4
 -42     4
— 40     4
 -38     3
 -36     3
 -34     3
 -32     4
— 30     4
 -28     4
 -26     4
 -24     4
 -22     4
— 20     4
 -18     5
 -16     6
 -14
 -12
— 10     8
 -8
 -6
 -4
 -2
— 0      13
```

Total Score	Client Measure	Standard Error
44	100	13
43	91	8
42	85	6
41	81	5
40	78	5
39	75	4
38	73	4
37	70	4
36	67	4
35	64	5
34	61	5
33	58	5
32	55	5
31	52	4
30	49	4
29	47	4
28	45	4
27	43	4
26	41	4
25	39	4
24	38	3
23	36	3
22	34	3
21	33	3
20	31	4
19	29	4
18	27	4
17	26	4
16	23	4
15	21	4
14	18	5
13	15	6
12	9	8
11	0	13

Client Measure ____ **42**

Standard Error ____ **4**

Figure 13.5 OPHI-II Keyform.

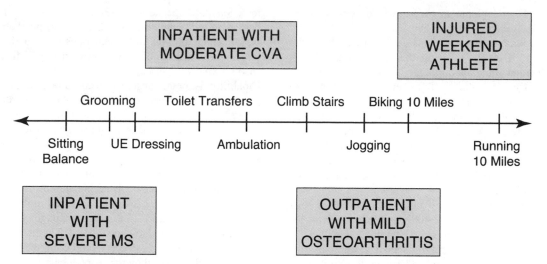

Figure 13.6 Hypothetical continuum of function with associated items in hierarchical order of difficulty from left to right. Framed boxes relate where on the continuum each of these clients could be located and the items most appropriate for testing these clients.

the relative widespread use of CAT in educational testing, its use in health care is in its infancy. Cella and his colleagues have developed CATs to monitor quality of life outcomes in oncology (Webster, Cella, & Yost, 2003) and Ware and colleagues have developed a CAT to assess the impact of headaches (Ware, Cella, & Yost, 2003; Ware et al., 2003). At present, we are aware of two CATs being development in the area of rehabilitation and disability. Haley and his colleagues are presently field testing their Activity Measure for Post Acute Care (AM-PAC) (Haley, Coster, Andres, & Kosinski, 2004) and Velozo and his colleagues are presently field testing the ICF Activity Measure, a self-report assessment of physical disability (ICFmeasure.com).

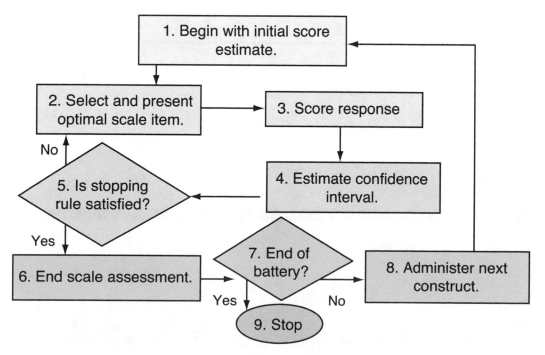

Figure 13.7 Algorithm for computer adaptive testing. (Adapted from Wainer et al., 2000.)

The development of the ICF Activity Measure was funded by the Department of Education, National Institute of Disability and Rehabilitation (H133G000227). Using the International Classification of Functioning, Disability, and Health (ICF) as a theoretical framework, an initial item bank was developed that focused on movement challenges for individuals with upper extremity injuries, lower extremity injuries, back pain, or spinal cord injury. The bank was edited on the basis of focus groups and interviewing of individuals with disabilities as well as a professional advisory panel.

A paper-and-pencil field test of the item bank was completed with 408 participants across the four diagnostic groups to produce the data for Rasch analysis. Item fit statistics were used to identify erratic items and principle components analysis was used to identify separate constructs within the item bank. The result was an item bank of 264 questions representing six constructs: (1) positioning/transfers, (2) gross upper extremity, (3) fine hand, (4) walking and climbing, (5) wheelchairs/scooters, and (6) self-care activities.

The computerized aspect of the ICF Activity Measure was built using unix/linux operating system. Standard apache web server and PHP server side scripting technology was used to design Web pages which present individual questions to the respondent via a standard Web browser (e.g., Microsoft Explorer, Netscape, Mozilla). Data storage capability is being designed using PostgreSQL. The system is upward scalable (e.g., questions can be added, deleted, and changed) and the administrator can select a number administration criterion (e.g., initial item calibration, amount of randomness in selecting the initial item) and exit criterion (e.g., confidence interval, maximum number of questions). Since the CAT is administered using a standard Web browser, it can be accessed globally via the Internet. Figure 13.8 presents a page of the CAT as it is presented to a respondent. The investigators are using touch screen laptop computers to administer the CAT, allowing respondents to use a pencil-like probe or their finger to select an answer instead of a computer mouse.

Since computerized adaptive testing is relatively new in health care, there are few studies presenting its advantages and feasibility. Initial findings are promising. Haley and colleagues (2004) with CAT simulations of their 101-item AM-PAC have shown that measures derived of

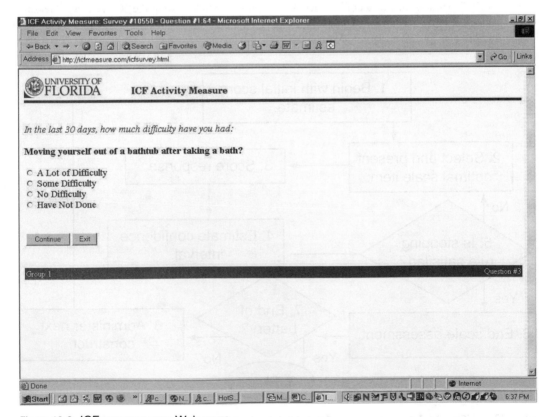

Figure 13.8 ICFmeasure.com Web page.

four- or five-item CAT presentations correlate with measures derived from the total item bank (101 items) between .90 and .95, and measures derived from 10 item CAT presentations correlate between .96 and .98 with measures derived from the total item bank. These findings suggest abbreviated CAT-based assessments can be administered without losing the accuracy of administering full tests. This decrease in respondent burden should be welcomed by patients and study participants and should represent considerable cost-savings in administering instruments as part of clinical and research protocols.

Linking Existing Measures

A third potential application of IRT methodologies is the capability of linking healthcare measures (Velozo et al., 1999). As presented earlier in this chapter, a measure is not confined to a specific scale or specific set of items, but instead can be presented by large banks of items that represent the measure. Considering that as many as 85 instruments measuring functional ability exist, it is possible that these individual instruments do not each measure a unique aspect of functional ability but are simply subsets of items representing the unidimensional construct of functional ability. Examples from the physical sciences (e.g., the ability to easily convert across the many instruments used to measure time), and Thurstone's (1926) requirement that measures must be "test free," imply that similar measures in health care can be linked. The possibility of linking measures of functional ability was underscored when the difficulty order of ADL/motor items on the FIM, Patient Conference Evaluation Conference System (PECS) and Level of Rehabilitation Scale-III (LORS-III) were found to be virtually identical (Linacre et al., 1994; Silverstein et al. 1991; Velozo et al., 1995). These initial findings provided evidence that the scales were measuring the same underlying functional ability, despite differences in item definitions and rating methodology.

While the above studies suggest that translation across functional measures is feasible, actual instrument linking can be accomplished through common-sample equating (Fisher, Harvey, Taylor, Kilgore, & Kelley, 1995). For this methodology, the items from both instruments are calibrated on a common sample of persons (i.e., subjects must be assessed with both instruments). Data from both instruments are "co-calibrated" in a single Rasch analysis, producing item measures using the same scaling unit. Comparisons across the two instruments can then be accomplished by analyzing the

data from each instrument in separate Rasch analyses while "presetting," or anchoring, items at the cocalibrated item measures.

Fisher and colleagues (1995) were the first to use common-sample equating to link two global measures of function, the FIM and PECS. Using the methodology described above, they showed that the 13 FIM and 22 PECS ADL/motor items could be scaled together in a 35-item instrument. The authors found that separate FIM and PECS measures for 54 rehabilitation patients correlated .91 with each other and correlated .94 with the cocalibrated values produced by Rasch analysis. Furthermore, these authors demonstrated that either instrument's ratings were easily and quickly converted into the others via a table that used a common unit of measurement, which they referred to as the "rehabit." This common unit of measurement allows the translation of scores from one instrument to another. Since the results of Rasch analysis are sample free, these tables can be used for all future and past instrument-to-instrument score conversions.

A number of more recent studies support the potential of linking functional measures. Recently, Smith and Taylor (2004) replicated the FIM-PECS linking with a more substantial sample of 500 patients with similar results. Fisher, Eubanks, and Marier (1997) used common-sample equating to link the 10 physical function items of the Medical Outcome Scale (MOS) SF-36 (the PF-10) and the Louisiana State University Health Status Instrument. Difficulty estimates for a subset of similar items from the two instruments correlated at .95, again indicating that the items from the two scales were working together to measure the same construct. McHorney and Cohen (2000) applied a two-parameter IRT model to 206 physical functioning items (through 71 common items across samples), and in a similar study McHorney (2002) linked 39 physical functioning items (through 16 common items) from three modules of the Asset and Health Dynamics Among the Oldest Old study. Both studies demonstrated successful linking of item banks through sets of common items, allowing placement of all items on a common metric.

Preliminary studies by Velozo and colleagues are designed to investigate the validity of linking functional measures. Using the FIM and MDS with common sample data on 290 veterans, these investigators created a crosswalk between the measures using the Rasch common-person linking method described above. Using an independent sample of 2,600 veterans, Velozo and colleagues compared the converted FIM and converted MDS raw scores to actual FIM and MDS raw scores. Distributions of converted and actual scores did not differ significantly and showed moderate correlations (.73–.74). While the strength of these correlations may not support using converted scores to monitor individual patients, these preliminary findings suggest that that converted scores may be feasible for population-based studies (e.g., predictive studies).

Conclusion

While classical test theory has produced numerous useful assessments, it does not address aspects of objective measurement. This chapter provided an overview of item response theory and its potential for objective measurement in occupational therapy. The chapter discussed how this new methodology provides tools to identify and correct limitations of existing instruments and to develop new measures that meet the requirements of objective measurement.

The chapter also discussed emerging applications of IRT in instantaneous measurement and computer adaptive testing. These approaches allow for new levels of efficiency and precision in occupational therapy and healthcare measurement. Finally, the chapter discussed the process of linking measures that could allow the comparison of results from different studies and tracking outcomes of clients across the continuum of care. While the use of these modern measurement techniques are in their infancy in occupational therapy, they promise to have great value in improving how our clients are measured for clinical and research purposes.

REFERENCES

Baron, K., Kielhofner, G., Iyenger, A., Goldhammer, V., & Wolenski, J. (2006). *The Occupational Self Assessment (OSA)* (version 2.2). Model of Human Occupation Clearinghouse, Department of Occupational Therapy, College of Applied Health Sciences, University of Illinois at Chicago, Chicago, IL.

Bates, B. E., & Stineman, M. G. (2000). Outcome indicators for stroke: Application of an algorithm treatment across the continuum of post acute rehabilitation services. *Archives of Physical Medicine and Rehabilitation, 81,* 1468–1478.

Bland, J. M., & Altman, D. G. (1997). Statistics notes: Cronbach's alpha. *British Medical Journal, 314,* 572.

Braveman, B., Robson, M., Velozo, C., Kielhofner, G., Fisher, G., Forsyth, K., & Kerschbaum, J. (2005). *Worker Role Interview (WRI)* (Version 10.0). Model of Human Occupation Clearinghouse, Department of Occupational Therapy, College of Applied Health

Sciences, University of Illinois at Chicago, Chicago, IL.

Campbell, N R. (1920). *Physics: The elements.* London: Cambridge University Press.

Fisher, A. G. (1993). The assessment if IADL motor skills: An application of many faceted Rasch analysis. *American Journal of Occupational Therapy, 47,* 319–329.

Fisher, W. P. (1997). Physical disability construct convergence across instruments: Towards a universal metric. *Journal of Outcome Measurement, 1*(2), 87–113.

Fisher, W. P., Eubanks R. L., & Marier, R. L. (1997). Equating the MOS SF36 and the LSU HSI physical functioning scales. *Journal of Outcome Measurement, 1,* 329–362.

Fisher, W. P., Harvey, R. F., Taylor, P., Kilgore, K. M., & Kelley, C. K. (1995). Rehabits: A common language of functional assessment. *Archives of Physical Medicine and Rehabilitation, 76,* 113–122.

Forsyth, K., Lai, J., & Kielhofner, G. (1999). The Assessment of Communication and Interaction Skills (ACIS): Measurement properties. *British Journal of Occupational Therapy, 62*(2), 69–74.

Forsyth, K., Salamy, M., Simon, S., & Kielhofner, G. (1998). *The Assessment of Communication and Interaction Skill (ACIS)* (version 4.0). Model of Human Occupation Clearinghouse, Department of Occupational Therapy, College of Applied Health Sciences, University of Illinois at Chicago, Chicago, IL.

Guttman, L. (1950). The basis for scalogram analysis. In Stouffer et al. *Measurement and prediction* (Vol. 4, pp. 60–90). Princeton, NJ: Princeton University Press.

Haley, S. M., Coster, W. J., Andres, P. L., Kosinski, M., & Ni, P. (2004). Score comparability of short forms and computerized adaptive testing: Simulation study with the activity measure for post-acute care. *Archives of Physical Medicine and Rehabilitation, 85,* 661–666.

Haley, S. M., Coster, W. J., Ludlow, L., Haltiwanger, J., & Andrellos, P. (1992). *Pediatric Evaluation of Disability Inventory (PEDI).* Boston: Boston University Center for Rehabilitation Effectiveness.

Haley, S. M., McHorney, C. A., & Ware, J. E., Jr. (1994). Evaluation of the MOS SF-36 physical functioning scale (PF-10): I. Unidimensionality and reproducibility of the Rasch item scale. *Journal of Clinical Epidemiology, 47,* 671–684.

Hambleton, R. K., & Jones, R. W. (1993). Comparison of classical test theory and item response theory and their applications to test development. *Educational Measurement: Issues and Practice, 12,* 38–47.

Institute of Objective Measurement (2000). *Definition of objective measurement.* Retrieved September 3, 2004 from http://www.rasch.org/define.htm.

Kielhofner G., Dobria, L., Forsyth K., & Basu, S. (2005). The construction of keyforms for obtaining instantaneous measures from the occupational performance history interview rating scales. *Occupational Therapy Journal of Research: Occupation, Participation and Health, 25*(1), 1–10.

Kielhofner, G., Mallinson, T., Crawford, C., Nowak, M., Rigby, M., Henry, A. & Walens, D. (2004). *Occupational Performance History Interview II (OPHI-II)* (version 2.1). Model of Human Occupation Clearinghouse, Department of Occupational Therapy, College of Applied Health Sciences, University of Illinois at Chicago, Chicago, IL.

Kielhofner, G., Mallinson, T., Forsyth, K., & Lai, J-S. (2001). Psychometric properties of the second version of the Occupational Performance History Interview (OPHI-II). *American Journal of Occupational Therapy, 55*, 260–267.

Lai, J-S., Velozo, C. A., & Linacre, J. M. (1997). Adjusting for rater severity in an unlinked functional independence measure database: An application of the many facets Rasch model. In R. M. Smith (Ed.), *Physical Medicine and Rehabilitation. State of Arts Reviews, 11*, 325–332.

Linacre, J. M. (1997). Instantaneous measurement and diagnosis. *Physical Medicine and Rehabilitation, 11*, 315–324.

Linacre, J. M. (1998). Detecting multidimensionality: Which residual data-types work best? *Journal of Outcomes Measurement, 2*, 266–283.

Linacre, J. M., Heinemann, A. W., Wright, B. D., Granger, C. V., & Hamilton B. B. (1994). The structure and stability of the Functional Independence Measure. *Archives of Physical Medicine and Rehabilitation, 75*, 127–132.

Linacre, J. M., & Wright, B. D. (1989). The "length" of a logit. *Rasch Measurement Transactions, 3*(1), 3–5.

Lord, F. M. (1953). The relation of test score to the trait underlying the test. *Educational and Psychological Measurement, 13*, 517–548.

Marino, R. J., & Graves, D. E. (2004). Metric properties of the ASIA motor score: subscales improve correlation with functional activities. *Archives of Physical Medicine and Rehabilitation, 85*, 1804–1810.

Martin, J. T., McBride, J. R., & Weiss, D. J. (1983). *Reliability and validity of adaptive and conventional tests in a military recruit population.* (Research Report 83-1). Minneapolis: University of Minnesota.

McHorney, C. A. (2002). Use of item response theory to link 3 modules of functional status items from the Asset and Health Dynamics among Oldest Old Study. *Archives of Physical Medicine and Rehabilitation, 83*, 383–394.

McHorney, C. A. (2003). Ten recommendations for advancing patient-centered outcomes measurement for older persons. *Annals of Internal Medicine, 139*, 403–409.

McHorney, C. A., & Cohen, A. S. (2000). Equating health status measures with item response theory: Illustrations with functional status items. *Medical Care, 38* (Suppl. II), 1143–1159.

Merbitz, C., Morris, J., & Grip, J. C. (1989). Ordinal scales and foundations of misinference. *Archives of Physical Medicine and Rehabilitation, 70*, 308–312.

Olsen, J. B., Maynes, D. D., Slawson, D., & Ho, K. 1986). *Comparison and equating of paper-administered, computer-administered, and computerized adaptive tests of achievement.* Paper presented at the annual meeting of the American Educational Research Association, San Francisco.

Rasch, G. (1960). *Probabilistic models for some intelligence and attainment tests* [Danish Institute of Educational Research 1960, University of Chicago Press 1980, MESA Press 1993]. Chicago: MESA Press.

Silverstein, B., Fisher, W. P, Kilgore, K. M., Harley, J. P., & Harvey, R. F (1991). Applying psychometric criteria to functional assessment in medical rehabilitation: II. Defining interval measures. *Archives of Physical Medicine and Rehabilitation, 73*, S3–S23.

Smith, E. V., Jr. (2002). Detecting and evaluating the impact of multidimensionality using item fit statistics and principal component analysis of residuals. *Journal of Applied Measurement, 3*, 205–231.

Smith, R. M. (1992). *Applications of Rasch measurement.* Maple Grove, MN: JAM Press.

Smith, R. M., & Taylor, P. (2004). Equating rehabilitation outcome scales: Developing common metrics. *Journal of Applied Measurement, 5*, 229–242.

Stone, M. H. (1997). Steps in item construction. *Rasch Measurement Transactions, 11*, 559.

Streiner, D. L., & Norman, G. R. (1989). *Health measurement scales: A practical guide to their development and use.* New York: Oxford University Press.

Thurstone, L. L. (1926). The scoring of individual performance. *Journal of Educational Psychology, 17*, 446–457.

Thurstone, L. L. (1928). Attitudes can be measured. *American Journal of Sociology, 23*, 529–554.

Thurstone, L. L. (1931). Measurement of social attitudes. *Journal of Abnormal and Social Psychology, 26*, 249–269.

Thurstone, L. L., & Chave, E. J. (1929). *The measurement of attitude.* Chicago: University of Chicago Press.

Velozo, C. A., Kielhofner, G., & Lai, J-S. (1999). The use of Rasch analysis to produce scale-free measurement of functional ability. *American Journal of Occupational Therapy, 53*, 83–90.

Velozo, C. A., Magalhaes, L. C., Pan, A-W., & Leiter, P. (1995). Functional scale discrimination at admission and discharge: Rasch analysis of the Level of Rehabilitation Scale–III. *Archives of Physical Medicine and Rehabilitation, 76*, 706–712.

Velozo, C. A., & Peterson, E. W. (2001). Developing meaningful fear of falling measures for community dwelling elderly. *American Journal of Physical Medicine and Rehabilitation, 80*, 662–673.

Wainer, H., Dorans, N. J., Eignor, D., et al. (2000). *Computerized adaptive testing: A primer* (2nd ed.). Mahwah, NJ: Lawrence Erlbaum Associates.

Ware, J. E., Jr, Kosinski, M., Bjorner, J. B., Bayliss, M. S., Batenhorst, A., Dahlof, C. G., Tepper, S., & Dowson, A. (2003). Applications of computerized adaptive testing (CAT) to the assessment of headache impact. *Quality of Life Research, 12*, 935–952.

Webster, K., Cella, D., &Yost, K. (2003). The Functional Assessment of Chronic Illness Therapy (FACIT) measurement system: Properties, applications, and interpretation. *Health Quality of Life Outcomes, 1*, 79.

Weiss, D. J. (1985). Adaptive testing by computer. *Journal of Consulting and Clinical Psychology, 53*, 774–789.

Wright, B. D. (1997a). A history of social science measurement. *MESA Memo 62*, http://www.rasch.org/memo62.htm.

Wright, B. D. (1997b). Fundamental measurement for outcome evaluation. *Physical Medicine and Rehabilitation: State of the Art Reviews, 11* (2), 261–288.

Wright, B. D., & Linacre, J. M. (1989). Observations are always ordinal; measurements, however, must be interval. *Archives of Physical Medicine and Rehabilitation, 70*, 857–860.

Wright, B. D., & Linacre, J. M. (1994). Reasonable mean-square fit values. *Rasch Measurement Transactions, 8*, 3.

Wright, B. D., & Masters, G. (1982). *Rating scale analysis.* Chicago: MESA Press.

Wright, B. D., & Stone, M. H. (1979). *Best test design.* Chicago: MESA Press.

RESOURCES

Books

This book is an excellent introductory/intermediary textbook about Rasch measurement theory and applications of Rasch analysis:

Bond, T. G., & Fox, C. M. (2001). *Applying the Rasch model: Fundamental measurement in the human sciences*. Mahwah, NJ: Lawrence Erlbaum.

This brief manual provides explanations of WINSTEPS and FACETS software output:

Smith, R.M. (2003). Rasch measurement models: Interpreting WINSTEPS and FACETS output. Maple Grove, MN: Journal of Applied Measurement Press.

Software

This software can be used to run the Rasch, 1-parameter model to analyze dichotomous and rating scale data A free student/evaluation version of the software called MINISTEPS can be downloaded from the same site:

Linacre, J. M. (2004). *WINSTEPS Rasch measurement computer program*. http://winsteps.com

This software can be used to run the Rasch, 1-parameter model to analyze additional facets such as rater severity. A free student/evaluation version of the software called MINIFAC can be downloaded from the same site:

Linacre, J. M. (2001). *FACETS Rasch measurement computer program*. http://winsteps.com

Web Sites

This Web site provides extensive information, resources and access to software on the Rasch measurement model and Rasch analysis. Of particular note is the search engine of this site that provides access to the Rasch Measurement Transactions – extensive short and mid-size reports on the many aspects of Rasch theory and analysis:

Institute of Objective Measurement, http://www.rasch.org/

Evaluating the Use of Assessments in Practice and Research

Wendy J. Coster

Typical research texts spend considerable time addressing research design issues such as sample size and power, the degree to which threats to internal validity such as rater bias or inappropriately matched comparison groups have been controlled, or the appropriate selection of statistical analysis methods. In comparison, content related to questions of measure validity is often quite limited. While research designs typically are subjected to very critical evaluation, critique of the choice of measures and interpretation of results from their use is often surprisingly superficial. Yet, the usefulness of the entire clinical research enterprise rests on the extent to which the measures used to examine whether the experimental group has "improved" or whether persons who received occupational therapy "function" better in their homes really do measure what they say they do.

An example from the stroke literature illustrates this point (Duncan, Lai, & Keighly, 2000). Stroke is a major health event that often results in long-term disability; thus considerable research has been devoted to examining the extent to which rehabilitation can decrease the likelihood or extent of disability or improve the degree or rate of recovery of function. In this study, the authors examined the impact of using different measures and different cutoff points to define successful recovery after stroke. The results indicated that the percentage of both the treatment and placebo groups considered "recovered" varied quite significantly depending on which measures and cutoff points were used. For example, shifting the definition of "recovered" by one level on the modified Rankin Scale (a commonly used disability severity measure) (Rankin, 1957) changed the percentage of those classified as recovered from < 25% to 53.8%, a substantial difference. Thus, a study that used the more lenient cutoff to classify someone as recovered would report more successful results than one using the more conservative cutoff.

A related paper (Duncan, Jorgensen, & Wade, 2000) reported that, across 27 drug trials for treatment of stroke that used the Barthel Index (an index that measures need for assistance while performing activities of daily living [ADLs]), seven different cutoff scores had been used to differentiate favorable and unfavorable outcomes. As the authors note, in a comment that could be applied to many areas of rehabilitation research, "Clearly, when there is so much variability in the methods used for outcome assessment ... it is difficult to know what to make of the results" (Duncan et al., 2000, p. 1435). This uncertainty affects not only the investigators, but also practitioners searching for sound evidence to guide clinical decision-making and consumers seeking information about effective intervention options.

The purpose of this chapter is to provide a framework for practitioners and clinical researchers for thinking about the choice of assessment instruments and interpretation of evidence from clinical research and practice. It is organized around a series of important questions that need to be asked and answered in all assessment situations.

What Assumptions Are Reflected in This Measure?

The very process of using an assessment from which one derives a score rests on an important assumption, which is that functional skills, capability, emotional experience, or whatever construct is the focus of the assessment can be quantified. When we observe behavior in the natural environment, it typically appears fluid and seamless, but when we use a scale such as the Functional Independence Measure (FIM) (Guide for the uniform data set for medical rehabilitation, 1997) we accept for the moment that meaningful differences between people in their dressing, bathing, or walking can be described using one of seven distinct categories of assistance.

Similarly, when we ask a parent to complete the Functional Skills section of the Pediatric Evaluation of Disability Inventory (PEDI) (Haley, Coster, Ludlow, Haltiwanger, & Andrellos, 1992), we accept for the moment that there is a clear

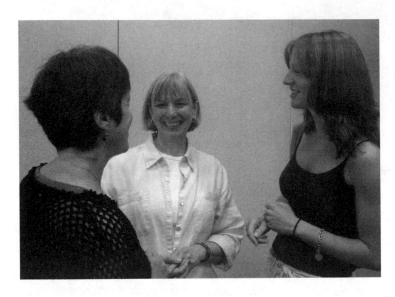

Figure 14.1 Dr. Coster chats with colleagues following a presentation on assessments at the annual American Occupational Therapy Association (AOTA) meeting.

(observable) difference between children who are and are not capable of "using a fork well" and that this difference can be represented by a score of 1 or 0. This assumption is necessary in order to conduct any kind of quantitative measurement of behavior. However, like all assumptions, the plausibility of its application in a particular measurement situation should be carefully evaluated.

A second assumption is that a sample of a person's behavior, thoughts, or opinions taken at one point in time can serve as a legitimate representation of his or her "true" situation or experience. This assumption rests on the interesting proposition, strongly reflected in Western culture, that there is such a thing as the person's "true" situation or experience. In other words, an investigator who had the correct methods would be able to pinpoint the person's "true" level of function, understanding, judgment, and so forth. Some form of this assumption is also necessary in order to engage in measurement. However, assessment developers and users may vary in how they interpret the meaning of information derived from a particular sample of behavior.

Until the past decade or so, users of measures of skill performance or ability (both clinicians and researchers) accepted that administration under standard, controlled conditions yielded the best approximation of the person's "true" capability. This assumption confounds two important but distinct issues. By having persons perform under standard conditions we do help ensure that the scores for each person were obtained under reasonably similar conditions, which is necessary for a fair comparison. However, it does not follow

that this standard performance context necessarily reveals more about the person's abilities than his or her performance in a different context, for example, in one that is more familiar. That is separate issue, which we will discuss later in the chapter.

What Social Forces Have Affected the Design and Use of This Assessment?

Other chapters in this text address in depth a variety of social and cultural influences that shape the inquiry process. To the extent that "knowing" in the quantitative tradition involves information derived from assessments, these influences also must be considered here. Consider how the outcomes of intervention methods are currently evaluated in physical rehabilitation practice and research. A large proportion of studies use measures of body function/body structure or impairment, such as strength, range of motion, or endurance. Why? The reasons are complex; however, at least one factor is the continuing influence of the medical model paradigm, which assigns a higher scientific value to physical or biological indicators that can be measured precisely using well-calibrated equipment. Within this paradigm, it has been traditionally assumed that improved function will follow directly from reduced impairment. Therefore, demonstration of change in impairment is considered sufficient evidence of a meaningful outcome and additional measures of function are not necessary. However, function, as measured by activity and participation, is a complex phenomenon, and the relationship between discrete impairments and function in daily life is not straightforward.

A second large group of studies use measures of basic ADL performance, in particular the Barthel (Mahoney & Barthel, 1965) and the FIM (Guide for the UDS, 1997), to examine outcomes. Both of these instruments measure function in terms of the amount of assistance needed. Why? Again, the reasons are very complex; however at least one factor is the influence of reimbursement systems in the United States. ADLs such as eating, toileting, and bathing must be performed regularly in order to regain and/or maintain physical health. Therefore, inability to complete these activities without help (sometimes referred to as the burden of care) has significant cost implications for payers. In contrast, the health implications of inability to do grocery shopping or to get together with friends are not as immediate or obvious. Cost is a legitimate concern; however, it is important to question whether the extent of improvements in basic ADL performance should be the primary *scientific* criterion for evaluation of rehabilitation effectiveness (Wade, 2003).

What Is Really Being Measured?

Assessments are often named according to the major construct they are thought to measure, for example, the *School Function Assessment* (SFA)

> Validity is not an attribute of the test itself, but rather it is evidence that supports interpretation or application (i.e., the meaning) of the test scores.

(Coster, Deeney, Haltiwanger, & Haley, 1998) or the *Stroke Impact Scale* (Duncan et al., 1999, 2003). Ideally, the authors provide a definition of this construct (and, possibly, its relevant dimensions) and cite theoretical and research work to support the validity of their definition in a manual or in published papers. However, the items and measurement scales constitute the actual operational definition of the construct. Any inferences that practitioners or researchers want to draw from results of using the instrument are restricted to those that can be drawn appropriately from this operational definition. Therefore, it is important to examine that definition independent of what the authors describe.

For example, consider the Barthel index used in the studies of stroke outcomes described earlier. The Barthel index was used by researchers as a measure of functional recovery, and inferences about rates of recovery were made based on these scores. The Barthel's operational definition of recovery is that the person can complete a specific set of basic ADLs with minimal to no assistance (depending on the cutoff score that is used). However, this is only one of many possible operational definitions of the construct of functional recovery. The person who no longer needs physical help with ADLs, but still cannot do the grocery shopping, return to work, or drive a car may not describe himself as "recovered." (See Lai, Perera, Duncan, & Bode, 2003; Lai, Studenski, Duncan, & Perera, 2002 for an example). Thus, when reviewing research results, or reporting results from an assessment, it is critically important to know the item content of the assessment in order to set the appropriate boundaries around conclusions.

It is also important to be familiar with the scale used to quantify degrees of the construct being measured because this scale is also part of the operational definition. For example, asking the person if he or she *needs physical help* to get dressed in the morning is not the same as asking if he or she *has difficulty getting dressed* (e.g., Laditka & Jenkins, 2001). A person who gets the maximum score on an assistance scale (does not need help) may not achieve the maximum score on a difficulty scale; according to one scale he is "recovered," while on the other scale he is experiencing "continuing limitations." In studies in which we have

---

What social forces affected the design and use of this assessment?

Who (what group of users) was the measure intended for?

What purpose was the measure designed for?

How has this purpose affected the content and design of the assessment?

What values are reflected in this measure?

Are these values and purpose consistent with *my* purpose and values?

compared items with similar content from different functional assessment instruments, we have found repeatedly that these different operational definitions may result in very different pictures of the person's function (Coster et al., 2004; Coster, Haley, Ludlow, Andres, & Ni, 2004).

What Evidence Supports the Congruence Between the Conceptual Model and the Actual Measure?

When we are examining what an assessment actually measures, we are considering questions of *validity* (see Chapters 12 and 13 for further discussions of validity). Validity is not an attribute of the test itself, but rather it is evidence that supports interpretation or application (i.e., the meaning) of the test scores (Messick, 1995; Morgan, Gliner, & Harmon, 2001). Because interpretations may vary according to *who* is being assessed, or the *context* in which he or she is being assessed, or the *purpose* of conducting the assessment, validity examination is an ongoing process from which evidence is accumulated over time. Two related areas of validity investigation are discussed here:

- Investigations that support interpretation of the assessment as a valid indicator of the underlying construct, and
- Investigations of the extent to which scores reflect factors or processes that are irrelevant to the construct.

What does this assessment actually measure?
What domain do the authors identify as the focus of the measure?
What is this definition based on?
  Does this definition derive from a theoretical or a conceptual model?
  Is there evidence to support this model?
What is the *operational definition* of the construct, as defined by the items and rating or scoring system?
  Are there aspects of the construct that are *not represented* by this operational definition?
  Does this operational definition cover the phenomenon that is important for *my* current purpose?
Are the authors' conclusions appropriate, based on this operational definition?

What Is the Model of the Underlying Construct?

As noted earlier, the authors of an assessment should provide a definition and conceptual model of the attribute they are trying to measure. In the behavioral sciences, a theoretical model is typically cited to support the construction of the assessment; however, it is not uncommon in the rehabilitation sciences to find that an assessment was designed based simply on pragmatic considerations; for example, the items selected are a set of "typical daily activities." A theoretical model lends itself to testing through research because it contains a series of propositions about how certain elements of performance should relate to other elements, or how performance on the assessment should differ according to age, functional status, or other factors. By testing these propositions, data are obtained that either do or do not support the interpretation of test scores in the way the authors proposed. For example, the function/disablement model that guided the development of the School Function Assessment (SFA) (Coster et al., 1998) proposes that functional performance of students with disabilities is context dependent. If this proposition is correct, then ratings on the SFA Participation Scale should vary across school settings. This proposition was supported by findings from the standardization data, which indicated that performance did vary significantly across settings and, furthermore, that there was a hierarchy of settings, with students likely to participate more in some settings than others (Mancini & Coster, 2004).

Do Subscales Represent Distinct Dimensions of the Construct?

Many assessments used by occupational therapy practitioners include subscales for which individual scores can be obtained, as well as overall summary scores. This kind of structure implies that the construct being measured has several distinguishable dimensions and evidence should be provided to support this proposition. Factor analysis is used frequently to test this aspect of the model, by looking to see if the items really do group themselves into separate factors that correspond to the subscales of the test (e.g., Jette et al, 2002; Ronen, Streiner, Rosenbaum, & the Canadian Pediatric Epilepsy Network, 2003). If they do not, this result contradicts the authors' model and suggests that the subscale scores do not reflect different dimensions of the attribute, ability, or skill, or that the dimensions are different from what the authors identified. This information is important for users of the assessment, because it has implications for the appropriate interpretation of subscale scores. Without evidence to support the distinctiveness of the subscales, interpreting differences among subscale scores as describing a profile of strengths and weaknesses has no sound basis.

On the other hand, if the assessment provides a meaningful summary score by averaging or summing subscale scores, then evidence should be provided to support this aspect of the model as well (e.g., see Young, Williams, Yoshida, & Wright, 2000). In this case, the authors are proposing that even though there may be some differences across subscales, there will also be meaningful consistency across them that can be represented by a summary score. Various kinds of analyses may be conducted to provide this evidence. For example, correlations may be conducted between subscale scores and summary scores to show the extent of association between them. Although it is unlikely that all subscale scores would be equally correlated with the summary score, major discrepancies in the size of the correlations may indicate that it is dominated by one or more subscales, or, conversely, that the summary score does not accurately reflect the performance, ability, or experience measured by that subscale. Factor analysis results may also be examined as evidence. If there is very little overlap in the factors (i.e., each item loads on one and only one factor), this weakens the basis for aggregating these factors in a summary score. More recently, scale dimensionality has been examined using the IRT methods discussed in Chapter 13 (for examples, see Duncan et al., 2003; Young et al., 2000).

These validity questions are complex and are not resolved by a single study. The developer of an assessment may have examined the factor structure in a sample of typically developing children, but that does not ensure that the conclusions can be applied to a sample of children with cerebral palsy or Down syndrome. Many clinical conditions affect one area of performance abilities more than another, which can result in very different profiles across subscales of complex tests by different groups, and may yield summary scores whose meaning is very unclear.

Are Scores Affected by Irrelevant Factors?

The example just described is one where there is substantial construct-irrelevant variance (Messick, 1995), meaning that too much variance in scores may be due to factors that are not part of the construct. There are many other types of irrelevant variance that may affect the validity of score inter-

Some readers may have noticed that I have not used terminology they have encountered in other discussions of assessment (see Chapter 12), such as *content validity, discriminant validity,* or *concurrent validity* (Gregory, 2000; Morgan, et al., 2001). These terms really all refer to different ways of *obtaining evidence* related to construct validity, which is the overarching concern we have been examining, rather than to separate categories of validity. From this perspective, content validity refers to evidence that the assessment adequately covers the relevant domains of the construct (*content coverage*) and that all of the content is relevant to the construct (*content relevance*). *Discriminant validity* refers to evidence that the assessment differentiates between groups who should behave or perform differently on a measure of this particular construct. *Concurrent* or *criterion validity* refers to evidence gathered by examining the relation between the assessment and other measures administered to the same persons at a similar point in time. If the assessment in question is a good measure of its intended construct, then scores from the measure should correlate with scores from other measures of that construct (*convergence*). It is also important to demonstrate that the assessment does *not* correlate with other measures of different constructs (*divergence*). Although this evidence is obtained by administering *concurrent* measures, the results speak to the meaning of the scores obtained from each, in other words, to *construct validity*.

pretation as well (see Baum, Perlmutter, & Dunn, 2001). Of course, the definition of "irrelevant" depends on the construct of interest and the population being assessed. If one is interested in measuring elders' knowledge about community resources, then factors such as a survey's small print size and advanced reading level may introduce irrelevant variance in responses. On the other hand, if one is assessing functional literacy, then print size may be highly relevant to determining the limits of what the person can and cannot do in natural settings. Practitioners can apply their knowledge about the clients they work with to identify these threats to valid interpretation of assessment scores, whether they are in a research report or in a clinical assessment report.

Whose Voice Is Represented?

A researcher or practitioner selecting an assessment must also think about what source of infor-

> **What evidence supports the congruence between the conceptual model and the actual measure?**
> What methods were used to group items into scales? Are these methods based in evidence?
> What evidence supports the distinctions among subscales and/or the creation of an aggregate (summary) score?
> Was this evidence derived from a population similar to mine? If not, how might differences between these populations affect my application of these results?
> Are there characteristics of my client group that could be sources of construct-irrelevant variance on this measure?
> What evidence has been presented to support validity of the measure as an indicator of the underlying construct? Does this evidence apply to my client population?

mation is appropriate for the question being asked. The source should be congruent with the definition or model of the construct, as well as with the purpose of the assessment. For example, in her discussion of *participation* as defined in the International Classification of Functioning, Disability, and Health (World Health Organization, 2001) Law (2002) notes that a person's preferences for and satisfaction with engagement in occupations are important dimensions of this construct. To be consistent with this definition, the only appropriate respondent for assessment of these aspects of participation is the person him- or herself.

However, an assessment also reflects the developer's idea of *what's important to measure about another person*. Therefore, decisions are not just conceptually based, but are also value based. Often, the values behind these decisions are implicit and may go unexamined for a long period of time. For example, the child development literature contains many studies that describe themselves as reporting on *parents'* effects on development, or *parents'* perceptions of their children's behavior, or *parents'* beliefs. A closer examination of the studies reveals that most or all of the *parents* providing this information are mothers, and that fathers (even in two parent families) often are not included. This design decision may have been made for practical reasons (e.g., fathers were less available during working hours than mothers; the project did not have sufficient funds to interview both parents). However, the value implicit in the studies' titles and descriptions is that mothers' voices are more important to listen to, and that they can speak for both parents' experience.

Thus, when we are evaluating evidence to incorporate into practice decisions, we want to look at where that evidence comes from (Brown & Gordon, 2004). We need to think about: Whose voice are we hearing? Is that the appropriate voice? Are we using the correct vehicle to bring us that voice? These questions have been asked with much more frequency in recent years. As discussed below, there are some excellent examples in the literature that illustrate the importance of, for example, making more effort to include the consumer's voice in the design of instruments or including the voices of children and others with more limited communication skills rather than substitute proxy respondents

Meyers and Andresen (2000) have critiqued the design of instruments and data collection methods from a universal design perspective. They note that population survey research (the kind of research, for example, used to identify the health status or service needs for a city, state, or nation's population) often relies on random digit dialing methods, with specific restrictions on number of rings allowed before terminating a call and against leaving messages. What impact does this methodology (which is quite rigorous in the traditional sense) have on obtaining the perspective of persons with mobility limitations (who may take a longer time to reach the phone), or of persons who communicate through assistive technology?

Other limitations may be less conspicuous. For example, many health status questionnaires ask the respondents to make statements about their general health over a specific time period, such as "in the past 12 months" or "in the past month." How will a person with a variable condition such as multiple sclerosis or Parkinson's disease, whose ability to engage in various life activities may have varied dramatically over the period in question, respond to such an instrument? Or, how should a middle-aged man who sustained a spinal cord injury as an adolescent respond to a question that asks: "As a result of your health, have you been limited in your ability to complete your tasks at work?" This question probably was written by someone without a disability whose definition of *health conditions* includes all variations from "typical," including the mobility limitations that follow spinal cord injury. That may not be the perspective of the person with the disability, who may reserve the term *health condition* for more acute physiological conditions such as flu or pressure sores, and may view limitations at work as resulting from inadequate accommodations in that environment. Finally, if the highest item on a scale (i.e., the item that would identify those with the greatest health) is the ability to *walk* a mile, how will the scale give voice to the experiences of those who may have skied, whitewater-rafted, or traveled extensively without ever *walking* a mile?

Researchers who have begun the measurement development process by asking consumers about their perspectives often hear different issues than what is represented on available instruments. For example, Laliberte-Rudman, Yu, Scott, and Pajouhandeh (2000) conducted a qualitative study using focus groups on the perspectives of persons with psychiatric disabilities of what constitutes *quality of life*. The participants identified key themes of managing time, connecting and belonging, and making choices and having control, each of which had several subthemes. The authors compared the themes identified by the participants to the content of existing quality of life instruments and identified a number of gaps. Interestingly, not only were some areas identified as important by the participants with disabilities not represented in the instruments, but even when certain content was included, the instrument often did not emphasize the aspects that were important to the participants. For example, many instruments ask about the number of friends a person has, or how frequently the person interacts with others, but the participants indicated that the important element to them was the *quality* of the interactions they had and whether it enhanced their sense of connectedness and belonging. Other authors have also questioned the use of *quantity* as an appropriate indicator of the *quality* of a person's social life (Dijkers, Whiteneck, & El-Jaroudi, 2000).

One group whose voice was heard very little until recently is children. Instead, we have heard the voices of concerned adults—parents, teachers, clinicians—who reported on the activities and participation of the children. However, studies have shown that by age 7 and up children can respond to many of the typical response formats used in self-report instruments (e.g., Juniper et al., 1996), that they can reliably report on their own functional performance (e.g., Young, Yoshida, Williams, Bombardier, & Wright, 1995), and that they can identify meaningful dimensions of their quality of life (e.g.,

> If the highest item on a scale (i.e.,, the item that would identify those with the greatest health) is the ability to *walk* a mile, how will the scale give voice to the experiences of those who may have skied, white-water-rafted, or traveled extensively without ever *walking* a mile?

Ronen, Rosenbaum, & Law, 1999). As has been reported for adults, children's own perceptions of their function, distress, or difficulties may differ significantly from the perceptions of adult proxies (e.g., Achenbach, McConaughy, & Howell, 1987; Ronen et al., 2003) and reports of children's function may also differ as a function of the context in which they are observed (Haley, Coster, & Binda-Sundberg, 1994).

Not surprisingly, populations with developmental or intellectual disabilities have also been excluded frequently from having a "voice," often because persons with disabilities were assumed to be unable to report reliably on their own experience. However, this assumption is being challenged increasingly as new, better adapted methods are used for the design of measures (e.g., see Cummins, 1997).

How Do We Know if the Information From Our Measures Is Trustworthy?

As noted earlier, our use of assessments rests on the assumption that the sample of behavior we gather at one point in time can be treated as a legitimate representation of a person's situation or experience. Reliability data provide one source of evidence regarding the validity of this assumption (Gliner, Morgan, & Harmon, 2001), specifically whether the information obtained at one point in time or from one particular source is likely to be replicated on another occasion (test–retest) or when provided by a different source (inter-rater). As discussed in Chapters 12 and 17, the most common form for estimates of reliability is the correlation coefficient (r).

Whose voice is represented?
Whose perspective guided the selection of content and the scoring metric of the instrument?
Who is the respondent? If someone other than the client is the respondent, is this an appropriate source of information for the purpose?

Reliability is a feature of a measurement, not of an instrument; thus it is more appropriate to talk about *score* reliability rather than *test* reliability. This distinction is often overlooked in the literature, but is important for practitioners to keep in mind. A study of an instrument's test–retest reliability is actually an examination of the reproducibility of the scores under specific conditions. The practitioner must decide whether the conditions in which he or she wants to use the instrument are similar enough to those conditions that the estimate can be generalized. For example, if an instrument has been tested only with healthy middle-aged adults, would scores be equally reliable when the instrument was administered to young men with traumatic brain injury? If the assessment is typically administered by having the person fill out the survey independently, will the scores be equally reliable if the information is gathered by having a clinician ask the questions in face-to-face interview? The research to answer these questions may not be available, in which case practitioners will need to use their clinical expertise to think these questions through carefully before making a decision. (For some provocative commentary on reliability, see Rothstein, 2001, 2002, 2003).

Should We Always Expect Consistency in Scores?

Inter-respondent (or inter-rater) comparisons raise additional questions. First, for survey measures or judgment-based assessments such as the PEDI (Haley et al., 1992), is client–therapist (or clinician–parent, or teacher–parent) agreement really a *reliability* estimate? If the ratings are different, does this mean that one of the respondents is wrong or unreliable? Not necessarily. It may be that each person is responding based on different information or perspectives. For example, using meta-analysis to examine agreement between respondents on children's behavioral and emotional problems, Achenbach, McConaughy, and Howell (1998) found that the mean correlation between pairs of informants varied depending on whether they usually saw the child in the same situation or not. Rogers et al. (2003) examined agreement between self and proxy reports, and in-hospital and in-home observed performance of ADL and IADL activities by community-dwelling older women. They concluded that cognitively intact respondents provided a reasonably accurate indication of the functional tasks they could do at home, and that clinical judgment (estimates based on client

impairment information) and performance in the occupational therapy clinic were less concordant with in-home performance.

Could the Change on This Measure Be Due to Measurement Error?

Standard reliability estimates provide evidence about reliability of scores for a *group*. This evidence is very useful when evaluating a test for possible use; however practitioners may be less concerned with scores for a group than with the reliability of the score of a particular *individual*. That is, we need an estimate of the likely *consistency of that individual's score*, which would let us know how confident we should be that the score we obtained is a good indicator of the individual's "true" ability or performance level. The standard error of measurement (SEM) (Portney & Watkins, 2000) is used for this purpose.

For assessments developed using classical test theory (CTT), the standard error of measurement is calculated from a reliability coefficient and applies to an entire scale. However, one of the advantages of assessments developed using IRT methods (discussed in Chapter 13) is that they yield separate standard error estimates for each possible score on the scale, which are therefore more precise. The SEM indicates how much variability is expected around a given summary score and is used to construct confidence intervals around scores. Use of these confidence intervals cautions us that our measures are not perfect and that the best we can do is identify the *range* within which the person's score is likely to fall.

Thus, when using a cutoff score to make a diagnostic or eligibility decision, we should be sure that the person's score is not only below the *cutoff* point, but is below the *lower* confidence interval. If we are examining whether a person has made significant progress, we should be sure that the amount of improvement on the reassessment extends beyond the *upper* confidence interval of the initial score. Otherwise, we are exaggerating

---

How do we know if the information from our measures is trustworthy?

How has reliability been examined and what were the results?

Has reliability been examined with clients/conditions similar to mine?

What is the standard error of measurement? How wide (how many points) is the confidence interval around an individual score?

the accuracy of our instruments and, potentially, drawing inaccurate conclusions about the effects of intervention.

If Reassessment Shows "No Change," Does That Mean the Intervention Didn't Work?

In practice and in research, assessments may be used for a variety of purposes, including describing a person's current status (e.g., cognitive development; motor skills), identifying deficit or clinical disorder, or predicting the likelihood of a future outcome. Another major use of assessment in health and rehabilitation is to examine whether change has occurred over time as a result of intervention, natural development, or recovery processes (Kirshner & Guyatt, 1985). This particular application of assessments requires support from another type of evidence, which is evidence that the instrument is sensitive enough to detect meaningful change over time. Evaluation of that evidence requires application of clinical expertise as well as knowledge about the relevant research methods.

Can This Measure Capture the Kind of Change That Is Likely?

When considering the use of an assessment to measure change over time, one of the first questions that must be asked is how much change is likely in the situation one will be examining. If a practitioner is planning to measure changes in function in a student with cerebral palsy receiving in-class intervention, what degree and type of change is reasonable to expect over the course of a school year (based on experience or research literature)? Are the items and scoring system of the assessment designed to record those changes? To illustrate, suppose items on my test are scored with a 4-point scale, and that, in order to obtain a rating higher than "0," the student must perform the activity described with no physical help. If the student I am working with has moderate cerebral palsy, and my intervention is focused on enabling the student to complete some part of each activity on his own, so that physical help is needed only for the final, more difficult parts, then, even if the student achieves this amount of progress on all the items, his summary score will not change. The

scale is not *sensitive* to this degree of change in performance.

Do Lower Scores Always Mean That No Gains Were Made?

Reassessment with norm-referenced tests is common practice (sometimes even a requirement) within some settings (e.g., schools). It is not uncommon to find that children with disabilities obtain *lower* scores on these tests as they get older, which may be misinterpreted as a lack of overall progress or even as a worsening of the condition (see Garwood, 1982). This interpretation is valid only in the very narrow sense that the child is not performing the items expected for his age group. Norm-referenced scores reflect a comparison to same-age peers; thus, the performance or behavior on which the scores are based changes as children's development proceeds. A very young child with a developmental disorder may acquire many of the basic skills measured for that age group and, therefore, obtain an average or "slightly delayed" score. However, if the child's pace of skill acquisition does not match the very rapid pace that is typical of nondisabled children during the toddler and preschool period, then, at the next assessment, the comparison-based score will drop. The child may have continued to make steady progress; however, it wasn't enough to obtain an "average" score.

Criterion-referenced scores are better suited to indicate whether progress has occurred in situations in which one doesn't expect "catch-up" with a comparison group (Haley, Coster, & Ludlow, 1991). These types of scores, which may be designed for a specific age group but are not norm-referenced, provide a clearer indication of whether the person being assessed has continued to move toward the positive end of the continuum represented by the measure, for example, functional skill acquisition (see the PEDI, Haley et al., 1992; and SFA, Coster et al., 1998 for examples).

Can This Measure Capture Meaningful Change?

An instrument's ability to detect change (sensitivity), however, does not guarantee that the change detected has clinical or "real life" meaning, which is referred to as responsiveness. Responsiveness requires evidence that changes on the measure relate to some external criterion of usefulness, value, or meaning. There are two important issues to consider. The first involves the distinction between statistical and clinical differences. Given a large enough sample, even a small difference on a measure (e.g., change in scores from the first to the second test administration, or the difference between two groups' scores) may achieve *statistical* significance. This result only reflects the probability that the average amount of change detected is greater than might be expected due to chance variation. The result says nothing about whether this amount of change is large enough to have any sort of clinical or "real life" impact or meaning. To illustrate, in certain circumstances changes of a few degrees in range of motion may be *statistically* significant, but the likelihood that this amount of change altered the person's ability to accomplish daily activities, i.e., that it is *clinically significant*, is probably slim.

Responsiveness studies are needed to determine whether the amount of change on a measure has value or meaning (Liang, 2000). The basic design of such studies is a comparison of change measured on the assessment to some other, valid indicator of change in the attribute. Unfortunately, there are no real "gold standards" we can use for this purpose in rehabilitation, so most studies use a combination of other methods to judge change such as client or clinician visual analog ratings of how much overall change has occurred or performance observations by raters who do not know the client's score on the assessment (i.e., "masked" or "blinded" raters) (e.g., Bedell, Haley, Coster, & Smith, 2002). These data are also sometimes used to calculate the "minimal clinically important difference (MCID), which is the minimum amount of change on the assessment (e.g., number of points) needed before an externally observable difference is detected (see Iyer, Haley, Watkins, & Dumas, 2003, for an example). The MCID is particularly useful information for the practitioner who is trying to translate assessment scores into "real-life" implications.

Conclusion

This chapter has discussed a series of important questions to ask about the assessments used in practice and reported in clinical research. They all, in some way, concern *validity*, that is, the meaning that can justifiably be assigned to numbers generated by our instruments. None of these questions

> **Is this measure responsive to change in the clients and context I am interested in?**
> Is the method for scoring items likely to detect the degrees or types of change seen in my clients over the usual assessment period?
> Is there evidence that summary scores are sensitive to changes in clients like mine?
> Is there evidence about how much change on the measure is needed to be clinically meaningful?

can be answered by the application of formulas or concrete rules because they require careful analysis and synthesis of multiple factors including the question of interest, the clients being assessed and the conditions of assessment, the features of the instrument itself, and the interactions among all of these. A thorough evaluation of these questions also requires integration of knowledge derived from clinical experience with knowledge about measurement so that our conclusions are guided by what we know from our interactions with the real people whose lives may be affected by the numbers applied to them by our assessments.

> An instrument's ability to detect change…does not guarantee that the change detected has clinical or "real-life" meaning.

REFERENCES

Achenbach, T. M., McConaughy, S. H., & Howell, C. T. (1987). Child/adolescent behavioral and emotional problems: Implications for cross-informant correlations. *Psychological Bulletin, 101*, 213–232.

Baum, C., Perlmuttter, M., & Dunn, W. (2001). Establishing the integrity of measurement data: Identifying impairments that can limit occupational performance and threaten the validity of assessments. In M. Law, C. Baum, & W. Dunn (Eds.), *Measuring occupational performance* (pp. 43–56). Thorofare, NJ: Slack.

Bedell, G. M., Haley, S. M., Coster, W. J., & Smith, K. W. (2002). Developing a responsive measure of change for pediatric brain injury rehabilitation. *Brain Injury, 16*, 659–671.

Brown, M., & Gordon, W. A. (2004). Empowerment in measurement: "Muscle," "voice," and subjective quality of life as a gold standard. *Archives of Physical Medicine and Rehabilitation, 85* (Suppl. 2), S13–S20.

Coster, W. J., Deeney, T., Haltiwanger, J., & Haley, S. M. (1998). *School function assessment*. San Antonio, TX: The Psychological Corporation/Therapy Skill Builders.

Coster, W. J., Haley, S. M., Andres, P., Ludlow, L., Bond, T., & Ni, P. (2004). Refining the conceptual basis for rehabilitation outcome measurement: Personal care and instrumental activities domain. *Medical Care, 42* (Suppl. l), I-62–I-72.

Coster, W. J., Haley, S. M., Ludlow, L. H., Andres, P. L., & Ni, P. S. (2004). Development of an applied cognition scale for rehabilitation outcomes measurement. *Archives of Physical Medicine and Rehabilitation, 85,* 2030–2035.

Cummins, R. A. (1997). Self-rated quality of life scales for people with an intellectual disability: A review. *Journal of Applied Research in Intellectual Disabilities, 10,* 199–216.

Dijkers, M. P., Whiteneck, G., & El-Jaroudi, R. (2000). Measures of social outcomes in disability research. *Archives of Physical Medicine & Rehabilitation, 81* (Suppl 2), S63–S80.

Duncan, P. W., Jorgensen, H. S., & Wade, D. T. (2000). Outcome measures in acute stroke trials: A systematic review and some recommendations to improve practice. *Stroke, 31,* 1429–1438

Duncan, P. W., Lai, S. M., Bode, R. K., Perera, S., DeRosa, J. & the GAIN Americas Investigators. (2003). Stroke Impact Scale-16: A brief assessment of physical function. *Neurology, 60,* 291–296.

Duncan, P. W., Lai, S. M., & Keighley, J. (2000). Defining post-stroke recovery: implications for design and interpretation of drug trials. *Neuropharmacology, 39,* 835–841.

Duncan, P. W., Wallace, D., Lai, S. M., Johnson, D., Embretson, S., Laster, L. J. (1999). The Stroke Impact Scale Version 2.0: Evaluation of reliability, validity, and sensitivity to change. *Stroke, 30,* 2131–2140.

Garwood, S. G. (1982). (Mis) use of developmental scales in program evaluation. *Topics in Early Childhood Special Education, 1*(4), 61–69.

Gliner, J. A , Morgan, G. A., & Harmon, R. J. (2001). Measurement reliability. *Journal of the American Academy of Child & Adolescent Psychiatry, 40*(4), 486–488.

Gregory, R. J. (2000). *Psychological testing* (3rd ed.). Boston: Allyn & Bacon. *Guide for the uniform data set for medical rehabilitation (Including the FIM instrument)*, Version 5.1 (1997). Buffalo: State University of New York at Buffalo.

Haley, S. M., Coster, W. J., & Binda-Sundberg, K. (1994). Measuring physical disablement: The contextual challenge. *Physical Therapy, 74,* 443–451.

Haley, S. M., Coster, W. J., & Ludlow, L. H. (1991). Pediatric functional outcome measures. In K. Jaffe (Ed.), *Pediatric Rehabilitation. Physical Medicine & Rehabilitation Clinics of North America, 2*(4), 689–723.

Haley, S. M., Coster, W. J., Ludlow, L., Haltiwanger, J., & Andrellos, P. (1992). *Pediatric Evaluation of Disability Inventory (PEDI).* Boston, MA: Boston University Center for Rehabilitation Effectiveness.

Iyer, L. V., Haley, S. M., Watkins, M. P., & Dumas, H. M. (2003). Establishing minimal clinically important differences for scores on the Pediatric Evaluation of Disability Inventory for inpatient rehabilitation. *Physical Therapy, 83,* 888–898.

Jette, A. M., Haley, S. M., Coster, W. J., Kooyoomjian, J. T., Levenson, S., Heeren, T. et al. (2002). Late Life Function and Disability Instrument: I. Development and evaluation of the disability component. *Journal of Gerontology: Medical Sciences, 57A,* M209–M216.

Juniper, E. F., Guyatt, G. H., Feeny, D. H., et al. (1996). Measuring quality of life in children with asthma. *Quality of Life Research, 5,* 35–46.

Kirshner, B., & Guyatt, G. H. (1985). A methodological framework for assessment of health and disease. *Journal of Chronic Disease, 38,* 27–36.

Laditka, S. B., & Jenkins, C. L. (2001). Difficulty or dependency? Effects of measurement scales on disability prevalence among older Americans. *Journal of Health & Social Policy, 13*(3), 1–15.

Lai, S. M., Perera, S., Duncan, P. W., & Bode, R. (2003). Physical and social functioning after stroke: Comparison of the Stroke Impact Scale and Short Form-36. *Stroke, 34,* 488–493.

Lai, S. M., Studenski, S., Duncan, P. W., & Perera, S. (2002). Persisting consequences of stroke measured by the Stroke Impact Scale. *Stroke, 33,* 1840–1844.

Laliberte-Rudman, D., Yu, B., Scott, E., Pajouhandeh, P. (2000). Exploration of the perspectives of persons with schizophrenia regarding quality of life. *American Journal of Occupational Therapy, 54,* 137–147.

Law, M. (2002). Participation in the occupations of everyday life. *American Journal of Occupational Therapy, 56,* 640–649.

Liang, M. H. (2000). Longitudinal construct validity: establishment of clinical meaning in patient evaluative instruments. *Medical Care, 38,* 84–90.

Mahoney, F. I., & Barthel, D. W. (1965). Functional evaluation: The Barthel Index. *Maryland State Medical Journal, 14,* 61–65.

Mancini, M. C., & Coster, W. J. (2004). Functional predictors of school participation by children with disabilities. *Occupational Therapy International, 11,* 12–25.

Messick, S. (1995). Validity of psychological assessment: Validation of inferences from person's responses and performances as scientific inquiry into score meaning. *American Psychologist, 50,* 741–749.

Meyers, A. R., & Andresen, E. M. (2000). Enabling our instruments: Accommodation, universal design, and access to participation in research. *Archives of Physical Medicine & Rehabilitation, 81* (Suppl. 2), S5–S9.

Morgan, G. A., Gliner, J. A., & Harmon, R. J. (2001). Measurement validity. *Journal of the American Academy of Child & Adolescent Psychiatry, 40*(6), 729–731.

Portney, L. G., & Watkins, P. (2000). *Foundations of clinical research* (2nd ed.). Upper Saddle River, NJ: Prentice-Hall.

Rankin, J. (1957). Cerebral vascular accidents in patients over the age of 60. II. Prognosis. *Scottish Medical Journal, 2,* 200–215.

Rogers, J. C., Holm, M. B., Beach, S., Schulz, R., Cipriani, J., Fox, A., & Starz, T. W. (2003). Concordance of four methods of disability assessment using performance in the home as the criterion method. *Arthritis & Rheumatism, 49,* 640–647.

Ronen, G. M., Rosenbaum, P., & Law, M. (1999). Health-related quality of life in childhood epilepsy: the results of children participating in identifying the components. *Developmental Medicine and Child Neurology, 41,* 554–559.

Ronen, G. M., Streiner, D. L., Rosenbaum, P., & the Canadian Pediatric Epilepsy Network. (2003). Health-related quality of life in children with epilepsy: Development and validation of self-report and parent proxy measures. *Epilepsia, 44,* 598–612.

Rothstein, J. M. (2001). Sick and tired of reliability? *Physical Therapy, 81,* 774–775.

Rothstein, J. M. (2002). Switching from autopilot. *Physical Therapy, 82,* 542–543.

Rothstein, J. M. (2003). Living with error. *Physical Therapy, 83,* 422–423.

Wade, D. T. (2003). Outcome measures for clinical rehabilitation trials: Impairment, function, quality of life, or value? *American Journal of Physical Medicine and Rehabilitation, 82* (10, Suppl.), S26–S31.

World Health Organization (2001). *International Classification of Functioning, Disability, and Health.* Geneva, Switzerland: Author.

Young, N. L., Williams, J. I., Yoshida, K. K., & Wright, J. G. (2000). Measurement properties of the Activities Scale for Kids. *Journal of Clinical Epidemiology, 53,* 125–137.

Young, N. L., Yoshida, K. K., Williams, J. I., Bombardier, C., & Wright, J. (1995). The role of children in reporting their physical disability. *Archives of Physical Medicine & Rehabilitation, 76,* 913–918.

RESOURCES

Listings and Samples of Assessments

Asher, I. E. (1996). *Occupational therapy assessment tools: An annotated index* (2nd ed.). Bethesda, MD: American Occupational Therapy Association.

*Dittmar, S. S., & Gresham, G. E. (1997). *Functional assessment and outcome measures for the rehabilitation health professional.* Gaithersburg, MD Aspen.

*Finch, E., Brooks, D., Stratford, P. W., Mayo, N. E. (2002). *Physical rehabilitation outcome measures: A guide to enhanced clinical decision making* (2nd ed.) (with CD-ROM). BC Decker: Hamilton, Ontario.

Law, M., Baum, C., & Dunn, W. (2001). *Measuring occupational performance: supporting best practice in occupational therapy.* Thorofare, NJ: Slack.

Law, M., King, G., MacKinnon, E., Russell, D., Murphy, C., & Hurley, P. (1999). *All about outcomes* (CD-ROM). Thorofare, NJ: Slack.

*These resources include actual assessments.

Structured Review Forms for Evaluating Assessments

M. Law (Ed.), (2002). *Evidence-based rehabilitation: a guide to practice.* Thorofare, NJ: Slack.

Forms are also available on the CanChild web site: http://www.fhs.mcmaster.ca/canchild

CHAPTER 15

Making Meaning From Numbers: Measurements and Descriptive Statistics

Machiko R. Tomita

Numbers are tools for making meaning. They are the basic tools of mathematics and represent formal ways of characterizing and making sense of the world. Statistics, a branch of mathematics, involves systematically converting observations into numbers, and then using those numbers to characterize and to draw inferences about the world. Because the procedures for translating observations into numbers and for manipulating numbers to answer questions and make decisions are formal and systematic, they are especially useful in achieving an objective approach to conducting science. The purpose of this chapter is to introduce the use of statistics in research and to overview basic concepts of statistics.

Researchers in occupational therapy are always a bit discouraged when they hear therapists or students comment that, when reading research articles, they skip the statistical analysis section, or find it difficult to understand. Nonetheless, it is recognized that many who are drawn to occupational therapy because of its humanistic and pragmatic orientation find mathematics and statistics both distant and obscure. The intent of this and subsequent chapters is to illustrate that statistics are simply pragmatic tools and that their use can help us understand phenomena and make important decisions that address humanistic ends.

Statistics are not only central tools of quantitative science; they are also important for informing decision making in occupational therapy practice. That is, statistical analysis is also the basis on which therapists may decide such things as whether one practice approach is better than another, how much confidence to have in the results of an assessment, whether a client's performance is sufficient for a particular functional task, and how long a therapist may need to continue an intervention to achieve certain results.

For the new researcher who uses statistics it is no longer necessary to calculate difficult math.

User-friendly computer software now handles this task. Moreover, for complicated statistics, most investigators collaborate with statisticians and biostatisticians.

It is important for both consumers and users of statistics to have a good understanding of:

- Which statistics should be used to answer research questions or test hypotheses,
- How the statistic goes about reaching conclusions (i.e., what is the underlying logic of the statistic), and
- How statistical results should be interpreted.

For these reasons, this and subsequent chapters dealing with statistics will emphasize the conceptual formulas of statistical tests, not the calculation formulas. Moreover, the discussions will focus on the underlying logic of each statistic, what kinds of information the statistic gives, and how to make sense of the statistic's results.

A good basic grasp of statistics is necessary for even simple quantitative research. When one grasps the underlying logic of statistical analysis, it is possible to design better research, to ask better questions, and to formulate correct hypotheses. Understanding the basics of statistics is also essential to being able to read research articles critically and to draw conclusions about what the research findings mean for one's practice.

What Is Statistics?

Simply said, statistics is a method for generating the best information from available data. Statistics is a branch of applied mathematics that deals with the collection, description, and interpretation of quantitative data, and with the use of probability theory, estimates population characteristics from samples. In a quantitative study, the investigator ordinarily wants to draw conclusions about all the people who share certain characteristics. However, it is usually impossible to study all of them, so investigators study only a selected subgroup of these people.

The larger group of people about whom an investigator wants to draw conclusions is called the population and the measures of their characteristics are called parameters. The subgroup of people who are actually studied is called the sample, and the measures of their characteristics are called statistics. In most studies, the population parameters are unknown; therefore, they must be estimated from the sample statistics. When investigators objectively collect some type of information from the sample (i.e., data), they can apply a statistical procedure to the data to estimate the population parameter.

How Do Investigators Use Statistics?

Statistics are used in three ways. The first is to describe information of the sample meaningfully and efficiently by using smaller sets of data. For this, one uses descriptive statistics, and one can typically find them in a demographic table or a summary table of most published quantitative research articles. The second is to generalize the observed information of the sample to the population with a degree of confidence. For this one uses inferential statistics, and this process is explained in Chapters 16 and 17. The third is to identify associations, relations, and differences among the sets of observations, and inferential statistics are also used for this purpose. Various statistical methods for this purpose are described in Chapter 17. The primary purpose of quantitative research is to estimate the population parameters; therefore, the investigators report the sample statistics that the generalization is based on and the accuracy of the sample that represents the value of the population parameter.

Measurement Scales

What Is Measurement?

Investigators collect data from the sample for a research study to answer the research question. Therefore, data should provide the information necessary for answering the question. Data consist of variables; a variable is a characteristic being measured that varies among the persons, objects, or events being studied. For example, age is a variable because it can have many values. If age is measured as "Young" or "Old," one can say the age has two levels: young and old. Functional ability is a variable because it may vary from "Completely Independent" to "Completely Dependent." If an investigator introduces two types of occupational therapy interventions and compared them with a control group, then the intervention is a variable and it has three levels: "occupational therapy intervention 1, occupational therapy intervention 2, and no intervention."

Although the levels of all variables described in the preceding paragraph use words, they can be expressed as numerals. For instance, it is possible to assign a "1" for "Young" and a "2" for "Old." In this case, the numerals are used to indicate to which category of young or old the person belongs. Similarly, numbers could be assigned to indicate where a person falls on the continuum from completely independent to completely dependent. Therefore, measurement is the process of assigning numerals to observed people, objects, or events according to a set of rules for the purpose of understanding them objectively without ambiguity. These rules designate how numbers are to be assigned, reflecting amount or values and units of measurements.

Types of Measurement Scales

The rules that define how numbers are assigned to observed people, objects, or events determine the levels (scale) of measurement. There are four levels, or scales, of measurement: nominal, ordinal, interval, and ratio. Whenever a variable is measured it requires using one of the four scales. Among the four measurement scales, nominal and ordinal scales are called categorical scales since they use only discrete numbers. A discrete variable can be described only in whole units for data collection. Examples are the number of children in a family, the number of times a person has been hospitalized, and the number of mistakes a person makes on a test of cognition, which are expressed as 1, 2, 3, etc. When categorical scales are used to

> The word *statistics* originally came form the phrase "lecture about state affairs," meaning the analysis of data about the state. In the early 19th century it became the collection and classification of data.

> The traditional classification of levels of measurement was developed by Stevens (1946) and is still widely used: nominal, ordinal, interval, and ratio.

measure a dependent variable, nonparametric statistics are used.

Interval and ratio scales are called continuous scales; they can use discrete numbers or continuous numbers. A continuous variable can take on any value along a continuum within a defined range. For instance, a person's weight could be 60.455 kg and blood pressure can be 120.051. Parametric statistics are used for a dependent variable measured by a continuous scale.

Nominal Scale

A nominal scale is a categorical scale and is the lowest scale of measurement used to classify variables. Although numerals are assigned for each category, they have no numerical values in that they "name" the characteristic but do not suggest an order, an amount, or value. For example, investigators may code types of disability as (1) physical, (2) cognitive, and (3) mental, or assign male = 1 and female = 2, but the numbers are merely labels and it does not make sense, for example, to add these numbers, or to calculate an average. Finally, nominal data cannot be converted to any other scales whereas other scales can be converted to nominal scales.

Further examples of nominal scales are type of occupation (work, play, or self-care), race (African-American, Caucasian, Hispanic, Native American, etc.), work status (full time, part time, retired, etc.), and the dichotomous answer, "Yes" or "No." Nominal scale categories have to be mutually exclusive so that no person or object can be assigned to more than one category.

Most demographic tables in research studies include variables measured by a nominal scale. Table 15.1 illustrates hypothetical nominal data for the characteristics of two groups of assistive technology workshop participants. The variables measured by a nominal scale in this table are sex, race, and group affiliation.

When a variable is a construct that is an abstract variable such as pain, physical functioning level, and cognition, a series of nominal level items may be used together to provide a measure of the variable. In this case, each item may have a dichotomous choice to indicate the presence or absence of some characteristic. Each item is thus measured by a nominal scale. However, to interpret the variable, a total score based on all items is calculated. The resulting total score is ordinarily considered to be an interval scale because of its wide range of scores. Examples are the Observed Tasks of Daily Living-Revised (OTDL-R) (Diehl, Marsiske, Horgas, & Saczynski, 1998) and Sickness Impact Profile (Gilson et al., 1975). The OTDR-L is a behavioral measure of everyday competence that requires a client to perform a number of observable actions in response to a question by the tester. Scores are recorded as correct or incorrect. Then a score of 1 is given to a correct response and 0 to an incorrect response; the possible total score range of 0 through 26.

Sometimes instruments use weighted items to arrive at a total score; weighting allows items to contribute different amounts to the total score based on some criterion such as their importance, severity, or difficulty. For example, The Sickness Impact Profile (SIP)-Dysfunction consists of 45

Table 15.1 Characteristics of Assistive Technology Workshop Participants for Each Group ($N = 37$)

	Group A		Group B	
	n	%	n	%
Sex				
Men	4	19	4	25
Women	17	81	12	75
Race				
Caucasian	8	38	9	56
African-American	5	24	1	6
Hispanic	8	38	6	38
	Mean	SD	Mean	SD
Other variables				
Age	56.0	(10.0)	44.7	(8.5)
Years since onset	10.7	(3.3)	12.1	(6.3)
Fatigue Severity Scale Score	5.3	(.9)	5.3	(.9)

items that use dichotomous scales to determine a physical functioning level. A client will answer yes/no for each item and items have been assigned various weights to indicate the severity of the physical problem. For example, for the statement "I am getting around only within one building" if a subject answers "Yes" the score of 86 is given, and if the response is "No" the score of 0 is given. Moreover, for the statement "I walk shorter distances or stop to rest often" the "Yes" response weighs 48. The total weighted scores for all 45 items divided by all weights together determine the physical functioning level.

Ordinal Scale

An ordinal scale requires one to rank-order the categories. This is considered the second lowest scale and the data measured using an ordinal scale can be converted to that of a nominal scale. Data are organized into adjacent categories in a linear fashion, ascendant or descendant. Two examples are health status ranked as (1) Very Poor, (2) Poor, (3) Fair, (4) Good, and (5) Very Good, and pain levels ranked as (1) No pain, (2) Mild, (3) Moderate, and (4) Severe (Jette, 1980). When numbers are used to indicate ranking, they refer only to the relative position of the category along the continuum. The distances between the ranks are not necessarily equal. Using the example of the pain level, the distance between (1) No pain and (2) Mild may not be the same as the distance between (3) Moderate and (4) Severe. Investigators often tabulate ranking of an item and report the mean rank. For instance, Mitcham, Lancaster, and Stone (2002) reported a study of the effectiveness of occupational therapy faculty development workshops. In this study, 106 participants ranked eight elements of the workshop on a 10-point scale. For example, the mean rank for teaching skills of leader was 9.1 (the highest score); handouts, 8.4; and opportunity for career development, 7.7 (the lowest score).

Strictly speaking, if a dependent variable is measured by an ordinal scale, the data should be analyzed by nonparametric statistics. However, there are research studies in which data gathered by ordinal scales were treated as interval scale data, and parametric statistics were applied. When the intervals between adjacent ranks can be assumed reasonably equal and there are many items within the variable, the ranking of each item can be summed to produce many rankings. In this case, many investigators will consider the total score to "approximate" a continuous (interval) scale. An example is a depression instrument called the Center for Epidemiology Study for Depression (CES-D) (Gilson et al., 1975). This scale requires frequency of the feelings experienced during the past week. It consists of 20 items, and for each item there are four choices: Rarely (less than 1 day), Some of the time (1 to 2 days), Moderately (3 to 4 days), and Mostly (5 to 7 days). These choices have rankings assigned of 0, 1, 2, and 3 respectively. To interpret the depression level, the total scores of 20 items will be calculated, producing rankings 0 to 60. The total score is considered to be continuous (interval), thus allowing arithmetic calculations.

Other investigators prefer not to consider such scales as interval in nature since they are composed of only ordinal rankings. A method called Rasch analysis that converts items that were measured by an ordinal scale to interval scale (Bond & Fox, 2001) is discussed in Chapter 13. Increasingly, investigators prefer to use Rasch methods to convert scores based on ranked items to true interval scales rather than assuming they "approximate" an interval scale. The Functional Index Measure (FIM) that measures Activities of Daily Living (ADL) is an example of an instrument created using Rasch analysis (Wright & Linacre, 1989).The FIM uses the following ordinal scale for each of 18 items: (7) complete independence, (6) modified independence, (5) supervision, (4) minimal assist, (3) moderate assist, (2) maximal assist, and (1) total assist (Center for Functional Assessment Research/Uniform Data System for Medical Rehabilitation, 1994). Rasch analysis converts the ordinal data generated from completing the scale to an interval measure. However, in practice, many persons continue to use the raw total score to avoid the necessity of computer analysis of the raw scores to generate a true interval measure. Linacre (1995, 1997) developed an alternative to computer scoring for obtaining measures. He introduced the idea of a keyform—a paper-and-pencil method that generates interval measures from the ordinal raw data of the FIM (Linacre, 1997). More recently Kielhofner, Dobria, Forsyth, and Basu (2004) used this same methodology to create keyforms for the Occupational Performance History Interview—2nd version (OPHI-II). These keyforms allow occupational therapists to obtain instantaneous measures from raw rating scale data. The availability of such methods for achieving interval scores from raw data may make it less common in the future that investigators will treat data generated from ordinal rankings as "approximately" interval.

Nonetheless, there have been long statistical debates on appropriateness of treating ordinal data as interval data (Guildford, 1954; Kerlinger, 1973; Nunally, 1978; Merbitz, Morris, & Grip, 1989; Velleman & Wilkinson, 1993). Portney and Watkins (2000) take a stand that investigators should treat ordinal data as such, but if the investigator can make a reasonable argument that the ordinal scale approximates an interval scale, the error involved is defensible.

Interval Scale

An interval scale is the second highest measurement scale; therefore, the data measured by an interval scale can be converted to a nominal or an ordinal scale. The distance between any two adjacent units of measurements or intervals is the same, but not their proportionate magnitude, since there is no meaningful zero point. Zero can be used on interval scales, but it does not mean nonexistence or absence. A good example is temperature, either in Fahrenheit or Centigrade. Zero degrees Centigrade is 32 degrees Fahrenheit, and zero degrees Fahrenheit is negative 17.8 degrees Centigrade. Zero is merely a line on the thermometer. Therefore, temperature is an interval scale and does not indicate absolute magnitude of an attribute. Within the Fahrenheit or Centigrade temperature scale, the distance between 21 and 31 degrees is the same as that between 61 and 71 degrees. However, it is incorrect to say 60 degrees is three times hotter than 20 degrees, since zero does not represent the absence of temperature. A dependent variable measured using an interval scale can be analyzed using parametric statistics if other statistical assumptions are met.

> The higher levels of measurement can always be converted to lower levels of measurements, if necessary, but the converse is not possible.

Ratio Scale

The ratio scale is the highest measurement scale and the data gathered using a ratio scale can be converted to other lower measurement scales. It is a scale in which any two adjacent values are the same distance apart (just like an interval scale) and in which there is a true zero point (unlike an interval scale). All arithmetic computations are possible with a ratio scale and if the dependent variable is measured by a ratio scale, and if other statistical assumptions are met, parametric statistics can be applied. Some examples of ratio level scales are height, weight, age, range of motion, distance, strength, blood pressure, duration of exercise, handwriting speed, amount of food consumed, and number of falls. In Table 15.1, "Age" and "Years since onset" are measured by ratio scales. Variables measured by interval and ratio scales are generally called continuous variables. However, strictly speaking, among variables measured by ratio or interval scales, there are two types of variables: continuous variables (e.g., duration of exercise) and discrete variables (e.g., number of falls). All nominal and ordinal scales are discrete variables.

It is useful to remember that if possible, investigators should use a higher level measurement scale to measure people, objects, and events. The higher levels of measurement can always be converted to lower levels of measurements, if necessary, but the converse is not possible.

For instance, an investigator who collects data on age using a nominal scale such as "old" and "young" will never be able to categorize them further or recategorize them. If on the other hand, the investigator uses a ratio scale (i.e., years of age) this data could be converted to ordinal scales (e.g., below 10, 11–20, 21–30, etc.) or to nominal scales (young versus old). As a final point, although researchers use measurement scales to measure both independent and dependent variables, the type of scale used to measure the dependent variable, not the independent variable, is one of the determining factors for the use of parametric versus non-parametric statistics.

Types of Statistics in Relation to Measurement Scales

The scale that measures the dependent variable together with other statistical assumptions determines which of two types of statistics are used: parametric statistics versus nonparametric statistics. Here, without explaining much detail, it can be pointed out that many researchers prefer to use parametric statistics over nonparametric statistics for two reasons:

• With use of parametric statistics, a researcher can be more confident to say one group's characteristics are significantly different from the others, and

• There are more parametric statistics than non-parametric statistics, so in that sense, parametric statistics represent a wider range of tools for answering research questions.

The details of these statistics are explained in the following chapters. Figure 15.1 summarizes the relationship between use of types of statistics and measurement scales.

Descriptive Statistics

When data are collected, the initial form of the data is called raw data. To understand characteristics of people, objects, and events, the raw data must be organized. Even though the main purpose of performing statistical analyses is to infer population characteristics that are likely to be the nature of entire people for your inquiry (which involves inferential statistics), it is important to summarize the sample characteristics on which the inferences are based. This involves descriptive statistics. Presentation of descriptive statistics includes graphs and frequency distribution tables as well as measures of central tendency and variability.

> The type of scale used to measure the dependent variable, not the independent variable, is one of the determining factors for the use of parametric versus non-parametric statistics.

Frequency Distribution

Data summarized using a frequency distribution typically present individual percentages and cumulative percentages as well. The notation of frequency is (f). Table 15.2 is a Statistical Package for the Social Sciences (SPSS) (version 12.0, 2003) printout of frequency distribution of the total number of medications taken among 72 home-based frail elderly. The capital N indicates the total sample size and lowercase n indicates the sample size of each subcategory.

The first column contains the number of medications taken, the second column is number or frequency of people who reported the number of medications taken, the third column is percentage of the frequency of the total sample size, and the last column is a cumulative percentage up to the particular value. Note in this data no one took 2 or 11 medications; therefore 2 and 11 are absent in the first column.

The same data can be grouped into classes in which each class represents a unique range of scores within the distribution. The classes are mutually exclusive or there are no overlapping values and are exhaustive within the range of scores obtained. If the range of each class is two, the grouped frequency distribution of Table 15.2 will form five classes (0–2, 3–5, 6–8, 9–11, and 12–14)

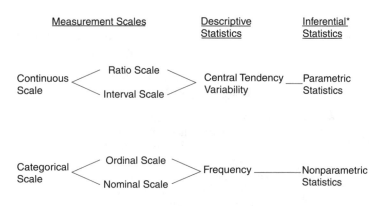

*Type of inferential statistics to be used for analysis is determined by:
  • Type of measurement scale used for the dependent variable,
  • Type of distribution of scores of the dependent variable, and
  • Homogeneity of groups in terms of dependent variable.
In addition, a random selection or assignments of sample is an assumption.

Figure 15.1 Relationship between measurement scales and types of statistics for descriptive and inferential statistics.

Table 15.2 **Frequency Distribution of Total Number of Medications Taken Among Home-Based Frail Elderly (*N* = 72)**

	n	Frequency	Percentage	Valid Percentage	Cumulative Percentage
Valid	0	6	8.3	8.3	8.3
	1	2	2.8	2.8	11.1
	3	9	12.5	12.5	23.6
	4	9	12.5	12.5	36.1
	5	12	16.7	16.7	52.8
	6	5	6.9	6.9	59.7
	7	7	9.7	9.7	69.4
	8	8	11.1	11.1	80.6
	9	6	8.3	8.3	88.9
	10	4	5.6	5.6	94.4
	12	2	2.8	2.8	97.2
	13	1	1.4	1.4	98.6
	14	1	1.4	1.4	100.0
	Total	72	100.0	100.0	

and the frequencies are 8, 30, 20, 10, and 4, respectively. When the intervals of the classes are the same, the comparisons of classes are easy. Investigators will typically report intervals of classes when individual classes contain a few or zero frequency. In this case classes are clustered to reveal a more meaningful interpretation of the data. For example, in the study titled, "Development of a standardized instrument to access computer task performance," (Dumont, Vincent, & Mazer, 2002) the table of sample characters consists only of frequencies and percentages. Some of the types of information included are age in five classes (17–19, 20–29, 30–39, 40–49, and 50+), occupation in three categories (homemaker or retired, student, and employed), frequency of computer use (rarely, occasionally, and regularly), touch-typing method (yes and no).

Graphical Presentation of Frequency Data for Discrete Variables

There are several ways to graphically present a frequency distribution of data. Since the number of medications a person takes is a whole number, it is a discrete value such as three or five medications. Discrete variables are presented using a bar graph or chart. A space separates each bar to emphasize the noncontinuous nature of the data. All nominal and ordinal data and some interval and ratio data use the bar graph. For instance, the information contained in Table 15.2 can be presented in a bar

graph as shown in Figure 15.2a. The *x*-axis (horizontal) is the number of medications taken and the *y*-axis (vertical) is the measured variable (i.e., frequencies of persons who take the number of medications). The advantage of this graphical presentation is the obvious efficiency in identifying the shape and characteristics of distribution. The largest number of elders (*n* = 12) took five medications and the fewest number of elders (*n* = 0) took 2 or 11 medications.

The pie graph, an alternative to the bar graph, is a circle that has been partitioned into percentage distribution and presented in Figure 15.2b. For detailed information on constructing a pie chart, refer to Wallgren, Wallgren, Persson, Jorner, and Haaland (1996).

Graphical Presentation of Frequency Data for Continuous Variables

There are several ways to present frequency data for continuous variables. They are a histogram, a frequency polygon, and the stem-and-leaf plot. A histogram is a bar graph without space between bars. A frequency polygon is a line plot, where each point on the line represents frequency or percentage. Figure 15.3 is a SPSS (2003) printout of a frequency polygon of grip strength by sex of frail elders in kilograms. In this figure, the two lines represent females and males.

The stem-and-leaf plot is most useful for presenting the pattern of distribution of a continuous variable. There are two parts in this plot: stem and

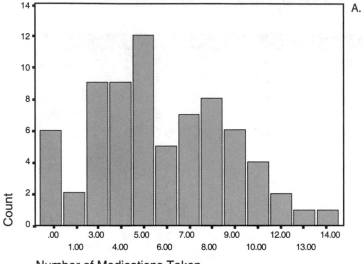

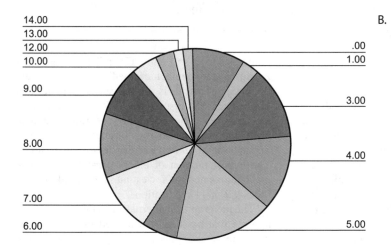

Figure 15.2 (a) Bar graph of frequency of medications taken. (b) Pie chart of frequency of medications taken.

leaf. Table 15.3 shows raw data of age of veterans with spinal cord injury and its stem-and-leaf plot. The stem in this plot is segmented by every 10 years and the leaf represents additional ages. Examples of interpretation of this plot are the following: there are two veterans with spinal cord injury who are in the teens, 18 and 19 years old. Therefore, in the stem of 10, 8 and 9 are listed in the leaf. Similarly, there are six veterans who are in the 40s. Since the leaf contains two zeros, two veterans are 40 years old, and others are 42, 44, 45, and 47 years old.

Measures of Central Tendency

When a variable is measured using an interval or ratio scale, measures of central tendency or averages are often used to describe the typical nature of the data. There are three indices: the mean, the median, and the mode.

Mean

The mean is the sum of individual scores (X) divided by the number of sample size (n). The symbol used to represent a population mean is the Greek letter, μ (read as mu) and a sample mean is represented by $\overline{X}$ or M. The formula for calculating the sample mean from raw data is

$$\overline{X} = \frac{\sum X}{n}$$

where $\sum$ (read as sigma) indicates summation. If the values of X are 2, 4, 5, 6, 3, 7, 4, and 10, the sum of all values is 41 and dividing it by the number of cases, 8, equals 5.125. The mean is the most useful average because it is most reliable among measures of central tendency. When samples are drawn randomly and repeatedly from the population, the means of those samples would fluctuate

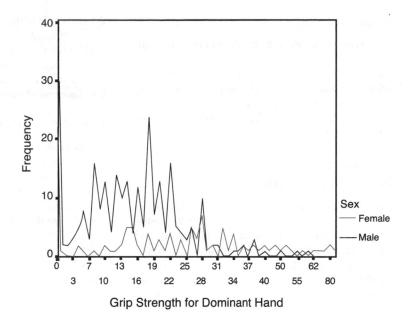

Figure 15.3 Frequency polygon for grip strength by sex (*N* = 319).

less than the mode or median. The mean can be used for arithmetic calculations and is used most often for statistical analyses.

Median

The median is the middle position of measurement in a set of ranked scores. Therefore, the values should be arranged in an ascending or descending order. Using the same preceding example, the values are rearranged: 2, 3, 4, 4, 5, 6, 7, and 10. The midpoint is between 4 and 5. When the number of

scores is even, there is no single middle score. In that case, the median is calculated by taking the average of the two middle scores. Therefore, the median for the value is 4.5 ($= \dfrac{4 + 5}{2}$). When there is an extreme score in a dataset, the median is a better index than the mean because the median is not influenced by the score. In the preceding example, if 100 replaces the value 10, the new mean will be 16.375 owing to the extreme score of 100, but the median is still 4.5.

Table 15.3 Age of Veterans with Spinal Cord Injury (Age 18–50): Raw Data and Stem-and-Leaf Plot

Raw Data in Chronological Order								Stem-and-Leaf Plot	
18	24	27	29	30	32	34	37	Stem	Leaf
19	25	27	29	30	32	34	37	10	89
20	25	27	29	30	32	34	37	20	0122333444445555556677
21	25	27	29	30	32	35	38	20	7777777778888888999999
22	25	27	29	30	32	35	38	20	99999
22	25	28	29	30	32	35	39	30	000000000001111122222
23	26	28	29	30	33	35	39	30	2233333334444555555666
23	26	28	29	31	33	35	40	30	77778899
23	27	28	29	31	33	35	40	40	002457
24	27	28	30	31	33	36	42		
24	27	28	30	31	33	36	44		
24	27	28	30	31	33	36	45		
24	27	29	30	32	34	37	47		

Mode

The mode is the score that occurs most frequently in a dataset. In the example discussed in the previous paragraph, the mode is 4. In the set, there is only one mode; therefore, the data is unimodal. If there are two modes, the distribution is considered bimodal. Some distributions of variables do not have a mode.

Location of Central Tendency in Various Distributions

Locations of central tendencies are affected by the distribution of values in the data. When the distribution of values is normal, the mean, median, and mode are all in the center of the distribution of the values (Figure 15.4a). A normal distribution is unimodal, and both sides of the mean have symmetrical shapes (a more detailed discussion of normal distribution occurs later in this chapter). When the distribution is skewed to positive (positively skewed distribution), the tail is toward the right side of the graph. In this type of distribution, the mode is located in the far left among the three central tendencies, the median is in the middle, and the mean is toward the tail (Figure 15.4b). When the distribution is skewed to negative (negatively skewed distribution), the tail is toward the left side of the graph, the mode is located in the far right,

the median is in the center, and the mean is toward the tail (Figure 15.4c). The median is always in the middle between the mean and the mode, and the mean is pulled toward the tail. Therefore, if two central tendencies are reported, one can identify the skewness of the data distribution.

Measures of Variability

To understand the sample characteristics, in addition to the distribution and the central tendency, it is important to understand variability. Variability is the dispersion of values of any variable in a dataset. For example, consider a study that aims to identify the difference in effectiveness in teaching methods for statistics: in class A the instructor used a conventional teaching style only, and in class B the instructor used an interactive method. The scores for the final exam in statistics in class A ($n = 7$) were: 98, 72, 85, 88, 65, 93, and 79. Therefore, the mean was 82.9 and the median was 85. In class B ($n = 7$) the scores were: 89, 86, 79, 78, 92, 71, and 85; therefore, the mean was also 82.9 and the median was 85 as well. Since there is no mode in both classes, values of the central tendency in these classes are identical. Therefore, both methods appear to be equal in their effectiveness. However, scores in class A are more widely spread than the scores in class B; therefore, there is a difference in variability. There are five meas-

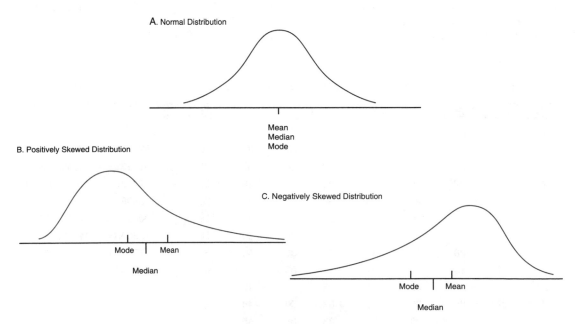

Figure 15.4 Types of distribution and location of the central tendency. (A) Normal distribution. (B) Positively skewed distribution. (C) Negatively skewed distribution.

ures to describe variability: range, percentiles, variance, standard deviation, and coefficient of variation.

Range

The range is the difference between the highest and lowest values in the dataset. Using the preceding example, the range for class A is $98 - 65 = 33$, and the range for class B is $92 - 71 = 21$. Therefore, the range in class A is larger than that of class B, indicating more variability in scores of class A. Since range is merely the difference between two extreme values and ignores other values, it is a rough descriptive measure of variability. Many research papers report the highest or maximum value and the lowest or minimum value, rather than providing the range.

Percentiles

Percentile is a value above and below which a certain percentage of values in a distribution fall and describes a score in relation to other scores in a distribution. Percentiles are symbolized by the letter P, with a subscript indicating the percentage below the score value. Therefore, P_{75} refers to the 75th percentile, which indicates that the particular value is higher than 75% of values in the dataset.

Quartiles divide a distribution into four equal parts, or quarters. The 25th percentile is called the first quartile, the 50th percentile the second quartile, and the 75th percentile the third quartile. The most commonly used interpercentile measure is the interquartile range (IQR), which is the distance between the 25th and 75th percentiles. In the previous example, arranging the scores from the minimum to the maximum in class A, the scores are: 65, 72, 79, 85, 88, 93, 98. The 50th percentile is the median, 85. There are three values below 85 (65, 72, and 79). Their median is 72. Their median of three values above 85 (88, 93, and 98) is 93. Therefore, the interquartile range is 72 to 93. For class B, the interquartile range is 78 to 89. This indicates that class B is less variable or more homogeneous than class A. These interquartile ranges, like the median, are not sensitive to extreme values and if a distribution is severely skewed, it is an appropriate method to indicate variability.

When comparing two very different subgroup characteristics, one eliminates the participants that fall in the interquartile range and instead compares the participants below the first quartile and above the 3rd quartile.

Variance

Variance is the variability of the individual cases away from the mean. It is one of the most important concepts for statistical analysis, such as Analysis of Variance (ANOVA). A group with a larger variance has scores that are more dispersed or scattered (i.e., is less homogeneous) than a group with a smaller variance. The sample variance is symbolized as s^2. The population variance is noted as σ^2 and read as sigma squared. The formula to identify the sample variance is the sum of the squared deviation from the mean scores divided by the degrees of freedom (i.e., the number of cases minus 1):

$$s^2 = \frac{\sum(X - \bar{X})^2}{N - 1} = \text{SS/df}$$

The numerator is called sum of squares and its abbreviation is SS. The deviation from the mean is squared because otherwise the sum of deviations from the mean becomes zero. The denominator is called degrees of freedom and is denoted as df. The degrees of freedom are identified as the sample size minus 1. If one is dealing with the population, the denominator is N but when one is dealing with a sample, $N–1$ provides a more accurate value of variability.

The process to calculate variance is shown in Table 15.4 using the final exam scores from the statistics classes that were presented in an earlier example found in this chapter. For class A, the variance is 135.81 while for class B, it is 52.48, indicating class A is more diverse in the scores than class B. Class B is more homogeneous than class A.

Standard Deviation

Standard deviation is the most widely used measure of variability. It indicates the average variability of the individual scores from the mean. Therefore, the greater the standard deviation, the greater the variability in a dataset. The standard deviation is symbolized as SD, Sd, sd, or s for a sample. The sample SD is defined as the square root of variance:

$$s = \sqrt{s^2} = \sqrt{\frac{\sum(X - \bar{X})^2}{n - 1}}$$

The standard deviation of population is symbolized as σ (read as sigma) and the denominator in the square root is N, the sample size. The advantage of the standard deviation over the variance is that the standard deviation has the same unit of measurement as the mean, since it is the square

Table 15.4 Process of Calculating Variance for Final Exam Scores in Statistics Classes

Raw Score	Deviation from the Mean $(X - \bar{X})$	Squares of the Deviation from the Mean $(X - \bar{X})^2$	Sum of Squares $\sum(X - \bar{X})^2$	Variance $(X - \bar{X})^2/n\text{-}1$	Standard Deviation $\sqrt{\dfrac{\sum(X - \bar{X})^2}{n\text{-}1}}$
For Class A					
98	98 − 82.9 = 15.1	228.01			
72	72 − 82.9 = − 10.9	118.81			
85	85 − 82.9 = 2.1	4.41			
88	88 − 82.9 = 5.1	26.01			
65	65 − 82.9 = − 17.9	320.41			
93	93 − 82.9 = 10.1	102.01			
79	79 − 82.9 = − 3.9	15.21			
SS and S²			814.87	814.87/6 = 135.81	$\sqrt{135.81} = 11.76$
For Class B					
89	89 − 82.9 = 6.1	37.21			
86	86 − 82.9 = 3.1	9.61			
79	79 − 82.9 = − 3.9	15.21			
78	78 − 82.9 = − 4.9	24.01			
92	92 − 82.9 = − 9.1	82.81			
71	71 − 82.9 = − 11.9	141.61			
85	85 − 82.0 = 2.1	4.41			
SS and S²			314.87	314.87/6 = 52.48	$\sqrt{52.48} = 7.24$

root of the squared value (variance). Using the example of final scores in two statistics classes described earlier, the standard deviation for class A is $\sqrt{135.81} = 11.76$ and that for class B is $\sqrt{52.48} = 7.24$ (see Table 15.4). Therefore, class B is more homogeneous than class A in terms of final scores.

The standard deviation of sample data should be reported with the mean so that the data can be summarized according to both central tendency and variability.

Many studies report them in one of the two following formats: 82.9 ± 11.76 or 82.9 (11.76). The value of standard deviation is always positive but if it is zero, it means there are no variations in distribution, or all values are the same. When the value of standard deviation is large, it indicates heterogeneity among the group. Standard deviation is a continuous value. When reporting a standard deviation next to a mean in descriptive statistics, one uses 1 standard deviation. Using the example above, 2 standard deviations for class A is 23.52. The standard deviation is an important statistic in its own right and is also used as the basis of other statistics such as correlations, standard errors, and z-scores.

In the study titled "Impact of pediatric rehabilitation services on children's functional outcomes" (Chen, Heinemann, Bode, Granger, & Mallinson, 2004), three summaries of descriptive statistics are presented. One is a summary table titled "Sample characteristics" in frequencies and percentages (Table 15.5) and the second one is a summary table titled "Descriptive

> The standard deviation of the sample data should be reported with the mean so that the data can be summarized according to both central tendency and variability.

Table 15.5 **Sample Characteristics**

	n	(%)[a]
Gender[b]		
Male	465	(57)
Female	346	(43)
Race		
Caucasian	522	(64)
African-American	182	(22)
Hispanic-American	65	(8)
Admit From		
Home	255	(31)
Acute—Own	151	(19)
Acute—Other	380	(47)
Pre-Rehabilitation Setting		
Home	773	(95)
Acute—Own	7	(1)
Acute—Other	8	(1)
Discharge Setting		
Home	745	(91)
Nursing Home	4	(.5)
Rehabilitation Facilities	18	(2)
Acute Units	23	(3)
Discharge Live With		
Two Parents	314	(39)
One Parent	199	(24)
Relatives	37	(5)
Foster Care	12	(2)
Other (or missing)	252	(31)
Primary Payer		
Medicaid	263	(32)
Commercial	286	(35)
HMO	216	(27)
Private Pay	16	(2)

$N = 814$

[a]*Note.* Total percentages may not add up to 100 due to "other" or "missing"

[b]Three participants are missing; percentages are rounded to nearest whole number

From Table 2 in Chen, C.C., Heinemann, A.W., Bode, R.K., Granger, C.V. & Mallinson T. (2004). Impact of pediatric rehabilitation services on children's functional outcomes. *American Journal of Occupational Therapy,* 58, 44–53, with permission.

statistics by impairment groups" in means, standard deviations, and ranges (Table 15.6). The last summary is a graph titled, "Mean therapy units (15-minute) by impairment" in multiple bars (Figure 15.5). The length of therapy is compared among four therapies (occupational therapy, phys-ical therapy, speech pathology, and psychology) for five types of diagnoses (cerebral palsy, non-traumatic brain injuries, traumatic brain injuries, major multiple trauma, and other impairments). This type of visual presentation allows efficient simultaneous comparisons for two independent variables (in the study mentioned earlier, they are types of therapy and types of diagnoses).

Coefficient of Variation

The coefficient of variation (CV) is an indicator of variability that allows comparisons of different variables. The CV is the ratio of the standard deviation to the mean, expressed as a percentage:

$$CV = (\frac{SD}{\overline{X}}) \times 100$$

The CV is independent of the units of measurement.

In a study to develop a standardized instrument to assess computer task performance (Dumont et al., 2002), the authors described the sample size, the mean, the standard deviation, the range using the minimum and maximum scores, and the coefficient of variation for the impaired group and the nonimpaired group in terms of tasks involved in a keyboard and a mouse. For keyboard use, the CV for the nonimpaired group is constantly lower (32.8–68.5) than the CV for the impaired group (40.9–92.2), indicating the impaired group is more variable in physical capacity than the nonimpaired group. It should be noted that the CV cannot be used when the variable mean is a negative number, since CV is expressed as a percentage.

Graphical Presentation of Central Tendency and Variability

Box Plot

A box plot, or a box-and-whiskers plot, is a graphical presentation that uses descriptive statistics based on percentiles. It employs the median, the interquartile range (IQR), and the minimum and the maximum values in the dataset. The box plot is illustrated in Figure 15.6. The length of box corresponds to the IQR ($P_{75}- P_{25}$); that is, the box begins with the 25th percentile and ends with the 75th percentile. Then, it determines the extreme outlying values by multiplying the IQR ($P_{75}- P_{25}$) value by 3. Individual scores that are more than three times the IQR from the upper and lower edges of the box are the extreme outlying values and are denoted by a symbol, *E*. Minor outlying values are determined by multiplying the IQR by

Table 15.6 **Descriptive Statistics by Impairment Group**

	CP (n=91)	NTBI (n=114)	TBI (n=336)	MMT (n=57)	Other (n=216)	Total (N=814)
			Impairment[1]			
			Mean (SD) Range			
Age (in months)	87 (48) 16–222	104 (62) 12–237	133 (63) 12–220	157 (55) 21–231	137 (63) 12–239	126 (64) 12–239
Onset Days[2]	845 (1554) 0–6782	96 (415) 0–3978	35 (171) 0–2780	29 (60) 1–407	199 (768) 0–5207	178 (723) 0–6782
Length of Stay	27 (16) 5–85	30 (22) 5–123	33 (26) 5–145	40 (31) 7–119	28 (21) 5–120	31 (24) 5–145
			Raw FIM Scores[3] Mean (SD)			
Admission Total FIM	41 (20)	41 (26)	40 (25)	44 (24)	58 (26)	45 (26)
Discharge Total FIM	56 (25)	62 (37)	84 (30)	90 (21)	82 (31)	78 (32)
FIM Gain	15 (14)	22 (23)	44 (26)	45 (22)	24 (17)	32 (25)
FIM Efficiency	.60 (.65)	1.08 (1.26)	2.11 (1.72)	1.79 (1.33)	1.24 (1.26)	1.54 (1.52)
			Rasch-Transformed Measures Mean (SD)			
Admission Self-Care	18 (19)	21 (22)	22 (22)	24 (20)	34 (20)	25 (22)
Discharge Self-Care	36 (18)	39 (28)	56 (24)	57 (13)	52 (21)	50 (24)
Self-Care Gain	18 (18)	17 (19)	33 (21)	33 (18)	18 (15)	25 (20)
Admission Mobility	14 (11)	21 (18)	23 (16)	19 (13)	26 (17)	22 (16)
Discharge Mobility	24 (14)	39 (27)	55 (22)	52 (19)	45 (20)	47 (23)
Mobility Gain	15 (11)	18 (18)	32 (18)	33 (18)	20 (14)	25 (18)
Admission Cognition	52 (26)	31 (26)	31 (24)	45 (31)	65 (31)	43 (31)
Discharge Cognition	54 (25)	44 (29)	57 (21)	71 (18)	74 (27)	60 (26)
Cognition Gain	2 (16)	13 (18)	26 (20)	26 (20)	9 (14)	17 (19)

[1]CP = Cerebral Palsy, NTBI = Nontraumatic Brain Injuries, TBI = Traumatic Brain Injuries, MMT = Major Multiple Trauma, Other = Other impairments

[2]Interquartile range of onset (time from diagnosis of impairment to rehabilitation admission): CP 3–1525 days, NTBI 1–38 days, TBI 6–19 days, MMT 7–23 days, Other 8–42 days

[3]FIM = WeeFIM® (Functional Independence Measure of Children) (UDSMR, 1993)

From Table 3 in Chen, C.C., Heinemann, A.W., Bode, R.K., Granger, C.V. & Mallinson.T. (2004). Impact of pediatric rehabilitation services on children's functional outcomes. *American Journal of Occupational Therapy*, 58, 44–53, with permission.

1.5. Individual scores between 1.5 times the IRQ and three times the IQR away from the edges of the box are minor outlying values and indicated by *O*. Finally, whiskers of the box indicate the maximum and the minimum values that are not minor or extreme outlying values.

Using as an example the final scores for class A discussed previously, the 25th percentile is 72 and 75th percentile is 93; therefore the IQR is 21. The extreme outlying values should be over the value of 156 ($= 93 + 21 \times 3$) or under the value of 9 ($=$

$72 - 21 \times 3$). The minor outlying values should be between the values of 124.5 ($= 93 + 21 \times 1.5$) and 156 or between the values of 40.5 ($= 72 - 21 \times 1.5$) and 9. In the example, no values fall into the minor or extreme outlying value ranges. The largest value that is not an outlier is 98 and the smallest value that is not an outlier is 65.

A box plot is useful for comparisons among several groups. Gagné and Hoppers (2003), in the study titled "The effects of collaborative goal-focused occupational therapy on self-care skills: a

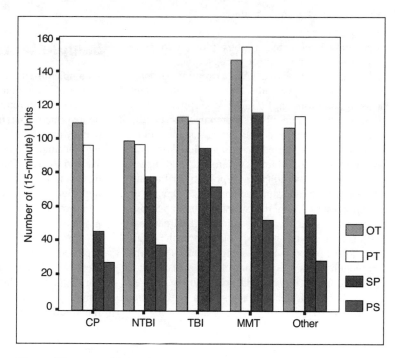

Figure 15.5 Mean therapy units (15 minute) by impairment. (From Figure 1 in Chen, C.C., Heinemann, A.W., Bode, R.K., Granger, C.V., & Mallison, T. (2004). Impact of pediatric rehabilitation services on children's functional outcomes. *The American Journal of Occupational Therapy, 58*(1), 44–53. Reprinted with Permission from *The American Journal of Occupational Therapy*.)

Mean Therapy Units (15-Minute) by Impairment.
N = 814
CP = Cerebral Palsy, NTBI = Nontraumatic Brain Injuries, TBI = Traumatic Brain Injuries, MMT = Major Multiple Trauma, Other = Other impairments

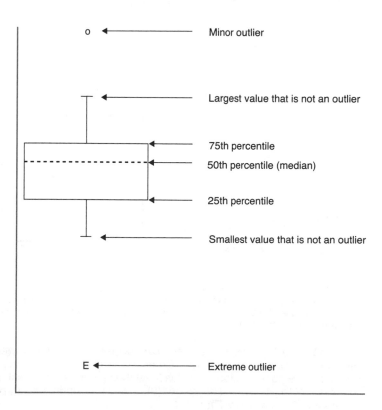

Figure 15.6 Box plot.

pilot study," presented 12 box plots, two plots (experimental and control groups) each for six activities of daily living (ADLs) (eating, grooming, bathing, upper-body dressing, lower body dressing, and toileting) (Gagné & Hoppers, 2003) (Figure 15.7). For visual comparisons of the change in FIM scores across the ADLs, the unit of scale (vertical axis) needs to be considered. In their presentations, for eating, grooming, and upper body dressing, the unit was .5 points; for bathing and lower body dressing the unit was 1.0; and for toileting it was 2.0. In this study, the main purpose of the presentation was to compare the treatment and control groups within, not across, the ADL tasks. If the purpose of the comparisons is to identify which tasks show more changes than other tasks, the unit of the dependent variable (Changes in FIM Scores) for each graph should be the same for all graphs.

Sample Distributions

A sample distribution not only describes the distribution of data characteristics but also determines the type of inferential statistics (parametric versus nonparametric statistics) one should use. Frequency distributions of samples can be categorized into normal, positively skewed, and negatively skewed distributions. Whichever shape it takes, a distribution is a ranking, from lowest to highest, of the values of a variable and the resulting pattern of measures or scores. Often these are plotted on a graph.

If something in a sample is measured that is representative of the population and has a sufficient size, the results tend to form a distribution curve that is similar to a normal (or a bell-shaped) curve. Most scores will fall around the mean, and the frequency will be less as distance from the

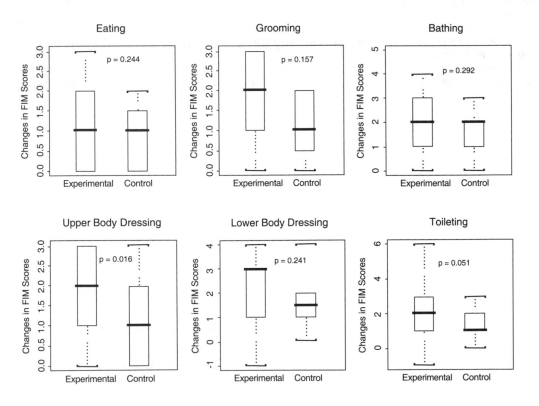

Participants' gains in self-care scores on the FIM between measurements at admission and 2-week follow-up. Note. The heavy horizontal bar represents the median change. The box represents the middle 50% of the change data. The dashed lines represent the range of the data within 1.5 times the interquartile range. The stand-alone bar represents possible outliers.

Figure 15.7 Participants' gains in self-care scores on the FIM between measurements at admission and 2-week follow-up. (From Figure 1 in Gagne, D. E., & Hoppes, S. (2003). The effects of collaborative goal-functional occupational therapy on self-care skills: A pilot study. *The American Journal of Occupational Therapy, 57*(2), 215–219. Reprinted with permission from *The American Journal of Occupational Therapy.*)

mean increases, with relatively few extreme scores. The normal distribution is important for two reasons:

• Many of inferential statistics called parametric statistics assume that the populations are normally distributed, and
• The normal curve is a probability distribution that helps to determine the likelihood of occurrence of the group difference by chance.

Normal Distributions

Normal distributions are continuous distributions with bell-shaped (normal) frequency curves that are unimodal and symmetrical. There are many different normal distributions, one for every possible combination of mean and standard deviation. A normal distribution is sometimes called Gaussian distribution.

Normal Standard Distribution

Sometimes investigators report scores in terms of standard deviation units (i.e., standardized scores or z-scores). The distribution of these scores is called the normal standard distribution (Z-distribution). It is a normal distribution that has a mean equal to 0 and a standard deviation equal to 1. The horizontal axis of this distribution is expressed using standard deviation units. The mean, mode, and median should equal zero; therefore, 0 has the highest peak and both sizes of 0 are symmetrical. Theoretically, there are no boundaries to the curve, that is, scores potentially exist with infinite values. Therefore, the tails of the curve will never touch the baseline. The normal standard distribution is illustrated in Figure 15.8.

Since these properties are constant or standard, one can determine the proportion of the area under the curve by the standard deviations in a normal distribution. If the area under the curve is 100%, the area between 0 (mean) and 1 standard

The normal distribution was originally studied by DeMoivre (1667–1754), who was curious about its use in predicting the probabilities in gambling. The first person to apply the normal distribution to social data was Adolph Quetelet (1796–1874).He collected data on the chest measurements of Scottish soldiers, and the heights of French soldiers, and found that they were normally distributed. His conclusion was that the mean was nature's ideal, and data on either side of the mean were a deviation from nature's ideal. Although his conclusion was absurd, he nonetheless represented normal distribution in a real-life setting.

deviation is 34.13% or 0.3413. The area between −1 standard deviation and 1 standard deviation (± 1 sd) is 68.26% or 0.6826. Similarly, (± 2 sd) will cover 95.44% and (± 3 sd), 99.74% of the area under the curve.

z-Score

A z-score (a lowercase z is used for this statistic) is the most commonly used standard score. It gives the distance in standard deviation units from the mean. It is calculated by dividing the deviation of an individual score from the mean by the standard deviation:

$$z = \frac{X - \overline{X}}{s}$$

A z-score of −2.0 means the particular score is two standard deviations below the mean of 0. z-scores are useful for comparing several measures that have different means and standard deviations.

The following is an example; it is illustrated in Figure 15.9. If a child's weight is 29 kg where the mean is 25 kg and the standard deviation is 3.8 kg, then the z-score is 29 − 25/3.8 = 1.05. If one refers to Appendix A, Table A [areas under the normal

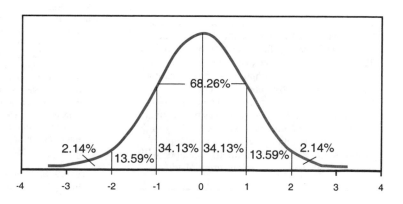

Figure 15.8 Normal standard distributions.

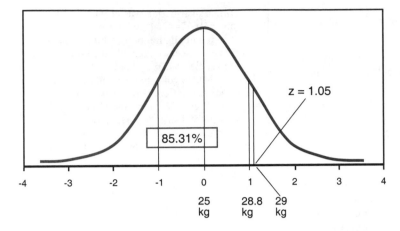

25
kg

28.8
kg

29
kg

Figure 15.9 z-score for 29 kg.

curve (z)], the area between 0 and the $z = 1.05$ is 0.3531 and the area above $z = 1.05$ is 0.1469. From this information one can calculate that 85.31% (0.3531 + 0.50 = 0.8531 or 1.00 − 0.1469 = 0.8531) of children are lighter than the child's weight of 29 kg and 14.69% of children are heavier than the child. Moreover, if the sample size is 200, one could further calculate that about 171 children (200 × 0.8531) were lighter than the child and 29 are heavier (200 × 0.1469 = 29 or 200 − 171 = 29).

Conclusion

This chapter discussed how researchers measure people, objects, and events when conducting quantitative research. It also discussed how measurement scales and descriptive statistics are the basis of statistics for all quantitative inquiry. In occupational therapy, many quantitative studies aim to identify relationships among variables or are experiments designed to identify causal relationships. For those types of studies, the investigator uses inferential statistics. Chapter 16 introduces inferential statistics.

> Parametric statistics assume that data are normally distributed in the population being studied. Therefore, if the sample distribution is skewed, even after a random sampling, a transformation of the data is usually done if one does not wish to use nonparametric statistics. The transformed scales are not in the same metric as the original; therefore, interpretations should be made with caution. On the other hand, Glass and Hopkins (1996) argue that many parametric methods will work even if their assumptions are violated.

REFERENCES

Bond, T. G., & Fox, C. M. (2001). *Applying the Rasch model*. Mahwah, NJ: Lawrence Erlbaum.

Center for Functional Assessment Research/Uniform Data System for Medical Rehabilitation (1994). *Guide for the use of the uniform data set for medical rehabilitation*. Buffalo, NY: Center for Functional Assessment Research.

Chen, C. C., Heinemann, A. W., Bode, R. K., Granger, C. V., & Mallinson, T. (2004). Impact of pediatric rehabilitation services on children's functional outcomes. *The American Journal of Occupational Therapy, 58* (1), 44–53.

Diehl, M., Marsiske, M., Horgas, A. L., & Saczynski, J. (1998). *Psychometric properties of the revised observed tasks of daily living (OTRL-R)*. Poster session presented at the 51st Annual Scientific Meeting of the Deontological Society of America, Philadelphia.

Dumont, C., Vincent, C., & Mazer, B. (2002). Development of a standardized instrument to assess computer task performance. *The American Journal of Occupational Therapy, 56*(1), 60–68.

Gagné, D. E., & Hoppers, S. (2003). The effects of collaborative goal-focused occupational therapy on self-care skills: A pilot study. *The American Journal of Occupational Therapy, 57*(2), 215–219.

Gilson, B., Gilson, M., Bergner, R., Bobbit, S., Kressel, W., Pollard, W., et al. (1975). Sickness Impact Profile: Development of an outcome measure of health care. *American Journal of Public Health, 65*, 1304–1325.

Glass, G. V., & Hopkins, K. D. (1996). *Statistical methods in education and psychology* (3rd ed.). Boston: Allyn and Bacon.

Guildford, J. (1954). *Psychometric methods* (2nd ed.). New York: McGraw-Hill.

Jette, A. (1980). Functional Status Index: Reliability of chronic disease evaluation instrument. *Archives of Physical Medicine and Rehabilitation, 61*, 395–401.

Kerlinger, F. N. (1973). *Foundations of behavioral research*. New York: Holt, Rinehart & Winston.

Kielhofner, G., Dobria, L., Forsyth, K., & Basu, S. (2004). Construction of keyforms for obtaining instantaneous measures from the Occupational Performance History Interview rating scales. *Occupation and Participation: An Occupational Therapy Journal of Research, 25*, 23–32.

Linacre, J. M. (1995). KeyFIM—Self-measuring score form. *Rasch Measurement Transactions, 9*, 453–454.

Linacre, J. M. (1997, June). Instantaneous measurement and diagnosis. *Physical Medicine and Rehabilitation: State of the Art Reviews, 11*(2), 315–324.

Merbitz, C., Morris, J., & Grip, J. C. (1989). Ordinal scales and foundations of misinference. *Archives of Physical Medicine and Rehabilitation, 70,* 308–312.

Mitcham, M. D., Lancaster, C. J., & Stone, B. M. (2002). Evaluating the effectiveness of occupational therapy faculty development workshops. *The American Journal of Occupational Therapy, 56* (3), 335–339.

Nunally, J. C. (1978). *Psychometric theory* (2nd ed.).New York: McGraw-Hill.

Portney, L. G., & Watkins, M. (2000). *Foundations of clinical research* (2nd ed.). Upper Saddle River, NJ: Prentice-Hall.

Statistical Package for the Social Sciences (SPSS) (2003). Version 12.0 [software]. Chicago: SPSS, Inc.

Stevens, S. S. (1946). On the theory of scales of measurement. *Science, 103,* 677–680.

Velleman, P. F., & Wilkinson, L. (1993). Nominal, ordinal, interval and ratio typologies are misleading. *American Statistician, 47,* 65–72.

Wallgren, A., Wallgren, B., Persson, R., Jorner, U., & Haaland, J. (1996). *Graphing statistics & data.* Thousand Oaks, CA: SAGE Publications.

Wright, B. D., & Linacre, J. M. (1989). Observations are always ordinal; measurements, however, must be interval. *Archives of Physical Medicine and Rehabilitation, 70,* 857–860.

RESOURCES

For a Web site on definition of statistics, go to http://www.wordiq.com/definition/Statistics.

For information to draw a pie chart, refer Wallgren, A., Wallgren B., Persson, R., Jorner, U., & Haaland, J. (1996). *Graphing statistics & data.* Thousand Oaks, CA: SAGE Publications.

To understand Rasch Analysis, refer Bond, T. G. & Fox, C.M. (2001). *Applying the Rasch model.* Mahwah, NJ: Lawrence Erlbaum Associates..

For a Web site on normal distribution, go to http://cnx.rice.edu/content/m11164/latest/

For detailed information on data transformation, read:

Tabachnic, B. G., & Fidell, L. S. (1996). *Using multivariate statistics* (3rd ed.). New York: Harper Collins College.

Glass, G. V., & Hopkins, K. D. (1996) *Statistical methods in education and psychology.* Boston: Allyn and Bacon.

Concepts of Inferential Statistics: From Sample to Population

Machiko R. Tomita

Inferential Statistics

Investigators conduct quantitative research with the aim of generalizing their results from the sample studied to the population that sample was selected to represent. The population is usually a theoretical concept in research. For instance, if an investigator wants to measure the effectiveness of a sensory stimulation versus a play-oriented intervention for children in the United States with developmental disabilities whose ages are between 3 and 8 years, the population of interest would be all children with the aforementioned characteristics. However, it is impossible to access that entire population and test two types of occupational therapies on them. Therefore, the investigator must infer the population parameter from the results obtained from the sample.

Inferential statistics are used to estimate population parameters based on data from a sample. The accuracy of the estimation depends on the extent to which the sample is representative of the population. In estimating population parameters from a sample, two statistical concepts are used: probability and sampling error.

Probability

Probability is the likelihood that a particular event will occur in the long run. Therefore, the probability is predictive in that it reflects what should happen over many instances, but not necessarily what will happen for any given event.

· For example, an occupational therapist concludes from many studies that 80% of clients with chronic mental illness who receive a structured program designed to enhance their motivation and habits show increased activity levels after the program. While this conclusion predicts that 80% of people with chronic mental illness who receive such a program will demonstrate increased activity levels, it does not mean that every person has an 80% chance of increased activity level. Twenty percent of the population (for unknown reasons) will not increase activity level following such a program. Whether a single individual belongs to the 80% or the 20% category is not known.

Although the probability of interest is always population probability, it is unknown. Therefore, the sample probabilities are used to estimate population parameters. Values of statistical probability range from 1.0 (always) to 0 (never). They cannot take on a negative value. The probability of an event, denoted by $P_{(Event)}$, is given by:

$$P_{(Event)} = \frac{\text{Number of observations for which the event occurs}}{\text{Total number of observations}}$$

Consider a sample of 100 frail elders who are living at home. In this sample of 100 persons, four are placed in a nursing home and five die over a 3-month period. Therefore, the sample probability that frail elders will be placed in a nursing home in 3 months is $P_{(Institutionalization)} = 4/100 = .04$ (or 4%), and the probability that frail elders will die is $P_{(Death)} = 5/100 = .05$ (or 5%). The probability that frail elders survive and live at home is $P_{(Survival)} = 91/100 = .91$ (or 91%). These three events are mutually exclusive and complementary events because they cannot occur at the same time and because they represent all possible outcomes.

> Probability is the likelihood that a particular event will occur in the long run. Therefore, the probability is predictive in that it reflects what should happen over many instances, but not necessarily what will happen for any given event.

Therefore, the sum of their probabilities will always equal 1.00 (or 100%). These probabilities are good estimates of population probabilities if samples were selected at random.

Suppose, for instance, an investigator wanted to test the effectiveness of an occupational therapy intervention on fatigue among individuals with various levels of chronic fatigue syndrome. If the investigator chooses only study participants whose symptoms were mild and assigned them to the treatment and control groups, the results of the study could not be generalized to the population as a whole. While they could be generalized to persons with mild symptoms they may not reflect what the outcome would be with persons with severe symptoms. Therefore, the result of such a study would not be a true reflection of the population (which includes persons with both mild and severe symptoms) because bias was introduced in the process of sampling. Consequently, the estimation of population characteristics from sample data is based on the assumption that the samples are randomly chosen and are valid representatives of the population. Below is a brief overview of random sampling; a more detailed discussion can be found in Chapter 31.

Two criteria for random sampling are:

- Every person, object, or event must have an equal chance to be chosen, and
- Each choice must be independent of other choice.

The notion of independence means that the occurrence of one event does not influence the probability of another event. For instance, in a study of children with developmental problems, if an investigator randomly chooses a child with autism, that choice does not affect the probability of choosing another child with the same condition.

Sampling Error

In research, investigators use probability not only to decide how well the sample data estimates the population parameter, but also to determine if the experiment or intervention differences are likely to be representative of population differences or if they could have happened by chance. For most statistics this probability is represented as the *p*-value (presented as a lowercase *p*). For example, $p = 0.04$ means that there is a 4% probability that the

statistic will occur by sampling error or by chance alone. Traditionally, psychosocial and health researchers often use a cutoff point of $p \leq .05$ (5%) and biomedical investigators tend to use a cutoff of $p \leq .01$ (1%). Even though investigators do random sampling from the population, the sample mean and sample standard deviation are not exactly the same as the values of population. The tendency for sample values to be different from values of population is called sampling error. The characteristics of a larger sample are likely to be closer to those of the population than that of a smaller sample. This is because the larger the sample, the less likely it is that an unusual occurrence will bias the entire sample. For instance, consider a population in which three out of every 1000 persons have an unusual characteristic. If by chance one of the people with that characteristic is selected, that subject will have a much larger biasing influence on a sample of 20 than on a sample of 100. Sampling error cannot be avoided but its magnitude can be reduced by increasing sample size.

> Sampling error cannot be avoided but its magnitude can be reduced by increasing sample size.

Sampling Distribution

When many samples are drawn from a population, the means of these samples tend to be normally distributed. The larger the number of samples, the more the distribution of their means approximates the normal curve. The distribution of means from many samples is called a sampling distribution (the distribution of raw data is called a sample distribution). A sample size of 30 or more usually will result in a sampling distribution of the mean that is very close to a normal distribution (Vaughan, 1998). Sampling error of the mean is the difference between the sample mean and the population mean, and this difference happens by chance. The Central Limit Theorem explains why sampling error is smaller with a large sample than with a small sample and why one can use the normal distribution to study a wide variety of statistical problems. The Central Limit Theorem consists of three statements:

1. The mean of the sampling distribution of means is equal to the mean of the population from which the samples were drawn.
2. The variance of the sampling distribution of means is equal to the variance of the population from which the samples were drawn divided by the size of the samples.

3. If the original population is distributed normally (i.e., it is bell shaped), the sampling distribution of means will also be normal. If the original population is not normally distributed, the sampling distribution of means will increasingly approximate a normal distribution as sample size increases (i.e., when increasingly large samples are drawn) (Kallenberg, 1997).

Sampling Error of the Mean

Drawing on the second statement, the variance of the sampling distribution can be expressed as s^2/n (variance divided by the sample size). More frequently, investigators use the standard deviation of the sampling distribution which is called the standard error of the mean. It is calculated as:

$$S_{\bar{X}} = s/\sqrt{n}$$

Therefore, the standard error of the mean indicates how much, on average, the sample mean differs from the population mean. If the standard deviation is 5 and the sample size is 10, then the standard error of the mean is 1.58; with the same standard deviation and an increased sample size of 30, the standard error of the mean is 0.91. As this example demonstrates, the larger the sample size, the smaller the difference between the sample mean and the population mean. Both the sample mean and the standard error of the mean can allow us to estimate the population characteristics.

Confidence Intervals

There are two ways to use the sampling distribution to estimate population parameters. One is a point estimate using a sample mean ($\bar{X}$) to estimate a population mean (μ). The other is to use an interval estimate, which specifies an interval within which the population mean (parameter) is expected to fall. A confidence interval (CI) is a range of scores with specific boundaries or confidence limits that should contain the population mean. The degree of confidence is expressed as a probability percentage, such as a 95% or 99% CI, meaning one is 95% or 99% sure that the population mean will fall within the interval. The formula to obtain the confidence limits is:

$$CI = \bar{X} \pm (Z) S_{\bar{x}}$$

For 95% confidence interval, $z = 1.96$ (from Appendix A, Table A).

For the mean = 5 and the standard error of the mean = 1.58, the limits of a 95% CI are:

$$95\%CI = 5 \pm (1.96)(1.58)$$
$$= 5 \pm 3.10$$
$$95\%CI = 1.90 \text{ to } 8.10$$

One can be 95% confident that the population mean falls between 1.90 and 8.10. Therefore, there is a 5% chance that the population mean is not included in the interval.

If one wants to be confident 99% of the time, thus, allowing a 1% risk, one uses $z = 2.596$. For the mean = 5 and the standard error of the mean = 1.58, the limits of a 99% CI are:

$$99\%CI = 5 \pm (2.596)(1.58)$$
$$= 5 \pm 4.10$$
$$99\%CI = 0.90 \text{ to } 9.10$$

The confidence interval becomes wider (a difference of 6.20 to 8.20) with an increased confidence level (95% to 99%). Clinical research tends to use the confidence interval more often than the point estimate.

When the sample size is smaller than 30, use of the standard normal curve is not considered an adequate representation and an alternate sampling distribution, called the *t*-distribution, should be used. The *t*-distribution is unimodal and symmetrical but flatter and wider at the tails than the normal curve. In order to calculate the CI, instead of the *z*-score, the *t*-value is used. To identify the *t*-value, degrees of freedom (df), that is $n - 1$, is used. (Refer to Appendix A, Table B). Therefore, the formula to calculate confidence intervals for small sample sizes is:

$$CI = \bar{X} \pm (t) S_{\bar{x}}$$

Use of a 95% confidence interval is illustrated in a study comparing typically developing children with children who have Asperger's syndrome reported by Dunn, Smith-Myles, and Orr (2002). In their report, the authors provide descriptive statistics for sections and factors of the sensory profile for typically developing children and children with Asperger's syndrome. These statistics include the mean, the standard deviation, and the 95% CI. For 13 of the 14 sections and for all nine factors, the higher limit of the 95% CI for the children with

Most researchers in health care use 5% for the alpha level. It is mainly due to tradition that Ronald Fisher, the influential statistician at that time, started in 1926 and even now it is used by many journals as the general standard (Moore, 1991).

Asperger syndrome was lower than the lower limit of the 95% CI for the typically developing children. This finding indicated that the two groups have separate characteristics when measured by the sensory profile.

The information provided by the CI is useful especially when two mean values are close to each other. Using an example from Table 16.1, the mean of "Items indicating threshold for response" for typical children was 13.53 (SD = 0.32) and that for children with Asperger syndrome is 11.08 (SD = 0.40). In this study, the investigators wanted to ask: "Can 11.08 be considered typical?" Since the 95% CI for the typical children was 12.89 and 14.16, the score of 11.08 falls outside that CI. Thus, the answer is "No." Since this type of question is frequently asked in clinical research, the confidence interval is widely used.

Hypothesis Testing

In addition to estimating population parameters, inferential statistics are used to answer questions regarding the relationships among variables such as comparisons of group means, proportions, correlations, and associations.

Null Hypothesis and Alternative Hypothesis

Since sampling error is unavoidable, its effect on a study must always be taken into consideration. For example, if in a study comparing two different occupational therapy treatment approaches there are no true differences in the dependent variable, one, nevertheless, would expect to find some differences solely due to chance (i.e., sampling error).

Table 16.1 Means, Standard Deviations, and 95% Confidence Intervals for Groups on Each Section

Section	Typical *M (SD)*	Asperger *M (SD)*	Typical CI	Asperger CI
Auditory processing	34.28 (0.63)	23.73 (0.78)	33.03–35.52	22.18–25.28
Visual processing	38.80 (0.71)	31.50 (0.89)	37.37–40.23	29.73–33.27
Vestibular processing	52.53 (0.73)	44.54 (0.90)	51.08–53.98	42.74–46.34
Touch processing	83.50 (1.22)	61.31 (1.52)	81.06–85.94	58.28–64.33
Multisensory processing	30.88 (0.50)	22.81 (0.62)	29.88–31.87	21.58–24.04
Oral sensory processing	54.85 (1.18)	42.65 (1.46)	52.50–57.21	39.73–45.58
Sensory processing related to endurance/tone	42.28 (0.89)	31.27 (1.11)	40.49–44.06	29.05–33.49
Modulation related to body position and movement	46.48 (0.70)	38.92 (0.87)	45.08–47.87	37.19–40.66
Modulation of movement affecting activity level	27.45 (0.56)	20.00 (0.69)	26.34–28.56	18.62–21.38
Modulation of sensory input affecting emotional responses and activity level	18.43 (0.36)	12.46 (0.45)	17.71–19.14	11.57–13.35
Modulation of visual input affecting emotional responses and activity level	17.45 (2.21)	16.65 (2.74)	13.04–21.86	11.19–22.12
Emotional/social responses	72.03 (1.23)	49.81 (1.52)	69.57–74.48	46.68–52.85
Behavioral outcomes of sensory processing	26.13 (0.48)	16.12 (0.59)	25.18–27.07	14.94–17.29
Items indicating thresholds for response	13.53 (0.32)	11.08 (0.40)	12.89–14.16	10.29–11.87

Note. CI = 95% confidence interval. Lower scores indicate poorer performance; that is, the children engage in the difficult behaviors more often (always = 1, never = 5). Children without disabilities (typical) have a low rate of the behaviors on the Sensory Profile; fewer behaviors yield a higher score.

From Table 3 in Dunn, W., Smith Myles, B., & Orr, S. (2002). Sensory processing issues associated with Asperger Syndrome: A preliminary investigation, *American Journal of Occupational Therapy, 56,* 97–106, with permission.

Therefore, one needs to be able to determine when differences found in a study reflect the true differences in the population under study. The mechanism for determining this is called a process of hypothesis testing.

Sorting out whether an observed difference in the dependent variable between the two groups has occurred by chance due to sampling error is the concern of the statistical hypothesis. The statistical hypothesis is also called the null hypothesis (noted as H_0). The null hypothesis states that the observed difference between the groups is due to chance (i.e., that there is no true difference between the groups). In a study comparing different treatment approaches, the investigator is really asking whether one approach is more effective than the other (e.g., whether the mean of the dependent variable for one group will be different than the mean for the other group). This research question is represented by the alternative hypothesis (also called the research hypothesis), and it is the opposite of the null hypothesis. By either rejecting or not rejecting the null hypothesis, the investigator, in effect, accepts or rejects the alternative (research) hypothesis.

> One can never prove the existence or nonexistence of the true differences because researchers cannot simply test all possible cases (members of a population).

The null hypothesis is concerned with the population parameter, so the mean is expressed using a Greek letter. The null hypothesis can be stated in one of the following two formats:

- The population mean of group A and the population mean of group B are the same, or
- The population mean of group A minus the population mean of group B is equal to zero.

These two options are written as follows:
- H_0: $\mu_A = \mu_B$ or
- H_0: $\mu_A - \mu_B = 0$

Usually, the researcher's intention is to reject the null hypothesis. By rejecting the null hypothesis, the investigator concludes that it is unlikely that the observed difference occurred by chance; therefore the researcher concludes that there is a significant effect. When the null hypothesis is not rejected, the investigator concludes that the observed difference is probably due to chance and, thus, that the difference is not significant. When a difference is not significant, it does not necessarily mean that there is no true effect, or no difference. Rather, it means that the evidence is too weak to substantiate the effect. One can never "prove" the existence or nonexistence of true differences because one cannot test all members of the population.

Since research involves a sample drawn from the population to which the investigator wants to generalize the results, it is only possible to reject or not reject the hypothesis based on a chosen level of confidence (typically a 5% or 1% chance of error).

When reporting the results of a study, researchers usually present the alternative (or research) hypothesis or the research question. For example, King, Thomas, and Rice (2003, p. 517) stated the following alternative hypothesis: "There will be a difference in range of shoulder motion and quality of movement..... when wearing the orthosis compared to the free hand condition." Other investigators present a research question such as "Is there a difference between learning the functional living skill of cooking for people with serious and persistent schizophrenia when it is taught in a clinic or in their homes?" (Duncombe, 2004, p. 272). Either way, the null hypothesis (which is typically not stated in a research report) is implied.

Types of Alternative Hypothesis

An alternative (research) hypothesis can be stated as either directional or nondirectional. The two examples given in the previous paragraph are both nondirectional hypotheses because they do not state which group is expected to obtain a higher dependent variable mean. If, on the other hand, the alternative hypothesis indicates that one group mean will be higher than the other, it is a directional hypothesis. An example of a directional hypothesis is, "...the program would lead to an overall reduction in symptom severity and improvements in quality of life over time for individuals in the program as compared to controls..." (Taylor, 2004, p. 35). In this case, the difference being compared is a difference in amount of change as opposed to a sample mean but the principle is the same.

The notation for a nondirectional hypothesis is:

$$H_1: \mu_A \neq \mu_B \text{ or } H_1: \mu_A - \mu_B \neq 0 \text{ for } a,$$

whereas the notation for directional hypotheses are either:

$H_1: \mu_A > \mu_B$ or $H_1: \mu_A - \mu_B > 0$ or

$H_1: \mu_A < \mu_B$ or $H_1: \mu_A - \mu_B < 0$.

depending on the direction the mean is expected to move toward.

Although most research reports will state that the (research) hypothesis was accepted, statistically the investigators are dealing only with the null hypotheses, not alternative hypotheses. (That's why a null hypothesis is called a statistical hypothesis.) That is, they have either rejected or not rejected the null hypothesis.

Types of Errors in Testing Hypothesis

When one draws a sample from which to infer the population parameter, there is always sampling error. Therefore, there is always a possibility of making a wrong inference. Since one either rejects or does not reject the null hypothesis when drawing a conclusion, each conclusion can be either right or wrong, allowing for four possible outcomes as shown in Table 16.2.

Drawing the wrong conclusion is called an error of inference. There are two possible types of error: type I error and type II error. If one rejects the null hypothesis and states there is a significant difference when in actuality the difference does not exist and the null hypothesis is true, concluding there is a difference, one has made a type I error. In this situation, the difference was due to chance. This type of error should be avoided because often it is a serious mistake.

> Although most research reports will state that the (research) hypothesis was accepted, statistically the investigators are dealing only with the null hypotheses, not alternative hypotheses. That is, they have either rejected or not rejected the null hypothesis.

If one accepts the null hypothesis when it is true, concluding there is no difference when in actuality there is no difference, one made a right decision. If one accepts a null hypothesis that is false (i.e., conclude there is no difference when there is an actual difference), a type II error is made. Figure 16.1 describes the relationship between the two types of null hypothesis and two types of error.

Type I Error

The probability of committing a type I error is called alpha (α) level. The α level of .05 or .01 is usually used and it indicates the maximum amount of type I error that can be committed if one rejects a true null hypothesis, 5% or 1%, respectively. If α is .05, it means that one will accept up to a 5% chance of falsely rejecting the null hypothesis.

Alpha is the level of significance that determines whether the observed difference is due to sampling error or real and is denoted as p (lowercase). If $p = .24$, it means that there is a 24% probability that the difference occurred by chance, or there is a 24% chance of committing a type I error if the researcher decides to reject the null hypothesis. However, when one has set $\alpha = .05$ (5%) a priori, 24% is beyond the set 5%; in this instance one cannot reject the null hypothesis and must accept it instead, concluding that there is no difference. On the other hand, if $p = .03$, one would reject the null hypothesis, concluding there is a significance difference.

Table 16.2 Four Possible Decision Outcomes in Null Hypothesis Testing

Results of Testing H_0	Null Hypothesis (H_0) (There is no difference between groups)	
	True	False
Reject H_0	Type I error (α)	Correct decision Statistical power (1-β) (There is difference between groups.)
Accept H_0	Correct decision (There is no difference between groups)	Type II error (β)

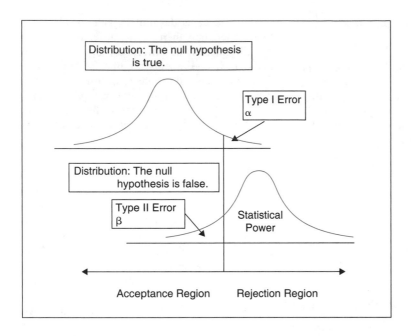

Figure 16.1 Two types of null hypotheses and type I and type II error.

Interpretation of a *p*-value requires caution. It is a common mistake, when α = .05, to say a smaller *p*-value (e.g., *p* =. 001) is "more significant" than a larger *p*-value (e.g., *p* = .01). The magnitude of *p* is not an indicator of the degree of validity of the alternative hypothesis. Once the *p*-value is judged against the set α level, the decision is dichotomous: either yes, significant or no, not significant.

> The magnitude of *p* is not an indicator of the degree of validity of the alternative hypothesis. Once the *p*-value is judged against the set α level, the decision is dichotomous: either yes, significant or no, not significant.

Type II Error

If an investigator does not reject the null hypothesis when it is false, a type II error is committed. This type of error is of great concern in clinical research. For example, in a study whose aim was to determine whether an occupational therapy intervention was better than a control condition, a type II error would mean concluding that the intervention does not produce better outcomes when, in fact, it does.

A type II error is denoted by beta (β). Thus the value of β represents the likelihood that one will be unable to identify real differences (however, there is no direct mathematical relationship between type I and type II error). Decreasing the likelihood of type II error by increasing α would only increase the chance of type I error.

The solution to decreasing the chances of type II error is to increase statistical power (i.e., the probability that a test will lead to rejection of the null hypothesis). Statistical power is represented as 1 – β. The power of .80 is considered reasonable because 80% of the time an investigator would correctly identify a statistical difference and reject the null hypothesis (Cohen, 1988). Conventionally, then, β is set at .20 or 20%.

Statistical Power and Effect Size

There are four factors that influence the statistical power:

- Significance level (α),
- Variance of data (s^2),
- Sample size, and
- Effect size.

The effect size is an indicator of magnitude of the observed difference in the dependent variable. Said another way, it is the impact made by the independent variable and if the impact is strong, the effect size will be large. So, for example, consider a study that was designed to determine the extent to which a new occupational therapy intervention was more effective than a traditional intervention for increasing functional capacity. In this instance, the effect size would refer to the amount of difference observed between the two groups in the functional outcomes.

The first method to increase the power is to increase the significance level (α) for example, from .05 to .10. Then β will be decreased and that will increase the power. However, as noted earlier, doing so increases the chance of type I error (from 5% to 10%). This is always undesirable since type I error is often a serious mistake to commit.

The second method to increase power is to decrease the dependent variable's variance within groups. Achieving a reduction in within group variance can be accomplished by selecting a more homogeneous sample that will show less variability in the dependent variable. It can also be achieved by selecting a more accurate measure of the dependent variable. Since observed variance is a function of true variance plus error variance, increasing within-group homogeneity and measurement accuracy are both ways of reducing observed variance.

The third method to increase the power is to increase a sample size. When small samples are used, power is reduced. Increasing sample size is the only way to increase power once a study design has been finalized (i.e., when the independent and dependent variable and the measure of the dependent variable have already been determined).

The last method used to increase power is to increase effect size (often called clinical significance). There are different ways to calculate effect size. One common way to calculate the effect size between two groups is to use a d-index. d is calculated as the difference between the two means (or the mean difference) divided by the common standard deviation (i.e., the square root of the mean of the two groups' variance when sample size is the same for the two groups). If the mean difference is a half size of the common standard deviation, then $d = .50$ and it is interpreted as medium effect size. The effect size of $d = .30$ is considered small and $d = .80$ is large. Since effect size is the degree to which the null hypothesis is false, the large effect size means more power.

In a study comparing two different treatment approaches, increasing effect size means widening the observed difference between the two groups' dependent variable means. One of the most common ways of doing this is increasing the length or frequency of the interventions when the treatment that is expected to produce better outcomes improves with greater intensity. Another means of

doing this is comparing independent variables that are more clearly differentiated from each other so that a larger difference of the dependent variable is more likely to be observed.

Power Analysis

One of the largest concerns when planning any study is determining the necessary sample size. Investigators use power analysis to estimate the sample size needed to obtain a desired level of power. This should be done before one finalizes the study plan.

To determine the sample size, one first decides a significance level (usually either .01 or .05) and desired power (usually .80). Effect size should be calculated on the dependent variable that is the focus of the primary study question or hypothesis. Effect size should be calculated based on the past studies or preliminary data, using the appropriate statistical analysis for the study. (For calculation of effect size for various statistics, see Chapter 17.)

Power analyses can also be used when a study's results are not statistically significant. In this case, it may be that a type II error was committed. This can be determined based on the significance level, observed effect size, and sample size. Nonsignificant findings may have occurred because of a small sample size and not because of the true effectiveness of the treatment (effect size). Suppose observed effect size was $d = .40$ at $\alpha = .05$, and the sample size in each group was 20. Then the power is only .23. With the same effect size, if the sample size in each group was 100, the power becomes .80. In this instance, even though results are not statistically significant, it is worth reporting the medium effect size with the hope that a similar study will be conduced in the future with a larger sample size. Therefore, whenever results are not significant, the effect size should be reported.

Critical Value

To find the difference between the means of two groups, one uses a test statistic called a t-test to calculate the t-value. Then, one identifies whether or not the null hypothesis can be rejected at a given α level (e.g., $\alpha \leq .05$) using a t-distribution. In doing this, one identifies the critical value (i.e., the value determining the critical region [5%] in a sampling distribution) by looking it up on a t-distribution table (Appendix A, Table B). The critical region is the area wherein one can reject the null hypothesis.

To find the critical value for *t*-tests, one must first identify the degrees of freedom (df). The df indicates how much data are used to calculate a particular statistic. For *t*-tests, df $= (n_1 - 1) + (n_2 - 1)$, where n_1 and n_2 are sample sizes for each group. For instance, if one has 15 subjects in each group, the df is 28. When $\alpha_1 \leq .05$ (the subscript, 1, indicates the hypothesis is directional and one-tailed test is used), the critical value is 1.701 from the *t*-distribution table. A *t*-test can be one-tailed (for when there is a directional hypothesis) or two-tailed (for when there is not a directional hypothesis), as will be discussed in more detail later. If the calculated *t*-value is 1.90, it is larger than the critical value 1.701; therefore, it is within the rejection region (of the null hypothesis). Then one can say the difference between the two groups is significant. If the *t*-value is smaller than the critical value, one cannot reject the null hypothesis. Therefore, the difference between two groups is not considered significant. This explanation is presented in Figure 16.2a and b. The step-by-step process of hypothesis testing is described later in this chapter.

> Degrees of freedom (df) is the number of values that are free to vary when the sum is predetermined. For example, when there are five numbers in a group that sums up to 15, the first four numbers can vary but once the first four numbers are determined, the last number does not have freedom to vary. Therefore, df = 4.

One-Tailed and Two-Tailed Tests

The word "tail" refers to the end of the probability curve. Many researchers use a one-tailed test of significance when a research hypothesis is directional and a two-tailed test for a nondirectional research hypothesis. When researchers use a one-tailed test there is more power than two-tailed test as illustrated in Figure 16.2. To return to the previous example, a directional hypothesis indicated the use of a one-tailed test ($\alpha \leq .05$), with df = 28. According to Appendix A, Table B, the critical value for a two-tailed test is 2.048. Since the calculated *t*-value, 1.90, is smaller than the critical

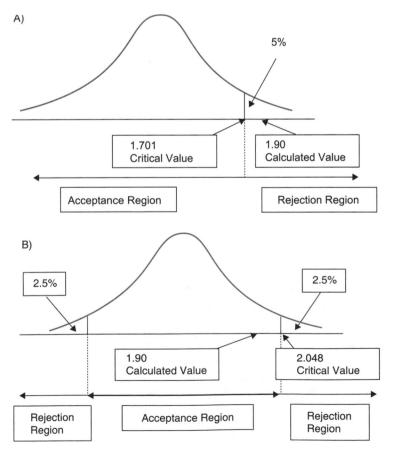

A)

5%

| 1.701 Critical Value | | 1.90 Calculated Value |

Acceptance Region | Rejection Region

B)

2.5% | 2.5%

| 1.90 Calculated Value | | 2.048 Critical Value |

Rejection Region | Acceptance Region | Rejection Region

Figure 16.2 (A) Critical value and critical region: One-tailed test. (B) Critical value and critical region: Two-tailed test.

value for a two-tailed t-test, the researcher cannot reject the null hypothesis. With a two-tailed test, the 5% of rejection region is divided into two regions of 2.5% each. In order to reject the null hypothesis when the alternative hypothesis is nondirectional (two-tailed), the calculated value needs to be much larger than the calculated value for the directional (one-tailed) hypothesis. Thus the one-tailed test has more power than two-tailed test.

Steps of Hypothesis Testing

Given the previous discussions, the following are recommended steps for hypothesis testing after stating the alternative (research) hypothesis, and collecting data.

Step 1. Decide the alpha level such as $\alpha \leq .05$.

Step 2. Use an appropriate test statistic such as a t-test and identify a calculated value, a t-value.

Step 3. Identify the critical value on a t-distribution table and compare it with the calculated t-value. (If one is using statistical software, it will calculate the p-value for the calculated t-value, such as $p =. 234$ or $p < .000$.)

Step 4. Decide whether to reject the null hypothesis (H_0) or not. If the calculated value is larger than the critical value, one can reject the null hypothesis, saying the mean difference was significant. (When using statistical software, if the p-value of the calculated value is equal to or less than .05 ($\alpha \leq .05$), then one can reject the null hypothesis.)

Step 5. When the results do not allow one to reject the null hypothesis (i.e., the critical value is greater than the calculated t-value), it is a good idea to calculate effect size to determine the strength of the effectiveness of intervention and the level of type II error (β).

When the sample size is very large (for example, 2500 subjects), the result may be statistically significant ($p \leq .05$) even if the effect size is small (e.g., $d = 10$). Consequently, one must be aware of what statistical significance means. It simply means that the observed difference is rare (i.e., occurring 5 out of 100 times) when the null hypothesis is true. In occupational therapy research, the more important significance is clinical significance and that is identified by the effect size. For example, when reporting their findings from a study of the effects of an energy conservation course on fatigue impact for persons with progressive Multiple Sclerosis, Vanage, Gilbertson, and Mathiowetz, (2003) reported effect size regardless the significance of t-tests for subcategories and total score of the Fatigue Impact Scale (Table 16.3).

Table 16.3 Means and Standard Deviations of Difference Scores Between Various Assessment Times[a], One-Sample t Tests for All Subjects ($N = 37^b$) and Cohen's d Effect Sizes.

FIS	M	(SD)	df	t	d
Pre-EC Course vs. Post-EC Course #1					
Cognitive	4.0	(6.8)	36	3.6*	.82
Physical	4.2	(7.9)	36	3.2*	.75
Psychosocial	7.5	(12.7)	36	3.6*	.83
Total	15.7	(25.0)	36	3.8*	.89
Post-EC Course #1 vs. Post-EC Course #2					
Cognitive	−.4	(7.2)	27	−.3	−.08
Physical	1.0	(8.1)	27	.6	.17
Psychosocial	1.0	(13.3)	27	.4	.11
Total	2.1	(23.7)	27	.5	.13

[a]Pre-EC Course scores were those recorded prior to the course. Post-EC Course #1 scores were recorded immediately following the completion of the course. Post-EC Course #2 scores were recorded 8 weeks after the completion of the course.

[b]$n = 28$ Available for Post-EC Course #2.

*$P < .01$.

FIS = Fatigue Impact Scale

EC = Energy conservation

From Table 5 in Vanage, S.M., Gilbertson, K.K., & Mathiowetz, V. (2002). Effects of an energy conservation course on fatigue impact for persons with progressive multiple sclerosis. *American Journal of Occupational Therapy, 56,* 315-323, with permission.

The differences between the pretests and the posttests resulted in large effect sizes (d is close to or larger than .80) across categories, indicating the occupational therapy intervention had a definite and effective impact. The report of the effect sizes made the study more meaningful than only stating the statistical significance. Reporting the effect size is the only way to indicate the clinical significance for occupational therapy intervention studies.

Conclusion

This chapter discussed the estimation of population characteristics based on the sample statistics. It concluded with discussions of statistical power and effect size, two important statistics for occupational therapy research and practice. The next chapter discusses inferential statistics in two parts: univariate analysis and multivariate analysis.

REFERENCES

Cohen, J. (1988). *Statistical power analysis for the behavioral science* (2nd ed.). Hillsdale, NJ: Lawrence Erlbaum.

Duncombe, L. W. (2004). Comparing leaning of cooking in home and clinic for people with schizophrenia. *The American Journal of Occupational Therapy, 58* (3), 272–278.

Dunn, W..Smith Myles, B., & Orr, S. (2002). Sensory processing issues associated with Asperger syndrome: A preliminary investigation. *The American Journal of Occupational Therapy, 56*(1), 97–106.

Kallenberg, O. (1997). *Foundations of modern probability.* New York: Springer-Verlag.

King, S., Thomas, J. J., & Rice, M. S. (2003). The immediate and short-term effects of a wrist extension orthosis on upper-extremity kinematics and range of shoulder motion. *The American Journal of Occupational Therapy, 57*(5), 517–524.

Moore, D. S. (1991). *Statistics: Concepts and controversies* (3rd ed.). New York: W. H. Freeman.

Taylor, R. R. (2004). Quality of life and symptom severity for individuals with chronic fatigue syndrome: Findings from a randomized clinical trail. *The American Journal of Occupational Therapy, 58*(1), 35–43.

Vange, S. M, Gilbertson, K. K., & Mathiowetz, V. (2003). Effects of an energy conservation course on fatigue impact for persons with progressive multiple sclerosis. *The American Journal of Occupational Therapy, 57*(3), 315–323.

Vaughan, E. D. (1998). *Statistics: Tools for understanding data in the behavioral sciences.* Upper Saddle River, NJ: Prentice-Hall.

RESOURCES

For relationship between confidence interval and p-value, read:

Munro, B. H. (2001). *Statistical methods for health care research* (4th ed.) Philadelphia: Lippincott.

For sampling distribution, refer to:

Kallenberg, O. (1997). *Foundations of modern probability.* New York: Springer-Verlag.

For power analysis, refer to:

Cohen, J. (1988). *Statistical power analysis for the behavioral science* (2nd ed.). Hillsdale, NJ: Lawrence Erlbaum Associates.

For Central Limit Theorem, visit:

http://mathworld.wolfram.com/CentralLimitTheorem.html.

Methods of Analysis: From Univariate to Multivariate Statistics

Machiko R. Tomita

This chapter discusses inferential statistics, which are statistical techniques used to draw conclusions about a population on the basis of data describing a sample. These statistical procedures can be categorized into:

• Parametric statistics, and
• Nonparametric statistics.

The statistics discussed in this chapter can also be categorized into the following approaches:

• Univariate,
• Bivariate,
• Multivariable, and
• Multivariate approaches.

Finally, these statistics can be differentiated by the use of either independent samples or correlated samples. This chapter considers all these distinctions and explains the statistics characterized by these categories. Throughout the chapter, the formulas for these statistics are given. In most instances, these statistics are calculated in statistical packages. Nonetheless, the formulas are given here, and examples of how they are calculated are provided, as they help develop a conceptual understanding of the statistics.

Parametric and Nonparametric Statistics

Parametric statistics are for estimating population parameters (characteristics) and for testing hypotheses based on population parameters. Parametric statistics can be used if the following statistical assumptions are met:

• The sample is normally distributed (normal distribution),
• The dependent variables are measured using an interval or ratio scale, and
• The variance of the dependent variable is the same across all levels of the independent variable. That is, the groups in the sample are homogeneous (referred to as homogeneity of variance assumption).

If the sample size is large ($N > 30$), those assumptions are usually met. Ideally, samples are randomly selected or assigned to groups. When the data do not present a normal distribution, the variables are measured using a nominal or ordinal scale, and/or they are not homogeneous across the groups, in general, nonparametric statistics will be used. When the sample size is small, data characteristics are such that one may have to use nonparametric statistics.

Nonparametric tests, in usual instances, have less power for finding statistical significance than parametric tests. However, with very small sample sizes (six or less), the power of nonparametric tests becomes equal to that of parametric tests.

Independent and Correlated Samples

Both nonparametric and parametric statistics can be further categorized to statistics for independent samples and those for dependent or correlated samples. This is important since statistical procedures are different for independent samples and correlated or dependent samples.

Samples are independent when they are not related to one another in terms of the dependent variable. For example, consider an investigator studying the effects of an occupational therapy program for people with chronic mental illness. This investigator could compare the outcomes of a treatment group that receives occupational therapy to those of a control group that does not receive therapy. In this case, the samples are independent because the people in the two groups are mutually exclusive and, thus, the outcome measures taken on the two groups will not be related to each other. On the other hand, the investigator might investigate the effects of the occupational therapy program by measuring the dependent variable before and after the therapy on the same group. Since the investigator is comparing data collected from the same sample, it is called dependent or correlated.

This notion of independent and correlated samples is sometimes not so clear. For example, consider a study in which an investigator is testing strength in different shoulders (right extension or left extension). In this case, the shoulders can be considered independent groups, even though they belong to the same person, since the strength in one shoulder is not affected by the other. On the other hand, consider a study that aims to determine parents' attitudes about an affordable price range for a child's powered wheelchair. In this case, the opinion of the mother and father are based on the same financial resources. Therefore, they can be considered a correlated sample.

It is inappropriate to mix a dependent (correlated) sample and an independent sample in a statistical analysis. For example, take a study designed to identify whether parents of nondisabled children differ in their opinions about appropriate toys from parents of children with physical disabilities. It would be incorrect to include two mothers of two children and both parents of a third child in the same sample. This is because the toy preference of the mother and father of the third child are likely correlated, while those of the mothers of the different children are not. To include both parents of the third child in this sample means that they are counted as two different opinions, just as the two opinions of the mothers of the first and second child. Although it is possible to analyze both a correlated sample and an independent sample in one study using a mixed design, it is still required that independent samples are analyzed by statistics for independent samples and the correlated samples analyzed by statistics for correlated samples (see repeated measures analysis of variance [ANOVA] with a between-factor discussed later in this chapter).

Univariate, Bivariate, Multivariable, and Multivariate Analyses

Another way of classifying statistics is based on the number of variables in the study. This classification is as follows:

- Univariate statistics deal with one dependent variable and one independent variable,
- Bivariate statistics handle two variables regardless of direction of influence in the analysis,
- Multivariable statistics manage one dependent and several independent variables together, and

- Multivariate statistics, strictly speaking, deal with more than one dependent variable simultaneously.

Table 17.1 summarizes the statistical methods presented in this chapter according to the classifications just discussed.

Nonparametric Statistics: Chi-Square

There are many nonparametric statistics but in this section only Chi-square (read as kai) will be introduced. Other types of nonparametric statistics are explained in the following sections together with the parametric statistics they parallel.

Chi-square can be used when:

- There is only one categorical variable with more than one level (group), or
- There are two categorical variables.

For the former, goodness of fit tests are used, and, for the latter, tests of independence are used.

Either way, Chi-square is the difference between the expected and observed frequencies and is denoted as χ^2. The formula to calculate Chi-square values is:

$$\chi^2 = \sum \frac{(O - E)^2}{E}$$

where O represents the observed frequency and E represents expected frequency.

The Chi-square value is the sum of squared difference between the observed and expected values divided by the expected values. To use Chi-square, categories should be mutually exclusive and exhaustive.

Goodness of Fit Test (a Nonparametric Test)

The goodness of fit test compares an observed frequency with a uniform, known, or normal distribution.

Uniform Distribution

A uniform distribution expects the same frequency counts across all categories. For example, suppose an investigator wishes to identify the number of fall occurrences across three time periods (morning, afternoon, and evening) among older psychiatric inpatients. The null hypothesis is that an equal number of falls will occur across the three

Table 17.1 **Types of Inferential Statistics (Introduced in this chapter)**

Types of Statistics	Independent Sample	Correlated Sample
Frequency analysis		
Nonparametric (only)	Chi-square	McNemar test
Comparison of two group means		
Parametric	Independent-test	Paried t-test
Nonparametric	Mann-Whitney U test	Wilcoxon Signed rank test
		The sign test
Comparision of more than two group means		
One dependent variable and one independent variable		
Parametric	One-way ANOVA	Repeated measures ANOVA
Nonparametric	Kruskal-Wallis one-way ANVOA	Friedman test
One dependent variable and more than one independent variables		
Parametric (only)	Two-way ANOVA	Repeated measures ANOVA
	Multi-way ANOVA (more than 2)	
	Mixed design	Same as independent sample
	ANCOVA	Same as independent sample
More than one dependent variables and one or more independent variables		
Parametric (only)	MANOVA	Same as independent sample
	MANCOVA	Same as independent sample
Associaion between variables		
Two variables		
Parametric	Pearson correlation	Same as independent sample
Nonparametric	Spearman rank order correlation	Same as independent sample
More than two variables		
Parametric (only)	Multiple correlation	Same as independent sample
Predication		
One criterion and one predictor variable		
Parametric (only)	Simple linear regression	Same as independent sample
One criterion and more than one predictor variable		
Parametric (only)	Multiple regression	Same as independent sample
	Logistic regression	Same as independent sample
Classification		
Parametric (only)	Exploratory factor analysis	Same as independent sample
Causal relationship establishment		
Parametric (only)	Path analysis	Same as independent sample
	Confirmedly factor analysis	Same as independent sample

time periods. For example, if a total of 90 falls were observed, one would assume that 30 falls occurred in each period; thus, that is the expected value. If the observed falls occurred 0, 60, and 30 times in each period, then the Chi-square value would be:

$$\chi^2 = (0 - 30)^2/30 + (60 - 30)^2/30 + (30 - 30)^2/30 = 60$$

In a uniform distribution, degrees of freedom (df) are the number of categories (k) minus 1. Therefore, in this example, df $= 3 - 1 = 2$. If α is set at .05, then the critical value is $_{(.05)}\chi^2_{(2)} = 5.99$

(see Appendix A, Table C). To use this table, one looks up the degrees of freedom and selects the set α (or significance) level to see the critical value for χ^2. In this example, for there to be a significant difference between categories, the χ^2 value must be greater than the critical value of 5.99. The calculated value of 60 is larger than 5.99; therefore, one finds that the observed value is significantly different from the expected value and concludes that the number of falls varied across the periods. The next step is to identify which category is contributing to the significant difference. For that, standardized residuals (SR) should be calculated. SR is determined by the absolute value of the difference between the observed and expected values divided by the square root of the expected value:

$$\text{Standardized Residual} = \frac{|O - E|}{\sqrt{E}}$$

Residuals close to or greater than 2.00 or smaller than –2.00 are considered important (Haberman, 1984). Returning to the example, the standardized residuals for the first and second zones are 5.477 for both. Therefore, zones 1 and 2 are both contributing to the significant value of χ^2.

Known Distribution

When the distribution within a population or underlying population is known, then the observed frequency counts can be compared against this known distribution. For example, if the number of people with disabilities in several age categories in the United States is known, and one wants to compare that with those in a particular state, the former frequencies will serve as expected values and the latter, observed values. The calculation method is exactly the same as for the uniform distribution, and the degrees of freedom is $k - 1$. If the difference is significant, then the sample distribution is different from the known distribution.

Normal Distribution

The goodness of fit test can be used to determine if the sample distribution is significantly different from a normal distribution by dividing the normal distribution into eight sections. From the Z-distribution (see Appendix A, Table A), one knows the area under the curve is 1.00 or 100%. The area between $Z = 0$ and $Z = 1$ SD is .3413; 1 SD and 2 SD, .1359; 2 SD and 3 SD, .0215; and more than 3 SD, .0013. Since the shape is symmetrical, the negative side of the mean has the same area respectively. The expected frequency can be determined by multiplying the total sample size by the area. To make the calculation simple, if the sample size is 100, the expected value between 0 and 1 would be 34.13, between 1 and 2 it would be 13.59, and so on. Therefore, the observed frequencies should be classified into the eight sections and the Chi-square value can be determined using the formula. For example, if 50 cases were observed in the area of $Z = 0$ and $Z = 1$, the difference between the observed and the expected value would be $50 - 34.13 = 15.87$. Then it will be squared ($15.87 \times 15.87 = 251.86$), and divided by 34.13 ($251.86/34.13 = 7.38$). In the same manner, the remaining of seven sections can be calcu-

lated and the sum of calculated values for the eight categories will be the χ^2 value. In this case, the degrees of freedom are $(k - 3)$ or $8 - 3$; therefore, df = 5. Three degrees of freedom are subtracted because in addition to the usual 1 degree of freedom, two additional degrees of freedom are lost because of the known mean score and the known standard distribution in the normal distribution (Snedecor & Cochran, 1991).

Tests of Independence (Nonparametric Tests)

The more common use of Chi-square in occupational therapy research is for tests of independence. These tests are used to examine the association of two categorical variables. When data are arranged in a two-way matrix, it is called a contingency table or a cross-tabulation. For this test, the null hypothesis is: the two variables are independent (i.e., not associated). Therefore, if the resulting Chi-square value is statistically significant, one concludes that the two variables are associated. Usually the rows (R) are for the dependent variable and the columns (C) are for the independent variable.

Consider an investigation of whether being a veteran with combat experience is associated with a diagnosis of depression. In the survey of 80 adults with 40 combat-exposed veterans, 16 veterans are diagnosed with depression. Among the 40 non-veterans, 8 are diagnosed as depressed. The null hypothesis states that veteran status is independent of the presence of a depressive diagnosis. As shown in Table 17.2, observed frequency of Cell A (Veterans who are depressed) is 16; Cell B (Non-Veterans who are depressed), 8; Cell C (Veterans who are not depressed), 24; and Cell D (Non-Veterans who are not depressed), 32. Expected values are calculated using the total frequency counts for each row and column. The formula for the expected frequency (E) is:

$$E = \frac{f_R f_C}{N}$$

where f_R indicates the total frequency of the row, and f_C indicates the total frequency of the column.

In the example above, the expected value of veterans who are depressed (Cell A) is $E = 40 \times 24/80 = 12$. Once one finds an expected value of a cell in a 2×2 table, other expected values can be easily identified by subtracting the expected value from the total in the row or the column. Thus, expected values of veterans who are not

Table 17.2 Chi-Square for Veteran's Status and Depression ($N = 80$)

	Veterans	Non-veterans	Total
Depressed	(A) $O = 16$ $E = (40 \times 24)/80 = 12$ SR $= \|16 - 12\| / \sqrt{12} = 1.15$	(B) $O = 8$ $E = 24 - 12 = 12$ SR $= \|8 - 12\| / \sqrt{12} = 1.15$	24
Not depressed	(C) $O = 24$ $E = 40 - 12 = 28$ SR $= \|24 - 28\| / \sqrt{28} = 0.76$	(D) $O = 32$ $E = 56 - 28 = 28$ SR $= \|32 - 28\| / \sqrt{28} = 0.76$	56
Total	40	40	80

SR = Standardized residual.

depressed are found by subtracting 12 from the total of the row, 40, $E = 40 - 12 = 28$. The expected frequency of non-veterans who are depressed is identified by $E = 24 - 12 = 12$. Non-veterans who are not depressed are found by subtracting 8 from the total of the row, 40; therefore, 32. Below those values are plugged in the Chi-square formula:

$$\chi^2 = \frac{(16 - 12)^2}{12} + \frac{(24 - 28)^2}{28} +$$

$$\frac{(8 - 12)^2}{12} + \frac{(32 - 28)^2}{28} = 3.82$$

This yields a Chi-square value of 3.82. Degrees of freedom are obtained by $(R - 1) \times (C - 1)$. Therefore, $(2 - 1) \times (2 - 1) = 1$. From Appendix A, Table C, the critical value of $_{(0.5)}\chi^2_{(1)} = 3.84$. Since χ^2 is always positive (defined by the squared term divided by a positive value), the Chi-square distribution is always a one-tailed test and the significance value should be estimated based on a one-tailed test.

In this instance, the calculated value is smaller than the critical value at $p = 05$.[1] Therefore, the investigator cannot reject the null hypothesis and must conclude that the two variables are not associated.

When there is a small sample size (an expected frequency is less than 1 in each cell, and less than 20% of the cells have observed frequencies of less than 5), one should collapse the table to have fewer

cell categories if possible. If it is not possible, Yates' correlation for continuity can be used, but it has less power. If the table is 2 × 2 (two by two), the Fisher Exact test should be used. Both are discussed later in this chapter.

McNemar Test for Correlated Samples (a Nonparametric Test)

When the sample is correlated and the dependent variable has only two levels, such as Yes and No, then the table is 2 × 2 and the McNemar test can be used. This is often used for pre- and posttests on the same sample to identify if the change is significant or not.

The calculation formula is (A and D are locations of cells. See Table 17.2 to see how cells are labeled):

$$\chi^2 = \frac{(A - D)^2}{(A + D)} \text{ with df} = 1$$

Power Analysis

Chapter 16 discussed the importance of examining the effect size. For a contingency table, the effect size (ω, omega) for 2 × 2 and larger numbers of cell categories are obtained respectively by:

$$\omega = \sqrt{\frac{\chi^2}{N}}, \text{ or } \omega = \sqrt{\frac{\chi^2}{N(q - 1)}} \left(\sqrt{q - 1}\right)$$

where q = the number of rows or columns, whichever is smaller.

The interpretation of the effect size is:

- $\omega = .10$ is small,
- $\omega = .30$ is medium, and
- $\omega = .50$ is large.

---

[1] The α level is the probability or p-value one is willing to accept as the amount of error, therefore, $\alpha = .05$ is the same as $p = .05$. If α is set at 5%, in order to reject the null hypothesis, the p-value has to be equal to or smaller than $p = .05$.

Using the example of veterans and depression,

$$\chi^2 = 3.82, \omega = \sqrt{\frac{3.82}{80}}$$, and the effect size is .22,

which is small to medium. By referring to Appendix A, Table G, one can see that the power is approximately .50. To increase the power to conventional .80, with the effect size, one needs a sample size of about 200.

Comparisons of Two Group Means: t-Tests

This section deals with statistics to compare two group means. When comparing of two group means, the null hypothesis is:

$$H_0: \mu_1 = \mu_2$$

Complementing the null hypothesis is the alternative (research) hypothesis:

$$H_1: \mu_1 \neq \mu_2 \text{ (for nondirectional hypothesis), or}$$
$$H_1: \mu_1 > \mu_2 \text{ or } \mu_1 < \mu_2 \text{ (for directional hypothesis)}$$

These hypotheses are tested, for independent samples, by using one of the following two statistics:

- The parametric independent t-test, or
- The nonparametric Mann-Whitney U-test.

For dependent or correlated samples, investigators use:

- The parametric paired t-test,
- The nonparametric Wilcoxon Signed Rank Test, or
- The nonparametric Sign test.

Each is discussed below.

Independent t-Test (a Parametric Test)

Independent t-tests are used to compare two group means of independent samples. Because the t-test is a parametric test, one must ensure that the normality assumption of the data is met and the dependent variable is measured by either an interval or a ratio scale. Since the t-test is robust, the assumption of homogeneity is not really an issue, but the calculation methods of the t-value vary depending on whether the two groups are homogeneous or not. The test of homogeneity can be performed using either a Levene's test or a Bartlett's

test (both of these tests use an F-statistic). When the F-value is significant ($p < .05$), it means that two group variances are considered dissimilar, and thus the homogeneity assumption has not been met. In this case, the formula for the t-test must be adjusted (many statistical software packages will perform this calculation automatically.) If the F-value is not significant, it means that the two group variances are considered similar or homogeneous. The formula for the t-test will not have to be adjusted.

The formula for the t-test below is used with groups that have similar or homogenous variance:

$$t = \frac{\overline{X}_1 - \overline{X}_2}{S_{\bar{x}_1 - \bar{x}_2}}$$

with df $= N - 2$, where N is the total sample size or $(n_1 - 1) + (n_2 - 1)$, and where n_1 and n_2 are the sample sizes for two groups.

In this equation, the numerator is the difference between the two group means. The denominator is called the standard error of the difference between the means. This indicates how much the difference between the mean of the sample is different than that of the population. It is calculated as follows:

$$S_{\bar{x}_1 - \bar{x}_2} = \sqrt{\frac{S^2_P}{n_1}} + \sqrt{\frac{S^2_P}{n_2}} \text{ where}$$

$$S^2_P = \frac{S^2_1 (n_1 - 1) + S^2_2 (n_2 - 1)}{n_1 + n_2 - 2}$$

The t-test for groups with unequal variances is:

$$t = \frac{\overline{X}_1 - \overline{X}_2}{\sqrt{\frac{s^2_1}{n_1} + \frac{s^2_2}{n_2}}}$$

In both forms of the t-test, the calculated value is compared to the critical values in Appendix A, Table B.

When t-tests are performed in a statistical package, output is generated that includes all the steps and information noted above. For example, a comparison of Instrumental Activities of Daily Living (IADL) scores between elders who remained at home and those who were institutionalized was made using the Statistical Package for the Social Sciences (SPSS). The output from this analysis is shown in Tables 17.3a and 3b.

Table 17.3a indicates that there are 234 elders who were still living in their own home and 42 elders who were institutionalized. For those living at

Table 17.3 Independent *t*-Test for IADL Scores for Home Living and Institutionalized Elders: SPSS Output

(a) Descriptive Statistics

	FINAL	N	Mean	Std. Deviation	Std. Error Mean
IADL total score	Living at own home	234	9.91	3.265	.213
	Institutionalized	42	5.38	3.682	.568

(b) Independent *t*-Test

	Levene's Test for Equality of Variances		*t*-test for Equality of Means					95% Confidence Interval of the Difference	
	F	Sig.	t	df	Sig. (two-tailed)	Mean Difference	Std. Error Difference	Lower	Upper
Equal variances assumed	2.980	.085	8.122	274	.000	4.53	.558	3.435	5.633
Equal variances not assumed			7.469	53.204	.000	4.53	.607	3.316	5.751

home, the mean of the total IADL scores was 9.91 (SD = 3.265). For those who went to a nursing home, the mean was 5.38 (SD = 3.682). As shown in Table 17.3b, Levene's test indicated that two groups were homogeneous ($p > .05$). Therefore, one examines the statistics given in the row labeled "Equal variances assumed." The *t*-value of 8.122 was determined by the Mean Difference (4.53) over the Standard Error Difference (.558). The degrees of freedom (df) (274) were calculated by (234 – 1) + (42 – 1). The *t*-value was significant at $p < .001$. The 95% confidence interval of the difference is between 3.435 and 5.633. The SPSS printout shows the probability of $p = .000$ (see Table 17.3b) using a two-tailed test (nondirectional hypothesis). If an alternative hypothesis is directional, one should use a one-tailed test. If that is the case, one can divide the *p*-value by 2. For example, if $p = .064$ for a two-tailed test, the *p*-value would be .032 for a one-tailed test.

Mann-Whitney U-Test (a Nonparametric Test)

The Mann-Whitney *U*-test (also called Wilcoxon rank-sum test) is a powerful nonparametric test that is used in place of the independent *t*-test when the data do not meet the statistical assumptions required for parametric statistics.

If the dependent variable is measured on a ratio or interval scale, the raw scores have to be converted to rank orders across both groups (not within a group) and the *U* statistic is calculated as follows:

$$U_1 = R_1 - \frac{n_1 (n_1 + 1)}{2} = \text{ and}$$

$$U_2 = R_2 - \frac{n_2 (n_1 + 1)}{2}$$

where n_1 is the smaller sample size, n_2 is the larger sample size, and R_1 and R_2 are the sum of ranks for each group.

The smaller of these values (U_1 or U_2) is designated to be the calculated *U* value. This calculated value should be smaller than the critical value to be statistically significant. This is opposite to what is done in parametric statistics. For parametric statistics, the calculated value should be larger than the critical value to be statistically significant. When the sample size is larger than 25, *U* is converted to *z* and tested against the Z-distribution. The article by Parush, Winokur, Goldstand, and Miller (2002) used the Mann-Whitney *U* for testing their rank order data. Since they had a sample size of 30, they used z-scores for reporting. Most statistical software packages automatically convert the raw scores to rank orders when using the Mann-

Whitney U-test. This is available in many statistical software packages.

Paired t-Test (a Parametric Test)

For dependent or correlated samples, one uses a paired t-test to analyze the difference scores (d) or change scores within each pair. The formula to calculate a paired t-test is:

$$t = \frac{\bar{d}}{s_{\bar{d}}}$$

where $\bar{d}$ is the mean of the difference scores and $s_{\bar{d}}$ is the standard error of the difference scores.

The degrees of freedom are $n - 1$, where n represents the number of pairs of scores. Tables 17.4a, b, and c contain an SPSS printout of changes in two FIM scores in a single sample of 59 people over a period of 4 years.

Table 17.4a shows that the mean of the FIM Motor scores of 59 people was about 76.4, but 4 years later it became about 71.0. Therefore, the difference between the two mean scores is almost 5.3 (Table 17.4c). For the paired t-test, the statistical assumption is whether there is significant correlation or not between the first or pretest scores and the second or posttest scores. Since Table 17.4b tells that there is a very high correlation

($r =. 893$) between the two scores that is significant ($p<.001$), one can use a paired t-test. The t-value of 6.301 was calculated by the mean difference (5.339) over the standard error of the mean (.84739) and it is significant ($p<.001$). The degrees of freedom (df) are 58 (59 − 1). The conclusion is that the FIM Motor score declined by about 5.3 and the decline was significant over 4 years.

The Sign Test and Wilcoxon Signed Rank Test (Nonparametric Tests)

There are two nonparametric tests that can be used in place of a paired t-test. They are:

- The Sign Test, and
- The Wilcoxon Signed Rank Test.

The Sign Test is used when changes in the direction of the data are of primary interest (i.e., pluses and minuses, or data changing in either a positive or a negative direction). Suppose an investigator wanted to find out what effect an occupational therapy intervention had on some behavior (e.g., using proper body mechanics during activity) among 15 people. An increase of such behaviors can be recorded as "+," a decrease as "−," and no changes as "0." The null hypothesis is that

Table 17.4 Paired t-Test for Changes in FIM Scores: SPSS Output

(a) Descriptive Statistics

		Mean	N	Std. Deviation	Std. Error Mean
Pair 1	FIMYEAR1	76.3559	59	14.34040	1.86696
	FIMYEAR5	71.0169	59	13.58180	1.76820

(b) Paired Samples Correlation

		N	Correlation	Sig.
Pair 1	FIMYEAR1 and FIMYEAR5	59	.893	.000

(c) Paired-test

		Paired Differences					t	df	Sig. (two-tailed)
		Mean	Std. Deviation	Std. Error Mean	95% Confidence Interval of the Difference				
					Lower	Upper			
Pair 1	FIM YEAR1 FIM YEAR5	5.3390	6.50891	.84739	3.6428	7.0352	6.301	58	.000

the number of occurrences of negative and positive change are equal. The alternative hypothesis is that there are more positive changes than negative changes. Suppose there were 10 positive and 3 negative changes, ignoring two people who had a sign of "0." One takes the smaller number of changes (i.e., 3). From Appendix A, Table L, the Probabilities Associated with Values of X in the Binomial Test, the probability of having three pairs indicating a negative change among 13 pairs is $p = .046$. Therefore, the investigator would reject the null hypothesis and conclude that there are more positive changes than negative behavioral changes after exposure to the intervention. This test should be used only when the Wilcoxon Signed Rank Test cannot be used for most instances.

The Wilcoxon Signed Rank Test is similar to the Sign test, but it uses the T (capital T) statistic that identifies the relative magnitude of differences and the direction of changes. The T will be the smaller sum of ranks of scores for one direction of change. Both Wilcoxon Signed Rank Test and Sign test are available in a statistical software SPSS.

Power Analysis

To calculate an effect size for t-tests, one uses a d-index. This is the most commonly referred effect size because it is easy to understand. It examines the mean difference in terms of the standard deviation. For example, if the mean difference is half the value of the standard deviation, it is considered to have a medium effect size.

For independent t-tests with equal variances assumed, the formula is:

$$d = \frac{\overline{X}_1 - \overline{X}_2}{s}$$

For independent t-tests with equal variances not assumed, it is:

$$d = \frac{\overline{X}_1 - \overline{X}_2}{\sqrt{\dfrac{S^2_1 + S^2_2}{2}}}$$

For paired t-tests, the formula is

$$d = \frac{\overline{d}}{s_d}\sqrt{2}$$

The interpretation of the effect size index is:

- Small is $d = .20$,
- Medium is $d = .50$, and
- Large is $d = .80$.

Effect sizes are often reported in the occupational therapy literature. Although in this chapter and the previous chapter, power analyses developed by Cohen (1988) are described, some occupational therapy researchers use the effect size recommended by Stratford, Binkley, and Riddle (1996). When a paired t-test is used, the latter produces a more conservative effect size than Cohen's. Power tables for the t-tests are presented in Appendix A, Table H.

Comparison of More Than Two Group Means (ANOVA)

When comparing three or more group means (or levels of a single independent variable), investigators use the analysis of variance (ANOVA). For the ANOVA, groups represent levels of the independent variable, and the scores for each group on an outcome are the values for the dependent variable. For example, consider a study in which an investigator compares the quality of life of individuals with chronic fatigue syndrome according to time since onset (more than 10 years since onset, between 5 and 10 years, and less than 5 years). In this instance, quality of life is the dependent variable and the independent variable is time (duration since the onset can be broken down into three groups and therefore has three levels). In this case, only one independent variable is being tested; thus, the proper name for this test is called a One-way ANOVA. It is possible to use an F-test (i.e., a one-way ANOVA) when there are only two groups. This will produce the same results as a t-test (i.e., $F = t^2$).

It is rare and not methodologically rigorous for researchers to use multiple t-tests instead of an ANOVA to compare more than two group means. When one sets $\alpha = .05$, and the comparisons are repeated using multiple t-tests, there is a potential cumulative type I error. This accumulated error can be calculated, using the following formula:

$$\alpha = 1 - (1 - \alpha)^e$$

where e is the number of possible comparisons.

For example, if there are four levels in the independent variable, then six comparisons should be made (Groups A vs. B, A vs. C, A vs. D, B vs. C, B vs. D, and C vs. D). When one uses t-tests for six comparisons, the type I error would be .26. Thus, the cumulative error is 26% (not the original 5%).

In order to keep the type I error at a 5% level, investigators use the F-statistic. When investigators use an ANOVA, and an *F*-value is statistically significant, a multiple comparisons test or a post-hoc test is typically used thereafter. Commonly, these tests are used to identify which pairs within the three or more groups being compared are significantly different from the determined minimum mean difference.

Because it is a parametric test, the statistical assumptions for an ANOVA are that the sample groups are randomly drawn from a normally distributed population with equal variances among the groups. When the sample sizes for each group are similar, minor violations of normality and homogeneity of variance do not seriously affect the population estimate. However, if the sample sizes are different, and gross violations of homogeneity of variance are present, this violation may increase the chances of a type I error. In that case, a nonparametric test would be used.

One-Way ANOVA (A Parametric Test)

The term "one-way" indicates that there is one independent variable, or a factor, with three or more levels or groups. If there are two independent variables involved in one analysis, it is called a two-way or two-factor analysis of variance and it is one of the multivariable tests that will be explained in the following section. ANOVA involves only one dependent variable.

The null hypothesis of a one-way ANOVA is that all group means are equal. It is denoted as:

$$H_0: \mu_1 = \mu_2 = \mu_3 = \ldots\ldots = \mu_k$$

where μ (mu) is the population mean, and k is the level or group.

The alternative hypothesis can vary. For example, it can be:

$$H_1 : \mu_1 \neq \mu_2 \neq \mu_3, \text{ or } (\mu_1 = \mu_2) \neq (\mu_3 = \mu_4)$$

The *F*-test is used to determine how much of the total variability in the sample is explained by the differences among group means (between-groups) and the variability among subjects in each group (within-groups). Therefore, the *F* ratio is determined by comparing the between groups variances to the within groups variances. The former variability is explained by the independent variable, meaning the differences in the group mean are due to the independent variable or intervention. The latter variability is unexplained (by the independent variable) and is, therefore, referred to as error variance. The assumption is that individual scores in each group are the same due to the same

intervention they receive. In ANOVA, the variance is called mean square (MS). As discussed in Chapter 16 variance is the ratio of the sum of squares (SS) and degrees of freedom. The following is an example of a One-way ANOVA and compares visual motor integration scores among three groups. As shown in Table 17.5a, the group means are 4.58, 7.89, and 8.22. The grand mean (the mean of all cases) is 6.90. The conceptual formula to derive the F ratio is illustrated Table 17.5b.

The total SS (the last row in Table 17.5b) is the sum of squared differences between an individual score and the grand mean. It is expressed as:

$$SS_{total} = \Sigma(X - \overline{X}_G)^2$$

where X denotes each individual score and $\overline{X}_G$ is the grand mean.

The between-groups SS is the sum of the sample size in the group multiplied by squared differences between the group mean and the grand mean.

$$SS_{between} = \Sigma n (\overline{X}_J - \overline{X}_G)^2$$

where *n* is the sample size for the group, and $\overline{X}_J$ is the group mean.

The within-groups SS is the Sum of Squared differences between the individual score and the group mean.

$$SS_{within} = \Sigma(X - \overline{X}_J)^2$$

The degrees of freedom for the total sample are: $(N - 1)$; for between-groups are: $(k - 1)$; and for within-groups are $(N - 1) - (k - 1)$, $N - k$, or $k(n - 1)$. The MS is determined by the sum of squares divided by the degrees of freedom (SS/df) for each source. Finally, the *F*- value is derived by dividing the between-groups MS by the within-groups MS ($MS_{between}$ /MS_{within}).

As shown in Table 17.5c, the resulting *F*-value is 32.371. The degrees of freedom for the total sample is one less than the total number, so df_{total} = 30 – 1 = 29. For the between-groups, it is one less than the number of groups ($k - 1$), thus, df_b = 3 – 1 = 2. Finally, for the within-groups or error, the degrees of freedom is the total sample size minus the number of groups ($N - k$), or df_e = 30 – 3 = 27. The degrees of freedom (df) for the *F*-value include both df_b and df_e. Then the critical value of *F* can be obtained from Table for Critical Values of *F* at α = .01 in Appendix A, Table D. If the α level has been set at .05, looking at df of 2

Table 17.5 One-Way ANOVA for Independent Samples: Visual Motor Integration for Three Groups ($N = 30$)

(a) Raw Scores, Group Means, and Grand Mean

	Group 1 ($n = 10$)	Group 2 ($n = 10$)	Group 3 ($n = 10$)	Total ($N = 30$)
Raw score	2.50	7.80	7.00	
	3.50	5.80	6.50	
	4.70	6.80	8.30	
	2.90	7.50	7.80	
	5.80	8.80	9.20	
	6.30	9.00	9.90	
	4.80	7.90	8.00	
	5.20	8.50	7.40	
	4.90	8.00	9.60	
	5.20	8.80	8.50	
Mean	4.58	7.89	8.22	6.90 (Grand mean)

(b) Conceptual Formula

Source of Variance	Sum of Squares	df	Mean Square (SS/df)	F
Between groups	$\sum n(\overline{X}_j - \overline{X}_G)^2$	$k - 1$	SS (between group)/$k - 1$	$\dfrac{\text{MS (between group)}}{\text{MS (within group)}}$
Within groups	$\sum(X - \overline{X}_j)^2$	$k(n - 1)$ or $N - k$	SS (within group)/$k(n - 1)$	
Total	$\sum(X - \overline{X}_G)^2$	$N - 1$		

(c) ANOVA Summary Table

Source of Variance	Sum of Squares	df	Mean Square (SS/df)	F
Between groups	81.05	2	40.52	32.37
Within groups	33.80	27	1.25	
Total	114.85	29		

and 27, the critical value of F is 3.35. Since the calculated value is 32.37, and larger than the critical value, one would conclude that there is a significant difference among the three group means. However, one does not yet know which group difference is contributing to the significant F. In fact, an F-test is known as an omnibus test for this very reason. It is an overall test that specifies whether there are significant differences but it does not specify what kinds of differences exist among which groups.

Therefore, post-hoc tests are used to identify which differences between the two mean score are contributing the significant F. They are called post-hoc analyses because they will be performed once an ANOVA has been completed and it has revealed significant results.

Multiple Comparison Tests for One-Way ANOVA

Multiple comparison tests are classified as:

• Post-hoc (done with an ANOVA procedure), and
• A priori test (planned comparisons).

Post-hoc Tests

Post-hoc tests are completed after an investigator conducts a one-way ANOVA and finds a significant F-value. These tests are done in the following way. First, the groups are arranged in the order of the size of the mean. Second, the difference between these two means is obtained, and third, the difference is compared with a minimum significant difference (MSD). If the absolute difference between the two group means is equal to or greater than the minimum significant difference, then the difference is considered significant. The ways to identify the minimum significant difference vary depending on the methods, but there are only two types of error rates that different methods use:

• Per comparison error rate, and
• Familywise error rate.

The former (per comparison) uses a 5% or a 1% margin for a type I error for each single comparison. The latter (familywise) sets a type I error of 5% or 1% for all comparisons in one experiment. The latter may be the more conservative and preferred approach for multiple comparisons for the same reason discussed earlier (i.e., performing multiple comparisons to answer a single study question increases the margin for a type I error).

One of the most widely used post-hoc tests is Tukey's honestly significant difference (HSD) test. This approach uses a familywise error rate. Its minimum significant difference is identified by:

$$MSD = q \sqrt{\frac{MS_e}{n}}$$

where q is the critical value of the studentized range statistic, MS_e is mean square for error or within-groups from the ANOVA output summary table (see Table 17.5c), and n is a sample size in each group.

From Table 17.5a, the means of Groups 1, 2, and 3 are 4.58, 7.89, and 8.22, respectively. The difference between Groups 1 and 2 is (7.89 – 4.58 =) 3.31, that of 2 and 3 is (8.22 – 7.89 =) 0.33, and that of 1 and 3 is (8.22 – 4.58 =) 3.64. Using $\alpha = .05$, and MS_e from Table 17.5c,

$$MSD = 3.51 \sqrt{\frac{1.25}{10}} = 1.24$$

Therefore, the differences between Groups 1 and 2 (3.31) and Groups 1 and 3 (3.64) are larger than the MSD (1.24) and are significant, but the

Table 17.6 Multiple Comparisons: SPSS Output

(a) Tukey's Honestly Significant Difference

(I) Group	(J) Group	Mean Difference (I–J)	Std. Error	Sig.	95% Confidence Interval	
					Lower Bound	Upper Bound
1.00	2.00	−3.31000(*)	.50038	.000	−4.5506	−2.0694
	3.00	−3.64000(*)	.50038	.000	−4.8806	−2.3994
2.00	1.00	3.31000(*)	.50038	.000	2.0694	4.5506
	3.00	−.33000	.50038	.789	−1.5706	.9106
3.00	1.00	3.64000(*)	.50038	.000	2.3994	4.8806
	2.00	.33000	.50038	.789	−.9106	1.5706

*The mean difference is significant at the .05 level.

(b) Scheffé Comparison**

(I) GROUP	(J) GROUP	Mean Difference (I–J)	Std. Error	Sig.	95% Confidence Interval	
					Lower Bound	Upper Bound
1.00	2.00	−3.3100(*)	.50038	.000	−4.6060	−2.0140
	3.00	−3.6400(*)	.50038	.000	−4.9360	−2.3440
2.00	1.00	3.3100(*)	.50038	.000	2.0140	4.6060
	3.00	−.3300	.50038	.806	−1.6260	.9660
3.00	1.00	3.6400(*)	.50038	.000	2.3440	4.9360
	2.00	.3300	.50038	.806	−.9660	1.6260

*The mean difference is significant at the .05 level.
**Dependent variable: SCORE.

difference between Groups 2 and 3 (0.33) is not significant.

Many other post-hoc tests are available in statistical software. Table 17.6a shows the SPSS output of a post-hoc analysis of the data of visual–motor integration (which was presented Table 17.5a), using Tukey's HSD. The results indicate that Group 1 is significantly different from Group 2 and Group 3 (both $p = .001$) but Group 2 and Group 3 are not ($p = .789$).

Another frequently used post-hoc procedure is the Scheffé comparison. This is a more rigorous method than Tukey's HSD. This method also uses a familywise error rate. The calculation formula for the Scheffé comparison is:

$$MSD = \sqrt{(k-1)F}\sqrt{\frac{2MS_e}{n}}$$

Using the results of MS_e from the Visual–Motor Integration example shown in Table 17.5c, and F is the critical value of F from Appendix A, Table D for 2 and 27 degrees of freedom at

$$MSD = \sqrt{(3-1)3.35}\sqrt{\frac{2 \times 1.25}{10}} = 1.29$$

Using this method, although the results are the same in this particular example, the MSD is larger, requiring a larger mean difference. An SPSS printout of this post-hoc test is presented in Table 17.6b.

A discrepancy between the results of the F-test and post-hoc tests sometimes occurs because two different statistical procedures are used. Even if the F-value is significant, there may be no significant differences between pairs or vice versa. In these instances, investigators may report both results.

Planned Comparisons

In some cases, investigators will decide which pairs should be compared before data collection takes place. This is called an a priori or planned comparison. In this instance, even if the F-value is not significant, the specific comparison will take place because prior to the data analyses, the investigator decided that the comparisons should be done. For example, the investigator may be mainly interested in knowing the difference between Group 2 and Group 3 in the preceding example. Then, the statistical procedure is an independent t-test. The results of an a priori test are usually presented together with the results of an omnibus test or the F-test. For multiple comparisons, the Bonferroni t-test (also called Dunn's multiple comparison procedure) is used (see later section).

Kruskal–Wallis One-Way ANOVA (a Nonparametric Test)

When it is not possible to use a parametric test for three or more group comparisons (such as when the measurement is made using an ordinal scale, the groups are not normally distributed, or group variance is not homogeneous) investigators use the Kruskal-Wallis nonparametric procedure. If this test is used in a study in which the measurements are done using a ratio or interval data, the data must be converted to ordinal rank data. For example, if there were 15 cases in total, the ranks would be between 1 and 15. In the case of ties, one would use the mean ranks. For example, if two cases scored the same after the case ranked 2, they would be ranked 3.5 by dividing the sum of rankings 3 and 4 by 2.

The Kruskal-Wallis H statistics is calculated as follows:

$$H = \frac{12}{N(N+1)} \sum \frac{R^2}{n} - 3(N+1)$$

where N is the number of total cases, n is the number of cases in each individual group, and R^2 is the squared sum of ranks for each group.

H is distributed as Chi-square with df $= k - 1$. Therefore the critical value is obtained from Appendix A, Table C. The numbers 12 and 3 are treated as constants in the equation. Suppose the data in Table 17.5a are analyzed using the Kruskal-Wallis test; then the total ranks are 56.5, 197.0, and 211.5 for each group. Therefore, $H = 18.939$. The critical value for degrees of freedom $= 2$ at $\alpha = .05$ is 5.99. Since the H-value is larger than the critical value, one concludes that there is a significant difference for at least one of the pair.

Multiple Comparisons for the Kruskal-Wallis ANOVA

To calculate multiple comparisons for the Kruskal-Wallis ANOVA, investigators estimate the pairwise difference among the mean rankings: $\bar{R} = \frac{R}{n}$. The number of pair wise comparisons is determined by $k(k-1)/2$. If there are three groups, three comparisons should be made. This is calculated by $3(3-1)/2$ and it tests Group 1 vs. Group 2, Group 2 vs. Group 3 and Group 3 vs. Group 1. The computational formula for the post-hoc procedures is:

$$|\bar{R}_1 - \bar{R}_2| \geq z \sqrt{\frac{N(N+1)}{12}\left(\frac{1}{n_1} + \frac{1}{n_2}\right)}$$

where N is the total number of cases and n_1 and n_2 are the number of cases in each group of comparisons. The z-score at $\alpha = .05$ is obtained from Table 17.7 in this chapter. Using the example from the previous section (Table 17.5a), the mean ranks are 4.58, 7.89, and 8.22. The difference between Groups 1 and 2 is 3.31; Groups 1 and 3, 3.64, and Groups 2 and 3, 0.33. To find the significant difference, these mean rank differences should be larger than

$$2.394 \sqrt{\frac{30(30 + 1)}{12} \left(\frac{1}{10} + \frac{1}{10} \right)} = 9.425$$

Therefore, one concludes that none of the group rank means are significantly different.

Repeated Measures ANOVA (a Parametric Test)

Study designs in which subjects are correlated and measurements are taken more than two times are called repeated measures designs or within-subjects designs. The statistical test that is used for these designs is a repeated measures ANOVA. The statistical advantage of using a repeated measures ANOVA over a series of one-way ANOVAs is that the repeated measures ANOVA reduces the error variance (i.e., variability that is not due to the independent variable or the treatment effect). This is because the repeated measures ANOVA controls for individual differences by subtracting the variances of individual differences from within-group variances in one-way ANOVA. This reduced error variance results in a larger F-ratio. Thus, the single-factor repeated measures ANOVA is more powerful than one-way ANOVA with independent samples. However, the choice of statistical procedures should be based on a study design and whether subjects are independent or correlated rather than on issues involving statistical power.

The repeated measures ANOVA does not require the statistical assumption of homogeneity among groups because it involves only one group. Rather, it requires that the variances of the score difference among each group are similar and correlated. This is called the assumption of sphericity. Statistical software packages will present the assumption of sphericity. If this assumption is violated, the test will have an inflated type I error rate and significant differences may be found when none actually exists.

The repeated measures ANOVA uses the F-ratio. The numerator of the F-ratio is the variance between treatment groups. The denominator of the F-ratio is the error variance. A repeated measures design removes individual differences from the within-group variance (in one-way ANOVA) because the same people are in all treatments. Expressed numerically, the error term is the residual of the total variances minus the sample variance (the error term is smaller than the error term of the one-way ANOVA). The conceptual formula is presented in Table 17.8a.

One can illustrate the repeated measures ANOVA using the same example of visual motor integration that was used above for the one-way ANOVA. To do so, one must assume that the three groups are the three measurements over time for the same persons (rather than three different groups of subjects as was assumed earlier when presenting the one-way ANOVA in Table 17.5a). In this case, the calculation is presented in Table 17.8b.

The conceptual formula for F is $MS_{between}/MS_{error}$ presented in Table 17.8a, and they are as follows:

$$SS_{total} = \Sigma (X - \overline{X}_G)^2$$
$$SS_{between} = \Sigma n(\overline{X}_j - \overline{X}_G)^2$$
$$SS_{subject} = \Sigma k(X_s - \overline{X}_G)^2$$
$$SS_{error} = SS_{total} - SS_{between} - SS_{subject}$$

where X is an individual score, $\overline{X}_j$ is the group mean, $\overline{X}_G$ is the grand mean, $\overline{X}_S$ and is the mean of each person across interventions.

Using the same data presented in Table 17.5a, Table 17.8b shows the calculated values in the ANOVA summary table. The degrees of freedom for between-group variances are $k - 1 = 2$ and that for error is $(n - 1)(K - 1) = (10 - 1)(3 - 1) = 18$.

Table 17.7 Critical Values of z for Multiple Comparison with H Statistics and X_r^2

Number of Comparisons	z at $\alpha = .05$
1	1.960
2	2.241
3	2.394
4	2.498
5	2.576
6	2.638
7	2.690
8	2.734

Adapted from Table A$_{II}$ of Siegel, S., & Castellan, N.J. (1988). Nonparametric statistics for the behavioral sciences (2nd ed.). New York: McGraw-Hill, with permission.

Table 17.8 Repeated Measures ANOVA

(a) Conceptual Formula

Source of Variance	Sum of Squares	df	Mean Square (SS/df)	F
Between groups	$\sum n(\bar{X}_j - \bar{X}_G)^2$	$k - 1$	SS (between group)/$k - 1$	$\dfrac{\text{MS (between group)}}{\text{MS (error)}}$
Subject	$\sum k(\bar{X}_s - \bar{X}_G)^2$	$(n - 1)$		
Error	Total SS − Between group SS − Subject SS	$(n - 1) \times (k - 1)$	SS (error)/$(n - 1)$ $(k - 1)$	
Total	$\sum(X - \bar{X}_G)^2$	$N - 1$		

(b) ANOVA Summary Table: Constructed from SPSS Output

Source of Variance	Sum of Squares	df	Mean Square (SS/df)	F
Between groups	81.049	2	40.524	98.245
Subject	26.376	9	2.931	
Error	7.425	18	.412	
Total	114.85	29		

The mean square (MS) for each group is calculated by SS/df; therefore, MS $_{between}$ is 81.049/2 = 40.524 and MS $_{error}$ is 7.425/18 = .412, thus F = 40.524/.412 = 98.245. The F-value for the repeated measures ANOVA is much larger than the F for the one-way ANOVA (32.37).

Multiple Comparison Tests for Repeated Measures ANOVA

After finding the significant F, the investigator is often interested in knowing when the significant change occurred. In this instance, one uses a Bonferroni correction. This method reduces the type I error by dividing the α level by the number of comparisons. For example, in the above case with three pair comparisons, the alpha level becomes .05/3 = .0167. To use this method, the investigator performs three paired t-tests and each p-value is compared with .0167. When a computer statistical package is used, this multiple comparison procedure is called contrast. The results show that Group 1 is significantly different from Groups 2 and 3.

Friedman Two-Way Analysis of Variance of Ranks Test (a Nonparametric Test)

The nonparametric test that is commonly used in place of the repeated measures ANOVA is the Friedman test. If an investigator measures three fatigue levels of five persons with multiple sclerosis before exercise (time 1), right after exercise (time 2), and 1 hour after exercise (time 3), the Friedman test would be appropriate, owing to the small sample size. It uses rank orders within a subject. In this instance the ranks range between 1 and 3 for all subjects (i.e., when they had the most, least, and intermediate levels of fatigue). When there is a tie, ranks are averaged. Then, ranks are summed within each column (measurement/time). The null hypothesis is that the rank sums for all measurements are the same. If the null hypothesis is rejected, then at least one pair of measures will show a difference.

The formula to calculate the Friedman (chisquare r) value is:

$$X^2_r = \frac{12}{nk(k + 1)} \sum R^2 - 3n(k + 1)$$

where n is the number of subjects and k is the number of measurements/times (groups), and R^2 is the squared sum of rankings in each group.

The critical value for Chi-square r is found in the Chi-square r distribution with k minus 1 degrees of freedom. The critical values are presented in Table 17.7 in this chapter. The post-hoc test uses a familywise error rate. The formula to determine the minimum significant difference (MSD) for all pair differences is:

$$|R_1 - R_2| \geq z \sqrt{\frac{nk(k + 1)}{6}}$$

where R_1 and R_2 are the rank sums, n is the number of subjects, k is the number of measurements within a person, and the z is from Table 17.7.

Power Analysis

For the ANOVA, the effect size index is f and it is defined by:

$$f = \sqrt{\frac{SS_b}{SS_e}}$$

where SS_b is the sum of squares of the between-groups and SS_e is the sum of squares of the error that are obtained from the summary table of ANOVA. Using the data provided in Table 5c, f is

$$\sqrt{\frac{81.05}{33.80}} = 1.55.$$

The interpretation of f is:

• Small $f = .10$,
• Medium $f = .25$, and
• Large $f = .40$.

Therefore, 1.55 is very large. An effect size can be very large such as more than 1.0. The f index can be applied to independent samples and repeated measures ANOVA also. The sample sizes needed for ANOVA with various effect sizes for the power of .80 at $\alpha = .05$ are found in Appendix A, Table I.

Multifactorial Analysis of Variance: Comparison of Group Means for Two or More Independent Variables

When there are more than two independent variables and one dependent variable in an analysis, and when the purpose of the analysis is to compare group means, one uses a multifactorial design or multiway ANOVA. This is called a multivariable approach and there are no corresponding nonparametric statistics.

This section focuses only on the two-way ANOVA and mixed design where there is a within-groups factor and a between-groups factor. Also, simple cell effects are discussed to compliment omnibus factorial analyses.

Two-Way ANOVA

A two-way analysis of variance (ANOVA) or a two-factor ANOVA involves two independent variables (i.e., A and B). In this analysis, there are three possible questions:

• What is the main effect of variable A, independent of B,
• What is the main effect of variable B, independent of A, and
• What is the joint effect or interaction of variables A and B?

The main effects are effects of two separate independent variables.

A two-way ANOVA will be illustrated using a hypothetical study of the dependent variable, instrumental activities of daily living (IADLs) (scale score range = 0–14). The two independent variables are: (A) living status (two levels, i.e., living alone versus with someone), and (B) sex (two levels). The means for each cell and the means for levels of the main effects, called marginal means, are presented in Table 17.9. The standard deviations for each are presented in parentheses. In a two-way ANOVA, one compares marginal means, not the means in cells for the main effects.

Therefore, for sex, one compares 7.6 for males with 8.5 for females. For living status, one compares 9.4 for living alone with 6.9 for living with someone. In addition to main effects, one examines combined effects (interaction effects) of levels of independent variables on a dependent variable. Using the mean values in four cells from the data in Table 17.9, Figure 17.1a shows that there is no interaction because the two lines (Living Alone and Living with Someone) are not crossing and are almost parallel. Figure 17.1b indicates an interaction.

An interaction effect occurs when the relationship between two variables differs depending on the value of a third variable.

Table 17.9 Total IADL Score by Sex and Living Status Categories ($N = 758$)

Sex	Living Alone	Living With Someone	Total (Marginal Means)
Male	9.6 (2.9)	6.0 (4.1)	7.6 (4.0)
Female	9.4 (2.8)	6.9 (4.0)	8.5 (3.5)
Total (marginal means)	9.4 (2.8)	6.9 (4.0)	8.3 (3.6)

A)

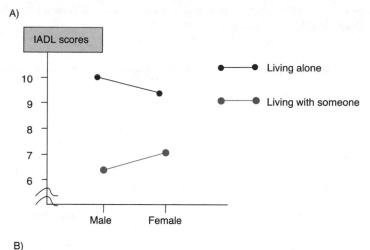

B)

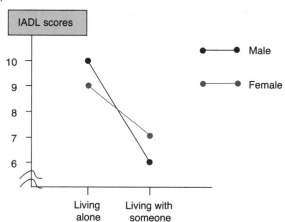

Figure 17.1 Types of Interaction.
(A) No interaction. (B) Possible interaction.

Using the example above, the null hypotheses are:

1. $H_0: \mu_{A1} = \mu_{A2}$
2. $H_0: \mu_{B1} = \mu_{B2}$
3. $H_0: \mu_{A1B1} = \mu_{A1B2} = \mu_{A2B1} = \mu_{A2B2}$

Where $A1$ is male, $A2$ is female, $B1$ is living alone, $B2$ is living with someone, $A1B1$ denotes males who live alone, $A1B2$ denotes males who live with someone, $A2B1$ indicates females who

live alone, and $A2B2$ indicates females who live with someone.

The statistical assumptions are that the independent variable must be comprised of mutually exclusive groups and the dependent variable must be normally distributed and demonstrate homogeneity of variance across groups.

A hypothetical summary table for a two-way ANOVA is shown in Table 17.10. This table is based on an analysis of the impact of two inde-

Table 17.10 Hypothetical Summary Table for Two-Way ANOVA

Source of Variance	Sum of Squares	df	Mean Square (SS/df)	F
Sex (M or F)	120.98	1	120.98	10.37
Living regions	105.03	2	52.515	4.50
Interaction	128.37	2	64.185	5.5
Error	8770.53	752	11.67	
Total	9910.64	757		

pendent variables, region in which a person lives (East, West, and South) and sex (male versus female) on daily activity level. The α level was set at .01.

From the degrees of freedom in this table, one can tell there are 758 subjects in the study ($df_{total} = N - 1 = 757$), sex has two levels ($df_{sex} = k - 1 = 1$), and living regions have three levels ($df_{living\ regions} = k - 1 = 2$). The degrees of freedom for the interaction is $1 \times 2 = 2$ and that of error is obtained by $df_{total} - df_{sex} - df_{living\ regions} - df_{interaction} = 757 - 1 - 2 - 2 = 752$. All mean square values are determined by dividing the sum of squares for each effect by its associated degrees of freedom. The F-ratio for sex is determined by $MS_{sex}/MS_{error} = 120.98/11.67 = 10.37$. The F-ratio for living regions is found by $52.515/11.67 = 4.50$. The F-ratio for the interaction is calculated by $64.185/11.67 = 5.5$. Note that the error term is the same for all main effects and interaction effects. The critical value for each effect is obtained from

Appendix A, Table D. For sex, the critical value is $_{(.01)}F_{(1,752)} = 6.63$ and that for living regions and interaction is $_{(.01)}F_{(2,\ 752)} = 4.61$. Therefore, the main effect of living regions is not significant, but the main effect of sex and the interaction effect (living regions x sex) are significant. Since the interaction effect is significant, Figures 17.1c and 17.1d show almost and complete crossing lines.

In two-way ANOVA, before examining the two main effects, one should examine the interaction effect. If it is not significant, then one can report the main effects as shown in the results. If the interaction is significant, the next step is to examine the type of interaction, which can be ordinal or disordinal. In an ordinal interaction, one effect is not affected by the other effects. Figure 17.1c shows an ordinal interaction in that regardless of living regions, males are more active than females. Therefore, lines for male and female do not cross. The rank order of activities for East is one for males (more active) and two for females. This

C)

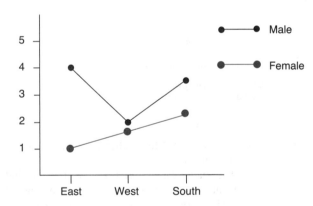

D)

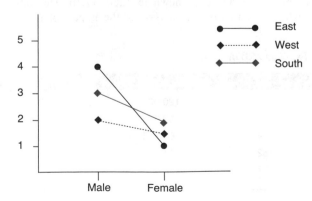

Figure 17.1 (C) Ordinal. (D) Disordinal.

order is the same for West and South; therefore, it is called ordinal interaction, and one can say that males are always active than females. For the conclusion, one can look at the F-value of sex, a main effect.

In contrast, Figure 17.1d shows a disordinal interaction, presenting crossed lines. Among males, residents in the East are the most active, then residents in the South. Residents in the West are most inactive. This order is not the same for females. Females living in South are most active, followed by West, and then East. When the order of the dependent variable scores for levels of one independent variable is not the same across levels/groups of another independent variable in the X-axis, a disordinal interaction occurs. When it happens, it is meaningless to compare mean scores across the first independent variable (Living regions). The F-value for the main effect is often not significant.

The next step is to examine males and females separately. These separate effects are called simple effects. Since six comparisons are made using independent t-tests, the type I error must be controlled; using a Bonferroni correction. The α level can be set to $\alpha = .05/6 = .0083$.

Mixed Design

When a single experiment involves at least one independent factor (between-groups) and one repeated factor (within-groups), the design is called a mixed design and it is analyzed using a repeated measures ANOVA with a between-factor. A mixed design is the most often used design in occupational therapy experimental research studies.

This design combines a one-way ANOVA for the between-factor and a repeated-measures ANOVA for the within-factor. For example, in a study designed to identify the effects of school-based occupational therapy services on students' handwriting (Case-Smith, 2002) a mixed design was used. The within-factor was time (i.e., pre- and posttest scores). The between-factor was intervention (i.e., students who received an occupational therapy intervention and a control group that did not receive the intervention). There were three separate dependent (outcome) variables: handwriting legibility, speed, and associated performance components. For all components of legibility scores, posttest scores were higher than pretest scores regardless of occupational therapy intervention. Also, the control group always scored higher than the treatment group. Therefore, there were no significant interaction effects ($p = .054$). The main

effect for time (a within-factor) was significant but the main effect for intervention, the between-factor, was not. Then, pre- and posttest scores for the treatment group were compared using only paired t-tests. The results of t-values, p-values, and effect sizes (d-index) were reported. One of the dependent variables, visual–motor control, showed significant interaction effects ($p = .004$). The pretest scores of the treatment and control groups were 9.14 and 15.44, respectively, and the posttest scores were 11.25 and 16.67, respectively. Note that the interactions were ordinal (the control group always scores higher than the treatment group and the posttest scores are always higher than the pretest scores). Therefore, both main effects were considered valid ($p = .111$ for the within-factor and $p = .715$ for the between-factor).

Since the main interest of the research was the effect of intervention, pre- and posttest scores of visual–motor control for only the treatment group were analyzed, using a paired t-test. The result was statistically significant ($p = .039$) with a moderate effect size ($d = .58$).

There is no comparable nonparametric test for multifactor analyses such as two-way ANOVAs, mixed designs, and multiway ANOVAs. The ANOVA is robust, and thus minor violations of statistical assumptions might not alter the results significantly. However, the same does not apply to the repeated measures ANOVA.

Since a mixed design reflects the combination of the two statistical methods, when dealing with a small sample size, one may not be able to use a repeated measures ANOVA with a between-factor. One solution is to conduct separate analyses for the between-factor and the within-factor.

Simple Cell Effect

Because of their omnibus nature, significant main effects for a two-way ANOVA and a mixed design simply indicate that at least one pair of marginal means is significantly different. Using the example of Figure 17.1c, the ANOVA compares marginal means of Male (activity mean is 3) and Female (activity mean is 1.5), and indicate that the F-value for sex is significant. Since this analysis compares only two different levels (Male and Female), there is no post-hoc procedure. However, the investigator may be interested in knowing the difference between Male and Female in East and West. In this case, the next step is to examine the simple cell effects, such as the difference between the mean of Male (4) and that of Female (1) for East and the mean of Male (2) and that of Female (1.5) for West, using independent t-tests. It is best to determine the intention of particular simple cell analysis prior to conducting an ANOVA. This process is called an a priori test or a planned comparison. Actually, in such a case, one may not even be interested in conducting an *F*-test to find overall effects. Therefore, regardless of the significance of the *F*-value, one would conduct a priori tests. This procedure involves a Bonferroni correction or Dunn's multiple comparison procedure. It requires one to set the α level by dividing the set α level by the number of comparisons. For example, if one sets the α level as .05 and wants to compare three sets of means, then the altered α level would be .05/2 = .025. While this approach reduces the likelihood of the type 1 error, it does make it more difficult to find significant results.

Correlation

Correlation is the extent to which two or more variables are related to one another, and does not necessarily mean that one causes another although often the causal relationship may be obvious, such as age up to 20 years or so and height. Height does not cause age, but as a boy becomes older, he becomes taller; therefore, age is a cause of height. Nevertheless, the purpose of correlation analysis is to identify the association between two variables, not to identify a causal relationship. Height and weight often have a high correlation, which means, if a person is tall, he or she tends to be heavier than a short person. In this case, the two variables are denoted by *X* and *Y* (height and weight, respectively) and when the variable (*X*) increases one unit, the variable (*Y*) also increases. This is referred to a bivariate correlation (or zero-order correlation), since the relationship between only two variables is of concern. There is another type of correlation, such as a multiple correlation, where the relationship between one dependent variable and several independent variables is examined. It is discussed in the next section. In this section two correlations are explained:

- Pearson (or Pearson's) correlation, in which both variables should be measured by a continuous scale, and
- Spearman (or Spearman's) rho in which variables are measured by rank orders.

Correlation Coefficient

Pearson Correlation uses the correlation coefficient to express the strength of the relationship between two variables. The strongest correlations are 1.00 or –1.00, and if there is no correlation, the correlation coefficient is 0. In some instances, two variables have a curvilinear relationship, such as a U-shape or an arch-shape. This occurs when one variable follows the pattern of another variable up until a certain point and then it reverses direction. For example, half of variable *X* might have a strong positive correlation with variable *Y*, but the other half of variable *X* might have a strong negative correlation with variable *Y*. In this case, the correlation coefficient will be close to 0. This means there is no linear correlation but has a curvilinear relationship. To find the nature of the relationship between the two variables, it is best if one plots them.

Pearson Product Moment Correlation

Definitional Formula

The Pearson Product Moment correlation coefficient is the most often used measure of correlation. The symbol for the coefficient is r and it is used when both variables are normally distributed and measured using an interval or ratio scale. It is called "product-moment" because it is calculated by multiplying the *z*-scores of the two variables to get their "product" and then calculating the average, which is called a "moment," of these products. The conceptual formula is:

$$r = \frac{\sum Z_X Z_Y}{N}$$

where $z = (X - \overline{X})/SD$ and *N* is the number of pairs. The degrees of freedom are $N - 2$.

The second formula is:

$$r = \text{Covariance}/SD_x SD_Y$$

where covariance is a measure of the joint variances of two variables and calculated by:

$$\frac{\sum (X - \overline{X})(Y - \overline{Y})}{N - 1}$$

and $SD_x SD_Y$ is the product of the standard deviation of the two variables.

A correlation can be easily identified by creating a scattergram or scatter plot. In Figures 17.2a through 17.2d, various patterns of correlation are shown. The first graph (17.2a) presents a perfect positive correlation ($r = 1$); the second graph (17.2 b) is a perfect negative correlation ($r = -1$); the third (17.2c) shows a moderate relationship ($r = .60$); and the fourth (17.2d) illustrates a pattern in which there is no correlation ($r = 0$).

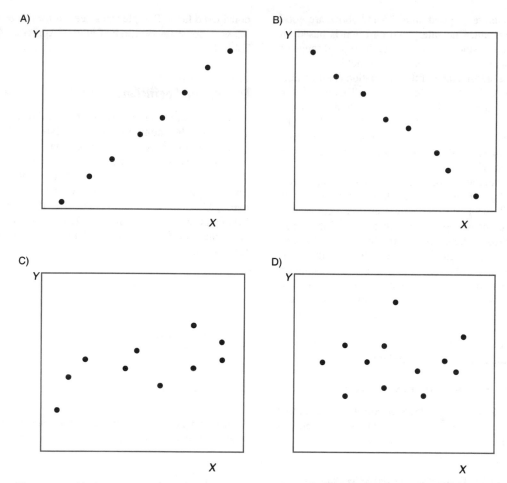

Figure 17.2 Various patterns of correlation. (A) Perfect positive correlation. (B) Perfect negative correlation ($r = -1.0$). (C) Moderate correlation ($r = .60$). (D) No correlation ($r = 0$).

Correlation Matrix

When an investigator uses many variables in one study, it is often useful to identify bivariate correlations among them. Then, one uses a correlation matrix such as the one shown in Table 17.11. In this matrix, there are five variables: age, number of illnesses, Body Mass Index (BMI), physical disability level, and Mini Mental State Exam (MMSE) score. As shown in the table, the correlation of each variable with itself is 1. The correlation coefficients on either side of the diagonal are the same. For example, the correlation between age and MMSE ($-.240$) is found in two places: one in the bottom of the first column and the other in the top of the last column. Therefore, one can look at either at the upper or the lower side of the matrix that is separated by ones. The highest correlation in the matrix is $r = -.290$ between age and BMI. This correlation is interpreted to mean that the

older they are, the lower the BMI score. The lowest correlation is $r = -.026$ between age and number of illnesses. In this matrix there is a negligible correlation between age and number of illnesses.

Strength and Significance of the Correlation Coefficient

The interpretation of the correlation coefficient is the strength of the relationship. The following is how values are typically interpreted:

- 0–.20 suggests a negligible correlation,
- .20–.40 is a low correlation,
- .40–.60 is a moderate correlation,
- .60–.80 is a high correlation, and
- .80–1.00 is a very high correlation.

Other researchers interpret the values of 0–.25 as little or no relationship .25–.50 as fair, .50–.75

as moderate or good, and .75 and above are good to excellent. The interpretation often is based on the area of study and it reflects the typical range of correlations demonstrated in that field.

The significance of the correlation coefficient is expressed as the probability (p). Therefore, if it is set as $\alpha = .05$, then the interpretation is that it is either significant or not. The p-value should not be interpreted as reflecting the strength of the relationship. Critical values of r are found in Appendix A, Table F.

Correlation is very sensitive to the sample size. Therefore, if one has a very large sample size such as in Table 17.11 ($N = 389$), even if a correlation coefficient is negligible such as $r = .145$, the p-value is significant at $\alpha = .01$. In this case, the correlation is significant; but its magnitude is negligible and does not indicate a meaningful association between the two variables. The coefficient of determination (r-square) accurately describes the strength of a bivariate correlation. It represents the percentage of variance of one variable that is explained by the variance of the other variable in a bivariate correlation.

Effect Size of Pearson Correlation

The effect size for Pearson correlation is simple because r is the same as the effect size. When $r = .10$, it is small, $r = .30$ is medium, and $r = .50$ is considered large. Sample sizes needed for r at $\alpha = .05$ with power $= .80$ can be found in Appendix A, Table J.

Spearman Rank Correlation Coefficient

When the correlation is between two rank-ordered variables, the nonparametric statistic, called Spearman rank correlation, or Spearman's rho (r_s), is used. To calculate r_s, one ranks the scores within the variable X and Y separately. A rank of 1 is given to the smallest value and ties are given the average of their ranks. Then the difference between the rank X and the rank $Y(d)$ is calculated and squared (d^2) for each pair. The computational formula is:

$$r_s = 1 - \frac{6\sum d^2}{n(n^2 - 1)}$$

where n is the number of pairs. As most nonparametric statistics, this has less power than Pearson correlation.

Regression

Regression is a statistical technique used to ask whether it is possible to predict some variables by

Table 17.11 **Correlation Matrix: SPSS Printout**

		Age	Number of Illness	BMI	Physical Disability Level	MMSE
Age	Pearson Correlation	1	−.026	−.290(**)	.145(**)	−.240(**)
	Sig. (two-tailed)	.	.613	.000	.004	.000
	N	389	389	389	389	389
Number of illness	Pearson Correlation	−.026	1	.128(*)	.287(**)	.069
	Sig. (two-tailed)	.613	.	.011	.000	.172
	N	389	389	389	389	389
BMI	Pearson Correlation	−.290(**)	.128(*)	1	.038	.158(**)
	Sig. (two-tailed)	.000	.011	.	.461	.002
	N	389	389	389	389	389
Physical disability level	Pearson Correlation	.145(**)	.287(**)	.038	1	−.213(**)
	Sig. (two-tailed)	.004	.000	.461	.	.000
	N	389	389	389	389	389
MMSE	Pearson Correlation	−.240(**)	.069	.158(**)	−.213(**)	1
	Sig. (two-tailed)	.000	.172	.002	.000	.
	N	389	389	389	389	389

**Correlation is significant at the 0.01 level (2-tailed).
*Correlation is significant at the 0.05 level (2-tailed).

knowing other variables. It is used to answer questions, such as can a parent's stress level (Y) be predicted based on the infant's length of stay in a hospital (X)? If there is a strong correlation between X and Y, the prediction would be easier than if the correlation is weak.

In this case, infant's length of hospital stay is the independent variable (X) and the parent's stress level is the dependent variable (Y). In regression analysis, some researchers use the term "a predictor" for the independent variable and "a criterion variable" or an "outcome variable" for the dependent variable.

To answer the question of whether one variable predicts another, one can use a simple linear regression. If there are several independent variables, then one needs to use multiple regression. In this section, in addition to these two linear regression analyses, logistic regression is also discussed. Logistic regression is a type of regression technique in which the dependent variable is measured by nominal scale. In addition, analysis of covariance (ANCOVA) is discussed. ANCOVA uses a combination of ANOVA and regression.

Simple Linear Regression

Simple linear regression assumes that two variables are linearly correlated and the line that best describes the relationship is called a regression line. To determine this line, one uses a regression analysis. The regression line is expressed by the regression equation:

$$Y' = a + bX$$

where Y' or $\hat{Y}$ is the predicted value of Y, a is the Y-intercept (the value of Y when X is 0), and b is the slope of the line (the rate of change in Y' for each unit change in X). The variable a is the regression constant and b is the regression coefficient. When b is positive, the Y' line goes higher as X increases, indicating a positive correlation. When b is negative, the Y' line goes lower as X increases, indicating a negative correlation. If a is 3, b is 2, and X is 5, then $Y = 3 + (2)(5) = 13$.

The regression line is called the line of best fit, because it is the line that best describes (fits) the pattern of the data. The errors determined by the differences between observed values and predicted values ($Y - Y'$) are called residuals. The regression line is the line for which the residuals are smallest. The squared term of residuals is used to avoid the negative values; therefore, the smallest sum of squared residuals is the line of best fit. The method to identify this best fit line is called the method of least squares.

The calculation of the regression equation starts with that of b.

b = the ratio between the standard deviation of Y to that of X, SD_y/SD_x

$$a = \overline{Y} - b\overline{X}$$

Therefore, the observed value, Y is calculated by $a + bX$ + residual or error, but typically, the regression equation is expressed as Y (not Y' or $\hat{Y}$) $= a + bX$.

For statistical inferences about the regression equation (i.e., to verify that the relationship between X and Y did not occur by chance), one analyzes the variance of regression. The null hypothesis is H_0: $b = 0$. It means there is no slope and the best bet to predict the Y score is based on the mean of Y for any value of X.

The Assumptions for Regression Analysis

In regression analysis, for any values of X, a random distribution of Y scores exists. Therefore, theoretically, the mean of each distribution of Y lies on the regression line. Each distribution is normal and its standard deviation is homogeneous. These statistical assumptions are illustrated in Figure 17.3 on p. 266. This figure illustrates a theoretical regression line, which theoretically contains a series of normal distributions running across it. The mean of each normal distribution is shown to fall directly onto the regression line.

In regression analysis, these assumptions can be examined by plotting residuals (the difference between observed and predicted scores). Usually the residuals are plotted on the Y-axis and the predicted scores are on the X-axis. When the linear regression model is a good fit, the residuals will be randomly dispersed around $Y = 0$ with similar width above and below the horizontal line (Figure 17.4 on p. 266).

If the plot of residuals deviates from this pattern, a transformation of the data may be necessary. Transformations use a constant to covert the data to a more normal distribution. For transformation methods, read Tabachnick and Fidell (1996).

In regression, outliers should be examined. If one determines that the outlier is due to a data entry error, it can be eliminated. Some researchers consider the score an outlier if it is beyond three standard deviations. However, if it is a true score, one has to consider whether it should be discarded or not. Since outliers can greatly influence the results of a regression, they can distort the overall picture of how well X predicts Y.

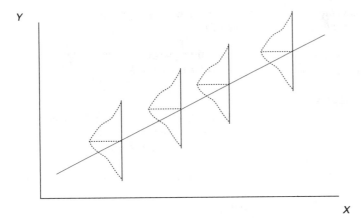

Figure 17.3 A statistical assumption of linear regression: Normal distribution of predicted scores and their means being on the linear regression.

Accuracy of Prediction

To examine the accuracy of prediction (how well X predicts Y), one examines the coefficient of determination (r-square for simple linear regression and R-square for multiple regression and the standard error of the estimate (SEE). The coefficient of determination is a measure of proportion: the percentage of the total variance in the dependent variable that can be explained by the independent variable; therefore, indicating the accuracy of prediction based on the independent variable. The correlation of $r = .30$ means $r^2 = .09$; that is, 9% of the variances of Y is explained by the variances of X. On the other hand, $1 - r^2$ is the unknown variances; therefore, the higher the values of coefficient of determination, the more accurate of the prediction based on the independent variable.

The standard deviation of the distribution of errors is called the standard error of the estimate. The SEE indicates the average error of

prediction of the regression equations and is calculated by:

$$ SEE = \sqrt{\frac{\sum(Y - Y')^2}{(n - 2)}} $$

where $\sum (Y - Y')^2$ is the sum of the square residuals and n is the number of pairs of scores.

Analysis of Variance for Regression

There are three variance components in analysis of variance for regression:

- The sum of squared distance between the mean of all Y scores ($\overline{Y}$) and the observed scores (Y) are total SS (SS_{total}),
- The sum of squared distance between the mean of all Y scores ($\overline{Y}$) and the predicted scores (Y') are explained by regression SS (SS_{reg}), and
- The sum of squared distance between observed score (Y) and predicted value (Y') is residual SS (SS_{res}).

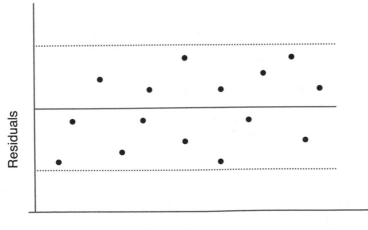

Predicted Scores

Figure 17.4 Residuals indicating the assumption of linear regression is being met.

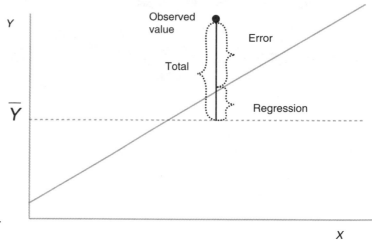

Figure 17.5 Components of variances in regression.

These components are illustrated in Figure 17.5 and summarized in Table 17.12 (Analysis of Variance Table for Regression).

An F-distribution is used for testing the significance of the relationship between X and Y but not the strength between the two variables. The interpretation of the strength relies on R^2 (multiple correlation) or r^2 for a simple linear regression.

The definitional formula to derive F value is as follows:

$$SS_{total} = \sum(Y - \overline{Y})^2$$
$$SS_{regression} = \sum(Y' - \overline{Y})^2$$
$$SS_{residual} = SS_{total} - SS_{regression}$$

where Y is the observed value, $\overline{Y}$ is the mean of all Y values, and Y' is the predicted Y value.

Degrees of freedom (df) for total is $N - 1$, df for regression is the number of independent variables ($= 1$ for a linear regression), and df for residual is $df_{total} - df_{regression}$. Mean Square (MS) is obtained by dividing SS by df and the F-value is $MS_{regression}/MS_{residual}$.

Using the example of correlation between Age and BMI in Table 17.11, a regression analysis was performed. The results of the SPSS output are shown in Tables 17.13 a, b, and c on p. 268.

In Table 17.13a, the R is the multiple correlation coefficient (i.e., the correlation between all independent variables altogether and the dependent variable). In simple linear regression analysis, there is only one independent variable; therefore, R is the same as r, and $r = .290$ in Table 17.13a. The next column, R-square, indicates the shared variance and explains how much of the variance of the dependent variable is explained by that of the independent variables (8.4%). Table 17.13b shows that $F = 35.506$ and it is significant at $p < .001$, indicating that the regression line is a good fit (Appendix A, Tables D and E).

As shown in Table 17.13c, a t-test is applied to find out whether b (the regression coefficient and B in the SPSS printout) is significantly different from 0 degrees (angle of the slope) or not. If it is close to 0, the regression line will be horizontal or parallel to the X-axis, indicating there is no correlation between the two variables. Since t (-5.959) is significant, it can be interpreted that the value of Y can be predicted by value of X. In this case the regression equation ($Y = a + bX$) is:

$$Y = 48.722 - .268X.$$

Since b (B in SPSS printout) is negative, it is indicated that as people become older, the BMI score will be less. This is true since the sample is

Table 17.12 Conceptual Definitions of Analysis of Variance Table for Regression

Sources of Variance	SS	df	MS	F-value
Regression	$\sum(Y' - \overline{Y})^2$	No. of IV	SS/df	MS reg./MS residual
Residual	$\sum(Y - Y')^2$	$(N - 1) -$ No. of IV	SS/df	
Total	$\sum(Y - \overline{Y})^2$	$N - 1$		

Table 17.13 **Regression Analysis: SPSS Printout**

(a) Model Summary

Model	R	R^2	Adjusted R^2	Std. Error of the Estimate
1	.290*	.084	.082	7.10929

*Predictors: (Constant), age.

(b) ANOVA Table for Regression*

Model		Sum of Squares	df	Mean Square	F	Sig.
1	Regression	1794.526	1	1794.526	35.506	.000**
	Residual	19559.746	387	50.542		
	Total	21354.272	388			

*Dependent variable: BMI.
**Predictors: (Constant), age.

(c) Coefficients*

Model		Unstandardized Coefficients		Standardized Coefficients	T	Sig.
		B	Std. Error	Beta		
1	(Constant)	48.722	3.427		14.216	.000
	dem1b	−.268	.045	−.290	−5.959	.000

*Dependent variable: BMI.

65 years old or over. For example, if a person is 70 years old, his/her BMI can be predicted as 48.722 − .268 × 70 = 29.962.

Power Analysis for Linear Regression

For a simple regression analysis and multiple regression analysis, the effect size is calculated using f^2. The calculation formula for the effect size for the example above uses multiple correlation and it is calculated by:

$$f^2 = \frac{R^2}{1 - R^2}$$

The interpretation of the effect size index is:

• Small is $f^2 = .02$,
• Medium is $f^2 = .15$, and
• Large is $f^2 = .35$

To obtain the statistical power for regression analyses, one more step is necessary, using λ (lambda). The lambda is calculated by:

$$\lambda = \frac{R^2}{1 - R^2} \times \begin{array}{l}\text{(the number of independent} \\ \text{variables + the number of df} \\ \text{for the error variance + 1)}\end{array}$$

The power can be obtained from the Appendix A, Table K. For the detailed power analysis, consult Cohen's (1998).

Multiple Regression

The true benefit of using regression is best realized in use of multiple regression. The main purpose of multiple regression is to predict the value of a dependent variable based on several independent variables. Other purposes of regression analysis are to:

• Identify the strength of association (R^2) between the dependent variable and several independent variables together, and
• Identify variables that significantly contribute to predicting the values of the dependent variable.

In addition to the statistical assumptions for simple linear regression, one more thing that has to be considered for multiple regression is muticolinearity among independent variables in a regression equation. Multicolinearity means that the independent variables in the regression equations are highly correlated. If those variables have correlation of .80 or higher, the one that has a lower unique correlation with the dependent variable should be removed from the equation.

There are three major methods in selecting variables for a multiple regression: the standard method, the hierarchical method, and the stepwise method. Usually, one wants to find the smallest group of variables that will account for the greatest proportion of variance in the dependent variable.

Standard Method

In the standard method, all independent variables are entered into the regression equation at once. In this instance, if two independent variables overlap in accounting for the variance of the dependent variable, as indicated by the unshaded variances in Figure 17.6a, the effects of neither of these independent variables are not accounted for. This is illustrated in Figure 17.6a.

Hierarchical Method

This method is best illustrated through an example. Suppose one wants to know whether depression is a predictor of assistive device use. In this case, there are already some variables that are known to affect assistive device use (i.e., fixed factors known to influence the dependent variable), such as disability levels, age, socioeconomic status, and medications taken. Therefore, in a hierarchical regression, one wants to know whether depression makes a difference over and above these fixed factors. In such a case, one may enter the fixed factors first (so they can explain the most variance of the dependent variable) and add depression last. The variables may be entered one at a time or in subsets, but there should always be a theoretical rationale for their order of entry. Within each subset, variables may be entered in standard format as a group, or in a stepwise fashion (see the next section). Tomita, Mann, Fraas, and Stanton (2004) used this approach in predicting the number of use of assistive devices to address physical disabilities among home-based frail elders. After adjusting the effects for physical disability, number of medications taken, race, living regions, living arrangement, and education, depression was an important predictor for assistive device use.

In hierarchical regression, the variance in the dependent variable are considered to be explained by the independent variable that was entered into the regression equation prior to the other independent variables. Thus, when two variables overlap in accounting for the variance of the dependent variable, the first variable entered receives credit for predicting the variance shared between the first

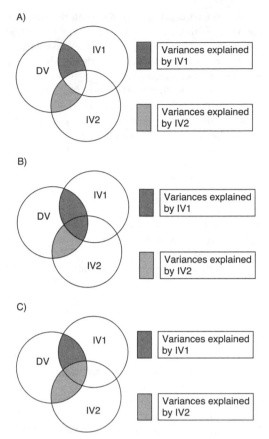

Figure 17.6 Regression methods. (A) Standard method: Shared Variances by IV1 and IV2 are not accounted for by either one of the independent variables. (B) Hierarchical method: The investigator decided to enter IV1 into the regression equation first before IV2, so the shared variance among the DV, IV1, and IV2 are explained by IV1. In this way, the investigator tests whether IV2 can explain any additional variance in the DV over and above the effects of IV1. (C) Stepwise method: The first variable entered into the regression equation was decided statistically (rather than theoretically) because it had the highest correlation with the dependent variable. Therefore, the variance that is shared by the DV, IV1, and IV2 is explained by IV2.

and second variables. This is illustrated in Figure 17.6b.

Stepwise Method

The stepwise method is generally used to identify important predictors when the field of study is still exploratory (i.e., an investigator is not testing a highly specific, theoretically grounded hypothesis). Stepwise selection is a combination of forward and backward procedures. With the stepwise solution, variables are entered using a method called the forward solution. They are assessed at each step using the backward method to determine whether their contribution is still significant, given the effect of other variables already in the equation (see Figure 17.6c). Dudek-Shriber (2004) used this approach to identify predictors among parent and infant characteristics for parent's stress level in the neonatal intensive care unit. One of the dependent variables was total stress. The most important predictor was infant cardiovascular diagnosis ($b = .504$) and the second predictor was gender of the parent ($b = -.337$), the variance accounted for was 7.4% ($R^2 = .074$), and corrected variance was 6.3% (Adjusted $R^2 = .063$). The Standard Error of Estimate was also reported (SEE = .709). In addition, the author reported the standardized beta (β) to identify which independent variables contributed more to explaining the variable of the dependent variable. The figures and their interpretations are in Table 17.14.

In Table 17.14, there are two predictors in the regression equation (presence or absence of cardiovascular diagnosis, and gender of parent, such as mother or father). The intercept (a) is 2.660, the regression coefficient for cardiovascular diagnosis is .504, that for gender is –.337. The author coded 1 for "Having cardiovascular diagnosis" and 0 for "Not having the diagnosis," and 1 for "Father" and 0 for "Mother."

The equation model to predict total means stress occurrence is 2.660 + .504 (cardiovascular diagnosis = 1 or 0) – .337(0 = mother or 1 = father). Therefore, the stress level that is found for the mother who has an infant with cardiovascular diagnosis is 3.164. The presence of cardiovascular diagnosis is a more important predictor than the gender of the parent because:

- The former was entered into the model (regression equation) first due to the highest bivariate

correlation with the dependent variable when a stepwise method is used, and
- The standardized beta weight (β), .222 is larger than the gender standardized beta, .183 (the sign is ignored) for the cardiovascular diagnosis. In the SPSS output β is called beta but the regression coefficient (b) is also a beta weight.

Absolute standardized beta weight (ignoring the positive or negative sign) is used to compare the magnitude of contribution in accounting for the variances of the dependent variable. It ranges 0 (no contribution) to 1 (total contribution). The squared multiple correlation R^2 indicates how much the variance of the dependent variable is explained by the variances of these two independent variables (i.e., cardiovascular diagnosis and gender of parent). $R^2 = .074$, which is 7.4%.

The adjusted multiple correlation represents R^2 that is corrected due to a chance occurrence. Therefore, the adjusted R^2 reflects a more accurate figure for the population, and some researchers prefer reporting the adjusted R^2 to R^2. The standard error of the estimate (SEE) indicates the accuracy of the equation model for the prediction. A smaller SEE is indicative of higher accuracy.

The stepwise solution is less popular today. Some of the reasons are: R- square values tend to be inflated, regression coefficients for some variables are inflated, and therefore, the possibility of making a type I error expands dramatically with increased numbers of independent variables. To avoid this, some statisticians say that this method requires a larger sample size than hierarchical methods. However, more serious problem is that p-values sometimes do not have the proper meaning and its correction is very difficult and increasing the sample size does not correct this problem. The preferable solution may be combine stepwise and hierarchical approaches by entering a block of variables to the regression equation hierarchically but use a stepwise regression within each block.

Table 17.14 Final Regression Model to Predict Parent's Total Means Stress Occurrence

Source	Constant a	The Most Contributing Variable b (β)	The Second Most Contributing variable b (β)	R^2	Adjusted R^2	Standard Error of Estimate
Total Means Stress Occurrence	2.660	Infant Cardiovascular Diagnosis .504 (.222)	Sex −.337 (−.183)	.074	.063	.709

Adapted from Table 7 in Dudek-Shriber, L. (2004). Parent stress in the neonatal intensive care unit and the influence of parent and infant characteristics. *The Journal of American Occupational Therapy, 58*(5), p. 516, with permission.

Analysis of Covariance

The main purpose of analysis of covariance (ANCOVA) is to control for extraneous factors (i.e., independent variables that are not a part of the theoretical model) that may influence the dependent variable. By doing so, one hopes that the variances of the dependent variable can be explained by that of the independent variables that are of particular interest. ANCOVA is a combination of ANOVA and linear regression. By removing the effect of the unwanted variables (called covariates) that are affecting the variability of the dependent variable prior to computing the group means of the dependent variables, one can achieve a more valid explanation of the relationship between the theoretically relevant dependent and independent variables.

In a study of the effects of assistive technology and environmental interventions in maintaining independence and reducing home care costs for the frail elderly Mann, Ottenbacher, Fraas, Tomita, and Granger (1999) used an ANCOVA to control for the difference in baseline (pretest) scores on the FIM motor scale between the treatment and control groups. After the intervention (i.e., providing necessary assistive devices and home modifications), the 18th month follow-up found that the difference between the two groups was significant at $p = .01$ (71.6 and 66.4, respectively). The process of adjusting the covariate (pretest scores in the example above), is illustrated in Figures 17.7a and b using hypothetical data. For the treatment group, pretest FIM Motor score was 70.83, and for the control group it was 70.83. For posttest, the treatment group was 81.25 and the control group

A)

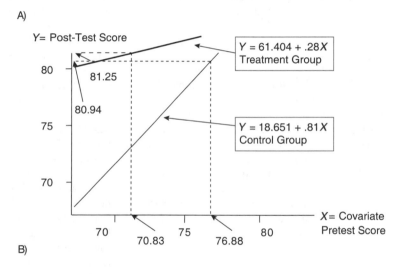

B)

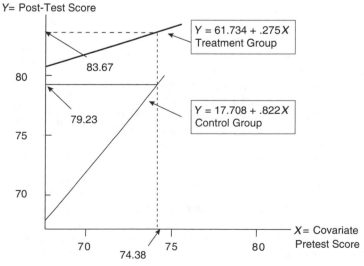

Figure 17.7 Process of ANCOVA. (A) Regression lines explaining the relationship between the initial FIM motor score (covariate) and the follow-up FIM Motor Score (dependent variable). (B) Adjusted means for follow-up FIM motor score, based on initial FIM motor score as covariate.

was 80.94. The difference of posttest scores for the two groups is statistically not significant ($p = .904$).

First, the regression lines for both groups (where the X-axis is the covariate, pretest FIM Motor score, and the Y-axis is the dependent variable, FIM Motor scores posttest) are drawn (see Figure 17.7a). The regression equation for the treatment group is $Y = 61.404 + .28X$ and that for the control group is $Y = 18.651 + .81X$. The mean score for X for the treatment group is 70.83 and that for the control group is 76.88. To eliminate the difference, one statistically equated the two groups on the pretest scores, using the mean of the total sample (74.38). One assigned this value as the mean pretest FIM Motor score for each group, and used the regression lines to predict the mean score for the posttest FIM Motor score (= dependent variable). By moving the treatment group up by 3.55 (= 74.38 − 70.83) and moving the control group down by 2.50 (= 76.88 − 74.38), one artificially made the initial scores equal. Then, the mean of the posttest ($\overline{Y}$) for the treatment group became 83.67 and that for the control group, 79.23. These are called adjusted means. This process is illustrated in Figure 17.7b. The adjusted mean score for the treatment group is higher than the actual follow-up score of FIM Motor, and that for the control group is lower than the actual follow-up of FIM Motor, thus, making a larger difference. The result is the significant difference between posttest scores of the two groups ($p = .007$). This process may work in the opposite direction, resulting in no significant difference between the two groups.

Logistic Regression

In multiple regression, the dependent variable should be measured using a continuous variable. In logistic regression, the dependent variable is a dichotomous outcome, such as "Yes" for presence and "No" for absence of a particular condition. The independent variable can be categorical or continuous. Therefore, logistic regression allows us to predict the probability (i.e., likelihood of "Yes") of an event occurring (target group) based on several independent variables. For that one uses the logarithm of the odds:

$$Z = a + b_1X_1 + b_2X_2 + b_3X_3 .... + b_kX_k$$

where Z is the natural logarithm of the odds, called a logit; a is a constant; and b is the regression coefficient or a slope. (Note: this is the usual linear regression equation.)

The probability that an individual belongs to the target group uses the logit, and is computed by:

$$\text{Probability} = \frac{e^z}{1 + e^z}$$

where e is a log of 1 (= 2.718).

Therefore, the difference between multiple regression and logistic regression is that the linear portion of the equation ($a + b_1X_1 + b_2X_2 + b_3X_3 .... + b_kX_k$) is not the end purpose, but is used to identify the odds of belonging in one of categories.

Logistic regression does not minimize the error by the least square method that is used for linear regressions. Instead, logistic regression estimates the maximum likelihood that results in the accurate prediction of group membership.

This approach is illustrated in a study that aimed to predict home-based living (the target group) or institutional living (the reference group) within a year among 276 home-based frail elders, based on their Mini Mental State Exam (MMSE) total score and Body Mass Index (BMI). Table 17.15a shows the classification table for community living and 17.15b shows logistic regression results for selected important predictors.

In Table 17.15a, step 1 is based only on the MMSE total score. As seen in the table, this score predicts 97.4% of home-based living and 40.5% of institutionalization accurately. The overall accuracy is 88.8%. Step 2 is based on the MMSE total score and the BMI. Although the accuracy for home-based living is the same, for the nursing home, the classification accuracy increased by 2.4%, resulting in 89.1% of overall accuracy. The uniqueness of logistic regression involves the use of the odds ratio. The odds ratio indicates how much more likely it is that an individual belongs to the target group than the reference group.

If the odds ratio is 1, then it does not predict classification at all. If the odds ratio is greater than 1, the change of one unit in the independent variable increases the likelihood of being classified in the target group than in the reference group. In an SPSS printout, the odds ratio is designated as Exp B. In Table 17.15b for MMSE, odds is .744, indicating if a person decreases one unit of MMSE (1 of 30), the person is .744 times more likely to be living at home than being institutionalized. Likewise, if a person exhibits one unit decrease in BMI, then the person is .890 times more likely to live at home rather than in an institution. When the coding (0 and 1) is flipped for the dependent variable, the same data would show that the odds for

Table 17.15 **Logistic Regression: SPSS Printout**

(a) Classification Table

Observed					Predicted	
				NHHOME		Percentage Correct
				1.00	2.00	
Step 1	NHHOME	1.00		17	25	40.5
	Home Based	2.00		6	228	97.4
	Overall percentage					88.8
Step 2	NHHOME	1.00		18	24	42.9
	Home Based	2.00		6	228	97.4
	Overall percentage					89.1

The cut value is .500

(b) Variables in the Equation

		B	SE	Wald	df	Sig.	Exp(B)
Step 1*	MMSE TOTAL	−.292	.046	40.474	1	.000	.74 7
	Constant	5.961	1.217	24.001	1	.000	387.936
Step 2**	BMI	−.117	.040	8.708	1	.003	.890
	MMSE TOTAL	−.296	.048	37.304	1	.000	.744
	Constant	9.299	1.788	27.059	1	.000	10931.603

*Variable(s) entered on step 1: MMSE TOTAL.
**Variable(s) entered on step 2: BMI.

the MMSE is 1.344 and that for the BMI is 1.124. They should be interpreted that when the MMSE increases one unit, the person is 1.344 times more likely to be living at home than being institutionalized and when the BIM increases one unit, they are 1.124 times more likely to be living at home than being institutionalized. Among frail elders, a lower BMI is a predictor for institutionalization. This study used a binary logistic regression. However, logistic regression can also be used when the dependent variable has more than two categories (i.e., multinominal categories). This is referred to as multinomial logistic regression. Many researchers prefer binary or dichotomous outcomes because the interpretation using odds ratios is clearer than in multinominal logistic regression.

Since logistic regression can be used for a multinominal function, this approach is becoming more popular than discriminant analysis where the statistical assumptions are more rigid than for logistic regression.

Multivariate Analysis

Multivariate analysis is conducted when there is more than one dependent variable in the analysis. In this section, factor analysis, path analysis, and multivariate analysis of variance (MANOVA) are explained.

Factor Analysis

The purpose of factor analysis is to find structure among data by reducing it. It is a statistical technique applied to a single group of variables to determine which combinations of variables in the group form unique and coherent subsets that are relatively independent from each other. Factor analysis is often used to establish construct validity of an instrument, meaning one creates or validates an instrument to describe its construct, such as depression, self esteem, quality of life, and so forth, by identifying underlying different concepts or factors. Factor analysis does not compare group means, such as ANOVA, identify the correlation between two variables, such as Pearson correlation, or predict values of the dependent variable based on several independent variables, such as multiple regression or logistic regression. Instead, this analysis produces factors that consist of a grouping of variables that are highly correlated with each other but are poorly correlated with other factors. There are two types of factor analysis: exploratory and confirmatory. In exploratory factor analysis that is this section's focus, one seeks to describe and summarize data by grouping together variables that are correlated, and it is usually performed in the early stage of research. The results are often used to generate hypotheses about underlying processes. On the other hand, confirmatory factor analysis is a much more sophisticated technique, and is used in the advanced stages of research to test a theory about latent processes.

There are two major different methods for factor analysis: principal component analysis (PCA) and factor analysis (FA). These two approaches share major procedures, and even problems. For example, both PCA and FA take steps in the following order:

1. Select and measure a set of variables,
2. Prepare the correlation matrix,
3. Extract a set of factors from the correlation matrix,
4. Determine the number of factors, rotating the factors to increase interpretability, and
5. Interpret the results.

The problems are discussed later in this section. The difference between PCA and FA is that PCA produces components and FA produces factors. In PCA, all variance in the observed variable is analyzed, while in FA, only shared variance, called covariance or communality, is analyzed. The goal of PCA is to extract maximum variance from a data set with a few independent components, while the goal of FA is to reproduce the correlation matrix with independent factors. Very often, both components and factors are referred as factors. The choice between PCA and FA depends on many things, but as a rule of thumb, if one is interested

in a theoretical solution uncontaminated by unique and error variability, FA is the choice, while one wants an empirical summary of the data set, PCA is the choice.

In this chapter, FA is explained, using the Functional Index Measure (FIM) as an example. Tables 17.16 a, b, and c show some of the steps involved in factor analysis. In this example, FIM 1 is self-care, FIM 2 is sphincter control, FIM 3 is transfer, FIM 4 is locomotion, FIM 5 is communication, and FIM 6 is social cognition.

The first step in a factor analysis is based on the observed correlation matrix, meaning the matrix created by observed variables. This correlation matrix was explained in the earlier section in this chapter. Then, the correlation matrix is used to identify the factors of the data by the process called extraction. In the beginning, the number of factor extracted is the same as the number of variables. An eigenvalue reflects the amount of the total variance accounted for by each factor. Then, the number of factors are reduced by using the eigenvalue cutoff that is conventionally 1.0. The first factor in the SPSS printout in Table 17.16a accounts for the largest variance in the data (61.754%).The second factor accounts for the second largest variance from the remaining variance (17.037%). The factor analysis presented in Table 17.16a shows only two factors, and these explain 78.791% of the total variance. The factor matrix in Table 17.16b shows the factor loadings for each of the six FIM variables and their correlations with each of the two identified factors (i.e., factors 1 and 2). Factor loadings greater than .30 are generally considered to be indicative of some degree of relationship. Two of the factor loadings for the FIM scores for both of the factors are above .30, and it is not clear as to which factors some variables such as FIM 5 and 6 belong to.

The next step is to maximize the likelihood that each variable relates highly to only one factor (i.e., that the FIM variables that show factor loadings of .30 or above for factor 1 will be different than the FIM variables that show factor loadings of .30 or above for factor 2). This is accomplished by rotating the X- and Y-axes. Although there are several ways to rotate, the most commonly used method is varimax rotation. A varimax rotation means that the two axes stay as perpendicular to each other as possible (orthogonal) as they are rotated. The results of this rotation are shown in Table 17.16c. Following rotation, it is now much clearer that FIM variables 1 to 4 belong to factor 1 and variables FIM 5 and 6 belong to factor 2. As evident in table 16c, FIM variables 1 and 2 also have factor loadings above .30 in factor 2. However, because

Table 17.16 **Factor Analysis: SPSS Printout**

(a) Total Variance Explained:

Factor	Initial Eigenvalues			Extraction Sums of Squared Loadings			Rotation Sums of Squared Loadings		
	Total	% of Variance	Cumulative %	Total	% of Variance	Cumulative %	Total	% of Variance	Cumulative %
1	3.906	65.093	65.093	3.705	61.754	61.754	2.653	44.216	44.216
2	1.166	19.427	84.520	1.022	17.037	78.791	2.074	34.574	78.791
3	.461	7.689	92.209						
4	.245	4.088	96.297						
5	.135	2.243	98.539						
6	.088	1.461	100.000						

Extraction method: Principal Axis Factoring.

(b) Factor Matrix*

	Factor	
	1	2
FIM1	.904	−.199
FIM2	.698	−.073
FIM3	.843	−.397
FIM4	.709	−.429
FIM5	.779	.557
FIM6	.762	.572

Extraction method: Principal Axis Factoring.
*Two factors extracted. Eight iterations required.

(c) Rotated Factor Matrix*

	Factor	
	1	2
FIM1	.829	.412
FIM2	.590	.380
FIM3	.906	.219
FIM4	.821	.110
FIM5	.259	.922
FIM6	.236	.923

Extraction method: Principal Axis Factoring. Rotation method: Varimax with Kaiser Normalization.
*Rotation converged in three iterations.

the factor loadings for FIM 1 and 2 are higher in factor 1, the investigator decided that FIM variables 1 and 2 should remain a part of factor 1. In cases like these when the same variable has a factor loading above .30 for more than one factor, an investigator must make a judgment call regarding where to place the variable (e.g., factor 1 versus factor 2). This judgment is made by placing the variable in the factor for which it has the higher of the two factor loadings. In our example (Table 17.16c), the factor loading for FIM 1 and 2 are higher in factor 1 (.829 and .590, respectively) than in factor 2 (.412 and .380, respectively) so the variables are placed in factor 1.

Once an investigator has identified factors within the group of variables being examined, the investigator usually gives the factors unique names or labels. These labels should reflect the unique characteristics of the cohesive variables that comprise the factor or component. Using our example, one sees that the FIM variables that comprise the first factor (component 1) include FIM 1 to 4. Since all of these share motor characteristics, this factor was named "FIM Motor." FIM 5 and 6 comprise factor 2 and it was named "FIM Cognition."

As to the required sample size, there are various opinions. Munro (2001) states that a ratio of at least 10 subjects for each variable is desirable to generalize from the sample to the population. Knapp and Brown (1995) argue that only three subjects are required for each variable. However, this estimate is on the low side and likely to increase the chances of type 1 error, particularly in a factor analysis in which issues of multicollinearity are involved. In terms of total sample size, Tabachnic and Fidell (1996) say at least 300 subjects are required to perform a factor analysis. When there are high loadings such as .80, only 150 cases may be required, according to Guadagnoli and Velicer (1988).

Since factor analysis can be subjective and judgmental owing to many choices of extraction methods and rotation methods, one should consult an experienced statistician to perform a factor analysis. Factor analysis and principal components analysis should not be confused with confirmatory factor analysis, which is an application of structural equation modeling (SEM). Confirmatory factor analysis is used when there is a theory about factors. Further explanation of confirmatory factor analysis is beyond the scope of this chapter. For a more detailed discussion, readers are referred to Tabachnick and Fidell (1996).

Path Analysis

Path analysis is a procedure that is associated with multiple regression. It is a diagram-based statistical approach used to test the strength and direction of relationships among several variables, and it enables an investigator to identify direct and indirect causal pathways among the variables. To use a path analysis, all variables should be measured on a continuous (i.e., interval or ratio) scale. For the sample size, it is recommended that there are 30 subjects per independent variable to be generalized. Path analysis can be used with cross-sectional or longitudinal study designs, but because it tests causal relationships, it is best used for longitudinal designs.

There are a number of theoretical and statistical assumptions that need to be considered in a path analysis. Theoretically, the dependent variable and the independent variable should be correlated, the dependent variable should occur later than the independent variable, and the relationship between the two variables exists even with the presence of another variable. The statistical assumptions are in addition to those of regression analysis, so the flow of causation in the model is unidirectional and the measurement error is zero.

In a path analysis, there are direct and indirect effects. The direct effects are drawn using straight lines connecting two variables and indicating the cause and effect by an arrow head. Indirect effects are indicated by lines not connecting two variables. All variables are either endogenous or exogenous. Endogenous variables are ones that are being influenced by other variables in the model. One needs to apply a regression analysis for every endogenous variable. Exogenous variables are ones that are independent of any influence.

In the study titled, "After rehabilitation: an 18-month follow-up of elderly inner-city women" (Lysack, Neufeld, Mast, MacNeill, & Lichtenberg, 2003), the authors presented a path diagram. The modified path diagram is presented in Figure 17.8.

In the diagram, there are two endogenous variables (IADL and living status) and three exogenous variables (dementia, comorbidity, and ADL). Their sample consisted of 125 older women who were living alone prior to their hospitalization, and who were then followed up 18 months after discharge. The path coefficients, seen adjacent to the lines connecting the four figures, are the same as the standardized regression coefficients (beta weights) described in regression analyses. Based on the model, the dementia is the most influential variable for IADL. ADL has a positive relationship with IADLs, comorbidity has a negative relationship with IADLs, and IADLs have a negative relationship with the status of living alone (0 = living alone and 1 = not living alone). A higher level of IADL is indicative of being able to live alone. In this diagram, all paths are direct paths, and it is an overidentified model in that there are more measured variables than the number of paths. If the numbers of variables and paths are the same, it is called an identified model, and if the number of paths is more than that of variables, it is an underidentified model.

Originally, direct paths from all four exogenous variables (depression was also integrated) to IADL were included. However, the path from depression to IADL was statistically not significant; therefore, it was removed after the analysis. Until recently,

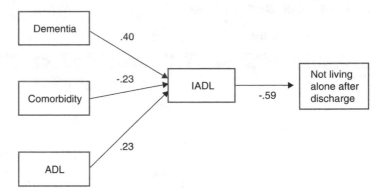

Figure 17.8 Path diagram for living alone status 18 months after discharge. (Adapted from Lysack, Neufeld, Mast, MacNeill & Lichtenberg, 2003. *The American Journal of Occupational Therapy, 57*(3), p. 303, with permission.)

investigators used regression analysis and manual calculations for path models, but currently a number of software packages are available, such as AMOS (produced by the manufacturers of SPSS). For a more complete understanding of path analysis, readers are referred to Munro (2001).

Multivariate Analysis of Variance

Multivariate analysis of variance (MANOVA) is similar to an ANOVA, but unlike an ANOVA, which is designed to manage only one dependent variable, MANOVA allows an investigator to examine outcomes for more than one dependent variable. MANOVA is used when there are several dependent variables that are theoretically and statistically correlated. When comparing group means, one considers the overall effect of the independent variable on all dependent variables together; this is called a vector $(\overline{V})$. If a score for one dependent variable changes based on an independent variable (e.g., an intervention), then the scores of the other dependent variables should also change. Suppose, for example, that there are two groups (elders who are living at home and elders living in nursing homes) and two dependent vari-

ables (number of illnesses and physical disability level), and the Pearson correlation between the two dependent variables is $r = .326$. Vectors for home-based elders are written as $\overline{V}_1 = (6.2, 27.6)$ and that for nursing home residents are $\overline{V}_2 = (5.8, 39.5)$. The vector values are shown in Table 17.17a on p. 278 in the column labeled "Mean." When the two groups are drawn, there are center points in these groups that are called group centroids. They represent the intersection of the means for both dependent variables that are the spatial location of the mean vector (Figure 17.9). The goal of the MANOVA is to determine if there is a significant difference among the group centroids. In MANOVA, the total variance in the sample is divided into parts that represent between-groups and error, variability is measured against centroids while in ANOVA, variability is measured against group means.

The null hypothesis for a MANOVA is:

$$H_0: \overline{V}_1 = \overline{V}_2 = \text{.......} = \overline{V}_k$$

Table 17.17b shows multivariate test results. Since there are two groups, Hotelling's Trace (T^2) should be used. Other statistics such as Pillai's

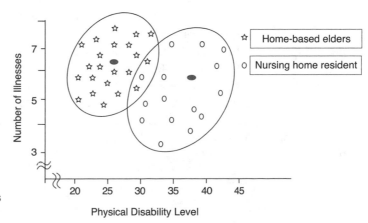

Figure 17.9 Representation of physical disability level and number of illnesses in nursing home residents and home-based elders for logistic regression.

Table 17.17 **MANOVA: SPSS Printout**

(a) Descriptive Statistics

	Living Status	Mean	Std. Deviation	N
Number of illnesses	Home-based	6.2051	2.77338	234
	Nursing home	5.8333	3.39236	42
	Total	6.1486	2.87238	276
Physical disability level				
	Home-based	27.6130	14.02267	234
	Nursing home	39.4981	16.72233	42
	Total	29.4216	15.05276	276

(b) Multivariate Tests*

Effect		Value	F	Hypothesis df	Error df	Sig.
Intercept	Pillai's Trace	.790	513.568**	2.000	273.000	.000
	Wilks' Lambda	.210	513.568**	2.000	273.000	.000
	Hotelling's Trace	3.762	513.568**	2.000	273.000	.000
	Roy's Largest Root	3.762	513.568**	2.000	273.000	.000
Living status	Pillai's Trace	.102	15.568**	2.000	273.000	.000
	Wilks' Lambda	.898	15.568**	2.000	273.000	.000
	Hotelling's Trace	.114	15.568**	2.000	273.000	.000
	Roy's Largest Root	.114	15.568**	2.000	273.000	.000

*Design: Intercept + FINAL.
**Exact statistic.

(c) Tests of Between-Subjects Effects

Source	Dependent Variable	Type III Sum of Squares	df	Mean Square	F	Sig.
Corrected model	Number of illnesses	4.922*	1	4.922	.596	.441
	Physical disability	5029.931**	1	5029.931	24.060	.000
Intercept	Number of illnesses	5160.574	1	5160.574	624.561	.000
	Physical disability	160377.932	1	160377.932	767.156	.000
Living status	Number of illnesses	4.922	1	4.922	.596	.441
	Physical disability	5029.931	1	5029.931	24.060	.000
Error	Number of illnesses	2263.987	274	8.263		
	Physical disability	57281.093	274	209.055		
Total	Number of illnesses	12703.000	276			
	Physical disability	301224.961	276			
Corrected Total	Number of illnesses	2268.909	275			
	Physical disability	62311.024	275			

*R^2 = .002 (Adjusted R^2 = −.001).
**R^2 = .081 (Adjusted R^2 = .077).

Trace, Wilk's Lambda, and Roy's Largest Root should be used when more than two groups are compared. Since it is significant ($p < .001$), the two vectors are significantly different. However, when two dependent variables are explained separately, it produces a slightly different result.

When the MANOVA demonstrates a significant effect, follow-up analyses are usually based on either univariate ANOVA or discriminant analysis. The latter may be preferable because it is still a multivariate analysis. The univariate analyses are produced by SPSS MANOVA automatically and presented in Table 17.17c. The number of illnesses is not significantly different for the two groups, but the physical disability levels are different. Nursing home residents are considerably more disabled.

Some researchers use MANOVA instead of repeated measures ANOVA with one between-factor (mixed design) because a repeated measures ANOVA has more rigid statistical assumptions than a MANOVA. If the measurements are done three times (pre-, post-, and follow-up), one can conduct a repeated measure ANOVA with three levels and one-between factor, or one can use a MANOVA with three dependent variables with one-between factor. However, many researchers use a repeated-measures ANOVA because it is more conservative and interpretable. For a MANOVA, a large sample size is required. A sample size of 20 in the smallest cell in a univariate case may be adequate.

In a study titled "Sensory processing issues associated with Asperger syndrome: A preliminary investigation" (Dunn, Smith-Myles, & Orr, 2002), 42 children with Asperger syndrome and 42 children without the syndrome were compared on both section and factor scores of the instrument, called Sensory Profile, using MANOVA. In the MANOVA results tables, the authors reported F-value, p-value, effect size (η^2), and power. Among 14 sections, 13 were statistically significant and all 9 factors were also significant, indicating that children with Asperger's syndrome have clearly different sensory processing patterns from peers without the syndrome.

Finally, when one wants to control for intervening variables, a MANCOVA will be used. A MANCOVA is similar to ANCOVA in that it combines MANOVA and regression analysis, and that treats one or more of the independent variables as covariates in the analysis. Simply stated, a MANCOVA allows an investigator to consider the effects of multiple independent and dependent variables in a single analysis, controlling for intervening vari-

ables. For more information on this topic, readers are referred to Tabachnick and Fidell (1996).

Conclusion

This chapter discussed major inferential statistics that are frequently used in occupational therapy research. The basic logic of each of the statistical approaches was discussed and illustrated. While this discussion should serve as an introduction to understanding these statistics, there are often many subtleties involved in their use. Thus, investigators are referred to more detailed treatments of the sophisticated statistics.

REFERENCES

Case-Smith, J. (2002). Effectiveness of school-based occupational therapy intervention on handwriting. *The American Journal of Occupational Therapy, 56*(1), 17–33.

Cohen, J. (1988). *Statistical power analysis for the behavioral sciences* (2nd ed). Hillsdale, NJ: Lawrence Erlbaum.

Dudek-Shriber, L. (2004). Parent stress in the neonatal intensive care unit and the influence of parent and infant characteristics. *The American Journal of Occupational Therapy, 58* (5), 509–520.

Dunn, W., Smith-Myles, B., & Orr, S. (2002). Sensory processing issues associated with Asperger syndrome: A preliminary investigation. *The American Journal of Occupational Therapy, 56* (1), 97–102,

Guadagnoli, E., & Velicer, W. F. (1988). Relation of sample size to the stability of component patters. *Psychological Bulletin, 103*, 265–275.

Haberman, S. J. (1984). *The analysis of residuals in cross-classified tables. Biometrics, 29,* 205–220.

Knapp, T. R. & Brown, J. K. (1995). Ten measurement commandments that often should be broken. *Research in Nursing & Health, 18*, 465–469.

Lysack, C., Neufeld, W., Mast, B., MacNeill, S., & Lichtenberg, P. (1993). After rehabilitation: An 18-month follow-up of elderly inner-city women. *The Journal of American Occupational Therapy, 57*(3), 298–306.

Mann, W. C., Ottenbacher, K., Fraas, L., Tomita, M., & Granger, C. (1999). Effectiveness of assistive technology and environmental interventions in maintaining independence and reducing home care costs for the frail elderly. *The Archives of Family Medicine, 8,* 210–217.

Munro, B. H. (2001). *Statistical methods for health care research* (4th ed.). Philadelphia: Lippincott Williams & Wilkins.

Parush, S., Winokur, M., Goldstand, S., & Miller, L. J. (2002). Prediction of school performance using the Miller Assessment for Preschoolers (MAP): Validity study. *The American Journal of Occupational Therapy, 56*(5), 547–555.

Siegel, S., & Castellan, N. J. (1988). *Nonparametric statistics for behavioral science* (2nd ed.). New York: McGraw-Hill.

Snedecor, G. W., & Cochran, W. G. (1991). *Statistical methods* (8th ed.). Ames, A: Iowa Sate University Press.

Stratford, P. W., Binkley, J. M., & Riddle, D. L. (1996). Heath status measures:

Strategies and analytic methods for assessing change scores. *Physical Therapy, 76,* 1109–1123.

Tabachnick, B., & Fidell, L. (1996). *Using multivariate statistics* (3rd ed.). New York: HarperCollins.

Tomita, M. R., Mann, W. C., Fraas, L., & Stanton, K. (2004). Predictors of the use of assistive devices that address physical impairment among community-based frail elders. *Journal of Applied Gerontology, 23*(2), 141–155.

RESOURCES

Web site that does statistical calculations including power analyses, visit http://members.aol.com/johnp71/javastat.html

For history of *F*-test, go to World of Visual Statistics (2004). Retrospect and prospectus. http://www.visual-statistics.net/

For the list of publication of effect size and power analyses, go to http://www.kuleuven.ac.be/psystat/power-training/References.pdf

For review of statistical power analysis software, go to http://www.zoology.ubc.ca/~krebs/power.html

CHAPTER 18

Meta-Analysis

Kenneth J. Ottenbacher • Patricia Heyn • Beatriz C. Abreu

The dramatic expansion of research in health care over the past 20 years is well documented (Institute of Medicine, 2001). Primary studies published in the healthcare research literature routinely recommend further investigation of the topic so that the findings can be corroborated. These calls for additional research are based on the belief that scientific knowledge should be cumulative. Ideally, cumulative scientific findings lead to valid knowledge that can be integrated into practice to improve health-related outcomes. In the current climate of accountability and evidence-based practice, this cumulative approach to determining scientific knowledge is extremely powerful (Abreu, 2003).

Evidence-based practice emerged in the 1990s and continues to provide a strong incentive for increased research designed to refine and guide practice in clinical fields including occupational therapy (Evidence-Based Medicine Working Group, 1992; Tickle-Degnen, 1998). Chapter 41 of this text provides a detailed description of the history and methods of evidence-based practice. The focus of evidence-based practice over the past 10 years has been to develop strategies to translate research findings into information that can be used to justify and improve clinical decision-making (Sackett, Straus, Richardson, Rosenberg, & Haynes, 2000). A sophisticated system of evaluating quantitative studies has been established to identify those investigations that provide the best evidence for determining treatment effectiveness. The system is often referred to as "levels of evidence," and provides a hierarchy of research designs and grades of evidence. Figure 18.1 includes an overview of the levels of evidence hierarchy currently used by the Center for Evidence-Based Medicine (Sackett et al., 2000; University Health Network, 2004). Inspection of the figure indicates that the strongest level of evidence is a systematic review or meta-analysis of randomized trials. The terms meta-analysis and systematic review are often used interchangeably, but there is an important difference. A systematic review does not need to contain a *statistical* synthesis of the results from the included studies. This might be impossible if the designs of the studies are too different for a statistical average of their results to be meaningful, or if the outcomes measured are not sufficiently similar, or if the studies reviewed are qualitative in nature. If the results of the individual studies are statistically combined to produce an overall quantitative outcome, this is usually called a meta-analysis. The remainder of this chapter describes the procedures used to conduct a meta-analysis. These same procedures, with the exception of computing a common statistical metric (effect size), are used to conduct a systematic review. Therefore, they can be taken as relevant to the review of qualitative research publications.

There are several systems for defining the strongest or best evidence for integrating research findings with clinical practice. Some disciplines, such as nursing, have developed variations of the levels of evidence hierarchy currently used by the Center for Evidence-Based Medicine. The vast majority of the different "levels of evidence" frameworks used in healthcare research rate meta-analyses or systematic reviews as providing the best or highest level of research evidence.

Why are the results from meta-analyses studies considered the highest level of evidence in making evidence-based decisions to improve clinical practice? Traditional quantitative studies are based on a model of hypothesis testing using statistical tests. The results of these tests provide estimates of the probability that a research hypothesis is valid and should be supported. Whenever a researcher conducts a statistical test and makes a decision about whether to accept or reject the null hypothesis, there is a chance of making an error. In a typical research study, the investigator may report a statistical value followed by $p < .05$. This means the researcher has found a statistically significant result and will reject the null hypothesis and accept the research hypothesis (i.e., that there is a difference between the groups or conditions compared). In making this decision, the researcher is usually correct, but there is also a probability of being wrong. The probability of being wrong in this case is 5% ($p < .05$). The fact that even the best controlled and most rigorously conducted study may come to an incorrect conclusion (type I or type II error) is why replication and corroboration of research findings are so important.

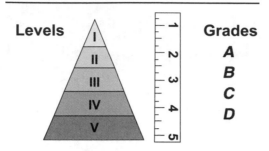

Evidence-based practice research design rating system

Levels of Evidence Based on Research Design	
Level 1*	a. Systematic review (meta-analyses) of randomized trials with narrow confidence intervals b. Individual randomized trial with narrow confidence intervals
Level 2	a. Systematic review (meta-analyses) of homogenous cohort studies b. Individual cohort studies and low-quality randomized trials (e.g. trials with <80% follow-up)
Level 3	a. Systematic review (meta-analyses) of homogenous case-control studies b. Individual case-control studies
Level 4	Case series and poor quality cohort and case-control studies
Level 5	Expert opinion without explicit critical appraisal, or based in physiological or bench research.

*Developed by Centers for Evidence-Based Medicine (http://www.cebm.net/). Not all grades are shown for each Level of Evidence.

Figure 18.1 A description of levels of evidence hierarchy used in evidence-based clinical medicine.

The details of statistical hypothesis testing are not the topic of this chapter, but are discussed elsewhere (see Chapter 17). The important point is that evidence from one study is not sufficient to draw conclusions about the outcomes of a health intervention. To determine the effectiveness of a treatment, or the validity of a scientific finding, multiple studies are required that address the same research question and produce consistent findings. Meta-analysis is a systematic method of combining the results of multiple individual research studies to answer a scientific question. The ability to obtain a statistical consensus across many studies is why meta-analysis pro-

> To determine the effectiveness of a treatment, or the validity of a scientific finding, multiple studies are required which address the same research question and produce consistent findings.

duces the highest level or best evidence in making evidence-based decisions.

The capacity to synthesize multiple research studies is at the heart of the evidence-based practice movement and philosophy. Narrative reviews of aggregated investigations have traditionally been used to synthesize information from individual quantitative research studies. These narrative reviews have been shown to be biased, subjective, and often lead to conflicting conclusions (Glass, McGaw, & Smith, 1981; Whitehead, 2002). For example, two narrative reviews were published in *Neurology* in 1989 examining the effectiveness of stroke rehabilitation programs. One paper was

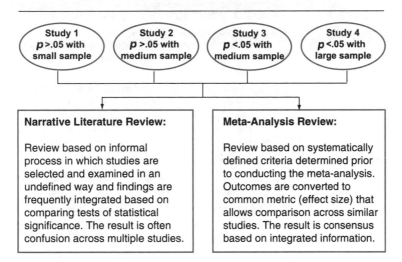

Figure 18.2 Schematic diagram of meta-analysis process including comparison of narrative review and meta-analysis methods.

titled "Focused stroke rehabilitation programs improve outcomes" (Reding & McDowell, 1989) and the second article was titled "Focused stroke rehabilitation programs do not improve outcomes" (Dobkin, 1989). Both papers were written by respected researchers and appeared in a prestigious journal. From the titles there was a clear difference in the conclusions. These two narrative reviews generated confusion rather than consensus.

The subjective and biased outcomes of narrative reviews led to the development of methodologies and techniques in the 1970s to systematically integrate findings from many individual research studies (Glass et al., 1981; Rosenthal, 1978). The procedures associated with meta-analysis are designed to treat the review process as a unique type of research endeavor that produces an objective quantitative synthesis of research results (Cooper & Hedges, 1994; Lipsey & Wilson, 2001). The procedures provide a mechanism for investigating variation in study characteristics such as sampling, design procedures, and type and number of dependent and independent variables (Cooper, 1998). Variance in these variables is then related to study outcome. This type of comparison is not possible in traditional literature reviews based on narrative descriptions of published studies. Figure 18.2 presents a comparison of the characteristics of narrative reviews of the research literature and meta-analysis.

Cooper (1989) argues that integrating separate research projects involves scientific inference. He has conceptualized meta-analysis as a unique type of research endeavor with a series of distinct steps. In the remainder of this chapter we present:

- Steps involved in conducting a meta-analysis,
- An example of a meta-analysis relevant to occupational therapy, and
- Advantages and disadvantages of meta-analysis as a research method in occupational therapy.

Steps in Meta-Analysis

Meta-analysis typically follows the same steps used in a primary research design. The investigator first defines the research question or problem, the inclusion criteria, the selection method, and the data collection process. Sample selection in meta-analysis consists of applying procedures for locating studies that meet the specified criteria for inclusion. Data are collected from studies in two ways:

- Major study features are coded according to the objectives of the review, and
- Study outcomes are transformed to a common metric called an effect size (ES), so that they can be compared.

Table 18.1 **Steps Involved in Planning, Conducting, and Reporting a Meta-Analysis Review of Published Research**

Steps	Description
1. Problem formulation	A topic that can be addressed by meta-analysis is selected followed by a formulation of a research question relevant to the topic of interest. It includes identification of the problem and formation of the research questions.
2. Data collection	A comprehensive, sensitive, and extensive search strategy is developed to compile possible reports. Key words and variables determine sources of potentially relevant reports. The inclusion criteria are defined and eligibility criteria are set for the meta-analysis. Construct definitions to distinguish relevant from irrelevant studies.
3. Data evaluation and coding	Includes three areas: 1. *Study Quality Assessment*: Assessment of the methodological quality and validity of the studies. 2. *Data Identification and Quantification*: Outcome variables are identified and extracted into a coding system. The group's contrasts and effect sizes calculations are performed. 3. *Characteristics of Interest*: General information regarding study/trial design should be standardized into a coding system for further analysis, such as treatments and sample characteristics.
4. Analysis and interpretation	It includes two areas: 1. *Statistical Procedures*: Compiling the data for quantitative synthesis and summary effect sizes by using appropriate methods and effects models (random or fixed) should be clearly stated. Effect models should explore the sources of variation if variability i present (e.g., differences in study quality, participants, treatments, or outcomes). 2. *Interpretation of Results*: Translating the results with caution and reanalyzing the data due to the robustness or uncertainty of results is desired. Results could be uncertain due to imperfections in original study reports or missing data.
5. Reporting the results	Key aspects of all of the above stages should be clearly stated in the final report in order to allow replication and critical appraisal of the meta-analysis. The process of reporting should be rigorous and explicit. Methodological limitations of both original studies and the meta-analysis should be highlighted. Implications for future research should be included.

Effect size is the name given to a family of indices that measure the magnitude of a treatment effect. Unlike significance tests, these indices are independent of sample size. They are calculated by taking the difference between control and experimental group means and dividing that difference by the standard deviation of the scores of both groups combined. It is also called delta or *d*.

The procedures necessary to conduct a meta-analysis study are summarized in Table 18.1.

Problem Formation

The first task in any research endeavor is to identify the focus or formulate the problem to be stud-

ied. In its most basic form, the research problem includes definitions of relevant variables and a rationale for relating the variables to one another. Two levels of definition are commonly associated with variables included in the problem formation step; these levels are conceptual and operational.

The independent variable or treatment must first be defined conceptually. Both primary researchers and research reviewers must choose a conceptual definition and a degree of abstractness for variables contained in the problem. The conceptual definitions employed by reviewers using quantitative methods tend to be rather broad to include all relevant instances of a particular construct. For instance, in the example described earlier the problem question might be stated as: "Do rehabilitation programs improve functional outcome for persons who have had a stroke?"

After the variables have been identified conceptually, they must be linked to empirical reality. This is accomplished by the formulation of an operational definition that relates the concept under study to concrete events. The operational definition allows the investigator to determine whether a concept is present in a particular situation.

Primary research usually involves only one or two operational definitions of the same construct. In contrast, meta-analysis reviews may involve many empirical versions of a concept. For instance, in a meta-analysis of sensory integration, the variable "sensory integration therapy" may be operationalized in a number of ways across the studies that are reviewed.

As a consequence of the variety of operational definitions of a construct, the evidence retrieved by reviewers typically contains more method-generated variance than evidence collected as primary data. The fact that a particular concept or construct may be operationally defined in a variety of ways across different studies is referred to as operational multiplicity. The presence of multiple operationalizations in a meta-analysis represents an important source of variance. Two reviewers using an identical label for a construct may employ different operational definitions. For example, in a meta-analysis on the effectiveness of rehabilitation for stroke described later in this chapter, the authors looked at the impact of rehabilitation programs for stroke on functional outcomes. Functional outcomes were operationally defined as measures of activities of daily living (ADLs), length of stay (LOS), language/cognitive tests, and motor/reflex tests. Other investigators have included physiological measures such as muscle strength, sensation, and/or proprioception as functional outcomes. A meta-analysis that operationally defines functional outcomes as only ADLs will produce different results than a meta-analysis that operationally defines functional outcomes as including measures of ADLs, LOS, and language/cognitive and motor/reflex tests.

In the problem formation stage, it is important for the researcher to provide a clearly stated research question. This question must include detailed operational descriptions of how the concepts will be defined. This, in turn, determines which studies will be included in the meta-analysis.

Data Collection

Research reviewers have multiple methods at their disposal to identify and retrieve research studies relevant to the research problem or question. As discussed in Chapter 27, the most popular and efficient method is the online computer or Internet search. The computer search is a time-saving technique that allows the reviewer to exhaustively scan several retrieval sources at a rapid rate. The fact that different electronic resources contain different journals and document indicators or descriptors is a limitation of online databases. Bibliographic searches using the same terms as descriptors or keywords may produce different results depending on the database searched.

A related retrieval approach is to employ a descendency search using the *Science* or *Social Science Citation Indexes* (Web of Science). Because the citation indexes are primarily organized by author (not topic), they are most useful when particular investigators or research papers are closely associated with an area of investigation. In contrast to the descendency approach, a reviewer may employ the ancestry method in which the reviewer retrieves information by tracking citations from one study or research report to another. Most reviewers are aware of several studies related to their problem before they formally begin the literature search. These studies provide bibliographies that cite earlier research reports that may be related to the topic under study. The most informal method of retrieving research reports occurs when researchers who are working in a particular area exchange reprints and study information (Crane, 1969).

The investigator conducting a meta-analysis samples completed studies. Reviewers may attempt to retrieve an entire population of studies rather than draw a representative sample of the studies on a particular topic. The multiple methods of study retrieval may affect the results of various reviews. Research reports available may differ from one source to another. Two reviewers who use different retrieval techniques to locate studies may end up with different sets of research reports and potentially different evidence. Diversity in information retrieval methods represents a procedural variation that may affect review conclusions. Therefore, reviewers should specify the various retrieval sources or methods they employed just as a primary researcher would report the procedures used to select subjects to include in their sample.

Data Evaluation and Coding

Each research report retrieved is examined carefully to determine whether it meets certain predetermined criteria. These criteria are formulated to eliminate studies:

• Not related to the problem under investigation, or
• Not meeting particular operational parameters.

Reviewers may differ in the identification of criteria for evaluating the relevancy of a particular research report. For instance, some reviewers may decide to include only studies published in peer-reviewed journals. Other investigators may attempt to be more inclusive and obtain research reports presented at professional meetings or in nonpublished sources such as master's theses or doctoral dissertations.

Decisions about which studies to include depend upon:

• The availability of research reports,
• How many studies there are in total,
• How many are published,
• The frequency and quality of research designs used, and
• The research question that is being examined (Petitti, 2000).

In making decisions regarding which studies to include two important questions must be addressed:

• What are the criteria for choosing studies?
• What are the implications for a particular selection strategy?

An area that requires special attention in making an evaluation decision is the type of research design used in the study (Lipsey & Wilson, 2001). There is considerable disagreement in the literature on meta-analysis regarding this issue. One approach widely used in the biomedical research literature is to include only reports published in peer-reviewed journals that are based on randomized clinical trials (RCTs). The argument supporting this approach is that these studies use designs that reduce bias and have the greatest ability to ensure that any effects are the result of the treatment (independent variable) as opposed to some uncontrolled or unknown factors (Light & Pillemer, 1984). In addition, studies appearing in scientific journals have undergone a rigorous review process and this helps ensure the validity and accuracy of the findings.

In contrast, Glass and colleagues (1981) suggest that all potentially relevant studies be included in the meta-analysis and that no prior judgments about the quality of a study design be made. They argue that the question of study "quality" and how quality variables impact on the outcome of a study can be addressed using the appropriate quantitative reviewing methodology. Previous research has reported mixed results regarding the impact of

The Cochrane Collaboration

The Cochrane Collaboration (2004) was started in 1993 and is the largest organization in the world engaged in the production and maintenance of systematic reviews and meta-analyses related to health care. There are 50 Cochrane Collaboration Review Groups responsible for reviews within particular areas of health care. The groups review and evaluate published meta-analyses from existing journals. They synthesize this evidence and then present it in a standard structured way. The reviews and summaries are available online as part of the Cochrane Library (http://www.cochrane.org/). The Cochrane Collaboration only includes randomized trials in its database of clinical or therapeutic outcome studies.

study design on outcomes. In some research areas, the design is associated with a higher probability of achieving a positive or negative outcome (Colditz, Miller, & Mosteller, 1989). Generally, the poorer or lower level designs (see Figure 18.1) are associated with a higher likelihood of a positive outcome. Other studies have found no relationship between design characteristics, such as random assignment of subjects, and study outcome (Concato, Shah, & Horwitz, 2000). The researcher conducting a meta-analysis must make a decision regarding which approach to use in evaluating whether to include a study in the final group of articles to be examined.

Once the evaluation decisions have been clearly specified, information is extracted from the individual studies. In a primary research study, data are collected from the individual subjects participating in the investigation. In a meta-analysis, information is gathered by coding the characteristics of the individual studies. Systematic coding frames are developed to record information and outcomes from each individual study. An example of a coding frame used in a recent meta-analysis examining the effects of exercise programs on physical, behavioral, and social outcomes in older adults with dementia or Alzheimer's disease (Heyn, Abreu, & Ottenbacher, 2004) is in Figure 18.3.

The accuracy and reliability of the coding process and information recorded on the coding frame must be determined. This is accomplished by having more than one rater record information from the study and then comparing their independent ratings.

The reliability and accuracy of collecting information from the primary studies included in a

UTMB/TLC Interventions Trial Quality Form
Systematic Review of Exercise Training & Physical Activity for Elderly People with Dementia and Cognitive Impairments

SINGLE STUDY QUALITY SCORE

Study Quality Points (%)
___ ≥22 points (≥95%) = Very High
___ 19–21 points (81-92%) = High
___ 16–18 points (70-81%) = Medium
___ ≤15 points (≤69%) = Low

Grade of Evidence
___A ___B ___C ___D ___E
Level of Evidence
___1 ___2 ___3 ___4 ___5
___a ___b ___c

Rater Name: ______________________________ **Date** ________

Study Author and Year: ______________________________

Study Title: ______________________________

Recommendation for analysis: ☐ Yes ☐ No ☐ Unclear

IVS: ☐ 3 ☐ 2 ☐ 1 **EVS:** ☐ 3 ☐ 2 ☐ 1

A. Descriptions	**Yes**	**No**	**Unclear**	
♦ Was the study population well described (time, place, & person)?	1. ☐	☐	☐	
Was the intervention well described (what, how, who, where)?	2. ☐	☐	☐	Total
	+____ / 2	-____ / 2	0 ____ / 2	____ / 2
Comments:				

B. Sampling	**Yes**	**No**	**Unclear**	
♦ Did the authors specify the sampling frame or universe of selection for the study population?	3. ☐	☐	☐	
♦ Did the authors specify the screening criteria for study eligibility (MMSE of † 25; or CI descriptions as stated by primary study author)?	4. ☐	☐	☐	
♦ Was the population that served as the unit of analysis the entire eligible population?	5. ☐	☐	☐	
Are there other selection bias issues not otherwise addressed (high refusal, inappropriate control, restricted sampling) ?	6. ☐	☐	☐	TOTAL
	+____ / 4	-____ / 4	0 ____ / 4	____ / 4
Comments:				

C. Measurement	**Yes**	**No**	**Unclear**	
♦ Did the authors attempt to measure exposure to the intervention?	7. ☐	☐	☐	
♦ Was the exposure variable:				
o Valid (Cronbach's alpha)?	8. ☐	☐	☐	
o Reliable (consistent, reproducible, Interrater, ICC, Kappa)?	9. ☐	☐	☐	
♦ Where the outcome and other independent (or predictor) variables:				
o Valid?	10. ☐	☐	☐	
o Reliable (consistent & reproducible)?	11. ☐	☐	☐	TOTAL
	+____ / 5	-____ / 5	0 ____ / 5	____ / 5
Comments:				

D. Data Analysis	**Yes**	**No**	**Unclear**	
♦ Did the authors conduct appropriate statistical testing by:				
o Conducting statistical testing (when appropriate)?	12. ☐	☐	☐	
o Reporting which statistical tests were used?	13. ☐	☐	☐	
o Controlling for design effects in the statistical model?	14. ☐	☐	☐	
o Controlling for repeated measures in populations that were followed over time?	15. ☐	☐	☐	
o Controlling for differential exposure to the intervention?	16. ☐	☐	☐	

(continued)

Figure 18.3 An example of a coding frame used in a recent meta-analysis examining the effects of exercise programs on physical, behavioral, and social outcomes in older adults with dementia or Alzheimer's disease (Heyn, Abreu, & Ottenbacher, 2004).

		Yes	No	Unclear	
o	Using a model designed to handle multi-level data when they included group-level and individual co-variates in the model?	17. ☐	☐	☐	
o	Are there other problems with the data analysis? Describe.	18. ☐	☐	☐	Total
		+ _____ 7	- _____ 7	0 _____ 7	_____ 7

Comments:

E. Interpretation of Results	**Yes**	**No**	**Unclear**	
♦ Did at least 80% of enrolled participants complete the study?	19. ☐	☐	☐	
♦ Did the authors assess the confounding variables?				
o Whether the units of analyses were comparable prior to exposure to the intervention (report p values and ICC for demographic age & gender)?	20. ☐	☐	☐	
o Correct for controllable variables or institute study procedures to limit bias appropriately (e.g., randomization, restriction, matching, stratification, or statistical adjustment)?	21. ☐	☐	☐	Totals
	+ _____ 3	- _____ 3	0 _____ 3	_____ 3

Comments:

F. Reporting of Biases or Confounders	**Yes**	**No**		
♦ Check yes if authors reported all or most potential biases or unmeasured/contextual confounders.	22. ☐	☐	☐	Total
	+ _____ 1	- _____ 1	0 _____ 1	_____ 1

Comments:

				TOTAL
				_____ 22

22A. Grade for Internal Validity

	Definition (after Portney & Watkins, 2000)
Internal Validity	Represents the degree of confidence that the results of a study can be attributed to the intervention rather than to flaws in the research design (confidence in the relationship between the independent and dependent variables). 10 areas that can lower the confidence are: selection, history, maturation, repeated testing, instrumentation, regression to the mean, experimental mortality, selection —maturation interaction, and experimenter bias. A variable is an observed and measurable characteristic or concept: the independent variable is the causal intervention or manipulation, and the dependent variable is the outcome measure.
3	High internal validity: no alternate explanation for outcome.
2	Moderate internal validity: attempt to control for lack of randomization.
1	Low internal validity: 2 or more serious alternative explanations for outcome.

Internal Validity Score (IVS): _____

22B. Grade for External Validity

	Definition (after Portney & Watkins, 2000)
External Validity	Refers to the degree to which the findings of the study are useful and generalized outside the experimental participants, setting and times. It is the heterogeneity of the sample that allows you to generalize well. (i.e. age range, one gender, a specific diagnosis, one level of function).
a (3)	High external validity: S's represent population – AND – treatments represent current practice. If the participants, settings and times are all varied the level is High
b (2)	Moderate external validity: between high and low. If 2 of 3 (participants, settings, or times) are varied the level is Moderate.
c (1)	Low external validity: heterogenous sample without being able to understand whether effects were similar for all diagnoses – OR – treatment does not represent current practice. If only 1 of 3 (participants, settings, or times) is varied the level is Low.

External Validity Score (EVS): _____

Figure 18.3 *(Continued)*

Confounders for Internal Validity
(From the 1st Measure to the 2nd Measure)

1. History: The potential effect that participation in specific events that may be responsible for change in the outcome (dependent) variable. (i.e. participation in other therapies, or global event state law mandating specific behaviors)

2. Maturation: The potential effect that passage of time affecting subjects or measures that may be responsible for change in the outcome (d)v. (i.e. growing older, stronger, healthier, more experience, weaker, tired, or bored)

3. Attrition: The potential effect that (also called experimental mortality) the loss of study subjects by dropout or death may be responsible for changing the randomness. (i.e. group with unequal variances)

4. Testing: The potential effect that the pretest or repeated measure may be responsible for change in the outcome (dependent) variable. (i.e. coordination tests may be reactive measures)

5. Instrumentation: The potential effect (non-reliable testing) that the calibration, observer or tester experience and skill may be responsible for the change in the outcome (dependent) variable.

6. Statistical Regression: The potential effect of a (non-reliable) test to tend to extreme scores on pretest to regress toward the mean of the post-test and be responsible for the change in the outcome

7. Selection: The potential effect that the difference between the groups (control vs treatment) cannot be balanced out.

8. Interaction: The potential effect that the interaction between any combination of selection, maturation, history, and/or instrumentation may be responsible for the change in the outcomes.

9. Treatment: The potential effect that ambiguity of cause-effect, diffusion of treatment, imitation of treatment, compensatory equalization of treatments, compensatory rivalry and resentful demoralization of participants receiving less desirable treatment causes the differences in outcomes.

10. Experimental Bias: The potential effect that the experimenter or subjects expectation or best presentation: is not representative of natural behavior.

Grade of Recommendation	Level of Evidence	Therapy/Prevention, Aetiology/Harm
A	1a	SR (with homogeneity) of RCTs
	1b	Individual RCT (with narrow Confidence Interval)
	1c	All or none
B	2a	SR (with homogeneity) of cohort studies
	2b	Individual cohort study (including low quality RCT; e.g., <80% follow-up)
	2c	Outcomes Research
C	3a	SR (with homogeneity) of case-control studies
	3b	Individual Case-control Study
D	4	Case-series (and poor quality cohort and case-control studies)
E	5	Expert opinion without explicit critical appraisal, or based on physiology, bench research or first principles

Figure 18.3 *(Continued)*

meta-analysis is improved when the definitions for treatments, outcomes, study design, subject characteristics, and other variables are clearly and completely described.

Another potential problem in extracting information from studies is coder bias. Strategies have been developed to help reduce coder bias including training and pilot testing the coding forms. One method to reduce bias is to have examiners code the introduction, demographics, and methodology sections of the article without knowledge of the findings. The results and discussion section of the article are rated independently so that they will not be influenced by the knowledge of the study design and type of subjects participating or by knowledge of the investigators or institution where the research was conducted. A comprehensive discussion regarding how to evaluate coding decisions and reduce error and bias are available in the literature (Orwin, 1994; Stock, 1994).

Analysis and Interpretation

The traditional criterion for gauging the importance of quantitative research findings is statistical significance. Significance testing is strongly influenced by the size of the sample and various authorities have questioned its continued use in empirical research (Carver, 1978). Significance testing, which compares an observed relation to the chance of no relation, becomes less informative as evidence supporting a phenomenon accumulates (Hunter & Schmidt, 1994).

The question turns from whether a treatment effect exists to how much of an effect exists. Effect size measures can play an important role in determining the degree to which a treatment exerts an influence on different outcomes. As noted earlier, the use of a summary statistical measure such as an effect size is what distinguishes meta-analysis from systematic reviews.

Two primary methods were originally advocated to statistically integrate results across multiple studies:

- Combining probabilities by adding z-scores and
- Explaining variation in study effect sizes.

The technique of combining probabilities, referred to as the Stouffer Method, is easy to compute when probability levels are reported. However, the method of combining probabilities has two major inadequacies:

- Studies with significant p-levels are more likely to be published than are studies with nonsignificant p-levels.
- The technique does not tap the wealth of information contained in the variation of results found in multiple studies.

As a consequence, the method of combining probabilities is rarely used in current meta-analysis investigations.

Quantitative procedures capable of uncovering systematic variation in study outcomes were pioneered by Cohen (1988). He defines an effect size

measure as the "degree to which the null hypothesis is false." Cohen developed and cataloged effect size measures appropriate for use with most types of research design and statistical analysis. Three types of effect sizes are used in most meta-analyses conducted in occupational therapy research:

- The standardized mean difference,
- The odds ratio, and
- The correlation coefficient.

Table 18.2 contains a brief description of each of these measures of effect size.

There are other types of effect size measures available to investigators conducting a meta-analysis and these effect sizes are described in many excellent publications available on meta-analysis (Cooper & Hedges, 1994; Petitti, 2000). The standardized mean difference or d-index is among the most widely used effect size in meta-analysis studies reported in occupational therapy. For example, Vargas and Camilli (1999) used d-indexes to compare the effects of sensory integration therapy to conditions in which the subjects either received no therapy or a comparison therapy. The d-index is a number that tells how far apart two group means are in terms of their common standard deviation. If a d-index equals 0.3, it indicates that 3/10 of a standard deviation separates the average person in the two groups being compared. This effect size transforms the results from any two-group comparison into a standardized metric, regardless of the original measurement scales.

The d-index can be computed from t and F ratios when means and standard deviations are not reported in an article. Friedman (1968) has provided formulas and a rationale for transforming t and F values to d-indexes. In cases where t and F ratios are not reported, they may be estimated from the significance level and sample size. When nonparametric statistics or percentiles are reported, effect sizes can be computed using procedures described by Glass and others (Glass et al., 1981; Hedges & Olkin, 1985).

Cohen (1988) presents several measures of distribution overlap meant to enhance the interpretability of effect size indexes. The overlap measure most often employed in meta-analysis is called U_3.

> The reliability and accuracy of collecting information from the primary studies included in a meta-analysis is improved when the definitions for treatments, outcomes, study design, subject characteristics, and other variables are clearly and completely described.

Table 18.2 **Description of Effect Size Measures Commonly Used in Occupational Therapy Meta-Analysis Studies**

Effect Size	Formula	Description	Range
d-Index	$$\overline{ES} = \frac{\overline{X}_{G1} - \overline{X}_{G2}}{S_{pooled}}$$	The d-index represents a standardized group for a contrast *continuous* measure. It is commonly used for designs where two groups or conditions are compared. X represents mean of groups and S_{pooled} is the pooled standard deviation (some situations use control group standard deviation). Sometimes referred to as "g."	0.20–0.49 small 0.50–0.79 medium > 0.80 large
Odds ratio*	$$\overline{ES} = \frac{ad}{bc}$$	The odds ratio is based on a 2 × 2 contingency table, such as the one below. The odds ratio is the odds of success in the treatment group relative to the odds of success in the control group.	1.50–2.49 small 2.50–4.29 medium > 4.30 large
r-index	$$\overline{ES} = r$$	Represents the strength of association between two continuous measures. Generally reported directly as "r" (the Pearson product moment coefficient).	0.10–0.24 small 0.25–0.39 medium > 0.40 large

*2 × 2 Table used to compute odds ratio.

		Frequencies	
		Success	**Failure**
	Treatment group	a	b
	Control group	c	d

The U_3 value indicates the percentage of the population with the smaller mean (generally control groups) that is exceeded by the average person in the population with the higher mean (generally treatment groups). Figure 18.4 presents the overlapping distributions for two groups of subjects being compared in a meta-analysis investigation. The U_3 associated with a d-index of 0.30 is 61.8. This means that the average performance of subjects in the higher meaned (treatment) groups is

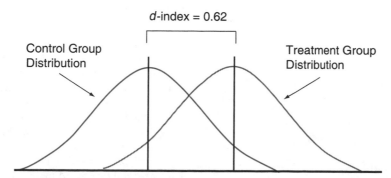

Figure 18.4 Overlapping distributions of effect sizes from the control group and treatment group. The U_3 associated with a d-index of 0.62 is 0.73. The U_3 value indicates that the average performance of subjects in the higher meaned (treatment) groups is "better" than 73% of the subjects in the lower meaned (control or comparison) groups not receiving the intervention.

"better" than 61.8% of the subjects in the lower meaned (control or comparison) groups not receiving the particular intervention or independent variable.

Once the type of effect size to be used has been determined, there are several other analysis concerns that the investigator must address. One of the most important is dealing with potential sampling bias and error in the studies examined. It is generally accepted that effect sizes should be weighted based on the number of participants included in the individual study. This is because large samples will produce more accurate population estimates. For example, a *d*-index or *r*-value based on a sample of 500 subjects will give a more precise estimate of the true population effect size than a sample of 50 subjects. Effect sizes from the studies included in the meta-analysis should reflect this fact. Various sample size weighting systems have been developed for different effect size measures.

Another sampling related concern is the degree of variability present in the sample of effect size values included in the meta-analysis study. This is tested by what is called a homogeneity analysis. The sample of effect size values generated by a meta-analysis will vary due to normal sampling error. The researcher wants to know if the amount of variability in the effect sizes is greater than would be expected by chance (sampling error). The homogeneity analysis asks the question: Is the observed variance in effect sizes significantly different from that expected by sampling error? If the answer is "No," then some statisticians would argue the analysis should stop, since sampling error is the simplest explanation for why effect sizes differ. If the answer is "Yes," that is, the variance in effect size values is larger than would be expected from sampling error, then the investigator begins to examine whether study characteristics, such as research design are associated with differences in effect sizes. The sophistication of statistical procedures to examine this variation has increased dramatically over the past decade and is beyond the scope of this introductory chapter. Information on statistical methods used in meta-analysis to test the homogeneity of effect sizes is provided in a number of excellent sources (Cooper & Hedges, 1994; Hedges & Olkin, 1985).

Reporting Results

Cooper (1989) observed that reviewers using traditional narrative methods have no formal guidelines describing how to structure the final report of their findings (see Figure 18.2). Narrative reviewers have traditionally followed informal guidelines

provided by previous reviews on the same or related topics. In most cases, the reviewer chooses a format that is convenient for the particular review problem. Cooper (1989) proposed that reviewers employing quantitative methods report their results using a format similar to that employed by investigators conducting primary research studies. The results of a meta-analysis should include Introduction, Methods, Results, and Discussion sections.

In the Introduction, the investigator identifies the problem under review and discusses the results of previous research and traditional literature reviews. The need for a meta-analysis is established in the Introduction. The Methods section describes the procedures the reviewer used to retrieve research reports and the sources searched. Information on the number of studies selected, criteria used for inclusion, and coding of studies (i.e., what information was extracted from each research report) is also included in this section of the meta-analysis. The Results section includes the findings of the quantitative synthesis and should contain information on the type of effect size used, how it was computed, the basic unit of analysis, and the actual statistical outcomes. Finally, the Discussion section allows the reviewer to summarize the findings, compare them to previous narrative reviews and primary research studies, and suggest areas in need of further investigation.

Table 18.3 lists a number of meta-analyses that have been published on topics directly relevant to occupational therapy. These studies provide examples of how to conduct and report the findings of meta-analyses in the professional and research literature.

An Example Relevant to Occupational Therapy

The narrative reviews regarding stroke rehabilitation referred to in the introduction were published in 1989 and did not include meta-analysis procedures. They led to confusion regarding the effectiveness of stroke rehabilitation programs. In 1993, a meta-analysis was published in *Neurology* titled "Results of clinical trials in stroke rehabilitation research" (Ottenbacher & Jannell, 1993). This meta-analysis involved 36 clinical trails examining stroke rehabilitation and included a total of 3,717 patients. The overall quantitative results suggested that the average patient in the treatment group receiving a focused program of stroke rehabilitation had a better outcome than 65.5 percent of the patients in the control groups not receiving reha-

Table 18.3 **Occupational Therapy Related Meta-Analysis Articles**

Year	Author(s)	Topic
1985	Ottenbacher & Peterson	Vestibular stimulation research
1986	Cusick, A.	Research in occupational therapy
1993	Ottenbacher & Jannell	Clinical trials in stroke
1996	Carlson et al.	Occupational therapy for older patients
1997	Lin, Wu, Tickle-Degnen, & Coster	Occupational embedded exercise
1998	Wu	Context and CVA
1998	Tickle-Degnen	Collaborative treatment
1999	Vargas & Camilli	Sensory integration treatment
2000	Sudsawad	Kinesthetic training and handwriting in children
2000	Dennis & Rebeiro	Occupational therapy and mental health
2002	Horowitz	Geriatric rehabilitation
2002	Reid et al.	Seated mobility devices and performance of users and caregivers
2002	Trombly & Ma	Occupational therapy for stroke, part 1
2002	Ma & Trombly	Occupational therapy for stroke, part 2
2002	Deane et al.	Paramedical therapies and Parkinson's disease
2002	Steultjens et al.	Occupational therapy for rheumatoid arthritis
2003	Mulligan	Sensory integration and children
2003	Handy et al.	Upper limb function after stroke
2003a	Steultjens et al.	Occupational therapy for multiple sclerosis
2003b	Steultjens et al.	Occupational therapy for stroke (cognition)
2004	Steultjens et al.	Occupational therapy for children with cerebral palsy
2004	Kielhofner et al.	Outcomes research

bilitation (d-index of 0.40). The 65.5% represents an example of the U_3 value described earlier.

All primary research studies included in the meta-analysis involved a comparison between a group of persons who received a focused program of rehabilitation following a stroke and a group that received standard medical care on a neurological or medical unit within the hospital. The outcome measures in this meta-analysis were categorized as ADLs, visual/perceptual, language/cognition, length of stay, motor/reflex, and other. The consistency and accuracy of the coding for all study characteristics were examined by having three raters independently review and complete the coding form for 20 randomly selected studies. The intraclass correlation coefficient values ranged from 0.77 to 1.00, indicating good to excellent agreement for the items on the coding form used in the analysis.

The meta-analysis found the largest effect size (d-index) for measures labeled as ADL and the smallest average effect size for language/cognition measures. An important variation in study results was found related to the type of research design. The type of research design was coded in each study as experimental, quasi-experimental, or pre-experimental. There was a significant difference in the average effect size (d-index) based on whether the outcome measure was blindly recorded. Blind recording means that the persons collecting the outcome information did not know if the individual subject was a member of the treatment or control group. The impact of blind recording, however, was only found for research designs in which subjects were not randomly assigned to a treatment or control group (pre- and quasi-experimental designs). Figure 18.5 displays the interaction between research design and how the outcome measures were recorded.

In contrast to the narrative literature reviews published in 1989 (Dobkin, 1989; Reding & McDowell, 1989) that reported conflicting findings regarding the effectiveness of stroke rehabilitation programs, the stroke rehabilitation meta-analysis illustrates how quantitative reviewing procedures can produce consensus by systematically combin-

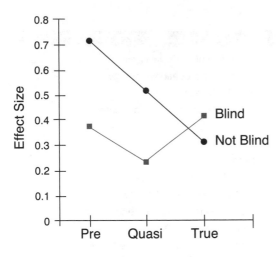

Figure 18.5 Interaction between type of research design and method of recording outcome measure (blind versus not blind). (Reprinted with permission from Ottenbacher, K.J., & Jannell, S.J. [1993]. The results of clinical trials in stroke rehabilitation research. *Neurology*, 50, 37–44.)

ing the results of multiple studies. This meta-analysis also illustrates how study design characteristics can be examined in unique ways not possible in a single or primary research investigation. The meta-analysis on stroke rehabilitation outcomes found an interaction between blind recording of the outcome measures and type of study design. This information is important to the interpretation of existing research investigations in this area, but is also important to researchers planning future studies.

Advantages and Limitations of Meta-Analysis

Light and Pillemer (1984) have identified four specific advantages in the use of meta-analysis to integrate studies. These advantages include:

• Increased statistical power,
• Obtaining an estimate of the magnitude of experimental effects,
• Greater insight into the nature of relationships among variables, and
• The ability to objectively explore contradictions in a group of studies.

Statistical power is related to the sensitivity or ability of a study to find a true difference between

groups (treatment and control groups) when a difference actually exists. Statistical power is directly influenced by sample size; the larger the sample size, the greater the statistical power when all other factors remain the same. Statistical power is also associated with type II errors. A type II error occurs when a researcher mistakenly rejects a null hypothesis (indicating no difference between groups) although a difference actually does exist (see Chapter 17).

Meta-analysis increases statistical power by increasing the sample size used in making comparisons between groups. For example, in the meta-analysis examining the effectiveness of stroke rehabilitation the combined sample size for the 36 studies was 3,717. This sample size is much larger than the sample size included in any individual primary research study and ensures that the results generated from the meta-analysis will not be a type II error.

The second advantage is the ability to determine the magnitude of a treatment effect. This advantage is related to the distinction between findings that are statistically significant versus findings that are clinically or practically important. Statistical significance is an all-or-none determination based on a probability level, usually $p < .05$. Effect sizes, in contrast, allow for a range of interpretations. The interpretations require judgments on the part of the researcher or reader. As implied earlier, statistical significance is closely related to sample size, such that with large sample sizes small differences between groups may be statistically significant. These small differences may have limited practical importance. In contrast, large differences that are practically important may not be statistically significant if the sample size is small.

Measures of effect size provide a more direct indication of treatment impact. Effect size measures can be converted to percent differences using indexes such as the U_3 value described earlier. For example, the d-index of 0.40 reported for the stroke rehabilitation meta-analysis described earlier can be converted to a U_3 value of 65.5% (Cohen, 1988). This U_3 value means that the average person in the treatment groups receiving stroke rehabilitation did 15.5% better than the average person in the control or comparison group who received standard medical care. Using this information, the reader is able to make a judgment regarding whether a 15.5% increase in performance is clinically or practically important.

The third advantage of meta-analysis is the ability to better understand the relationship between study subject characteristics and study outcome. Since multiple studies are included in a meta-analysis, there is greater variability in study design and subject characteristics than are found in an individual primary research study. This variability allows the researcher conducting a meta-analysis to examine questions that cannot be asked in a primary study. The meta-analysis on stroke rehabilitation provides an example of such a question. As noted in the previous section, an interaction was found between the type of research design (per-experimental, quasi-experimental, and true-experimental) and how the outcome measures were recorded (blind recording versus not blind) (see Figure 18.5). This relationship could not have been found in a primary research study.

> Meta-analysis is particularly relevant to disciplines such as occupational therapy that are in the early stages of developing theory and research to support clinical practice.

The final advantage is the potential to explore contradictions across a series of primary research studies. Meta-analysis allows the investigator to systematically examine moderating or confounding variables that may explain contradictory outcomes in primary studies. For example, if age is a variable that impacts the outcome of interest so that a treatment is more likely to work for subjects older than 60 years of age than for those younger than age 60, this can be detected in a meta-analysis; a meta-analysis may help explain why previous studies including younger subjects produce results different or contradictory to studies using the same treatment, but that include older subjects.

Meta-analysis procedures also have limitations that must be recognized and acknowledged. Meta-analysis methods contain aspects of both art and science, as does all research. The science is revealed in the systematic application and definition of a research approach related to literature reviewing. The art refers to the judgments that need to be made in the application of the procedures. Like all research methods, meta-analysis involves assumptions that must be made explicit, and if these assumptions are not clear to the user or reader, misleading conclusions may occur.

The ability of meta-analysis procedures to test certain interactions or relationships contained within aggregated studies does not mean that all problems of conceptualization or methodological artifact can be resolved in this manner. As in evaluating a single study, alternate conceptualizations of included treatment variables may rival the one offered. In addition, some readers may judge that the quantitative synthesis of results from mul-

tiple studies may create an illusion of statistical objectivity that is not justified by the data obtained from the review. Related to the issue of statistical precision is the fact that multiple hypotheses tests may be included in a single research report and effect sizes generated from these multiple hypotheses are not independent data points. This introduces the problem of non-independence, which may affect the results of inferential statistical procedures used to analyze the data. The role of inferential statistical procedures in the data analysis stage of meta-analysis is controversial and beyond the scope of this introductory chapter (Lipsey & Wilson, 2001).

Qualitative Methods and Meta-Analysis

Researchers using qualitative methods have proposed applying the concepts associated with systematic reviews to synthesize findings from multiple qualitative studies (Paterson, Thorne, Canam, & Jillings, 2001). Upshur (2001) suggested that there are two different definitions of evidence from the qualitative perspective. The first narrative evidence he describes as primarily Qualitative/Personal and the second as Qualitative/General. Qualitative/Personal evidence is concrete, particular, and historical while Qualitative/General evidence is historical and social.

Occupational therapists have embraced qualitative methodologies in search of a better understanding of the social and personal aspects of heath care (Clark, 1993; Krefting & Krefting, 1991), in conducting individual studies; however, we were unable to find examples of systematic reviews of qualitative research in the occupational therapy literature. Examples do exist in the broader healthcare literature (Clemmens, 2003; McCormick, Rodney, & Varcoe, 2003; Varcoe, Rodney, & McCormick, 2003; Sandelowski, Lambe & Barroso, 2004).

Qualitative systematic reviews are a new research methodology and the procedures and technology are not well developed (Schreiber, Crooks, & Stern, 1997). Qualitative research has informed healthcare practitioners for decades, it deepens our understanding of human experience and of phenomena that illustrate that experience (Morse, 1997). Standards for assessing the rigor of qualitative research methods for conducting and disseminating systematic reviews need to be developed and tested (Davies & Dodd, 2002; Whittemore, Chase, & Mandle, 2001). There is also a lack of agreement regarding how to assess the quality and usefulness of qualitative studies for evidence-based practice (Marks, 1999; Morse, 1997; Morse, Swanson, & Kuzel, 2001; Paterson et al, 2001).

Practitioners traditionally combine the art and science of occupational therapy to determine the quality of clinical care. This integrative perspective requires the use of qualitative studies to improve our understanding of occupational therapy and occupational science (Giacomini, 2001). The contributions to occupational therapy evidence are complemented by both methodologies; they both can enhance client and caretaker empowerment and the quality of occupational therapy and occupational science. One of the challenges facing researchers in occupational therapy is to collectively integrate the information from multiple qualitative investigations.

In spite of the limitations and challenges cited earlier, meta-analysis represents a significant advance over the traditional narrative methods of reviewing quantitative research. Meta-analysis is particularly relevant to disciplines such as occupational therapy that are in the early stages of developing theory and research to support clinical practice. The use of meta-analysis represents an important shift in scientific thinking in which the literature review is conceptualized as a form of scientific inquiry in its own right. The continued evolution and application of meta-analysis should help researchers establish a scientifically respected foundation for evidence-based practice in occupational therapy.

REFERENCES

Abreu, B. C. (2003). Evidence-based practice. In G. L. McCormack, E. Jaffe, & M. Goodman-Lavey (Eds.), *The occupational therapy manager* (4th ed.) (pp. 351–373). Bethesda, MD: AOTA Press.

Carlson, M., Fanchiang, S. P., Zemke, R., & Clark, F. (1996). A meta-analysis of the effectiveness of occupational therapy for older persons. *American Journal of Occupational Therapy, 50,* 89–98.

Carver, R. P. (1978). The case against statistical significance testing. *Harvard Educational Review, 48,* 378–399.

Clark, F. (1993). Occupation embedded in a real life: Interweaving occupational science and occupational therapy. 1993 Eleanor Clarke Slagle Lecture. *American Journal of Occupational Therapy, 47*(12), 1067–1078.

Clemmens, D. (2003). Adolescent motherhood: A meta-synthesis of qualitative studies. *The American Journal of Maternal/Child Nursing, 28*(2), 93–99.

Cochrane Reviews. (2004). Cochrane Collaboration Website [Online]. Retrieved November 15, 2005 from http://www.cochrane.org

Cohen, J. (1988). *Statistical power analysis for the behavioral sciences* (2nd ed.). Hillsdale, NJ: Lawrence Erlbaum.

Colditz, G. A., Miller, J. N., & Mosteller, F. (1989). How study design affects outcomes in comparisons of therapy, Part 1: Medical. *Statistics in Medicine, 8,* 441–454.

Concato, J., Shah, N., & Horwitz, R. I. (2000). Randomized, controlled trials, Observational studies, and the hierarchy of research designs. *The New England Journal of Medicine, 342,* 1887–1892.

Cooper, H. M. (1989). *Integrating research: A guide for literature reviews.* Newbury Park, CA: SAGE Publications.

Cooper, H. M. (1998). *Synthesizing research: A guide for literature reviews.* Thousand Oaks, CA: SAGE Publications.

Cooper, H. M., & Hedges, L. V. (1994). *The handbook of research synthesis.* New York: Russell Sage Foundation.

Crane, D. (1969). Social structure in a group of scientists: A test of the invisible college hypothesis. *American Sociological Review, 34,* 335–352.

Cusick, A. (1986). Research in occupational therapy: Meta-analysis. *Australian Occupational Therapy Journal, 33,* 142–147.

Davies, D., & Dodd, J. (2002). Qualitative research and the question of rigor. *Qualitative Health Research, 12*(2), 279–289.

Deane, K. H., Ellis-Hill, C., Jones, D., Whurr, R., Ben Shlomo, Y., Playford, E. D., & Clarke, C. E. (2002). Systematic review of paramedical therapies for Parkinson's disease. *Movement Disorders, 17,* 984–991.

Dennis, D. M., & Rebeiro, K. L. (2000). Occupational therapy in pediatric mental health: Do we practice what we preach? *Occupational Therapy in Mental Health, 16,* 5–25.

Dobkin, B. H. (1989). Focused stroke rehabilitation programs do not improve outcome. *Archives of Neurology, 46,* 701–703.

Evidence-Based Medicine Working Group. (1992). Evidence-based medicine: A new approach to teaching the practice of medicine. *Journal of the American Medical Association, 268,* 2420–2425.

Friedman, H. (1968). Magnitude of experimental effect and a table for its rapid estimation. *Psychological Bulletin, 70,* 245–251.

Giacomini, M. K. (2001). The rocky road: Qualitative research as evidence. *ACP Journal Club, 134* (1), A11–A13.

Glass, G. V., McGaw, B., & Smith, M. L. (1981). *Meta-analysis in social research.* Beverly Hills, CA: SAGE Publications.

Handy, J., Salinas, S., Blanchard, S. A., & Aitken, M. J. (2003). Meta-analysis examining the effectiveness of electrical stimulation in improving functional use of the upper limb in stroke patients. *Physical and Occupational Therapy in Geriatrics, 21,* 67–78.

Hedges, L. V., & Olkin, I. (1985). *Statistical methods for meta-analysis.* Orlando, FL: Academic Press.

Heyn, P., Abreu, B. C., & Ottenbacher, K. J. (2004). The effects of exercise training on elderly persons with cognitive impairment and dementia: A meta-analysis. *Archives of Physical Medicine and Rehabilitation, 85,* 1694–1704.

Horowitz, B. P. (2002). Rehabilitation utilization in New York state: Implications for geriatric rehabilitation in 2015. *Topics in Geriatric Rehabilitation, 17,* 78–89.

Hunter, J. E., & Schmidt, F. L. (1994). Correcting for sources of artificial variation across studies. In H. M.Cooper & L. V. Hedges (Eds.), *The handbook of research synthesis* (pp. 323–336). New York: Russell Sage Foundation.

Institute of Medicine. (2001). *Crossing the quality chasm: A new health system for the 21st century.* Washington, DC: National Academy Press.

Kielhofner, G., Hammel, J., Finlayson, M., Helfrich, C., & Taylor, R. R. (2004). Documenting outcomes of occupational therapy: the center for outcomes research and education. *American Journal of Occupational Therapy, 58,* 15–23.

Krefting, L., & Krefting, D. (1991). Leisure activities after a stroke: An ethnographic approach. *American Journal of Occupational Therapy, 45*(5), 429–436.

Light, R. J., & Pillemer, D. B. (1984). *Summing up: The science of reviewing research.* Cambridge, MA: Harvard University Press.

Lin, K., Wu, C., Tickle-Degnen, L., & Coster, W. (1997). Enhancing occupational performance through occupationally embedded exercise: A meta-analytic review. *Occupational Therapy Journal of Research, 17,* 25–47.

Lipsey, M. W., & Wilson, D. B. (2001). *Practical meta-analysis* (Vol. 49) Thousand Oaks, CA: SAGE Publications.

Ma, H. I., & Trombly, C. A. (2002). A synthesis of the effects of occupational therapy for persons with stroke, Part II: Remediation of impairments. *American Journal of Occupational Therapy, 56,* 260–274.

Marks, S. (1999). Qualitative Studies. In A. McKibbon (with Eady, A. & Marks, S.). (Eds.), *PDQ evidence-based principles and practice* (pp. 187–204). Hamilton, Ontario: B. C. Decker.

McCormick, J., Rodney, P., & Varcoe, C. (2003). Reinterpretations across studies: An approach to meta-analysis. *Qualitative Health Research, 13*(7), 933–944.

Morse, J. M. (Ed.). (1997). *Completing a qualitative project: Details and dialogue.* Thousand Oaks, CA: SAGE Publications.

Morse, J. M., Swanson, J. M., & Kuzel, A. J. (2001). *The nature of qualitative evidence.* Thousand Oaks, CA: SAGE Publications.

Mulligan, S. (2003). Examination of the evidence for occupational therapy using a sensory integration framework with children: Part one. *Sensory Integration Special Interest Section Quarterly, 26,* 1–4.

Orwin, R. G. (1994). Evaluating coding decisions. In H. M.Cooper & L. V. Hedges (Eds.), *The handbook of research synthesis* (pp. 139–162). New York: Russell Sage Foundation.

Ottenbacher, K. J., & Jannell, S. (1993). The results of clinical trials in stroke rehabilitation research. *Archives of Neurology, 50,* 37–44.

Ottenbacher, K. J., & Petersen, P. (1985). A meta-analysis of applied vestibular stimulation research. *Physical and Occupational Therapy in Pediatrics, 5,* 119–134.

Paterson, B. L., Thorne, S. E., Canam, C., & Jillings, C. (2001). *Meta-study of qualitative health research: A practical guide to meta-analysis and meta-synthesis* (vol. 3). Thousand Oaks, CA: SAGE Publications.

Petitti, D. B. (2000). *Meta-analysis, decision analysis, and cost-effectiveness analysis: Methods for quantitative synthesis in medicine.* New York: Oxford University Press.

Reding, M. J., & McDowell, F. H. (1989). Focused stroke rehabilitation programs improve outcome. *Archives of Neurology, 46,* 700–701.

Reid, D., Laliberte-Rudman, D., & Hebert, D. (2002). Impact of wheeled seated mobility devices on adult users' and their caregivers' occupational performance: A critical literature review. *Canadian Journal of Occupational Therapy, 69,* 261–280.

Rosenthal, R. (1978). Combining results of independent studies. *Psychological Bulletin, 85,* 185–193.

Sackett, D. L., Straus, S., Richardson, S., Rosenberg, W., & Haynes, R. B. (2000). *Evidence-based medicine: How to practice and teach EBM* (2nd ed.) Edinburgh, UK: Churchill Livingstone.

Sandelowski, M., Lambe, C., & Barroso, J. (2004). Stigma in HIV-positive women. *Journal of Nursing Scholarship, 36*(2), 122–128.

Schreiber, R., Crooks, D., & Stern, P. N. (1997). Qualitative meta-analysis. In J. M. Morse (Ed.), *Completing a qualitative project: Details and dialogue* (pp. 311–326). Thousand Oaks, CA: SAGE Publications.

Steultjens, E. M., Dekker, J., Bouter, L. M., Cardol, M., van de Nes, J. C., & van den Ende, C. H. (2003a). Occupational therapy for multiple sclerosis. *Cochrane Database Systematic Reviews,* CD003608.

Steultjens, E. M., Dekker, J., Bouter, L. M., van de Nes, J. C., Cup, E. H., & van den Ende, C. H. (2003b). Occupational therapy for stroke patients: A systematic review. *Stroke, 34,* 676–687.

Steultjens, E. M., Dekker, J., Bouter, L. M., van de Nes, J. C., Lambregts, B. L., & van den Ende, C. H. (2004). Occupational therapy for children with cerebral palsy: A systematic review. *Clinical Rehabilitation, 18,* 1–14.

Steultjens, E. M., Dekker, J., Bouter, L. M., van Schaardenburg, D., van Kuyk, M. A., & van den Ende, C. H. (2002). Occupational therapy for rheumatoid arthritis: A systematic review. *Arthritis Rheumatism, 47,* 672–685.

Stock, W. A. (1994). Systematic coding for research synthesis. In H. M. Cooper & L. V. Hedges (Eds.), *The handbook of research synthesis* (pp. 125–138). New York: Russell Sage Foundation.

Sudsawad, P. (2000). The effect of kinesthetic training on handwriting performance in grade one children with handwriting difficulties. [Dissertation Abstract: 2000-95010-344]. *Dissertation Abstracts International: Section B: The Sciences & Engineering, 60* (11-B), 5472. US: University Microfilms International.

Tickle-Degnen, L. (1998). Communicating with clients about treatment outcomes: The use of meta-analytic evidence in collaborative treatment planning. *American Journal of Occupational Therapy, 52,* 526–530.

Trombly, C. A., & Ma, H. I. (2002). A synthesis of the effects of occupational therapy for persons with stroke, Part I: Restoration of roles, tasks, and activities. *American Journal of Occupational Therapy, 56,* 250–259.

University Health Network. (2004) Center for Evidence-Based Medicine [Online]. Available at: http://www.cebm.utoronto.ca/

Upshur, R. E. G. (2001). The status of qualitative research as evidence. In J. M. Morse, J. M. Swanson & A. J. Kuzel (Eds.), *The nature of qualitative evidence* (pp. 5–26). Thousand Oaks, CA: SAGE Publications.

Varcoe, C., Rodney, P., & McCormick, J. (2003). Health care relationships in context: An analysis of three ethnographies. *Qualitative Health Research, 13*(7), 957–973.

Vargas, S., & Camilli, G. (1999). A meta-analysis of research on sensory integration treatment. *American Journal of Occupational Therapy, 53*, 189–198.

Whitehead, A. (2002). *Meta-analysis of controlled clinical trials. Chichester: John Wiley & Sons.*

Whittemore, R., Chase, S. K., & Mandle, C. L. (2001). Validity in qualitative research. *Qualitative Health Research, 11*(4), 522–537.

Wu, C. Y. (1998). Effects of context on movement kinematics in adults with and without cerebral vascular accident. [Dissertation Abstract: 1998-95002-215]. *Dissertation Abstracts International: Section B: The Sciences & Engineering. 58* (7-B), 3593. US: University Microfilms International.

APPENDIX A

Statistical Reference Tables

Machiko R. Tomita

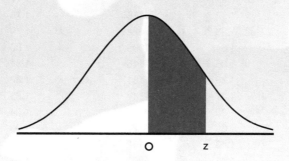

Table A Areas Under the Normal Curve Between Mean and z-Score

z	Area Between 0 and z	z	Area Between 0 and z	z	Area Between 0 and z
0.00	.0000	0.25	.0987	0.50	.1915
0.01	.0040	0.26	.1026	0.51	.1950
0.02	.0080	0.27	.1064	0.52	.1985
0.03	.0120	0.28	.1103	0.53	.2019
0.04	.0160	0.29	.1141	0.54	.2054
0.05	.0199	0.30	.1179	0.55	.2088
0.06	.0239	0.31	.1217	0.56	.2123
0.07	.0279	0.32	.1255	0.57	.2157
0.08	.0319	0.33	.1293	0.58	.2190
0.09	.0359	0.34	.1331	0.59	.2224
0.10	.0398	0.35	.1368	0.60	.2257
0.11	.0438	0.36	.1406	0.61	.2291
0.12	.0478	0.37	.1443	0.62	.2324
0.13	.0517	0.38	.1480	0.63	.2357
0.14	.0557	0.39	.1517	0.64	.2389
0.15	.0596	0.40	.1554	0.65	.2422
0.16	.0636	0.41	.1591	0.66	.2454
0.17	.0675	0.42	.1628	0.67	.2486
0.18	.0714	0.43	.1664	0.68	.2517
0.19	.0753	0.44	.1700	0.69	.2549
0.20	.0793	0.45	.1736	0.70	.2580
0.21	.0832	0.46	.1772	0.71	.2611
0.22	.0871	0.47	.1808	0.72	.2642
0.23	.0910	0.48	.1844	0.73	.2673
0.24	.0948	0.49	.1879	0.74	.2704

(continued)

Table A Areas Under the Normal Curve Between Mean and z-Score (continued)

z	Area Between 0 and z	z	Area Between 0 and z	z	Area Between 0 and z
0.75	.2734	1.23	.3907	1.70	.4554
0.76	.2764	1.24	.3925	1.71	.4564
0.77	.2794	1.25	.3944	1.72	.4573
0.78	.2823	1.26	.3962	1.73	.4582
0.79	.2852	1.27	.3980	1.74	.4591
0.80	.2881	1.28	.3997	1.75	.4599
0.81	.2910	1.29	.4015	1.751	.4600
0.82	.2939	1.30	.4032	1.76	.4608
0.83	.2967	1.31	.4049	1.77	.4616
0.84	.2995	1.32	.4066	1.78	.4625
0.85	.3023	1.33	.4082	1.79	.4633
0.86	.3051	1.34	.4099	1.80	.4641
0.87	.3078	1.35	.4115	1.81	.4649
0.88	.3106	1.36	.4131	1.82	.4656
0.89	.3133	1.37	.4147	1.83	.4664
0.90	.3159	1.38	.4162	1.84	.4671
0.91	.3186	1.39	.4177	1.85	.4678
0.92	.3212	1.40	.4192	1.86	.4686
0.93	.3238	1.41	.4207	1.87	.4693
0.94	.3264	1.42	.4222	1.88	.4699
0.95	.3289	1.43	.4236	1.881	.4700
0.96	.3315	1.44	.4251	1.89	.4706
0.97	.3340	1.45	.4265	1.90	.4713
0.98	.3365	1.46	.4279	1.91	.4719
0.99	.3389	1.47	.4292	1.92	.4726
1.00	.3413	1.48	.4306	1.93	.4732
1.01	.3438	1.49	.4319	1.94	.4738
1.02	.3461	1.50	.4332	1.95	.4744
1.03	.3485	1.51	.4345	1.96	.4750
1.04	.3508	1.52	.4357	1.97	.4756
1.05	.3531	1.53	.4370	1.98	.4761
1.06	.3554	1.54	.4382	1.99	.4767
1.07	.3577	1.55	.4394	2.00	.4772
1.08	.3599	1.56	.4406	2.01	.4778
1.09	.3621	1.57	.4418	2.02	.4783
1.10	.3643	1.58	.4429	2.03	.4788
1.11	.3665	1.59	.4441	2.04	.4793
1.12	.3686	1.60	.4452	2.05	.4798
1.13	.3708	1.61	.4463	2.054	.4800
1.14	.3729	1.62	.4474	2.06	.4803
1.15	.3749	1.63	.4484	2.07	.4808
1.16	.3770	1.64	.4495	2.08	.4812
1.17	.3790	1.645[1]	.4500	2.09	.4817
1.18	.3810	1.65	.4505	2.10	.4821
1.19	.3830	1.66	.4515	2.11	.4826
1.20	.3849	1.67	.4525	2.12	.4830
1.21	.3869	1.68	.4535	2.13	.4834
1.22	.3888	1.69	.4545	2.14	.4838

[1]$z = 1.645$. Area between $0-z = .4500$ indicates the area above $z = .05$.

Table A Areas Under the Normal Curve Between Mean and z-Score (continued)

z	Area Between 0 and z	z	Area Between 0 and z	z	Area Between 0 and z
2.15	.4842	2.58	.4951	3.03	.4988
2.16	.4846	2.59	.4952	3.04	.4988
2.17	.4850	2.60	.4953	3.05	.49886
2.18	.4854	2.61	.4955	3.06	.49889
2.19	.4857	2.62	.4956	3.07	.49893
2.20	.4861	2.63	.4957	3.08	.49896
2.21	.4864	2.64	.4959	3.09[3]	.49900
2.22	.4868	2.65	.4960	3.10	.49903
2.23	.4871	2.66	.4961	3.11	.49906
2.24	.4875	2.67	.4962	3.12	.49910
2.25	.4878	2.68	.4963	3.13	.49913
2.26	.4881	2.69	.4964	3.14	.49916
2.27	.4884	2.70	.4965	3.15	.49918
2.28	.4887	2.71	.4966	3.16	.49921
2.29	.4890	2.72	.4967	3.17	.49924
2.30	.4893	2.73	.4968	3.18	.49926
2.31	.4896	2.74	.4969	3.19	.49929
2.32	.4898	2.75	.4970	3.20	.49931
2.326[2]	.4900	2.76	.4971	3.21	.49934
2.33	.4901	2.77	.4972	3.22	.49936
2.34	.4904	2.78	.4973	3.23	.49938
2.35	.4906	2.79	.4974	3.24	.49940
2.36	.4909	2.80	.4974	3.25	.49942
2.37	.4911	2.81	.4975	3.26	.49944
2.38	.4913	2.82	.4976	3.27	.49946
2.39	.4916	2.83	.4977	3.28	.49948
2.40	.4918	2.84	.4977	3.29	.49950
2.41	.4920	2.85	.4978	3.30	.49951
2.42	.4922	2.86	.4979	3.31	.49953
2.43	.4925	2.87	.4979	3.32	.49955
2.44	.4927	2.88	.4980	3.33	.49957
2.45	.4929	2.89	.4981	3.34	.49958
2.46	.4931	2.90	.4981	3.35	.49960
2.47	.4932	2.91	.4982	3.36	.49961
2.48	.4934	2.92	.4982	3.37	.49962
2.49	.4936	2.93	.4983	3.38	.49964
2.50	.4938	2.94	.4984	3.39	.49965
2.51	.4940	2.95	.4984	3.40	.49966
2.52	.4941	2.96	.4985	3.45	.49972
2.53	.4943	2.97	.4985	3.50	.49977
2.54	.4945	2.98	.4986	3.60	.49984
2.55	.4946	2.99	.4986	3.70	.49989
2.56	.4948	3.00	.4987	3.80	.49993
2.57	.4949	3.01	.4987	3.90	.49995
2.576	.4950	3.02	.4987	4.00	.49997

[2]z=2.326. Area between 0-z = .4900 indicates the area above z = .01.
[3]z=3.09. Area between 0-z = .4990 indicates the area above z = .001.

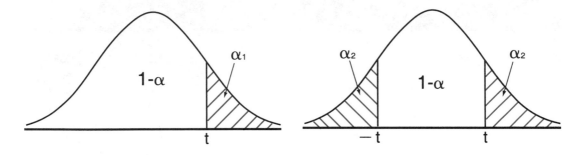

Table B Critical Values of t

df	α_1	0.10	0.05	0.025
1		3.078	6.314	12.706
2		1.886	2.920	4.303
3		1.638	2.353	3.182
4		1.533	2.132	2.776
5		1.476	2.015	2.571
6		1.440	1.943	2.447
7		1.415	1.895	2.365
8		1.397	1.860	2.306
9		1.383	1.833	2.262
10		1.372	1.812	2.228
11		1.363	1.796	2.201
12		1.356	1.782	2.179
13		1.350	1.771	2.160
14		1.345	1.761	2.145
15		1.341	1.753	2.131
16		1.337	1.746	2.120
17		1.333	1.740	2.110
18		1.330	1.734	2.101
19		1.328	1.729	2.093
20		1.325	1.725	2.086
21		1.323	1.721	2.080
22		1.321	1.717	2.074
23		1.319	1.714	2.069
24		1.318	1.711	2.064
25		1.316	1.708	2.060
26		1.315	1.706	2.056
27		1.314	1.703	2.052
28		1.313	1.701	2.048
29		1.311	1.699	2.045
30		1.310	1.697	2.042
40		1.303	1.684	2.021
60		1.296	1.671	2.000
120		1.289	1.658	1.980
∞		1.282	1.645	1.960
	α_2	.20	.10	.05

For independent t-tests $df = (n_1 - 1) + (n - 1)$
For paired t-tests $df = n - 1$
Calculated value must be greater than or equal to critical value to reject H_o.
Source: Adapted from Table 12 in Pearson and Hartley (Eds.) (1970). *Biometrika tables for statisticians.*
   New York: Cambridge University Press, with permission of Biometrika Trustees.

Table B Critical Values of t (continued)

df α_1	0.01	0.005	0.0025	0.0005
1	31.821	63.657	127.322	636.590
2	6.965	9.925	14.089	31.598
3	4.541	5.841	7.453	12.924
4	3.747	4.604	5.598	8.610
5	3.365	4.032	4.773	6.869
6	3.143	3.707	4.317	5.959
7	2.998	3.499	4.029	5.408
8	2.896	3.355	3.833	5.041
9	2.821	3.250	3.690	4.781
10	2.764	3.169	3.581	4.587
11	2.718	3.106	3.497	4.437
12	2.681	3.055	3.428	4.318
13	2.650	3.012	3.372	4.221
14	2.624	2.977	3.326	4.140
15	2.602	2.947	3.286	4.073
16	2.583	2.921	3.252	4.015
17	2.567	2.898	3.222	3.965
18	2.552	2.878	3.197	3.922
19	2.539	2.861	3.174	3.883
20	2.528	2.845	3.153	3.849
21	2.518	2.831	3.135	3.819
22	2.508	2.819	3.119	3.792
23	2.500	2.807	3.104	3.768
24	2.492	2.797	3.091	3.745
25	2.485	2.787	3.078	3.725
26	2.479	2.779	3.067	3.707
27	2.473	2.771	3.057	3.690
28	2.467	2.763	3.047	3.674
29	2.462	2.756	3.038	3.659
30	2.457	2.750	3.030	3.646
40	2.423	2.704	2.971	3.551
60	2.390	2.660	2.915	3.460
120	2.358	2.617	2.860	3.373
∞	2.326	2.576	2.807	3.291
α_2	.02	.01	.005	.001

For independent t-tests $df = (n_1 - 1) + (n - 1)$
For paired t-tests $df = n - 1$
Calculated value must be greater than or equal to critical value to reject H_o.
Source: Adapted from Table 12 in Pearson and Hartley (Eds.) (1970). *Biometrika tables for statisticians.*
New York: Cambridge University Press, with permission of Biometrika Trustees.

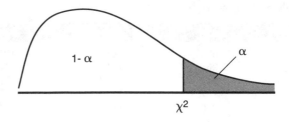

$1-\alpha$ α

χ^2

Table C Critical Values of Chi-square (χ^2)

df α_1	.05	.025	.01	.005	.001
1	3.84	5.02	6.64	7.88	10.83
2	5.99	7.38	9.21	10.60	13.82
3	7.82	9.35	11.35	12.84	16.27
4	9.49	11.14	13.28	14.86	18.47
5	11.07	12.83	15.09	16.75	20.52
6	12.59	14.45	16.81	18.55	22.46
7	14.07	16.01	18.48	20.28	24.32
8	15.51	17.53	20.09	21.96	26.13
9	16.92	19.03	21.67	23.59	27.88
10	18.31	20.48	23.21	25.19	29.59
11	19.68	21.92	24.73	26.76	31.26
12	21.03	23.34	26.22	28.30	32.91
13	22.36	24.74	27.69	29.82	34.53
14	23.69	26.12	29.14	31.32	36.12
15	25.00	27.49	30.58	32.80	37.70
16	26.30	28.85	32.00	34.27	39.25
17	27.59	30.19	33.41	35.72	40.79
18	28.87	31.53	34.81	37.16	42.31
19	30.14	32.85	36.19	38.58	43.82
20	31.41	34.17	37.57	40.00	45.32
21	32.67	35.48	38.93	41.40	46.80
22	33.92	36.78	40.29	42.80	48.27
23	35.17	38.06	41.64	44.18	49.73
24	36.42	39.36	42.98	45.56	51.18
25	37.65	40.65	44.31	46.93	52.62
26	38.89	41.92	45.64	48.29	54.05
27	40.11	43.19	46.96	49.65	55.47
28	41.34	44.46	48.28	50.99	56.89
29	42.56	45.72	49.59	52.34	58.30
30	43.77	46.98	50.89	53.67	59.70
40	55.76	59.34	63.69	66.77	73.40
50	67.51	71.42	76.15	79.49	86.66

For one-sample test, df = $k - 1$. For two sample test, df = $(R - 1)(C - 1)$ where R is number of cells in row and C is number of cells in column. Calculated value must be greater than or equal to critical value to reject H_0.

Source: Adapted from Table 8 in Pearson and Hartley (Eds.) (1970). *Biometrika Tables for Statisticians.* New York: Cambridge University Press, with permission of the Biometrika Trustees.

Table D Critical Values of F, at α = .05

| | df for Between-Groups | | | | | | | | | | | | | | | |
df for Error	1	2	3	4	5	6	7	8	9	10	12	15	20	30	60	∞
1	161.4	199.5	215.7	224.6	230.2	234.0	236.8	238.9	240.5	241.9	243.9	245.9	248.0	250.1	252.2	254.3
2	18.51	19.00	19.16	19.25	19.30	19.33	19.35	19.37	19.38	19.40	19.41	19.43	19.45	19.46	19.48	19.50
3	10.13	9.55	9.28	9.12	9.01	8.94	8.89	8.85	8.81	8.79	8.74	8.70	8.66	8.62	8.57	8.53
4	7.71	6.94	6.59	6.39	6.26	6.16	6.09	6.04	6.00	5.96	5.91	5.86	5.80	5.75	5.69	5.63
5	6.61	5.79	5.41	5.19	5.05	4.95	4.88	4.82	4.77	4.74	4.68	4.62	4.56	4.50	4.43	4.36
6	5.99	5.14	4.76	4.53	4.39	4.28	4.21	4.15	4.10	4.06	4.00	3.94	3.87	3.81	3.74	3.67
7	5.59	4.74	4.35	4.12	3.97	3.87	3.79	3.73	3.68	3.64	3.57	3.51	3.44	3.38	3.30	3.23
8	5.32	4.46	4.07	3.84	3.69	3.58	3.50	3.44	3.39	3.35	3.28	3.22	3.15	3.08	3.01	2.93
9	5.12	4.26	3.86	3.63	3.48	3.37	3.29	3.23	3.18	3.14	3.07	3.01	2.94	2.86	2.79	2.71
10	4.96	4.10	3.71	3.48	3.33	3.22	3.14	3.07	3.02	2.98	2.91	2.85	2.77	2.70	2.62	2.54
11	4.84	3.98	3.59	3.36	3.20	3.09	3.01	2.95	2.90	2.85	2.79	2.72	2.65	2.57	2.49	2.40
12	4.75	3.89	3.49	3.26	3.11	3.00	2.91	2.85	2.80	2.75	2.69	2.62	2.54	2.47	2.38	2.30
13	4.67	3.81	3.41	3.18	3.03	2.92	2.83	2.77	2.71	2.67	2.60	2.53	2.46	2.38	2.30	2.21
14	4.60	3.74	3.34	3.11	2.96	2.85	2.76	2.70	2.65	2.60	2.53	2.46	2.39	2.31	2.22	2.13
15	4.54	3.68	3.29	3.06	2.90	2.79	2.71	2.64	2.59	2.54	2.48	2.40	2.33	2.25	2.16	2.07
16	4.49	3.63	3.24	3.01	2.85	2.74	2.66	2.59	2.54	2.49	2.42	2.35	2.28	2.19	2.11	2.01
17	4.45	3.59	3.20	2.96	2.81	2.70	2.61	2.55	2.49	2.45	2.38	2.31	2.23	2.15	2.06	1.96
18	4.41	3.55	3.16	2.93	2.77	2.66	2.58	2.51	2.46	2.41	2.34	2.27	2.19	2.11	2.02	1.92
19	4.38	3.52	3.13	2.90	2.74	2.63	2.54	2.48	2.42	2.38	2.31	2.23	2.16	2.07	1.98	1.88
20	4.35	3.49	3.10	2.87	2.71	2.60	2.51	2.45	2.39	2.35	2.28	2.20	2.12	2.04	1.95	1.84
21	4.32	3.47	3.07	2.84	2.68	2.57	2.49	2.42	2.37	2.32	2.25	2.18	2.10	2.01	1.92	1.81
22	4.30	3.44	3.05	2.82	2.66	2.55	2.46	2.40	2.34	2.30	2.23	2.15	2.07	1.98	1.89	1.78
23	4.28	3.42	3.03	2.80	2.64	2.53	2.44	2.37	2.32	2.27	2.20	2.13	2.05	1.96	1.86	1.76
24	4.26	3.40	3.01	2.78	2.62	2.51	2.42	2.36	2.30	2.25	2.18	2.11	2.03	1.94	1.84	1.73
25	4.24	3.39	2.99	2.76	2.60	2.49	2.40	2.34	2.28	2.24	2.16	2.09	2.01	1.92	1.82	1.71
26	4.23	3.37	2.98	2.74	2.59	2.47	2.39	2.32	2.27	2.22	2.15	2.07	1.99	1.90	1.80	1.69
27	4.21	3.35	2.96	2.73	2.57	2.46	2.37	2.31	2.25	2.20	2.13	2.06	1.97	1.88	1.79	1.67
28	4.20	3.34	2.95	2.71	2.56	2.45	2.36	2.29	2.24	2.19	2.12	2.04	1.96	1.87	1.77	1.65
29	4.18	3.33	2.93	2.70	2.55	2.43	2.35	2.28	2.22	2.18	2.10	2.03	1.94	1.85	1.75	1.64
30	4.17	3.32	2.92	2.69	2.53	2.42	2.33	2.27	2.21	2.16	2.09	2.01	1.93	1.84	1.74	1.62
40	4.08	3.23	2.84	2.61	2.45	2.34	2.25	2.18	2.12	2.08	2.00	1.92	1.84	1.74	1.64	1.51
60	4.00	3.15	2.76	2.53	2.37	2.25	2.17	2.10	2.04	1.99	1.92	1.84	1.75	1.65	1.53	1.39
120	3.92	3.07	2.68	2.45	2.29	2.17	2.09	2.02	1.96	1.91	1.83	1.75	1.66	1.55	1.43	1.25
∞	3.84	3.00	2.60	2.37	2.21	2.10	2.01	1.94	1.88	1.83	1.75	1.67	1.57	1.46	1.32	1.00

Calculated value must be greater than or equal to critical value to reject H_o.

Table E Critical Values of F, $\alpha = .01$

df for Error	df for Between-Groups															
	1	2	3	4	5	6	7	8	9	10	12	15	20	30	60	∞
1	4052	5000	5403	5625	5764	5859	5928	5982	6022	6056	6106	6157	6209	6261	6313	6366
2	98.50	99.00	99.17	99.25	99.30	99.33	99.36	99.37	99.39	99.40	99.42	99.43	99.45	99.47	99.48	99.50
3	34.12	30.82	29.46	28.71	28.24	27.91	27.67	27.49	27.35	27.33	27.05	26.87	26.69	26.50	26.32	26.13
4	21.20	18.00	16.69	15.98	15.52	15.21	14.98	14.80	14.66	14.55	14.37	14.20	14.02	13.84	13.65	13.46
5	16.26	13.27	12.06	11.39	10.97	10.67	10.46	10.29	10.16	10.05	9.89	9.72	9.55	9.38	9.20	9.02
6	13.75	10.92	9.78	9.15	8.75	8.47	8.26	8.10	7.98	7.87	7.72	7.56	7.40	7.23	7.06	6.88
7	12.25	9.55	8.45	7.85	7.46	7.19	6.99	6.84	6.72	6.62	6.47	6.31	6.16	5.99	5.82	5.65
8	11.26	8.65	7.59	7.01	6.63	6.37	6.18	6.03	5.91	5.81	5.67	5.52	5.36	5.20	5.03	4.86
9	10.56	8.02	6.99	6.42	6.06	5.80	5.61	5.47	5.35	5.26	5.11	4.96	4.81	4.65	4.48	4.31
10	10.04	7.56	6.55	5.99	5.64	5.39	5.20	5.06	4.94	4.85	4.71	4.56	4.41	4.25	4.08	3.91
11	9.65	7.21	6.22	5.67	5.32	5.07	4.89	4.74	4.63	4.54	4.40	4.25	4.10	3.94	3.78	3.60
12	9.33	6.93	5.95	5.41	5.06	4.82	4.64	4.50	4.39	4.30	4.16	4.01	3.86	3.70	3.54	3.36
13	9.07	6.70	5.74	5.21	4.86	4.62	4.44	4.30	4.19	4.10	3.96	3.82	3.66	3.51	3.34	3.17
14	8.86	6.51	5.56	5.04	4.69	4.46	4.28	4.14	4.03	3.94	3.80	3.66	3.51	3.35	3.18	3.00
15	8.68	6.36	5.42	4.89	4.56	4.32	4.14	4.00	3.89	3.80	3.67	3.52	3.37	3.21	3.05	2.87
16	8.53	6.23	5.29	4.77	4.44	4.20	4.03	3.89	3.78	3.69	3.55	3.41	3.26	3.10	2.93	2.75
17	8.40	6.11	5.18	4.67	4.34	4.10	3.93	3.79	3.68	3.59	3.46	3.31	3.16	3.00	2.83	2.65
18	8.29	6.01	5.09	4.58	4.25	4.01	3.84	3.71	3.60	3.51	3.37	3.23	3.08	2.92	2.75	2.57
19	8.18	5.93	5.01	4.50	4.17	3.94	3.77	3.63	3.52	3.43	3.30	3.15	3.00	2.84	2.67	2.49
20	8.10	5.85	4.94	4.43	4.10	3.87	3.70	3.56	3.46	3.37	3.23	3.09	2.94	2.78	2.61	2.42
21	8.02	5.78	4.87	4.37	4.04	3.81	3.64	3.51	3.40	3.31	3.17	3.03	2.88	2.72	2.55	2.36
22	7.95	5.72	4.82	4.31	3.99	3.76	3.59	3.45	3.35	3.26	3.12	2.98	2.83	2.67	2.50	2.31
23	7.88	5.66	4.76	4.26	3.94	3.71	3.54	3.41	3.30	3.21	3.07	2.93	2.78	2.62	2.45	2.26
24	7.82	5.61	4.72	4.22	3.90	3.67	3.50	3.36	3.26	3.17	3.03	2.89	2.74	2.58	2.40	2.21
25	7.77	5.57	4.68	4.18	3.85	3.63	3.46	3.32	3.22	3.13	2.99	2.85	2.70	2.54	2.36	2.17
26	7.72	5.53	4.64	4.14	3.82	3.59	3.42	3.29	3.18	3.09	2.96	2.81	2.66	2.50	2.33	2.13
27	7.68	5.49	4.60	4.11	3.78	3.56	3.39	3.26	3.15	3.06	2.93	2.78	2.63	2.47	2.29	2.10
28	7.64	5.45	4.57	4.07	3.75	3.53	3.36	3.23	3.12	3.03	2.90	2.75	2.60	2.44	2.26	2.06
29	7.60	5.42	4.54	4.04	3.73	3.50	3.33	3.20	3.09	3.00	2.87	2.73	2.57	2.41	2.23	2.03
30	7.56	5.39	4.51	4.02	3.70	3.47	3.30	3.17	3.07	2.98	2.84	2.70	2.55	2.39	2.21	2.01
40	7.31	5.18	4.31	3.83	3.51	3.29	3.12	2.99	2.89	2.80	2.66	2.52	2.37	2.20	2.02	1.80
60	7.08	4.98	4.13	3.65	3.34	3.12	2.95	2.82	2.72	2.63	2.50	2.35	2.20	2.03	1.84	1.60
120	6.85	4.79	3.95	3.48	3.17	2.96	2.79	2.66	2.56	2.47	2.34	2.19	2.03	1.86	1.66	1.38
∞	6.63	4.61	3.78	3.32	3.02	2.80	2.64	2.51	2.41	2.32	2.18	2.04	1.88	1.70	1.47	1.00

Adapted from Table 18 in Pearson and Hartley (Eds.) (1970). *Biometrika Tables for Statisticians*. New York: Cambridge University Press, with permission of Biometrika Trustees.

Table F Critical Values of r

df	α_1	.05	.025	.01	.005	.0005
1		.988	.997	.9995	.9999	.9999
2		.900	.950	.980	.990	.999
3		.805	.878	.934	.959	.991
4		.729	.811	.882	.917	.974
5		.669	.755	.833	.875	.951
6		.622	.707	.789	.834	.925
7		.582	.666	.750	.798	.898
8		.549	.632	.716	.765	.872
9		.521	.602	.685	.735	.847
10		.497	.576	.658	.708	.823
11		.476	.553	.634	.684	.801
12		.458	.532	.612	.661	.780
13		.441	.514	.592	.641	.760
14		.426	.497	.574	.623	.742
15		.412	.482	.558	.606	.725
16		.400	.468	.543	.590	.708
17		.389	.456	.529	.575	.693
18		.378	.444	.516	.561	.679
19		.369	.433	.503	.549	.665
20		.323	.381	.445	.487	.597
25		.360	.423	.492	.537	.652
30		.296	.349	.409	.449	.554
35		.275	.325	.381	.418	.519
40		.257	.304	.358	.393	.490
45		.243	.288	.338	.372	.465
50		.231	.273	.322	.354	.443
60		.211	.250	.295	.325	.408
70		.195	.232	.274	.302	.380
80		.183	.217	.257	.283	.357
90		.173	.205	.242	.267	.338
100		.164	.195	.230	.254	.321
	α_2	.10	.05	.02	.01	.001

df = $n - 2$.
Calculated value must be greater than or equal to critical value to reject H_o.
Source: Adapted from Table 13 in Pearson and Hartley (Eds.) (1970). *Biometrika Tables for Statisticians.*
   New York: Cambridge University Press, with permission of Biometrika Trustees.

Table G Power of the Chi-Square Test at $\alpha = .05$ for df $= 1$

	Effect size (ω)								
N	.10	.20	.30	.40	.50	.60	.70	.80	.90
10	.062	.097	.158	.244	.353	.475	.600	.716	.812
15	.067	.117	.213	.341	.491	.642	.774	.873	.937
20	.073	.146	.269	.432	.609	.765	.879	.947	.981
25	.078	.170	.323	.516	.705	.851	.938	.979	.995
30	.085	.195	.376	.591	.782	.908	.970	.992	.999
35	.091	.220	.427	.658	.841	.944	.985	.997	
40	.096	.244	.475	.716	.885	.967	.993	.999	
45	.102	.269	.521	.765	.9184	.981	.997		
50	.108	.293	.564	.807	.942	.988	.999		
60	.121	.341	.642	.873	.972	.996			
70	.133	.387	.709	.917	.9869	.999			
80	.145	.432	.765	.947	.994				
90	.157	.475	.812	.967	.9973				
100	.170	.516	.851	.979	.999				
120	.194	.591	.907	.9923					
140	.219	.658	.944	.997					
160	.243	.716	.967	.999					
180	.268	.765	.981						
200	.293	.807	.990						
300	.410	.934							

Power of the Chi-Square Test at $\alpha = .05$ for df $= 2$

	Effect size (ω)								
N	.10	.20	.30	.40	.50	.60	.70	.80	.90
10	.058	.081	.124	.188	.274	.378	.495	.614	.723
15	.061	.098	.164	.264	.392	.537	.678	.799	.887
20	.065	.115	.207	.341	.504	.669	.807	.904	.959
25	.069	.133	.250	.415	.603	.771	.890	.957	.986
30	.073	.151	.293	.487	.688	.846	.940	.982	.996
35	.077	.169	.336	.553	.758	.899	.968	.993	.999
40	.081	.188	.378	.614	.815	.935	.984	.997	
45	.085	.207	.420	.669	.861	.959	.992	.999	
50	.090	.226	.46	.718	.896	.975	.996		
60	.098	.264	.537	.79	.944	.991	.999		
70	.107	.302	.606	.859	.971	.997			
80	.115	.341	.669	.904	.985	.999			
90	.124	.378	.723	.935	.993				
100	.133	.415	.771	.957	.997				
120	.151	.487	.846	.982	.999				
140	.169	.553	.899	.993					
160	.188	.614	.935	.997					
180	.207	.669	.959	.999					
200	.226	.718	.975						
300	.322	.883	.998						

Power of the Chi-Square Test at $\alpha = .05$ for df = 3

N	Effect size (ω)								
	.10	.20	.30	.40	.50	.60	.70	.80	.90
10	.056	.075	.109	.161	.233	.325	.433	.548	.660
15	.059	.088	.142	.225	.338	.472	.613	.742	.845
20	.062	.102	.176	.291	.441	.603	.752	.865	.937
25	.065	.116	.213	.359	.537	.711	.848	.934	.977
30	.068	.130	.250	.424	.623	.796	.911	.970	.992
35	.071	.145	.287	.488	.698	.859	.950	.987	.997
40	.075	.161	.325	.548	.761	.905	.972	.994	.999
45	.078	.176	.363	.603	.814	.937	.985	.998	
50	.081	.192	.400	.654	.856	.959	.992	.999	
60	.088	.225	.472	.742	.917	.983	.998		
70	.095	.258	.540	.812	.954	.994			
80	.102	.291	.603	.865	.975	.998			
90	.109	.325	.660	.905	.987	.999			
100	.116	.359	.711	.934	.993				
120	.130	.424	.796	.970	.998				
140	.145	.488	.859	.987					
160	.161	.548	.905	.994					
180	.176	.603	.937	.998					
200	.192	.654	.959	.999					
300	.275	.840	.996						

Power of the Chi-Square Test at $\alpha = .05$ for df = 4

N	Effect size (ω)								
	.10	.20	.30	.40	.50	.60	.70	.80	.90
10	.055	.071	.099	.144	.207	.290	.389	.499	.611
15	.058	.082	.128	.200	.301	.426	.563	.696	.808
20	.060	.093	.158	.259	.396	.553	.706	.831	.916
25	.063	.106	.189	.320	.488	.664	.812	.912	.966
30	.065	.118	.222	.381	.573	.754	.884	.957	.987
35	.068	.131	.255	.441	.649	.824	.931	.980	.996
40	.071	.144	.290	.499	.716	.877	.961	.991	.999
45	.073	.158	.324	.553	.773	.916	.978	.996	
50	.076	.172	.358	.605	.820	.943	.988	.998	
60	.082	.200	.426	.696	.891	.975	.997		
70	.088	.229	.492	.771	.936	.990	.999		
80	.093	.259	.553	.831	.964	.996			
90	.099	.290	.611	.877	.980	.999			
100	.106	.320	.664	.912	.989				
120	.118	.381	.754	.957	.997				
140	.131	.441	.824	.980					
160	.144	.499	.877	.991					
180	.158	.553	.916	.996					
200	.172	.605	.943	.998					
300	.244	.802	.994						

Source: For permission to reprint, contact T & T Pacific Communications, Buffalo, NY or the author of this Appendix, Machiko R. Tomita.

Table H Power of the t-Test for $\alpha_1 = .05$

					Effect size (d)						
n	.10	.20	.30	.40	.50	.60	.70	.80	1.00	1.20	1.40
8	.073	.103	.142	.189	.244	.308	.377	.451	.601	.738	.845
9	.075	.108	.150	.203	.265	.335	.412	.492	.650	.785	.884
10	.076	.112	.159	.217	.285	.362	.445	.530	.694	.825	.914
11	.078	.117	.167	.230	.304	.388	.476	.566	.732	.858	.936
12	.080	.121	.176	.243	.324	.413	.507	.600	.767	.885	.953
13	.081	.125	.184	.257	.342	.437	.536	.632	.797	.908	.966
14	.083	.129	.192	.270	.361	.461	.563	.661	.824	.926	.975
15	.084	.133	.200	.282	.379	.483	.589	.689	.848	.941	.982
16	.086	.137	.207	.295	.396	.505	.614	.714	.868	.953	.987
17	.087	.141	.215	.307	.414	.527	.638	.738	.886	.962	.991
18	.088	.145	.223	.320	.431	.547	.660	.760	.902	.970	.993
19	.090	.149	.230	.332	.447	.567	.681	.781	.916	.976	.995
20	.091	.153	.238	.344	.463	.587	.702	.799	.928	.981	.997
30	.103	.190	.310	.455	.606	.743	.850	.922	.985	.998	1.000
40	.115	.224	.376	.551	.716	.845	.928	.971	.997	1.000	1.000
50	.125	.257	.438	.634	.799	.909	.966	.990	1.000	1.000	1.000
100	.174	.407	.681	.880	.970	.995	.999	1.000	1.000	1.000	1.000
200	.259	.637	.911	.991	1.000	1.000	1.000	1.000	1.000	1.000	1.000

Power of the t-Test for $\alpha_2 = .05$

					Effect size (d)						
n	.10	.20	.30	.40	.50	.60	.70	.80	1.00	1.20	1.40
8	.0532	.0631	.0803	.1054	.1393	.1828	.2360	.2983	.4440	.5991	.7386
9	.0538	.0655	.0857	.1154	.1555	.2066	.2684	.3398	.5009	.6621	.7961
10	.0544	.0678	.0912	.1255	.1717	.2302	.3003	.3798	.5532	.7163	.8416
11	.0550	.0702	.0967	.1356	.1879	.2537	.3315	.4184	.6011	.7626	.8774
12	.0555	.0726	.1022	.1458	.2041	.2769	.3619	.4553	.6447	.8020	.9055
13	.0561	.0750	.1078	.1560	.2202	.2998	.3916	.4906	.6842	.8353	.9274
14	.0567	.0774	.1133	.1662	.2363	.3224	.4205	.5243	.7200	.8634	.9444
15	.0573	.0797	.1189	.1763	.2523	.3447	.4484	.5563	.7522	.8870	.9575
16	.0579	.0821	.1245	.1865	.2682	.3666	.4755	.5866	.7810	.9067	.9676
17	.0584	.0845	.1301	.1967	.2840	.3881	.5017	.6183	.8069	.9232	.9754
18	.0590	.0869	.1357	.2069	.2996	.4091	.5269	.6424	.8300	.9369	.9814
19	.0596	.0893	.1413	.2171	.3151	.4298	.5512	.6679	.8506	.9487	.9859
20	.0602	.0918	.1470	.2272	.3305	.4500	.5746	.6919	.8689	.9577	.9894
30	.0660	.1161	.2035	.3267	.4742	.6258	.7595	.8613	.9668	.9948	.9994
40	.0719	.1407	.2597	.4204	.5966	.7546	.8710	.9417	.9924	.9994	1.000
50	.0778	.1654	.3149	.5062	.6963	.8438	.9336	.9767	.9984	.9999	1.000
100	.1066	.2888	.5594	.8041	.9410	.9884	.9985	.9999	1.000	1.000	1.000
200	.1685	.5136	.8494	.9790	.9988	1.000	1.000	1.000	1.000	1.000	1.000

Source: For permission to reprint, contact T & T Pacific Communications, Buffalo, NY or the author of this Appendix, Machiko R. Tomita.

Table I Sample Sizes Needed for the ANOVA at $\alpha = .05$ and Power $= .80$

df	Effect size (f)																		
	0.05	0.1	0.15	0.2	0.25	0.3	0.35	0.4	0.45	0.5	0.55	0.6	0.65	0.7	0.75	0.8	0.85	0.9	0.95
1	1571	394	176	100	64	45	34	26	21	17	15	12	11	10	9	8	7	6	6
2	1286	323	144	82	53	37	28	22	17	14	12	10	9	8	7	7	6	6	5
3	1092	274	123	70	45	32	24	19	15	12	11	9	8	7	6	6	5	5	5
4	956	240	108	61	40	28	21	16	13	11	9	8	7	6	6	5	5	5	4
5	857	215	96	55	36	25	19	15	12	10	9	7	7	6	5	5	4	4	4
6	780	196	88	50	33	23	17	14	11	9	8	7	6	5	5	5	4	4	4
7	719	181	81	46	30	21	16	13	10	9	7	6	6	5	5	4	4	4	3
8	669	168	76	43	28	20	15	12	10	8	7	6	5	5	4	4	4	4	3
9	627	158	71	40	26	19	14	11	9	8	7	6	5	5	4	4	4	3	3
10	592	149	67	38	25	18	13	11	9	7	6	5	5	4	4	4	3	3	3

Source: For permission to reprint, contact T & T Pacific Communications, Buffalo, NY or the author of this Appendix, Machiko R. Tomita.

Table J Sample Sizes Needed for Correlation at $\alpha_1 = .05$ and Power $= .80$

Effect size (f)																		
0.05	0.1	0.15	0.2	0.25	0.3	0.35	0.4	0.45	0.5	0.55	0.6	0.65	0.7	0.75	0.8	0.85	0.9	0.95
2472.897	618.116	274.618	154.371	98.688	68.413	50.130	38.233	30.047	24.159	19.769	16.394	13.729	11.572	9.783	8.261	6.925	5.696	4.459

Sample Sizes Needed for Correlation at $\alpha_2 = .05$ and Power $= .80$

Effect size (f)																		
0.05	0.1	0.15	0.2	0.25	0.3	0.35	0.4	0.45	0.5	0.55	0.6	0.65	0.7	0.75	0.8	0.85	0.9	0.95
3138.315	783.639	347.570	194.925	124.248	85.831	62.639	47.559	37.190	29.741	24.197	19.943	16.592	13.888	11.655	9.762	8.110	6.603	5.101

Source: For permission to reprint, contact T & T Pacific Communications, Buffalo, NY or the author of this Appendix, Machiko R. Tomita.

Table K Power of the F-Test for Regression Analysis at α = .05

		Lambda (λ)														
K	df_{res}	2	4	6	8	10	12	14	16	18	20	24	28	32	36	40
1	20	.268	.473	.640	.763	.848	.906	.942	.966	.980	.988	.996	.999	1.00	1.00	1.00
	50	.283	.500	.670	.792	.873	.924	.956	.975	.986	.992	.998	.999	1.00	1.00	1.00
	150	.290	.511	.682	.802	.881	.931	.961	.978	.988	.994	.998	1.00	1.00	1.00	1.00
2	20	.195	.355	.506	.634	.737	.816	.873	.915	.944	.963	.985	.994	.998	.999	1.00
	50	.214	.393	.555	.688	.788	.861	.911	.944	.966	.979	.993	.998	.999	1.00	1.00
	150	.222	.408	.575	.708	.807	.876	.923	.953	.972	.984	.995	.998	1.00	1.00	1.00
3	20	.159	.288	.418	.589	.644	.732	.801	.856	.897	.927	.965	.984	.993	.997	.999
	50	.179	.332	.481	.613	.721	.805	.867	.911	.942	.962	.985	.994	.998	.999	1.00
	150	.188	.350	.506	.641	.749	.829	.887	.927	.954	.972	.990	.996	.999	1.00	1.00
4	20	.137	.242	.354	.464	.565	.653	.729	.791	.842	.881	.936	.966	.983	.992	.996
	50	.158	.290	.427	.554	.664	.754	.824	.877	.916	.943	.975	.990	.996	.999	.999
	150	.167	.310	.456	.589	.700	.788	.854	.902	.935	.958	.983	.994	.998	.999	1.00
5	20	.121	.209	.304	.402	.495	.581	.658	.725	.781	.828	.897	.940	.966	.982	.990
	50	.143	.260	.385	.506	.615	.707	.783	.842	.888	.921	.963	.984	.993	.997	.999
	150	.152	.281	.417	.546	.658	.750	.822	.876	.916	.944	.976	.991	.996	.999	1.00
10	20	.081	.118	.160	.205	.253	.302	.352	.401	.450	.500	.585	.663	.730	.787	.833
	50	.105	.177	.259	.348	.438	.525	.605	.677	.740	.794	.876	.928	.960	.779	.989
	150	.116	.202	.302	.407	.510	.605	.689	.760	.818	.865	.929	.965	.984	.993	.997
15	20	.062	.075	.088	.102	.116	.131	.146	.161	.177	.192	.224	.257	.289	.321	.353
	50	.089	.138	.195	.260	.328	.398	.468	.536	.599	.658	.758	.835	.892	.931	.957
	150	.100	.165	.243	.329	.418	.505	.588	.663	.729	.785	.872	.927	.961	.980	.990
20	20	—														
	50	.079	.114	.156	.202	.253	.307	.363	.419	.474	.528	.629	.716	.789	.846	.891
	150	.090	.143	.207	.278	.355	.433	.509	.582	.650	.711	.810	.882	.929	.960	.978

Source: For permission to reprint, contact T & T Pacific Communications, Buffalo, NY or the author of this Appendix, Machiko R. Tomita.

Table L Probabilities Associated with Values of x in the Binomial Test

n	x																
	0	1	2	3	4	5	6	7	8	9	10	11	12	13	14	15	16
4	.062	.312	.688	.938	—	—	—	—	—	—	—	—	—	—	—	—	—
5	.031	.188	.500	.812	.969	—	—	—	—	—	—	—	—	—	—	—	—
6	.016	.109	.344	.656	.891	.984	—	—	—	—	—	—	—	—	—	—	—
7	.008	.062	.227	.500	.773	.938	.992	—	—	—	—	—	—	—	—	—	—
8	.004	.035	.145	.363	.637	.855	.965	.996	—	—	—	—	—	—	—	—	—
9	.002	.020	.090	.254	.500	.746	.910	.980	.998	—	—	—	—	—	—	—	—
10	.001	.011	.055	.172	.377	.623	.828	.945	.989	.999	—	—	—	—	—	—	—
11	—	.006	.033	.113	.274	.500	.726	.887	.967	.994	—	—	—	—	—	—	—
12	—	.003	.019	.073	.194	.387	.613	.806	.927	.981	.997	—	—	—	—	—	—
13	—	.002	.011	.046	.133	.291	.500	.709	.867	.954	.989	.998	—	—	—	—	—
14	—	.001	.006	.029	.090	.212	.395	.605	.788	.910	.971	.994	.999	—	—	—	—
15	—	—	.004	.018	.059	.151	.304	.500	.696	.849	.941	.982	.996	—	—	—	—
16	—	—	.002	.011	.038	.105	.227	.402	.598	.773	.895	.962	.989	.998	—	—	—
17	—	—	.001	.006	.025	.072	.166	.315	.500	.685	.834	.928	.975	.994	.999	—	—
18	—	—	.001	.004	.015	.048	.119	.240	.407	.593	.760	.881	.952	.985	.996	.999	—
19	—	—	—	.002	.010	.032	.084	.180	.324	.500	.676	.850	.916	.968	.990	.998	—
20	—	—	—	.001	.006	.021	.058	.132	.252	.412	.588	.748	.868	.942	.979	.994	.999
21	—	—	—	.001	.004	.013	.039	.095	.192	.332	.500	.668	.808	.902	.961	.987	.996
22	—	—	—	—	.002	.008	.026	.067	.143	.262	.416	.584	.738	.857	.933	.974	.992
23	—	—	—	—	.001	.005	.017	.047	.105	.202	.339	.500	.661	.798	.895	.953	.983
24	—	—	—	—	.001	.003	.011	.032	.076	.154	.271	.419	.581	.729	.846	.924	.968
25	—	—	—	—	—	.002	.007	.022	.054	.115	.212	.345	.500	.655	.788	.885	.946
26	—	—	—	—	—	.001	.005	.014	.038	.084	.163	.279	.423	.577	.721	.837	.916
27	—	—	—	—	—	.001	.003	.010	.026	.061	.124	.221	.351	.500	.649	.779	.876
28	—	—	—	—	—	—	.002	.006	.018	.044	.092	.172	.286	.425	.575	.714	.828
29	—	—	—	—	—	—	.001	.004	.012	.031	.068	.132	.229	.356	.500	.644	.771
30	—	—	—	—	—	—	.001	.003	.008	.021	.049	.100	.181	.292	.428	.572	.708

Tabled probabilities are for one-tailed tests. Double values in table for a two-tailed test.

Adapted from Table D in Siegel S, Castellan NJ: *Nonparametric Statistics for the Behavioral Sciences* (2nd ed.). New York: McGraw Hill, 1988, with permission.

Summary of Common Research Statistics

Gary Kielhofner • **Machiko R. Tomita**

- Analysis of Covariance (ANCOVA)
- Chi-Square
- Cronbach's Coefficient Alpha (α)
- Factor Analysis (Exploratory Factor Analysis)
- Friedman Test
- Hierarchical Linear Models (HLM)
- Independent *t*-Test
- Intraclass Correlation Coefficient
- Kappa
- Kruskal-Wallis (One-Way ANOVA)
- Logistic Regression
- Mann-Whitney U-test (also called Wilcoxon Rank-Sum Test)
- McNemar Test
- Multifactor Analysis (Two-Way ANOVA, Three-Way ANOVA)
- Multivariate Analysis of Variance (MANOVA)
- Multiple Regression
- One-Way Analysis of Variance (ANOVA)
- Paired *t*-Test
- Path Analysis
- Pearson Product Moment Correlation
- Rasch Analysis
- Repeated Measures (ANOVA)
- Sign Test
- Simple Linear Regression
- Spearman Rank Correlation Coefficient
- Wilcoxon Signed Rank Test

Statistic	Purpose of the Statistic and How It Analyzes Data	Symbols and Numeric Values Reported for this Statistic and What They Mean	Things to Consider When Using/Drawing Conclusions from this Statistic	Where the Statistic is Discussed in this Text
Analysis of Covariance (ANCOVA)	Tests the main and interaction effects of categorical variables on a continuous dependent variable, controlling for the effects of other variables.	F, which is the test of significance of the main and interaction effect, of a single interval dependent and one or more independent variables. If p-value is smaller than the set α level, at least two group means are significantly different after adjusted to covariates.	Assumptions include: • Interval or ratio level dependent variable • Limited number of covariates • Low measurement error of the covariate • Covariates linearly related • Homogeneity of covariate regression coefficients • No covariate outliers • No high multicollinearity of the covariates • Independence of the error term • Independent variables orthogonal to covariates • Homogeneity of variances • Normal distribution within groups	Chapter 17, Section on Analysis of Covariance
Chi-Square	Two purposes: • Goodness-of-fit-test: Identifies whether one sample distribution (frequencies) differs from an expected/known distribution. • Test of independence: Measures whether two categorical variables have a relationship.	χ^2, which is the sum of the squared difference in observed and expected scores over the expected score. This concept applies for both types of Chi-square. Goodness-of-fit-test: If the p-value is smaller than the set α level, the observed frequencies are different from the expected/known frequencies. Test of independence: if the p-value is smaller than the set α level, the two variables are not independent or they are associated.	Goodness-of-fit test compares observed frequency with an expected (uniform or normal distribution) or known distribution. Tests of independence are used to examine the independence of two categorical variables.	Chapter 17, Section on Nonparametric Statistics

Statistic	Purpose of the Statistic and How It Analyzes Data	Symbols and Numeric Values Reported for this Statistic and What They Mean	Things to Consider When Using/Drawing Conclusions from this Statistic	Where the Statistic is Discussed in this Text
Cronbach's Coefficient Alpha (α)	Asks whether the items that make up a scale are homogeneous.	α, which like any correlation coefficient ranges from 0.0 to 1.0 and indicates the strength of relationship; in this case it indicates the extent to which all items are interrelated or constitute a homogeneous instrument	Alpha is the average of all split half reliabilities for the items that make up the instrument. Alpha values that approach .90 are indications of high homogeneity. Alpha is affected by the number of items; so, longer scales will tend to generate higher coefficients	Chapter 12, Section on Internal Consistency
Factor Analysis (Exploratory Factor Analysis)	Reduces items into fewer sets of the similar concepts (i.e., factors).	Eigenvalues, which reflect the amount of variance accounted for by each factor. Factor loadings, which represent the correlation between each item and each factor. Rotations are done to identify meaningful factors that include highly correlated items to the factor.	There are two major methods for factor analysis: • Factor analysis, and • Principal component analysis. Exploratory factor analysis should not be confused with confirmatory factor analysis, which is an application of structural equation modeling (SEM). Usually the factor loading of .30 or less is not meaningful.	Chapter 17, Section on Multivariate Analysis
Friedman Test	Compares the rank orders taken more than two times for correlated samples.	χ_r^2 which reflects the difference among three or more group rank orders. If the p-value is smaller than the set α level, at least one pair of rank orders is significantly different. A post-hoc test will follow to identify which pairs of mean ranks are significant.	This test is a nonparametric alternative to the repeated measures ANOVA. The raw data are converted into rank orders.	Chapter 17, Section on Comparison of More than Two Group Means

Statistic	Purpose of the Statistic and How It Analyzes Data	Symbols and Numeric Values Reported for this Statistic and What They Mean	Things to Consider When Using/Drawing Conclusions from this Statistic	Where the Statistic is Discussed in this Text
Hierarchical Linear Models (HLM)	Examine the growth trajectories (i.e., change in dependent variable over time) and study factors that may influence these trajectories. Nested type of data will be analyzed in two levels: • First-level data will use time as predictor variable to estimate individual growth trajectories. The estimated intercepts and regression coefficients can be used as dependent variables in the second model. • Second-level data can be modeled and uses the individual as the unit of analysis.	Symbols are not always the same across the published literature. Interpretation of intercepts and regression coefficients follow the same principles used in regression analysis.	Users must be cautious in setting up models as well as interpreting the results. Second level sample size has influence on the power of the test.	Chapter 17
Independent t-Test	Compares two group means when the samples are independent.	t, which reflects the difference between the two group means divided by the standard error of the difference. If the p-value is smaller than the set α, the two group means are significantly different.	The t-test is preceded by a test for homogeneity (either Bartlett's test or Levine's test) and if the two groups are not homogeneous, the formula for the t-test must be adjusted; this is done automatically in many statistical packages. Used for either a directional hypothesis or a nondirectional hypothesis but α is adjusted accordingly.	Chapter 17, Section on Comparisons of Two Group Means
Intraclass Correlation Coefficient	Calculates the reliability of an observed score in estimating the true score.	ICC, which is a correlation ranging from 0.0–1.0	Estimates reliability while taking into consideration error due to several factors such as variations in the raters and testing conditions, alternate forms, and administration at different times.	Chapter 12, Section on Generalizability Theory and Intraclass Coefficients

Statistic	Purpose of the Statistic and How It Analyzes Data	Symbols and Numeric Values Reported for this Statistic and What They Mean	Things to Consider When Using/Drawing Conclusions from this Statistic	Where the Statistic is Discussed in this Text
Kappa	Examines extent of rater agreement with categorical instruments; attenuates for chance agreement.	K, which indicates strength of relationship; values range from 0.0 to 1.0	Guidelines for interpretation of kappa values: • > 0.75 = excellent agreement • 0.40–0.75 = fair to good agreement • < 0.40 = poor agreement Is influenced by sample size, subject variability and the number of categories used; must be interpreted with care.	Chapter 12, Section on Assessing Inter-rater Reliability
Kruskal-Wallis (One-Way ANOVA)	Compares rank orders among three or more groups for independent samples.	H, which is distributed as Chi-square with df = $k - 1$. If the p-value is smaller than the set α level, at least two group means are significantly different. Then, a post-hoc test to identify which pairs of means are significantly different will follow.	This test is a nonparametric alternative to the one-way ANOVA. Used when dependent variable is measured with an ordinal scale, or when assumptions are not met if measured with an interval/ratio scale.	Chapter 17, Section on Comparison of More than Two Group Means
Logistic Regression	Examines the effect of several independent variables (categorical or continuous) on a categorical dependent variable.	Z, which is the logarithm of the odds. The odds ratio is how likely it is that an individual belongs to the target group rather than the reference group. If the p-value for each regression coefficient is smaller than the set α level, the relationship between the two variables is not likely to be due to chance. Classification accuracy indicates the rate of accurately predicted frequencies to actual observed frequencies.	Logistic regression estimates the maximum likelihood that results in the accurate prediction of group membership. Need fairly large number of cases, and avoid multicollinearity and outliers. There are direct and sequential logistic regressions.	Chapter 17, Section on Logistic Regression

Statistic	Purpose of the Statistic and How It Analyzes Data	Symbols and Numeric Values Reported for this Statistic and What They Mean	Things to Consider When Using/Drawing Conclusions from this Statistic	Where the Statistic is Discussed in this Text
Mann-Whitney U-test (also called Wilcoxon Rank-Sum Test)	Measures difference of rank orders between two groups.	U score for each group is calculated and the smaller of the two values (i.e., calculated U value) is compared to a critical value. When the calculated value is smaller than the critical value for the set α level, it is statistically significant (i.e., p-value is smaller than the set α level). A p-value smaller than the set α level indicates a significant difference in rank orders between the two groups.	Used in place of the independent t-test when the data do not conform to all or most of the normality assumptions required for parametric statistics. If the dependent variable is measured on a ratio or interval scale, the raw scores have to be converted to rank orders across both groups.	Chapter 17, Section on Comparisons of Two Group Means
McNemar Test	Compares correlated frequency distributions (i.e., pre- and post-measures) to see if there is a significant difference.	χ^2, which reflects the independence of frequencies. If the p-value is smaller than the set α level, there is a significant change or difference.	This test is used when: • The samples are correlated, and • The dependent variable has only two levels, such as Yes and No.	Chapter 17, Section on Nonparametric Statistics
Multifactor Analysis (Two-Way ANOVA, Three-Way ANOVA, etc.)	Tests the main effects (of more than one independent variable) and interaction effects (among independent variables) on the dependent variable.	F, which is the ratio of between-subjects variance to within-subjects variance. If the p-value is smaller than the set α level, the independent variable or interaction has significant effects on the dependent variable. Post-hoc analysis will follow to identify which independent variables/interaction account for differences.	Used for independent samples. To interpret the results, the interaction effects should be analyzed first. If significant, the type of interaction should be identified (ordinal vs. disordinal). If the interaction is disordinal, the variables causing the interaction should be examined separately.	Chapter 17, Section on Multifactorial Analysis of Variance

Statistic	Purpose of the Statistic and How It Analyzes Data	Symbols and Numeric Values Reported for this Statistic and What They Mean	Things to Consider When Using/Drawing Conclusions from this Statistic	Where the Statistic is Discussed in this Text
Multivariate Analysis of Variance (MANOVA)	Tests whether there is an overall effect of the independent variable(s) on all dependent variables together.	F for multivariate test which reflects the level of association among all dependent variables and the main effect(s) and interaction effect(s). F for between-subjects tests which reflects the level of association between each of the dependent variables and each of the independent variables and interaction effects. If the p-value is smaller than the set α level, the effect of independent variable or interaction is significant. The post-hoc analysis is performed by either one-way ANOVA or Discriminant Analysis.	Assumptions: • Multivariate normal distribution, • Linear relationships among all pairs of dependent variables, and • Homogeneity of variances and regression. • Multicollinearity and outliers should be avoided.	Chapter 17, Section on Multivariate Analysis
Multiple Regression	Examines ability of several independent variables to predict the value of a dependent variable.	R^2, which is the strength of the association between the dependent variable and all independent variables in the model. F, which reflects the ratio between the variance (Mean Square) of predicted values and the variance (Mean Square) of error. If the p-value is smaller than the set α level, it tells that the relationship between the two variables is not likely to be the result of chance.	Assumptions: • Same as for simple linear regression, • No multicollinearity (independent variables are highly correlated) or outliers. There are three major methods of selecting variables for multiple regression: • Standard (all independent variables entered at once), • Hierarchical (independent variables entered one at a time or in subsets based on a theoretical rationale) and • Stepwise method. Usually the smallest group of variables that will account for the greatest proportion of variance in the dependent variable is the goal.	Chapter 17, Section on Regression

Statistic	Purpose of the Statistic and How It Analyzes Data	Symbols and Numeric Values Reported for this Statistic and What They Mean	Things to Consider When Using/Drawing Conclusions from this Statistic	Where the Statistic is Discussed in this Text
One-Way Analysis of Variance (ANOVA)	Compares group dependent variable means for three or more groups representing different levels of a single independent variable.	F, which is the ratio of between-group variance to within-group variance. If the p-value is smaller than the set α level, it means at least two group means are significantly different. Then, a post-hoc multiple comparison test will follow to determine differences between means.	Assumes that the samples are randomly drawn from a normally distributed population with equal variances among the groups. If the statistical assumptions are not met, then Kruskal-Wallis nonparametric test should be used.	Chapter 17, Section on Comparisons of More than Two Group Means
Paired t-Test	Compares two group means when the samples are dependent/correlated (e.g., when comparing pre- and posttests on the same sample).	t, which is obtained by dividing the mean of the difference in scores by the standard error of the difference in scores. If the p-value is smaller than the set α level, there is a significant change or difference.	The paired t-test assumes a significant correlation between two dependent variables; if they are not correlated, an independent t-test may be used.	Chapter 17, Section on Comparisons of Two Group Means
Path Analysis	A diagram-based statistical procedure used to test the strength and direction of relationships among several variables as well as identifying direct and causal pathways among the variables.	Direct and indirect effects. Direct effects are drawn using straight lines connecting two variables and indicating the cause and effect by an arrowhead. Indirect effects are indicated by lines not connecting two variables. All variables are endogenous (ones that are influenced by other variables) and/or exogenous (ones that are independent of any influence). r, which indicates a correlation between two variables. $p_{y,x}$, which indicates a path coefficient from the variable x to the variable y. If the p-value is smaller than the set α level, the path will be exhibited.	Assumptions: • The dependent variable and the independent variable should be correlated, • The dependent variable should occur later than the independent variable in time, and • The relationship between the two variables exists even in the presence of another variable.	Chapter 17, Section on Multivariate Analysis

Statistic	Purpose of the Statistic and How It Analyzes Data	Symbols and Numeric Values Reported for this Statistic and What They Mean	Things to Consider When Using/Drawing Conclusions from this Statistic	Where the Statistic is Discussed in this Text
Pearson Product Moment Correlation	Measures the strength of the association between two continuous variables.	r, which represents the strength of association, and can range from 0 (no association) to ±1.0 (perfect association), and can be positive (indicating a parallel relationship) or negative (indicating an inverse relationship). p-value which indicates the likelihood the observed relationship occurred by chance	The r values are generally interpreted as follows: • 0–.2 negligible correlation • .2–.4 low • .4–.6 moderate • .6–.8 high • .8–1.0 very high The p-values for this statistic are sensitive to sample sizes.	Chapter 17, Section on Correlation
Rasch Analysis	Answers the following questions: • Do items on an instrument fit or conform to an underlying unidimensional construct? • Does a subject's pattern of scores fit with the underlying unidimensional construct? • Do raters use the instrument in a way that reflects the underlying unidimensional construct? (This question is not asked when the took is a self-report, since there is no separate rater or assessor.)	Mean Square Fit Statistic (MnSq): • 1.0 is the desired/ideal mean square; scores above 1.0 indicate proportion of error or noise (unexpected variability), e.g., 1.2 = 20% error or noise. • Scores lower than 1.0 indicate less variation than expected. • Standardized Mean Square (Zstd) = significance of MnSq; Zstd = 2.0 = .05 level of significance Zstd > 2.0 indicates < .05 level of significance. Separation index value indicates: • The number of strata into which subjects were separated by the instrument. • The number of strata into which items on the scale are separated.	A sample of 30 is considered a minimum. This statistic does not require random sampling. When multiple raters are examined, they must be linked via a common subject or subjects. Ordinary norm for interpreting the Mean Square (MnSq) is that values between .7 and 1.4 are considered acceptable for a clinical assessment. MnSq ≥ 1.4 with a Zstd ≥ 2.0 means: • Item is either poorly defined or doesn't fit (belong) to the same construct as the other items. • Subject's pattern of scores was unexpected (may mean subject was not validly assessed). • Rater's pattern of scores was unexpected (indicates rater is not using the scale in a valid way). MnSq ≤ 0.7 with a Zstd ≥ 2.0 means: • Item is too invariant, doesn't add much information about the true ability/ characteristic of the subjects.	Chapter 13

Statistic	Purpose of the Statistic and How It Analyzes Data	Symbols and Numeric Values Reported for this Statistic and What They Mean	Things to Consider When Using/Drawing Conclusions from this Statistic	Where the Statistic is Discussed in this Text
Rasch Analysis (continued)	• How well spread out are the items? (i.e. what range of the characteristic do they measure?) • How many groups does the instrument separate subjects into? (i.e., how sensitive is it?) • How much of the characteristic measured is represented by an item? (Where does this item fall on a continuum of less to more of the construct?) • How much of this trait does a given person have? • How much difference is there in the severity/ leniency of raters?	• The number of strata into which raters are separated. Note: also gives a coefficient that indicates the reliability with which items, subjects and raters are divided into their strata Item, person, and rater calibration: usually given in positive and negative numbers called logits; this is an interval level measure created through log transformation; hence logits refers to "log linear units." The meaning of the numbers is specific to the assessment being studied. (Note sometimes authors convert the logits to a 1–100 scale to make it easier to deal with the logit values.) Interpreted as: • Where the item falls on the continuum from less to more of the trait measured. • Where this person falls on the continuum of less to more of the trait measured. • How severe or lenient a rater is compared to other raters.	• Item may overlap with another item. • Subject tended to get same scores on all items irrespective of how much of the trait the item represented. • Rater tended to give same ratings to subjects irrespective of where the subject fell on the scale.	

Statistic	Purpose of the Statistic and How It Analyzes Data	Symbols and Numeric Values Reported for this Statistic and What They Mean	Things to Consider When Using/Drawing Conclusions from this Statistic	Where the Statistic is Discussed in this Text
Repeated Measures (ANOVA)	Compares changes or differences among three or more measures or groups in correlated samples.	F, which is the ratio between Mean Square of between-factors (group variance) and Mean Square of within-factors (error variance). If the p-values is smaller than the set α level, at least two group measures are significantly different or changes in at least two measures are significantly different. Then, identify which pairs of means are significantly different.	Since the sample is correlated, the statistical assumption of homogeneity among groups is not applicable. However, the similarity and correlation among variance of change scores should be tested. This is the assumption of sphericity.	Chapter 17, Section on Comparison of More than Two Group Means
Sign Test	Tests whether there are significant changes in directions (positive or negative) of a dependent variable.	Z, which reflects the ratio of the difference between the number of fewer changes and a half of the sample size to a half of the square root of the sample size. The probability (p-value) of the occurrence of the result is derived from the calculated z; if the p-value is smaller than the set α level there is significant change in direction.	Used when changes in the direction of the data are of primary interest (e.g., data changing in either a positive or a negative direction). This statistic provides the lowest level of statistical information. If possible, Wilcoxon signed rank test should be used.	Chapter 17, Section on Comparisons of Two Group Means

Statistic	Purpose of the Statistic and How It Analyzes Data	Symbols and Numeric Values Reported for this Statistic and What They Mean	Things to Consider When Using/Drawing Conclusions from this Statistic	Where the Statistic is Discussed in this Text
Simple Linear Regression	Asks whether a dependent variable can be predicted from an independent variable.	R^2 ($= r^2$), which reflects the variance of the dependent variable explained by the variance of the independent variable. F, which reflects the ratio between the variance (Mean Square) of predicted values and the variance (Mean Square) of error. If the p-value is smaller than the set α level, the relationship between the two variables is not likely to be the results of chance.	The dependent variable should be measured by either interval or ratio scale. Assumes that two variables are linearly correlated. Sensitive to outliers.	Chapter 17, Section on Regression
Spearman Rank Correlation Coefficient	Measures the strength of the association between two ranked variables.	r_s, which represents the strength of association. It ranges from −1 to +1.	The r_s values reflect the strength of the relationship between two variables and are generally interpreted as follows: • 0–.2 negligible correlation • .2–.4 low • .4–.6 moderate • .6–.8 high • .8–1.0 very high This test is a nonparametric alternative to Pearson correlation. Used when variables are measured by ordinal scales.	Chapter 17, Section on Correlation
Wilcoxon Signed Rank Test	Identifies the relative magnitude of differences and the direction of the change for correlated samples.	T, which is the smaller sum of the rank of scores for one direction of change. If the p-value is smaller than the set α level, there is a significant change or difference	This is a nonparametric alternative to the paired t-test when the sample is dependent. Used when the dependent variable is measured with an ordinal scale, or when groups are not normally distributed if measured with an interval/ratio scale.	Chapter 17, Section on Comparisons of Two Group Means

C H A P T E R   1 9

Overview of Qualitative Research

Mark R. Luborsky • Cathy Lysack

The aim of this chapter is to provide a broad overview of qualitative research. It considers the nature and uses of qualitative research, discussing its place and importance in scholarship in general and occupational therapy in particular. This chapter also introduces the major epistemologies or traditions of thought within qualitative research.

The Nature of and Need for Qualitative Research

Research is, simply, asking informed questions. The hallmark of all research is curiosity about the nature and functioning of the world including its peoples, and working to develop some generalizations about this world. In this quest for understanding, investigators make use of existing concepts and knowledge including wisdoms received from others while growing up as human beings and during professional training (deductive processes). Investigators also keep their eyes open to see in new ways and build up new ideas (inductive processes).

Both approaches are needed. Scholars continually move between studying things in terms of what is already known to be true about the world and studying things from a fresh point of view. The latter is especially important when received wisdoms seem not to apply to a new situation or cannot explain why things go poorly in certain circumstances.

The Nature of Qualitative Research

Qualitative study methods are needed when researchers ask certain kinds of questions. Qualitative research is a broad term for approaches to developing new knowledge that have as their main goal the

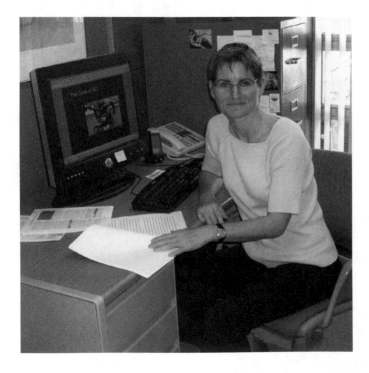

Figure 19.1 Dr. Lysack reflects upon questions arising from past research on the experience of living with spinal cord injury and identifies new qualitative research questions for future exploration.

naturalistic discovery, identification, and description of basic features of the worlds people live in and their experiences of those worlds. Qualitative methods are used when it's important to learn more about the kinds of features that are present, and about what are the salient contents and meanings of a phenomenon. Simply stated, qualitative methods are well suited to the task of discovering what needs to be measured or described, and how to measure it.

Questions Addressed by Qualitative Research

Occupational therapy contributes outstanding questions to the wider scientific research enterprise. These include, for example, questions about the impact of disability on occupation, meaningful activities, and habits. As a relatively young field, its scholars are continuing to develop the tools for answering these questions. Qualitative research is emerging as an important tool for answering many of the questions generated in the field.

First, qualitative methods enable discovery of the basic form of salient things to measure in situ-

---

Judge a man by his questions not his answers.

—Voltaire

Science is the belief in the ignorance of the experts.

—Richard Feynman, American physicist, 1985 Nobel Prize winner

These two scholars, widely separated in time, embody the basic scientific stance of active questioning and critical disbelief in taken-for-granted or official normative descriptions and explanations.

Good research is determined by what and whose questions are asked. A clearly focused important *question* that leads to new knowledge (if only to dissuade us from the complacency of taken for granted ideas) is more crucial than the methods investigators use. Just labeling or naming things by applying existing knowledge is not research, even if it leads to useful interventions and treatments. Such an approach only applies what is accepted as knowledge instead of challenging it. Using an established disease classification ("nosology") or behavioral checklist only assigns a place in an already established universal framework. Discovery is needed to establish new knowledge; it is not enough to merely apply an existing label or idea to something observed.

---

ations where there is insufficient prior work. In this case, qualitative research is often the first step for investigating a particular phenomenon. In addition, it is often the case that certain phenomena, experiences, or processes are inadequately captured by the preconceived concepts and predefined tools. This is the second major reason for qualitative research.

Many phenomena in occupational therapy are best studied with qualitative methods. For example, an investigator who wishes to learn about the evolution of occupational therapists' acquisition of professional competencies could count words or behaviors, or collect data on constructs such as independence, judgment, reasoning, and control. While such a strategy would answer certain questions, it would likely not capture the dynamic range of issues, dilemmas, and struggles that real occupational therapists grapple with as they seek to design and implement therapies and interventions to facilitate the recovery and well-being of their clients. A qualitative, narrative approach would be required to discover these aspects of professional development. Narratives discovered in qualitative research reflect the lived experience of therapists. They reveal layers of intention, emotion, and meaning, including complex contradictions that fixed questions may miss. The following are some additional examples of questions that require qualitative research.

Consider the question of what factors affect adherence to adaptive device use. Research shows that the answers to this question reside in the interface between the device and the person, the social settings of device use, and even within the person's ideals and expectations with respect to the perceived benefits afforded by the device. Research also shows that adaptation of environments can dramatically alter the need for assistive devices. Conducting qualitative research in naturalistic settings like people's homes and communities has been essential to discovering these factors (Gitlin, Luborsky, & Schemm, 1998; Luborsky, 1997).

Consider the question of what factors affect outcomes in stroke rehabilitation. In a series of studies, researchers have shown that rehabilitation after stroke is sometimes devalued by healthcare professionals, in contrast to the views of stroke patients (Becker & Kaufman, 1995; Kaufman & Becker, 1986). For patients, rehabilitation represented a hopeful opportunity for recovery if they worked hard enough, which resulted in feeling let down when full recovery did not occur. On the other hand, professionals' views were dominated by the idea that the potential to influence the illness trajectory is quite limited. As a result, rehabilitation professionals in stroke settings tend to divide patients into two categories: rehabilitation candidates and geriatric care patients. This practice is founded on culturally based assumptions about aging and notions of appropriate rehabilitation for older people which ultimately serve to limit costs. Tham and Kielhofner (2003) studied older women with stroke focusing on unilateral neglect. They found that how the women experienced neglect differed from professional conceptions of neglect. Consequently, the strategies that were most helpful in assisting these women to manage daily life were not those that emanated from professional conceptions of neglect treatment. Rather, as the women's experience of neglect changed over time, an evolving set of strategies helped them reclaim and occupy the neglected half of the world. Tham and Kielhofner concluded that occupational therapy interventions for persons with neglect as a consequence of stroke could become more effective by systematically incorporating the kinds of strategies identified in this study.

Consider the question of what it is like for clients and families to live every day with the physical and social consequences of chronic illness and disability. Understanding what that is like from their perspectives can provide invaluable insights. Examples of qualitative research that provide such understanding are abundant. For example, some research has centered on observations of a particular person or group, such as persons with cancer, autism, or mental retardation (c.f., Langness & Levine, 1986). In other instances, the researcher is simultaneously the author and the subject of the study, as in the case of Murphy's (1987) classic, *The Body Silent*, which powerfully illustrates living with a disabling and terminal disease.

Edgerton's (1967, 1993) *Cloak of Competence* reports research that showed how the stigma of mental retardation pushed individuals to hide and even deny their cognitive handicap in attempts to pass as normal in society, and thus escape the social inspection and surveillance that accompanied their disability. Edgerton also revealed the unexpected skills, resources, and insights of his study participants, dispelling myths about the public's sense of their incompetence. Finlayson's (2004) qualitative research illuminated the perspective of adults with multiple sclerosis, describing the challenges they encounter and fear as they enter older age. These are only a few illustrations of qualitative research that provided an insider's viewpoint on illness and disability. Such research offers important insights that can shape and improve occupational therapy practice.

The Features of Qualitative Research

All qualitative research is characterized by several aims. It seeks to discover:

- The insider's (emic) view and compare it to the observer's outsider (etic) view,
- Meanings, symbols, beliefs, and values in the language of the participants,
- The multiple perspectives of persons, groups, and organizations across the spectrum of positions in a social setting or culture, including those at the margins of society, not just the center, and
- Features of the worlds of everyday lived experience.

While these aims are common to all forms of qualitative inquiry, there are different epistemologies or traditions of thought within qualitative research. These are considered next.

Major Epistemologies or Traditions of Thought in Qualitative Research

Terms such as philosophical traditions and epistemology may seem abstract and unrelated to daily life. Yet everyone already has a philosophy and already does philosophy when thinking about and addressing questions about life, meaning, society, and morality. Philosophies, albeit at times unconsciously, underlay everyone's approaches to thinking and acting.

Qualitative research traditions are somewhat akin to social traditions. They are gestalt ways of seeing the world; they define events, practices, activities, ideals, and goals. Just as deeply held cultural values and beliefs shape the expression of peoples' lives, the perspectives of qualitative research traditions shape how researchers within those traditions see and act on the world in their studies.

The Diversity of Qualitative Research Epistemologies

Each epistemological approach presents a particular philosophical stance that directs investigators to certain questions and ideas about what counts as answers. Each stance involves contrasting ideas not only about how to go down the path to new

The Norms of Interest in Qualitative Research

There are two kinds of norms. Norms derived by statistical analyses of standardized measures describe the central tendency of a phenomena defined by researchers. In clinical practice, a patient's test results can be normal, meaning they fall within probabilistically defined normal categories. Social norms are the expected standards and ideals by which people orient their actions. Social norms both pattern social action and are used to evaluate right and wrong, and admonish deviations from the norm. These norms also operate powerfully in the clinical situation, though they are most often implicit and unacknowledged. It is this latter kind of norms that qualitative researchers seek to discover.

Consider the point of a master clinician when he wrote,

It happened the other morning on rounds, as it often does, that while I was carefully auscultating a patient's chest, he began to ask me a question. 'Quiet,' I said, 'I can't hear you while I'm listening' (Baron, 1985, p. 606).

He tells us how trained clinicians efficiently ignore the thinking person while listening for signs of anatomical parts. When clinical practitioners hear a patient's words, they often select only those that are relevant to a medical diagnostic model of norms. They typically do not attend to the social norms, meanings, concerns, and ways of interpreting experiences. In contrast, patients typically do not separate out the physical from the social disturbances.

Qualitative research aspires to learn the entire range of features characterizing a patient's experience and build up a picture and evaluate how existing trait systems (like those used in clinical practice) are useful, when they miss important phenomena, and even when they do harm. Medical and rehabilitation classifications are powerful and enable the control or management of impairment, the fixing of serious injuries, and the prevention of disease. Nonetheless, the next era of medical science and discovery needs methods and tools to better address patients' continuing lives within the social fabric of daily life in the community. For example, current quantitative research on the diagnosis of depression focuses on asking patients about the presence, duration, and effect of feelings of sadness and despair. To extend this knowledge base, qualitative research must also be undertaken to seek to learn about individual and group concepts of depression. Such research would ask whether the way lay persons understand depression is different from that of researchers and professionals. It would seek to understand their beliefs about the nature, causes, and natural course of depression. It would ask about their views of what should be done about depression. No doubt such research will yield unexpected insights. These insights will likely have direct and, perhaps, dramatic practice implications.

Occupational therapy has already recognized that the nosology it inherited from medicine and rehabilitation is too limiting. Recognition of the limitations of a narrow biomedical focus led Reilly (1962), Kielhofner (2001), and others (Zemke & Clark, 1996) to attempt to develop a more integrative conceptual framework for the profession that more properly includes human occupations, meaningful activities, and personal values. Occupational therapists increasingly are examining the embodied experiences of patients as socially and not only physically functioning beings and as intending and feeling persons. The notion of embodiment has at its core, the idea that substance and spirit are inseparable (Csordas, 1994; Kielhofner, 1995).

knowledge, but also about the destination. The rules of each epistemological tradition directly shape the type and style of research questions asked as well as the specific procedures used.

It is beyond the scope of this chapter to consider which stance best addresses a problem. Instead, the aim is to provide an appreciation of each stance, its basic principles, definition, and procedures. Occupational therapy researchers can benefit from learning the different stances that have shaped qualitative research epistemologies. People who adopt one stance are led to investigate particular problems that can be answered within the perspective of that stance. Those who adopt a different stance will be directed to other problems.

> The rules of each epistemological tradition directly shape the type and style of research questions asked as well as the specific procedures used.

The Place of Qualitative Research in Science

Because research in the behavioral sciences and health care was historically dominated by quantities methods, for many decades qualitative research was misunderstood and viewed as less rigorous. Fortunately, this circumstance has changed in most sectors of science. In many fields of knowledge there is a very complementary and interdependent relationship between quantitative and qualitative approaches. In occupational therapy, as in other fields, scholars are increasingly trained in both qualitative and quantitative traditions (although they may specialize in one or the other). There is growing recognition that rigorous criteria for qualitative data exist. These criteria are recognized increasingly, in top tier medical journals (e.g., *British Medical Journal*; Mays & Pope 1995a–c, 2000), and research funding agencies (National Institutes of Health 2001; Ragin, Nagel, & White, 2004). There has also been a rapid expansion of specialty journals and book series attending to qualitative research. It has been estimated that upwards of several hundred journals exists across disciplines that publish qualitative work (Wark, 1992).

Today in qualitative research, major epistemological traditions include:

• Participatory action research (PAR),
• Critical theory,
• Ethnography,
• Phenomenology, and
• Grounded theory.

The sections that follow will provide a sense of what each tradition posits and what it offers.

Participatory Action Research (PAR)

Participatory Action Research (PAR) is an approach to research used to confront pressing social problems. Although PAR can be combined

The Nature of Epistemology

Epistemology refers to the broad arena of philosophy concerned with the nature and scope of knowledge. Epistemology asks such questions as: What does it mean to know (the truth), and what is the nature of truth? What kinds of things can be known? Can we believe in knowledge that is outside the evidence of our senses, such as the lived experiences of others or events of the past? What are the limits of self-knowledge?

with quantitative designs (Taylor, Braveman, & Hammel, 2004), it most often employs qualitative research strategies. Moreover, because PAR involves important ideals and principles about how knowledge should be generated and used, it is viewed by many qualitative researchers as a particular epistemological tradition. This section provides a brief overview of PAR in qualitative research; Chapters 38 to 40 in this text provide detailed examinations of participatory research and its application in occupational therapy.

PAR combines both research efforts and active intervention within a single project. PAR is striking for how the research goal is formulated and pursued: it involves multiple stakeholders, including research participants, institutional representatives (e.g., teachers, doctors, service providers), and researchers as equal partners. In addition to concerns for research rigor, PAR adds concern with creating community trust and a sense of ownership of the project and findings. The people who conduct the study and the procedures, and forms of the findings and dissemination are collaboratively planned and conducted in order to ensure that the results both represent all the stakeholders and they are able to trust the processes by which it was developed.

Conducting a PAR Project

The aphorism, "Look, think, act," (Stringer, 1999) sums up the main features of PAR and highlights its socially engaged stance. When looking, investigators collect information to discover, define, and describe a phenomenon or setting. When thinking, they explore by interpreting, analyzing, and explaining. Finally, when acting, investigators develop, implement, and evaluate a purposeful plan formulated to meet a local need or change something in the context. These three steps provide PAR collaborators with a script of explicit orientations and goals. Looking, thinking, and acting can be repeated, iteratively, throughout the research process as new information, agendas, and questions emerge from the input and shared experiences of all the PAR partners.

Overall, the structure of PAR proceeds in the following steps. A project begins with the initial identification of a problem first by the researchers or the participants, or both together. Then, collaborative discussion and negotiations among all stakeholders serves to refine the sense of the problem. Next, the research partners review what is already known and published about the issue and/or attempts to address a problem. Afterwards, they work to redefine the problem more clearly and formulate an agenda for change. Next, the methods for research and evaluation are selected. Then, the partners implement the change, and collect and analyze data to evaluate their efforts. Finally, the results are prepared and disseminated with recommendations for wider audiences. Generally, the investigators will return to refining the problem, goals, and procedures as they make use of the emerging knowledge and experiences including evaluation of the changes.

Contributions of Participatory Action Research

Interest in PAR has grown rapidly. In part, this is because the collaborative design incorporates core progressive social ideals. PAR seeks to ensure that the interests of all the partners are on an equal footing; it is often described as "democratic" (Gitlin, Lyons, & Kolodner, 1994). Its popularity is also owing to the fact that the results of PAR are more likely to be trusted by consumers and professionals and are more likely to be used. Thus, the end result of PAR is not only new knowledge, but also changes in practices, organizations, and in governmental, legal, economic, or social rules. It is also socially progressive since it is designed to enhance the life of individuals and communities. While PAR is relatively new to occupational therapy, a number of projects using this approach have demonstrated how services can be improved and how therapists and clients can be empowered to achieve desired ends (Forsyth, Summerfield-Mann, & Kielhofner, 2005; Taylor et al., 2004).

Ethnography

Ethnography is a research approach that aims to discover and describe the point of view of a people or social scene. Ethnography is a dynamic tradition with a long history. From its early days in the late 1800s it was defined by a fieldwork tradition. Investigators, such as Franz Boas (1966), who first studied the Eskimo (Inuit) or Malinowski who studied the natives in the South Pacific Islands, lived among the people they studied and immersed themselves in the settings and events in those places. These investigators systematically learned and spoke the local language; they observed and described the material lives, activities, structures of social life, relationships, and cultural beliefs that they observed. By conducting such fieldwork to learn directly from the natives about their viewpoints, these early ethnographers developed a method of first-hand discovery.

Ethnography continues to evolve. For example, ethnographers now see researchers as instruments;

Resources on Participatory Action Research

In the United States, the federal Agency for Health Quality Research (AHQR) has published the results of a consensus conference and literature meta-analyses; it confirmed the positive outcomes of PAR, and summarized key design criteria (Viswanathan et al., 2004). PAR has been vital to the success of projects spanning from patient-centered mental health and substance abuse treatment to community-based health and in many primary health care and international development projects, including the community-based rehabilitation movement (Lysack & Kaufert, 1994). Several excellent studies using the PAR approach are featured in recent issues of the *American Journal of Public Health* (AJPH, 2003, August & September), Hart and Bond (1996), Stringer (1999), a report commissioned by the AHRQ (Viswanathan et al., 2004), and from Minkler and colleagues (2003). One of the most comprehensive reviews of the history, development, and international uses of PAR is Koning and Martin (1996). An excellent text published by the American Psychological Association with occupational therapy contributors discusses the use of PAR in community contexts (Jason et al., 2004). Finally, a new occupational therapy text (Crist & Kielhofner, 2005) illustrates the use of PAR in advancing practice.

their experiences and reactions are part of the process of gaining insight into the people and settings studied. What distinguishes ethnographic fieldwork from other methods conducted in field settings is a quest for the naturally occurring language, insider's viewpoint and values, and cultural patterns.

The term, ethnography, embraces a wide range of approaches that share an interest in learning:

• The patterns in how a people define and view the world,
• Habitual patterns and ways of life,
• Categories of thought,
• Symbols and meanings,
• Kinds of social relationships, and
• Systems of moral goals, values, and social structures.

It strives to gain an insider's view of the social scene (Spradley 1979, 1980). Geertz (1973) summed up the ethnographic task as figuring out what those under study think they are up to. This aim contrasts with trying to force fit a description of those under study into the language categories and values held by the researcher.

Ethnography is distinctive in several ways. Among these are its aims to:

- Describe the insider's view, categories of language, thought, rules for behavior and relationships, and symbols,
- Conduct studies in the natural settings of informants' lives by immersion and participation,
- Regard participants as informants who help to direct and interpret the topic of study, verify or refute conclusions, and
- Focus on exploring the particulars of the specific setting in time (historical, life course, developmental), people, and place (physical and culturally constructed).

Ethnography also aims to build, validate, and refute generalizations about human society. While ethnography focuses on the detailed case of a particular culture or setting, it does so with an eye to proposing larger patterns of human life by using what was already learned about the beliefs and structures of other societies. Generalizations grow from the accruing record of each society which reveals recurrent patterns of similarity and difference across systems of cultural values, relationships, and symbols. General theories about the sociocultural life of humans are built and constantly case tested by "the ethnographic veto," a term for the use of the rich record of empirical ethnographic studies of societies to provide counter examples to a theory or over-simplification. For example, to provide a newer model of stigma (the social labeling of a person as undesirably different) researchers used a comparative global perspective to reveal institutional practices that covertly perpetuate stigma (Das, 2001; Link & Phelan, 2001).

Ethnography's insider view also helps to dispel myths. For example, economic development experts engaged to help subsistence peasant farmers living high in the Andes Mountains believed the poverty was due to idleness and under-employment. These experts wanted to get more out of those they labelled as lazy peasants because they saw few were laboring to dig or work the fields, tasks associated with busy productivity to the economists' industrial models. Ethnographers used time allocation cultural methods (Gross, 1984) to observe and ask peasants what they did, when and why. Their findings showed that the crops required seasonal effort, not constant intense work. Moreover, of equal importance was that people must be posted to stand watch over the fields to protect the grain harvests from predation by birds and animals. Thus, crop watching was a very important economic routine. When understood and counted as productive activity (not idleness), the employment rate was 98% (Brush, 1977).

Conducting Ethnographic Research

Ethnographic research is conducted in a series of basic phases:

- Preparation and entry,
- Immersion using participation and observation,
- Exit, and
- Writing up.

Study participants are properly called "informants" as they inform and teach about their life and community; they are not "subjects" controlled by the researcher.

The start of immersion can take several forms, from preparation by reading in an archive or publications, to entry into the field site. As an outside participant, the ethnographer begins to learn the language and folk categories, how to ask and answer questions, the history, kinds, and structure of relationships, behavioral expectations, social and life values, and life as defined by the participants. Next, with continued immersion and increasing insider knowledge, the questions reach into deeper realms of cultural values and philosophy; they explore diversities in beliefs, and individual and group histories. Comparisons between observed actions and events and the informants' expressed beliefs and social rules become possible with extended time in the field. Keeping an ongoing field journal is used to monitor accruing insights and highlight gaps and questions. Lastly, ethnographers exit the setting to begin summarizing and interpreting their field data, but now at a distance. The distance allows them to mentally compare insider and outsider viewpoints to explore and analyze the fieldwork data.

The data collection toolkit for ethnography features:

- Direct interview and observation of people, events, and artifacts,
- Personal participation in the ongoing routine and special events of social life, and
- Interpreting the stories, symbols, and objects in the field site.

Nowadays the traditional handwritten journal notebooks and maps for collecting data, are replaced by a range of technology including digital audio or video recordings, GPS mapping, and computer software for taking field notes, indexing, and analyzing of observations and interpretations.

Contributions of Ethnography

Since ethnography can provide systematic data on people's own perceptions, meanings, expectations and needs, and structures for action, it is a powerful tool for the health and social service fields. Ethnography is used to study topics that range from the social structure and value systems in hospitals and rehabilitation facilities to patterns of practitioner-patient interactions. Such research has provided important insights to problems and practices. For example, ethnographic studies of the culture of nursing homes have shown that:

- Disruptive behavior by residents on a Alzheimer's care unit may be tied to the timing of nursing shift changes (e.g., during meals) (Stafford, 2003),
- Incontinence is defined and managed by nursing home staff as a wetness problem requiring diapers instead of a potentially reversible medical condition that can be treated (Schnelle et al., 1989), and
- Malnutrition is a major problem in American nursing homes (Kayser-Jones et al., 2003).

Without such sustained ethnographic field research, these important health issues would never have been identified.

The ethnographic tradition shares with occupational therapy the desire to work to learn, not predefine, people's own meaningful desired habits, values, and actual life settings as well as perceived challenges and resources. Perhaps this is why occupational therapists have looked to and welcomed ethnographic insights offered by anthropology researchers, and reciprocally, anthropologists have benefited from the insights of occupational therapy clinicians to guide and frame their own work on disability and rehabilitation (c.f., Mattingly, 1998).

Grounded Theory

Grounded theory is an inductive method designed to construct theory from qualitative data (Glaser & Strauss, 1967). It does so by following a defined set of procedures for data collection but without direction from existing constructs or theory about the phenomena. The term *grounded* refers to the aim to have the theory emerge from, or be grounded in, the data. The grounded theory approach seeks to ensure that the theory derives from the experiences of those on whom the study is focused. In this instance, the theory is a generalization about the empirical data. That is, the investigator seeks to explain the data from the specific study, not to propose a conceptual or philosophical model.

Conducting a Grounded Theory Study

The procedures for conducting a grounded theory study can be described individually, but are undertaken concurrently during the project rather than in a sequence. Researchers will use data collection methods such as narratives, focused interviews, informal discussion, participant observation, and field notes. Sample sizes often are not large, usually in the range from 20 to 50 participants at the most.

What distinguishes the grounded theory method from other qualitative methods is the structured formalized process for data collection and theory development. It specifies a continuous interplay between data collection and interpretation leading to a generalization that is project-specific for that data (Strauss & Corbin, 1990). The work of evolving a theory from the data is one of constant comparison by which each new piece of information (a belief, explanation for an event, experience, symbol or relationship) is compared to each other piece of data as it is gathered.

Investigators code the conditions, actions, strategies for interactions, and outcomes observed. Should the information be similar to other already existing information, it is assigned to that category and labeled, or coded with the descriptive word or phrase for that group. On the other hand, if the idea or phenomenon does not fit a category already created, then a new one is created.

Over time a set of categories emerge that are refined and confirmed and the resulting set of categories is used to make a more abstract generalization (i.e., the grounded theory) to explain the phenomenon. The published reports from grounded theory studies follow a similar design; they usually would not contain a detailed literature review (preexisting theory and data). The report is a descriptive discussion of the structured procedures followed and findings.

Contributions of Grounded Theory

Grounded theory studies have the potential to offer important understanding of how people live with the challenges of illness and disability. For example, the goal of a grounded theory study by Clements, Copeland, and Loftus (1990) was to learn how parents coped with the adversity of living and caring for a child with a chronic illness. This study included focused interviews with thirty families who attended a clinic where the children were treated. They found heightened challenges and resource needs at the critical changes in the child's condition. A grounded theory developed by the researchers focused specifically on the phenomena described by participants in that study. The theory they proposed was that the specific ways of coping developed by a family with a chronically ill child attempts to meet the needs of all the family members. A balance or equilibrium is reached if there are resources, but that can not be maintained if the demands rise or the support changes.

Critical Theory

Critical theory researchers take the stance that knowledge (and theory) is not universal and absolute. Instead, it starts with the basic premise that social reality is embedded in and constructed in specific historical times and places and that it is produced and reproduced by people. Simply stated, then, adherents of critical theory see social reality and knowledge as relative to particular people and times. They argue that multiple social realities exist distributed across the various segments of society and groups. Critical theory overlaps with the post-modern philosophical perspectives discussed in Chapter 2.

Critical theorists contrast starkly with "positivists" who assume there is but one objective reality which can be captured and measured by instruments that are independent of the observer. Positivist studies generally attempt to test theory, in an attempt to increase the predictive understanding of phenomena. On the other hand, critical theory's purpose is to enlighten people and make them critically aware.

The goal in critical theory research is to bring to light or become aware, or (i.e., critical) rather than passively acting according to the reigning sociopolitical structures and settings that shape ways of thinking. In this context, the term, critical, does not mean to demean or ridicule. Rather, it means to pose questions. The aim of critical theory is positive social and political transformation, including reducing social injustices. Thus, it focuses on taken for granted ways of thinking, insights gathered through heightened awareness of the diversity, and inequalities afflicting many segments of society. More fundamentally, critical theorists view human inaction in the face of social injustices as resulting from domination by the status quo.

Critical theory is reflected in the work of a wide range of scholars from Marx and Hegel to Foucault and Derrida. One of the best known proponents of critical theory, Habermas (1988), along with others, argue that scientific and philosophical constructs are enmeshed in and serve to recreate wider social-historical patterns.[1]

[1]More general critical theory programs are sometimes also described as critical research (Mishler, 1986) or analytic induction (Strauss & Corbin, 1990). Cogent reviews of the limits of critical theory are also available (Hammersley, 1992; Honneth, 1991).

Qualitative Research Is Not Only for Pilot or Preliminary Research

Although qualitative research is often used as the first or exploratory investigation in a new area, it is also used to address problems that other methods have not been able to unravel in a well researched area. For example, research has shown that persons' appraisals of their own health are one of the most powerful predictors of disability and death. For example, persons who rate their health as fair or poor have a three times greater likelihood of death than those who rate it as good or excellent. These findings emerged from the analyses of many large-scale secondary datasets on health services utilization. Yet, extensive replication in multiple international studies has revealed little about what people have in mind or how they go about reasoning on their way to such self-labels for their health. Consequently, epidemiologists have recently turned to a variety of qualitative interview methods to learn first hand what was in the minds of individuals as they provided these self ratings. Qualitative findings are beginning to shed light on this issue. For example, Idler and Benyamini (1997) reported that persons making self-rated health judgments are influenced not only by factors associated with their physical body and its maladies, but rather, include social aspects of the impact of their illnesses and disabilities too. Luborsky (2005) has found that self-appraisals and interpretations of health include complex belief systems related to the perceived moral consequences associated with labeling yourself as 'good' or bad'. The social fall-out associated with functional independence and the meaning associated with participation in roles, activities, and settings, exert an overwhelmingly powerful influence on how individuals rate their health, well-being, and overall life quality. None of these evaluations are or ever can be predicted by blood tests, medical diagnoses, or the severity of one's illness or injury. Similarly, research has shown that injury severity is not a useful predictor of either long term physical functioning or social participation and community integration (Dijkers, 1997, 1998; Lysack, Zafonte, Neufeld, & Dijkers, 2001; Mossey & Shapero, 1982).

Critical theory is less familiar to occupational therapy than some other qualitative epistemological traditions. Nonetheless, there are some examples of occupational therapy research that are directly informed by a critical theory perspective, such as the work of Whiteford and Wright-St. Clair (2004). A more critically informed occupational therapy will be reflective about the nature of the research questions it asks, their historical origins, and the forms for answers and solutions it allows. To the extent that occupational therapy is centrally concerned with practices that are "client-centered" (Law, 1998; Townsend, Langille, & Ripley, 2003) and morally concerned with their clients' social positions in society, they must be attentive to the diversity in their clients' desired goals and the methods by which occupational therapy practitioners can fully address their rehabilitation needs within that broader social context.

One limitation of this approach to research that is particularly relevant to occupational therapy is that in critical theory, the individual is not conceptualized as a willful autonomous person. Instead, individuals are viewed as social rule or norm bound; they are defined simply as the sum of family, work and community roles.

Conducting a Critical Theory Study

No formalized procedures exist for critical theory, compared to those for grounded theory. But, a generalized approach can be outlined (Luborsky & Sankar, 1993). The critical theory approach rests on the systematic pursuit of a set of clearly articulated questions.

There are four general components. First, a clear definition of a key concept or problem is presented. Second, a description of how the construct is currently conceptualized is stated, and that formulation's place in the continuing (past to present) thought on the issue is summarized, often as a literature review. Third, the current definition is critiqued to reveal gaps and limitations in the concept/problem formulation's ability to explain the phenomena it focuses on, and other problems that it does not highlight. Notably, one would ask in what ways the problems defined for study are consonant with the wider sociopolitical climate of that time, and in what ways they implicitly embody visions for continued re-creation of the existing social organization and values for human life. Fourth, the researcher conducts research and presents data that is informed by the analytical and historical critique. The form of results for critical theory research is new data as well as new questions and analytic frames for thought.

The Contributions of Critical Theory

Critical theory helps reveal how each culture and group has its own definitions for familiar scientific categories such as health, illness, ethnicity, family, or self. It points out that such familiar categories are not universal. For example, historically unrecognized ethnic and social class differences in how age relates to health, morbidity, and mortality have shaped the scientific portrait of what constitutes normal aging. While these intertwined social influences have always been present, they are only now coming to be understood (Dannefer & Sell, 1988; Longino, 1990).

In many respects, this is because it is difficult to be reflective about the times in which one lives. It is only afterwards, with the benefit of hindsight that investigators can see a historical period more clearly. For example, consider how clothing styles and fashions, tastes in music, and design of automobiles evolve over a period of years. The same is true for less visible attributes of a historical period. People during different decades hold very different attitudes and values than generations before, and afterwards.

A case in point is the public's attitudes toward people with disabilities. These attitudes have changed substantially over the last several decades. For examples, disabled persons are no longer systematically segregated in asylums and institutions. Moreover, while the status of persons with disability can still be much improved, there are disability rights laws, protections against disability discrimination in the workplace, more accessible buildings, and more public visibility and acceptance of disabled persons.

Occupational therapists are in a position to utilize the results of critical theory research to enhance their interventions and positively impact the occupational well-being of their clients. For example, occupational therapists are more aware of the disproportionate prevalence of disability among economically disadvantaged people (House, Kessler, Herzog, 1990; Townsend & Wilcock, 2003) and the exclusion of oppressed persons from opportunities or resources needed to engage in meaningful activity (Kronenberg, Simo-Algado, & Pollard, 2005; Whiteford & Wright-St. Clair, 2004). The promise of critical theory for occupational therapy is in examining and documenting underlying assumptions that reflect power imbalances and social injustices.

Phenomenology

Phenomenology is both a way of doing research (method) and a way of questioning and conceptualizing thought (philosophy). Like critical theory, phenomenology is a complex and multifaceted philosophy that is not easily characterized. Moustakas (1994) explains, "The understanding of meaningful concrete relations implicit in the original description of experience in the context of a particular situation is the primary target of phenomenological knowledge" (p. 14). Schwandt (1997) reminds us that phenomenology "rejects scientific realism and the accompanying view that the empirical sciences have a privileged position" (p. 114) in identifying and explaining features in our world.

At its most basic level, this approach focuses on the everyday life-world and gives great attention to the careful description of how the ordinary is experienced and expressed in the consciousness of individuals. This requires that phenomenology rests on an assumption that there is a structure and essence to personal experience that can be communicated to others in a systematic way, often using narratives. The primary question that is asked from this perspective is: what is the meaning of one's experience and how does one interpret it?

When William James appraised kinds of mental activity in the stream of consciousness (including their embodiment and their dependence on habit), he was practicing a form of phenomenology (James, 1967). So too are all analytic philosophers of the mind. Still, the discipline of phenomenology as we know it today is largely due to Edmund Husserl (2001) who launched the modern day movement with his seminal work, Logical Investigations. For Husserl, phenomenology integrates a kind of psychology with a kind of logic. It is psychological in the sense that it describes and analyzes types of subjective mental activity or experience, and it is logical in the sense that it describes and analyzes the objective contents of consciousness (i.e., experience). Other famous phenomenologists are Heidegger, Sartre, and Merleau-Ponty. Each hold different conceptions of phenomenology however, and use different methods to study human experience. The Encyclopedia of Phenomenology (Embree, 1997) is an excellent reference that comprehensively details the features of seven separate forms of phenomenology, including these prominent theorists.

Phenomenology contrasts with other qualitative research approaches in its stance toward the informant and the researcher. Phenomenological research regards the sense of lived experiences and meanings as fully knowable only by those who share the experience. That is, in ordinary life, people are somewhat limited in their ability to grasp and intuit the meanings of lived experiences of other individuals. This is because the meanings of experience must be transmitted and filtered from the person who has the experience to the other persons who wish to understand that experience (Luborsky, 1994a, 1994b, 1995). Of course, things can be lost in translation!

There are many forms of expressive media beyond words that are used to communicate expe-

rience with other people (e.g., body language, art, music, etc.). Nonetheless, it is not easy for one person to comprehend or appreciate another person's experience in exactly the same way that one does. Therefore, a critical element in phenomenological studies is the skill of the researchers in identifying an appropriate source of information about the experience they are choosing for study, a topic which will be addressed shortly.

There is a second major contrast with other qualitative approaches worthy of notice. In terms of the researcher, phenomenological research differs from ethnographic and grounded theory. In the latter forms of qualitative research, the meanings emerge through a back and forth unfolding exploration between the researcher and the researched, and are then further interpreted and explained during data analyses. In phenomenology, no structure or framework is imposed on the data by the researcher. Rather, the researcher must find and (re)present the experiences in the form they are expressed. This can be very challenging and considerable investigator effort must be devoted to the choice of sample to ensure that it can provide the fundamental insights into the experience that is the target of the investigation (Luborsky, 1994b; Luborsky & Rubinstein, 1995).

For example, if a phenomenological study is designed to understand the experience of surviving a hip fracture and returning to normal life in the community, then it would be imperative that an informed participant is selected for interview and perhaps even observation. Importantly, qualitative researchers must remember that in a study about the experience of hip fracture, the unit of study would be the individual with this injury, but the focus of research enterprise, or the units of analysis would be the experiences of hip fracture and the experiences of reconnecting to a personally meaningful life. The intent of a phenomenological researcher in such a study would be to gain understanding of what it is like to live with an altered body that limits mobility, and perhaps makes other people think of one as old. Phenomenological researchers would also want to know how these experiences shape the person's sense of themselves as a full adult person (Luborsky, 1994a).

As stated earlier, one's choice of informant is critical in phenomenology. Sampling in this tradition, as should be clear by now, must be purposive and theoretically driven, in an effort to maximize the range of experiential phenomenology of people with the experience of interest (Karlsson, 1993). Sampling in this tradition must also build on what is already known (Bertaux, 1981; Glaser & Strauss, 1967; Luborsky & Rubinstein, 1995). If phenomenological research is to be successful in capturing what particular experiences are like, it must gather their data from informed samples with first-hand access to the experience of interest. Only then can the investigation gain access and insight into the informant/participant's experiences.

Conducting a Phenomenological Study

Phenomenological researchers conceptualize the person and the environment as a whole. A central tenet of this perspective is that the only reliable source of information to answer questions about personal experience is the person with the experience, him or herself. Since each individual has his or her own unique reality, the task of the phenomenologist is to engage in lengthy discussions with participants about their experiences and then to locate and summarize common themes in their expressions of experiences that convey a central essential meaning. To begin to achieve this goal, four or more aspects of human experience need to be explored. These include:

> Just as quantitative researchers select from a toolkit of methods and frameworks, qualitative researchers have available a wide range of methods from which to select those best suited to their questions, the data required to answer the questions, and the forms of analyses suited to that data.

• The lived space (spatiality),
• The lived body (corporeal embodied experience),
• Lived social relationships (relationality), and
• Lived time (temporality).

Thus, phenomenology is simultaneously holistic and also relativistic to the particular experiences and situations of each person.

Understanding human experience also requires that the person with the experience must self-interpret these experiences for the researcher, and then the researcher must further interpret the individual's explanation provided by the person. Thus, the method of phenomenology is one of interactive dialogue and exchange, as the researcher seeks to know what the experience is like.

Typically, the data in phenomenological studies are collected by in-depth conversations in which the researcher and the informant are fully interactive. Analysis begins when the first data are collected. This analysis will guide decisions related to further data collection. The meanings attached to the data are expressed within phenomenological philosophy. The outcome of analysis is a theoretical statement responding to the research question. The statement is validated by examples of the data, often direct quotes from the subjects.

The procedures for phenomenological research involve biographical story telling and informal discussion, with encouragement to reflect on at least the four aspects of experience outlined above. Researchers listen for and inquire about the body, time, place, and settings of the phenomena, but the informant is entirely in charge of directing the narratives and story telling. In one example, occupational therapy researchers aimed to characterize the experiential features of engagement in creative activity as therapy for elderly people with terminal illness (la Cour, Josephsson, & Luborsky, 2005). Using extended discussions about the projects undertaken by older adults in Sweden, the researchers found how creative activity served as a medium that enabled creation of connections to wider culture and daily life which countered some of the more serious social consequences of terminal illness, such as isolation. The creation of connections to life experience in this study embodied three features: a generous perceptive environment as the foundation for meaningful activity, the creations as an unfolding evolving liberating process; and a reaching beyond the present for possible meaning horizons. The findings showed that creative activity fosters connections to meanings as an active person, even in the face of uncertain life-threatening illness.

Contributions of Phenomenological Research

As the previous example illustrated, powerful occupational therapy relevant insights are provided by this perspective. For example, Hasselkus (1998) used a phenomenological approach to illuminate the daily experiences of day-staff who cared for Alzheimer's patients on a dementia unit. Studies like this that deeply probe the experiences of care providers, be they professionals, family members, or others, are essential for the profession so that we can see how our interventions best fit to support the efforts of others.

A recent phenomenology method formulated by Karlsson (1993) is gaining use among occupational therapy researchers. For example, a compelling use of this phenomenological method is reported by Tham, Borell, and Gustavsson (2000). In this study of the experience of unilateral neglect post-stroke, research findings strongly supported the value of occupational therapy and clearly illustrate the links between research and effective practice. The following passage from the study illustrates the kind of insights that phenomenological research seeks to achieve (Tham & Kielhofner, 2003):

> *The study demonstrated that the participants needed to experience and ultimately come to a practical recognition of their own impairments and the consequences of those impairments during occupational performance, before they learned to handle them in everyday life. However, because neglect represents a particular life-world experience, people with neglect had to learn to stand outside their own experience. Specifically, because unilateral neglect is not directly experienced by the person who has it (e.g., the left half of the world is not "felt" to be absent from perception), persons with neglect must embark on a discovery process. This discovery process involves coming to understand that there exists a half of the world that is not part of their life-world. Once they can comprehend the existence of a part of the world that is outside their experience, they could begin to manage the consequences of their own unilateral neglect during occupational performance (p. 404).*

Conclusion

By now it should be clear that in qualitative research there is no single approach. As Patton (1990) suggests, investigators need to use the methods that are most appropriate for the research questions they confront. Just as quantitative researchers select from a toolkit of methods and frameworks, qualitative researchers have available a wide range of methods from which to select those best suited to their questions, the data required to answer the questions, and the forms of analyses suited to that data.

The reader should not expect to be able to neatly define and argue the merits and limits of each epistemological approach discussed in this chapter. It is sufficient to have begun to appreciate

the multiple kinds of stances and goals available to qualitative researchers. Chapters 20 to 22 provide more details of the nuts and bolts of undertaking qualitative research. They will illustrate in more practical ways how to implement the different frameworks outlined in this chapter.

REFERENCES

American Journal of Public Health. (2003, August). This issue focuses on public health advocacy and includes an article on challenges and strategies to obtain funding for Community-Based Participatory Research.

American Journal of Public Health. (2003, September). This issue focuses on the built environment and health. The article "Jemez Pueblo: Built and social-cultural environments and health within a rural American Indian community in the Southwest" describes a study that used participatory research to uncover sociocultural and environmental factors that indicate capacity for improving health.

Baron, R. J. (1985). An introduction to medical phenomenology. *Annals of Internal Medicine, 103*, 606–610.

Becker, G., & Kaufman, S. (1995). Managing an uncertain illness trajectory after stroke: Patients' and physicians' views of stroke. *Medical Anthropology Quarterly, 9*, 165–187.

Bertaux, D. (Ed.) (1981). *Biography and society: The life history approach in the social sciences*. Beverly Hills, CA: SAGE Publications.

Boas, F. (1966). *Kwakiutl ethnography*. Chicago, IL & London, England: University of Chicago Press & Toronto, Ontario: University of Toronto Press.

Brush, S. (1977). Myth of the idle peasant: Employment in a subsistence economy. In R. Halperin & J. Dow (Eds.), *Peasant livelihood* (pp. 60–78). New York: St. Martin's Press.

Clements D., Copeland L., & Loftus M. (1990). Critical times for families with a chronically ill child. *Pediatric Nursing, 16*(2), 157–161.

Crist, P., & Kielhofner, G. (2005). *The scholarship of practice: Academic and practice collaborations for promoting occupational therapy*. Binghamton, NY: Hayworth Press.

Csordas, T. (1994). *Embodiment and experience: The existential ground of culture and self*. Cambridge, UK: Cambridge University Press.

Dannefer, D., & Sell, R. (1988). Age structure, the life course and "aged heterogeneity": Prospects for research and theory. *Comprehensive Gerontology [B], 2*(1), 1–10.

Das, V. (2001). Stigma, contagion, defect: Issues in the anthropology of public health. Presented at "Stigma and Global Health: Developing a Research Agenda." An International Conference, September 5–7, 2001, Bethesda, Maryland. http://www.stigmaconference. nih.gov/papers.html (accessed June 20, 2005).

Dijkers, M. (1997). Quality of life after spinal cord injury: a meta-analysis of the effects of disablement components. *Spinal Cord, 35*, 829–840.

Dijkers, M. (1998). Community integration: conceptual issues and measurement approaches in rehabilitation research. *Topics in Spinal Cord Injury Rehabilitation, 4*, 1–15.

Edgerton, R. B. (1967, 1993). *The cloak of competence: Stigma in the lives of the mentally retarded*. Berkeley, CA: University of California Press.

Embree, L. (Ed.) (1997). *Encyclopedia of phenomenology.* Dordrecht and Boston: Kluwer Academic.

Finlayson, M. (2004). Concerns about the future among older adults with multiple sclerosis. *American Journal of Occupational Therapy, 58,* 54–63.

Forsyth, K., Summerfield-Mann, L., & Kielhofner, G. (2005). A scholarship of practice: Making occupation-focused, theory-driven, evidence-based practice a reality. *British Journal of Occupational Therapy, 68,* 261–268

Geertz, C. (1973). *The interpretation of cultures.* New York: Basic Books.

Gitlin, L., Luborsky, M., & Schemm, R. (1998). Emerging concerns of older stroke patients about assistive device use. *The Gerontologist, 38*(2), 169–180.

Gitlin, L., Lyons, K. J., & Kolodner, E. (1994). A model to build collaborative research or educational teams of health professionals in gerontology. *Educational Gerontology, 20*(1), 15–34.

Glaser, B., & Strauss, A. (1967). *The discovery of grounded theory: Strategies for qualitative research.* Chicago: Aldine.

Gross, D. (1984). Time allocation: A tool for the study of cultural behavior. *Annual Review of Anthropology, 13,* 519–558.

Habermas, J. (1988). *The logic of the social sciences.* Cambridge, MA: MIT Press.

Hammersley, M. (1992). *What's wrong with ethnography? Methodological explorations.* London, England: Routledge.

Hart, E., & Bond, M. (1996). Making sense of action research through the use of a typology. *Journal of Advanced Nursing, 23*(1), 152–159.

Hasselkus, B. R. (1998). Occupation and well-being in dementia: The experience of day-care staff. *The American Journal of Occupational Therapy, 52,* 423–434.

Honneth, A. (1991). *The critique of power: reflective stages in a critical social theory.* Cambridge, MA: MIT Press.

House, J., Kessler, R., & Herzog, A. (1990). Age, socioeconomic status, and health. *Milbank Quarterly, 68*(3), 383–411.

Husserl, E., (2001). *Logical investigations* (vols. 1 and 2), Trans. J. N. Findlay. Ed. with translation corrections and with a new Introduction by Dermot Moran. With a new Preface by Michael Dummett. London and New York: Routledge. A new and revised edition of the original English translation by J. N. Findlay. London: Routledge & Kegan Paul, 1970. From the second edition of the German. First edition, 1900–01; second edition, 1913, 1920.

Idler, E., & Benyamini, Y. (1997). Self-rated health and mortality: A review of twenty-seven community studies. *Journal of Health and Social Behavior, 38*(1), 21–37.

James, H. Jr. (1967). The Letters of William James (Boston: Atlantic Monthly Press, 1920). I:190 quoted in J. McDermott (Ed.), *The writings of William James* (p. xi). New York: Random House.

Jason, L. A., Keys, C. B., Suarez-Balcazar, Y., Taylor, R. R., Durlak, J., Davis M. & Isenberg, D. (Eds.) (2004). *Participatory community research: Theories and methods in action.* Washington, DC: American Psychological Association.

Karlsson, G. (1993). *Psychological qualitative research from a phenomenological perspective.* Stockholm: Almqvist & Wiksell International.

Kaufman, S., & Becker, G. (1986). Stroke: Health care on the periphery. *Social Science and Medicine, 22,* 983–989.

Kayser-Jones J., Schell, E., Lyons, W., Kris, A., Chan, J., & Beard, R. (2003). Factors that influence end-of-life care in nursing homes: The physical environment, inadequate staffing, and lack of supervision. *Gerontologist, 43*(2), 76–84.

Kielhofner, G. (1995). A meditation on the use of hands. *Scandinavian Journal of Occupational Therapy, 2,* 153–166.

Kielhofner, G. (2001). *A model of human occupation* (3rd ed.). Philadelphia, PA: Lippincott, Williams & Wilkins.

Koning, De K., & Martin, M. (1996). *Participatory research in health: Issues and experiences.* London: Zen Books.

Kronenberg, F., Simo-Algado, S., & Pollard, N. (2005). *Occupational therapy without borders.* UK: Churchill Livingstone.

la Cour, K., Josephsson, S., & Luborsky, M. (2005). Creating connections to life during life-threatening illness: Creative activity experienced by elderly people and occupational therapists. *Scandinavian Journal of Occupational Therapy, 12*(3), 98-109.

Langness, L., & Levine, G. (Eds.) (1986). *Culture and retardation.* Dordrecht: Reidel.

Link, B., & Phelan, J. (2001). Conceptualizing stigma. *Annual Review of Sociology, 27,* 363–385.

Luborsky, M. (1994a). The cultural adversity of physical disability: Erosion of full adult personhood. *Journal of Aging Studies, 8*(3), 239–253.

Luborsky, M. (1994b). The identification and analysis of themes and patterns. In J. Gubrium & A. Sankar (Eds.), *Qualitative methods in aging research* (pp. 189–210). Thousand Oaks, CA: SAGE Publications.

Luborsky, M. (1995). The process of self-report of impairment in clinical research. *Social Science & Medicine, 40*(11), 1447–1459.

Luborsky, M. (1997). Attuning assessment to the client: Recent advances in theory and methodology. *Generations, 21*(1), 10–16.

Luborsky, M., & Rubinstein, R. (1995). Sampling in qualitative research: Rationales, issues, and methods. *Research on Aging, 17*(1), 89–113.

Luborsky, M., & Sankar, A. (1993). Extending the critical gerontology perspective: Cultural dimensions. *Gerontologist, 33*(4), 440–444.

Lysack, C., & Kaufert, J. (1994). Comparing the origins and ideologies of the independent living movement and community based rehabilitation. *International Journal of Rehabilitation Research, 17,* 231–240.

Lysack, C., Zafonte, C., Neufeld, S., & Dijkers, M. (2001). Self-care independence after spinal cord injury: Patient and therapist expectations and real life performance. *Journal of Spinal Cord Medicine, 24*(4), 257–265.

Mattingly, C. (1998). *Healing dramas and clinical plots: The narrative structure of experience.* Cambridge, UK: Cambridge University Press.

Mays, N., & Pope, C. (2000). Qualitative research in health care: Assessing quality in qualitative research. *British Medical Journal, 320,* 50–52.

Mays, N., & Pope, C. (1995a). Observational methods in health care settings. *British Medical Journal, 311,* 182–184.

Mays, N., & Pope, C. (1995b). Reaching the parts other methods cannot reach: An introduction to qualitative methods in health and health services research. *British Medical Journal, 311*, 42–45.

Mays, N., & Pope, C. (1995c). Rigour and qualitative research. *British Medical Journal, 311*,109–112.

Minkler, M., Blackwell, A., Thompson, M., & Tamir, H. (2003). Community-based participatory research: Implications for public health funding. *American Journal of Public Health, 93*(8), 1210–1213.

Mishler, E. (1986). *Research interviewing*. Cambridge, MA: Harvard University Press.

Mossey, J., & Shapiro, E. (1982). Self rated health: A predictor of mortality among the elderly. *American Journal of Public Health, 72*, 800–808.

Moustakas, C. (1994). *Phenomenological research methods*. Thousand Oaks, CA: SAGE Publications.

Murphy, R. (1987). *The body silent*. New York: Henry Holt.

National Institutes of Health (2001). *Qualitative methods in health research: Opportunities and considerations in application and review*. Office of Behavioral and Social Sciences Research, National Institutes of Health. Bethesda, MD. NIH Publication No. 02-5046. (http://obssr.od.nih.gov/Publications/Qualitative.PDF)

Patton, M. (1990). *Qualitative evaluation and research methods*. Thousand Oaks: SAGE Publications.

Ragin, C., Nagel, J., & White, P. (Eds.) (2004). *Workshop on the scientific foundations of qualitative research*. National Science Foundation. Arlington, Virginia. Document Number: nsf04219. (also, http://www.nsf.gov/pubs/2004/nsf04219/start.htm accessed May 3 2005).

Reilly, M. (1962). Eleanor Clark Slagle Lecture: Occupational therapy can be one of the great ideas of 20th century medicine. *American Journal of Occupational Therapy, 16*, 1–9.

Schnelle, J. F., Traughber, B., Sowell, V. A., Newman, D. R., Petrilli, C. O., & Ory, M. (1989). Treatment of urinary incontinence in nursing home patients. A behavior management approach for nursing home staff. *Journal of the American Geriatrics Society, 37*, 1051–1057.

Schwandt, T. (1997). *Qualitative inquiry*. Thousand Oaks, CA: SAGE Publications.

Spradley, J. (1979). *The ethnographic interview*. New York: Holt, Rinehart and Winston.

Spradley, J. (1980). *Participant observation*. New York. Holt, Rinehart and Winston.

Stafford, P. (Ed.) (2003). *Gray areas: Ethnographic encounters with nursing home culture*. Sante Fe, NM: School of American Research Press.

Strauss, A, & Corbin, J. (1990). *Basics of qualitative research: Grounded theory procedures and techniques*. Newbury Park, CA: SAGE Publications.

Stringer, E. (1999). *Action research* (2nd ed.). Thousand Oaks, CA: SAGE Publications.

Taylor, R. R., Braveman, B., & Hammel, J. (2004). Developing and evaluating community services through participatory action research: Two case examples. *American Journal of Occupational Therapy, 58*, 73–82.

Tham, K., Borell, L., & Gustavsson, A. (2000). The discovery of disability of disability: A phenomenological study of unilateral neglect. *American Journal of Occupational Therapy, 54*, 398–406

Tham, K., & Kielhofner G. (2003). Impact of the social environment on occupational experience and performance among persons with unilateral neglect. *The American Journal of Occupational Therapy, 57*, 403–412.

Townsend, E. A., & Wilcock, A. A. (2003). Occupational justice. In C. Christiansen & E. Townsend (Eds.), *Introduction to occupation* (pp. 243–273). Thorofare, NJ: Prentice-Hall.

Viswanathan, M., Ammerman, A., Eng, E., Gartlehner, G., Lohr, K., Griffith, D., Rhodes, S., Samuel-Hodge, C., Maty, S., Lux, L., Webb, L., Sutton, S., Swinson, T, Jackman, A, & Whitener, L. (2004). *Community-based participatory research: assessing the evidence*. Summary, Evidence Report/Technology Assessment No. 99 (Prepared by RTI–University of North Carolina Evidence-based Practice Center under Contract No. 290-02- 0016). AHRQ Publication 04-E022-1. Rockville, MD: Agency for Healthcare Research and Quality. http://www.ahrq.gov/clinic/evrptpdfs.htm#cbpr.

Wark, L. (1992). Qualitative research journals. *The Qualitative Report, 1* (4): (pages not numbered) (http://www.nova.edu/ssss/QR/QR1-4/wark.html)

Whiteford, G., & Wright St. Clair, V. (2004). (Eds.) *Occupation and context in practice*. Sydney: Churchill Livingstone.

Zemke, R., & Clark, F. (Eds.) (1996). *Occupational science: The evolving discipline*. Philadelphia: F. A. Davis.

CHAPTER 20

Gathering Qualitative Data

Cathy Lysack • Mark R. Luborsky • Heather Dillaway

Qualitative research has become an increasingly important mode of inquiry for occupational therapy. Long dominated by techniques borrowed from the experimental sciences, occupational therapy has embraced many of the methods of the social sciences, particularly from anthropology and sociology, as an alternate means of studying and understanding social phenomena of relevance to the profession. While valuable in its own right, quantitative research differs substantially from qualitative research. Quantitative research describes phenomena using a single universal standardized language (numbers), and investigator-defined topics and issues. Based on statistical theories of probability, it seeks to discover and describe such things as statistically defined norms and central tendencies and averages in the distribution of the data.

> Irrespective of its particular disciplinary roots, qualitative studies ask questions that are rarely specifiable as conventional hypotheses, as is the case in quantitative research.

In contrast, qualitative methods use the local varieties of languages and words of the participants in the social settings studied. These methods work to discover and describe participant-defined topics of concern and socioculturally constructed worlds within which individuals pursue meaningful actions. In short, qualitative methods seek to discover and describe socioculturally constructed worldviews, values, and sociocultural norms and how these are instilled, enacted, reinforced, or resisted and changed in everyday life. Qualitative researchers go to the field to study the topic in the natural settings where people socially interact.

While it would be tidy if the phrase "qualitative research" denoted one single methodological approach, unfortunately this is not the case. There are many different forms of qualitative research, depending on the discipline and its assumptions about what counts as knowledge and how it is generated. Probably the best known approaches in the qualitative tradition come from anthropology and sociology. These disciplines provide a wide array of tools and approaches with which to gather qualitative data including ethnography, life histories, narrative analysis, symbolic interactionism, content analysis, discourse analysis, critical theory, semiotics, and action research, to name a few.

Each of these qualitative approaches is different with respect to the type of research designs commonly used, the methods used to gather data, data analysis approaches, and the form in which study findings are disseminated. In spite of their differences, there are some common characteristics and procedures for the conduct of qualitative research and several philosophical assumptions that are shared among them. Most basically, all qualitative researchers are intrigued with the complexity of social interactions as expressed in daily life. This interest takes them into natural settings as opposed to laboratories. This is why qualitative research is also sometimes called naturalistic inquiry. Rossman and Rallis (1998) have summarized the core features of qualitative research and qualitative researchers. Although they originally outlined eight features, we believe the following five are unique to qualitative work. Qualitative work is:

- Naturalistic,
- Emergent and evolving, rather than prefigured,
- Fundamentally interpretive,
- Characterized by a holistic view of social phenomenon, and
- Sensitive to the influence of investigators on the study and its findings.

In its broadest sense, qualitative research must be understood as the systematic study of social phenomena. Irrespective of its particular disciplinary roots, qualitative studies ask questions that are rarely specifiable as conventional hypotheses, as is the case in quantitative research. The ultimate goal of qualitative research is to go beyond the *what* of research to explain the *why* and *how*. This empirical pursuit requires concepts and tools that yield such information and approaches.

Major Data Gathering Strategies

The following are four main methods for gathering qualitative data:

• Participation in the setting,
• Direct observation,
• In-depth interviewing, and
• Analyzing documents and objects.

All of these methods fundamentally reflect the core qualities of qualitative research as identified by Rossman and Rallis (1998). This chapter provides a review and discussion of these four methods, highlighting their relative strengths and weaknesses. Given the key role of the qualitative researcher as a data collection instrument, the role and stance of the qualitative researcher are also critically examined.

Participation

Participation is both an overall approach to inquiry and a data gathering method. To some degree all qualitative research has a participatory element. Participation demands first-hand involvement in the social world chosen for study. Qualitative researchers work to gain access to modes of understanding and to approximate as closely as possible the lived realities of those studied, knowing that they will rarely (some would say never) truly experience the situation exactly as their participants do. The purpose of engaging in participation is not to become one of the group studied, but rather to use what is seen and heard to help identify what is important to learn about, and to discover issues and events that might not be obvious to an outsider who is using only preconceived ideas.

Ideally, as with the traditions of cultural anthropology and qualitative sociology, researchers will spend considerable time in the field. Depending on the study purpose and the size of the research project, this could mean anywhere from several weeks to a year or more participating in the routine activities of the group and setting. This immersion experience offers the qualitative researcher the opportunity to learn directly from his or her own experience. The implicit premise is that a truer understanding of the phenomenon studied will be obtained. This approach requires the researcher to be very self-aware and reflective, not only observing the actions and behaviors of others, but also appreciating and recording his or her own personal thoughts, experiences, and reactions.

The personal reflections gained from participation in the research setting, as well as the observations made, are systematically recorded and included as an essential part of the study data. Thus, simultaneously, the researcher using participation as a method is challenged to recognize and record how his or her presence in the field may or may not be influencing study participants' behaviors in the field. Major efforts to track the impact of the presence of the investigator in the field are a feature of this methodology. Journals and field-notes, recorded both during and after episodes of data collection, are a core source of study data.

Observation

Observation requires careful watching, listening, and recording of events, behaviors, and objects in the social setting chosen for study. The observation record, frequently referred to as field notes, is composed of detailed nonjudgmental, concrete descriptions of what has been observed. For studies relying exclusively on observation, the researcher makes no special effort to have a particular role other than simply being an unobtrusive observer.

Unlike participation methods, observational methods do not ask the researcher to become actively involved. Rather, the researcher takes a relatively outsider role. Observational studies of in-patient rehabilitation units are one example of this type of study. Of course, without other sources of data, the meaning of observations can only be inferred. That is why, when setting, interactions among persons, and their personal views are important, qualitative studies include both observation *and* participation.

Participant observation is a more active data gathering strategy and combines elements of both approaches. In this method, the investigator establishes and sustains a many-sided relationship with a social phenomenon in its natural setting for the purpose of developing a scientific understanding of that phenomenon. Participant observation thus allows qualitative researchers to see how things really are (observation) and also check in (participation) with knowledgeable insiders who can confirm, or not, the researchers' emergent insights, understandings, and explanations as they experience the the social phenomenon first hand.

There can be several degrees of participant observation, sometimes in sequence. In its earliest stages, the qualitative researcher using a participant observation approach enters the field with a broad topic of interest but no predetermined categories or strict observational checklists. At this stage, the investigator is intent on identifying and describing the actions of the participants in pursuit of meaningful goals, values, and ideals. Noting these patterns and reviewing them systematically over time leads to the development and use of more highly specified observational checklists and perhaps even some direct questions to key participants in the setting.

The ultimate goal of the qualitative researcher using participant observation is to understand and explain the sociocultural values, norms, and expectations that underlie the personal beliefs and individual actions observed. As time in the field proceeds, it is possible to understand more fully both what one is observing and what it all means. As stated at the beginning of this chapter, qualitative research is responsive to the changing conditions of the research setting and the topic studied. Thus, as new data are obtained and synthesized, the iterative process of uncovering and then confirming emergent understandings (that is, analysis) begins.

Many qualitative studies use observational methods, at least to some degree. For example, when conducting an in-depth interview, a qualitative researcher is engaged in a shared social scene with customs and expectations about how to interact, be respectful, and reciprocate. The nature of the social interaction is part of the data collection and the data to record. Also, investigators are attentive to the participants' body language and affect— not only their words. In whatever ways observation is used, it is demanding on the part of the researcher. Observational researchers confront psychological discomfort and fatigue, unexpected ethical dilemmas, and may even expose themselves to unanticipated danger. In addition, interviewers are required to responsibly and as completely as possible record the social happenings around them at the same time as they are trying to find the big picture analytically. This is a real challenge since studying human beings in their natural environments (e.g., in home settings, rehabilitation centers, schools, etc.) by definition implies complexity and a fast-paced and ever-changing social scene.

The following are key activities of qualitative researchers using participation and observation:

- "Gaining entry" to the setting,
- Negotiationg and establishing a social identity in the setting,
- Sustained engagement in the research setting over time and learning how to maintain good relationships in that community or group,
- Active and genuine involvement with group members,

- Development of useful observational measures,
- Accurate documentation of observations in distracting conditions,
- Managing requests to align oneself with one person or group versus another,
- Simultaneously participating with and recording observations of study participants at the same time as experiencing the phenomenon oneself and recording it in a complex and ever-changing environment, and
- Documenting additional fieldnotes, questions, quandaries, and complexities after each data collection episode.

It must be recognized that qualitative studies utilizing observation and participation have both strengths and weakness. Their greatest strength is that they provide very rich and detailed data in settings and situations in which subjects are observed. While other methods such as in-depth interviews would contribute information from one individual's point of view, observation and participation allow the investigator to study interactions between multiple persons and between persons in specific physical and/or social environments. Furthermore, observation and participation methods are necessary when individual interviews are not possible because of the limited capacity of the participants. For example, some research participants may not be able to provide full and complete information about their experiences owing to the nature of their disability or health condition. When this is the case, alternate or at least supplemental data gathering strategies are necessary. Clearly, participation and observation studies are very time- and labor-intensive. These types of studies also require a great deal of advance preparation, including, at times, special permissions to allow access to the setting and group members of interest. In addition, the presence of the researcher in both participation and observation studies can lead study participants to alter their behavior in order to "look good" in the eyes of the researcher or provide what they perceive to to be as "the right answer" (i.e., social desirability bias or Hawthorne effect). This can pose a serious threat to the validity of study findings.

Qualitative researchers must be aware of the potential for study participants to influence the events that transpire during data collection as well as the potential for those influences to impact the study findings. Fortunately, while individuals being studied may be conscious of the presence of the researcher and consciously edit or restrict their more extreme or controversial opinions and

An Example of Research in Which Both Observation and Participation Were Key Data Collection Methods

Siporin and Lysack (2004) were interested to know how the self-perceived quality of life (QOL) of women with developmental disabilities working in supported employment differed from those working in sheltered workshops. In this study, the principal investigator (Siporin) devoted weeks of inconspicuous observational data collection in the places of employment of her research participants. In the daytime, she accompanied her research participants as they worked in small enclaves as housekeepers in local hotels and as food preparation assistants in fast-food restaurants. In the evenings, she observed their leisure activities with their family and friends.

This design choice provided invaluable data about the structures and routines that characterized her subjects' work and home life. For example, the pace of work, chain of authority at work, and the complexity of numerous pieces of equipment in the workplace were far more evident to the investigator after observation than before. So were the stresses these women experienced because of unreliable transportation. Frequent but unpredictable disruptions in bus transportation wreaked havoc with the official work schedule to which they were supposed to adhere. This caused tensions and occasionally heated arguments and certainly reduced the more positive attitudes these women might have held toward the supported employment experience. A lack of available safe transportation also curtailed participants' leisure activities (e.g., shopping, going out to movies, bowling).

Other observations in the home setting provided essential data with which to understand these women's QOL. These data painted a picture about the love, respect, and acceptance these women enjoyed and what specific roles and responsibilities they assumed within their families. These data provided a valuable contrast or counterpoint against which to compare the workplace observations. Participant observation data in this study revealed how agency policies and governmental regulations impacted participants' QOL. For example, it was learned that if a supported employment worker actually improved her skills to the extent that she was promoted and received a pay raise, she would likely become Medicaid ineligible, thus putting in jeopardy insurance coverage for significant medical expenses including, for example, hospital care, durable medical equipment, prescription medications, and eyeglasses. This was not something these women (or their families) were prepared to do. Thus, despite their wishes and efforts to become more self-sufficient, the women with developmental disabilities stopped short of any "success" that would put their Medicaid eligibility at risk. Without the method of participant observation, these policies and regulations would not have been identified; nor would their consequences on the participants' perceived QOL be fully understood.

actions, over time study participants will become less concerned about the presence of the investigator and reveal their "true" thoughts and behaviors. As with all data collections methods, however, the investigator faces trade-offs with every methodological choice. Table 20.1 summarizes the strengths and weaknesses of participant observation. The most successful qualitative researchers will consider all aspects of their topic, its purpose, and the research setting they are in, and then choose their research methods accordingly.

In-Depth Interviews

In-depth interviews are most often conducted in face-to-face situations with one individual, although they can be conducted by telephone and in a group situation (see focus group interviews below). The goal of the in-depth interview is to delve deeply into a particular event, issue, or context. Interviews differ from participation and observation primarily in the nature of the interaction. In the in-depth interview, the purpose is to probe the ideas of the interviewees and obtain the

most detailed information possible about the topic at hand. Interviews vary with respect to their a priori structure and in the latitude the interviewee has in responding to questions.

Generally speaking though, in-depth interviews can be developed along a continuum. At one end of the continuum is the most open-ended and unstructured conversational approach, in which the interview proceeds more like a casual visit. Another, slightly more directed approach includes having some prepared but still unstructured topics about which to inquire. A semistructured interview provides even more structure by using a combination of fixed-response and open-ended questions. At the far other end of the continuum is the structured interview, in which the questions and response categories are virtually all predetermined.

Irrespective of their specific form, data gathered using in-depth interviewing methods are typically recorded using audiotapes and written notes, and sometimes even video recording when the study purpose demands. Audio and video recording is used to increase the amount of data available for later analyses and to provide verification of

Table 20.1 **Participant Observation: Relative Strengths and Limitations**

Strengths	Weaknesses
"Rich description," that is, detailed information about the social phenomenon studied.	Few opportunities to probe the specific meanings of participants' actions and behaviors if data are not supplemented by other methods such as interviews.
Very natural (i.e., valid) data are obtained in these normal (versus laboratory) settings.	
Only method that permits study of people's actual behaviors (versus merely their attitudes and beliefs) in a particular physical and social environment.	Responses may be influenced by social desirability bias.
	Can be complex to analyze these data without other data to confirm the observed and/or investigator experienced data.
May be the only form of data collection possible when study participants themselves cannot be interviewed because of their disability.	Often requires advance planning, special permissions, and more detailed IRB/ethics proposals before approval for the study is granted.

data accuracy. For example, audiotapes can be used to create data ranging from a paraphrase or summary of a conversation all the way to microscopically detailed data on tone and speed contours, including the length of pauses and speed of talking. Verbatim transcripts of interviews can be analyzed at a later point in the study, at varying amounts of detail.

Unstructured Interviews

Unstructured interviews resemble guided conversations. Such interviews typically include a relatively short list of "grand tour" general questions (sometimes referred to as an "interview guide"), and interviewers generally respect how the interviewee frames and structures their responses. For example, an unstructured interview about the adequacy of home care received by a recently discharged stroke patient may begin with a general question such as, "How is your home care going since you got out of the hospital?" The answer provided may be brief or lengthy, but no matter what the interviewee says, the interviewer accepts the words used and explanations as offered. Still, when appropriate, some gentle probe style follow-up questions may be used to delve more deeply into interviewees' initial responses, seeking examples, explanations, and rationales for expressed beliefs and behaviors. For example, an appropriate probe after a question such as, "Have you encountered any unexpected surprises with your home care?" might be something like "Could you describe one or two of these surprises?" Optimally, probes like this are value neutral and function simply to elicit more information. They are not meant to direct the respondent toward any particular topic or value judgment, but rather to encourage the respondent

to reveal more specific information about his or her personal experiences and circumstances. Other appropriate probes might be: "Can you tell me more about your reasons for this answer?" and "Could you give an example?" Most importantly, however, the unstructured or conversational interview conveys the attitude that the participant's views are valuable and useful, and the task of the researcher is to capture these views as completely and accurately as possible.

Semistructured and Structured Interviews

These types of interviews permit modest to maximum investigator control over the design and sequence of research questions. In structured interviews, interviewers are trained to ask each question precisely as written. This does not mean, however, that the interview consists only of fixed-response questions. All interviews, whether unstructured or structured, can include both fixed-response and open-ended questions. For example, a qualitative interview focused on the meaning of disability might include a fixed-response question such as, "Do you think of yourself as the same person you were before your injury?" for which the response set could be limited to "yes" versus "no." The response categories could also be categorical and ordered, for example, "Yes, just the same," Yes, somewhat the same," "No, not really the same," and "No, absolutely not the same at all." Finally, the question could be entirely open-ended. As their name suggests, semistructured interviews typically include a combination of fixed-response and open-ended questions with a variety of response categories, some of which border on the kinds of response categories typical of surveys. Structured interviews provide the least interviewer

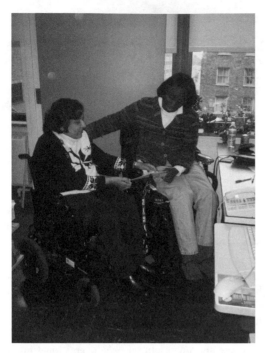

Figure 20.1 Research team members practice conducting a semistructured interview using an interview guide.

flexibility, as all of the questions are predetermined and the interviewer is encouraged not to deviate at all from the prescribed interview protocol. Table 20.2 summarizes the strengths and weaknesses of fixed-response versus open-ended interview questions.

Interviewing has strengths and limitations. Interviews involve personal interaction and cooperation; trust and rapport between interviewer and interviewee are essential. Interviewees may not be comfortable sharing all that the interviewer hopes to explore, or may be unaware of specific facts and experiences that are relevent to the study purpose but are not revealed in the interview.

Lack of skill and training on the part of the qualitative researcher may also lead to poorly developed questions, and inadequate interviewer training may lead to inadequate probing and follow-up questions during the interview itself. To be successful, qualitative interviewers must work to develop superb listening skills and be skillful at personal interaction, question framing, and gentle probing for elaboration. One of the great benefits of interviews is the volume of detailed data that can be obtained. However, even optimal interview data are time consuming to analyze, and depend-

Table 20.2 Fixed-Response Versus Open-Ended Interview Questions: Relative Strengths and Limitations

	Strengths	Limitations
Fixed-response questions		
	Quick to ask and answer.	Unclear if the respondent understands the question as the researcher intended.
	Large cohort of data can be obtained in a short time.	
	By forcing "one best answer" a respondent's basic position is clarified.	Relevant information may not be collected.
	Responses can be more easily compared across groups.	Responses may be influenced by social desirability bias.
	Statistical analysis can be conducted on numerical data.	
Open-ended questions		
	Respondents' interpretation of the question is more obvious.	Can be very time consuming to both gather data and analyze it.
	Issues of importance to the participant are more likely to be identified and described.	Respondents may not wish to reveal personal, sensitive, or provocative information.
	There is sufficient time and interviewer awareness to record nonverbal behaviors and emotional responses (e.g., tears, anger, confusion, etc.).	Data from open-ended questions are not easily comparable across groups.
	With a skilled interviewer, sensitive topics can be more easily probed and explored.	Without well-trained interviewers, too much of the data gathered may be "off-topic" and not adequately address the study aims.

ing on the expertise of the interviewer, too much of these data will not be central to the study aims and thus may not illuminate the study topic at hand. Transcribing and analyzing less relevent data is costly and time consuming.

Finally, there is the issue of the quality of interview data. When interviewing is the sole method of qualitative data collection, the qualitative researcher obtains the interviewees' perspectives on events and issues. This is usually absolutely appropriate. However, if the study aims require more objective confirmation of events and issues, the qualitative investigator may need to triangulate his or her interview data with data gathered through other methods. The process of triangulation (discussed further below) provides an additional methodological check on the validity and reliability of study data.

In certain circumstances, qualitative researchers will have to consider a wider array of factors when planning and carrying out interviews. This is true when interviewing special or vulnerable populations, for example, children or persons with specific types of disabilities. For example, interviews with children require greater care during the construction of interview questions to ensure they are not too complex for a child to understand. Depending on the topic, questions may also pose unique risks to the child. For example, particular interview questions about severe burns they sustained in a traumatic house fire, or injuries sustained in a serious car accident, may create emotional upset, fear, or even psychological distress, depending on circumstances associated with those events. Similarly, interviews with persons with specific types of physical and cognitive disabilties demand special consideration.

Qualitative interviewing in these contexts requires not only more careful interview item construction in advance of the interview, but also training to prepare the interviewer for a range of expected and unexpected challenges during data collection itself. For example, persons with stroke may have comprehension and speaking difficulties and it may be necessary to move from more open-ended to more fixed-response style questions. In addition, the choice of interviewer is a consideration, even if the answer is not. Sensitive topics about sexual function or victimization, for example, clearly require attention to who can best make the interaction comfortable, such as a same-sex or same-age person. Alternatively, choosing someone with the same ethnic background may not always provide better data. In studies of minorities there may be unstated assumptions about shared under-

standings or experiences (true or not) that make it harder to get an informant/participant to fully verbalize and explain experiences or beliefs that are "obvious" or taken for granted. Qualitative investigators conducting interviews with these special populations will need to address a wide array of considerations such as these in the institutional review board (IRB)/ethics approval process that is virtually always required in advance of approvals to conduct research studies sponsored by universities, whether these studies take place in a rehabilitation facility, or a person's home, school, or workplace, and so forth.

The following are key activities of qualitative researchers before and during in-depth interviews:

- Identifying an appropriate study sample,
- Logging communication during recruitment efforts,
- Establishing comfort, rapport, and trust with interviewees,
- Developing the interview guide (conversational style) or explicit interview protocol (structured style interviews),
- Skillful listening and question asking,
- Judging appropriately when and how and if to probe and pursue interesting turns in the interview (e.g., disclosure of unexpected information, controversial or provocative opinions and statements, etc.),
- Presentation of the self as a competent and skillful interviewer,
- Note taking comprehensively while astutely questioning and listening, and
- Writing-up summaries and notes about what the interviewee said as well as reflective personal observations.

Table 20.3 summarizes the strengths and weaknesses of qualitative interviewing. In addition, there are two other kinds of interviewing that deserve brief mention owing to their frequency of use and potential to contribute unique data to a qualitative research project. These are focus group interviews and key informant interviews. Table 20.4 summarizes their strengths and weaknesses.

Focus Group Interviews

The focus group interview emerged from consumer research in the 1950s. Consumer research showed that people tended to make decisions within a group context, and therefore, to understand consumer behavior, consumer preferences needed to be studied in a group setting. The same

Table 20.3 **Qualitative Interviewing: Relative Strengths and Limitations**

Strengths	Weaknesses
The researcher can gather detailed information on the topic of interest. This method also permits exploration of additional topics generated by individuals' responses. Optimal confidentiality. Assuming expert interviewers who establish a respectful and trusting relationship, more personal information is revealed in interviews than may be the case in focus group situations.	Lack of efficiency: It takes much more time to gather data from individuals than from groups. All data are "self-reported." There is no opportunity to confirm or disconfirm the personal values, attitudes, and beliefs or the related background and events related by participants, unless triangulation is used. Vast amounts of data are generated by interviews and they are very costly to transcribe. Data analysis is costly and time-consuming, even with excellent data.

principle holds in occupational therapy research. Occupational therapists recognize that many aspects of decision-making, especially decisions related to health and disability, are made with family members and other valued persons. Thus, the optimal context to gather data can sometimes be a context in which numerous and varied perspectives can be heard at the same time. This is what makes the focus group a popular method of gathering qualitative data.

Table 20.4 **Focus Group and Key Informant Interviews: Relative Strengths and Limitations**

	Strengths	Limitations
Focus groups	Efficiency: The researcher can gather data from multiple persons instead of only one. Because of the dynamic interactions across group members, there is the potential for contradictory opinions and not only consensual views to be shared. More valid data: Group interactions tend to hone in on the most salient issues, therefore making it relatively easy to identify a relatively consistent shared view among interviewees.	The number of questions asked must be minimized since it takes so much more time to gather multiple responses. With six people in a one-hour focus group, an interviewer would have difficulty asking any more than 10 questions. Responses may be overly "sanitized," that is, negatively influenced by social desirability bias. Difficult to control: Unexpected diversions, interpersonal conflicts, etc. can distract group members from its purpose. Skilled facilitators are essential to quality data. Difficult to take notes with so much going on. Limited ability to protect confidentiality.
Key informant interviews	Insight: Key informants are well informed and can shed considerable light on the history and policies of groups and organizations. They may be elites or simply ordinary informants who are identified for more intense in-depth follow-up.	Often requires a referral from a prestigious and respected "others" before access is achieved. Requires great skill and effort to "manage" the egos and personalities of these important leaders and spokespersons.

Focus group interviews are conducted with a small group of people on a specific topic. Typically four to six people participate in the interview, which lasts about 1 to 2 hours (although focus groups can include eight to twelve participants, or even more). Participants in focus group interviews are usually a homogeneous group who are selected because of their knowledge about the study topic. Participants in focus groups get to hear each others' responses and contribute their own responses in light of what others have said. Often the questions in a focus group are deceptively simple. The aim is to promote the focus group participants' expressions of their views through the creation of a supportive environment.

As with other methods, the focus group has countervailing strengths and weaknesses. To a great extent, the advantages of the focus group interview are the disadvantages of the individual interview and vice versa. The primary advantage of focus group interviews is their efficiency. A great deal of information can be gathered quickly. In addition, focus groups provide the opportunity for data to emerge as a result of the dynamic interactions between group members. However, it is a common misperception that focus groups are only, or best, for learning about shared opinions or main themes. Further, focus group interviews have high face validity because they are conducted in a natural social setting and under more relaxed circumstances than individual interviews.

The downside, of course, is their management. Particularly strong personalities can dominant the focus group and some individuals may not have an opportunity to express their views, especially if they are in disagreement with a dominant member of the group. Optimal data from focus groups require a skilled facilitator so that there are opportunities for all members to participate and contribute. Because the facilitator/interviewer has less control over what is discussed in the focus group, the interview can result in lost time as irrelevent and dead-end issues are discussed. It may also be difficult to manage the group conversation at the same time as recording people's opinions on the topic at hand, which is why a focus group convenor and a note-taker are often used. Finally, data gathered using this method can be very difficult to analyze because context is essential to understanding individual comments and it is simply not possible to delve into the background context for every opinion offered without the entire focus group grinding to a halt. The feature box on the next page illustrates the usefulness of focus group interviews.

Key Informant Interviews

Key informants are used in at least two ways. In one form, "elite" interviews are conducted with individuals considered to be influential, prominent, and/or well-informed people in an organization or community. Key informants (elites) are specifically selected for interview on the basis of their expertise in areas relevant to the research. In another approach, key informants are selected from the larger sample for more extended and in-depth discussion.

Key informant interviewing has many advantages. Valuable information can be gained owing to the positions these persons hold in social, political, or administrative realms. Key informants can also provide an overall view of the organization and its activities, policies, past history, and future plans from a particular perspective. The disadvantage of key informant interviewing is that is often difficult to gain access to this group. They are often very busy people and difficult to contact, especially initially. The interviewer may have to rely on an introduction or recommendation of another elite to gain access/entry to the study setting. Another disadvantage of interviewing key informants or elites is that the interviewer may have to radically adapt the interview to suit the wishes and predilections of the person interviewed. Although this is a possibility with all individual interviewing, elites may be especially bright, thoughtful, and articulate and will resent poorly conceived or ill-phrased questions.

Well practiced at public meetings and persuasive arguments, key informants may desire an active interplay with their interviewer and be unhappy and uncooperative if the interviewer is not superbly prepared or not capable of a pleasing intellectual exchange (see Table 20.4). Thus, conducting key informant interviews can put a considerable strain on the interviewer, who must demonstrate competence in inquiring about the subject matter at hand, and, at some level, be prepared to entertain his or her interviewee with shrewd questioning, and even sharp debate. This hard work can pay off, however, as elites are typically intelligent and quick-thinking people and are completely at home in the realm of ideas, policies, and generalizaitons.

Written Documents and Material Objects

Researchers may choose to gather their data using sources of already existing information, or secondary data. Analysis of available documents (as opposed to primary data newly collected by the

An Example of Focus Group Interviews

Dillaway and a research team from the Barbara Ann Karmanos Cancer Institute in Detroit recently conducted a study about African-American men and prostate cancer (Dillaway et al., 2005). The purposes of this study were threefold:

1. To explore African-American men's awareness of prostate cancer,
2. To determine the barriers to their participation in prostate cancer research trials, and
3. To begin to develop new ideas for recruitment strategies to encourage more African-American men to participate in research trials.

In the pilot stage of the research, focus group interviews were used since research team members wanted to make sure that they were exploring a large range of potential barriers to recruitment and were unsure what recruitment strategies would increase African-American men's participation in research.

Not wishing to assume they already knew the answers to these questions, focus groups were selected so the investigators could see how African-American men themselves conversed about these topics. Eight focus groups with 61 African-American men were conducted. Focus group participants highlighted a range of barriers to their participation in research trials, many of which were expected. For instance, in every focus group, participants highlighted their mistrust of doctors and researchers as a reason for their reluctance to participate, sometimes referring to the infamous Tuskegee experiment as a reason for this mistrust. In that experiment, which is discussed in detail in Chapter 29, African-American men with syphillis were not informed that they were taking part in a research study on the long-term consequences of untreated syphillis.

Since the investigators were well aware of the historical injustices perpetrated on this minority population in the name of health research, they expected participants to highlight such barriers. Yet, in the course of conversation, African-American men also highlighted reasons why they would participate in research trials. For instance, in all eight focus groups, participants discussed how important it was for African-American men to "step up" and be models for future generations. They also discussed how important it was to keep themselves healthy so that they could ensure their ability to finish raising their children. Finally, they highlighted the fact that, in order to remedy the lack of knowledge about African-American men's health, they knew they had to overcome their mistrust of research studies and participate in research, if only to make certain that their children would be healthier than they were.

As a result of the focus groups, the research team learned that individual participants had a higher awareness of prostate cancer and a greater desire for more research than anyone of the team expected. In addition, while the researchers expected participants to highlight barriers to participation in research, they did not expect participants to highlight so many reasons why they would be willing to participate. Because most existing research only highlights the barriers to African-Americans' participation in research, the researchers did not even ask any questions about why individuals might want to participate in research trials. Thus, if the researchers had not conducted focus groups, a method of data collection in which new meanings can be highlighted within group conversation, they may not have realized that individual African-American men have many reasons to participate in prostate cancer research and, more specifically, may not have realized that African-American men's connections to their families and to racialized communities could directly facilitate individuals' participation in research trials. These data would not have been identified without the focus group method.

researcher such as interview transcripts) can include diaries and personal journals, historical documents, minutes of meetings, Web sites, advertisements, annual reports, newspapers, magazines, or political speeches. Analysis can also utilize materials or cultural objects and artifacts.

Researchers who use as their primary or sole method a review of documents or studies of inanimate objects can be described as using an unobtrusive methodology. Observation, described earlier, is also an unobtrusive methodology. It is considered as such because there is minimal investigator disruption to the study participants and setting.

The use of documents often entails a special-ized analytic approach called content analysis. The raw material of content analysis may be any form of communication or text, although written forms are most common. Historically, content analysis emphasized systematic, objective, and quantitative counts and descriptions of content derived from researcher-developed categories. Today, content analysis can be exclusively numeric or exclusively interpretive—largely dependent on the theoretical traditions dominant within the researcher's discipline. For example, quantitative political scientists might rely exclusively on numerical counts of words in a political speech and use the evidence of the amount of particular forms of speech to argue that a particular politician holds a particular view. In contrast, an anthropologist or a historian will be far more interested in the meaning of the words conveyed by the text than by the number of times a phrase is spoken.

One can easily imagine an occupational therapy researcher designing a study using methods of document review and content analysis. For example, if a researcher was interested in understanding the meanings of mobility aids such as walkers, crutches, and wheelchairs to adults with mobility disabilities, they could design a study in which the family photographs of persons who have lived with mobility impairments all of their lives were reviewed and analyzed. The photographs would likely reveal a number of insights including how the devices were commonly used, and what activities these devices were helpful in facilitating.

The qualitative researcher in this type of study would also note who was in the photographs, in what locales the activities occurred, and whether there was any evidence of attempting to hide the mobility devices, perhaps related to embarrassment, shame, or stigma. Of course, a study that supplemented this analysis with individual interviews would result in potentially more useful data than relying on the photographs alone. When multiple methods of data collection are used in the same study, the approach is called triangulation. This is one way of increasing the rigor of a qualitative study, a technique that is discussed in more detail below.

Reviews of material and cultural objects are not restricted to those provided by individuals in one-on-one situations. Brochures, descriptions of program services, and historical documents developed by organizations, health programs, or social movements can be studied too. For example, in a study described in Lysack and Kaufert (1999), Lysack reviewed books, promotional, and educational materials used by activists within the independent living movement and professional proponents of international community-based rehabilitation. The goal of this research was to understand how consumer organizations and professional and policy bodies used the language and imagery of "community" to guide their disability-related educational and rehabilitation activities. Lysack used discourse analysis in this study, a specific method by which special attention is paid to the process of spoken and unspoken communication. This method revealed dramatic tensions between the service delivery models of the two groups, tensions that were directly linked to the fundamental views held about the meaning of community.

In another example, an ongoing study of com- munity integration after spinal cord injury, Lysack and Luborsky's (2004) research team is analyzing drawings made by its research participants depicting the meaning of this injury. While in many cases these drawings are only crude sketches, the visual representations offer a medium by which to express and represent experiences and ideas not readily put into words. Drawing allows participants a nonverbal way to "tap into" and express deeper feelings. Interviewers on this project are trained to ask questions after the drawing is completed to elicit responses about how and why the drawings were generated as they were. The drawings themselves, coupled with the participants' responses, shed considerable light on topics including the level of responsibility for the injury felt by participants; the degree of resentment and hostility aimed at those who have provided, or currently provide, medical treatment and care; and in a somewhat more abstract way, the existential place these persons occupy when they assume the label "disabled person" in an able-bodied world.

As stated earlier, methods that use written documents, visual materials, and cultural objects have their advantages. For example, they are usually more quickly moved through the human subjects IRB/ethical review process because they may be regarded as posing less "risk" of harm to the participant. On the downside, without supplementation with other data gathering methods, it may be difficult for the qualitative researcher to clarify the meanings of these materials and objects to those who possess them or are influenced by them. As mentioned previously, triangulation of data sources and data methods are two ways of increasing the methodological rigor of a qualitative study, issues that are discussed below.

The following are key activities of qualitative researchers engaged in document reviews and analysis of material and cultural objects:

- Selecting appropiate documents or objects,
- Gaining permissions to observe and study them,
- Selecting and using analytic methods best suited to the kind of data, and
- Identifying additional means by which to confirm their meanings.

Ways of Strengthening the Quality of Qualitative Data

In all research, the question must continuously be asked: "How trustworthy are these data? The trustworthiness of qualitative data, or how sure we can be that the data are accurate and reflect social, cultural, and lived reality, is essential since the goal of the qualitative researcher is to capture and communicate experiences, meanings, and social situations.

Several important methodological actions can be undertaken to enhance data trustworthiness, including:

• Interviewer training,
• Prolonged engagement in the field,
• Reflexivity,
• Triangulation,
• Stakeholder checks, and
• Audit trails.

These methods can be employed whether the data are collected via observation, participation, interviews, or review of existing documents, materials, and objects.

Interviewer Training

The importance of interviewer training should not be underestimated. The time and financial costs of interviews are great. Thus, significant time spent training interviewers is a critical investment to ensure that data are obtained most efficiently, without compromising quality.

Interviewer training includes technical skills on how to ask the interview questions and the use of follow-up probes to elicit more detailed explanations. It also includes training on appropriate behaviors needed to gain entry into the research context. The latter includes the interpersonal behaviors with research participants that occur during subject recruitment and data collection. Interviewers must also be carefully trained to ensure a consistent style of data collection across research participants. This requires an element of standardization in question asking and probing. At the same time, however, the interviewer needs to be flexible and responsive when the need arises.

These are skills that can be learned. For example, mock interviews under supervision are an excellent way to learn to ask questions skillfully, to listen carefully, and to pose appropriate follow-up questions. Interviewers especially must learn how to facilitate a somewhat conversational style during the interview at the same time that they communicate respect for the research participant. They must also learn to practice a quiet awareness of the trade-off between patience and efficiency.

Managing Bias in Qualitative Research

Bias is a type of prejudiced consideration or judgment. Several types of bias can negatively impact qualitative studies: (1) Over-reliance on accessible research participants or favoring more dramatic events and statements involving research participants and the context of study; (2) biasing effects produced by the presence of the investigator in the research site, that is, the Hawthorne effect; and (3) biases stemming from the influence of the participants and the research site on the investigator. In all of these situations, the investigator may be biased if he or she is unaware of the social influences that various players in the research enterprise exert and are subject to. In qualitative research, biases must be recognized and accounted for. Qualitative investigators have an onus to report on the reasons for having chosen their particular topic for study, their design choices, as well as decisions about sample and methods. All need to be transparent so that the reader of the study can judge for themselves the quality of the results.

Prolonged Engagement in the Field

Prolonged engagement is the phrase used to describe the period of time spent in the field observing the phenomenon of interest. The amount of time in the field varies, depending on:

• The nature of the inquiry and its scope,
• The design of the study,
• The time available to the investigator, and
• The time available to the research participants themselves.

> Trustworthiness in qualitative research is crucial since the primary contribution of qualitative research is to capture and convey the experiences, meanings, and events encountered in the field.

As a rule of thumb, however, data collection continues in the field until saturation is reached. Saturation is the point in the data collection period when the researcher is gaining little or no new information. Since the criteria are data-based and not time-based, there is no fixed standard duration of time in the field. Investigators need to evaluate their data for signs of diminishing gains or saturation. When investigators are no longer adding new insights, or no longer puzzled by what they observe and are able to predict what is going to happen next, saturation is likely being reached. This means that it is nearing the time to leave the field and begin writing up the results of the observations in the field.

Reflexivity

Reflexivity refers to a deliberate and systematic process of self-examination. It involves a continuous cycle of:

• Seeking insights from inward reflection on the experiences of working in the outside world, and
• Looking back at what is being learned outside in light of the inner experience.

This process is necessary in qualitative research because the investigator will encounter a wide array of thoughts, feelings, and reactions to people and events in the course of data collection. While such feelings and reactions are not a major concern of quantitative researchers, they are of great importance to qualitative researchers.

First, these data are important in and of themselves. Especially in observational and participation studies, these are the only data that will be collected and analyzed. Second, the reactions and views of the qualitative researcher—both gleaned as a direct result of participation in the study and brought to the study in the form of preexisting attitudes and values—have the potential to color the data collection and analyses processes. Qualitative researchers acknowledge that this sort of influence is real and has the potential to influence study findings.

They also know that while the "bias" cannot, and in fact, should not be eliminated, it is important to identify it and examine its influence on emerging interpretations. Personal diaries are frequently used by qualitative investigators to note these attitudes, feelings, and reactions. Later, the diaries themselves become a source of data and are an important check on the development of research conclusions.

Triangulation

Triangulation is another technique used to increase the accuracy (or trustworthiness) of data gathered. Triangulation refers to the use of two or more strategies to collect and/or interpret or analyze information. For example, in a single study triangulation may mean using interviews to learn what people say to investigators about using a wheelchair and observation to see what they actually do and tell to others, instead of relying on either one

method alone. The purpose of triangulation is to validate a particular finding. Triangulation of data methods increases the chances that the conclusions reached are better able to represent the whole set of relevant features, or are "true" due to the complementary strengths of the respective methods.

While triangulation of methods is the most common form of triangulation in qualitative inquiry, there are other forms of triangulation, including triangulation of data gatherers. Triangulation of data gatherers refers to the use of two or more individuals who have independently observed and recorded their own field notes of a phenomenon. Data quality is enhanced by comparing their observations afterwards, and resolving differences through discussion. The same process can be undertaken during the data analysis stage of a research project. Triangulation in this sense refers to the use of multiple persons to do the data analysis. Sometimes this is called peer debriefing. Irrespective of its title, the process is one of multiple investigators simultaneously but independently engaging in the analytic process.

Peer debriefing is very valuable in qualitative inquiry because it provides a means by which areas of disagreement and controversy are highlighted. Again, as in data collection, the use of multiple analysts provides a mechanism for contrary views to arise and receive careful review. Peer debriefing may be the only way for opposing opinions to be heard and contrary explanations for phenomenon aired. The use of peer debriefing sometimes leads to additional data collection as the need to clarify conflicting data and conflicting views becomes apparent. The entire process strengthens the legitimacy of the final version of study findings. It is an important point of departure from more standardized forms of data collection that rely on a standardized fixed set of measures conducted identically with each participant.

Stakeholder Checks

Also called member checking, stakeholder checks is the process whereby the investigators check out their assumptions and emerging interpretations about the data with the original stakeholders who provided the information. This is vitally important. Not only does it ensure accuracy of the facts and information gathered in the study, but it also helps ensure that the investigator's conclusions make sense from the perspective of the persons who experienced those events.

As with prolonged engagement in the field, there is no magic amount of stakeholder checking that is "right" for every study. In very small studies, it may be possible to return the interview transcript to every person interviewed for checks on accuracy of transcription and to return drafts of emerging research findings to the original participants too. In a large study, however, this is usually not possible and sometimes only a small portion of the data (commonly about 20%) are returned to the original stakeholders for this sort of check.

Audit Trail

An audit trail is a systematically maintained set of documentation, typically including:

- All data generated in the study,
- Explanations of all concepts and models that shaped the study design,
- Explanations of procedures used in data collection and analysis,
- Notes about technical aspects of data collection and analysis as well as decisions taken throughout the study to refine data collection procedures and interpretations,
- Personal notes and reflections, and
- Copies of all instruments and interview protocols used to collect study data.

The audit trail can be used by the researcher as a means of managing record-keeping and encouraging reflexivity about a project and its goals. It also permits a third-party examiner to review all aspects of the conduct of a qualitative study and attest to the use of dependable procedures. In this way, the audit trail functions as a means of reliability checking on both the procedures and conclusions of a study.

Project-Based Methods

Project-based methods include daily operational procedures that help to minimize errors in all processes related to data collection, data storage, and data management. Chapter 33 addresses these more technical and procedural aspects of actions taken to ensure optimal data quality and data security in detail. However, two final aspects of qualitative data gathering should be reviewed, namely entry and exit from the research setting.

Entering the Field Study Site

Textbooks on qualitative research do not often address the basic issues of entry and exit from the field, especially the relationships that must be created and then ended with the participants/informants and stakeholders who support access to the research setting. Neglecting these processes can ruin even the best developed scientific design. Thus, entering and exiting relationships with participants at the field site requires careful and full consideration of practical details.

Adequate preparation is necessary to ensure that all members of the research team (subject recruiters, interviewers, etc.) present themselves and treat others professionally. This includes, for example, one's style of dress and behavior, since appearance and verbal communication send very important messages to the research participants about the importance of the study, and the investigator's respect for them as human beings. A reasonable rule of thumb is to dress conservatively but professionally. It is important to be attentive to the values and style of the individuals and organizations where the data are gathered. This can require "dressing up" in studies conducted in more formal settings, as well as "dressing down" in studies with teenagers or where circumstances dictate.

The hazards associated with being both too formal and too informal can be overlooked by qualitative researchers. When project staff misjudge the impression required to be taken seriously in the research setting, the entire study can be put in peril. In those cases, organizations will be impossible to penetrate and informants impossible to recruit for the simple reason that participants perceive the research is not sufficiently "in tune" with them to reward the project with their participation.

If research participants do not accept the legitimacy of the researchers or do not take the research endeavor seriously, they may not participate, or, alternatively, provide only very limited data. Ongoing effort is needed to remind project staff of the importance of appearance and professionalism and to take care to represent the project to others appropriately. Only in this way can the highest quality of data be collected.

Gaining entry to the field of a qualitative study can be difficult and challenging for other reasons. For example, an organization or group may have had a negative experience with a previous project. For example, in the study of community integration after spinal cord injury described earlier, research staff realized that potential study recruits had several misperceptions about what participation in the study really meant. They learned, for example, that for some recruits spinal cord research meant being "stuck with needles" or "strapped to a machine." Interest and willingness to participate increased significantly, once it was understood that the study involved being interviewed and no invasive procedures would be used.

Another reason that gaining entry into the field can be difficult is because the gatekeepers to the research setting are important and busy people. They may view research participation as less important than many of their other activities. In such a situation, gaining access will require considerable persistance, tact, and possibly assistance from someone who is respected in the setting. At this preliminary level, gaining access requires the investigator to negotiate with those who control access to the research setting, or access to the documents or objects that wish to be studied. The investigator must also balance the needs of the study against the concerns of the host group.

Where the investigator expects cooperation, gaining entry may be largely a matter of establishing trust and rapport. A mainstay of the qualitative investigator is saying something like: "I'm here because I would like to understand X better and because we believe your opinions and experiences will help us to learn more about Y and help to improve Z". When access is expected to be more difficult, often the best tack is through the known sponsor approach. In this approach, the qualitative researcher is vouched for by an already familiar and respected person. If truly trusted and respected, the qualitative researcher can rely on his or her introduction to facilitate entry and to facilitate if or when unanticipated bumps arise in the data collection process over time.

A useful technique in participant observation studies in particular is to begin observations/fieldwork at the same time that new members begin the activity of study interest or join the group. By using timing to one's advantage, investigators can minimize the disparity between their level of knowledge and that of the study participants.

A closely related challenge is obtaining high-quality data once in the field (Dillaway, 2002). Although achieving excellent data quality is not directy linked to gaining access to the research site, it too is a topic not often addressed in qualitative methods textbooks. If measures are not taken to ensure smooth operations, data quality will suffer. As mentioned earlier, challenges to data occur when participation in the research is difficult for participants, for whatever reason. This may be due to research questions that participants consider too private, provocative, or controversial. In situations like this, participants may be too embarrassed to reveal their true attitudes and describe their experiences in full detail, even to a well-trained and empathetic interviewer. When participants feel the questions they are answering are too personal or intimate or find the topics studied too emotionally difficult, they may drastically restrict the information they share. Superficial data is the result.

On the other hand, the interviewer may cause poor quality data. An interviewer who is perceived to be overly comfortable or overly intrusive and who creates an unwelcome sense of familiarity with participants, can have negative consequences. These interviewer problems can best be avoided by thorough staff training, clearly written recruitment materials, and prepared interview scripts and responses to frequently asked qestions to use verbatim when answering the most common queries of prospective research recruits. With complete descriptions of the study purpose, information about the kinds of the questions that will be asked, and honest evaluations about the time and effort required of participants provided before data collection, most problems of data collection can be avoided.

Collecting qualitative data can be challenging for reasons beyond the practical issues reviewed above. A qualitative interviewer or qualitative participant-observer is always at some risk of being pulled into the lives of study participants (Dillaway, 2002). This pull can come in the form of requests for assistance and advice, and emotional support, for example. For occupational therapists who are also researchers, the dual role of clinician and researcher can be especially challenging. For example, in the study of community integration after spinal cord injury mentioned earlier, office staff and interviewers were frequently asked for advice on the following: where to obtain better home care services, where to socialize in order to meet someone of the opposite sex, how to find a better medical specialist, where to buy an adapted motor vehicle, how to obtain funding to return to school, how to find research projects that paid more, and how to find a better job. Of course, these requests for advice were predicated on the reasonable assumption that the staff possessed a higher degree of expertise in some of these areas than participants did themselves, although this is not always true. When researchers are also clinicians, they may find themselves in conflict about which hat they are wearing and what ethical and practical obligations they have to both the project and the research participants. Thus, qualitative researchers should be aware that while they must develop sufficient rapport and closeness to research participants to elicit useful research data, there will be times when the relationship becomes too close with the potential for negative consequences to participant and researcher alike.

To be clear, it is commonplace and expected that qualitative researchers will give back to their study participants in at least a modest way. The provision of helpful answers, advice, and assistance are some immediate ways of doing this and providing the reciprocity that researchers feel they owe their research participants given their generous contributions of data. Reciprocating research participation (e.g., simple assistance, thank you cards, educational handouts) can become substantial and frequent, placing more serious demands on the qualitative researcher. When this occurs, the psychological resources of the interviewer/researcher can be stretched and even ethically compromised. In some instances, it can drain the financial, social, and tangible resources of the entire project.

In such situations, team meetings and discussions with the principal investigator of the study are imperative to ensure guidelines are set and followed to clarify what does and does not constitute appropriate action. These guidelines will involve issues of practicality but will also bear directly on a variety of ethical issues and responsibilities, not only to research participants, but also to project staff, the university, and even the agency that funded the research (Stern, 2005, November). Regular debriefing sessions with project peers, particularly after difficult data collection episodes, are essential to provide emotional support to data gatherers who can and do face surprising and stressful events during qualitative interviews.

When the interviews take place in the homes and communities of the research participants, the range of unexpected events can be rather remarkable. These surprises can inlcude such diverse things as insect infestations, angry family members, unhealthy pets, and instances of negligent care or abuse. Thus, thorough staff supervision and leadership by the principal investigator of the study is essential to provide guidance in dealing with such situations. This guidance is necessary to ensure that the actions of the staff are:

- As scientifically sound as possible,
- Ethically appropriate,
- Adequate to protect the research staff and the participants in the encounter, and
- In compliance with legal requirements (e.g., reporting abuse and neglect).

Since qualitative research can involve deep investigations of social experiences and meanings on personal and emotionally difficult topics there will be occasions when qualitative researchers encounter a study participant who becomes upset or tearful, or more rarely, expresses severe depressive symptoms or suicidal thoughts. Although these instances are infrequent, the qualitative researcher must be knowlegeable and prepared to exercise skill and resourcefulness. On such occasions, qualitative researchers must be appropriately emphathetic, but also be prepared to offer referrals to professionals for counselling and to relevent agencies for more tangible resources. Confronting these types of challenging interpersonal circumstances repeatedly and over a sustained time frame can lead to fatigue, stress, and potential burnout. Thus, the principal investigator must address such circumstances at their earliest evidence because they not only adversely affect the health and well-being of research staff, but also compromise optimal data quality.

Leaving (Exiting) the Field Study Site

Lofland and Lofland (1995) report that leaving the field is one of the most difficult aspects of research for the qualitative researcher. Leaving the field reminds the qualitative researcher of the unequal power relationships that exist between the researcher and the researched. Not uncommonly, leaving creates feelings of guilt since the researcher walks away with valued data and the participants appear to receive little or nothing at all. Of course, this is not completely true. The give backs mentioned above including small measures of assistance and advice can have a real and lasting impact on some study participants. Even sending out simple thank you cards might be appreciated. Beyond these tokens of appreciation, it is important to realize that many informants welcome the opportunity to not be seen as helpless, but rather to be seen as valued and useful to others through their role as research participants. In the end, however, all researchers must say thank you and goodbye.

One important reward to research participants is a methodologically rigorous study that yields important new findings that are disseminated to audiences where changes and improvements can be made. In this way, although the benefits of the research do not accrue directly to the individuals who originally contributed the data, and they are hardly immediate, there are meaningful benefits to others who share the same health condition, social circumstances, or experience. For all these reasons, qualitative reserch increasingly involves utilization of participatory approaches (see Chapters 38 to 40) that seek in the course of the study to empower participants to effect desired changes in their own circumstances.

Conclusion

As noted at the outset, qualitative research is a naturalistic, emergent and evolving, and interpretive endeavor (Rossman & Rallis, 1998). Qualitative data collection reflects these characteristics. In part, it means that the data collection process is intimately interwoven with the analysis and interpretation processes discussed in Chapters 21 and 22. Morover, qualitative researchers view social phenomena holistically, and are sensitive to their own influence on the study and its findings (Rossman & Rallis, 1998). These two elements always guide how the data collection strategies discussed in this chapter are undertaken in a given study.

REFERENCES

Dillaway, H. E. (2002). *Menopause in social context: Women's experiences of reproductive aging in the United States.* Unpublished doctoral dissertation, Michigan State University, East Lansing, MI.

Dillaway, H., Stengle, W., Miree, C., St. Onge, K., Berry-Bobovski, L., White, J., King, S., & Brown, D. (2005). *Community as paradox: Understanding both barriers and incentives to African American men's participation in prostate cancer prevention trials.* Manuscript submitted for publication.

Lofland, J., & Lofland, L. (1995). *Analyzing social settings: A guide to qualitative analysis and observation.* Belmont, CA: Wadsworth.

Lysack, C., & Kaufert, J. (1999). Disabled consumers' perspectives on provision of community rehabilitation services. *Canadian Journal of Rehabilitation, 12* (3), 157–166.

Lysack, C., & Luborsky, M. (2004). *Community living after spinal cord injury: Models and outcomes.* (R01 #1HD43378, funded by NIH / NICHD / NCMRR).

Rossman, G. B., & Rallis, S. F. (1998). *Learning in the field: An introduction to qualitative research.* Thousand Oaks, CA: SAGE.

Siporin, S., & Lysack, C. (2004). Quality of life and supported employment: A case study of three women with developmental disabilities. *American Journal of Occupational Therapy, 58* (4), 455–465.

Stern, E. (2005, November). American Occupational Therapy Foundation and American Occupational Therapy Association's "Promoting Integrity in the Next Generation of Researchers: A Curriculum for Responsible Conduct of Research in Occupational Therapy (Web-based curriculum)." Retrieved November 28, 2005 from http://www.aotf.org/html/rcrgraduateeducation.shtml

RESOURCES

Web Sites Relevant to Gathering Qualitative Research

http://www.socialresearchmethods.net/kb/

http://www.vanguard.edu/faculty/dratcliff/index.cfm?doc_id=4258

Recommended Readings for Gathering Qualitative Research

Creswell, J. C. (1998). *Qualitative inquiry and research design: Choosing among five traditions.* Thousand Oaks, CA: SAGE Publications.

Denzin, N. K., & Lincoln, Y. S. (2000). *Handbook of qualitative research* (2nd ed.). Thousand Oaks, CA: SAGE Publications.

Gubrium, J. F., & Holstein, J. A. (Eds.)(2002). *Handbook of interview research: Context and method.* Thousand Oaks, CA: SAGE Publications.

Lincoln, Y. S., & Guba, E. G. (1985). *Naturalistic inquiry.* Beverly Hills, CA: SAGE Publications.

Lofland, J., & Lofland, L. (1995). *Analyzing social settings: A guide to qualitative analysis and observation.* Belmont, CA: Wadsworth.

Marshall, C., & Rossman, G. B. (Eds.) (1999). *Designing qualitative research.* Thousand Oaks, CA: SAGE Publications.

Shaffir, W. B., & Stebbins, R. A. (Eds.) (1991). *Experiencing fieldwork: An inside view of qualitative research.* Newbury Park, CA: SAGE Publications.

Spradley, J. (1979). *The ethnographic interview.* New York: Holt, Rinehart and Winston.

Qualitative Methods In Health Research: Opportunities and Considerations In Application and Review. Office of Behavioral and Social Sciences Research National Institutes of Health. http://obssr.od.nih.gov/Publications/Qualitative.PDF

Contemporary Tools for Managing and Analyzing Qualitative Data

Nadine Peacock • Amy Paul-Ward

In any research endeavor, "raw" data must be transformed into coherent, believable, and meaningful findings. In qualitative studies, this transformation requires that the investigator make a number of strategic decisions about data management and analysis, including whether to use specialized technology. These decisions ordinarily require consideration of the following factors:

- The amount of time and funds allocated to the analysis process,
- The volume and structure of the data,
- One's comfort level with computer use and learning new software, and
- Epistemological stances guiding one's research.

Qualitative studies can range from those that are very exploratory to those designed to test or confirm hypotheses or findings from prior research. They can be performed by an individual investigator using participant observation in extended ethnographic fieldwork, or by a team doing rapid assessment with structured check lists and interview guides. The data can take many forms including:

- Loosely structured, lengthy narratives derived from interviewers,
- Short-answer responses to open-ended survey questions,
- Field notes taken by participant observers,
- Sound or video recordings, and
- Secondary data (e.g., documents, brochures, minutes of meetings) created by persons other than the investigators.

The data from a given study may range from a handful of documents to hundreds of them. Management and analysis of qualitative data can be done by an individual researcher or by a team, and can take a low-technology approach such as reading through data and making note of passages that illustrate useful themes, or a high-technology approach that makes use of sophisticated and specialized software. Finally, analysis and interpretation of qualitative data can reflect a broad spectrum of epistemological stances, from the strongly positivist to constructivist and interpretivist.

The aim of this chapter is to identify key elements shared by a range of approaches to qualitative data analyses, and to describe some of the varied software programs and other types of technological support (such as transcription and editing systems) that are useful for managing and analyzing qualitative data. This chapter will not provide an exhaustive list or review of software programs, as there are a number of publications and Internet resources that do this quite nicely (see Resources).

Common Features of Qualitative Research

Though qualitative research approaches are many and varied as discussed in Chapter 19, they tend to share certain commonalities. First, qualitative studies tend to have a less formal, less structured purpose. A qualitative study is often built around what Mason (1996) calls an intellectual puzzle—that is, a general question about a social phenomenon that the investigator hopes to understand better. This puzzle can then be expanded into a number of more specific research questions, which are usually best addressed by observing, listening, and interpreting rather than measuring and testing. Thus, qualitative research tends to be more inductive than deductive, and leans more toward theory building than theory testing.

A corollary to the inductive nature of the research is the blurring of boundaries among the tasks of data collection, data management, and data analysis. In other words, qualitative research is an iterative process, wherein some data are collected, interim analyses are performed, and research instruments are modified before further data are collected and analyzed. Because of the fluid, nonlinear nature of this process, it becomes particularly important to establish an audit trail, in which study design, data collection and management procedures, and analytic decisions are carefully documented.

Another key feature of qualitative data analysis is the creation of meta-data (i.e., data about data). These are new text and/or graphic products created by the researcher to represent key themes, constructs, and relationships that emerge from and are applied to a body of qualitative data. As such, they are tools for as well as products of data analysis. The following are examples of meta-data in qualitative research:

• Memos,
• Codes,
• Data matrixes,
• Concept maps, and
• Case summaries.

These are discussed in more detail in this chapter.

Management and Analysis— General Principles

One might think of coding and the production of other meta-data as features of computer-assisted qualitative data analysis. However, it is important to realize that qualitative analysis software simply adds a layer of technology to a process that was a well-established component of qualitative inquiry for decades before the widespread use of computers for these purposes.

To illustrate this point, consider a study undertaken at the University of California at Los Angeles (UCLA) in the 1970s to investigate the experiences of adults with developmental disabilities who were deinstitutionalized from state hospitals into community residential facilities. This study was funded through the Maternal and Child Health Division of the U.S. Public Health Service and undertaken by a team of anthropologists, sociologists, and occupational therapists. The investigators in this study were interested in how successfully these adults integrated into community life, what types of occupational routines they established, and how the organization structures and practices of the residential settings affected their lives (Bercovici, 1983; Goode, 1983; Kielhofner, 1979, 1981; Kielhofner & Takata, 1980).

In this study, participant observation was selected as the key method of data collection. The occupational therapists and social scientists accompanied and observed these adults going through their normal activities in the residential facilities and the neighborhoods where they lived. They took special note of:

• Interactions and conversations between the adults with developmental disabilities and staff in the facilities,
• Interactions between these adults and persons in the neighborhood,
• The daily routines of the participants, and
• The perspectives of participants on their everyday lives.

They also conducted interviews with these adults with developmental disabilities and with staff in the facilities. Observations were recorded as handwritten field notes, which were later typed up with additional descriptive detail. Interviews were audiotaped and later transcribed into typewritten documents. Occasionally, events or interviews were video-recorded; scripts of some of these videotapes were produced that included not only transcribed records of what was said, but also descriptions of behaviors that took place.

The researchers also routinely included the following in their expanded notes:

• Parenthetical comments and explanations that help fill in the picture of what was going on during the observations, and
• Reflexive notes on the investigators' reactions in the field and their role in generating and interpreting the data.

Qualitative research is an iterative process, wherein some data are collected, interim analyses are performed, and research instruments are modified before further data are collected and analyzed.

The activities described so far (typing and expanding field notes and transcribing interviews) are data management tasks as well as early steps in analysis, whereby the investigators began to extract meaning from and make sense of their qualitative data.

There are other important data management tasks that involved identifying the body of products that constituted the investigators' data. In this instance the data included not only typewritten information from participant observation, interviews, and videotaping, but also:

• Documents produced in the residential facility (e.g., mission statements, policies, notices, advertising brochures and reports),

- Medical records of some of the developmentally disabled adults, and
- Photographic and video records of events.

Decisions had to be made about where and how these varied types of data were stored, who had access to them, and what role they played in addressing the intellectual puzzle and research questions.

Once the investigators had begun to amass typed field notes, interview transcriptions, and other documents, they were ready to delve further into the analytic process. Recall that desktop computers were not widely available in the 1970s when this study took place. Although mainframe computers were commonly used in the social and behavioral sciences, their use for qualitative data analysis at this time was rather rare. How then did the systematic management and analysis of this data set proceed?

> Qualitative analysis software simply adds a layer of technology to a process that was a well-established component of qualitative inquiry for decades before the widespread use of computers for these purposes.

First, the investigators made multiple photocopies of each set of typed field notes and transcripts. An original copy with complete provenance information (such as the date and location the observation or interview took place, who gathered the data, who transcribed the tape, etc.) was kept in a reference file that was arranged chronologically and by site. The photocopies of the data were working copies that team members marked up in a process of active reading of the data—a key early step in the analysis process.

As the investigators first read through the data, they routinely made free-form margin notes, commenting on things that struck them as important and noting consistencies or contradictions in different observations or interviews. This process was facilitated by leaving a wide margin when notes were typed, so that there was ample room for such secondary note-taking. When more room was needed, notes were stapled to the pages to which they pertained. On examining these notes, one would notice that they fell into two broad categories (Figure 21.1):

- Conceptual labels, which were words or short phrases that serve as a kind of tag for segments of text, categorically describing information the segments contained. These would eventually evolve into a list of index codes used to label and retrieve segments of text that relate to a common theme (see the next heading).

- Analytic memos, which were reflective notes through which the investigators began to organize their thoughts about the data. These were the raw materials for later interpretations and findings.

In this study, because several investigators worked together they routinely presented and discussed the conceptual labels and analytic memos. These discussions led to the identification and elaboration of important emerging themes which were captured in additional analytic notes. They also guided the focus of future data gathering sessions, in that special attention could be paid to data that were relevant to these emerging concepts and themes. Clearly, the active reading and working discussions described here served as early stages of data analysis.

Conceptual Labels and Index Codes

As these investigators proceeded with multiple readings through the data, descriptive conceptual labels tended to become more systematic and consolidated, eventually culminating in a fairly comprehensive set of what can be called index codes. Such codes function much like the index to a book, in that they indicate places in the text where one can retrieve information on a particular topic.

Codes in this study included labels for different types of social behaviors (e.g., approaching, avoiding, staring, demeaning, reproaching, punishing); cognitive/affective states (embarrassment, frustration, anger, fear); subjective experiences (e.g., helplessness, agency, being "frozen in time"); and issues over which there was often misunderstanding between mainstream culture and those who were the focus of study (e.g., privacy, personal space, scheduling time). The early creation of codes such as "stigmatizing behavior" and "time use" reflects the fact that the study was conceptually grounded in the field of occupational therapy (e.g., Kielhofner, 1977), and that it built on previous research on deinstitutionalization (e.g., Edgerton, 1971).

Index codes then can be derived from findings of prior studies or from an initial conceptual framework, and additional codes can be added as new concepts emerge from the data. As codes are

Daniel and Michelle had brought their guitars, so naturally Doris was asked to play. Doris began to play and sing with Michelle accompanying her both playing guitar and singing. I was sitting on top of a picnic table a few feet away and Tim sat beside me. From where I sat I could see not only Doris and Doreen, Bill, Shereen, Jess and the UCLA folks, but also the many kids in the background who had noticed us and were curiously looking on. Finally one brave soul (a young man who appeared 10 years old) approached the corner of the area and ~~unobu~~ unobtrusively watched.

He appeared almost mesmerized by the whole scene which included: a toothless lady with funny red skin and very obese, wearing a red wig playing a guitar and singing her soul out; Buddy, a 50 year old with Down Syndrome whose appearance approximates a buddha figure, Doreen whose appeances approximate Doris's but who appears older in a black wig. Everyone else could possibly pass for "normal" on appearances alone. Probably the presence of these folks and the 5 UCLA people make the whole scene a little ~~lss~~ less threatening.

After the first young man had ventured into "our territory" more and more children began to approach. Those who were younger held expressions of curiosity, fear and intensity. They appeared nervous and cautious but inexorably drawn toward the scene. Two little girls looked at Buddy (A downs-syndrome phenotype) whispered to each other, giggled with their hands over their mouths, stopped, stared for a while and so forth over and over. Bobby seemed unaware of their attention; he did not appear to look at them. Most of the others focused on Doris and Doreen (who were doing the singing and ~~guiart~~ guitar playing). Responses were obviously age graded. The younger ones in the group seemed not to know what to make of it. The few who were older recognized that it was a spectactle and laughed obviously, with only mild attempts to hide their response such as turning away sometimes when they laughed harder. Something about their laughter was interesting- it was nervous laughter, not the open enjoyable laughter of a harmless joke, but laughter which betrayed some sort of ambivalence about the whole ~~sene~~ scene.

Most of the Picadilly people were unaffected by the presence of the children. Doris and Doreen seemed to definitely like them as an audience. Jim ~~is~~ was laughing about their presence and I think he saw them as just an audience to the music. Tim, however, got very nervous from the beginning. More than anyone else from Picadilly, so I think Tim knew what was going on. he turned to me with a mortified look on his face and said he was going to leave the area and join Nancy and Sheryl and Lolita who were playing tennis. I asked him if what was happening was making him nervous and he said yes. I knew that Tim knew and that he clearly wished not to accrue guilt by association. Later when Lisa, and the others joined us from the tennis area, Tim came along. I noted later that he was singing along with the music and appeared much more comfortable and there was definitely less tension ~~on~~ in the air.

Note, there is a legitimizing affect that those who "appear normal" have in being associated with those who have obvious physical characteristics that lead to stigma.

(Physical features that make stigma obvious)

Note; an interesting feature of the age differences is that children appear to become increasingly aware with age that it is okay (perhaps normative) to make fun of people who are different and their sense of shame in responding to stigma seems to correspondingly, disappear

(attracting "spectators")

Personal reflection: I was uncomfortable initially and then became aware of this. Let me elaborate. The feeling I had was one of "guilt by association" There was this automatic feeling of self protectiveness that arose with the thought that the children would "think ther was something wrong with me too" When I realized this I was ashamed of the feeling

(Differential awareness of others reaction to stigma)

Figure 21.1 Field notes from a 1970s UCLA study with index labels and analytic notes.

developed, a code directory or codebook is constructed, which includes operational definitions, as well as inclusion and exclusion criteria—instructions about circumstances under which the code should or should not be applied (MacQueen, McLellan, Kay, & Milstein, 1998). Code definitions tend to evolve over time, meaning that with increasing use, the definitions and the inclusion and exclusion criteria become more precise. Codes that represent broad themes may be broken down to component parts, and conversely codes that are conceptually very closely related may be merged. Investigators should keep careful records of when codes are created, split or merged, and when their definitions or application criteria are refined. (This is one component of the "audit trail" discussed previously). Investigators may need to go back and recode earlier coded portions of the data set in light of evolving code criteria.

In the UCLA study, the investigators eventually developed a fairly exhaustive indexing system, consisting of a comprehensive list of concepts grouped together into various themes. For example, one emergent theme was "temporal adaptation" (Kielhofner, 1979). This pertains to how the deinstitutionalized adults experienced time, and the ways in which their unique experience of time differed from the mainstream culture. Within this broad conceptual theme of temporality were nested subcategories, such as:

- Time-related behaviors (e.g., waiting, dealing with appointments, filling time),
- Temporal perspectives (e.g., how people talked about the future), and
- Temporal misunderstandings (i.e., problematic interactions that emanated from non-normative views of time held by the participants).

These and other index codes were written in the margin of clean copies of the typed field notes.

Recall that a main purpose of coding is to allow the investigators to retrieve all relevant passages on a given theme so that their content can be further explored. The index code "Time-related Behaviors" is used to indicate where in the texts one can find participants' comments about making appointments, waiting, and so forth. To conduct a more in-depth analysis of this content area, the investigators needed to find all passages labeled with this code, and look in detail at the selected passages. This could prove difficult, given that any single page of data (field notes, transcribed interview, or other document) can have numerous codes and margin notes, and a single passage might be coded for more than one concept. Looking through hundreds of pages of codes and margin notes would be

a quite cumbersome way of finding all the passages containing information on time-related behaviors.

The investigators chose instead to physically group together all the text segments dealing with the topic of interest. Any passage labeled with the relevant code was physically cut from a photocopy of the original page, tagged with information on its source location, and placed along with all other such text segments in a folder as shown in Figure 21.2. Typically multiple copies of a coded page needed to be made, since more than one code was often associated with a given text passage, and therefore the passage would be filed in more than one folder.

By flipping through any folder, the investigators were able to read, grouped together, all the passages in the data where participants discuss these issues. Passages gathered from different parts of the data set (thus "de-contextualized") were used to build an explanation about various ways the participants behaved with reference to time, and how this behavior was related to their life experiences and perspectives, and to the organization of the settings where they lived.

Of course it was also important to preserve information on where in the document a passage was originally located, since appreciating its full meaning often required viewing it in the context of the surrounding text. Thus, de-contextualizing and re-contextualizing of data are important components of the qualitative analysis process.

As data accumulated in the folders representing various concepts, the reading and processing of that material sometimes resulted in the contents of a folder being divided into two or more component concepts. At other times, two folders were collapsed into one. In this way, the coding scheme was continuously being refined as the data analysis unfolded.

Memos

Recall that the margin notes contain not only index labels, but also longer annotations we referred to as memos. Rather than serving primarily an indexing function, memos are methodological and analytic notes from which explanations and findings are built. While these memos may start as notes in the margin, they commonly become longer and more complex as analysis proceeds.

Over time, the investigators in the UCLA study started recording these memos in a larger format, using separate sheets of paper that were filed along with text passages in topic folders. Eventually, these memos were integrated together into working drafts of the analysis. These working papers

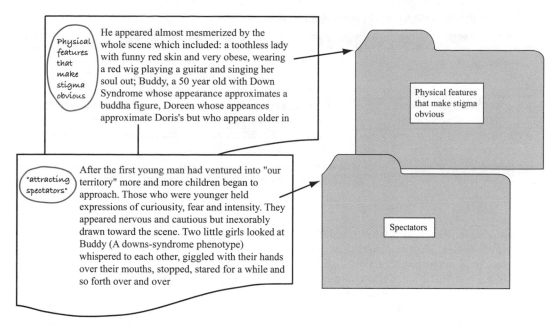

Figure 21.2 An example of "decontextualizing" data by grouping text passages related to a common theme.

were shared in meetings of the research team which led to discussion, critique, and new insights. These developing ideas were also recorded as memos. Individual team members or small groups had primary responsibility for generating explanations on a given theme, but the group process allowed for other team members to write memos and share their thoughts on the topic. In this way the analysis was organic and collaborative, unfolding in constant interaction with the data.

Interdependence of Codes and Memos

While indexing is fairly simple and mechanical, and memo-writing is more complex and analytic, they are quite interdependent and coordinated. As analysis proceeds, the coding scheme may be elaborated, and perhaps made hierarchical, with some index terms reflecting conceptual domains. These domains serve as cover terms for more detailed analytic categories, which commonly emerge after the investigator spends time intellectually processing the data and writing memos. The coding scheme may be used to develop a concept map in which relationships among categories are defined and graphically illustrated.

Summary

This section provided an overview of some of the major steps or processes involved in qualitative

data analysis. These are summarized in Table 21.1. These steps, of course, primarily refer to the more "procedural" aspects of data analysis. How one actually goes about the more "conceptual" aspects of data analysis depends on the particular form of qualitative research one is doing. These conceptual aspects of data analysis are covered in detail in Chapter 22.

Quality Assurance in Qualitative Data Analysis

Methods for ensuring the quality or trustworthiness of qualitative data were introduced in Chapter 20. These methods include interviewer training, prolonged engagement in the field, reflexivity, triangulation, stakeholder checks, and audit trails. Since qualitative inquiry is an iterative process involving successive rounds of data collection and interim analyses, these methods are as relevant to data analysis as to data collection.

Coding and Retrieving

There are additional quality assurance measures that are specific to data analysis, particularly to the process of coding. The creation of a code directory with clear operational definitions is an important first step in ensuring that the coding process is rig-

Table 21.1 **Qualitative Data Analysis Procedures and Their Functions**

Analysis Procedure	Function
Active reading	The process by which investigators immerse themselves in their qualitative data, reading and re-reading while making marginal notes about important themes and constructs
Index codes/conceptual labels	Words or short phrases that serve as a kind of tag for segments of text, categorically describing information the segments contain
Analytic memos	Reflective notes through which the investigators began to organize their thoughts about the data
Code directory	A list of all codes with clear operational definitions to ensure that the coding process is rigorous and reliable

orous and reliable. Particularly when multiple investigators are coding, analyzing, and/or interpreting the data, it is important that these activities take place in a systematic and consistent way.

This is not to say that all investigators working on a project should arrive at the same interpretations and explanations of qualitative data. Indeed, the possibility that investigators will bring different perspectives to analysis (in other words, investigator triangulation) is an important reason for conducting collaborative research. However, the mechanics of analytic tasks such as coding and retrieval of text segments must be systematic and consistent across researchers and documents. Otherwise, the results are simply a series of independent, individually conducted analyses rather than a coordinated research effort.

Inter-Rater Reliability

There are a number of steps investigators can take to assess and improve inter-rater reliability in the application of codes. This generally involves some form of redundant coding, where two researchers code the same text passages and compare their results. One can then quantitatively assess the level of agreement between the coders by calculating some kind of agreement statistic. The simplest approach is to calculate the proportion of instances in which the two coders agree on the coding of given text passages. This method, however, can overestimate agreement for codes that are commonly applied, because some degree of agreement by pure chance is likely. An alternative approach is to calculate a statistic such as kappa, an agreement statistic discussed in Chapter 12 that takes chance agreement into account (Carey, Morgan, & Oxtoby, 1996). A separate kappa statistic is calculated for each code, and a range of kappa values can be reported for the entire set of codes.

In contrast to this quantitative approach, many researchers prefer discussion and reconciliation as a means of ensuring reliability of the coding process. This begins the same way—with the redundant coding of texts by two or more analysts. Differences are identified and discussed. Eventually, the parties reconcile their differences and agree on one set of codes for the document. Many qualitative researchers use only this approach, and reject any use of statistical measures, seeing those as a needless and even inappropriate since borrowed from positivist, quantitative paradigms.

The authors maintain that both approaches are useful and important. When code-by-code agreement statistics are collected and scrutinized, the investigators can detect patterns in which types of codes are more or less easily agreed on. For example, they may find that codes that represent affective states are much more difficult to apply consistently than those that capture overt behaviors. Discussions in which coders explain their rationale for applying codes in a particular way can lead not only to reconciliation, but also to more careful crafting of operational definitions that will make future disagreements less likely. This can be documented by assessing agreement statistics before reconciliation, and then again using a new subset of the data after code criteria have been refined.

Computer-Assisted Qualitative Data Analysis (CAQDAS)

This chapter has so far presented a very basic view of the qualitative data analysis process. Though the low-technology example of qualitative data analysis has not been discussed in its full complexity, this is nonetheless a good place to pause, review what the ULCA investigators did, and begin to talk about high-technology or computer-assisted versions of these activities.

Table 21.2 **Hard/Analog-to-Digital Data Conversion for Computer-Assisted Analysis**

	Hard/Analog	Digital
Text	Handwritten or typed field notes, observation records, pencil-and-paper surveys, brochures/small media	Word-processing files, spreadsheet data, text files, pdf files, etc.
Sound	Audiotape recordings	Word-processing files; digital recordings
Images	Photographs, drawings, etc.	Scanned images, pdf files, Web pages, etc.
Image and sound	Videotape, film	Digital film, streaming video/sound files, multimedia Web pages, etc.

Recall that the first thing that was done to facilitate systematic analysis was the conversion of data from one format (handwritten field notes) to another (multiple copies of typed and expanded notes). Likewise, computer-assisted qualitative data analysis almost always requires a preparatory step of data conversion. In this case, the conversion is from data stored in a "hard" or analog form to a digital form. For example, verbatim transcripts of audiotaped interviews are generally prepared by typing them in a word processing program. Other examples of such conversions are listed in Table 21.2 (read further for discussion of technologies that permit the automation or elimination of conversion steps).

If the UCLA study data were being analyzed in 2005 rather than the 1970s, how might the work proceed in a way that takes advantage of advances in computer technology? First of all, the observers' handwritten notes would likely be typed in a word processing program such as Microsoft Word or WordPerfect, and then imported into a qualitative data analysis (QDA) software program. The first commercially available QDA program, called The Ethnograph®, was introduced in the early 1980s. Since then, the selection has greatly expanded, with products such as N6® (originally marketed under the name NUD.IST®), NVivo®, and ATLAS.ti® being among the most popular. Newer on the scene are AnSWR® and EZ-Text®, programs that were developed by the Centers for Disease Control and Prevention (CDC), and that have the distinct advantage of being distributed free to the public.[1]

Depending on the program used, the data may need to be converted from a word processing format to a "text only" file. However, the latest versions of most QDA software programs can directly utilize word processing files, most typically rich text (.RTF) files, which maintain their formatting features across multiple software programs and platforms. Once files are imported into the QDA program, a variety of data management and analysis tasks can be performed. Some key tasks are described below, including data storage and management, tag-and-retrieval functions, memo writing, theory building, and quality assurance. Ways that software programs support team-based analysis and mixed-method approaches are also described.

Data Storage and Management

Recall that in the low-technology type of analysis described in the preceding text, a clean copy of all typed documents is kept in a master file organized on some selected criteria. For example, the project data might include transcripts of interviews, filed sequentially by their unique alpha-numeric ID numbers, which carry information about the particular data gathering event. For example, the ID number D022677_3M indicates that this interview was done in a facility labeled "Facility D" on the 26th of February, 1977. It was the third interview done at that site on that day, and the respondent was a male. No other interview could have exactly that constellation of attributes; thus the ID number is unique. Transcripts can be filed by a primary criterion (i.e., the setting), and within that grouping they can be ordered by a secondary criterion (i.e., the date of the interview).

Labeling Data in QDA Systems

How does computer-assisted data storage and management differ from the process described above? One major advantage in terms of computer applications is that one can easily use the software

[1]When illustrating computer-assisted qualitative data analysis in this chapter, examples from the ATLAS.ti program are used in most cases. This should not be considered an endorsement of a particular product over others, but is used simply because this is the program most familiar to the authors. Where we know of significant differences between programs, these are pointed out.

to categorize the data files in multiple ways. For example, the data may be entered and retrieved by any number of criteria such as sex, age, ethnic group, or disability status.

Text-Based Searches

All the major QDA programs allow for text-based searches, in which words or strings of text can be searched for in the original data. Most also have the capability to conduct word counts—calculation of the frequency with which different words appear in the text. Some programs have more specialized features for conducting various types of quantitative content analysis.

Codebook Development

All major QDA programs support the creation of a list of codes to be applied to textual data. The programs vary, however, in the extent to which full codebook development is supported. In ATLAS.ti, the investigator creates codes that are displayed in a drop-down list. Code definitions, instructions for application, examples, etc. must either be stored in a generic "comment" window attached to each code, or in a separate document such as a spreadsheet or word processing file. N6 is similar, with each code having a "description" window in which code definitions, application criteria, etc. can be recorded. CDC's AnSWR has more fully developed codebook features, with separate fields for the code name, a brief definition, a full definition, inclusion criteria, exclusion criteria, and examples.

Tag-and-Retrieval

Recall that in the "low-tech" coding example, investigators labeled passages of text with index codes, after which like-labeled passages were extracted and placed together in a folder. QDA software uses the same logic, but accomplishes the tasks with much greater efficiency by using hypertext connections, whereby noncontiguous text or images are electronically linked to one another. Codes stored in a code list can be linked electronically to segments of text. The text passage is selected and the relevant code or codes are attached through keystroke commands, drop-down menus, buttons, or a "drag-and-drop" function. This is the "tagging" part of tag-and-retrieval. In ATLAS.ti and AnSWR, text passages of any size, from a single character to the entire document, can be highlighted and designated as a "text segment" (in AnSWR) or a "quotation" (in ATLAS.ti) (see the feature box on QDA Software Coding).

In N6, the minimal "text unit" must be defined in advance as a line, a sentence or a paragraph, though the boundaries of a segment can be modified after creation (this reflects the influence on program developers of classic Grounded Theory methodology, with its signature line-by-line coding). In all of these programs, text segments can overlap with or be embedded within other segments.

QDA programs also include one or more search tools, which constitute the "retrieving" part of tag-and-retrieval. These tools allow the investigator to retrieve all text segments labeled with a particular code, so that passages on a given topic or theme can be grouped and viewed together, just as in the topic folders in the "low-tech" example. The QDA programs can go much further though, allowing for complex search commands that combine two or more codes, or other search criteria. This can be particularly useful with large data sets, when searching on a code that is heavily used may result in a very large volume of retrieved data, not all of which may be relevant to the question at hand. In such cases, the search can be narrowed by retrieving only a subset of the coded segments, either by combining one code with another, or by imposing other restrictions on what is retrieved.

Boolean Connectors. A common way to perform these more complex searches is by using Boolean connectors (e.g., "and," "or," "not") to combine codes. For example, the investigators might be interested in examining accounts of disability-related stigma in the community, but only when the stigma involves some kind of discriminatory behavior. The search string "stigma AND discrimination" would retrieve the desired material, while ignoring accounts of stigma not associated with discrimination, as well as discrimination linked to race or ethnicity but not disability. Chapter 27 has a more extended discussion of Boolean logic and how it can be used to search for information.

Semantic Connectors. Complex searches can also be conducted using semantic connectors. Recall from the discussion above that codes reflecting broad conceptual domains can serve as cover terms for more detailed analytic categories. In QDA software programs, semantic relationships can be created that indicate hierarchical or other types of relationships between codes. For example, "waiting," "filling time," and "being stuck in time" can be defined as types of "temporal experience." "Temporal experience" therefore serves as a parent term for the other three, and the three types of experiences are related to one another as sibling terms. This semantic relationship is illustrated in Figure 21.3.

Since these semantic relationships are specified in the software, one can issue a simple search command that says in effect "retrieve any passage coded with 'Temporal experience' *or* any of its daughter terms." Some programs also allow the

grouping of related codes without defining a semantic relationship. In ATLAS.ti, codes can be grouped together in units called "families," which can also be used as search terms. Families of other objects, such as documents and memos, can also be used in searches.

Proximity Connectors. A third kind of complex search uses proximity connectors, which analyze

QDA Software Coding Example—*Enabling Self-Determination*

Investigators at the University of Illinois at Chicago are carrying out a project to develop and test a new model of independent living services for persons living with HIV/AIDS (Kielhofner & Braveman, 2001). The project is based on a participatory research model that recognizes the importance of input and collaboration from clients and facility staff for achieving program goals. In an early project activity, investigators conducted a series of focus group discussions with clients and staff of service organizations, in which participants identified barriers to community living and

employment. Data are being analyzed with the assistance of ATLAS.ti, one of the QDA software programs described in this chapter. In the screen shot below, one can see how the QDA program permits the linking of index codes and memos to text segments in a manner that parallels the "low-tech" method described earlier.

Investigators on the ESD project are also using ATLAS.ti's theory-building functions to develop conceptual models that are grounded in the qualitative data. The next page provides an example of a Network View showing code–code relationships.

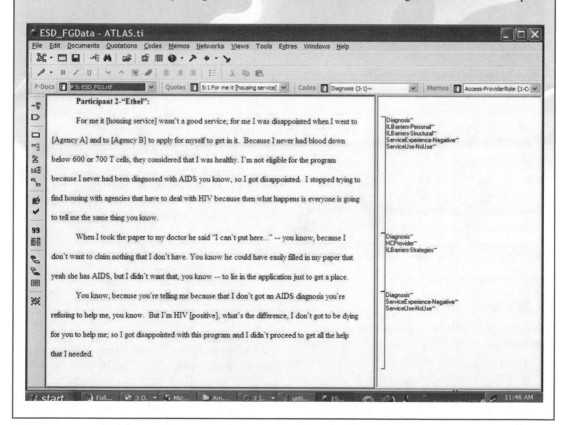

(continued)

QDA Software Coding Example—*Enabling Self-Determination* (continued)

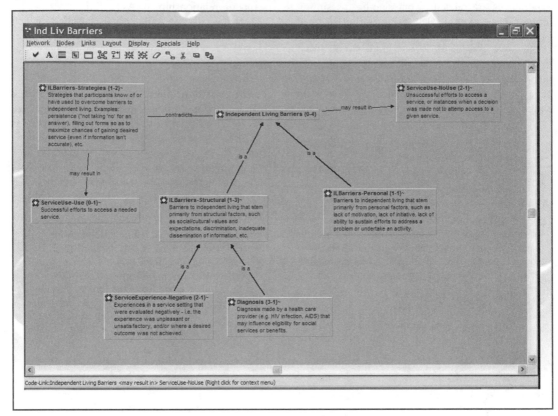

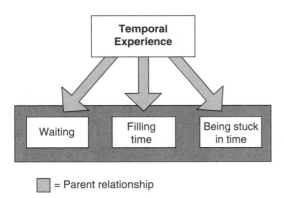

Figure 21.3 An illustration of semantic connectors.

spatial relationships between coded segments. Continuing with the preceding example, imagine that the data contain a passage describing a stigmatizing event in the community. This account itself may have had no overt reference to discrimination, but in the text segment immediately following it, an instance of discrimination may be reported. This co-occurrence would not be picked up using semantic connectors because the "stigma" and "discrimination" codes are not attached to a single text segment. Using proximity connectors, however, one could search for all "stigma" segments that are adjacent to (or overlapping or embedded within) a segment coded with "discrimination."

Memo-Writing

All major QDA programs have a mechanism for writing notes and memos, through which the investigators can record impressions about the data, methodological insights, developing interpretations and theory, and so forth. ATLAS.ti has two mechanisms for such annotations. Memos are one of the four major objects in the program (along with documents, codes, and quotations). These objects have a special status, and can be ordered, sorted, and displayed in special ways. "Comments" are a more general category of annotation, and serve as a kind of "sticky note" that can be attached to any object, including the entire project, a document, a code, or a "family." In N6, memos can be attached to both documents and codes. Comments on particular passages of text are recorded as "annotations," which are imbedded in the text when it is viewed within the program.

Theory Building

The most popular QDA programs go beyond simple tag-and-retrieval and memoing functions, and support theory-building. Theory-building functions allow the construction of explanations that are grounded in the qualitative data, and include mechanisms for defining relationships among data elements, including original text, codes, memos, and documents. ATLAS.ti has a tool called a Network Editor, which is a graphic space in which data and meta-data elements can be imported and linked to one another through semantic relationships, as described earlier. These "network" views can evolve into formal analytic products such as conceptual models or concept maps. In ATLAS.ti these connections can take the form of hypertext links between text segments in a project, even if they are not in the same document. For example, a staff member in a residential facility may comment that it is all right to let oneself into a resident's room unannounced since "they don't really care about privacy." Other passages in the dataset could be linked to this statement, with a semantic relationship such as "supports" or "contradicts."

Teamwork

All of the major QDA software programs provide some level of support for team-based analysis. Login names can be assigned to multiple users working on the same project so that their contributions can be tracked. Users can be assigned different levels of access, so that only those in supervisory positions have the ability to alter or delete data. There are "bundling" procedures to facilitate moving files between users, computers, and networks. Partial analyses performed by different researchers can be combined through merge procedures. The CDC programs (AnSWR and EZ-Text) include a tool for calculating Cohen's kappa, the inter-rater reliability statistic discussed in the preceding text.

Multimedia Capabilities

Several QDA programs allow for importing and coding not only text files, but also graphic files, HTML Web pages, and digital audio and video files. Of the general QDA programs, ATLAS.ti and another called HyperResearch® provide the most sophisticated handling of audio and video files. There are also specialized programs specifically designed for audio and video editing, some of which include tag-and-retrieval functions (e.g., Transana®).

Support for Mixed-Method Analyses

For those interested in incorporating quantitative methods into their qualitative studies, tools are available in some QDA software programs to support a variety of approaches including calculating and graphing code frequencies, creating code-by-document tables and other data matrixes, exporting data to statistical analysis or spreadsheet programs, and quantitative content analysis. Beyond basic functions, however, specialized programs may be needed. For example, programs such as Wordstat®, Alceste®, and Concordance® are specialized content analysis programs, used for tasks like concordance and cluster analyses of word distributions within texts. Programs such as AnthroPak® are used for analysis of data gathered through systematic elicitation techniques used to explore cultural domains. Examples are free lists (in which a respondent is asked to list items in a domain, such as types of discrimination), pile sorts (in which respondents sort a set of printed cards or items into piles from which taxonomies are built), and paired comparisons (in which items in a domain are ranked along some dimension by having respondents compare pairs of items in the domain). Complex quantitative procedures that often build on qualitative research are also supported by specialized software. For example, decision analysis is a kind of modeling exercise that attempts to predict behavioral choices under specified circumstances. Preliminary models are generally inductively constructed based on exploratory qualitative data, then refined based on new data that focuses more specifically on decision criteria for the behavior of interest. Models are iteratively tested and revised until an acceptably predictive model is reached. Another example is the Q-method, which is discussed in Chapter 23.

Other Tools and Software that Facilitate QDA

With new technological advances, some of the analog-to-digital conversion steps described earlier can be automated or even eliminated. Optical scanning can quickly convert written or typed material to machine-readable text or image files. Voice-recognition software programs can be used to convert taped interviews to text files. Audio and video data can be directly recorded in digital format with digital recorders and cameras. Interview responses may be typed directly into a computer by the investigator, or even by the respondent, as is done with Audio CASI technology, an interview method in which respondents use a computer keyboard to enter responses to prerecorded questions. Audio CASI is most often used with closed-ended questionnaires (often in order to deal with literacy as well as privacy issues), but can be used with open-ended questions as well.

> To make the best use of QDA software programs, qualitative researchers must first and foremost understand the fundamentals of qualitative inquiry.

Conclusion

Although increasingly common, the use of computers has not been universally embraced by qualitative researchers. Some simply have well-established work habits using manual techniques, and see no need to change them. There may be concern among some that the programs will be too difficult to learn or not worth the effort for the type of analysis planned. Some, particularly those working within participatory research (as discussed in Chapter 38), may fear that the computers distance the researchers too much from the voices and lived experiences of research participants and make it more difficult for the latter to participate in the data analysis. Still others have a basic philosophical opposition to using technological tools associated with positivist paradigms that they see as antithetical to the spirit of qualitative research.

Some of these concerns are not without merit. For very small projects it may arguably not be worth a researcher's while to learn a complex QDA program, when the same results could be achieved with low-technology approaches. Some researchers are tempted to use software inappropriately, for example, performing individual-level statistical analyses on focus group data. Some investigators become so wrapped up in their coding schemes and diagrams that they fail to stay close to the texts that are the true heart of their research findings. Such examples notwithstanding, computer-assisted analysis is appropriate and useful for many types of qualitative research.

As Weitzman (2000) notes, there are software tools to support a wide variety of research and analysis methods and not just those that are positivist or quasi-positivist in nature. Moreover, there is no single best program to meet all needs and no program will do the data analysis for an investigator. To make the best use of QDA software programs, qualitative researchers must first and foremost understand the fundamentals of qualitative inquiry. They must take time to think about and articulate their intellectual puzzles, research questions, and the type of inquiry needed to answer those questions. Finally, the researcher should take advantage of the considerable volume of resources available to help select an appropriate program. Some of those resources are listed at the end of this chapter.

REFERENCES

Bercovici, S. (1983). *Barriers to normalization*. Baltimore: University Park Press.

Carey, J. W., Morgan, M., & Oxtoby, M. J. (1996). Intercoder agreement in analysis of responses to open-ended interview questions: Examples from tuberculosis research. *Cultural Anthropology Methods 8*(3), 1–5.

Edgerton, R. (1971). *The cloak of competence: Stigma in the lives of the mentally retarded*. Berkeley: University of California Press.

Goode, D. (1983). Who is Bobby? In G. Kielhofner (Ed.), *Health through occupation: Theory & practice in occupational therapy*. Philadelphia: F. A. Davis.

Kielhofner, G. (1977). Temporal adaptation: A conceptual framework for occupational therapy. *American Journal of Occupational Therapy, 31*, 235–242.

Kielhofner, G. (1979). The temporal dimension in the lives of retarded adults: A problem of interaction and intervention. *American Journal of Occupational Therapy, 33*, 161–168.

Kielhofner, G. (1981). An ethnographic study of deinstitutionalized adults: Their community settings and daily life experiences. *Occupational Therapy Journal of Research, 1*, 125–142.

Kielhofner, G., & Braveman, B. (2001). Enabling Self Determination for people living with AIDS. Department of Occupational Therapy, University of Illinois at Chicago. Grant proposal submitted to and funded by the National Institute of Disability and Rehabilitation Research, U.S. Department of Education (H133G020217-3).

Kielhofner, G., & Takata, N. (1980). A study of mentally retarded persons: Applied research in occupational therapy. *American Journal of Occupational Therapy, 34*, 252–258.

MacQueen, K. M., McLellan, E., Kay, K., & Milstein, B. (1998). Codebook development for team-based

qualitative analysis. *Cultural Anthropology Methods,*
10(2), 31–36.

Mason, J. (1996). *Qualitative researching.* Thousand Oaks,
CA: SAGE Publications.

Weitzman, E. A. (2000). Software and qualitative research.
In N. K. Denzin & Y.S. Lincoln (Eds.), *Handbook of*
qualitative research (2nd ed.) (pp. 803–820). Thousand
Oaks: SAGE Publications.

RESOURCES

The past decade has seen a dramatic proliferation of books,
journals, Web sites, and listservs dealing with various
aspects of qualitative research. The following is a small
selection of resources the reader might find useful for
learning about computer-assisted qualitative data analysis. Though several of the books contain helpful advice
on selecting software programs, developments in these
products occur so quickly that it is best to consult
Internet resources that are more frequently updated for
help with selecting a program. The Web sites listed
below contain links to many software sites in addition
to those listed here. The software sites in turn contain
links to product-specific listservs.

Books

Denzin, N. K., & Lincoln, Y.S. (2000). *Handbook of quali-*
tative research (2nd ed.). Thousand Oaks, CA: SAGE
Publications.

Glaser, B., & Strauss, A. (1967). The discovery of
grounded theory: Strategies for qualitative research.
Chicago: Aldine.

Lofland, J., & Lofland, L. (1995). *Analyzing social settings*
(3rd ed.). Belmont, CA: Wadsworth.

Miles, M. B., & Huberman, A. M. (1994). *Qualitative data*
analysis (2nd ed.). Thousand Oaks, CA: SAGE
Publications.

Weitzman, E. A., & Miles, M. B. (1995). *Computer pro-*
grams for qualitative data analysis: A software source-
book. Thousand Oaks, CA: SAGE Publications.

Web Sites—General

CAQDAS Networking Project—a project housed at the
University of Surrey in the U.K., and funded to support
the use of software in qualitative data analysis.
http://caqdas.soc.surrey.ac.uk/

Web Sites—Product-Specific

AnSWR, EZ-Text: CDC, http://www.cdc.gov/ hiv/
software.htm

ANTHROPAC: Analytic Technologies, http://www.
analytictech.com/

ATLAS.ti: Scientific Software Development, http://www.
atlasti.com/

Ethnograph: Qualis Research Assoc., http://www.qualisre-
search.com/

Hyper-Research: ResearchWare, http://www.researchware.
com/

N6, NVivo: QSR International, http://www.qsrinterna-
tional.com/

Listservs

QUALRS-L—Qualitative Research for the Human
Sciences, University of Georgia: http://www.listserv.
uga.edu/archives/qualrs-l.html

ATLAS.ti Mailing List: http://www.atlasti.com/maillist.
shtml

QSR Forum (N6, NVivo): http://www.qsrinternational.
com/resources/qsrforum/qsr_forum.htm

CHAPTER 22

Qualitative Approaches to Interpreting and Reporting Data

Heather Dillaway • Cathy Lysack • Mark R. Luborsky

There are many ways in which qualitative approaches to data analysis are unique. This chapter outlines some of the basic purposes and stages of qualitative analysis. It also discusses how qualitative analyses can be reported to a broader audience after they are completed.

While there are many different qualitative approaches to analysis, this chapter does not deal with the specific nuances between them. Rather, it covers the broad themes and major characteristics of qualitative analysis and reporting. It aims to provide an understanding of the general philosophies behind and steps within any type of qualitative data analysis or reporting strategy. Interested readers may wish to explore grounded theory, narrative analysis, phenomenological analysis, discourse analysis, semiotic analysis, and other specific data analysis strategies themselves after reading this chapter.

This first section of this chapter defines the qualitative approach to interpreting or analyzing data, and discusses some major differences between qualitative data analysis and quantitative data analysis. It identified what makes qualitative data analysis unique. The sections that follow explain the process of completing qualitative analysis and reporting qualitative data once analysis is complete. The chapter concludes with reminders about qualitative approaches to analysis and reporting.

The Qualitative Approach to Data Analysis: The Uniqueness of Qualitative Data Analysis

In broad terms, the qualitative approach to interpreting and analyzing data has to do with interpreting words, not numbers.[1] The words that are analyzed are either in the form of observations

(from ethnographic field notes, for example), interviews, or documents (Miles & Huberman, 1994). Reading through observational field notes, interview transcripts, or examining documents, the researcher looks for:

• Patterns or common expressions of people's perceptions or understandings of their world,
• The meanings they attach to aspects of the settings in which they live or the behaviors in which they engage,
• The reasons why people think particular things,
• The ways in which people account for or come to particular actions, or
• How they organize their day-to-day situations.

At base, then, qualitative analysis is about understanding meanings, processes, people and their thoughts and actions, through the interpretation of people's words.

While qualitative researchers easily could reduce participants' words to numbers, it is important that they do not in most cases. The reasons for this can be found in the purposes of qualitative research. That is, qualitative researchers aim to describe and explore a particular topic, group, or culture. Qualitative research is useful when a particular topic or group has not been explored before, but it can also be used when much is already known about a topic and deeper understanding and explanation is needed to fully comprehend the phenomenon at hand. In both situations, people's presentations or constructions of their own worlds are very important since the central concern of the researcher is to describe and gain new insights.

Quantitative analysis addresses cause-and-effect, that is, how one independent variable or multiple independent variables may affect a dependent variable. The goal, then, of quantitative research is often more about explanation than description. In this latter case, numerical analyses become fruitful as they can help the researcher explain or predict relationships between two variables. But because qualitative researchers aim to describe and explore and understand, they need to preserve people's voices and the context that sur-

---

[1]There are some qualitative researchers who analyze images (moving or still) as their data, but we do not deal with this form of qualitative analysis in this chapter. In fact, we restrict most of our discussion to qualitative interviewing and observations.

rounds their voices. Ultimately this means that qualitative researchers preserve the original format of their data (or stay as close to the original as possible) so that readers of their analyses can see or experience for themselves as much of the participants' world as possible.

An Inductive Process

Qualitative analysis is deeply inductive. This is a characteristic of several steps and stages in the overall qualitative research enterprise. Thus, it was also emphasized in Chapter 20, which discussed the gathering of qualitative data. The idea behind an inductive approach is to allow research insights to emerge over the course of the study without being limited to predefined factors or predetermined theories. Miles and Huberman (1994) suggest that the researcher "attempts to capture data on the perceptions of local actors from the inside, through a process of deep attentiveness, of empathetic understanding…, and of suspending or 'bracketing' preconceptions about the topic under discussion" (p. 6). Emerson, Fretz, and Shaw talk about this same process as being one of "ethnographic participation." For these authors, qualitative research requires the investigator to achieve a "deeper immersion in others' worlds in order to grasp what *they* experience as meaningful and important" (1995, p. 2). Mishler (1979) has described this process as being more fundamental still. He wrote that any meaning that is extracted out of the interactions between the researcher and the researched is fundamentally social, and cannot exist without the context from which it was generated. Mishler argues the researcher and the researched are inextricably intertwined: the phenomenon studied cannot even have objective characteristics independent of the observer's perspectives and methods. Therefore, a researcher using an inductive naturalistic approach is not only centrally concerned with the identification of key themes and findings, but also concerned with epistemology, or what counts as knowledge.

The following example illustrates some of these fundamental differences between quantitative and qualitative research. In the area of adherence to medications, quantitative approaches have largely been used to measure a small set of

> In broad terms, the qualitative approach to analysis centers on the meanings, actions, and values embedded in social life.

patient characteristics (e.g., sociodemographic, psychosocial) or health behaviors (e.g., drug use, risk profile) in order to determine the statistical relationship between these factors and patient medication adherence, where adherence is generally specified as a percent (e.g., 90% adherent). In the literature, adherence has been variably operationalized as the number of pills or doses taken over a specified period of time, numbers of days with no missed doses, or patient self-report of percent adherence (e.g., "how adherent have you been in the last month?") and so on. Although many patient characteristics and health behaviors have been shown to be statistically correlated with adherence, their explanatory value is low (only small amounts of the variance in patient adherence is explained) and therefore it remains difficult to accurately predict who will not comply, based on patient characteristics.

A qualitative approach to medication adherence, in contrast, focuses on the understandings, meanings, and experiences of living with a particular disease and adhering to medications. An example is a study of adherence to HIV anti-retroviral medications among African Americans in Detroit. One finding is that patients hold a different understanding of how to be adherent than their doctors do. Patient understanding of the notion of being completely adherent often means "managing all aspects of one's illness the best one can given the circumstances," which may mean skipping doses of the prescribed medications (Sankar, Neufeld, & Luborsky, 2005)!

Thus, the power of qualitative research in this case is to explicate the variety of meanings of adherence held by patients and uncover reasons for patients' behaviors in relation to compliance with therapeutic medication regimens. As evident from this example, qualitative studies focus on uncovering how specific behaviors like taking medications are understood by patients in the context of their daily lives. This type of research is a powerful way to interrogate taken for granted assumptions about what constructs, like adherence, really mean on the ground in real people's lives.

The Goals of Description and Explanation

Another significant way in which qualitative research differs from quantitative research is in its ultimate goal. The goal of qualitative analysis is not to come up with conclusions that could be generalized to populations. In many cases, the qualitative researcher's goal is simply to describe his or her particular sample and/or the small group that he or she studied. This description begins an often new and in-depth understanding of the topics under study or people under study, and often spurs on larger, future research projects that could be more population-based. In other instances, as in the example on HIV medication adherence described earlier, the goal is to gain deeper insight into human behavior across a larger sample, in an effort to achieve full understanding across a wide range of study subjects.

As another related example from the same study, it has long been observed that many individuals with HIV are diagnosed only when they are very ill and hospitalized, and this has been attributed to a failure of public health education to properly teach people about HIV risk groups and behaviors. Qualitative research asks the "why" questions such as, "Why do some people wait so long to get tested for HIV?" Answers such as, "because I didn't think I was at risk," generate follow-up questions such as, "Why didn't you think you were at risk?" Results show that individuals have learned the health messages (i.e., they know what risky behavior is and precautions needed to avoid HIV infection), but they don't fit the risk categories defined by the experts (e.g., injection drug users, gay) (Neufeld, Berry, & Sankar, 2005).

Without this very systematic work to interview individuals with HIV and follow their logic, these insights and understandings would not be uncovered. This type of research is clearly essential in the areas of health-related behaviors and services.

In keeping with its purpose, qualitative researchers depend on nonprobability purposive sampling procedures to recruit the most informative people possible to illuminate the topic of interest. Again, the value of qualitative research lies in the "thick description" (Geertz, 2001), or deep understanding gained. Depth of understanding and proximity to people's worlds cannot be found in more structured, deductive, quantitative, population-based research.

Data Collection and Analysis Intertwined

Another extremely important characteristic of qualitative analysis is that it begins during data collection and then continues after data collection is completed. Thus there is a "zigzag" or back-and-forth process of data gathering and analysis, especially in the early stages. At times, especially in grounded theory studies, data analysis might also be interrelated with sampling and with the choice of setting for the research, as researchers try to find people or settings that will garner them more information about particular themes arising in early field notes, journals, and interview transcripts.

In qualitative research, several steps in the research process (i.e., sampling, recruitment, entry

---

Contributions of Qualitative Research to Understanding People's Worlds

Qualitative research is particularly valuable in providing an understanding of the unique circumstance of different groups of people. For instance, we would never know as much about how poor communities share resources (e.g., cars, childcare, money, etc.), if it were not for ethnographies such as *All Our Kin* by Carol Stack (1974). Although this research is not generalizable in the quantitative sense, it is nonetheless very valuable if our goal is to understand the role of kin and community resource networks among poor, racially disadvantaged groups. There are many other seminal contributions of qualitative research of relevance to the health sciences and to occupational therapy.

Many of these qualitative studies are ethnographic in nature and represent relatively prolonged periods of research time in the field. When this is the case, the reporting of the study often takes the form of a book. For example, Sue Estroff documented the lives of the mentally ill in *Making*

It Crazy (1981, 1985) and revealed how our society and even medical professionals stigmatize and discriminate against this group. Howard Becker and colleagues (1961, 1991) *Boys in White*, is another classic ethnography in book form. In this study, Becker and his team conducted interviews with a cohort of medical students as they moved through their medical school training. This research focused on the cultural rites of passage and rituals of professional indoctrination that transform medical students into doctors. Another excellent ethnography that focuses on cultural practices is *Everyone Here Spoke Sign Language* (Groce, 1985). This book is the result of a study of the islanders on Martha's Vineyard and how they worked to include those with congenital deafness. All of these examples enter the life worlds of social and cultural groups and explore their practices and rituals that help explain how and why things come to be the way they are.

into the field, data collection, analysis, etc.) may be intertwined. For example, in qualitative studies, interviewers might realize early in data collection that a particular theme is arising, and may vary the main questions and probes that they use in later interviews so that they can explore this theme more fully. In her study of menopausal women, Dillaway (2005) discovered in early in-depth interviews that women did not feel "old" upon this life stage. Because she began analysis of these early interviews before data collection was over she was able to explore the reasons why women felt this way overall, finding that many women distinguished between reproductive aging and other types of aging. That is, according to her later interviewees, menopause was positive because it allowed women to let go of a function that they were ready to give up, whereas other aging conditions (e.g., losing eyesight, Alzheimer's disease, etc.) meant the loss of a function they desired to keep (Dillaway, 2005). This theme was fully developed only during data analysis because data collection strategies were altered to explore menopausal women's perceptions more deeply through probing and follow-up questions.

In another example, recent studies have found that older adults may not adopt a mobility aid such as a scooter or a walker just because their occupational therapist tells them it will make them safer and more independent. Issues like their sense of being seen and treated as a disabled person and "less" than a full adult person actually weigh more heavily on their decision to acquire and utilize a mobility aid than many people, including therapists, realize (Gitlin, Luborsky, & Schemm, 1998; Luborsky, 1997). The fact that individuals' meanings of mobility aids differ from occupational therapists' perceptions is something that might be discovered only through a back-and-forth relationship between data collection and analysis. In early data collection, an occupational therapy researcher might not be inclined to ask older individuals about their own perceptions and, rather, may begin by asking about their contact with therapists and their recommendations. Yet, if analysis starts during data collection, a researcher could quickly pick up on the fact that they might not be exploring this issue in full, and that individuals' perceptions of mobility aids may be more important than the recommendations they are given by their occupational therapist.

Finally, it is useful to return once more to the HIV adherence study described above, since it very ably demonstrates how the results obtained from one set of qualitative research questions drive an entirely new set of questions. It should be noted that most, if not all, of these second round questions are impossible to identify and plan for in advance. For example, in responding to questions about their medication adherence, many patients reported their number of missed doses (during some specified period of time), but later in the interview or in "side-talk" revealed that the meaning of a missed dose may not be straightforward (e.g., "I missed that dose because I did not take it until later"). As a result, a new set of questions about the meaning of a missed dose was developed and given to patients and their clinicians. Results revealed large variability in the understanding of "missed dose," and what to do about missed doses, among both patients and clinicians and substantial differences between the two groups (Sankar, Nevedal, Neufeld, & Luborsky, 2005). The results have implications for the measurement of self-reported adherence, for patient–doctor communication, and for medication adherence itself.

Steps in the Analytic Process: Carrying Out Qualitative Data Analysis

While this section focuses on analysis and not on data collection, the reader should keep in mind that the two processes are not separate, and thus what was discussed in Chapter 20 should be kept in mind. A key to good qualitative analysis is that it is not a time-bound process, and that data collection and analysis are not partitioned from each other. At base, there is a reflexivity that develops between data collection and analysis in qualitative research. And this reflexivity specifically creates the ability to achieve new and deeper understandings of particular perceptions, behaviors, and ways of human living.

The Importance of Data Processing

Data processing must occur for data analysis to begin; in some ways it is the first step one takes in interpreting and reporting data. Chapter 21 covered many of the mechanics of data processing, so they are briefly noted here. Data processing includes making permanent records of interviews, field notes, or other documents that count as data (Rubin & Rubin, 2005). For example, data processing might be turning hand-written field notes into typed computer notes or transcribing audio-recorded (and/or video-recorded) data from in-depth interviews. Transcribing is the process by

Rigor, Flexibility, Challenge, and Reward in Qualitative Analysis

Qualitative analysis—and qualitative research in general—should be thought of as both a flexible and rigorous process. What qualitative researchers select to analyze in their data is not set in stone, and how qualitative researchers interpret these data can depend on many things (e.g., existing literature, the research questions or research problem he or she begins the project with, the kinds of themes that arise in early interviews or early analytic notes, or a combination of all of these). Yet, at the same time, there are particular systematic steps that a qualitative researcher goes through in order to arrive at a final interpretation of the data that can be reported.

While qualitative research is often touted for its flexibility and subjectivity, it is as important to think about how qualitative research is simultaneously precise, detailed, and valid or trustworthy because of the process that researchers undertake in data collection and analysis.

Qualitative researchers follow particular steps and verify their findings. At the same time, they adapt to the data that is arising in front of them.

Qualitative data analysis is a complex process that can be both time-consuming and exhausting; thus, it can be challenging. In qualitative research, and largely because data collection does not occur in controlled situations, data collection and especially data analysis will take considerable energy and time. The important thing to remember is that, at the same time as qualitative analysis can be challenging and time-consuming, it is a rewarding process as one sees participants' voices and lives come into focus as one shares these voices with a larger audience. Those who engage in qualitative research will acknowledge the difficulties that others have in qualitative analysis, but these difficulties do remain somewhat hidden from those who do not engage in this research.

which one listens to taped recordings of interviews, and types verbatim what is said during the interview so that the original data is preserved. Many researchers also take handwritten notes during in-depth interviews or as part of textual analysis in addition to audio recordings, so those notes would need to be typed as well. Data processing might also include making paper copies of all original data files stored in a computer so that original data is not lost during data collection, data analysis, or afterwards.

When analysis starts, one's analytic work should take place with or on a duplicate copy of the original data so there is no chance to ruin the original data; this also allows one to backtrack and start an analysis over if need be. At base, numerous attempts should be made to preserve data in its original format in multiple copies (and stored in multiple, safe locations) so that the researcher can always find and access it. This is particularly true of computer files—backing up data means not only peace of mind but also assurance against corrupted files, computers that crash and ruined files, stolen or damaged computers, and the like.

Just as importantly, data processing should at least begin alongside data collection, so that important themes in early interviews are not lost and the benefits of the reflexive, back-and-forth process between data collection and analysis can be captured. The earlier data processing is completed, the earlier one can begin the analysis process. Moreover, the earlier one starts the analysis process, the more likely one is able to grasp and

gain a deep understanding of the themes that might be arising out of the sample. With early data processing, one makes the best use of the strengths of the qualitative approach to interpreting and analyzing data.

Regardless of the fact that data has been processed, when starting one's analysis, one should be looking at and interpreting collected data in its original form. Thus transcriptions and typed notes should be as precise as possible. Certain types of qualitative analysis in particular (e.g., phenomenology, narrative analysis, or semiotic analysis) require that processed data mirror exactly what was said in an interview or what was typed in an original field note, but all qualitative analysis should be initiated with data in as close to its original format as possible. When and how an interviewee laughs during a conversation, for example, may be important in telling the researcher about their feelings of nervousness when discussing about a particular topic or about the level of trust the researcher has gained during the interview. How quickly an interviewee answers a particular interview question may tell the researcher how strongly that person feels about a particular topic. For those using semiotics or a linguistic approach to data analyses, even more detailed attention to the level of words and even syllables is undertaken. Thus, interview transcriptions, depending on the question, might even record laughs, hesitations, interruptions, emphases, and other speech patterns as much as possible, alongside the actual words of the conversation.

Riessman (1993) also notes that when an interviewee or informant appears to be going off on a side topic or tangent in conversation, one must make every effort to follow and keep records of that side conversation, because later on a researcher might realize that conversation was an entry into a story that is relevant for and answers one's research questions. Particular care should be taken during data processing so that all of these data are completely and systematically captured so that original data is maintained.

As noted in Chapters 20 and 21, researchers can and do expand upon their primary data (e.g., handwritten field notes, audiotaped interview data) by keeping informal notes, memos, or a field journal during data collection. Notes could be about important ideas that interviewees or participants are suggesting about the topic or their culture or their experiences, or their behavior, as well as general ideas that the researcher begins to have about what they are observing and hearing and would like to analyze as complex themes later in analysis (after they are out of the field). They might also record key quotes from interviews or conversations that researchers overhear that might be important in the data analyses later on. Notes could detail researcher's personal assessments or opinions about how interviews or field observations are going and the ways in which data collection needs to be altered in order to secure a deep understanding of the topic/group at hand. In addition, notes include one's reactions to being in the field if one is doing participant observation, or feelings about the course of any type of data collection experience.

The purpose of this extra data can be twofold; they can:

- Highlight key events during observations or interviews and thereby serve as a check on one's primary data source, and/or
- Serve as the first step to data analysis by getting one's main ideas out on paper to propel more advanced analytic thinking about the study topic.

For these reasons, all qualitative researchers should keep some sort of informal notes or a journal as they engage in qualitative data collection. These notes or journal entries will help in the interpretation and documentation of one's research experiences and one's data (Emerson, Fretz, & Shaw, 1995; Rubin & Rubin, 2005). They can be typed or handwritten, but optimally, should be made immediately after one leaves the research setting for the day. One may also have thoughts about how data collection is proceeding, or about the types of patterns arising in interviews, and

these thoughts may occur at random times (e.g., in the shower, lying in bed at night, driving). Thus, keeping a journal or a set of informal computer notes that can be accessed easily at all times is a way of documenting such thoughts, no matter when they occur. These informal notes or journals become important sources for ideas of how to analyze and report about the pile of data that one accumulates over time. This informal data source can make the analysis stage less cumbersome, especially at the beginning.

Next Steps After Accumulating a Pile of Processed Data

Rubin and Rubin (2005) suggest that it is helpful to think about data sources being broken down into data units, or blocks of information that will eventually be examined together. Investigators must begin their analysis by figuring out what blocks of information are appropriate to analyze. These blocks of information could be:

- Stories that interviewees tell that span several typed pages,
- A paragraph of typed text from an interview or field note in which an individual describes a particular encounter with a therapist, or discussion of a particular health condition and its meaning, or
- A phrase or term used over and over by interviewees or informants or members of a particular organization, clinical team, or profession.

The characteristic of these blocks of information is that they signify a key concept or theme. Thus, initial analyses consist of multiple readings of one's data sources, to look for the blocks of information that might be worth analysis. Once the researcher finds a block of information that seems to emerge as important, then she or he might look to see if a similar block of information exists in a second data source, whether that data source is an individual or a large group of individuals. Then, the researcher begins a process of comparing and contrasting across data sources, to see whether this data unit is important across a particular sample, as well as how and why it is important to the people interviewed or observed.

Four Steps in the Data Analytic Process

The analytic or interpretive process is discussed as four separate steps in this section. What follows is only one, albeit a common approach to data analysis. While data analysis frequently does begin with a singular data source as discussed below, it can also begin with responses to an entire set of inter-

Qualitative Results versus Qualitative Interpretation

Qualitative results are not useful until they are interpreted in order to gauge their credibility, importance, and meaning. The term "analysis" is avoided by some qualitative researchers because it is used to refer to quantitative standardized approaches. Thus, some qualitative researchers prefer to describe all the tasks of extracting meaning from the data as "interpretation" to better characterize their meaning-centered, naturalistic, interpretive paradigm. Nonetheless qualitative researchers are encouraged to be aware of the two separate stages and goals in the research process. In multidisciplinary collaboration, the rigor and value of qualitative research are reinforced when investigators clearly describe these steps separately, however they are labeled.

Thus, the following distinctions are made:

• The *results* of analyses are simply what an investigator finds out or produces by conducting procedures for processing and analyzing the data (e.g., those procedures discussed in Chapter 21). Hence, results are just an intermediate, internal step in the research process and have no inherent meaning or value. For example, listing three themes does not locate those findings within the larger framework of what we already know. It also does not reveal anything about the credibility of these particular results.

• *Interpreting* the results establishes the value or importance of the data analytic results. Only after the analytic results are interpreted can they be evaluated to determine if, how, and how much they contribute new knowledge.

Qualitative researchers interpret results by evaluating the resulting product of the analytic procedures in at least two ways:

• First, investigators gauge the results in two ways, in order to be clear about how credible they are. This is done in light of internal issues concerning the "epistemological" status (see Chapter 20) of the data to gauge its strengths and limitations (e.g., trustworthiness, validity, reliability, sample adequacy). In addition, with an eye to how credible the data are, investigators assess the findings in light of what was already known before starting the research, and answer the question of how the results add new knowledge by contradicting or confirming existing knowledge or by contributing new information.

The following are recommended strategies for interpreting results:

1. Tie the findings into one or more major contemporary theories related to the research topic. For example, Deppen-Wood, Luborsky, and Scheer (1997) have studied and written about post-polio syndrome. In this case study research, the investigators interpreted the results of one older African-American woman's life-long accommodations to mobility disability. The authors considered the multiple jeopardy hypotheses, a well known theory that suggests that disadvantage can create a cumulative burden. Specifically, in this case, the multiple jeopardy hypothesis suggests that visible minorities, women, and persons with disabilities are more disadvantaged than nondisabled white men. The authors of this study assessed this hypothesis in their analysis but through careful review of their data ultimately rejected this idea, in favor of an alternative interpretation. In this way, the authors framed the results of their study within a larger context and body of literature and theory. To find out more about this case, one should read the case study and see why this woman preferred to use a cane instead of a walker in public even though it provided much lower objective functional mobility.

2. Connect the analysis to a substantive or controversial issue; that is, compare the results of the qualitative analysis to those of prominent researchers on the topic or link the analysis to a high-profile issue or controversial debate in the field of study. For example, in rehabilitation research it has long been believed that the duration, intensity, and focus of physical rehabilitation is the primary cause of functional recovery. This has been generally accepted in stroke and orthopedic rehabilitation. More recently, however, researchers have found that the presence of key social relationships may be as critical if not more critical to long-term functional independence and community integration after stroke, hip fracture, and a wide array of other physical impairments as well (Dijkers, 1999; Glass, Matchar, Belyea, & Feussner, 1993; Magaziner et al., 2000).

view questions across a group of study participants. Furthermore, when the latter is the case, "codes and coding" refer to an analytic category and not merely the words of one single study participant. These distinctions are drawn below.

Step One: Formal Analysis or Interpretation of One Data Source

Formal analysis or interpretation of qualitative data often begins with one data source. This may be one interview or one field note, for example. The researcher reads through this data source multiple times, gaining comfort with what it includes. Rubin and Rubin (2005) explain how, in this step, one gains recognition of the concepts, events, feelings, and behaviors recorded, as well as the patterns within that particular data source. For instance, an investigator may ask whether an interviewee continually referred back to family history, situating the disability experience within the context of the extended family, or whether the informant characterized the disability experience as owing very little to the extended family.

Once researchers are familiar with the initial data source, they should begin coding it. That is, investigators should come up with brief terms that can be written in the margins or recorded within a computer program that summarize blocks of information in that data source. Schwandt (1997) defines coding as "a procedure that disaggregates the data, breaks it down into manageable segments and identifies or names those segments" (p. 16). It is impossible to undertake coding without at least some conceptual structure in mind. Nonetheless, coding can be undertaken in a more descriptive mode or in a more analytic mode, depending on the level of interpretation involved.

The most troublesome tendency in the act of coding according to Strauss (1987) is to code too much at the descriptive level instead of coding for the purposes of explaining or developing an understanding of what is going on. This understanding is the heart of data analysis for thoughtful, reflective, and critical qualitative researchers. It is very easy to be mechanical in the coding process but much more difficult to address the theoretical understandings that are involved in understanding social phenomena. Returning to the example alluded to briefly above, descriptive coding could thus take place every time a person refers to his or her family history during an interview, for instance, "family history" (even "fam. hist." or "FH") could be recorded or "coded" next to that data unit. At this descriptive level, the goal is to find a way to track similar blocks of information through a coding system, finding brief terms that categorize multiple areas of text. Miles and Huberman (1994) refer to this process as within-

> It is very easy to be mechanical in the coding process but much more difficult to address the theoretical understandings that are involved in understanding social phenomena.

case analysis, in that one is doing all one can to master an understanding of a particular interview transcription or a set of observational field notes.

If, on the other hand, the research is less exploratory and more conceptual (i.e., theory and literature driven), qualitative investigators may utilize more semistructured interviews, and as a result be in a position to focus on a clearly defined set of data provided in response to a clearly delineated subset of interview questions. In this case the single data source is somewhat more broadly construed. When this is the case, the researchers undertake a systematic process of comparisons across study participants simultaneously. They are also engaging in a deeper level of explanatory coding. In essence, the researchers are looking beyond the words and descriptions of their interview subjects to understand more fundamental conceptualizations of how people experience what they do.

Geertz (2001) has referred to this process as inscribing social discourse; it is a deliberate act to ensure that interactional details are fully captured. This level of detail in both the collection of data in fieldnotes and in the interpretive process of data analysis is demanding, but holds the potential to explain categories of meaning in a way that more superficial attention to words alone cannot.

Irrespective of the stance taken, it is generally accepted that one should code everything in the data source that is relevant to one's research questions or research problem. However, this does not mean that one will code everything within a data source (Rubin & Rubin, 2005). One must make a great many decisions about what data units are related to one's initial goals in the research project, and whether/how particular data units address the research questions one sets out to answer. Certainly, some research questions take on greater priority, as is the case when a particular manuscript on a specific topic is planned. Thus, at times, coding must be strategically undertaken in response to practicalities such as available time and energy.

Once data are coded, important and related blocks of information are easy to find and access for further analysis and for reporting. Codes essentially flag patterns or themes that rest within the data. By defining and labeling one's codes, and through the acting of assigning codes to their data, qualitative researchers begin to identify salient analytical connections among data units (even within the same data source). Thus, regardless of whether coding is undertaken on an informant by informant basis, or is done across subjects simultaneously at a more conceptual level, coding must be done with great care since it forms the bedrock of subsequent interpretations.

For example, an investigator may wish to know how interviewees understand and describe a particular health problem such as hip fracture in old age. The investigator may further be interested to determine whether particular symptoms of a hip fracture are more salient than others or whether certain meanings of having a hip fracture manifest over and over again in the same data source. To address these concerns, a specific code should be created for each issue to detail what is important about each data unit. A researcher may go back and recode this data source at a later point, but these initial analytic steps are essential to establishing a systematic and theoretically informed analytic strategy and for selecting particular data units to explore further.

Step Two: Selecting a Particular Code for Further Analysis

After the researcher completes the coding of one particular data source, the next step is to select a particular code (and thus, a particular set of data

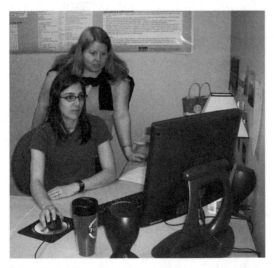

Figure 22.1 Members of a qualitative research team discuss their coding and analysis of an interview transcript.

units or pattern among data units) for further analysis. How one selects a particular code/pattern in the data for this second step of analysis is variable. Researchers could select a particular code to analyze based on their reading of literature on their topic of study, or based on the research questions with which they began their project. However, qualitative researchers need to know about past research but not let it dictate the specific data units they'll analyze. Over-reliance on past literature and preconceived research questions can constrict the ways in which one is reading the data source as a whole and/or how one interprets particular blocks of information (Emerson, Fretz, & Shaw, 1995; Miles & Huberman, 1994; Riessman, 1993).

Thus, investigators should pay attention to codes/patterns that simply emerge out of the data source themselves, upon the investigators' critical reflection. For example, Siporin and Lysack (2004) studied the work settings of women with developmental disabilities. They relied on prolonged engagement in the field and in-depth interviews to illuminate how different the experience of working in a sheltered workshop was from working in more community-based supported employment programs. This study relied on prolonged periods of observation in the workplace of clients to show how factors in the physical and social environment operated to enhance or limit the quality of life perceived by the clients.

Specifically, the investigators learned that the type of work characteristic of sheltered workshops as opposed to supported employment settings accounted for only a small amount of the clients' subjective quality of life. This finding contradicted the investigators' expectations that type of work would matter much more. Other factors such as the personalities of agency staff and life coaches, and the types of social opportunities linked to each distinctive type of worksite, turned out to be more powerful influences on clients' expressed quality of life. If these investigators had not paid attention to codes they attached to these other aspects of the work environment they may have overlooked a range of personally meaningful interactions with agency staff and fun opportunities outside of work as key contributors to self-rated quality of life.

Other things may also influence what analytic strategy an investigator chooses to pursue. For instance, the way in which current media is framing an issue/topic/cultural group may be important in shaping one's analytic strategy. A qualitative researcher engaged in a study on aging may note that aging is sometimes characterized negatively by the mainstream media, and will, in response, develop and assign one or more of codes that speaks to this issue. On the other hand, ideas from one's informal notes or field journal may generate some new codes. There are numerous ways in which researchers select the codes and data units they analyze. Qualitative investigators must be aware and open to a range of different strategies when developing their approach to data analysis and coding.

An important strategy for simplifying the complex task of data analysis is picking only one code to analyze at a time. This strategy can be particularly useful advice for novice qualitative researchers. Because qualitative data include many different patterns and themes a good strategy for the novice is to keep one's attention on one pattern in the data at a time. There is always time to go back and analyze other sets of data units at other times. As will be discussed later, the process of qualitative analysis is never completely over. Thus, researchers might as well dedicate themselves to just one specific analytic task and carry it through to completion before undertaking another.

Step Three: Compare and Contrast Data Sources Utilizing a Particular Code

After one has read and coded one particular data source and has selected one code or pattern to highlight in further analysis, the next step is to compare and contrast data sources utilizing a particular code. Miles and Huberman (1994) call this step, cross-case analysis. In this step one asks whether it is possible to:

- Move to the next data source and find similar ideas or topics, and
- Code that second data source in similar ways (i.e., using the same code selected in Step Two).

In this step, the researcher is essentially clarifying what is meant by a particular data unit or coded block of text (Rubin & Rubin, 2005). As one compares blocks of information in the first and second data source, one begins to understand the similar and different ways interviewees or field notes discuss a particular topic. Thus the information stored within each code is analyzed for nuances and the meaning of the original code becomes clearer than it was in previous steps.

Going back to the example of how people might talk about the role of their family history in explicating their disability experience, the researcher might find that one interviewee felt that fam-

ily history led directly to his or her own health condition. Therefore, such an interviewee might characterize the impact of family history as negative. However, a second interviewee might also talk about family history, but consider his or her own health problems to be an anomaly. In this second data source, then, the interviewee may have characterized family history more positively. In this example, the comparison of similarly coded text across two data sources leads to a greater understanding of how individuals attach importance or meaning to their family histories. It may become clearer as one compares and contrasts similarly coded text that, while importance is placed on family history across interviewees, the particular meanings they attach to family history vary. In such an instance, the codes may be adjusted to fit the new understanding of these data units as they are compared and contrasted. This is a repeated process, as one compares and contrasts each data source to others until one has analyzed all cases in a sample (Miles & Huberman, 1994).

The decisions one makes during initial coding and coding revisions shape what a researcher will be able to conclude at the end of the analysis. Thus, the process of coding and then comparing, contrasting, and revising one's understanding of codes is key to the analytic or interpretive process. One's emphasis should be on either finding ways of relating coded blocks of data together (similarities) or finding differences in the way data units uphold a particular code, so that the nuances underneath a code can be brought to the surface.

Step Four: Drawing Some General Conclusions About What a Coding Strategy or Arising Data Pattern Means

In a final step of analysis, investigators stop specific cross-case comparisons and zoom out, so to speak, on what has been found thus far. In this step, the investigator will draw some general conclusions about what a coding strategy or arising data pattern means. This allows both the consistencies and differences among a particular set of data units to be described and understood. Therefore, this step is about arriving at a kind of final synthesis (Rubin & Rubin, 2005) or a thematic narrative (Emerson, Fretz, & Shaw, 1995) that illuminates the theme or pattern that has been recognized or identified in the cross-case analyses completed in Step Three.

The goal of this step is to develop a way to refer to the theme or pattern, and the subthemes and subpatterns beneath it (if one has created subcodes underneath a main code, which is often the case). This is very much a reflective analytic step, one in which the researcher must step back and find a way to evaluate all data units underneath a specifically coded theme. The key questions[2] one needs to answer in this step are:

- What am I going to call this theme as I move into a reporting stage?
- How am I going to define the nuances I found within it as I looked at different data units and in different data sources?
- What are the examples of variations under the umbrella of this coded theme, and how can I explain them? Why do these variations matter?
- What are examples of the commonalities across all data units I have labeled with a given theme, and how do I explain them? Why do they matter?
- What is the significance of this theme overall for my research topic, and how might my analysis of this particular topic/theme add to previous literature on this subject?

If one's coding strategy and previous levels of analysis can hold as one answers these questions, then it is probably the case that one has arrived at what resembles a complete analysis. Perhaps the most important question in the above list is the last one. A researcher must think about the broader significance of the analysis just completed, and whether or not there are general implications of what one has learned. Thus, one should ask how far the thematic analysis (and thus codes/coding strategies one has developed) might extend.

For example, Lysack and Seipke (2002) found that oldest-old women often defined "aging well" differently than policymakers and healthcare providers. They defined their well-being in terms of whether they could still complete gendered household tasks rather than in terms of established health and independence scales used by therapists or policymakers to determine need for services. While individuals' definitions of aging well were interesting as findings in and of themselves, Lysack and Seipke (2002) found their results had policy and healthcare implications. Moreover, they suggested that traditional notions of successful aging and independence among the elderly need to be rethought at the national as well as local level. Thus, while qualitative research is not generalizable in that it cannot speak to a heterogeneous population's attitudes or behaviors, qualitative analyses can still hint at ideas that must be explored

further and broader implications that might have meaning outside of any particular research sample.

While this is a final step in analysis, it should be acknowledged that an investigator may return again and again (often in response to reviewers', editors', and particular audiences' comments) to clarify what is meant by particular data units explained by particular themes. Investigators may also add further nuances to the understanding of how data units fit (or do not fit) together at a later date.

It is also important to note that researchers typically move back and forth among these major steps as they attempt to make sense of the data units relevant to their research question or research problem. In the grounded theory tradition, this iterative process is called the constant comparative method (Glaser & Strauss, 1967).

Irrespective of the specific approach, just as data collection and analysis can be a back-and-forth process, so too is the analysis process. Investigators will move back and forth between looking at individual data sources and multiple data sources, and the tentative interpretations attached to the data. Only at the point when researchers are finding no more new interpretations or no new similarities and differences should they move to conclude that saturation has been reached, and begin to write up the findings. When one can draw a small set of conclusions about the interpretations that help to answer one's initial research questions (and that would be endorsed by the people studied as reflecting their views) the analysis is complete.

Enhancing Rigor Through the Steps of Qualitative Data Analysis

Emerson, Fretz, and Shaw (1995) urge qualitative researchers to utilize a variety of organizational strategies to enhance the rigor of their analyses. These authors and others (Strauss, 1987) devote entire chapters to strategies undertaken in the field to capture scene depictions, to communicate dialogue and interpersonal exchanges, to elucidate indigenous meanings with and without verbal data, to develop and analyze integrative memos, and many other tasks in the qualitative data collection and analysis process. All such measures contribute to achieving greater quality in the end product of qualitative research.

There are various ways to check oneself during the analysis process, or verify the patterns or themes one is finding in the original data. First, some researchers have multiple coders and/or analysts on their research projects to ensure that they

[2]This list of questions is based loosely on a list of questions found in Rubin & Rubin (2005: 216).

are reading data units in similar and valid ways. This is a check on the reliability of the emerging interpretations. Second, qualitative researchers may return copies of their initial analyses to their interviewees or informants in the field, to assess how closely they have captured what participants' voices and worlds are. This is called member checking in some qualitative traditions. Third, one can look to previous literature to evaluate whether one's initial results make sense (although this does not mean that one's findings need to mirror the results of past studies!). Fourth, one might reflect on whether, intuitively, initial findings make sense. Finally, within the analysis process itself, if one's coding holds up across multiple data sources and back-and-forth processes of within-case and cross-case analysis, then one probably has some reasonable grounds to conclude that the coding strategy undertaken and larger analytic strategy are valuable and the results generated from the qualitative data analysis are worth reporting.

How and Where to Report Findings

Researchers should make the transition from analysis to reporting by thinking about why they initiated their projects and what their goals were. For instance, qualitative research may be undertaken with:

- A purely basic science goal of adding to existing knowledge on the topic or group, or
- A more applied goal of coming up with ways to make a particular groups' lives better in some way.

Investigators also need to consider what form the results need to be in, in order for one to achieve their goals. This may include, for instance:

- A peer-reviewed journal article,
- A book or other lengthy manuscript,
- A policy brief,
- An oral presentation,
- A conference poster,
- A consumer magazine or newspaper article, and/or
- A TV interview.

Based on the initial goals, one should also determine the audience—that is, the group of people who will be reading and reacting to the findings. Different audiences will find different presentations of the analysis more or less impor-

tant, and will require different kinds of information. For instance, if one has a goal of influencing policy for the developmentally disabled, one needs to think critically about the policy implications in the final steps of analysis and make them understandable and believable to policymakers who are typically not well versed in academic literature or research methodology. Presentations to consumers also take on a very different shape. On the other hand, if one has an academic audience, it will be more important to spend time reporting on methodologic details, and linking findings to the results of prior studies. Thus, the audience of one's report will determine how the analysis is communicated.

Another important issue to think about, as one begins the reporting process, is how best to retain participants' voices and/or the original data as one communicates themes in the data. As noted earlier, one of the key goals of qualitative research is to report what a group's thoughts, behaviors, and lives look like from the inside (Miles & Huberman, 1994). To stay close to this goal, the researcher must maintain a commitment to reporting original data. This means, for instance, reporting participants' actual words from interview conversations or verbatim field notes so that readers can immerse themselves in the original research setting alongside the researcher.

Since the qualitative researcher is the research instrument, great care must be taken to include both what is observed or heard, alongside what is thought and interpreted by the researcher. This means that, within a report, examples of original data must be provided along with interpretations of these data. Thus, while a researcher may provide an interpretation of how to read or make sense of the data, the actual data is also in the report for readers to interpret on their own.

How to Go About Reporting the Analysis

Typically qualitative researchers select a broad pattern or theme to introduce in their report. This theme is directly related to the codes that are analyzed first in one data source, then across data sources. How one presents this theme is usually related to how one answers the questions presented under Step Four of the analysis. That is, one must first name and define what the finding or theme is. This is often about defining one's coding strategy. After one presents and summarizes a theme, one should present an example of original data.

For instance, in reporting the quality of nursing care in their report, Williams and Irurita (1998) discuss how nurses initiate rapport with their patients;

"initiating rapport" was a code they defined during the analysis stage of their research. In their report, they first define this concept: "Rapport was established by informal, social communication that enabled the nurse and the patient to get to know each other as persons" (p. 38). Then they present an example, stating: "One of the nurses interviewed described this interaction:

> *'Just by introducing yourself, by chatting along as you're doing things ... with the patient. Asking them ... questions about themselves...like 'how are you feeling about being in hospital? How are you feeling about the operation tomorrow?' And then they'll sort of give you a clue...and actually then tell you how they're feeling about things...just general chit chat... (Nurse).' (Williams & Irurita, 1998, p. 38)*

The sequence used by Williams and Irurita (1998) to describe and elaborate on the data patterns they analyzed is an effective format for reporting qualitative analyses. This format consists of:

• A name or label for the category,
• The authors' description of the meaning attached to the category, and
• A quotation from the raw text or original data to elaborate on the meaning of the category and to show the type of text coded into the category.

After presenting this sequence of information, the researcher goes on to present the nuances underneath each thematic category. This includes, perhaps, presenting the ways in which particular data sources grouped together under that category or theme during analysis. If one found, for example, that the way in which interviewees talked about family history varied depending on whether or not they felt family factors determined a current health condition, one could present first those who felt positively about their family history (defining this group and then presenting examples of original data), and subsequently present those who felt negatively about the same. Then one might speculate about the reasons why there were differences in the meanings attached to family histories.

The presentation of nuances underneath a theme or code illustrates the rigorous process by which the researcher arrived at conclusions about the important aspects of their data, and also helps shape a deeper understanding of the topic at hand. By presenting nuances underneath a theme, one shows how thorough the analysis has been and

brings the reader into the description as much as possible. The presentation of a theme or coding strategy begins broadly, and then becomes more specific. This pattern of reporting qualitative data is widely accepted and well understood as an adequate way to present complex analyses and, at the same time, remain as close as possible to participants' voices.

The novice researcher should be mindful of presenting a clear and complete description rather than presenting every theme. This means presenting very few themes or findings in each report. The definition and discussion of qualitative analyses is a lengthy process:

• The definition and discussion of the finding,
• The presentation of original data,
• The presentation of nuances within that finding, and
• The presentation of more original data (to provide evidence of these nuances).

Thus, there is often not enough room within any one written document or oral presentation to communicate more than one or a very few themes or findings. Thus, qualitative researchers should keep reports simple so that they can report specific findings in full, following the format of starting with a broad theme and then defining its specific nuances.

Regardless of the type of reporting qualitative researchers produce (e.g., poster, oral presentation, published paper or written report), they must stand ready to explain the qualitative approach and its benefits, as many questions about it are always raised by quantitative researchers. Thus, when making a report of qualitative analyses and/or responding to audience members' or readers' questions, one should be ready to discuss the following issues:

• Why one chose to do qualitative over quantitative research,
• The unique benefits of qualitative data, or why one might engage in qualitative research,
• The rigor of one's qualitative data collection and analysis strategies and the specific steps one completed to arrive at results, and
• The implications and/or significance of one's results—that is, how one's results can be used to promote future research, advocacy efforts, or policy efforts, even if one's analyses are based on a limited sample. In other words, why do one's results matter even if they are not generalizable and/or based on a random sample and numerical data?

Presenting Qualitative Analyses in Poster Form

Poster presentations can be made easily in software programs such as PowerPoint or Microsoft Word. Although various styles and formats for organizing one poster are possible, typically, the poster layout should permit the reader to move from left to right as they view the poster, as if he or she were reading a book. Thus, on the left, one should start with a small introduction of one's topic/study, and some brief information about the research methods undertaken. As a reader moves in front of the middle area of the poster, she or he should be confronted with information about basic results or findings—that is, a presentation of the broad themes found within the analysis. A reader of the poster should be presented with the name and definition of the theme/code and then original data examples to back up the definitions. As readers move to the right-hand side of the poster, they should then see the presentation of the specific nuances within the findings, or ways in which particular groups of one sample or groups of data sources allowed for a deeper understanding of that theme/code. The following is an illustration of how a poster might be organized:

	Title of Poster Author & Affiliation	
Introduction (perhaps 1-2 paragraphs)	Definition of Broad Theme/Code	Definition of Specific Nuances
Methods (perhaps 1-2 paragraphs and charts/graphs)	Examples of Original Data	Examples of Original Data
		Some Basic Conclusions

One variation to this basic example is to place the key research question and the main study findings and conclusions in the top center of the poster. This can be eye-catching and effective. Another variation might be undertaken to address particular needs of one's audience. That is, if this is a poster presented in an academic setting, one might want to present more details on prior research literature on the topic on the left-hand side of the poster, after the introductory section and before the presentation of methods. If this poster is for an advocacy organization's event or for a group of healthcare providers or policymakers, it might be less important to provide the results of prior research and instead highlight more salient take-home messages for policy decision-makers.

Oral Presentations of Qualitative Analyses

In presenting one's results orally, one would usually report the same data as in a poster format. The only variation may be based on one's audience, and this is very similar to our discussion of poster presentations: academic audiences are accustomed to hearing more about past literature than policy audiences or consumer/lay audiences. Thus, the researcher should know both the disciplinary backgrounds of her or his audience and the level of interest they might have in the components of one's presentation. Novice researchers should query prior conference participants on facts like these to ensure that their presentation "hits the mark" with respect to the audience's needs.

Typically, 10 to 20 minutes are allotted for an oral presentation at a scholarly or professional conference or other public forum, followed by 5 to 10 minutes of audience questions. The researcher should determine the allocated length of time and assure their presentation is of appropriate length. Oral presentations of qualitative data analyses are often quite difficult to complete in a short amount of time. Introducing the topic and discussing the research methods are needed, but you must allocate more time to describe your findings and their contribution. Moreover, since one often needs to read examples of original data out loud (or at least summarize what pieces of original data suggest) for the audience, time is quickly spent. Thus, to skillfully complete an oral presentation of qualitative analyses, one must prepare for the specific time allotted and present few findings. Keeping things simple and presenting as few themes/findings as possible is extremely important. One should expect that in a 10-minute presentation, for example, one might be able to present only two or three examples of original data to illustrate a broad theme and then may only be able to present one or two nuances under that theme.

(continued)

Common Ways to Report Qualitative Data: A Basic Guide (continued)

Formal Written Reports of Qualitative Analyses for Academic Audiences

When completing a thesis dissertation, or a funded report, or when publishing in an academic forum, one can present a fuller picture of the topic under study, the past literature on the topic, a broad description of one's research methods, and more detail on actual findings. In a formal written report, there is also considerably more emphasis on formalizing conclusions and the implications of completed analyses. Thus, this type of report is the most complete version of a qualitative analysis. The standard format for a formal written report, especially for an academic audience is as follows:

- An introduction to the topic or group under study, including a discussion of the research purpose and the relevance of the research,
- A literature review or "background" section, illustrating past research on the topic, including a discussion of any gaps in this past literature that might be filled by the current analyses,
- A methods section that details the sample, data collection and processing procedures, analytic strategies, and potential biases/limitation of the research,

- A findings section, detailing one or a few broad findings and all the specific nuances found within these findings. For both broad and specific sets of findings, numerous examples of original data should be presented and explained in full,
- A discussion and/or conclusion section, summarizing what was found in the results and the implications of the findings. Attention may be paid to avenues for future research, especially based on particular limitations of the current study,
- Any tables, charts, graphs, or other appendices that make the discussion of methods or findings clearer to the reader, and
- References to past research on the topic.

The above sections may vary in length, depending on the audience for the written report. If one follows this standard format, there is a greater chance that one's qualitative research and analytic procedures will be considered credible or believable. This is particularly important when presenting qualitative analyses to audiences who value numerical results more than original data, or people's voices, or who value explanation over description and exploration.

If one prepares statements or answers in response to these issues before finalizing the report, one can guarantee a better reception of the qualitative analyses and conclusions. Laypersons both value quantitative research for the autonomy of numbers, while they value qualitative research for its sense of authenticity of real people. Thus, qualitative researchers need to be prepared to deal with these societal views in public forums.

Conclusion

This chapter illustrated how both qualitative analysis and reporting of qualitative research findings are multilayered enterprises. Investigators start with a particular data unit in a particular data source and then connect it to other data units in other data sources during a complex, flexible yet rigorous, analytic process. Once connections are found (i.e., patterns or themes across multiple interviews or observations), investigators think about what those patterns mean and create a way to not only understand, but also to talk about those

connections (i.e., a reporting strategy). Qualitative reporting then involves sharing information about the research process and about both broad and specific information found in the research.

Qualitative analysis and reporting are ongoing as well. While one may come to the end of a cycle of analysis or the end of a particular report, there are always more data to analyze and more analyses to report. The researcher should be ready to continue analyzing the same data sources over and over again for more and deeper insights and explanations. Qualitative researchers should also be ready to go back and analyze the very same coded themes and patterns, for there is always more one can discover about previously coded data units. Each time the researcher starts a particular analysis or reporting cycle, she or he makes choices about what to concentrate on, which, ultimately, means some analysis and reporting is left for later.

This means, then, that the conclusions qualitative researchers discuss are partial, and always warrant further exploration. Thus, researchers should always be thinking about how they can extend the data they have with just a bit more data analysis. One should think about ways in which to push the boundaries of interpretation and understanding to facilitate insights that are needed to answer the range of study questions. This may include a search for ways of broadening the analytic strategy but it can also mean finding ways to be more specific and insightful. Finally, because data collection and analysis should always be reflexive and iterative, one should never stop thinking about the next steps that could be taken in data collection. Such reflection can lay the groundwork for yet another new phase of the research project.

While this chapter discussed the major steps or processes that all qualitative researchers complete in order to interpret and report qualitative data, there are necessarily and inevitably variations in how each researcher moves through the analysis and reporting processes. By no means does everyone analyze or report their data in the same way. Nor should they. As highlighted many times, a benefit to qualitative research is the flexibility that characterizes it. Thus, while this chapter detailed particular ways in which qualitative analyses and reports can be completed, they should be seen only as a guide. They should not be taken as a prescription for how to complete qualitative analysis and reporting.

Finally, qualitative research is time-consuming and conceptually demanding. The goals of qualitative research—to describe, to explore, to present people's voices—can be realized only if individuals are dedicated to the complexities involved in data collection, analysis, and reporting. Researchers should be mindful of this during the arduous process of qualitative analysis and reporting.

Qualitative research has contributed understanding about the wide range of factors that contribute to individuals' health and disability, about individuals' use of particular therapeutic treatments, and about the processes by which occupational therapists facilitate health and wellness through their interventions. Consequently, *the initiation of more qualitative research in occupational therapy settings is critical*. While there have been important qualitative studies in recent years in occupational therapy, there is a need for much more description and exploration of both clients' conditions, and of both clients' and therapists' attitudes and behaviors.

REFERENCES

Becker, H. S., Geer, B., Hughes, E. C., Strauss, A. L. (1961, 1991). *Boys in white: Student culture in medical school*. Somerset, NJ: Transaction.

Deppen-Wood, M., Luborsky, M., & Scheer, J. (1997). Aging, disability and ethnicity. In J. Sokolovsky (Ed.), *Cultural context of aging: Worldwide perspectives* (2nd ed., pp. 443–451). New York: Bergin & Garvey.

Dijkers, M. (1999). Correlates of life satisfaction among persons with spinal cord injury. *Archives of Physical Medicine and Rehabilitation, 80*(8), 867–876.

Dillaway, H. E. (2005). Menopause is the "good old": Women's thoughts about reproductive aging. *Gender & Society, 19*(3), 398–417.

Emerson, R. M., Fretz, R. I., & Shaw, L. (1995). *Writing ethnographic fieldnotes*. Chicago: University of Chicago Press.

Estroff, S. (1981, 1985). *Making it crazy: An ethnography of psychiatric clients in an American community*. Berkeley, CA: University of California Press.

Geertz, C. (2001). Thick description: Toward an interpretive theory of culture. In R. M. Emerson (Ed.), *Contemporary field research* (2nd ed., pp. 55–75). Long Grove, IL: Waveland Press.

Gitlin, L., Luborsky, M., & Schemm, R. (1998). Emerging concerns of older stroke patients about assistive device use. *The Gerontologist, 38*(2), 169–180.

Glaser, B., & Strauss, A. (1967). *The discovery of grounded theory: Strategies for qualitative research*. Chicago: Aldine Press.

Glass, T. A., Matchar, D. B., Belyea, M., & Feussner, J. R. (1993). Impact of social support on outcome in first stroke. *Stroke, 24*, 64–70.

Groce, N. (1985). *Everyone here spoke sign language: Hereditary deafness on Martha's Vineyard*. Cambridge, MA: Harvard University Press.

Luborsky, M. (1997). Attuning assessment to the client: Recent advances in theory and methodology. *Generations, 21*(1), 10–16.

Lysack, C., & Seipke, H. (2002). Communicating the occupational self: A qualitative study of oldest-old American women. *Scandinavian Journal of Occupational Therapy, 9*, 130–139.

Magaziner, J., Hawkes, W., Hebel, J. R., Zimmerman, S. I., Fox, K. M., Dolan, M., Felsenthal, G., & Kenzora, J. (2000). Recovery from hip fracture in eight areas of function. *The Journals of Gerontology: Series A. Biological Sciences and Medical Sciences, 55*(9), 498M 507.

Miles, M. B., & Huberman, A. M. (1994). *Qualitative data analysis: An expanded sourcebook* (2nd ed.). Thousand Oaks, CA: SAGE Publications.

Mishler, E. G. (1979). Meaning in context: Is there any other kind? *Harvard Educational Review, 49*, 1–19.

Neufeld, S., Berry, R., & Sankar, S. (2005). Pathways to HIV diagnosis among African Americans. Manuscript submitted for publication.

Riessman, C. K. (1993). *Narrative analysis*. Thousand Oaks, CA: SAGE Publications.

Rubin, H., & Rubin, I. (2005). *Qualitative interviewing: The art of hearing data* (2nd ed.). Thousand Oaks, CA: SAGE Publications.

Sankar, A., Neufeld, S., & Luborsky, M. (2005a). The meaning of adherence to HIV anti-retroviral medications. Manuscript submitted for publication.

Sankar, A., Nevedal, D., Neufeld, S., & Luborsky, M. (2005). What is a missed dose? Implications for construct validity and patient adherence. Manuscript submitted for publication.

Schwandt, T. A. (1997). *Qualitative inquiry: A dictionary of terms*. Thousand Oaks, CA: SAGE Publications.

Siporin, S., & Lysack, C. (2004). Quality of life and supported employment: A case study of three women with developmental disabilities. *American Journal of Occupational Therapy, 58*(4), 455–465.

Stack, C. (1974). *All our kin: Strategies for survival in a Black community.* New York: Harper & Row.

Strauss, A. (1987). *Qualitative analysis for social scientists.* Cambridge, UK: Cambridge University Press.

Williams, A. M., & Irurita, I. F. (1998). Therapeutically conducive relationships between nurses and patients: An important component of quality nursing care. *Australian Journal of Advanced Nursing, 16*(2), 36–44.

CHAPTER 23

Exploring Perceptions About Services Using Q Methodology

Susan Corr

Q methodology (also known as operant subjectivity) provides a complementary approach to quantitative and qualitative methods. It maintains the subjectivity of participants and has a rigorous and objective process of doing so (Smith, 2001). It is a tool for exploring and generating a greater understanding of people's perspectives and beliefs. Q methodology uses a unique method of data collection and statistical analysis techniques (Brown, 1996). It has been used in the United States, and to a lesser extent in Britain, by a broad range of researchers, including psychologists, social scientists, educators, and political scientists. The method is increasingly being used in healthcare studies. The following are some examples:

> Q methodology allows individuals to measure themselves rather than being measured by researchers (Smith, 2001).

- Exploring stress and coping strategies in community psychiatric nurses (Leary et al., 1995),
- Understanding reasons for pharmacy students entering this profession (Wigger and Mrtek, 1994),
- Explaining how patients with irritable bowel syndrome understand the nature and causality of their illness (Stenner, Dancey, & Watts, 2000),
- Assessing nurses' job satisfaction (Chinnis, Summers, Doerr, Paulson, & Davis, 2001), and
- Identifying priorities and barriers to primary health care in post-conflict Serbia (Nelson et al., 2003).

The use of Q methodology by occupational therapists is just developing. For example, one study used Q methodology as an aspect of an evaluation of a day service for adults post-stroke (Corr, Phillips, & Capdevila, 2003). Another used the method as part of an investigation of former service users'[1] perspectives of occupational therapy (Corr, Neill, & Turner, 2005). Both of these studies will be discussed later to illustrate the processes and use of Q methodology in service evaluation. In addition, this chapter outlines the theoretical assumptions of the method, the processes involved and gives an indication of its potential use in establishing views relating to occupational therapy services.

History of Q Methodology

William Stephenson first introduced Q methodology in the 1930s (Stephenson, 1935; Wigger & Mrtek, 1994). He had the "desire to understand what made the individual person unique rather than what characteristics could be found across large populations of individuals" (Wigger & Mrtek, 1994, p. 9). In developing both the concepts and techniques of Q methodology, Stephenson drew from both quantitative and qualitative research traditions. Q methodology allows individuals to measure themselves rather than being measured by researchers (Smith, 2001). How individuals felt about issues was the focus of his concern and the method he developed.

One of Stephenson's students, Steve Brown, was instrumental in providing a breadth of expertise about Q methodology. His publications, conference presentations, email discussion list, and seminars (see Resources section) have increased awareness of Q methodology.

[1]Service user is the preferred term for clients or consumers of occupational therapy in the United Kingdom where this study was conducted.

Theoretical Bases and Assumptions

Q methodology is based on Stephenson's (1978) view of subjectivity and his belief that an objective account of this viewpoint can be obtained through an operant process. It draws on quantitative and qualitative approaches for its data collection, analysis, and interpretation processes.

Subjectivity

The key to Q methodology is that the self is central to all else (Brown, 1972). Stephenson considered subjectivity to be a point of view that the individuals were willing to say, either to themselves or to others (Smith, 2001). He argued that since the individual holds the subjective viewpoint, he or she must be the center of the investigation (Brown, 1972).

> The key to Q methodology is that the self is central to all else (Brown 1972).

> Through Q methodology, an expression of feeling or opinion is identified through concrete behavior.

Operant Subjectivity

Q methodology establishes participants' viewpoints through individuals undertaking an operant procedure (behavior) (i.e., sorting statements that relate to the concept under investigation. Stephenson considered this process to produce an expression of the participants' subjectivity (Wigger & Mrtek, 1994). According to Brown (1980), behavioral and social scientists have assumed that feelings, preferences, and thoughts are traits that can be measured only indirectly by tests and scales. However, through Q methodology, an expression of feeling or opinion is identified through concrete behavior. This process can be measured and studied in a scientific manner, allowing a construct to develop (Smith, 2001). Thus, participants' viewpoints lead to theoretical interpretations of the emerging constructs (Cordingley, Webb, & Hillier, 1997). Brown (1980) acknowledges that the subjective opinions identified in a Q methodology study are not provable, but they can be shown to have structure and form.

Comparison with Qualitative and Quantitative Methods

As previously noted, Q methodology draws on both qualitative and quantitative approaches. Table 23.1 indicates the differences between these for ease of comparison. Although Q methodology like many qualitative approaches, aims to explore subjective phenomena from the individual's own perspective, a significant difference is that in Q methodology individuals are given specific statements to which they are asked to respond (Cordingley et al., 1997). In some cases these statements may originate from qualitative approaches such as semi- or unstructured interviews. A second difference is the fact that in Q methodology, the viewpoints (factors) that emerge from the data are derived statistically (Cordingley et al., 1997). This process of data analysis is more akin to that of quantitative studies and therefore limits researcher bias. The similarity with qualitative approaches emerges again when considering the interpretation of the analyzed data. The researcher needs to describe and interpret the emerging viewpoints. Although Q methodology allows each individual to reflect his or her own viewpoint through how he or she arranges the statements, the factor analysis process allows researchers to view clusters or patterns of responses to uncover perceptions even within small groups (Donner, 2001; Robinson, Popovich, Gustafson, & Fraser, 2003). Researchers may describe typical patterns of perceptions rather than average perceptions and will name or label distinct points of view and provide some interpretation of these (Robinson et al., 2003).

Steps to Conducting Q Methodology

Q methodology has the following four distinct phases, each of which is outlined in this chapter:

- Developing the Q-sort pack,
- Administering the Q-sort,
- Factor analyzing the data, and
- Interpreting factors.

Developing a Q-Sort Pack

The first, and according to Donner (2001) the most challenging, step in Q methodology is the development of the Q-sort pack. As in traditional survey techniques, discussed in Chapter 8, this early step involves creating items or statements that will be used to examine the topic of investigation (Chinnis

Q methodology can be used to:

* Make discoveries but not predictions.
* Examine emerging factors of the phenomenon of interest.
* Examine life as lived from the standpoint of the person living it.
* Identify characteristics of individuals who share common viewpoints.
* Measure arrays of attitudes at a certain point in time.
* Measure attitudinal changes over time.
* Study subjective preferences, sentiments, ideals, the nature of beauty, tastes.
* Understand individuals as complex, holistic beings.
* Discover unexpected characteristics.
* Discover what was previously unknown as opposed to testing a theory.

(Brown, 1972, 1996; Cordingley et al., 1997; Dennis, 1986; Mrtek et al. 1996; Smith, 2001; Wigger & Mrtek, 1994).

et al., 2001). The Q-sort pack ideally consists of between 40 and 80 statements related to the research topic (Dennis, 1986). These statements can be generated from several sources including preliminary interviews with potential participants, relevant literature or any sources that provide information, and opinions connected to the study (Brown, 1996; Dennis, 1986; Wigger and Mrtek, 1994). According to Barbosa, Willoughby, Rosenberg, and Mrtek (1998), there should be enough statements with a variety of opinions to cater to the widely different subjective feelings the participants may have about the research topic. Donner (2001) suggests that the statements can be assumed to be simply a subset of the possible concepts that may be important to the issue at hand.

The statements do not have to be lengthy (Donner, 2001). Pictures or images, simple phrases, or single words can be used and may be more appropriate for certain populations such as children. Donner (2001) suggests that to create a good set of statements researchers should try to choose statements that have distinct meanings and are not merely repetitive, overlapping, or the exact inverse of each other. He also recommends avoiding statements that are so extreme that all participants could be expected to either agree or disagree with them, to the exclusion of prioritizing other

> The factor analysis process allows researchers to view clusters or patterns of responses to uncover perceptions.

items. Therefore, statements need to "be plausible competitors with one another, such that some participants may be attracted to them and others disinclined to choose them" (Donner, 2001, p. 27). The statements should also be similar in style (e.g., either as full sentences or just phrases). These statements should be clear and without double negatives.

Two Case Examples

In a study conducted by Corr et al. (2003) to establish perceptions of benefit from a day service for young adults with stroke, group interviews were carried out to generate statements of perceived benefits of the service. Groups consisted of some of the users of the service, their caregivers, volunteers, fund holders, and those who referred clients to the service. The literature, especially that relating to the provision of day services, was also explored to generate statements. Finally the service's own documentation that outlines its aims was considered and used as a source of statements. An advantage of creating statements in this manner is that the preconceived biases of the researcher can be minimized, since the statements come from the participants themselves (Chinnis et al., 2001).

The statements were then checked for duplication to eliminate overlap. Finally statements were examined to make sure they focused on the intended topic. For instance, those describing the process of the service as opposed to the benefits were removed.

The second study aimed to explore former service users' views of occupational therapy (Corr, Neill, & Turner, 2005). Creek (2003) originally conducted an ethnographic study to develop a conceptual framework about the nature and purpose of occupational therapy. The document she produced, "Occupational therapy as a complex intervention" (Creek, 2003), was used to generate the statements for this study. In total 32 statements were generated and an example of these are presented in Figure 23.1.

Administrating a Q Sort

The Q-sort pack consists of a pack of cards with each statement on a separate card. Participants are asked to sort the various statements according to a specific condition of instruction given by the

Table 23.1 **Comparison of Q Methodology with Qualitative and Quantitative Methods**

Issue	Quantitative Methods	Q Methodology	Qualitative Methods
Purpose	Identify changes or characteristics in large populations.	Identify ranges of viewpoints.	Explore individual experiences.
Constructs being explored	Researcher identifies these at the outset.	Researcher provides the broad framework; the process enables the constructs to emerge.	Constructs are usually unknown and they emerge through the research process.
Population	Large populations are usually required.	The population needs to represent those who have a view on the topic in questions (all stakeholders). Between 20 and 40 are common population sizes.	A small population is used, and may even just be one individual.
Tools	Measurable items such as interval score and objective measurement scales.	Statements (or similar materials) that reflect the research topic.	Free-flow conversation via interviews.
Data collection	Objective measuring and recording of data usually in a numerical format.	Statements are sorted by individuals using an ordinal scale.	Interviews are using unstructured or semistructured.
Analysis	Uses descriptive and inferential statistics to look for trends and comparisons.	Uses a statistical process (factor analysis) to identity range of viewpoints and differences and similarities of views.	Content or discourse analysis used seeking meaning units and themes.
Interpretation	Reports results as statistical findings indicating levels of significance.	The researcher tells the story of the emerging viewpoints and explains differences and similarities.	The researcher interprets the data but may use techniques such as member checking to aid this.

researcher (Cordingley et al., 1997). The most usual conditions involve sorting according to the degree of agreement they place on each of the statements, from "most disagree" through "neutral" to "most agree" (Brown, 1996; Dennis, 1986; Leary et al., 1995). It can also be "most unlike" to "most like" or other such conditions (Smith, 2001). Stainton Rogers (1995) suggests that it is easier to start by separating the statements under relevant headings such as "disagree," "neutral," and "agree" before sorting them more discriminately along the continuum. Prior to administering the Q-sort pack, the researcher needs to develop a sorting grid (i.e., a grid layout to indicate the shape of the distribution). There are usually an odd number of column values in order to allow for a middle neutral column (Donner, 2001). Figure 23.2 shows the grid for the Corr et al. (2005) study, which used 32 statements. From this grid it will be clear how many statements should be placed in each cate-

gory. For example, referring to Figure 23.2, the participant would place two statements in the extreme "most disagree" box, and the extreme "most agree" box and six statements in the neutral box and so on. This "flattened" normal distribution curve, that is, a curve that allows more points on the extremes, is usually used in Q methodology (Dennis, 1986).

In using this grid, important statements, with which the participant has strongly agreed and strongly disagreed, should first be placed at the extreme ends of the distribution pattern. Statements that hold less salience for the participant would be found near the midpoint of the grid (Mrtek, Tafesse, & Wigger, 1996). Participants are therefore forced into prioritizing which statements they wish to use to express their strongest attitudes or feelings (Cordingley et al., 1997). Even though this approach does force the distribution, the number of ways in which a sample can be sorted is still

1. It provides an opportunity for me to retrain for work.

2. The occupational therapist provides group activities for me to participate in.

3. Helps me to cope in my community.

4. I have to work in partnership with my occupational therapist.

5. During treatment the activities are adjusted so that they remain challenging and interesting.

6. Enables me to remain independent.

7. Teaches me new skills and helps me to relearn old ones.

8. Looks at all areas of need from looking after myself to my hobbies and my employment.

9. Provides adaptations to my home.

10. Occupational therapists offer support to my caregivers as well as to me.

Figure 23.1 Example of the statements. [Reprinted with permission from Corr, S., Neill, G., & Turner, A. (2005). Comparing occupational therapy definition and consumers' experiences: A Q-methodology study. *British Journal of Occupational Therapy, 68*(8), 338-346.]

huge. All statements can be moved about and exchanged until the participant is completely satisfied with his or her choices, as there are no right or wrong answers (Brown, 1980; Stainton Rogers, 1995).

The sample size for Q methodology can be small, as the study concerns the viewpoints of participants rather than the character traits of a specific population that the participants are chosen to represent (Mrtek et al., 1996). Therefore, as in qualitative research, individuals are chosen to participate in a study based on their relevance to the study's aim and question, rather than on the basis of their representativeness of a larger population (Chinnis et al., 2001; Cordingley et al., 1997). Since the researcher aims to establish a variety of perspectives, a key issue in choosing participants is to ensure that diverse selections of viewpoints are included (Cordingley et al., 1997).

Sampling can be illustrated by referring back to the two studies previously discussed. In the first instance, 37 participants took part in the day service evaluation study (Corr et al., 2003). Nineteen had used the service while the remaining 18 were

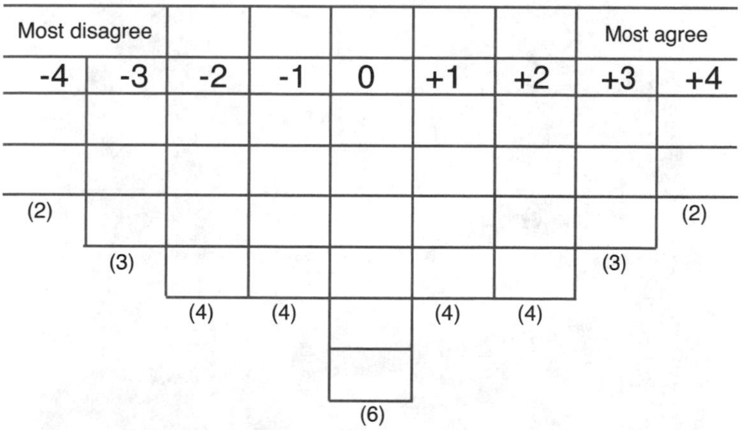

Figure 23.2 Sorting grid. [Reprinted with permission from Corr, S. Neill, G., & Turner, A. (2005). Comparing occupational therapy definition and consumers' experiences: A Q-methodology study. *British Journal of Occupational Therapy, 68*(8), 338-346.]

other stakeholders of the service such as caregivers of users, volunteers, and fund-holders. In the second instance, 16 former users were selected to give their views on occupational therapy (Corr et al., 2005).

The Q-sort pack can be administered in group or individual settings. The participants require enough space to sort the statements, visually view the entire sort (to make adjustments), and then record their answers without disturbing the sort (Donner, 2001). It takes on average 20 or 25 minutes for a sort of 30 statements. In addition, participants can be invited to add any comments they wish regarding the statements and sorting process. These should be recorded by the researcher and noted as complementary data for use in the interpretation of the factors.

> In this methodology it is the viewpoints that are important rather than the number of participants who held those viewpoints.

Analyzing the Data

Analysis of the data gathered by Q methodology can be carried out by a dedicated Q package such as PQMethod, which can be downloaded from the World Wide Web (see Resources section). The rank-ordering pattern (Q-sort) of each participant is entered into the statistical package. It is then factor analyzed for its meaning using principal component analysis and varimax rotation (Mrtek et al., 1996). Chapter 17 provides a discussion of factor analysis. The goal of factor analysis is to find the underlying factors that summarize the pattern of correlations among the Q-sorts undertaken by the participants (Cordingley et al., 1997).

The first stage of the analysis involves correlating each person's Q-sort with all the other Q-sorts, resulting in a matrix of correlation coefficients (Cordingley et al., 1997). The correlation coefficients indicate the extent to which pairs of Q-sorts resemble or are different from each other. If all participants sort the statements similarly, there will be a high correlation coefficient and only one factor (viewpoint) will be identified.

Factor analysis searches for groups of Q-sorts which, on the basis of their correlations, appear to go together as a view or factor. Participants are

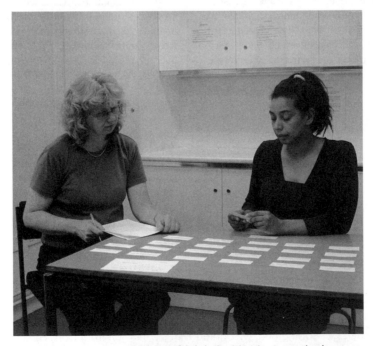

Figure 23.3 A study participant (right) decides how much she agrees or disagrees with statements about occupational therapy while Dr. Corr (left) notes any additional comments made and final positions of the statements.

grouped on the same factor when their Q-sorts are similar, that is, they have sorted the same statements that they most agree with and most disagree with (Dennis, 1986). Principal component analysis is used to provide eigenvalues for each factor (eigenvalues are an indication of the proportion of variance explained by each factor) (Kline, 1994). This information contributes to the decision making on the number of factors to identify. Factors with an eigenvalue greater than one explain more variance and therefore the maximum number of factors taken to the next stage (rotation) usually corresponds to the number of initial factors with eigenvalues greater than one (Donner, 2001). Varimax rotation clarifies the structure of the factors by maximizing the variance between each of the factors (Donner, 2001). It allows the researcher to identify those sorts that load cleanly on a single factor.

Usually, more than one but less than seven factors (viewpoints) are identified in Q methodology studies (Dennis, 1986). In this methodology, it is the viewpoints that are important rather than the number of participants who held those viewpoints. Once the factors are identified, Q-sorts are constructed in the arrangement of these views to facilitate interpretation. Figure 23.4 is the reconstructed sort of one factor for the study conducted by Corr et al. (2005). The researcher is then in a position to establish statistically how each individual's Q-sort relates (or loads) on to these identified factors (Cordingley et al., 1997).

Interpreting Findings

The final stage of a Q methodological study is to interpret the factors that have emerged. This is achieved by studying the analysis output and by looking at the reconstructed sorts representing each factor (Chinnis et al., 2001). The analysis output, as well as presenting the sorts for each factor, also allows comparisons to be made between the positioning of statements in each factor. It highlights contentious and consensus statements so that both differences and similarities can be noted.

At this stage often the factors are given labels that best describe the patterns of statements in the given factor (Corr, 2001). The researcher may use the additional interview data collected when the individual sorted the statements, or he or she may go back to the participants with the descriptions of the factors to confirm the interpretation (Cordingley et al., 1997). It is up to the researcher to infer the meaning of the factors (Donner, 2001). However, theory, previous research, and cultural knowledge may aid interpretation (Stainton Rogers, 1995). Interpretation of the factors according to Stephenson (1983) results in meaning or explanation and understanding of the factors. "Q factors point to the necessity for insights, hunches and guesses supported subsequently by facts" (Stephenson, 1998, p. 73).

As shown in the feature box below, six factors emerged in the study of views of occupational therapy (Corr et al., 2005). The 'story' for each factor was generated noting the placement of the "most agree," and "most disagree" statements and additional post-sort comments made by the participants. For example, it can be seen from Figure 23.3 that the "story" for this factor emerges from statements 20, 32, 28, 31, and 18 as well as 9, 13, 22, 1, and 2. This factor placed emphasis on occupational therapy as being beneficial for improving individuals' sense of self and adjusting to their disability and not about providing adaptations or assisting with returning to work. However, placing statement 22 in the −3 column raised questions about the consistency of the participants' experiences, as on the one hand they feel supported in adjusting to life after stroke while on the other they suggested that they are not supported in dealing with the emotional and psychological aspects of their stroke. The study found similarities in what the participants perceived as benefits of occupational therapy based on their experiences, compared to the professional view as noted in the definition document by Creek (2003). The study noted the importance of the individual within occupational therapy intervention, as a unique individual, for whom occupational therapy assists to retain his or her sense of self, and enables him or her to adjust to disability and to participate in society.

Potential Application in Occupational Therapy

Q methodology has the potential for use by occupational therapists as "the range of topics which can be studied using this technique is almost

Factors identified as views of service of occupational therapy services:
Factor 1: Improved sense of self
Factor 2: The importance of being heard
Factor 3: Practical assistance
Factor 4: Maintaining autonomy
Factor 5: Desire for involvement
Factor 6: General benefits
(Corr et al., 2005)

-4	-3	-2	-1	0	+1	+2	+3	+4
				19. I have to play an active role in my treatment.				
				23. I am able to freely express my feelings.				20. I am treated as an individual rather than as "just another patient."
		25. Occupational therapists help me to sort out my finanaces and benefits.	7. Teaches me new skills and helps me relearn old ones.	29. Enables me to pursue my leisure activities and hobbies.	21. Gives me a sense of achievement.	6. Enables me to remain independent.	28. Improves my quality of life.	
	22. Helps me to deal with the emotional and psychological effects of my stroke.	4. I have to work in partnership with my occupational therapist.	15. Provides equipment to enable to remain independent.	24. I am listened to rather than told what to do.	14. I am able to choose the goals of my treatment.	17. Helps me feel more able to participate in social activities.	31. It helps me to adjust to my disabilities.	32. Occupational therapy is concerned with how my stroke has affected me physically.
9. Provides adaptations to my home.	1. It provides an opportunity for me to retrain for work.	16. I am able to choose activities that are important and meaningful to me.	11. I am regularly asked how I feel about my treatment.	10. Occupational therapists offer support to my carers as well as to me.	12. The information given to me is easy to understand and helps me make decisions.	30. Uses activities to help me overcome my problems.	18. Helps me to gain a sense of identity.	
13. Carers are involved in my treatment.	2. The occupational therapist provides group activities for me to participate in.	8. Looks at all areas of need from looking after myself to my hobbies and employment.	3. Helps me to cope in my community.	27. Occupational therapy focuses on activities that help me look after myself, i.e., washing and dressing.	5. During treatment the activities are adjusted so that they remain challenging and interesting.	26. Occupational therapy treatment helps me to carry out everyday activities in my home.		
Least beneficial				Neutral				Most beneficial

Figure 23.4 Factor 1 Improved sense of self. [Reprinted with permission form Corr, S., Neill, G., & Turner, A. (2005). Comparing occupational therapy definition and consumers' experiences: A Q-methodology study. *British Journal of Occupational Therapy, 68*(8), 338-346.]

unlimited" (Stainton Rogers, 1995, p. 180). Wigger and Mrtek (1994) believe that whenever subjective matters are at the center of the research question, Q methodology can be used. It would help identify attitudes to illness and disability from a client's perspective and has already been used to attempt to explain health and illness (Stainton Rogers, 1991).

So far, occupational therapists have used Q methodology mainly in service evaluation. Service evaluation is considered key in providing effective and efficient services (Salmon, 2003) while Murphy, Dingwall, Greatbatch, Parker, and Watson (1998) consider it to be "an essential part of any intervention or program of action in health" (p. 215). Q methodology enables all relevant stakeholders to participate in service evaluation. However, historically it is the service users who have often been excluded from contributing to the development and change of services.

The aim of the day service evaluated by Corr et al. (2003) was to offer individuals between 18 and 55 years of age who had a stroke the opportunity to identify and pursue meaningful and realistic opportunities within the community. The purpose of the evaluation was to establish any benefits from attending the service including any perceived benefits to inform future planning and provision with respect to long-term care post-stroke (Corr et al., 2003; Corr, Phillips, & Walker, 2004). In addition to the Q methodology study, a randomized crossover design study was used to measure change objectively following attendance at the service for 6 months (Corr et al., 2004). The findings suggest that attending the service increased occupational performance and satisfaction with performance. However, there was no evidence that depression and anxiety were reduced, that quality of life and self-concept were improved, or that there was increased participation in community activities. Many unmet needs were also identified.

The Q methodology study generated a range of viewpoints with eleven factors identified, six from the service users and five from the nonusers (see feature box above). These factors suggested that the service provided new experiences, enabled individuals to feel valued, aided social recovery, provided security, prevented isolation, contributed to psychological gains, enhanced social confidence, encouraged communication, provided respite for caregivers, and engendered a sense of purpose.

The findings from both aspects of the evaluation suggested that the service provided some support to the individuals post-stroke although there were differences between what were perceived as

---

Factors Identified as Views of Users of Stroke Day Service

Factor 1: New experiences
Factor 2: Feeling valued
Factor 3: Social recovery
Factor 4: Security
Factor 5: Prevents isolation
Factor 6: General recovery

Factors Identified as Views of Nonusers

Factor 1: Psychological gains
Factor 2: Social confidence
Factor 3: Encourages communication
Factor 4: Respite for carers
Factor 5: Sense of purpose

(Corr et al., 2003)

---

benefits, what changes occurred, and the aim of the service. These findings allowed the stakeholders to review the service aims and therefore clarify whether the perceived benefits match the aim. They also enable the stakeholders to establish if new aims need to be set and to understand the various perceptions of benefits.

The factors and defining statements for the factors in a service evaluation, such as the example above, could be used to create a routine evaluation tool such as a Likert scale or questionnaire. The Q methodology study identified the relevant concepts through small-sample analysis. However, this can be useful in the development of questionnaires for administration to larger samples (Brown, 2002).

This previous example indicates the use of Q methodology in establishing perceptions of benefit to services. Q methodology could also be used to identify clients' attitudes both at the beginning and end of intervention. An additional use is as a single case study, in which the individual may be asked to sort the statements under a range of conditions of instruction (Smith, 2001). For example, an individual may be asked to sort according to how he felt when he was first referred to occupational therapy, how he feels now, and how he anticipates he will feel in the future.

Strengths and Limitations

Strengths

There are a number of benefits to using Q methodology. Most importantly, it allows people to express their own views (Corr, 2001). Turner

(2002) suggests that one element of the philosophy of occupational therapy is that "people are individuals of worth and inherently different from each other" (p. 5). If used with clients, occupational therapy researchers could establish the different views that individuals hold. Q methodology provides the opportunity for service users to have an active role in service evaluation, which is important (Martin, 1986).

Sorting the Q pack is a novel administration method that requires the active participation of the research participant. This, although not unique, is unusual in the research process. As a result of this active participation, it is rare to have missing data and undecided responses (Dennis, 1986). Donner (2001) has noted that participants want to see their opinions translated into factors and quantified. Also the ranking of the statements during the Q-sort requires participants to make fine discriminations they otherwise might not make (Dennis, 1986). In other research methods, such as Likert scales, participants are asked to indicate their levels of agreement on a range of statements. However, the advantage of Q methodology over one such as Likert is that participants have to identify their level of agreement with a statement in relation to all the other statements (Donner, 2001). It also allows researchers to clarify the range of constructs present in viewpoints on the research topic (Barbosa et al., 1998).

In Q methodology the content validity of each of the statements is derived from the rank order in which they are placed and the vicinity to other statements as determined by the participant (Wigger & Mrtek, 1994). The face validity of Q methodology relates to the degree of satisfaction a participant feels about how accurately his or her ranking of the statements reflects his or her personal feelings (Barbosa et al., 1998). Dennis (1986) suggests that the data tend to be highly reliable and this is supported by the studies of Fairweather (1981), who found test–retest correlations greater than .90 for short intervals and Kerlinger (1972), who found correlations of .81 for an 11-month period.

Another positive aspect of Q methodology is that only a small number of participants are needed (Mrtek et al., 1996). As few as a dozen participants may be used, while it is quite rare to have more than 100 participants in a study (Donner, 2001). Q methodology also reveals how many different viewpoints are present among the group of participants (Mrtek et al., 1996). It is like other qualitative methods in that it generates qualitative data. However, it is different in that it provides a way to quantify and analyze such information and allows differences as well as similarities between viewpoints to be easily identified (Cordingley et al., 1997; Mrtek et al., 1996).

Another more recent advantage related to Q methodology is the availability of free computer software such as PQMethod. This can perform the complex calculations associated with factor analysis and speedily identify the factors.

Limitations

Q methodology has several limitations, related mainly to the process involved. Time is required for each participant to sort the statements; this amount of time can add up depending on the number of participants in the study. Also, explaining the process to the participants can be time-consuming, as the instructions are comprehensive and participants may need to be shown how to proceed (Dennis, 1986). It is necessary to invest this time if participants are to represent their perspectives accurately and adequately. In the pilot for the day service study, those users of the service who had comprehension problems had some difficulties sorting the Q pack. Also, all service users took far longer than caregivers and volunteers and appeared to tire during the process. As a result, a smaller (33 statements) separate Q-sort pack and grid was developed for the service users to complete.

A second limitation is that it is not designed to show how many people in a study population have a specific viewpoint (Mrtek et al., 1996). Also, as Barbosa et al. (1998) point out, "no claim is made that other viewpoints do not exist in the broader population" (p. 1039). In essence, Q methodology cannot answer such questions so alternative methods should be considered. It is worth bearing in mind that a Q methodology study can provide the concepts for a larger questionnaire study that can allow inferences concerning the population to be made.

Validity can be compromised if the participants did not comprehend the Q-sort task, leading to a misrepresentation of his or her views (Dennis, 1986). Alternatively, there is the potential for participants to make mechanical rather than conceptual choices to complete the process, particularly if they find the process tiring, which may be the case with some client groups (Dennis, 1986). Participants have identified the forced nature of the sorting process as a difficulty (Chinnis et al., 2001). However, it ensures that participants systematically think about all of the statements in relation to each other and makes them identify the most strongly felt issues. It is important that the researcher clearly explains the instructions.

Another limitation is the fact that the meanings are given to factors by the researchers and therefore could be influenced by researcher bias (Barbosa et al., 1998). However, the analysis process aids objective reporting by indicating which statements define the factors.

REFERENCES

Barbosa, J., Willoughby, P., Rosenberg, C., & Mrtek, R. (1998). Statistical Methodology: VII. Q-Methodology, a structural analytic approach to medical subjectivity. *Academic Emergency Medicine, 5,* 1032–1040.

Brown, S. (1972). A fundamental incommensurability between objectivity and subjectivity. In S. Brown & D. Brenner (Eds.), *Science, psychology and communication* (pp. 57–94). New York: Teachers College Press.

Brown, S. (1980). *Political subjectivity. Applications of Q methodology in political science.* New Haven: Yale University Press.

Brown, S. (1996). Q methodology and qualitative research. *Qualitative Health Research, 6*(4), 561–567.

Brown, S. (2002). Q technique and questionnaires. *Operant Subjectivity, 25,* 117–126.

Chinnis, A., Summers, D., Doerr, C., Paulson, D., & Davis, S. (2001). Q methodology. A new way of assessing employee satisfaction. *Journal of Nursing Administration, 31*(5), 252–259.

Cordingley, L., Webb, C., & Hillier, V. (1997). Q methodology. Qualitative data analysis. *Nurse Researcher, 4*(3), 31–45.

Corr, S. (2001). An introduction to Q methodology, a research technique. *British Journal of Occupational Therapy, 64*(6), 293–297.

Corr, S., Neill, G., & Turner, A. (2005). Comparing occupational therapy definition and consumers experiences: A Q-methodology study. *British Journal of Occupational Therapy. 68*(8), 338–346.

Corr, S., Phillips, C., & Capdevila, R. (2003). Using Q methodology to evaluate a day service for younger adult stroke survivors. *Operant Subjectivity, 27*(1), 1–23.

Corr, S., Phillips, C., & Walker, M. (2004). Evaluation of a pilot service designed to provide support following stroke: A randomized cross-over design study. *Clinical Rehabilitation, 18,* 69–75.

Creek, J. (2003). *Occupational therapy defined as a complex intervention.* London: College of Occupational Therapy.

Dennis, K. (1986). Q methodology: Relevance and application to nursing research. *Advances in Nursing Science, 8*(3), 6–17.

Donner, J. (2001). Using Q-sorts in participatory processes: an introduction to the methodology. In R. Krueger, M. Casey, J. Donner, S. Kirsch, & J. Maack (Eds.), Social analysis. Selected tools and techniques (vol. 36, pp. 24–49). Washington: World Bank.

Fairweather, J. (1981). Reliability and validity of Q-method results: Some empirical evidence. *Operant Subjectivity, 5,* 2–16.

Kerlinger, F. (1972). Q methodology in behavioral research. In S. Brown & D. Brenner (Eds.), *Science, psychology and communication* (pp. 3–38). New York: Teachers College Press.

Kline, P. (1994). *An easy guide to factor analysis.* London: Routledge.

Leary, J., Gallagher, T., Carson, J., Fagin, L., Bartlett, H., & Brown, D. (1995). Stress and coping strategies in community psychiatric nurses: A Q-methodological study. *Journal of Advanced Nursing, 21,* 230–237.

Martin, E. (1986). Consumer evaluation of human services. *Social Policy and Administration, 20*(3), 185–200.

Mrtek, R., Tafesse, E., & Wigger, U. (1996). Q-methodology and subjective research. *Journal of Social and Administrative Pharmacy, 13*(2), 54–64.

Murphy, E., Dingwall, R., Greatbatch, D., Parker, S., & Watson, P. (1998). Qualitative research methods in health technology assessment: A review of the literature. *Health Technology Assessment, 2*(16).

Nelson, B., Simic, S., Beste, L., Vukovic, D., Bjegovic, V., & Van Rooyen, M. (2003). Multimodal assessment of the primary healthcare system of Serbia: A model for evaluating post-conflict health systems. *Prehospital and Disaster Medicine, 18*(1), 6–13.

Robinson, T., Popovich, M., Gustafson, R., & Fraser, C. (2003). Older adults' perceptions of offensive senior stereotypes in magazine advertisements: Results of a Q method analysis. *Educational Gerontology, 29,* 503–519.

Salmon, N. (2003). Service evaluation and the service user: A pluralistic solution. *British Journal of Occupational Therapy, 66*(7), 311–317.

Smith, N. (2001). *Current systems in psychology: History, theory, research and application.* Belmont CA: Wadsworth/Thomson Learning.

Stainton Rogers, W. (1991). *Exploring health and illness. An exploration of diversity.* New York: Harvester Wheatsheaf.

Stainton Rogers, R. (1995). Q methodology. In J. Smith & R. Harre & L. VanLangenhove (Eds.), *Rethinking methods in psychology* (pp. 178–207). Newbury Park, CA: SAGE Publications.

Stenner, P., Dancey, C., & Watts, S. (2000). The understanding of their illness amongst people with irritable bowel syndrome: A Q methodological study. *Social Science and Medicine, 51,* 439–452.

Stephenson, W. (1935). Technique of factor analysis. *Nature, 136,* 297.

Stephenson, W. (1978). Concourse theory of communication. *Communication, 3,* 21–20.

Stephenson, W. (1983). After interpretation. *Operant Subjectivity, 6*(3), 73–103.

Stephenson, W. (1998). Quantum theory media research: II. Intentionality and acculturation. *Operant Subjectivity, 21,* 73–91.

Turner, A. (2002). History and philosophy of occupational therapy. In A. Turner & M. Foster & S. Johnson (Eds.), *Occupational therapy and physical dysfunction: principles, skills and practice* (5th ed., pp. 3–24). Edinburgh: Churchill Livingstone.

Wigger, U., & Mrtek, R. (1994). Use of Q-technique to examine attitudes of entering pharmacy students toward their profession. *American Journal of Pharmaceutical Education, 58,* 8–15.

RESOURCES

The following are a range of resources available to anyone interested in Q methodology.

Web-Based Material

There is a Web site for Q methodology that contains a breadth of useful information for those interested in this method. It can be accessed at: http://www. qmethod.org

An e-mail discussion list is an active discussion forum regularly used by experts and novices alike to share ideas, recent publications, and solutions to problems. To join the list, send the command "subscribe Q-method <your name>" (without quotations or brackets) to Listserv@listerv.kent.edu

Computer Software

PQMethod is a factor analytic program, which is freely available on the Internet and is in the public domain. It was developed by Peter Schmolck, and is a software program specifically designed for Q methodology studies. This software can be downloaded for free at the following Web site: http://www.12.unibw-muenchen. de/p41bsmk/qmethod/

Journals

Operant Subjectivity is the quarterly journal of the International Society for the Scientific Study of Subjectivity. Details of subscribing are on the Q method Web site: http://www.qmethod.org

Conferences

The International Society for the Scientific Study of Subjectivity holds an annual meeting where research and theoretical papers are presented. For details check the Q methodology Web site: http://www.qmethod.org

Textbooks

A range of Q references are now available including those in this chapter's reference list. Two textbooks that are useful "manuals" are:

Brown, S. R. (1980) *Political subjectivity: Applications of Q methodology in political science*. New Haven: Yale University Press.

This somewhat weighty text covers all the steps and principles in undertaking a Q methodology study with examples drawn from political science.

McKeown, B. F., & Thomas, D. B. (1988). *Q methodology*. Newbury Park, CA: SAGE Publications.

This is a slim paperback that is user-friendly and contains the essentials of Q methodology.

CHAPTER 24

The Nature and Use of Consensus Methodology in Practice

Edward A. S. Duncan

Consensus methodology is the use of a structured approach to arrive at a single statement, or set of statements, that all participants accept; or to identify any central tendency and spread of opinion regarding an issue (Murphy et al., 1998). Consensus methods can make important contributions to the evidence base of occupational therapy and are increasingly used to assist in the development of clinical guidelines for practice. This chapter provides an overview of consensus methods and addresses what is important to consider when selecting and using a consensus methodology.

> While the findings of consensus studies are, to a certain extent, constructions of participants' own experiences, these representations can be valid and relevant to the population being studied.

The Philosophical Basis of Consensus Methodology: Subtle Realism

Consensus approaches comprise three separate methodologies:

• Delphi studies,
• Nominal group techniques (NGTs), and
• Consensus conferences.

Each of these three methodologies is presented and discussed later in the chapter. Consensus approaches embrace a mixed method philosophy and adopt a subtle realist perspective of knowledge (Duncan, 2004; Hammersley, 1992; Kirk and Miller, 1986). Subtle realists assert that all research involves subjective perceptions and observations and concede that different methods will produce different pictures of the participant(s) being studied (Pope & Mays, 2000). The subtle realist understands that researchers cannot claim to have absolute certainty regarding the findings of

their research (Hammersley, 1992; Kirk & Miller, 1986). Rather, as Murphy, Dingwall, Greatbatch, Parker, and Watson (1998a) argue, "...the objective should be the search for knowledge about which we can be reasonably confident. Such confidence will be based upon judgments about the credibility and plausibility of knowledge claims" (p. 69). While the findings of consensus studies are, to a certain extent, constructions of participants' own experiences, these representations can be valid and relevant to the population being studied.

Consensus methods are frequently employed to explore an area where there is a lack of empirical knowledge (Pope & Mays, 2000) or where consumer participation in the development of a clinical program is sought (Twible, 1992). Increasingly, the expert opinion of participants in consensus research is recognized as a valid form of developing evidence-based guidelines (Harbour & Miller, 2001).

Defining Features of Consensus Methodology

While each of the consensus approaches differs in its methods, all share four common themes (Pope & Mays, 2000):

• Anonymity,
• Iteration (i.e., the use of "rounds" that offer participants the opportunity to change their minds as the perspectives of other group members become known),
• Controlled feedback (i.e., the researcher shares the distribution of the group's response with the participants, and
• Statistical and qualitative analysis (i.e., each study contains statistical measures of agreement as well as a more qualitative analysis of the findings).

Table 24.1 A Comparison of Consensus Methods in Practice

	Delphi Methodology	Nominal Group Technique	Consensus Conferences
Participant Location	Remote	Local	Local
Time Scale	Different rounds are spread over weeks.	Approximately 60–90 minutes.	½–1 Day
Anonymity	Participant identification and study item prioritization.	Participant identification is not anonymous, but study item prioritization is.	Participant identification not anonymous and participant perspectives are also public.
Optimal Size	Variable, dependent on topic. Larger samples may be more open to high attrition rates.	Group sizes of between 6–9 participants are recommended. Several groups can be run and summative assessment occur.	Panel size of 10–15 people plus relevant conference delegates.
Analysis of Findings	Variable. Statistical or descriptive analysis is possible according to the study's design.	Both statistical and qualitative. Analysis can cease following an individual group or various groups can be combined for a summative analysis.	A consensus statement on the issues raised is prepared and is formally presented to relevant bodies and organizations.

Delphi Methodology

The Delphi study is an iterative, multistage form of survey designed to systematically gain, collate, and aggregate expert opinion and form a group consensus on a particular issue (Hasson, Keeney, & McKenna, 2000; Love, 1997). It is designed to:

• Create an environment in which each subject is anonymous—this enables people to share ideas and opinions, which they may not feel free to share if they are aware of other, possibly more dominant, opinions,

• Explore and expose assumptions and views,
• Gain the expertise of a larger number of people than possible through face-to-face gatherings,
• Educate the respondent group as to the consensus or diversity of their opinion, and
• Eliminate time-consuming but irrelevant discussion (Strauss & Ziegler, 1975).

Background

The Delphi technique was developed by Olaf Helmer-Hirschberg for the Rand Corporation. During the 1960s, the methodology was further developed within the scientific community as a method of predicting future trends. Today, Delphi studies have become an accepted methodology for the development of consensus within health care research (Cantrill, Sibbald, & Buetow, 1996; Love, 1997; Salmond, 1994). While Delphi studies have traditionally been paper-based, they are increasingly carried out in an electronic format (Duncan et al., 2004; Hasson et al., 2000; Jones & Hunter, 2000). This approach has the advantage of allowing for swift communication between the researcher and correspondent. However, it does require participants to be computer literate.

Methodological Considerations

Researchers, through time, have slightly modified the Delphi technique according to their own requirements. However, the basic format has remained unchanged and is outlined below. Within each of the stages various factors that impact on the methods integrity must be considered.

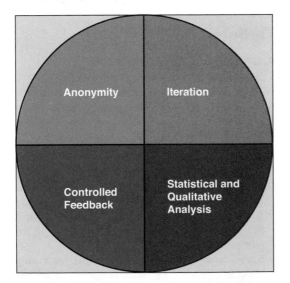

Figure 24.1 Features of consensus methodology.

Identification and Recruitment of Group Members

One of the benefits of Delphi methodology is the removal of geographical limitations encountered in other consensus methods (Jones & Hunter, 2000). Sample sizes of Delphi studies range broadly and should be viewed in light of the subject area under scrutiny. Samples tend to be smaller in a specialized area, while within a more general area there are generally greater numbers of participants. While large sample sizes may appear attractive, they tend to result in larger attrition rates in each round of the study, which can bias the final analysis (Reid, 1988).

To gain a meaningful consensus in an area, it is important to address the question to the correct audience. Participants in some Delphi studies should be those who are affected by the decision. In other Delphi studies it is vital that participants are experts in their area (Sweigert & Schabacker, 1974). Whatever the approach, the sampling method should be purposive or criterion based (Hasson et al., 2000). Purposive sampling assumes that the researcher's knowledge of the population can be used to choose the participants who will be approached to participate in the study (Polit & Hungler, 1997). However, such a sampling methodology is open to both researcher and participant bias (Hasson et al., 2000). An alternative method of purposive sampling is to employ a third party, who has knowledge of the population, but does not have a personal investment in the research.

Hasson et al. (2000) highlight the importance of carefully approaching and informing potential participants so that they are well prepared to consent and to maintain participation in the study. McKenna (1994) advocates that the initial contact should be face-to-face in order to increase response rates. However, this is obviously impractical if the sample is internationally dispersed and may raise ethical issues relating to consent. Whitman (1990) recommends that written information be given at initial contact and accompany the first round of the study, as an effective way to increase response rates. Reminder letters should be employed to attempt to increase response rates (Hasson et al., 2000).

Development, Analysis, and Presentation of Delphi Study Findings

The number of rounds of data collection during a Delphi study is not fixed. However, more than three rounds have been found to be ineffective in generating new information and greater consensus (Ludwig, 1997).

Construction and Distribution of Round One

Within a classical Delphi study, the first round consists of an open question aimed at generating ideas or statements for the participants to rank in subsequent rounds (Gibson, 1998). Some studies with large samples restrict the number of statements that can be generated in order to obtain a manageable amount of data (Schmidt, 1997). Other studies have adapted the standard Delphi process to include preexisting information for the purposes of ranking in round one (Duffield, 1993; Jerkins & Smith, 1994). However, this potentially introduces bias and limits participant options (Hassan & Barnett, 2002).

Responses are then collated and grouped together so that where several different terms are used to closely describe the same issue, the researcher groups them together in one universal description (Hassan & Barnett, 2002). Where terms are similar but with a different nuance, they are left separate. Hassan and Barnett (2002) emphasize the importance of verifying the process of groupings of statements to ensure that the data are fairly represented. Verifying is carried out by direct questioning of the participants about the research to ensure they have adequately understood what each term is communicating. Some researchers omit infrequently occurring items from future rounds of their Delphi studies (Green, Jones, Huges, & Williams, 1999; Whitman, 1990). However, such an approach may introduce bias to the results.

Construction and Distribution of Round Two

In the second round, the synthesized findings of the first round are presented to each participant in a manner that allows each item to be ranked. While ranking of items is a key component of the Delphi process, there is no standardized method of ranking (Love, 1997; Reid, 1988). Some typical approaches are to request that participants rank the findings according to a fixed Likert scale or to use categorical coding such as "Not important," "Slightly Important," "Important," and "Very Important."

Collation of Results and Round Three

The third round begins with providing the participants the collated results of the ratings given to statements in round two. The manner in which the results are presented will depend largely on the rating methods employed in round two.

Typically, within Delphi studies, only normative information (e.g., the mean ranking or average rating) is fed back to participants. However, it has been argued that providing each participant's rationale for giving each rating can enhance the responses and make the process more meaningful (Murphy et al., 1998b). Furthermore, providing purely normative data increases the tendency of participants to bow to group pressure (Kaplan & Miller, 1987).

Achievement of Group Consensus/Possible Further Rounds to Gain Consensus

There is little academic agreement regarding appropriate cutoff points for consensus in Delphi studies. Williams and Webb (1994) state that consensus can be defined only when there is 100% agreement among participants. Arguing that 100% agreement is often unrealistic, Love (1997) proposed 73% as the figure representing group consensus. Other studies have selected figures such as 51% (Loughlin & Moore, 1979), 70% (Sumison, 1998), and 80% (Green et al., 1999). Ultimately, the percentage chosen will depend on the sample size; one participant disagreeing in a sample size of 100 will result in a difference of 1%, while one participant disagreeing in a sample size of 15 will

result in a difference of more than 6%. Crisp, Pelletier, Duffield, Adams, and Nagy (1997) question the use of percentages and state that stability of ratings over time is a better indicator of consensus. However, such an approach diverges from the original methodology and has not been widely employed.

Anonymity

Reviews of the Delphi procedure highlight anonymity as one of its central positive features (Beech, 1999; Cantrill et al., 1996a; Jones & Hunter, 2000). Anonymity is not complete since the researcher must be aware of who has and has not responded in order to pursue nonrespondents and encourage their participation within the study. The term "quasi-anonymity" has been used to describe the situation within a Delphi study in which respondents will be known to the researcher and perhaps even to each other, but their individual responses and opinions will remain known to the researcher alone.

Nominal Group Technique

Nominal Group Technique (NGT) is an evaluative methodology that uses a structured group activity, designed to elicit the views of group members on

---

A Delphi Survey of Best Practice Occupational Therapy for Parkinson's Disease in the United Kingdom (Deane et al., 2003)

Deane et al. (2003) present a Delphi study that aimed to provide evidence for designing a best practice statement for occupational therapists working with people who have in the area Parkinson's disease. The study was also used to provide guidance for future randomized control trials of interventions for this population. Two hundred and forty-two individuals were invited to participate in the study and 69% ($n = 168$) responded.

As the Delphi study was a follow-up study of an earlier survey, the initial round of the research was formed from 30 practice statements and asked to rate these on a five-point scale. This procedure represents a modification of traditional Delphi studies that begin with the brainstorming of priorities prior to rating. However, a brainstorming of practice statements had recently been carried out by the authors and further statements were added on participants' suggestion.

The second round was sent out to 176 participants (as some had missed the deadline for first-

round data) and returned by 87% ($n = 153$) of participants. Before beginning the study, it was agreed that the criteria for consensus would be 80%. Consensus was reached on 82% ($n = 27$) of items (a total of 33 items were ranked in round two). The top 10 items in which participants strongly agreed that the specific expertise of occupational therapists should focus on improving on maintaining function were:

Eating and drinking (97%)
Domestic and kitchen skills (97%)
Washing and dressing (96%)
Home safety (93%)
Work activities (92%)
Leisure activities (90%)
Confidence (89%)
Cognitive skills (86%)
Transfers (85%)
Integration into society (78%)

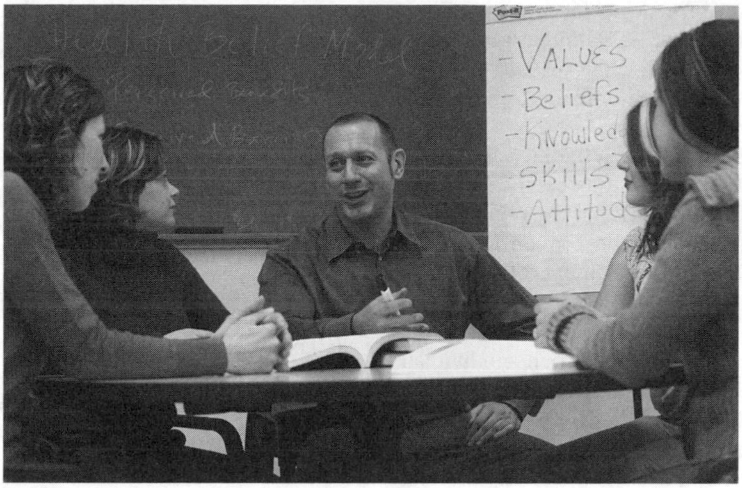

Figure 24.2 A researcher uses a nominal group technique with occupational therapy program graduates as part of a program evaluation.

a specific topic (Lloyd-Jones, Fowell, & Fligh, 1999).

Background

NGT was developed in the United States during the 1960s (Van de Ven & Delbacq, 1972). Initially it was applied to government services, education, and industry. Later, it became incorporated into the research repertoire of health care research, where the method was predominantly used for examining the appropriateness of clinical interventions, practice development, education, and priority setting (Cantrill et al., 1996; Pope & Mays, 2000).

Methodological Considerations

NGT has been compared with focus group methodology discussed in Chapter 20. However, in contrast to the open discussion used in focus groups, NGT tends to be strictly controlled and discussion is restricted to later stages of the data collection (Cantrill et al., 1996). Furthermore, NGT focuses on the study of a single topic rather than the range of ideas commonly associated with focus group methodology (Pope & Mays, 2000).

Several methodological issues must be considered when undertaking a nominal group study:

- Participant characteristics,
- Response rates, and
- Levels of validity and reliability (Cantrill et al., 1996; Pope & Mays, 2000).

Optimal size and composition of groups should be governed by the environment and purpose of the study (Cantrill et al., 1996). Hall (1983) recommends that the number of participants for each nominal group should range from six to nine, while Carney, McIntosh, and Worth (1996) suggest that groups with fewer than five participants may be mildly threatening. Ultimately, as Cantrill and colleagues (1996) state, "…the size of the eventual panel is determined by pragmatic considerations" (p. 69).

While Murphy and colleagues (1998b) argue that the personal characteristics of participants have little effect on the outcome, they suggest each nominal group panel should be interpreted in light of key characteristics such as the profession(s) represented (Cantrill et al., 1996; Murphy et al., 1998a). Hall (1983) suggests that heterogeneous groups, rather than homogeneous groups, generate a greater degree of high consensus outcomes. Regardless of the composition of the group, each participant should be selected on the basis of his or her expertise in the area (Pope & Mays, 2000). In health care studies, experienced clinicians are frequently viewed as experts (Cantrill et al., 1996) along with clients, who are viewed as experts of their own experience (Hares, Spencer, & Gallagher, 1992).

The level of response from participants partaking in a nominal group study will directly affect the reliability of the study's results. Not everyone who is invited to participate in a nominal group study will consent (Cantrill et al., 1996). One of the main disadvantages of NGT methodology is that participants must agree to come to a central meeting location, leading to a high level of nonresponse (Claxton, Ritchie, & Zaichkowsky, 1980). Lack of respondent interest is the most important factor influencing non-participation (Goyder, 1982; Heberlein & Baumgartner, 1978). Nominal groups can be biased, as they are likely to contain a disproportionate number of enthusiasts (Cantrill et al., 1996).

No specific assessment of reliability and validity of nominal group studies has been developed. Cantrill et al. (1996) suggest that the reliability of nominal group techniques can be considered by comparing the level of agreement of decisions between two or more groups. Twible (1992) has developed a twofold level of analysis of nominal group data, which reviews each group's individual ratings and combines the groups' responses in a form of summative analysis. The validity of a nominal group technique is also difficult to assess (Cantrill et al., 1996). Pope and Mays (2000) point out that agreement may reflect a consensus of ignorance, rather than wisdom. It is certainly important to appraise and report the validity and reliability of each NGT study.

Analysis and Presentation of Nominal Group Results

Frequently, studies that use nominal group methodologies use only one group for data collection (Crabb, Simpson, Hall, Beck, & Willard, 1981; Horton, 1980; Justice & Jang, 1990; Lloyd-Jones et al., 1999; McClusky, 2000; Sloan, 1999). Miller, Shewchuk, Eilliot, and Richards (2000) used two groups: Each group comprised differing experts (clinicians and patients) and was individually analyzed and then compared with the other. Two papers report data collection using several NGT groups and combining the results to form a summative analysis (Claxton et al., 1980; Twible, 1992).

Claxton et al. (1980) describe a four-stage process to analyzing the results of a series of nominal group interviews:

• Categorization of initial statements into themes,
• Calculation of a score or index reflecting the importance of each theme,
• Ranking of themes according to their index, and
• Regrouping of themes to form major dimensions.

Claxton et al. (1980) differentiate between statements, themes, and dimensions in the following manner:

> "...the purpose of identifying [themes] is to aggregate across NGT sessions statements that express essentially the same idea, a process conceptually similar to content

analysis. On the other hand, identification of dimensions is done for the purpose of providing a typology of themes i.e. grouping of themes that relate to a general problem area" (p. 311).

The process of indexing (or ranking) themes is carried out by aggregating the scores assigned to each statement. Therefore, themes that had been highlighted in the majority of sessions and rated highly receive a greater score than another theme that occurred less frequently and was rated lower (Claxton et al., 1980). The aggregation of statements to provide ranking of results is deemed as one of the advantages of the methodology (Claxton et al., 1980). This advantage is, however, tempered by the limitations of ordinal data.

Consensus Conferences

A consensus conference is a public hearing lasting 3 days. It is chaired with an audience. It involves active participation of 10 to 15 laypersons who are sometimes referred to as the jury or the panel and an equivalent number of experts, who may be from different disciplines and/or represent different viewpoints within a discipline. The purpose of a consensus conference is to develop an informed debate and report on a topic in which there is little developed knowledge. The debate is often developed using six to seven main questions to stimulate debate (Agersnap, 1992).

Background

Consensus conferences originated in the United States. They aim to provide a means by which members of specific professional groups and more broadly society become purposefully involved in influencing important decisions.

Methodological Considerations

The consensus conference engenders debate by means of a broadly based group of selected representatives. Experts present a variety of views on a subject and are open to questioning by the conference. Finally, the conference prepares a consensus statement on the issues raised and this statement is formally presented to the relevant bodies and organizations.

The conference is helped in its work by a moderator who ensures that the conference flows and functions efficiently. Background documentation is frequently sent to conference delegates regarding the focus of the conference so that delegates

Research Priorities in Forensic Occupational Therapy (Duncan et al., 2003)

Duncan et al. (2003) employed a Nominal Group Technique (NGT) as part of a an exercise for establishing research priorities for occupational therapists working with individuals who have mental illnesses or intellectual disabilities and are being cared for in secure (forensic) settings. In this case the NGT was selected as an appropriate consensus method. Since the data were gathered on a convenience sample of occupational therapists attending a national forensic occupational therapy conference, use of a method that could be completed in one session was advantageous.

All delegates ($n = 110$) were invited to attend the NGT session; however, only eight elected to participate in the session. Participants undertook a classic NGT process of idea generation, recording of ideas, discussion of ideas, and individual ranking of each individual's top six topics. The small number, coupled with the convenience sampling method, highlights the potential for participant bias in such a methodology. Despite this admitted weakness, the NGT study identified the following six clear research priorities for practice:

• Outcome measurement
• Evaluating interventions of effectiveness
• An examination of the efficacy of life-skills training
• The development of specific forensic risk assessments
• A multicentered study of AMPS
• Validation of current assessments in practice

These results correlated closely with those of a larger survey study that examined the same issue. Comparing the findings from these two studies with different methodologies provided important insights into research priorities in forensic occupational therapy.

come prepared for discussion. The experts should be given clear guidelines regarding their role in the proceedings. The technical and administrative requirements of such an event should not be underestimated as considerable input is required to synthesize the proceedings and produce a definitive consensus conference statement by its conclusion.

Methodological Considerations in Consensus Development Methodology

A wide variety of factors can influence the planning, development, and analysis of consensus studies. Several of these factors are discussed below.

Selection of Consensus Development Methodology

None of the three methods is innately superior to the others. Rather, the selection of an appropriate consensus method depends on a variety of factors such as participant availability, geographical dispersion, resources, and the overall aim of the consensus study.

Participant Selection

The main consideration in the selection of participants for consensus methods is their credibility as experts in the area (Fink, Kosecoff, Chassin, & Brook, 1984; Jones & Hunter, 2000; Lomas, 1991). Murphy et al. (1998b) highlight that the definition of an expert depends on the perspective being sought. For instance, clinicians are expert in the delivery of interventions; researchers bring scientific expertise; and clients have a unique expertise in experiencing the impact of interventions.

Group Composition: Heterogeneity vs. Homogeneity

When developing a consensus group, it is important to consider whether the characteristics of group participants should be similar (homogeneous) or mixed (heterogeneous). The following characteristics are typically considered:

• Age,
• Occupation,
• Cultural background,
• Abilities and expertise,
• Status, and
• Mix of initial opinions (Murphy et al., 1998b).

Neither heterogeneous nor homogeneous groups are considered superior. Rather, Cantrill et al. (1996) suggest that the "...composition of both Delphi and Nominal Group methodologies should be governed by the purpose of the investigation" (p. 69). Consensus conferences by definition include two distinct groups and, within each, consideration is given to issues of heterogeneity or homogeneity.

Social Environment

Time pressure and mood are two social environmental factors that have been highlighted as affecting the outcome of group decision-making. Karau and Kelly (1992) found that when time pressure was high, members' initial preferences had a greater influence than the overall group response. With moderate time pressure the groups became more focused and the quality of the output increased. Isen and Means (1983) demonstrated that participants who are more positive in mood engaged less thoroughly in a group process than participants who were neutral in mood.

> When rigorously applied, consensus methods offer the potential to develop an expert panel evidence base on which to develop best practice guidelines and provide the foundation for future research.

Characteristics of Group Facilitator

Wortman, Vinokur, and Sechrest (1988) found that a facilitative chairperson was crucial to a successful consensus conference. Clawson, Bostrom, and Anson (1993) suggest that the role of a group facilitator includes:

- Providing structure,
- Maintaining the agenda,
- Managing conflict, and
- Creating a positive environment.

Murphy et al. (1998b) state that the group facilitator will likely play a key role in each consensus method.

Limitations of Consensus Methodology

Consensus approaches contribute to the development of knowledge in health research, particularly in under-researched areas or where the geographical spread of experts restricts other methods of data collection (Harbour & Miller, 2001; Murphy et al., 1998b). Cantrill et al. (1996) suggest that "...when properly used, [consensus] techniques are powerful tools for increasing a group's capacity to generate critical ideas, understand problems and improve

the quality of group decisions" (p. 67). Cantrill et al. (1996) argue that consensus approaches are particularly suitable when individual judgments must be elicited and combined in order to form a rigorous understanding that cannot be made by a single person or random grouping of people.

Nonetheless, authors caution against over-reliance on the findings of consensus approaches and question the nature of consensus (Lomax & McLeman, 1984; Pope & Mays, 2000). Consensus approaches reflect issues on which the majority of the groups agree. However, agreement is affected by the particular methodology being applied which can skew the picture of the group response, concealing strong minority disagreement (Carney et al., 1996). Despite these drawbacks, consensus approaches have several advantages (Lomax & McLeman, 1984):

- They limit the influence and potential bias of the researcher,
- They avoid pressure on group participants to conform to other members' opinions,
- They incorporate the advantages of both qualitative and quantitative techniques, and
- They are economic and efficient methods for gathering data.

Summary

Consensus approaches to research are increasingly being used in health care research. They provide important methods for systematically structuring expert opinion in areas where the existing evidence base is sparse. However, these methodologies have been criticized (Sackman, 1975) and even proponents of the approach have recognized its limitations (Carney et al., 1996; Lloyd-Jones et al., 1999; Lomax & McLeman, 1984; Twible, 1992).

Pope and Mays (2000) have recommended that when carrying out studies using consensus methodology, the following criteria be used to examine the validity and relevance of the research:

- The emphasis should be on a clear justification for using such methods,
- The use of sound methodology, including the

selection of experts and a precise definition of target levels of consensus, should be described in detail,

• The findings should be presented in an appropriate and accessible manner, and

• The relevance of the findings to the topic area should be clearly articulated.

When rigorously applied, consensus methods offer the potential to develop an expert panel evidence base on which to develop best practice guidelines and provide the foundation for future research.

REFERENCES

Agersnap, T. (1992). Consensus Conferences for Technology Assessment. In: *Technology and democracy. The use and impact of technology assessment in Europe*. Proceedings of the 3rd European Congress on Technology Assessment, Copenhagen, November 4–7, 1992.

Beech, B. (1999). Go the extra mile-use the Delphi Technique. *Journal of Nurse Management, 7*(5), 281–288.

Cantrill, J. A., Sibbald, B., & Buetow, S. (1996). The Delphi and nominal group techniques in health services research. *International Journal of Pharmacy Practice, 4*(2), 67–74.

Carney, O., McIntosh, J., & Worth, A. (1996). The use of the Nominal Group Technique in research with community nurses. *Journal of Advanced Nursing, 23*(5), 1024–1029.

Claxton, J. D., Ritchie, J. R., & Zaichkowsky, J. (1980). The Nominal Group Technique: Its potential for consumer research. *Journal of Consumer Research, 7*(3), 308–313.

Clawson, V. Q., Bostrom, R. P., & Anson, R. (1993). The role of the facilitator in computer supported meetings. *Small Group Research, 24*, 547–565.

Crabb, L., Simpson, R., Hall, D., Beck, J. & Willard, D. (1981). Effective decision-making method for dentists: The nominal group technique. *General Dentistry, 29*(2), 129–132.

Crisp, J., Pelletier, D., Duffield, C., Adams, A., & Nagy, S. (1997). The Delphi method? *Nursing Research, 46*(2), 116–118.

Deane, K. H. O., Ellis-Hill, C., Dekker, K., Davies, P., & Clarke, C. E. (2003). A Delphi survey of best practice occupational therapy for Parkinson's disease in the United Kingdom. *British Journal of Occupational Therapy, 66*(6), 247–254.

Duffield, C. (1993). The Delphi technique: A comparison of results obtained using two expert panels. *International Journal of Nursing Studies, 30*(3), 227–237.

Duncan, E. A. S., & Nicol, M. M. (2004). Subtle realism and occupational therapy: An alternative approach to knowledge generation and evaluation. *The British Journal of Occupational Therapy, 67*(10), 453–456.

Fink, A., Kosecoff, J., Chassin, M., & Brook, R. H. (1984). Consensus methods: Characteristics and guidelines for use. *American Journal of Public Health, 74*, 979–983.

Gibson, J. M. (1998). Using the Delphi technique to identify the content and context of nurses' continuing professional development needs. *Journal of Clinical Nursing, 7*(5), 451–459.

Goyder, J. C. (1982). Further evidence on factors affecting response rates to mailed questionnaires. *American Sociology Review, 47*, 550–553.

Green, B., Jones, M., Hughes, D., & Williams, A. (1999). Applying the Delphi technique in a study of GPs' information requirements. *Health and Social Care in the Community, 7*(3), 198–205.

Hall, R. S. (1983). The Nominal Group Technique for planning and problem solving. *Journal of Biocommunication, 10*(2), 24–27.

Hammersley, M. (1992). *What's wrong with ethnography?* London: Routledge.

Harbour, R., & Miller, J. (2001). A new system for grading recommendations in evidence based guidelines. *British Medical Journal, 323*, 334–336.

Hares, T., Spencer, J., & Gallagher, M. (1992). Diabetes care: Who are the experts? *Quality in Health Care, 1*, 219–224.

Hassan, T. B., & Barnett, D. B. (2002). Delphi type methodology to develop consensus on the future design of EMS systems in the United Kingdom. *Emergency Medicine Journal, 19*(2), 155–159.

Hasson, F., Keeney, S., & McKenna, H. (2000). Research guidelines for the Delphi survey technique. *Journal of Advanced Nursing, 32*(4), 1008–1015.

Heberlein, T. A., & Baumgartner, R. (1978). Factors affecting response rates to mailed questionnaires: A quantitative analysis of the published literature. *American Sociology Review, 43*, 447–462.

Horton, J. N. (1980). Nominal group technique. A method of decision-making by committee. *Anaesthesia, 35*(8), 811–814.

Isen, A. M., & Means, B. (1983). The influence of positive affect on decision making strategy. *Social Cognition, 2*, 18–31.

Jerkins, D., & Smith, T., (1994). Applying Delphi methodology in family therapy research. *Contemporary Family Therapy, 15*, 411–430.

Jones, J., & Hunter, D. (2000). Using the Delphi and Nominal Group Technique in health services research. In C. Pope & N. Mays (Eds.), *Qualitative research in healthcare* (2nd ed.). London: BMJ Publishing Group.

Justice, J., & Jang, R. (1990). Tapping employee insights with the Nominal Group Technique. *American Pharmacy, 30*(10), 43–45.

Kaplan, M. F., & Miller, C. E. (1987). Group decision making and normative vs. informational influence: Effects of type of issue and assigned decision rule. *Journal of Personal and Social Psychology, 28*, 542–571.

Karau, S. J., & Kelly, J. R. (1992). The effects of time scarcity and time abundance on group performance quality and interaction process. *Journal of Experimental and Social Psychology, 28*, 542–571.

Kirk, J., & Miller, M. (1986). *Reliability and validity in qualitative research*. Beverly Hills, CA: SAGE Publications.

Lloyd-Jones, G., Fowell, S., & Bligh, J. G. (1999). The use of the nominal group technique as an evaluative tool in medical undergraduate education. *Medical Education, 33*(1), 8–13.

Lomas, J. (1991). Words without action? The production, dissemination, and impact of consensus recommendations. *Annual Review of Public Health, 12*, 41–65.

Lomax, P., & McLeman, P. (1984). The uses and abuses of Nominal Group Technique in polytechnic course evaluation. *Studies in Higher Education, 9*(2), 183–190.

Loughlin, K. G., & Moore, L. F. (1979). Using Delphi to achieve congruent objectives and activities in a pediatrics department. *Journal of Medical Education, 54*(2), 101–106.

Love, C. (1997). A Delphi study examining standards for patient handling. *Nursing Standard, 11*(45), 34–38.

Ludwig, B. (1997). Predicting the future: Have you considered the Delphi methodology? *Journal of Extension, 35.* Retrieved March 18, 2002, from http://www.joe.org/joe/1997october/tt2.html

McClusky, A. (2000). Collaborative Curriculum development: Clinicians views on the neurology content of a new occupational therapy course. *Australian Occupational Therapy Journal, 47*(1), 1–10.

McKenna, H. P. (1994). The Delphi technique: A worthwhile research approach for nursing? *Journal of Advanced Nursing, 19*(6), 1221–1225.

Miller, D., Shewchuk, R., Elliot, T. R. & Richards, S. (2000). Nominal group technique: A process for identifying diabetes self-care issues among patients and caregivers. *Diabetes Educator, 26*(2), 305–310.

Murphy, E., Dingwall, R., Greatbatch, D., Parker, S., & Watson, P. (1998a). Qualitative research methods in health technology assessment: A review of the literature. *Health Technology Assessment, 2*(16), vii–260.

Murphy, M. K., Black, N. A., Lamping, D. L., McKee, C. M., Sanderson, C. F. B. J., & Marteau, T. (1998b). Consensus development methods and their use in clinical guideline development. *Health Technology Assessment, 2*(3).

Polit, D. F., & Hungler, B. P. (1997). *Essentials of nursing research: Methods, appraisal and utilization.* New York: Lippincott, Williams & Wilkins.

Pope, C., & Mays, N. (2000). *Qualitative research in health care* (2nd ed.). London: British Medical Journal Publishing Group.

Reid, N. (1988). The Delphi technique: Its contribution to the evaluation of professional practice. In R. Ellis (Ed.), *Professional competence and quality assurance in the caring professions* (pp. 230–262). London: Chapman & Hall.

Sackman, H. (1975). *Delphi critique.* Boston, MA: Lexington Books.

Salmond, S. W. (1994). Orthopaedic nursing research priorities: A Delphi study. *Orthopaedic. Nurse, 13*(2), 31–45.

Schmidt, R. C. (1997). Managing Delphi surveys using non-parametric statistical techniques. *Decision Sciences, 28,* 763–774.

Sloan, G. (1999). Good characteristics of a clinical supervisor: A community mental health nurse perspective. *Journal of Advanced Nursing, 30*(3), 713–722.

Strauss, A. L., & Ziegler, L. H. (1975). The Delphi technique and its uses in social science research. *The Journal of Creative Behaviour, 9*(4), 253–259.

Sumsion, T. (1998). The Delphi technique: An adaptive research tool. *The British Journal of Occupational Therapy, 61*(4), 153–156.

Sweigert, R. L., & Schabacker, W. H. (1974). The Delphi technique: How well does it work in setting educational goals? Paper presented at the Annual Meeting of the American Educational Research Association. Chicago. (ERIC Document Reproduction Service No. ED 091 415)

Twible, R. L. (1992). Consumer participation in planning health promotion programmes: A case study using the nominal group technique. *Australian Occupational Therapy Journal, 39*(2), 13–18.

Van de Ven, A. H., & Delbacq, A. L. (1972). The nominal group as a research instrument for exploratory health studies. *American Journal of Public Health, 62,* 337–342.

Whitman, N. I. (1990). The Delphi technique as an alternative for committee meetings. *Journal of Nursing Education, 29*(8), 377–379.

Williams, P. L., & Webb, C. (1994). The Delphi technique: A methodological discussion. *Journal of Advanced Nursing, 19*(1), 180–186.

Wortman, P. M., Vinokur, A., & Sechrest, L. (1988). Do consensus conferences work? A process of evaluation of the NIH consensus development programme. *Journal of Health Politics Policy and Law, 13,* 469–498.

RESOURCES

The following resources are useful for people interested in conducting a consensus study:

General

Murphy, M. K., Black, N. A., Lamping, D. L., McKee, C. M., Sanderson, C. F. B. J., & Marteau, T. (1998). Consensus development methods and their use in clinical guideline development. *Health Technology Assessment, 2*(3).

Nominal Group Information

Claxton, J. D., Ritchie, J. R., & Zaichkowsky, J. (1980). The Nominal Group Technique: Its potential for consumer research. *Journal of Consumer Research, 7*(3), 308–313.

Dunham, R. B. (1998). Nominal Group Technique: A users guide. HYPERLINK "http://instruction.bus.wisc.edu/obdemo/readings/ngt.html" (28 April 2005).

Delphi Study Information

Greatorex, J., & Dexter, T. (2000). An accessible analytical approach for investigating what happens between rounds of a Delphi study. *Journal of Advanced Nursing, 32*(4), 1016–1024.

Hasson, F., Keeney, S., & McKenna, H. (2000). Research guidelines for the Delphi survey technique. *Journal of Advanced Nursing, 32*(4), 1008–1015.

Consensus Study Information

Anderson, I., & Jæger, B. (1999). Scenario Workshops and consensus conferences: Towards more democratic decision making. *Science and Public Policy, 26*(5), 331–340.

Slocum H (2005) Participatory Methods Toolkit: A practitioner's manual. Method: Consensus Conference. King Baudouin Foundation & Flemish Institute for Science and Technology Assessment. Belgium. Retrieved on November 29, 2005 from http://www.kbs-rb.be/files/db/EN/PUB_1540_Toolkit_4_ConsensusConference.pdf

CHAPTER 25

Using Mixed Methods Designs to Study Therapy and Its Outcomes

Mary A. Corcoran

Historically, only two major research traditions have been widely recognized in the global scientific community. These traditions are known by a number of terms, including post-positivist, experimental, and quantitative as opposed to constructionist, naturalistic, and qualitative. The quantitative–qualitative dichotomy may be most familiar since these terms differentiate the types of data primarily collected within each tradition. Chapter 3 discusses these two traditions and points out their differing epistemological modes (i.e., different underlying assumptions, focus, design, and methods of data gathering and analysis).

For years, scientists have informally combined designs or methods within or from both traditions. Usually, they did so by conducting a sidebar or secondary study within a larger one. These combinations are most often intended to generate in-depth information about the experiences or opinions of a group of people who have participated in an experimental study.

However, mixed methods as a legitimate design approach began to gain wide attention in the 1980s after Denzin (1978) introduced the concept of triangulation. Triangulation refers to the practice of gathering data from a number of different sources for the purposes of detaching the method of measurement from the phenomena being measured. For example, if a social behavior emerges in an interview *and* is observed in action, this finding may be regarded as particularly salient because two different data sources independently confirm it. The concept of triangulation fits well with a new paradigm of pragmatism that was emerging and taking root at the same time (Howe, 1988).

Pragmatism holds that qualitative and quantitative traditions are compatible and can be successfully combined in the same design. However, the mixed methods studies that followed were a hodgepodge of typologies, definitions, and proce-

dures. Prominent methodologists have called for conceptualizing mixed methods as a third tradition separate but equal to qualitative and quantitative traditions. They further support its development as a set of rigorous research tools for addressing complex questions.

The term *mixed methods* refers to a research design that integrates elements of both qualitative and quantitative methods so that the strengths of each are emphasized.[1] However, Tashakkori and Teddlie (2003) posit that mixed methods are more that just combinations of qualitative and quantitative procedures. Because qualitative and quantitative procedures stem from two separate (and in many ways, opposing) epistemologies, they must be combined as interdependent but separate procedures during data collection. This is usually accomplished by establishing one of the traditions (either qualitative or quantitative) as the core method. The underlying assumptions of the core method are prioritized and reflected in the study purpose, methodological decisions, and overall analytic approach. In implementing the portion of the study that is based on a secondary method, the investigator must guard against violating any of the assumptions of the core method while still maintaining the integrity of the secondary method. This requires careful planning and solid understanding of both traditions represented. During data analysis, the core method continues to dictate the overall approach, although data from the secondary method may be transformed and integrated with data from the core method.

This relatively new approach to scientific inquiry is growing in popularity owing to the flex-

> Prominent methodologists have called for conceptualizing mixed methods as a third tradition separate but equal to qualitative and quantitative traditions.

[1] Mixed methods should be distinguished from mixed designs, which are consistent with a quantitative tradition and involves "factorial designs in which the number of levels of the factors are not the same for all factors" (Vogt, 1993, p 140).

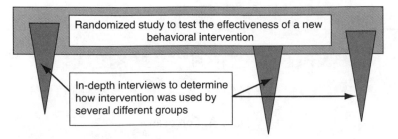

Figure 25.1 Illustration of a mixed methods design.

ibility it affords investigators. For example, a mixed methodologist has the ability to combine strict controls necessary for generalization with in-depth examinations of the study participants' experiences or perceptions on a particular topic. Figure 25.1 illustrates this combination of controlled quantitative design with a qualitative naturalistic design, graphically using a typical mixed method approach. In this figure, traditional quantitative methods, such as experimental and quasi-experimental designs, can be conceptualized as the wide, shallow box. This box in Figure 25.1 represents the broad scope of experimental studies regarding a very narrow topic. The narrow but deep triangle represents the in-depth but highly focused approach of qualitative studies. In Figure 25.1, a primarily quantitative study to test the effectiveness of a new behavioral intervention also contains in-depth interviews that allow the investigator to understand more about the experiences of those individuals who participated in this efficacy study. The investigator may want to hear from several types of participants, including those who were able to incorporate behavioral changes in their lives, those who had difficulty doing so, and those who were unable to make changes called for in the intervention. While investigators using such an approach can answer the question, "*What is the effect of the intervention on X?*", they can also gather information about how easy or difficult it was for participants to actually use the behavioral strategies from the intervention. This information can then be used to guide analysis, interpret study findings, and refine the intervention in future trials.

There are many ways to merge quantitative and qualitative procedures in new and unique ways. As research questions become more complex, mixed methods may emerge as a principal tradition in social science in years to come (Tashakkori & Teddlie, 2003). Mixed methods are particularly relevant for occupational therapy, a profession with firm foundations in a number of disciplines and that faces the challenge of blending many bodies of knowledge in the dynamic concept of occupation. Therefore, the purpose of this chapter is to introduce current thinking about mixed methods as a third methodological tradition with unique nomenclature, principles, designs, and procedures, and to apply that tradition to occupational therapy. The timing is perfect because Tashakkori and Teddlie (2003) have recently published the first *Handbook of Mixed Methods*, upon which this chapter draws heavily.

Mixed Methods Nomenclature and Typologies

The overarching typology of research designs that includes mixed methods is known as multiple methods designs (Tashakkori & Teddlie, 2003). Multiple methods designs refer to use of two or more data collection strategies or methods for a given research question. Multiple methods designs can be further divided into two subcategories, multimethod designs and mixed methods designs, which are defined below (Tashakkori & Teddlie, 2003).

Multimethod Designs

Multimethod designs incorporate two or more data collection techniques within only *one* tradition (qualitative or quantitative) (Taskakkori & Teddlie, 2003). For example, a study question regarding the effectiveness of an occupational therapy intervention may be best answered through a quantitative tradition, such as a randomized two-group design. However, an investigator using a multimethod approach may decide to triangulate his data with two different surveys to measure the dependent variable, independence in self-care. As shown in Figure 25.2, the dependent variable is measured by a self-report survey from the study participant and a proxy report from a caregiver.

Tashakkori and Teddlie (2003) make the observation that quantitative research designs have enjoyed a long tradition of commonly understood and well-defined terms. This has provided the quantitative tradition with a common language as a basis for developing and describing methodologies. The qualitative research tradition has been working toward a common lexicon only for the past two decades but during that time has made great strides in identifying and defining key concepts.

Mixed methods, as a tradition in its "adolescence" (Tashakkori and Teddlie, 2003), has only begun to consider whether a common language is needed, and if so, what system of terms and definitions should be adopted. Tashakkori and Teddlie (2003) provide a Glossary of terms in their *Handbook of Mixed Methods* that has been defined through consensus of several leading authors in the field and does not have alternative definitions. The serious student of mixed methods should be familiar with this new language.

Multimethod designs are powerful approaches to complex and nuanced research questions and an important strategy in the qualitative tradition for ensuring trustworthiness. However, because multimethod designs do not combine more than one research tradition, as do mixed methods designs, competing philosophies and underlying assumptions are not an issue. Therefore, the remainder of this chapter is devoted to discussing the unique methodological associated with mixed methods designs.

Mixed Methods Designs

In mixed methods designs, qualitative and quantitative traditions are used simultaneously or consecutively in the methods section (Tashakkori & Teddlie, 2003). Extending the above example, the investigator may suspect that an underlying cultural issue is mediating the effect of the intervention being tested. This investigator hypothesizes that the participants' culturally based definition of disability shapes the level at which they will enact the intervention procedures being studied.

A mixed methods design could be used in this case. To implement such a design, the investigator might conduct an ethnography subsequent to the field experiment to develop a better understanding of the relationship between definition of disability and self-care actions. By comparing Figures 25.1 and 25.2, one can see that the former is an illustration of a mixed methods design (using methods from both the qualitative and quantitative traditions), while the latter illustrates a multimethod design (using more than one method to collect data within a single quantitative design).

Other authors have recommended more complex typologies. For instance, Newman, Ridenour, Newman, and DeMarco (2003) suggest that the typology be organized by research purpose rather than design type. Interested readers are encouraged to consult other texts for additional ways of systematically classifying mixed methods designs, including Newman and Benz (1998), Tashakkori and Teddlie (1998, 2003), Creswell (2003), and Greene & Caracelli (1997).

Principles of Mixed Methods Designs

Morse (2003) warns strongly against using the "muddling method" of combining models (p. 189), which involves simply tossing together methods and models without adequate consideration for issues of validity. For example, the investigator who combines ethnography with a field experiment must avoid changing the intervention midstream to reflect what he has learned from the participants, and runs the risk of being unable to

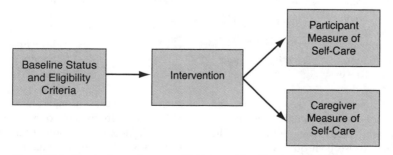

Figure 25.2 Illustration of a quantitative multimethod design.

maintain an unbiased and objective status. Neither of these actions would be a problem in a qualitative tradition, but would introduce threats to validity in the quantitative portion of the study.

As with all traditions of research, decisions must be made based on the conceptual framework, purpose, and research question(s) of the study. This may be even more important when combining qualitative and quantitative traditions, which have diametrically opposed philosophies on several fundamental points, including the shape of the research process (linear versus spiral), role of the investigator (objective versus subjective), and type of logic used (deductive versus inductive). If not carefully planned, an investigator may find that a number of threats to validity have been introduced in the process of mixing methods and models.

Principles of Mixed Methods Designs

Four principles are offered by Morse (2003) for a mixed methods design, and are discussed below.

Recognize the Theoretical Drive of the Project

Research projects fall broadly into two types of purpose: discovery or testing (i.e., inductive or deductive). Morse uses the term *theoretical drive* of a project to refer to whether the main reasoning process required for the purpose is inductive or deductive (1991). The investigator must remain clear as to the type of inquiry and reasoning process driving the project and how each component fits the whole.

In a mixed methods study, both the quantitative and qualitative components are introduced. However, there can be only one theoretical drive, either inductive or deductive. The following example is used to illustrate these decisions in action. An investigator is interested in describing the ways people with traumatic brain injury (TBI) handle information about their diagnosis and medical history on the job. Do they disclose their head injury, and if so, to whom and how? If they do not disclose, what barriers to they perceive as keeping them from doing so? The investigator plans to use both questionnaires and qualitative interviews drawing on both quantitative

> If not carefully planned, an investigator may find that a number of threats to validity have been introduced in the process of mixing methods and models.

and qualitative traditions. This is obviously a project with a *discovery* basis, so an inductive drive is appropriate.

Adhere to the Methodological Assumptions of the Core Method

Respecting the integrity of methods (i.e., do not violate the assumptions, philosophical foundations, and procedures of the core method) seems like a simple message when introducing other secondary methods. In actual practice, respecting methodological integrity requires continually linking the unique philosophical foundations with the research question(s) and maintaining one method as dominant over the other. When decisions are made throughout the project, methodological integrity is always among the first considerations, but an investigator using a mixed methods design cannot stop there. The investigator must begin with consideration for the integrity of the core method and then consider the implications of each decision for the integrity of the secondary method(s). Morse (2003) suggests keeping the core and secondary methods clear by using capital letters when referring to the core method (such as QUAL + quan to denote a study that is primarily qualitative with a secondary quantitative component).

For example, an investigator is interested in knowing how a school-based intervention affects both self-confidence and legibility of handwriting. The investigator decides to test intervention effects on the dependent variables in two ways, directly through a measure of self-confidence and handwriting samples of the participants, and indirectly through a proxy open-ended interview with the teachers on these variables (self-confidence and legibility). The type of mixed design would therefore be written so as to designate that the study is quantitative with a deductive theoretical drive plus an additional qualitative method (proxy open-ended interview) used simultaneously (i.e., QUAN + qual). If the secondary qualitative investigation were to be conducted sequentially the design would be written as: QUAN → qual, such as in the case of interviewing only those individuals who dropped out of an experimental study. For an in-depth discussion of this principle and its use in several multiple method studies, see Morse (2003).

Now, the investigator remains clear as to the order of each of the methods (quantitative and qualitative) and can make decisions that maintain the integrity of the core method. For example, the investigator using teachers' interviews to supplement direct observation and handwriting samples should gather the qualitative information at the same time data are collected from the children. Even though it would be logistically easier to get all the teachers together once in a focus group for the purposes of collecting information on all the study participants, to do so would introduce a problem of comparing two different timeframes for measuring the dependent variables.

Recognize the Role of the Imported Models to the Project

The core model of the project will determine the reasoning process of the entire project, but the secondary model must be understood to either supplement or inform the core model (Morse, 2003).

Using the earlier examples of a study of disclosure in the workplace among individuals with TBI, suppose the investigator notices midway through the investigation that individuals who appear to have an obvious residual physical impairment appear less reluctant to disclose. The investigator thus decided to pursue the heuristic that persons with less obvious impairment are more inclined to "pass" as nondisabled. However, this requires some kind of quantification of the extent to which a visible physical impairment is present. The investigator chooses a simple ordinal rating of:

• No obvious physical impairment,
• Marginally obvious physical impairment, and
• Obvious physical impairment.

The purpose of this secondary method is to further explore what is being discovered about individuals' perceptions regarding disclosure on the job. The project would be designated as QUAL → quan with an inductive drive and a subsequent collection of quantitative data.

Work with as Few Datasets as Possible

This principle refers to converting the datasets to forms that are consistent with the core method, when feasible. Converting datasets may not always make the most sense methodologically, especially in sequential designs (secondary methods implemented subsequent to the core method) described below. However, in concurrent designs (core and secondary methods implemented simultaneously) converting datasets can be a powerful way to approach analysis. That said, analysis of converted datasets must be approached carefully, however, to avoid violating the integrity of the core method. First, information about how to convert datasets will be presented, followed by an example of the decision making process involved when conducting the actual analysis.

Converting Datasets. In a primarily inductive study, quantitative data from the secondary method should be "qualitized"—collected quantitative data types converted to narratives that can be analyzed qualitatively (Tashakkori & Teddlie, 2003, p. 9). This is the approach used in the example above when ordinal data were treated as a "code" for sorting and examining information about disclosure attitudes. In the qualitized dataset, entire participant interviews are coded in terms of a quality (extent to which the physical impairment is obvious), which allows an investigator to sort all interview data according to whether the individual had obvious physical impairments or not. Conversely, in a primarily deductive study, qualitative data from the secondary method can be "quantitized"—that is, qualitative data types are converted into categorical or ordinal numerical codes that can be statistically analyzed (Tashakkori & Teddlie, 2003, p. 9). An example can be taken from the handwriting study mentioned earlier in which the investigator can code the teachers' open-ended interviews in terms of high or low self-confidence. A numerical code is assigned to the teachers' reports (1 = teacher reports child has high self-confidence; 2 = teacher reports child has low self-confidence) and the data are entered into a statistical software program for analysis. Converting data not only serves to reduce the number of datasets that must be handled, but also integrates the datasets.

Maintaining Methodological Integrity When Working With Converted Datasets. In a mixed methods study, an investigator must adhere to the methodological assumptions of the core method when deciding how to approach analysis. The implications of these decisions can be subtle, as illustrated in the TBI study mentioned previously. In that study, the investigator has ordinal data for a subset of participants (remember, he realized midway through the study that some participants may disclose based on how obvious their physical impairments were), which he has qualitized. As a result, for this subset of the sample, the investigator can sort narrative information according to how obvious the physical impairments are and analyze the data to describe how visibility of physical impairment interacts with the decision to disclose and other factors that influence thoughts about disclosure.

On the other hand, the investigator could decide to keep the ordinal data on the degree of residual physical impairment as numeric and quantitize the information on whether or not the person discloses (a dichotomous quantitative variable represented by 0 = does not disclose and 1 = discloses) in order to conduct a chi-square analysis. However, to do so could easily violate assumptions of the inductive theoretical drive by handling data analysis as though the purpose was deductive (i.e., testing the hypothesis of whether variable x is related to variable y). An inductive approach seeks to understand more about how differing levels of physical impairment interact with other factors to affect the way persons talk about disclosing, not to test a hypothesis about a specific relationship. Further, it is doubtful that number of informants in a qualitative study would be large enough to adequately power a statistical test of the differences, so assumptions of even the supplemental component are violated.

Design Types in Mixed Method Designs

Creswell, Clark, Gutmann, and Hanson (2003) identify six major designs in mixed methods research. These six designs can be organized into two larger categories:

• Sequential designs, and
• Concurrent designs.

Designs categorized as sequential introduce a secondary method subsequent to the core method. Designs in the concurrent category include secondary methods that are used simultaneously with the core method (Creswell et al., 2003). Each is described in more detail below and summarized in Table 25.1.

Sequential Explanatory Design

In a sequential explanatory design, an investigator first collects and analyzes core quantitative data used to explain or predict phenomena. This is followed by collection and analysis of in-depth information through the use of a qualitative tradition. The two approaches are analyzed separately. An example is a survey design to describe leisure performance patterns of adults who have survived a stroke that finds community access to be an identified issue, followed by in-depth interviewing of these individuals to fully describe their experiences.

Sequential Exploratory Design

A sequential exploratory design is identical to the one above (sequential explanatory design) except the sequence is reversed. The investigator first collects in-depth and nuanced information about a phenomenon using a qualitative tradition followed by collection and analysis of quantitative data. Again, the two models are analyzed and interpreted separately. An example of a study using this type of design is a qualitative project to determine the meaning of caregiving for spouses of individuals with dementia, followed by development and testing of a survey based on the results of the qualitative core. The qualitative component informs the interpretation of the psychometric findings of the survey, including the solution that best fits the factor analysis.

Sequential Transformative Design

As with the two sequential designs described in the preceding text, there are two separate and subsequent phases of data collection and analysis (Creswell et al., 2003). However, in this instance, rather than the first model being the core model, either model, qualitative or quantitative, can be used as the core model. Moreover, the purpose of a sequential transformative design is to use a clearly identified theoretical perspective to direct the research question toward change in policy, action, or ideology (Creswell et al., 2003). An example of a transformative design is an evaluation component of a service program with the main purpose being feedback for improvement in the service.

Concurrent Triangulation Design

Creswell et al. (2003) proposes that a concurrent triangulation design is the most familiar of all six types; it is often the design that comes to mind when the term "mixed methods" is raised. As in all concurrent designs, both qualitative and quantitative data are gathered simultaneously, and results are validated by virtue of having been confirmed through multiple data collection techniques. Neither tradition is designated as core or secondary, which frees the investigator to pursue interesting developments as they occur. The disadvantage is the need to make decisions that maintain the methodological integrity of both traditions simultaneously. Data from all sources are integrated in the analysis phase of the study, when feasible. An example of a concurrent triangulation design is a study that compared a self-report of caregiving strategies with an observation of caregiving in

Table 25.1 **Summary of Mixed Methods Designs**

Name	Notation	Description
Sequential explanatory design	QUAN → qual	Explanation or prediction followed by in-depth description
Sequential exploratory design	QUAL → quan	In-depth description followed by explanation or prediction
Sequential transformative design	QUAN → qual or QUAL → quan	First-phase core method used to direct second-phase change in policy or action
Concurrent triangulation design	Qual + quan or Quan + qual	Neither tradition is designated as "core" or "secondary." Data from each are collected simultaneously.
Concurrent nested design	QUAL + quan or QUAN + qual	Either tradition is designated as core. Data from each are collected simultaneously.
Concurrent transformative design	Either of the concurrent notations above	Data collected through use of both traditions simultaneously. May or may not have a designated core method. Purpose is to direct a change in policy or action.

action (Corcoran, 2004a). In this study, caregivers rated themselves on the Task Management Strategy Index (TMSI) (Gitlin et al., 2002) which recorded the caregivers' report of frequency with which specific strategies are used, such as "placing all items where they can be seen." Caregivers were then videotaped conducting a daily care task in which strategies on the TMSI may have been used. During a replay of the videotape, caregivers talked about their use of strategies in comparison to those reported on the TMSI, and these interviews were recorded and transcribed. During data analysis, the TMSI data were qualitized and interviews were coded according to the frequency of caregiver use of strategies (above or below median for the sample). The investigator then was able to sort according to frequency of strategy use and examine both the videotapes and interview data for these two groups. In addition, the sample size was large enough that the investigator could also conduct a chi-square test to examine the relationship between use of strategies and overall approach to care (quantitized data that emerged from the interviews and videotapes). This provided an opportunity to examine the data from multiple perspectives and to triangulate use of caregiving strategies from three sources, one quantitative (TMSI) and two qualitative (videotape and follow-up interview). This triangulation procedure served to strengthen the trustworthiness of the study by corroborating data from several sources (Creswell, 1998).

Concurrent Nested Design

A concurrent nested design differs from a triangulation design only in terms of the predominance of one tradition over another. In a concurrent nested design, the primary tradition determines how data from the secondary tradition will be handled.

Creswell et al. (2003) propose that a nested design can serve many purposes. Two different traditions may be used to answer two different but related questions. Other studies may wish to measure aspects of the same phenomena at different levels. For instance, managerial focus groups may be used for in-depth understanding of personnel practices, but a survey is a better choice to describe workers' agreement with these practices. One very common use of concurrent nested designs is seen in quantitative studies that illustrate a particularly salient finding with a case study.

One example of concurrent nested design is particularly important for occupational therapy. Like many professions, occupational therapy is challenged to validate practice with efficacy studies and has been making good progress in doing so. However, too little attention is paid to measuring the level at which the tested intervention is actually delivered to study subjects as designed. Several authors have promoted the use of treatment implementation, or treatment fidelity measures (Burgio et al., 2001; Lichstein, Riedel, & Grieve, 1994). Concurrent nested designs are very useful for devising strategies that collect valid treatment implementation data for the purposes of tracking the actual delivery, receipt, and enactment of an intervention as it was originally planned. Many issues can develop in an intervention study that threaten to change the treatment actually being tested. Problems with poorly defined protocols and lack of continual monitoring can result in a different form of the original intervention being delivered by each interventionist, and even changing over time as the interventionists gain more experience. Thus, each subject receives a different version of the original intervention plan. Further, subjects may actually receive and enact different versions of the intervention depending on their interpretation of what they are being told or shown. The result is that the investigator has little idea of what was actually being tested.

A concurrent nested design was used to measure and enhance treatment fidelity in the Resources for Enhancing Alzheimer's Caregiver Health (REACH), a large-scale, multisite study involving family caregivers of individuals with dementia (Schulz, Gallagher-Thompson, Haley, & Czaja, 2000; Wisniewski et al., 1999). In that study, each member of the research team was tested periodically for knowledge of relevant procedures (including those delivering the intervention), team meetings were analyzed for level of understanding regarding the intervention, and each interventionist was evaluated on-site frequently to monitor adherence to the protocol. In addition, each study site was assessed in terms of the accuracy of the intervention manual and use of handouts to ensure subjects actually received the intervention as designed. Finally, subject enactment of the intervention was assessed using a satisfaction survey that asked specifically the extent to which each component of the intervention was used (Burgio et al., 2001). Although time-consuming and associated with some additional costs, the treatment fidelity approach which used a concurrent nested design was vital to accurately interpreting and replicating the REACH intervention.

Concurrent Transformative Design

As with a sequential transformative design, the purpose of a concurrent transformative design is use of a theoretical perspective to enact change in a group or organization (Creswell et al., 2003, p. 230). Choices about the predominant tradition and whether methods are nested or triangulated are made based on the degree to which the theoretical perspective is facilitated. Thus, a transformative design may take on the characteristics of either a

nested or triangulated design, but the overall purpose is to promote change in the entity being studied. Participatory action research is usually based on a concurrent transformative design as investigators use the methods necessary to give all stakeholders a voice in identifying the problem, developing a solution, and evaluating the outcome of implementing the solution.

Conclusion

In this chapter, mixed methods has been examined as a flexible, yet rigorous approach to complex study problems that defy study with more traditional approaches. Mixed methods are used to strengthen the study and compensate for the weaknesses inherent in designs from both qualitative and quantitative traditions. Topics studied as part of occupational therapy seem well suited to the design types (sequential and concurrent) described in this chapter. Further, use of mixed methods is recommended as one way to ensure the treatment fidelity of occupational therapy interventions.

REFERENCES

Burgio, L., Corcoran, M. A., Lichstein, K. L., Nichols, L., Czaja, S., Gallagher-Thompson, D. E., Bourgeois, M., Stevens, A., & Ory, M. (2001). Judging outcomes in psychosocial interventions for dementia caregivers: The problem of treatment implementation. *The Gerontologist 41*, 481–489.

Corcoran, M. A. (2004a). *Understanding the care typologies of individuals providing care for a spouse with dementia*. American Occupational Therapy Association, annual meeting, Minneapolis, MN.

Corcoran, M. A. (2004b). Caregiving styles and strategies. In K. Dokar (Ed.), *Living with grief: Alzheimer's disease*. Washington, DC: Hospice Foundation of America.

Creswell, J. W. (1998). *Qualitative inquiry and research design: Choosing among five traditions*. Thousand Oaks, CA: SAGE Publications.

Creswell, J. W. (2003). *Research Design: Qualitative, Quantitative, and Mixed Methods Approaches (2nd Ed)*. Thousand Oaks, CA: SAGE Publications.

Creswell, J. W., Clark, V. P., Gutmann, M. L., & Hanson, W. E. (2003). Advanced mixed methods research designs. In A. Tashakkori & C. Teddlie (Eds.), *Handbook of mixed methods in social and behavioral research* (pp. 209–240). Thousand Oaks, CA: SAGE Publications.

Denzin, N. K. (1978). The logic of naturalistic inquiry. In N. K. Denzin (Ed.), *Sociological methods: A sourcebook*. New York: McGraw-Hill.

Gitlin, L. N., Winter, L., Dennis, M., Corcoran, M., Schinfeld, S., & Hauck, W. (2002). Strategies used by families to simplify tasks for individuals with Alzheimer's disease and related disorders: Psychometric analysis of the task management strategy index. *The Gerontologist, 42*, 61–69.

Greene, J. C., & Caracelli, V. J. (1997). *Advances in*

Mixed-Method Evaluation: The Challenges and Benefits of Integrating Diverse Paradigms (New Directions for Evaluation, No. 74). San Francisco: Jossey-Bass.

Howe, K. R. (1988). Against the quantitative-qualitative incompatibility thesis or dogmas die hard. *Educational Researcher, 17*, 10–16.

Lichstein, K.. L., Riedel, B. W., & Grieve, R. (1994). Fair tests of clinical trials: A treatment implementation model. *Advances in Behavior Research and Therapy, 16*, 1–29.

Morse, J.M. (1991). Approaches to qualitative-quantitiative metholdological triangulation. *Nursing Research, 40*(2), 120–123.

Morse, J. M. (2003). Principles of mixed methods and multimethod research design. In A. Tashakkori & C. Teddlie (Eds.), *Handbook of mixed methods in social and behavioral research* (pp.189–208). Thousand Oaks, CA: SAGE Publications.

Newman, I., & Benz, C. R. (1998). *Qualitative-quantitative research methodology: Exploring the interactive continuum*. Carbondale, IL: Southern Illinois University Press.

Newman, I., Ridenour, C. S., Newman, C., & DeMarco, G. M. P. (2003). A typology of research purposes and its relationship to mixed methods. In A. Tashakkori & C. Teddlie (Eds.), *Handbook of mixed methods in social and behavioral research* (pp. 167–188). Thousand Oaks, CA: SAGE Publications.

Schulz, R., Gallagher-Thompson, D. E., Haley, W., & Czaja, S. (2000). Understanding the intervention process: A theoretical/conceptual framework for intervention approaches to caregiving. In R. Schulz (Ed.), *Handbook of dementia caregiving interventions*. New York: Springer.

Tashakkori, A., & Teddlie, C. (1998). *Mixed methodology: Combining the qualitative and quantitative approaches (Applied Social Research Methods*, No. 46). Thousand Oaks, CA: SAGE Publications.

Tashakkori, A., & Teddlie, C. (2003). *Handbook of mixed methods in social and behavioral research*. Thousand Oaks, CA: SAGE Publications.

Vogt, P. W. (1993). *Dictionary of statistics and methodology*. Thousand Oaks, CA: SAGE Publications.

Wisniewski, S., Belle, S., Coon, D., Marcus, S., Ory, M., Burgio, L., Burns, R., & Schulz, R. (1999). The resources of enhancing Alzheimer's caregiver health (REACH) project design and baseline characteristics. *Psychology and Aging, 18*, 375–384.

RESOURCES

DePoy, E., & Gitlin, L. N. (2005). *Introduction to research: Understanding and applying multiple strategies* (3rd ed.). St. Louis: C. V. Mosby.

Newman, I., & Benz, C. R. (1998). *Qualitative-quantitative research methodology: Exploring the interactive continuum*. Carbondale, IL: Southern Illinois University Press.

Schwandt, T. A. (2001). *Dictionary of qualitative inquiry* (2nd ed.). Thousand Oaks, CA: SAGE Publications.

Tashakkori, A., & Teddlie, C. (2003). *Handbook of mixed methods in social and behavioral research*. Thousand Oaks, CA: SAGE Publications.

Vogt, P. W. (1993). *Dictionary of statistics and methodology*. Thousand Oaks, CA: SAGE Publications.

CHAPTER 26

Organizing the Components of Inquiry Together: Planning and Implementing a Coherent Study and Research Tradition

Gary Kielhofner • Marcia Finlayson • Renée R. Taylor

Implementing high-quality research is a multifaceted and challenging process. It requires planning, resources, careful implementation, documentation, and storage of data, analysis, and dissemination of findings in presentations and publications. Even a modest research project will take upwards of a year to implement from beginning to end. Typically, publication requires a year or more from the time a paper is submitted until it appears in the literature.

Therefore, conducting a quality study from planning to publication is ordinarily no less than a 2-year commitment. Most research projects extend much longer, with 3 to 5 years being the typical funding period for implementing major federally funded research projects, excluding dissemination efforts after the project is officially closed. Publication of a typical research article culminates a process that began years before with the initial planning of the research. By the time findings are in print, a great deal of time and effort has been expended.

Research involves commitment over a substantial period of time. Before embarking on a research project (even if it involves collaborating with one component of a study) one should have an appreciation of what the overall process entails. Taking responsibility for full collaboration or leadership in research requires a firm grasp of everything involved, something that takes training, mentoring from a seasoned investigator, and substantial experience.

The purpose of this chapter is to provide an overview of the major processes that are required to organize and complete a study from beginning to end. The steps in research that are overviewed in this chapter are covered in detail in the subsequent chapters. Our aim is to give the big picture of what a study entails from the time it is planned until the findings are disseminated. In addition, this chapter places the individual research study in the larger context of a tradition of inquiry.

Traditions of Inquiry

Conducting high-quality research is the outcome of a developmental process (Case-Smith, 1999) in which a variety of research strategies are integrated over time into a program of research. The following are some key elements of this process:

* Establishing a theoretical framework that frames the research,
* Refining the methods used in the research so that they become more sophisticated and suited to the topic under study,
* Establishing a track record in a defined area of research (through regular publication and dissemination of findings),
* Developing ongoing relationships with research collaborators and sites, and
* Securing funding to support the research.

When viewing research from a developmental perspective, the most productive context for research is a tradition of inquiry (Hammel, Finlayson, Kielhofner, Helfrich, & Peterson, 2002; Helfrich, Finlayson, & Lysack, in press; Kielhofner, Hammel, Helfrich, Finlayson, & Taylor, 2004; Taylor, Fisher & Kielhofner, 2005) A tradition of inquiry ordinarily encompasses the following elements:

* A line of inquiry defined by theoretical, substantive, and/or methodological interest, and
* A consistent stream of funding that supports the research.

A tradition of inquiry is ordinarily led by (a) principal investigator(s) and co-investigators and it involves the sustained effort of a team of research staff, including graduate students who are part of university-based research teams, community members, consulting or collaborating researcher from other organizations, and external agency personnel who are involved in the research.

A research tradition involves pursuing a line of inquiry over an extended period of time, so that those involved are continuously improving their skills and expertise. Within traditions of research, a given study never really stands alone. As part of a tradition of research each study picks up where a previous study has left off, generating new findings and new questions that inform and shape future lines of inquiry. A tradition of research takes many years to establish and typically extends over the entire career of a researcher.

> A research tradition involves pursuing a line of inquiry over an extended period of time, so that those involved are continuously improving their skills and expertise.

The Need for Planning

All studies, no matter the size and scope of the research, require a strong organizational plan. The planning process includes:

- Searching the literature,
- Identifying research questions, and
- Deciding the research methodology.

The Research Tradition as a Context for Learning Research

Research traditions are ideal learning contexts for graduate students who function within them as research apprentices (Hammel et al., 2002). Students learn research by participating in actual research procedures. Moreover, they typically have an opportunity to participate in informal interactions and to see how research actually unfolds. They gain an appreciation of what is being learned through the research and the inherent logic of the process.

The research tradition is also an ideal framework wherein students can select research topics, and complete masters' theses and doctoral dissertations. Rather than being expected to identify and pursue "original and independent" research, students working within such traditions engage in research that emanates from the ongoing research tradition. In this way, the directions for the research and the questions or hypotheses to be examined emanate from the previous round of research. Moreover, within traditions of research students learn not only from their research mentors, but also from project staff and peer students who have complementary knowledge and skills working.

Each of these processes is discussed separately below. However, it should be noted that they are not necessarily sequential steps. Rather, as shown in Figure 26.1, they are part of an interactive process with each element helping to refine the other. For instance, one may begin with a very broad research question, which guides the literature review. As one explores the literature, the research question may focus or go off in a somewhat different direction. Similarly, as one examines the methodological implications of asking a question, it may become apparent that the question is too broad or otherwise needs to be altered.

The Literature Search

A literature review involves the systematic and replicable process that identifies, evaluates, and interprets an existing body of recorded work on a particular topic or question. When one is planning an inquiry, the literature review serves two key objectives that include:

- Identifying the current level of theory and knowledge development, as well as gaps and areas of inconsistency, and
- Identifying the research methods that are commonly used, and their strengths and limitations.

By serving these objectives, the literature review allows the researcher to develop a sound rationale for his or her current project that is grounded in and builds upon existing knowledge. When planning a study, an often unappreciated secondary outcome of a good literature review is the identification of experts in the topic area that could be approached for consultation if that is deemed to be appropriate or necessary as the project develops.

A good literature review will be planned ahead of time, and guided by a specific question or series of questions. The search itself will be done in a systematic and methodical manner, taking into account the searching nuances and strategies relevant to the particular search method that is being used. There are four basic methods of searching the literature:

- Using electronic bibliographic databases such as MEDLINE, CINAHL, PSYCHinfo, ERIC, Science Citation Index, the Agency for Healthcare

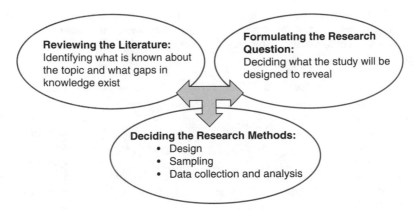

Figure 26.1 Mutually interactive components of planning a study.

Research and Quality Clinical Guidelines and Evidence Reports, British Medical Journal's Clinical Evidence, and the Cochrane Database of Systematic Reviews, AgeLine, and many others,
• Manually searching through specific journals, either hard-copy or through online tables of contents, for articles that are of interest,
• Reviewing articles listed in the reference lists of articles that were previously located on the topic of interest, and
• Searching the World Wide Web.

It is important to realize that searching an electronic bibliographic database and searching the WWW is not the same thing. Databases are compilations of published research, scholarly articles, books, government reports, newspaper articles, and so forth. There are many different databases, each with its own focus, purpose, and primary audience. For example, CINAHL indexes both peer-reviewed and "gray" literature (e.g., dissertations) from nursing and allied health, and focuses on serving this audience. Most electronic bibliographic databases are international in scope, and as a result, will provide publications that are written in English as well as other languages. In comparison, the WWW is a network of documents that are made available through the Internet. While some search engines can do complex searches, there are no standard search terms to use or thesauruses to assist when relevant materials are not being identified. Doing a WWW search may result in locating a relevant article, but many irrelevant materials will be found as well. In addition, it is often difficult to evaluate the credibility of a Web site, given that there are no restrictions as to who can post materials on the Web.

Regardless of the method used, a good literature review will be clearly documented, step by step, so that it is reproducible on subsequent days

or by other people. The initial steps in conducting a good literature review include:

• Writing a clear and focused question,
• Identifying the key concepts and relationships embedded within the question,
• Identifying the best search method or methods to use to address the question (e.g., electronic bibliographic databases and hand searching),
• Initiating the search, working through one method at a time, and
• Refining the search as needed, documenting changes in the question, terms, or method being used.

When searching the literature, one should be open to:

• The work of researchers in other disciplines, as they may have interesting new approaches or ideas that will inform the work that is being planned, and
• Literature that is more than 8 to 10 years old.

Some people consider reading older literature irrelevant, because it is out of date and potentially inaccurate. However, limiting searches to the most recently available work risks that important, classic pieces may be missed. Having a solid understanding of classic works is often integral to developing and refining ideas. Finally, reviewing the literature is not a once-only activity. Keeping up with the literature and new developments in a field is a critical part of building and organizing a program of inquiry.

Identifying Research Questions

All research sets out to generate new knowledge that fills a current gap. Such questions may have their origins in clinical experience. They might emerge from the literature. Or, they may have their origins in the findings of previous research. Articulating and refining the research question involves identifying:

- What it is that is not currently known, and
- What the investigation will address.

Research questions generally start out broad and are narrowed over time. For instance, an investigator might begin with the following types of questions:

- Why do so many persons who are hospitalized with serious mental illness tend to be rehospitalized?
- What kinds of characteristics predict which persons will be more successful following rehabilitation?
- What is the personal experience of persons following a cerebrovascular accident?
- What differentiates clients who tend to be motivated to get the most out of therapy and those who lack motivation?

The process of formulating a research question involves going from such broad formulations of the question to something that is much more specific and can be addressed in a single study. For example, the first question noted above might be narrowed into one of the following questions:

- Is functional level related to the frequency of hospitalizations over a 3-year period?
- Do persons who have family support have a lower rate of hospitalization in a year than those without family support?

As these examples illustrate, choosing a research question means that one must select an aspect of the broader question being studied that is manageable. Every research question has costs in terms of resources and time needed to generate a developing answer. Thus one should formulate the research question with an eye toward what will be feasible in the study being planned.

Formulating a research question usually involves the following steps:

- Reviewing the literature (as noted above) in order to identify what is already known about the topic, what type of questions have been asked in previous research on the topic, and how people have gone about asking those questions, and
- Consulting with others about the relevance, sig-

nificance, and timeliness of the research question/topic. Depending upon the objectives and scope of the study, this may involve:

- Talking to people who have done research in the area in order to receive their input about how to best formulate the problem (this can range from getting direct supervision or consultation from expert researchers in the topic area),
- Discussing the topic with practitioners or consumers in order to make sure the question has relevance and significance to contemporary practice,
- Obtaining information from public policymakers and potential grant funding agencies regarding their perspective on the significance, relevance, and timeliness of a given research question (within the field of occupational therapy, these may include members of public advisory boards, clinical organizations, hospital administrators, self-help or advocacy-based organizations, and governmental officials that provide funding for research and/or services), and
- Presenting an early version of the question to get feedback from others.

Developing a research question should be a public process that benefits from the input of people who know something about the problem from a research and/or practical perspective. Consulting with such people enhances the likelihood that the study will address an important and relevant question. Participatory approaches to research (see Chapters 38 to 40) stress the importance of involving stakeholders who will be influenced by or who would be expected to be consumers of the research.

Carefully deciding the research question is worth all the effort and time one can give it, since it influences all subsequent decisions and procedures and ultimately shapes the worth of the study. Moreover, choosing a research question involves creativity. Some of the best research is based on figuring out a new way to approach a problem or finding a different way to ask the question others have asked. Taking time to consider information from the literature and from others' perspectives is a wise investment for any research project.

> All research sets out to generate new knowledge that fills a current gap.

Deciding the Research Methodology

In deciding the methodology, one first needs to decide whether the study will be quantitative, qualitative, or a combination of these two methodological approaches. Once one has decided the broad type of methodology the study will employ, there are four critical methodological decisions:

• Design,
• Sampling,
• Data collection, and
• Analysis.

Each is briefly examined below. Although discussed separately, these four aspects of the methods must be considered together.

Design

Choosing a research design requires the investigator to decide how the research will be structured to answer the research question. Ordinarily, selecting the study design involves several layers of decision making. As noted earlier, one first decides whether the overall design will be qualitative or quantitative or combine facets of both. Then, one must select the details of the design. For quantitative studies one has to consider whether the overall design will be:

• A descriptive one in which quantitative data are collected to answer a broad question that characterizes a selected group or that explores relationships between variables,
• An experimental design (e.g., clinical trial) in which a variable will be manipulated to ascertain its effect on participants, or
• A prospective longitudinal or follow-up design in which data on a variable will be collected over time to determine how it changes naturally or in response to some event.

In the case of a qualitative study, the following types of broad design options are considered:

• Whether the study will involve naturalistic observation or participant observation,
• The number of different settings that will be examined in the study, and
• How data collection and analysis will be coordinated over time.

After such first level decisions are made then more detailed decisions must be made about the study design. At each level, the considerations that guide the design choices represent consideration of issues of rigor as they are conceptualized in the qualitative and/or quantitative traditions along with practical logistic considerations (e.g., what is possible to do in the study given constraints of resources, contexts, and other factors that influence the realistic parameters of choice). The following are some examples of the types of more detailed questions that will be asked in further delineating the study design:

• In the case of a longitudinal survey, how many times will participants be asked to respond and at what time points?
• If the study is an experimental study, how many different experimental conditions will be compared and what will be the control condition? What is the feasibility of assigning subjects to conditions randomly?
• If the study is qualitative and if it uses key informants, how will these be selected?

Most often, designing the study involves a number of iterative stages in which one:

• Examines how other investigators have approached the question one plans to address,
• Creatively considers ways to address the question,
• Compares ideas about the design to expected resources and research conditions to make sure the design is realistic, and
• Seeks consultation and feedback from other investigators and from persons who can provide information about logistics.

This same iterative process also applies to decisions about sampling, data collection, and analysis since they are all interrelated.

Sampling

Sampling refers to decisions about who will participate in the study and how they will best represent the larger population of interest. Deciding how to sample is a fairly complex process involving several parameters. It involves deciding:

• Who are appropriate potential subjects for the study (inclusion/exclusion criteria),
• How participants will be chosen for the study (selection),
• How many participants will be required for the study (sample size),
• What will be required of participants (participant burden), and
• How participants will be allocated to different conditions (assignment) if there are different conditions or situations on which subjects are compared.

Inclusion/exclusion criteria specify who will be included in the study and who will not. Participants are included based on the question to be asked. That is, if one wants to know about the experience of persons following cerebrovascular accident (CVA), then inclusion criteria might be persons who have experienced a CVA in the past 6 weeks. In occupational therapy studies, factors that are generally considered in inclusion criteria are the diagnosis/impairment, ethnicity, and age.

Exclusion criteria are generally decided on the basis of eliminating factors that may confound the research findings and excluding those who would not be capable of participating in the research protocol. Returning to the preceding example, an exclusion factor to eliminate confounding variables might be having another physical or psychiatric disability since the experience of a second disability would be difficult to sort out from the experience of the CVA. If the same study involved extensive interviewing of participants about their experiences, then one exclusionary criterion would be persons with expressive aphasia.

The method of selecting participants for a study depends on the study method and design. For example, a qualitative method generally uses a purposive sampling strategy that seeks out persons who are knowledgeable about the topic under study (i.e., key informants). In contrast, a large-scale survey may seek a sample that is randomly selected from the defined population so that findings can be generalized. Subject assignment is a concern when the study is an experiment. Random assignment is the most rigorous strategy in this situation to equalize the distribution of factors that might confound a research question across the groups that are being studied.

Sample sizes can vary widely and depend on the design of the study. Typically, qualitative research involves fewer participants from whom a great deal of information is collected over time. Some quantitative designs may involve large samples of participants who are contacted only once (e.g., to complete a written survey or respond to a structured interview), and in others (e.g., longitudinal studies) subjects may be contacted several times and evaluated using measures of the same variables over a period of time. In some cases the sample size will be determined by how many subjects are necessary to achieve a statistically significant finding. Experimental and longitudinal studies also have to account for attrition, or the likelihood that some subjects will drop out of the study, relocate, die, or go missing for some other reason. In this case, a power analysis (as discussed in Chapter 17) may be done to decide the number of subjects that are necessary.

Participant burden is generally defined as how much effort is required of the subject or how much the subject will be subjected to. Participant burden is a concern for two reasons. The first reason is ethical; that is, what is asked of subjects has to be weighed against the potential benefit of the study to the participants and to society in general. If the participant burden cannot be justified by the potential benefit then the study cannot be considered ethically warranted. Second, the more that is asked of subject, the more difficult it may be to recruit and retain subjects in the study.

Data Collection and Analysis

The answer(s) to the research question(s) of the study are dependent on the quality of data collected and how they are analyzed. Decisions about these two aspects of the study methods go hand in hand. First of all, the type of data collected and the type of analysis will depend on whether the study is qualitative and/or quantitative in nature. Qualitative data are ordinarily collected through observations or interviews that are recorded through field notes, audiotapes, or videotapes. Quantitative data are collected through observation, interview, and self-report forms that are generally recorded on paper or on computer.

Investigators are always concerned with the dependability of data, although this issue is considered differently within the qualitative and quantitative traditions. Briefly stated, qualitative concerns include such things as whether the experience and circumstance of those studied is faithfully represented while quantitative concerns are ordinarily couched in terms of data reliability (i.e., stability over time, method of data collection, and data collector) and validity (assurance that the data represent the intended concept). Most strategies for ensuring data dependability in qualitative research are dependent on how the investigator goes about gathering the data. Quantitative data dependability may be based on previous research that has demonstrated reliability and validity of the preexisting, standardized data collection tools that are chosen for the study. In cases where this type of research is not available on the data collection method chosen or where a data collection method has to be created for the study, data on the reliability and/or validity of the instrument may be gathered as part of the study itself or in a previous pilot study.

Data analysis also depends on whether the study is qualitative and/or quantitative. Qualitative data analysis ordinarily involves coding and classifying data to identify various themes that make up the findings. Qualitative data analysis tends to be more "organic." That is, the analysis is partly shaped by the research question and partly shaped by the nature of the data itself. Moreover, data collection and analysis in qualitative research is often a spiral process in which analysis of initial data shapes the kind of data that are collected next and the new data result in further analyses, and so on. Quantitative data analysis involves descriptive and inferential statistics. How the data will be analyzed depends on the type of data collected (nominal, ordinal, ratio, or interval), the research question, the sample size, and how the data are distributed.

Descriptive statistics can serve a number of purposes. For example, they can be used to describe the sociodemographic characteristics (e.g., sex, age range, and ethnicity) of a sample or to describe how a sample has scored or performed on a given measure. For example, consider a researcher who has obtained a sample of 60 women, 30 of whom have had a C-3 to C-6 spinal cord injury and 30 of whom have had a severe CVA. If the researcher is interested in describing fatigue severity in the two groups of individuals from a quantitative perspective, the researcher might utilize a measure of fatigue severity that provides a continuous fatigue score ranging from 0 (low) to 30 (high) and then provide statistics that show the variation and central tendency of fatigue in each of the two groups.

Descriptive statistics are most commonly reported in terms of frequency and percentage data (for categorical variables) or in terms of means and standard deviations (for continuous variables). Depending on the research question, other descriptive statistics that may be presented include medians, ranges, or modes. Descriptive statistics can also be presented visually in graphs such as histograms, scatterplots, or boxplots.

Statistics from the study sample can be compared to those from other sample groups within the same study, or to statistics from a normative reference group. If a researcher is interested in comparing scores between two groups, inferential statistics can be used. Inferential statistics allow the researcher to test a given hypothesis—or answer a research question that is comparative in nature, or probes the efficacy of a given intervention. In this case, the sample size and how the data are distributed must be considered.

For example, a direct comparison of means between the group of women with spinal cord injury and the group with CVA assumes that the data from the two study groups have adequate variability and are normally distributed. Whether data are distributed normally will, in part, be based on the sample size. Larger sample sizes (≥25 subjects) are more likely to be normally distributed than smaller sample sizes. However, sample size alone does not always predict normal distribution.

Descriptive statistics, such as measures of skewness, kurtosis, variability, and visual analysis of a scatterplot, can be used to determine whether data for a given group of individuals are normally distributed. If data are not normally distributed or if the sample size is small, then nonparametric statistics can be used.

Generally speaking, inferential statistics can be subclassified in terms of univariate and multivariate statistics. Univariate statistics are used to analyze a single dependent variable. Multivariate statistics are used to test the effects of one or more independent variables on more than one outcome variable. Considering the study example above, if a researcher wanted to compare the group of women with spinal cord injury to the group of women with CVA in terms of fatigue severity and hypothesized that the women with CVA would report more severe fatigue levels, the researcher would first check if the fatigue severity scores are normally distributed in both groups and then likely use a t-test to compare the mean fatigue severity scores between the two groups.

Integrating the Planning Components

As noted earlier, the three components of planning a study (literature review, formulating the question, and deciding the methods) are interrelated and influence each other. The kind of question one formulates will have implications for the literature search and research methodology. Moreover, the state of the literature and available methodological resources for implementing research will influence the types of questions that can or should be asked.

Consider, for example, the question posed earlier about the personal experience following cerebral vascular accident. Such a question will have certain implications for the research design depending on the state of the literature. If the literature indicates there is little to no information to answer this question, then a qualitative, exploratory design, or a quantitative pilot study that gathers information from a small sample is a good starting point. When such studies already exist, they may provide sufficient information for creating a large-scale survey research design. Such a study might enlist a larger sample of persons to see how much variability there is in their experience and then identify what demographic factors are associated with different experiences.

Similarly, if one explores the question about what accounts for recidivism and finds out little is known, then a qualitative research study may be indicated. However, if one finds out there is a large literature and quite a bit is known about a given topic, such as what causes rehospitalization in persons with mental illness, then the investigator may decide that the question needs to be reformulated to ask: "Can the rate of rehospitalization be reduced by offering follow-up services?" This type of question is best answered by a control group design in which some persons receive the service and others do not.

Writing the Research Plan

As one develops the research questions, completes the literature review, and plans the methodology of a study, it is typical that a research plan is written up. Writing up the plan helps to organize and record one's thinking processes. A research plan is ordinarily required before one can go on to implement research, since it is the basis for individuals or bodies who approve research (e.g., the research advisor in the case of research undertaken by a student or trainee, the ethical review board that approves the study on ethical grounds when human subjects are involved). Writing a good research plan not only helps one to systematically think about the study, it also provides some of the basic material that will be used later in writing a report of the research findings.

A research plan ordinarily includes:

- An introduction that indicates the general nature of the study and the rationale, or why it is important,
- A review of the literature that indicates what is already known in the area and that demonstrates the need for the question of the study to be asked,
- A statement of the overall aim(s) or objectives of the study,
- An indication of the specific questions to be answered and/or hypotheses to be tested, and
- A description of the planned methodology of the study including design, sampling strategy, data collection, and data analysis.

The actual format and length of the research plan will depend on a number of factors including the type of research planned and the intended audience for the plan.

Planning and Budgeting for Necessary Resources

Every study has financial implications. The cost of studies may range from small investigations that cost a few hundred dollars to large funded studies that require millions of dollars to implement. No matter what size the planned research, it is impor-

tant to think ahead about the funds and other resources that may be required to implement the research.

One important resource for any study is space. Even if the study is done in a natural setting, there needs to be a place where the investigator can store the data for the study and work on data analysis. Most studies require space for such things as:

- Housing research staff and equipment necessary for the research, and
- Conducting any procedures that are part of the research (e.g., experimental procedures, staff meetings, interviews with subjects).

It is important that space not only be adequate in size for the study but also that it can ensure confidentiality of subjects (e.g., private rooms for data collection and storage) and appropriate execution of any research procedure (e.g., quiet space for testing). In most cases research is conducted in existing space, so planning for the research involves requesting and securing permission for use of the space (exclusive or shared as needed) for the duration of the research. Space is ordinarily provided by the agency or organization sponsoring the research, but sometimes it is necessary to rent space for a study, in which case it can become part of the budget.

Other resources for research ordinarily are purchased specifically for the study. Therefore they fall under the process of planning and securing a budget for the research. In any research project the typical costs are:

- Personnel,
- Equipment,
- Supplies,
- Subject reimbursement,
- Travel, and
- Subcontracts.

The kinds of personnel who make up a research project are discussed below. Depending on the setting and size of the research project, some or all of the salaries of personnel involved in the study may be paid. Projects that require several persons ordinarily are supported by grants. Grants generally pay:

- Part of the salary of some persons who have other responsibilities,
- The full salary of persons who are employed solely for purposes of conducting the research, and
- Consultant or subcontract fees to people who are performing specific, limited tasks related to the study.

Equipment generally refers to objects that are durable while supplies refer to things that consumed by use (e.g., paper, office items). However, different granting agencies may specify different ways of deciding what is equipment and what are supplies. Within occupational therapy research, typical equipment needed for a study may range from motor and cognitive testing materials, to assistive devices, to therapeutic tools or toys, to splints, to highly specialized instruments that measure muscle strength, physical endurance, range of motion, or pain sensitivity. For qualitative research items such as tape recorders, transcription machines or video recorders may be needed. Other typical research equipment includes computers, fax machines, printers, telephones, and items used to enter and store data such as file cabinets. Supplies generally encompass office supplies, printing supplies, study brochures, postage, stationery, and software packages.

Many studies, particularly those that do not offer a service, reimburse subjects for the time, effort, or discomfort associated with participation. The extent of reimbursement depends on what the subjects are being asked to do. Subject reimbursement can be used as an "incentive" for subjects, but ethical concerns require that the amount of reimbursement not be so much that subjects feel compelled to participate in research in which they would not otherwise chose to participate.

Travel can include any costs incurred in conducting or reporting findings for a study. Travel may be the cost of investigators or data collectors traveling to subjects' homes. On the other hand, travel may include the cost of reimbursing subjects to travel to the research site. The cost of investigators traveling to scientific and/or professional conferences to present the research findings is also generally considered part of the cost of doing research.

Subcontracts are chunks of larger budgets that can be conceived as "sub-budgets." Based on a contractual agreement with a collaborator from a different institution, subcontracts are generally used to fund staff and research activities that occur outside of the main institution that houses the research.

Writing a Grant

The most typical way of obtaining resources for a study is to prepare a grant proposal. Proposals may be intramural or extramural. An intramural proposal is one submitted to the agency in which the investigator is employed and/or under whose auspices the research will be conducted. Intramural grants are generally smaller than extramural grants. The decision about funding may be made by an administrator or a committee who reviews that grant proposal and determines whether it merits funding. Intramural proposals may or may not be competitive (i.e., when several grant proposals are considered simultaneously and only the best ones are funded).

Extramural funding is provided by an agency outside the one where the researcher is employed or where the research will take place. There are two basic types of extramural funding agencies: private foundations and public (state or federal) agencies. Both types of agencies generally have published priorities indicating the type of research they wish to fund and both types of agencies typically have deadlines for submitting research proposals since their funding is generally competitive. The largest funder of research in the United States is the federal government. Since most agencies fund only a small proportion of the proposals they receive, a typical researcher will have to prepare substantially more grant proposals than projects that are actually funded.

A grant always includes a research plan. It also typically includes the other following elements:

- A management plan that includes discussion of the personnel necessary to implement the study, the objectives and tasks necessary to conduct the study, and a timeline for their completion,
- A budget indicating the necessary resources and justifying the proposed expenditures (most or all of which the granting agency will be asked to provide and some of which may be provided by the institution that houses the grant),
- An evaluation plan that indicates how the overall quality of the proposed project will be assessed,
- Evidence that ethical approval has been obtained or is being sought (when human subjects are involved), and
- Appendices that include such things as letters of commitment from individuals and organizations who will be essential to the study implementation, copies of instruments or procedures that will be used to collect and analyze data, and protocols describing procedures that will make up experimental and control conditions in experimental studies.

Depending on the granting agency and the nature of the study, a grant application may be only a few pages long or may contain several hundred pages of material.

Management Plan

Every research project requires a management plan that outlines:

- The major tasks necessary to complete the project,
- Who is responsible to accomplish those tasks, and
- When the tasks will be completed.

Generally the management plan is organized around the major objectives of the study, breaking down the tasks that are necessary to achieve those objectives. Table 26.1 shows a section of a management plan from a research project, Pathways to Self Determination (H133-G020-217). This control group study examines the effectiveness of an occupational therapy intervention in helping participants achieve independent living and employment. Since research projects unfold over long periods of time, the management plan is a useful way to monitor progress to make sure that critical tasks are being done on time.

Obtaining Ethical Review

Any study that involves human beings who participate in the research as subjects should undergo ethical review. In most countries it is required before a study funded by the government can be undertaken. Moreover, institutions that routinely receive government support for research are required to have all their human research ethically reviewed whether or not it is funded.

Ethical review is a process that is designed to protect those who participate as subjects from any harm and to ensure that their effort and any risk involved is warranted by the importance of the study. A fundamental principle governing ethical conduct of research involving human beings is informed consent. The elements of informed consent are:

- That the potential subject understands the purpose of the research, what is involved in being a subject of the study, and whether there are any potential risks to being involved, and
- That permission to participate is given freely without any form of coercion.

Institutions in which research is routinely conducted (e.g., universities and large medical or rehabilitation centers) maintain ethical boards [institutional review boards (IRBs) in the United States] that review and approve research as meeting ethical standards. Investigators must complete IRB applications that typically include:

- An explanation of the research, what it will address, why the research is needed/justified, and how the research will be done, especially how subjects will be recruited, selected, and what will be required of them,
- An explanation of how subjects will be informed about the study and how their consent will be obtained, and
- Letters that will be used to obtain/document subject informed consent.

Investigators cannot begin the process of recruiting subjects until ethical approval is obtained. This process can take several weeks or months depending on the institution and the nature of the study, so it should be set in motion as soon as the investigator has finalized the plan of the research.

Personnel (Staff) and Organizational Plan

Some research projects are simple enough to be conducted by a single person, without the support of additional staff. However, most research is sufficiently complex to require a diversity of research-related skills and the efforts of several personnel. To get the work done in the most accurate and efficient manner, it is often necessary to take a close look at the tasks that need to be completed, the skills necessary to complete these tasks well, and then identify what type of person can achieve them the best.

An array of different tasks is required for any given study. There is a research plan or proposal to be written, including the analyses sections. There may be a grant application to be completed, including the budget and budget narrative. An IRB application must be prepared and submitted if human subjects are to be involved. Data must be collected and managed in an appropriate and consistent way, and then they must be analyzed, interpreted, and prepared for dissemination.

Many people may be involved in such a series of efforts. Table 26.2 summarizes some of the key players on a research team, and their typical roles and responsibilities. Not every project will need all of these players. On the other hand, some projects may need multiple individuals within any of these categories. Regardless of size or setting of a research project, the same basic tasks must be accomplished. Consequently, it is important when planning a program of inquiry to think carefully about what needs to be accomplished, and the best ways to get the work done within the time frame and financial resources available.

Although having multiple people working

Table 26.1 Example Section of a Management Plan Excerpted from a Grant Entitled "Pathways to Self-Determination"

| PD-Project Director | CoPD-CoProject Director | OT-Occupational Therapist |
| RS Research Specialist | PM-Peer Mentor | RA-Research Assistant |

Aim 3: Rigorously study the impact of the ESD and its sustainability by implementing a three-group comparison study combined with Participatory Action Research

Goal	Objective	Primary Responsibility	Timeline (Yr/Mo)
3.1 Design system for data entry and storage.	3.1a Determine mechanism for providing data to RA for entry; check that data arecomplete/clean.	CoPD	1/1–1/2
	3.1b Monitor data collection, entry, and storage on an ongoing basis to ensure complete and timely data collection and storage; conduct bi–monthly reviews.	RS	1/2–3/1
3.2 Train staff in use of all data collection tools and methods of reporting; collect data.	3.2a Train program staff and research assistant in quantitative and qualitative data collection.	PD	1/1–1/2
	3.2 b Collect demographic and disability data for both baseline and outcomes.	RS	1/2, 1/8, 2/2
	3.2c Develop system for following clients who move out of the facilities to prevent missing data.	RS	1/1–1/3
3.3 Develop feedback systems for key stakeholders for continuous program improvement.	3.3a Establish formal mechanisms for program clients, facility staff and leadership, and employers to give feedback and suggestions for program improvements.	CoPD	1/1–1/11
	3.3b Routinely collect data from all key stakeholders and report to grant team at biweekly meeting.	RS	1/1–3/10
3.4 Analyze data to allow for program modification and continuous improvement.	3.4a Hold biweekly meetings of grant staff to review data collection systems, monitor program fidelity, and identify variances in program component implementation.	PD	1/1–3/1
	3.4b Meet quarterly to review evaluation findings with staff at the three facilities.	PD	1/3 and quarterly
	3.4c Produce semiannual and final reports with findings on project implementation and outcomes. Review with Advisory Council, staff, and leadership at the three facilities.	CoPD	1/7, 2/1, 2/7, 3/1, 3/7, 3/12
3.5 Identify and integrate changes and assess impact on outcomes.	3.5a Identify and implement strategies for program improvement, measure effect, and document results to aid with program replication and program fidelity.	PD	1/3–3/10
3.6 Evaluate effectiveness of staff intervention to maintain fidelity of program services.	3.6a Include facility staff in the development of the evaluation plan to empower participants.	PD	1/2–3/11
	3.6b Identify measures of program fidelity.	PD	1/1–1/2
	3.6c Develop data collection methods to measure of program effectiveness and program fidelity.	RS	1/1–2/1
	3.6d Evaluate services provided by facility staff.	RS	2/2–3/1

Table 26.2 Research Team Roles and Responsibilities

Team Member	Typical Roles and Responsibilities

Principal investigator	• Develops questions and research design.
	• Takes ultimate responsibility for the project, including:
	  • Writing proposal,
	  • Obtaining IRB approvals,
	  • Obtaining funds,
	  • Developing or selecting instruments and equipment,
	  • Hiring and training project coordinator and other staff,
	  • Supervising staff,
	  • Monitoring progress on all aspects of the project,
	  • Confirming accuracy of analysis, and
	  • Disseminating findings.

Co-principal investigator	• Works closely with the PI, often taking responsibility for a specific aspect of the project.

Project coordinator	• Works closely with the PI and Co-PI, under their supervision.
	• Fulfills a range of administrative and human resource responsibilities, including but not exclusive to:
	  • Participating in grant writing,
	  • Managing the day-to-day aspects of the budget (e.g., invoices, payments, etc.),
	  • Providing day-to-day supervision and coordination of research assistants,
	  • Coordinating data collection, entry, cleaning, and checking, and
	  • Participating in dissemination.

Research specialist	• Often a more senior member of the research team, and one with specialized skills or experience directly relevant to the project. • Often the primary data collector and/or interventionist, particularly when specialized skills are needed.
Research assistants	• Nature of responsibilities vary with project but are often the primary data collectors when specialized skills are not required (i.e., can be trained specifically for the project), e.g., interviewers, raters, testers. • May be involved in literature reviews, data coding and checking, data entry. • Exact nature and extent of their duties will depend on previous experience and education.
Statistician	• Can be a consultant or primary member of the team. • Typically works collaboratively with the PI, starting at the time of the study planning. • May take a role in data management, if other members of the team do not have the necessary skills.
Administrative assistant	• Common with large projects, particularly in center grants and other multiproject efforts. • Fulfills roles of receptionist and secretary; sometimes will be involved in coordinating data collection efforts.
Database manager	• Important for large projects, particularly ones that have multiple sources of data or are receiving data from multiple sites. • Maintains all computer files, and is often involved in running specific analyses. • Will have specialized computer and analytic skills (e.g., SAS).
Data entry specialists	• Convert raw data into electronic format.

together on a study can be invigorating and greatly enhance research productivity, supervising and coordinating research staff presents challenges. To manage these challenges, it is important to draw on knowledge from individuals who specialize in human resources management and supervision. Some of the basic tools that can be used to facilitate research team operations and the process of supervising staff include:

• Clear job descriptions that outline responsibilities, lines of authority, and required skills (the feature box below provides an example of a research assistant job description),
• Organizational charts, particularly for large and dispersed teams (Figure 26.2),

• Policy and procedure manuals that outline all aspects of the team's operations from contacting research participants, to entering and backing up data, and
• Regular team meetings to review progress and plan strategies to address challenges, and to celebrate achievements and keep team members motivated.

Recruiting and Retaining Subjects (Participants)

The success of every research project hinges on being able to recruit and retain adequate numbers of participants for the study. Since these subjects are volunteers who rarely receive much incentive

Job Description: Research Assistant

Project Title: Aging with Multiple Sclerosis: Unmet Needs in the Great Lakes Region

Principal Investigator: Marcia Finlayson, PhD, OTR/L

Name and Title of Direct Supervisor: Toni Van Denend, Project Coordinator

Summary of Job Character: The purpose of this position is to provide administrative and research support to Dr. Finlayson for the MS Health Care Delivery & Policy Research Grant. The research assistant will work under the direction of the Project Coordinator. Duties will include, but will not be exclusive to providing clerical support, assisting with data collection and entry, conducting basic statistical analyses, and communicating with other collaborators. The research assistant will be expected to work with minimal to moderate supervision, to meet deadlines, and to actively contribute to the efforts of the research team.

Under the direction of the principal investigator and/or the project coordinator, the research assistant will:

1. Assist in any logistical arrangements for the focus groups, as requested.
   a. Assist in the setup of office systems to manage focus group documents and data.
   b. Make telephone calls and send confirmations regarding focus group locations.
   c. Assist with notifications to focus group participants.
   d. Prepare audiotapes for the transcriptionist after the focus groups are completed.
   e. Assist in coding focus group transcripts, as requested.
2. Assist in the setup and maintenance of office systems to manage the sampling frame and the sampling process for both the older adult interviews and the caregiver interviews.

   a. Receive and organize return letters of individuals willing to participate under the direction of the project coordinator.
   b. Send letters to people chosen to participate to notify them of approximate date/time of interview call.
3. Assist in preparation of telephone interview guides for use.
   a. Participate in the pilot testing of the revised telephone interview guide for understandability and time using advisory group members and/or other volunteers.
   b. Transfer interview guide to SPSS Data Entry Builder.
   c. Pilot test interview guide using SPSS Data Entry Builder to confirm data entry process and make any necessary revisions.
4. Assist in telephone interviews with people with MS.
   a. Contact selected participants and conduct telephone interview.
   b. Complete data entry directly into SPSS Data Entry Builder program.
5. Assist in sample selection of caregivers.
   a. Maintain list of individual caregiver names and contact information provided by people with MS via the telephone interviews.
   b. Send letters to people chosen to participate to notify them of the study and upcoming telephone contact.
6. Assist in telephone interviews with caregivers.
   a. Contact selected participants and conduct telephone interview.
   b. Complete data entry directly into SPSS Data Entry Builder program.
7. Conduct literature reviews for dissemination activities.
8. Perform other duties as assigned.

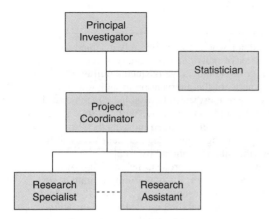

Figure 26.2 Simple organizational chart.

beyond the opportunity to contribute to science, it can be a challenge to secure adequate numbers. Subjects can be recruited for studies using a variety of approaches.

Within occupational therapy, samples are most commonly recruited from inpatient and outpatient clinics that house occupational therapy clients, from physicians and other healthcare providers, from schools, and from self-help and advocacy-based organizations to which individuals with impairments and chronic illness are members. Subjects can also be recruited through advertisements about the study in newsletters, local cable TV stations and newspapers, special interest magazines, and from special interest Web sites. However, placing advertisements in some of these venues can be very costly. Recruiting subjects for a study generally involves creating a recruitment plan. This plan involves five major steps:

• Locating the sample,
• Ensuring sample representativeness,
• Creating links to sample sources,
• Developing recruitment materials, and
• Funding recruitment efforts (recruitment materials and participant payment or incentive funds).

Locating the Sample

Developing a recruitment plan involves determining the most likely places where the intended sample exists. It also requires determining what is required in order to come into contact with the sample. Finally, it necessitates determining how best to make potential subjects aware of the study.

Ensuring Sample Representativeness

Ensuring that the sample is representative is important as a means of increasing the likelihood of generalizing findings from a given study to a larger population of interest. Ensuring representativeness involves a certain level of expertise and knowledge about the sociodemographic and impairment-related characteristics of a given population. Though clinical experience is helpful, it cannot always account for the wide ethnic and socioeconomic composition of a given sample. Moreover, clinical samples by definition do not include individuals without physical or economic access to health care because of low income, lack of insurance, or the nature and severity of the impairment. For these reasons, it is also important to gather knowledge about a population of interest from published epidemiological studies that describe the prevalence and incidence of a given condition and can include information about its geographic, racial/ethnic, sex, age, and socioeconomic distribution, among other variables.

Creating Links to Sample Sources

This step involves building relationships with the gatekeepers of the sample. Gatekeepers may take many forms and may include referring physicians, administrators of local outpatient rehabilitations centers, or presidents of self-help organizations. The stronger the relationships with these sources and the more incentive they have for allowing their clients or constituents to participate in the study, the more likely they will be to refer or allow access to participants.

Developing Recruitment Materials

Great care should be taken in developing recruitment materials, such as brochures and posters, that are clear, inviting, physically attractive, and in alternative, accessible formats (e.g., different languages). These materials should emphasize the benefits of the study and they should mention that incentives or payments will be available, if applicable.

Funding Recruitment Efforts

Recruitment is enhanced if there are sufficient economic resources to provide quality recruitment materials and incentives for participants. Incentives can range from direct cash payment to tokens such as gift certificates, raffle tickets, study pens, mouse pads, cups, candy, or stickers. Funding for these efforts is generally provided by the supporting institution or the supporting grant.

Collecting, Managing, Storing, and Analyzing Data

Research involves not only the actual process of collecting data, but also managing and storing

Statement of a Sampling Plan

The following is an excerpt from a federal grant proposal that describes plans to generate a sample of adults with chronic fatigue syndrome (CFS) for a randomized clinical trial. It illustrates the kind of detailed considerations that go into planning for a study sample.

To ensure that the sample is demographically representative of the general population of individuals with CFS, we will recruit participants so that *at least* 53% of individuals in our sample are from numerical minority backgrounds, and *at least* 72% of individuals are women. Consistent with our findings from a prior epidemiological study, we will also ensure that people of all ages over 18 years are represented, and that all levels of socioeconomic status are included, particularly those with the most limited resources. We will make concentrated efforts to ensure that as many participants who are ethnic minorities are recruited as possible using the following strategies: (1) our collaborating organization has a database of members that includes basic demographic information and research interest. We will actively recruit members who identified themselves on their initial membership application as being interested in research participation, and who identify as an ethnic minority; and (2) we will access our existing network of connections with Chicago-area physicians who treat individuals with CFS and practice in ethnically diverse neighborhoods and we will ask them to refer ethnic minority participants with CFS to the project. In general, we will also recruit participants by advertising the study in the newsletter produced by the collaborating association, in newsletters produced by larger national self-help organizations, and on listserves and Web sites dedicated to CFS.

In addition to these issues, we will also ensure that the sample is representative in terms of degree of disability of participants. Given that middle and higher functioning individuals may be more likely to participate than lower functioning individuals with CFS, we will actively recruit a sufficient number of lower functioning individuals by using a variety of approaches. First, we will target lower functioning individuals by asking referring physicians to refer their most disabled individuals with CFS to the intervention, and by asking the president of our collaborating organization to refer individuals who are most severely disabled from her roster of individuals seeking services. In addition, all of our study advertisements will emphasize the benefits of the intervention to individuals with CFS who are most severely disabled. Once referrals to the study are made, we will continue the recruiting of severely disabled individuals with CFS by highlighting issues related to easy accessibility to the intervention and by emphasizing the incentive value of the project, the provision of resource funds to support the opportunity to gain access to important resources (e.g., personal assistants, vocational rehabilitation evaluation and training). We will emphasize that the intervention is designed to accommodate people with CFS who use wheelchairs and/or are too ill to leave home via usual modes of car, taxi, or regular public transportation.

We will also add incentive value and make the intervention accessible to severely disabled individuals with CFS by informing prospective participants of our intention to provide the following alternative transportation options in order to provide transportation to and from the intervention: (1) renting wheelchairs to facilitate transportation to and from the CIL; (2) utilizing Chicago Transit Authority Special Services, which provides low-cost, door-to-door van service transportation with appointment and has the capacity to transport ambulatory individuals as well as individuals who use motorized scooters, motorized wheelchairs, and manual push wheelchairs; (3) utilizing taxi services operative within the Chicago area that accommodate standard wheelchairs and offer reduced fares with voucher for individuals with disabilities; or (4) utilizing private medical transportation companies (e.g., "Dial O Ride") that provide vans equipped to accommodate motorized wheelchairs with tilt-back features. When necessary, we will use grant resource funds to support the cost of these transportation options. In addition to these options, individuals too ill to attend group on any given day, but able to talk on the phone, will be encouraged to participate in the group via teleconference speaker hook-up. Our collaborating organization already owns this resource and is willing to provide it during the illness-management groups.

---

what is collected. Together, collecting, managing, storing, and analyzing data is referred to as data management. It involves:

- Documenting how all forms of data will be collected, handled, stored, and prepared for use,
- Developing tools and systems to operationalize the documentation, and

- Following through on the use of these tools and systems, refining and adding to them as the project evolves over time.

The purpose of data management is to:

- Ensure reliability of the information collected,
- Maintain data security,

• Facilitate research team communications, and
• Facilitate the preparation of the final reports.

Unfortunately, data management is a skill that most researchers learn through their own mistakes, which is why mentorship by senior investigators can save new researchers a great deal of time, and strengthen the rigor of their work.

Dealing with Typical Challenges in Study Implementation

As with any long-term undertaking, research projects are prone to encounter challenges. Three of the most typical challenges are:

• Participant recruitment and retention,
• Collaborative agencies, and
• Study staff changes.

Sometimes, despite the best intentions, plans for participant recruitment are unsuccessful, or come up short of the numbers needed to complete the work. In these situations, it is often necessary to reexamine the research questions, the recruitment strategies, and the data analysis plan and make revisions. These revisions will almost always need to be approved by the funding agency and the IRB before they can be implemented. To circumvent this challenge, it is best to plan recruitment strategies to take into account the worst-case scenario. It is better to have too many potential participants than not enough.

Challenges to research implementation can also arise when there are changes at collaborative agencies, such as changes in their organization or staffing that make it difficult to maintain their commitment to the project. To address this possibility, it is always wise to maintain close contacts with collaborators so that if problems are emerging, the researcher is not caught off-guard.

Given the length of many research projects, staff change is inevitable, particularly in a university environment where graduate students play a large role as research team members. Building in incentives to keep staff—for example, offering continuing education resources—can often help maintain a stable staff. Barring this, ensuring the project, tasks, and details of the study are well documented will aid in any transitions that a project must endure.

> No study is completed until it has been formally shared with other members of the scientific community and other interested constituencies.

Communication with Funding Agency (Progress and Final Reports)

Funders, whether intramural or extramural, want to know how a project is progressing as expected. Consequently, they will almost always provide a detailed schedule and a set of instructions about what reports to provide to them, and when. These instructions will include what information to include in the report, including updates on expenditures. It is critical that reports are completed on time, following the funder's specifications. Failure to do so can sometimes result in a revocation of funding.

Dissemination

No study is completed until it has been formally shared with other members of the scientific community and other interested constituencies. The usual vehicles for sharing research findings are:

• Presentations and posters at scientific/professional conference,
• Published papers in refereed journals, and
• Consumer-friendly dissemination products such as educational videos, resource manuals, booklets, and curricula.

Each of these venues of dissemination is briefly discussed below. Chapter 34 provides a detailed discussion of dissemination strategies.

Presentations and Posters

Presenting a study before peer scientists and/or professionals is an important form of sharing findings. Because presentations are face to face and involve opportunity for discussion of the findings, they can also provide an opportunity to help the investigator think about the implications of the study. Presentations and poster sessions are generally refereed—that is, one has to submit an abstract describing the presentation and then reviewers decide which of the abstracts will be selected for presentation. This selection process is designed to ensure that the presentations/posters meet some minimal criteria of scientific rigor. Depending on the type of conference, the referees may or may not be aware of the presenter's identity when abstracts are reviewed.

Publication

Refereed papers are by definition submitted to a journal editor for blind review (i.e., review by persons who are unknown to the author and to whom the author's identity is unknown). The process of blind review is designed to minimize bias and to maximize the degree of honesty in the feedback process. Scientific journals have published guidelines that specify the kinds of papers that are appropriate for the journal and that specify how the papers are to be submitted (electronic versus hard copy, number of copies, forms to be submitted with the article). Papers that are not judged to meet adequate standards or the purpose of the journal may be returned rejected. Depending on the journal, rates of acceptance may vary from a high proportion of submitted manuscripts to a very small percentage. It is also common for a paper to be returned with requests for substantial revision in which case the paper is typically re-reviewed by the original reviewers. Generally, even when submitted papers are accepted for publication, revisions are required before the paper goes into press. Different journals have different lead times for a journal to appear once accepted; these may be as short as a couple of months or longer than a year depending on the journal.

The process of submitting papers for publication requires a degree of patience and willingness to accept and use feedback. As challenging as the review process can be at times, it is necessary in order to help ensure the quality of papers that are published. Journals range in the degree of rigor they expect of papers and consequently some journals are much harder to publish in than others.

Consumer-Focused Dissemination

While presentations and publications are important ways to disseminate research findings to scientific and professional peers, there is increasing emphasis on sharing findings to other constituencies who might benefit from the information. These include consumers, their family members, and practitioners who are interested in using the procedures and tools that were developed or tested as part of the research process. Typical venues for dissemination include presentations or publications that are focused on the practical implications of the research findings, Web sites, and manuals.

Conclusion

As noted at the beginning of the chapter, the process of planning and implementing a study is long and complicated. Needless to say, it requires commitment, foresight, flexibility, and perseverance. Planning is key, and this process can be made significantly easier by connecting with more senior investigators, using co-investigators and collaborators, and being realistic about what can be accomplished. Like research itself, the process of doing research is developmental, with each new project building on the experiences and learning that took place during the previous project.

REFERENCES

Case-Smith, J. (1999). Developing a research career: Advice from occupational therapy researchers. *The American Journal of Occupational Therapy, 53*(1), 44–50.

Hammel, J., Finlayson, M., Kielhofner, G., Helfrich, C., & Peterson, E. (2002). Educating scholars of practice: An approach to preparing tomorrow's researchers. *Occupational Therapy in Health Care, 15*(1/2), 157–176.

Helfrich, C. A., Finlayson, M., & Lysack, C. (in press). Using a mentoring community to build programs of research: Lessons learned and recommendations from participating in a mentoring community. *Journal of Allied Health.*

Kielhofner, G., Hammel, J., Helfrich, C., Finlayson, M., & Taylor, R. R. (2004). Studying practice and its outcomes: A conceptual approach. *The American Journal of Occupational Therapy, 58*, 15–23.

Taylor, R. R., Fisher, G. & Kielhofner, G. (2005) Synthesizing research, education, and practice according to the scholarship of practice model: Two faculty examples. *Occupational Therapy in Health Care, 19*, 95–106.

CHAPTER 27

Searching the Literature

M. G. Dieter • Gary Kielhofner

Retrieving available information relevant to a topic is vital to both conducting and being a consumer of research. Two factors are rapidly transforming how investigators and practitioners search for knowledge. The first is an explosion of available information. For instance, in the year 2002, nearly five *exabytes* of information were newly created for storage in print, film, magnetic, and optical media. This new information would fill the equivalent of 500,000 new libraries equal in size to the Library of Congress print collection (Lyman & Varian, 2003). The second factor is how it is currently stored and made accessible. In the past, searching for information mostly involved accessing printed material stored in libraries. Over the last few decades information has become increasing available through information and communications technology (ICT).

While the exponential growth and ready availability of information is a substantial resource, it also means that one can easily be lost in too much information or fail to find all the information one needs. Effective identification and use of information requires a level of literacy. Information literacy is the ability to articulate one's information needs, and subsequently locate, retrieve, and critically evaluate information for its intended use (Association of College and Research Libraries [ACRL], 2000; Jenson, 2004; Saranto & Hovenga, 2004; Swanson, 2004). This chapter overviews what is involved in, and provides resources to enable readers to improve their information literacy.

Online Information Retrieval

All information retrieval (IR) activities are driven by information needs. Occupational therapists need information for purposes such as problem-solving, planning research, finding evidence to guide practice, and personal knowledge development. Information needs generally fall into two categories:

• Ready-reference, and
• Subject searching.

Ready-Reference

Ready-reference information requests are typically very specific, and usually resolved through a closed-ended search process. For example, an occupational therapist may wish to know the following kinds of things about a particular disease: its prevalence, etiology, prognosis, functional implications, and so on. In this instance, the IR task is to identify an appropriate information resource and to access the information (e.g., a text, Web site, and/or recent review article that contains the desired information). Ready-reference tends to be relatively straightforward.

Subject Searching

Subject searching is an iterative and ongoing information-seeking process. Subject searches use a querying method to transform abstract topic concepts into text search queries. These queries are inputted into the interface of online information retrieval tools, such as a bibliographic citation database search engine like PubMed or a Web search engine like Google. The resultant information retrieval is a set of information items ("hits") that have been identified by the search query, and organized or prioritized in some fashion.

Importantly, when one analyzes the retrieved set items, it is common that one will refine the subject. This, then, necessitates more search queries. Consequently, searching is essentially a sifting or

> Information literacy is the ability to articulate information needs, and subsequently locate, retrieve, and critically evaluate of information for appropriate use (Association of College and Research Libraries [ACRL], 2000).

filtering process intended to produce a core set of information items that are identified by a succession of specific search queries.

Searching allows one to integrate information into knowledge. This can take the form of an evidence-based search (as discussed in Chapter 42). The purpose of a search is to exhaustively identify all the information relevant to a topic. In some cases, the search may also put certain parameters on the kind of information one wishes to retrieve. For example, one may wish to limit information sources to published journal articles.

The Process of Information Retrieval

Most IR involves a combination of two broad search strategies, browsing and querying (Taylor, 2004). Each is discussed below:

Browsing

There are basically two browsing methods:

• A structured approach, and
• A serendipitous approach (Taylor, 2004).

Structured browsing involves a preplanned organization of a list of topics. These lists often take the form of a hierarchy in which there is a more general list of topics. Then, within each of these topics a sublist of more specific topics. In this approach, one follows a directed path to the information sought.

The serendipitous approach is more randomized. In this approach, the searcher travels a nonlinear path to information. For example, one might randomly follow an unfolding series of hyperlinks on the World Wide Web, picking up useful information along the way.

Querying

A querying method of information retrieval involves text phrase matching or keyword matching (Taylor, 2004). Phrase matching specifies a particular string of text that is used to reduce the quantity of retrieved items by increasing specificity. For example, an occupational therapist seeking to find appropriate assessments to use in a pediatric setting may begin with the phrase "occupational therapy assessment," proceed to "occupational therapy pediatric assessment," and then to "pediatric occupational therapy observational assessment."

Keyword searching generally involves using one or more words to retrieve information. Importantly, keywords can be logically combined and uniquely related to each other in search queries. This type of search strategy is discussed later in the chapter.

Online Access to Published Information

There are a number of possible ways to access the variety of information resources available online. One important source of access is through institutions that have access to online information resources, such as Web portals. An alternative is Web access through local public or community college libraries. Generally, there are three channels to online information retrieval that provide access to published information resources:

• Online public access catalogs (OPACs),
• Bibliographic citation databases, and
• The World Wide Web (WWW or Web).

In the following sections we focus mainly on strategies for subject query searching involving bibliographic citation databases, since these are the major sources for finding research publications used in evidence-based practice and in the literature review step of the research process.

Online Public Access Catalogs

Libraries and other repositories of information traditionally used catalogs as a point of access for locating their materials. Originally in print format as a book, catalogs later evolved into card catalog and microfilm formats. At present, both individual libraries and networks of libraries use an electronic database of their contents commonly known as an online public access catalog (OPAC). Consortia of OPACs may be networked to provide a wider range of information-locating possibilities. Although OPACs usually have subject searching functionality, OPAC searches tend to be more close-ended, seeking known items at a particular site, for example, a book by a specific author, or a title. OPAC records include bibliographic descriptions of physical items such as books, pamphlets, and periodicals, as well as electronically formatted materials.

Bibliographic Citation Databases

Bibliographic citation databases allow online access to the bibliographic records. Like OPACs, electronic citation databases group information content in certain ways, including by general subject. One example is the National Library of Medicine's (NLM) Medline bibliographic citation database, which offers access to predominantly biomedical information content. Unlike OPACs, the information items constituting a bibliographic citation database are not limited to resources that are located at a particular site or repository. Nonetheless, they may include information about institutions that own a particular book or journal, for instance.

Much of the information content represented by bibliographic citation databases has undergone some kind of review process that ensures its accuracy, originality, authority, rigor, and so on. For the kinds of information that occupational therapists generally seek, this review process ordinarily involves peer review, which is discussed in Chapter 29.

Bibliographic citation databases such as Medline, CINAHL, and the Cochrane Database of Systematic Reviews index research reports, practice guidelines, literature reviews, editorial comments, letters from subscribers, and other information into content groupings. What database one can use and what is available in the database depends on where one is searching from (e.g., through a university or a public library). Each institution has particular subscription arrangements that may provide access to citations only, or access to the full text of the publications.

> Ultimately, the *only* way to improve online searching skills is by continuing to actively perform and refine searches, and to evaluate information retrieval.

The WWW

The World Wide Web or WWW has made possible a wide variety of electronic publications. Unlike bibliographic citation databases, the Web currently lacks standardized indexing. While streamlining the processes of publication and dissemination, the WWW also bypasses traditional processes for evaluating the quality of the information included. Web search engines, along with WWW directories (e.g., Yahoo) that categorize Web information content, are a means of retrieving a wide variety of content published on the Web.

Subject Searching in Bibliographic Citation Databases

Subject Search Strategies

Selecting an online IR subject searching strategy depends on many factors, including:

• The scope and depth of one's information needs,
• The availability of information resources,

• The particular characteristics of the information resources one chooses,
• One's IR skills,
• Available time, and
• Resources to cover costs.

For subject querying bibliographic citation bases, there are two kinds of search processes:

• Concept expansion, and
• Concept contraction.

These are often combined in tandem as complementary iterative processes.

Concept expansion refers to broadening a search topic to include all its relevant dimensions. Concept expansion often originates from a specific item of information item, or a small set of such items. For example, one might receive a few specific research papers from a colleague, or find a previously completed literature review on a topic of interest. Alternatively, one might find a key source by browsing the Web and finding a Web site with a number of bibliographic references on a topic. In each of these instances, these resources are the initial context for conceptual expansion.

The goal of the complementary process, contraction, is to focus the retrieval into a more conceptually consistent, relevant, and manageable set of information. As noted earlier, one frequently alternates expansion and contraction techniques to modify the developing search concept, resulting in a search process that is dynamic and iterative.

In practice, expansion and contraction processes fine-tune the relationship between recall (the comprehensiveness or proportion of available information items available that are retrieved) and precision (i.e., the proportion of retrieved items that are relevant). In general, expansion strategies are aimed toward maximizing recall, while the goal of contraction strategies is precision.

For example, a search process may approach a figure of 100% recall, meaning that one has retrieved nearly every journal article in the bibliographic citation database that has any relevance to one's defined topic. However, if the topic for which one is searching is a well-researched area, one may retrieve more journal articles than one has resources to review and evaluate. Among them would be some that are extremely relevant to one's topic and others that are not particularly useful. To narrow the number of articles to those most relevant, one would use contraction strategies that maximize precision. This would generate fewer articles that more specifically address one's defined topic.

Precision is desirable, but can also be problematic if it results in too few articles and other resources. For instance, if one searches in an area of occupational therapy research for which there is more limited research, a precise search could result in too few articles. Thus, one can use expansion and contraction strategies to help identify just how specific the existing knowledge is, and to identify the right "pool" of articles and other resources to help one develop knowledge of a given topic.

Many online bibliographic citation database search engines and search interfaces have intrinsic search features and syntaxes. It is useful to read all Help screens, and print them out for future reference. The terms and concepts introduced in this chapter are found generally in most advanced search tools, and can save much time in defining a search.

Conducting Online Searches in Bibliographic Citation Databases

This section offers a generalized online IR framework for subject querying. The overall method involves making choices and decisions that lead to a manageable number of resources that can be examined, evaluated, retained or discarded, and used. An effective search strategy first requires that one:

- Transform concepts (topics) into words that will be used to search,
- Logically connect these words by specifying relationships between them, and
- Format them into search syntax appropriate for the bibliographic citation database being searched.

Next, one inputs the search queries into a database search engine interface to retrieve sets of information items. Then, one evaluates the information retrieved to ascertain if it is sufficiently relevant, detailed, and focused to the topic for which one was searching. The process is repeated to refine the search until the retrieved information items meet one's needs.

The overall search process can be guided by four key questions:

- *What* (am I looking for?),
- *Where* (can I find it?),
- *How* (do I access and retrieve it?), and
- *How Well:* (does it satisfy my information requirements?) (Figure 27.1).

Step One: What?

One must first identify one's information needs. Among other factors, this typically includes consideration of:

- Why the information is necessary,
- For whom/what it is intended,
- The format required (e.g., refereed journal articles), and
- The time frame.

This first step is crucial and not as simple as it may appear. How one initially chooses to define a subject influences:

- Later search decisions,
- Selection of which information items to include (e.g., articles, books, reports), and
- Examination and analysis of the information one retrieves (Rieh, 2002).

The ultimate goal of this step is to be clear about what one needs to retrieve so that it can be translated into search terms.

Step Two: Where?

Searching would be greatly simplified if there were a single comprehensive information resource that could be searched. Unfortunately, this is not yet reality. Bates (1989) originally described the process of information-seeking strategy as "berrypicking," since searchers typically go from

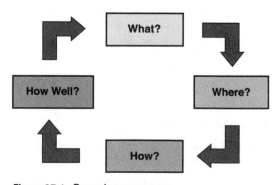

Figure 27.1 Search processes.

resource to resource in search of relevant information items.

A good search process is characterized by making good predictions of where relevant information will be and using retrieved information to further define and articulate the search concept and translate it into further search strategies. When making decisions about information resources, one should seek advice from knowledgeable peers, professors, mentors, colleagues, and reference librarians. General knowledge sources such as dictionaries, encyclopedias, and textbooks often are valuable as a point of entry into unfamiliar subject areas. Frequently, universities have created Web information portals where information resources are organized alphabetically or by subject grouping lists, often with appropriate thumbnail descriptions of the scope of each resource's information content. Figure 27.2 shows a page of the Web information portal found on the Web site of the University of Illinois at Chicago (UIC).

In addition to providing access points to bibliographic citation databases, some Web information portals will also suggest Internet Web sites that may have useful information content. For instance, Figure 27.3 shows UIC Library Internet Resources Page for Occupational Therapy.

Some institutions use metasearch engines that allow federated searching of multiple information resources. For example, Figure 27.4 shows the UIC Library's qUICsearch. It allows one to input a single set of search terms into the search interface that will be sent to many different information sources (mainly bibliographic citation databases) to retrieve a set of appropriate information items from each of them. These multiple sets can be combined, ordered, and sorted in a number of ways.

In general, selecting the appropriate information source depends on one's topic. This makes it difficult to apply a general rule for selecting appropriate information sources. For the purposes of this chapter, we have reduced the range of choices to several bibliographic citation databases that are clearly relevant to occupational therapy, for example, the Cochrane, Medline, and CINAHL bibliographic citation databases. These are not the only

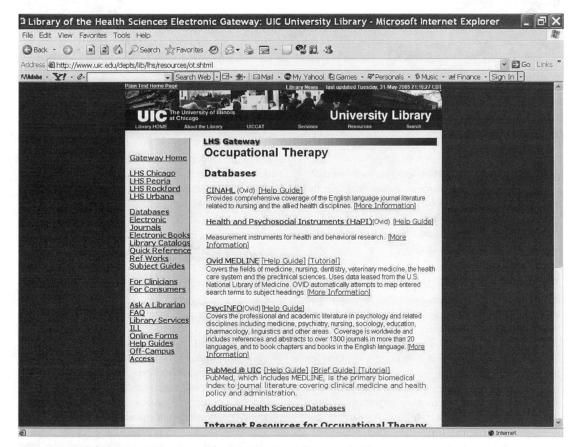

Figure 27.2 UIC library subject page for occupational therapy databases.

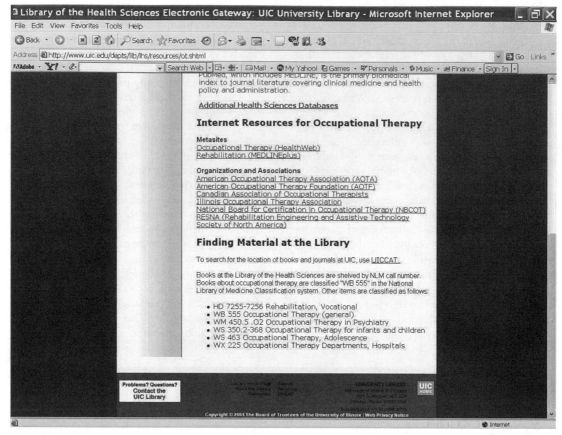

Figure 27.3 UIC library Internet resources page for occupational therapy.

citation databases that an occupational therapist might wish to use, but they are generally a good place to begin.

Once one selects a bibliographic citation database, search queries retrieve citations (i.e., the author, title, date of publishing, journal, etc.) of relevant information items. The citation may or may not be linked to an abstract or to the full text of the information item itself.

Citation Searching

Bibliographic citation analysis is another approach to subject searching. Citation searching means looking at the bibliographic citations or references at the end of articles. It offers another way to expand a search from a single article, chapter, book, or web resource, or from a few such resources. Such references represent the author's or Web creator's efforts to identify important writings from the work of earlier authors. A searcher can than ready-reference search these cited resources.

A prospective (forward-looking) form of citation searching requires access to a bibliographic

citation index database, such as the Thompson Corporation's Institute for Scientific Information (ISI) Web of Knowledge. Using this tool, one can look forward from the original item to identify publications that have subsequently cited it in their own references.

Step Three: How?

The decisions that searchers make during this stage are guided by the first two steps of the process. In this process, one must:

* Articulate and expand the topic into appropriate *search terms* using synonyms,
* Generate a *search query* defining logical relationships between the search terms,
* Apply appropriate *search syntax* to the search query as needed to expand and contract search retrieval in terms of precision and recall, and
* Analyze information content to evaluate how well it corresponds to one's intended topic.

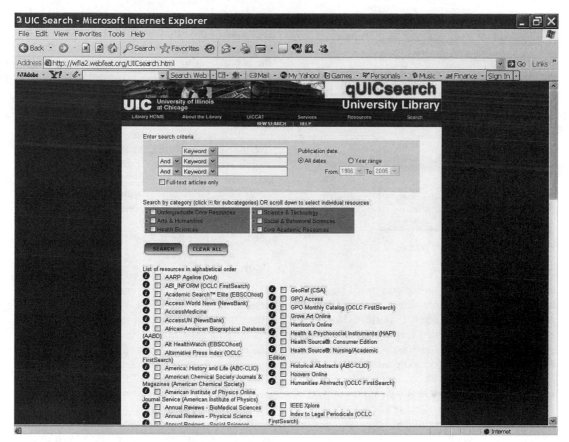

Figure 27.4 UIC's qUICsearch metasearch engine.

As shown in Figure 27.5, these activities are repeated in a cyclical process to refine the search process. These activities are elaborated in the discussion that follows.

Search Terms

The process of selecting search terms involves a process in which one uses information uncovered from the search to derive new search terms that yield the intended information (Dalrymple, 2001). Search terms are items used in search queries that connect the intended topic to text in information items that are retrieved. One continuously identifies new search terms to use to expand or contract the retrieval, improving recall and precision, respectively. For example, using synonyms for search terms is a common way to expand a search and, thus, maximize recall. When this results in irrelevant information being retrieved, one will subsequently use contraction strategies to improve precision. The most common search terms used are keywords and controlled language.

Keywords

Some bibliographic citation database search engines allow one to enter keyword search terms by providing a text box with a drop-down label specifying each text entry as belonging to one or more of the database's fields. These keywords are used to find information items in one of two ways. First, bibliographic citation databases sometimes index information items by selecting several key terms that describe the general scope of its content. In this instance, articles and other information items that have been assigned those keywords are retrieved. Second, keywords may be used to identify articles or other information items for which the keyword occurred in the title, author, subject, abstract fields, or full text.

Controlled Language

Some databases have features that allow one to retrieve specific kinds of information items. For example, the contents in a database may be organized according to a structured classification sys-

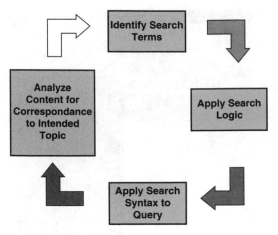

Figure 27.5 The search process.

tem. In this case, one can use controlled language terms to specify a more direct pathway to the information items one wants to retrieve. However, effective use of controlled language search terms requires one to understand how an information resource's content has been organized. Controlled language searches result in increased precision when the correct subject headings are used.

In some databases content is already organized (precoordinated) into controlled language classification systems that use subject headings, thesauri, and ontologies as means of classifying and locating content. In addition, controlled language systems provide cross-references and links between related terms to assist one in finding the appropriate subject heading.

The National Library of Medicine's Medline Medical Subject Headings system, (MeSH), and the Cumulative Index of Nursing and Allied Health Literature (CINAHL) Subject Headings are examples of controlled languages that are relevant for occupational therapists' information needs. Both are hierarchical arrangements of subject headings. Medline's content is predominately biomedical and clinical medicine, while CINAHL's is related to nursing and allied health. Both systems provide scope notes that explain the use of each subject heading, its position in the hierarchy, and the history of its use. Some bibliographic citation database search interfaces, like Ovid, map natural language terms to the correct subject headings, or present a list of near matches from which searchers can select a subject heading.

The Search Query

Skill in specifying logical relationships between search terms enhances one's ability to use expan-

sion or contraction strategies that maximize either the recall or precision. Both kinds of strategies can be incorporated into a single search query through the use of nesting, described in the section below on Boolean logic. One's competence in post-coordinating the logic of information retrieval processes will enhance the meaning and relevance of what one is able to retrieve.

Search query logic is arguably the most effective means of applying expansion and contraction search strategies to maximize retrieval recall and precision. When one configures precoordinated controlled language search terms using post-coordinated search logic one increases the likelihood of retrieving exactly the information one needs. This process is known as set searching.

Boolean Logic

The search logic that is commonly used in bibliographic citation databases is called Boolean logic, after 19th century English mathematician George Boole (Kluegel, 2001). Using Boolean logic, one can connect search terms, allowing more control over the information retrieved than when using individual search terms. While it may seem intimidating at first, it is well worth learning to increase the precision of searching.

Following the four-step search process described in this chapter, one enters search queries using syntax appropriate to the bibliographic citation database that is being used. The search engine then retrieves a set of information items that fit the requirements specified in the search query.

Boolean relationships specify the inclusion or exclusion of content that matches the text of search terms in search queries, as illustrated graphically in Figure 27.6. Each circle represents an information retrieval set that matches a text search term; each pair of circles represents the use of a different Boolean search operator to logically relate two search terms, changing what is retrieved. There are three main Boolean operators: AND, OR, and NOT.

Boolean AND. The Boolean AND logical condition creates an exclusive set of information items that match the specific text of both search terms. As shown in the left diagram in Figure 27.6, the relationship between "dogs AND cats" defines a retrieval set that includes only articles that are about *both* dogs and cats. By specifying dogs AND cats, one would not retrieve articles that are only about dogs or only about cats. As show in Figure 27.6, the shaded area representing the intersection of the two sets defines a set of articles mentioning both dogs and cats in their information content. As

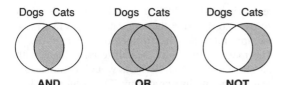

Figure 27.6 A Venn diagram of Boolean search logic.

this example illustrates, the Boolean AND operator can be used in contraction search strategies to increase the precision in retrieval sets.

Boolean OR. The Boolean OR logical condition creates a set of all information items that match the specific text of either of the search terms. As shown in the middle diagram in Figure 27.6, by specifying "dogs OR cats" one will retrieve articles about dogs, articles about cats, and articles about both dogs and cats. In the diagram, the shaded area represents the union of the two sets, a set of articles mentioning dogs, cats, and both dogs and cats. As this example illustrates, the Boolean OR operator can be used in expansion search strategies to increase recall.

Boolean NOT. The Boolean NOT logical condition creates an exclusive set of all information items that match only the specific text of one of the search terms. As shown the right diagram in Figure 27.6, specifying "cats NOT dogs" defines a retrieval set that includes articles about cats only. In this instance, any articles about cats that also contain information about dogs would be eliminated from the search set. In this case, the shaded area represents elimination of the dog set from the cat set; that is, articles about dogs, and articles about both cats and dogs are eliminated, leaving articles about cats only. The Boolean NOT operator can be used in contraction search strategies to increase precision.

Nesting

Nesting allows Boolean search term relationships to be combined with each other in a search query to improve control over the set of retrieval items. Parentheses are used to separate the search term relationships. For example, a nested statement would be "((cats OR dogs) AND pets) AND health." This search query would result in the retrieval of items about the health of cats and/or dogs that are pets. It is important to remember that leading and closing parentheses must enclose each logical set. One can readily see how much more precision is achieved by using this kind of search logic than simply searching for the key terms cats,

dogs, pets, and health. Among many other kinds of articles irrelevant to the intended topic would be those about pets that are not cats or dogs, and those about the health of humans.

Search Syntax

In general, each bibliographic citation database search interface has its own syntax or format rules specifying operations on search terms and queries. One should rely upon printouts of Help screens if one is unfamiliar with the commands. However, some generic syntax functions and commands that are common to many online information retrieval resources can be used to expand or contract retrieval.

Case Sensitivity

In general, most bibliographic citation database search engines are not case sensitive. The default condition is typically lowercase, and the retrieval includes lower- and uppercase occurrences.

Truncation

This is a useful search operator for expanding retrieval to account for multiple forms of a term, or when the exact spelling of the term is uncertain. The most frequent types of truncation functionality are termed "right-hand" and "left-hand"; most search engines offer right-hand (the end of the term). The specific operator varies, but often the "?", "#", or "*" character is used for truncation. An example of right-hand truncation is the search term "librar*." The retrieval would include items with "library," "libraries," "library's," "librarian," "librarians," and "librarianship." Left-hand truncation is situated at the leading end of a search term, and is used infrequently. Middle truncation functionality is less commonly available than right-hand truncation, but more so than left-hand truncation, for example, "wom#n" used for "woman" or "women."

Phrases

Some bibliographic citation databases allow phrase searching. Phrase searching searches for an exact string of text. This increases precision and reduces retrieval. For example, a search for "reduce tactile defensiveness" or "increase range of motion" would retrieve only information items in which those specific phrases occurred.

Proximity

Proximity searching (also called adjacency or positional searching) is a useful tool for specifying the relationship of terms by their nearness to each other in the text of the information item. For example, one might search for items about health care workers, and could search using the phrase "health care workers." This strategy might eliminate a number of useful information items that do not use the exact phrase "health care workers," such as "workers in health care" or "workers employed by health care providers." A proximity search operator allows one to expand the search, increasing the recall to include terms that are near each other in an article or other information item. Some bibliographic citation database search engines use "adj," "n," or "w" to specify proximity. The order of the search terms often specifies the order of occurrence in the text. More powerful search engines can specify the number of words that may occur between the terms in the item, or their order of occurrence. Proximity can be used as an expansion or contraction strategy.

Analyzing Information Content Evaluatively

When new information items are retrieved, one must evaluate them in terms of their relevancy to the topic for which one is searching. Also, one may use the retrieved information as feedback that can lead to broadening or narrowing of one's intended topic. This reflects the fact that the search process is iterative, with each step informing the next.

Sample Query

Prior to searching online, a good way to begin is by diagramming the terms one intends to use along with their logical relationships in a matrix. By doing this, one is constructing a nested search query from search terms that best represent the topic for which one is searching.

Figure 27.7 shows how a searcher might begin the process on paper with a search matrix for the research question: "What statistical methods might be used to describe the outcomes of occupational therapy interventions for persons with stroke?" The matrix rows show search terms related with the Boolean "AND," which would contract the search, facilitating precision. The columns relate terms with the Boolean "OR," which would expand the concept, facilitating recall.

Ideally one would employ an information resource that allows set searching, allowing one to use search terms related by Boolean logic. For the purpose of demonstration, Figure 27.8 illustrates and explains an example of a single search query that combines the matrix search terms according to the specified Boolean logic, using a generic syntax.

One should note that in the examples in Figure 27.8, lowercase and truncation functionalities were used to expand the terms further. In addition, positional syntax was substituted for phrase matching as a means of fine-tuning contraction. Truncation also reduced the number of search terms required for entry by accounting for variants of several terms (e.g., rehab* for rehabilitation, rehabilitate). In bibliographic citation databases such as CINAHL that use controlled language, there is pre-coordination of terms like "occupational therapy," which eliminates the need for positional syntax. Many variations of the query shown in Figure 27.8 are possible for querying the research question, as is true for all online subject search queries.

Post-Qualification and Limiting

At any point in the retrieval process, searchers can choose to further focus a retrieval set by limiting the retrieval to a certain time period, type of publication, language, or source. Typically, this is done near the final steps of the process. Searchers can also post-qualify terms by specifying occurrence

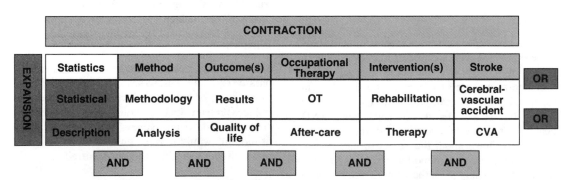

Figure 27.7 Initial topic expansion and contraction using Boolean relationships of search terms for the research question: "What statistical methods are used to describe the outcomes of occupational therapy interventions for persons with stroke?"

Note: Assume that "*" is used as a right-hand truncation symbol for 0 to *n* characters; and "*w*" is a proximity operator, where an optional number can be used to specify positional distance in number of words, e.g., the use of "*w2*" to specify the positional arrangement as shown in the example below. A logical representation of the relationships in the matrix could appear as below. In this case each "AND" separates text representing a column of the matrix.

(statistic* OR (descript* OR describe*)) AND (method* OR analy*) AND

(outcome* OR result* OR (quality*w **2)) AND ((occupational***w* **therapy) OR**

ot OR (aftercare OR (after*w* **care)) AND (intervent* OR rehab* OR therap*).**

This query contains the following elements:

- (statistic* OR (descript* OR describe*)) Inclusive expansion of column 1 of the matrix
- AND Used to contract the retrieval
- (method* OR analy*) Inclusive expansion of column 2 of the matrix
- AND Used to contract the retrieval
- (outcome* OR result* OR (quality *w2* life)) Inclusive expansion of column 3 of the matrix
- AND Used to contract the retrieval
- ((occupational *w* therapy) OR ot OR (aftercare OR (after *w* care)) Inclusive expansion of column 4 of the matrix
- AND Used to contract the retrieval by limiting inclusion
- (intervent* OR rehab* OR therap*) Inclusive expansion of column 5 of the matrix.

Figure 27.8 A sample search query derived from Figure 27.7.

in a particular database field, such as the title. This would reduce the amount of retrieval.

Step Four: How Well?

There are two levels of analysis at this stage; they concern:

- How well the information retrieved fulfills one's needs, and
- The reliability of the information items.

Although published literature often undergoes some form of a pre-publication review process (e.g., peer review), it is important for searchers to develop their criteria for critical thinking skills. For example, one may establish the criteria that all the articles one wants must employ random sampling of subjects or that they have a minimum sample size.

Critical evaluation requires that one select, weigh, and apply appropriate criteria to the information retrieved. For purposes of critically evaluating reports of research, the various discussions of methodological rigor in this text are a useful source of criteria. In the end, the criteria one uses

will vary by the purpose for which the information was retrieved. For example, in conducting a general literature review to refine a research question, one may include a wide range of studies that employ different research methods. For a meta-analysis (see Chapter 18) one may have very strict criteria related to sampling, the nature of the independent variable, presence of a control group, and so forth.

Searching the World Wide Web

Web Search Engines

Web search engines must comb a vast information space that grows larger every day. Unlike comparatively small, well organized, and well structured bibliographic citation databases, the WWW lacks a systematic schema of organization. Therefore, search engines used for searching the WWW have several distinguishing characteristics. Kluegel (2001) has suggested that Web search engines are in reality comprised of three parts:

- The crawler,
- The index, and
- The search engine itself.

The search engine crawler is a software tool that continually traverses the WWW looking for new information content and for information content changes. Information that the crawler locates is stored in an index. The search engine searches the index for query matches to terms that one enters. The way in which specific Web search engines identify, select, and prioritize information content for retrieval display is commonly proprietary knowledge, often patented by software designers. The most important thing to remember is that no one Web search tool has yet indexed or catalogued the entire WWW. An example of a Web search engine is Google (http://www.google.com/), one of the most extensively used search engines.

Web Search Tips. Like searching bibliographic databases, it is important to apply logical strategies for searching the Web. Here are some general considerations for using Web search engines to search the WWW:

- Utilize the Help function to identify search functionality and proper syntax.
- Use topic-appropriate keywords.
- Add more search terms to reduce retrieval.
- Check spelling; although some Web search tools may prompt for spelling errors, not all search engines have this function (this tip applies generally to all search queries).
- Look for an Advanced interface that gives more control to the searcher.
- Use phase searching to increase specificity and reduce retrieval size.
- Check for Boolean and nesting functionality; when entering multiple search terms, the default connector is usually "AND." Check if "+" and "−" can be used to force inclusion or exclusion of terms, respectively.
- Look for word stemming or truncation functionality to increase recall.
- Use the text search function in your browser to find text in the pages you select for examination; hit ctrl-f to open the search text box.

Metasearch Engines

Metasearch engines provide a single search interface for a cluster of individual search engines. The search terms one enters are transmitted to each of the component search engines. The resultant retrieval is usually categorized according to the component search tool. Additional processing of the information retrieval may eliminate multiple occurrences and organize the content in some fashion. Because individual search engines index only portions of the WWW, metasearch tools are a way to expand the scope of information retrieval, effectively improving the search recall. Examples of metasearch engines are Vivisimo (http://vivisimo.com/), metacrawler (http://metacrawler.com/), and DogPile (http://www.DogPile.com/).

Web Directories

Web directories are organized lists of WWW information content. The typical organizational structure is hierarchical. Unlike Web search engines, Web directories do not use crawlers to seek out or refresh information content, relying instead on Web authors to register their Web page or Web site with the directory. Most use a search engine to find a suitable subject point of access for searchers to subsequently browse from by clicking links. An example of a Web directory is Yahoo (http://www.yahoo.com/), a well known Web information portal, providing links to many different kinds of information and commercial sites.

Information Resources Relevant to Occupational Therapy

Ultimately, a wide range of resources are potentially relevant to occupational therapy. In this section, we discuss some of those most frequently used by occupational therapists.

Medline

Medline is a bibliographic citation database with more than 13 million references from 4800 biomedical journals and magazines covering the period from 1966 to present (plus some articles published between 1963 and present). This database can be searched free of charge using the National Library of Medicine (NLM) PubMed system at http://pubmed.gov. It is searchable using keywords or the (NLM) controlled language, MeSH (National Library of Medicine, 2004). The MeSH hierarchical tree structure includes "occupational therapy" as a precoordinated terminal subject heading under the subject heading "Rehabilitation," as shown in Figure 27.9. There are approximately 4,000 information items with an MeSH major topic focus of "occupational therapy" in Medline. The NLM provides free access to Medline via its Web-based PubMed search interface. Medline does not provide full text access online to information items, but specific institutions may offer links to electronic versions of journal articles indexed in Medline as part of publisher contractual arrangements.

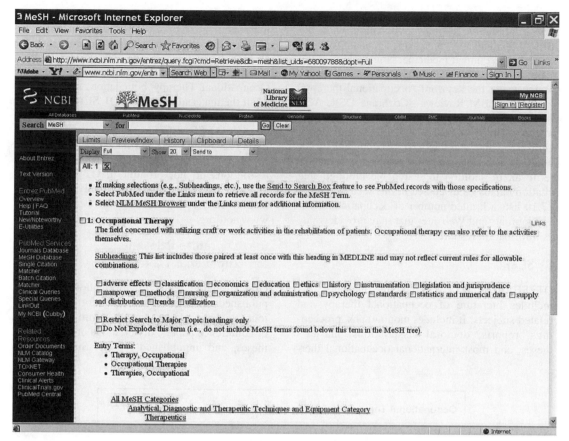

Figure 27.9 PubMed MeSH subject heading note for "Occupational Therapy."

CINAHL

The organizational structure of the CINAHL bibliographic citation database resembles Medline, but the focus of its information content lies in the fields of allied health. In addition to identifying "Occupational Therapy" as a CINAHL subject heading, there are nearly a dozen expanded OT variant subject headings that facilitate improved information retrieval selectivity. Altogether, controlled language terms with occupational therapy major subject headings translate into approximately 6,000 information items that are relevant to occupational therapy. In view of this, CINAHL should be considered a principal information resource for occupational therapy. Unlike Medline, CINAHL is a proprietary information resource that requires institutional access. Moreover, unlike Medline, CINAHL publication types include a number of formats other than journal articles, some with full text content. For the most part, links to electronic journal content are usually provided by institutions' contractual arrangements with journal publishers.

The Cochrane Library Databases

The Cochrane Collaboration prepares and disseminates systematic reviews of health care interventions, published in the Cochrane Library, that focuses mainly on controlled trials (Guyatt, Rennie, Evidence-Based Medicine Working Group, & American Medical Association, 2002). The main value of the Cochrane Library databases to occupational therapy is their potential as a resource to guide evidence-based practice. There are three main sections:

- The Cochrane Database of Systematic Reviews (CDSR), which contains reports on systematic reviews and protocols,
- The Database of Reviews of Effectiveness (DARE), which are searchable systematic reviews published outside Cochrane, and
- The Cochrane Controlled Trials Registry (CCTR), which includes economic and health technology assessments (Guyatt et al., 2002).

Some institutions package the Cochrane databases with *ACP Journal Club*, a publication of the

American College of Physicians, and *Evidence-Based Medicine*, a joint publication with the British Medical Journal Group. The main focus of Cochrane is clinical medicine. Nonetheless, at the time this chapter was being written, a simple search using the keyword "occupational therapy" in the All EBM Reviews—Cochrane DSR, ACP Journal Club, DARE, and CCTR database resulted in the retrieval of nearly 500 information items. Unlike Medline and CINAHL, Cochrane does not use a controlled language for selective information retrieval. In addition to searchable bibliographic citation databases discussed in this section, Figure 27.10 lists a limited number of occupational therapy journals and Web sites that may provide value as information resources.

OT SEARCH

OT SEARCH is a bibliographic database that includes literature of occupational therapy and related subjects. It includes monographs, proceedings, reports, doctoral dissertations, master's theses, and most international occupational ther-

apy journals (published in English) as well as journals related to the field. This database includes only bibliographic information and the abstract when there is one. The Wilma L. West (WLW) Library, which is part of the American Occupational Therapy Foundation, owns a copy of all the material indexed in OT SEARCH. If one is unable to otherwise locate material found through OT SEARCH, one can contact the WLW library to arrange an interlibrary loan or a photocopy (for a nominal charge) where copyright restrictions do not prohibit it. OT SEARCH is available on a subscription basis only. More information on the database can be found at http://www.aotf.org.

Gray Literature Relevant to Occupational Therapy

Gray literature refers to information that is not published or available in usual formats such as journals. Examples of gray literature are abstracts of conference papers, dissertations or unpublished theses, and unpublished reports. Such literature

---

Occupational Therapy Journals and Web Sites:

Journals and Periodicals

- *ADVANCE for Occupational Therapy Practitioners*
- *American Journal for Occupational Therapy*
- *Australian Occupational Therapy Journal*
- *British Journal of Occupational Therapy*
- *Canadian Journal of Occupational Therapy*
- *International Journal of Rehabilitation Research*
- *Irish Journal for Occupational Therapy*
- *Occupational Therapy in Health Care*
- *Occupational Therapy in Mental Health*
- *Occupational Therapy International*
- *Occupational Therapy Journal of Research*
- *Occupational Therapy Now*
- *Physical and Occupational Therapy in Geriatrics*
- *Physical and Occupational Therapy in Paediatrics*
- *Scandinavian Journal of Occupational Therapy*
- *South African Journal of Occupational Therapy*
- *Therapy Weekly*

Web Sites

- American Occupational Therapy Association (AOTA) http://www.aota.org/
- American Occupational Therapy Foundation (AOTF) http://www.aotf.org/
- Canadian Association of Occupational Therapists http://www.caot.ca/
- Illinois Occupational Therapy Association http://www.ilota.org/
- National Board for Certificaltion in Occupational Therapy (NBCOT) http://www.nbcot.org
- British Association of Occupational Therapists/College of Occupational Therapists http://www.cot.co.uk
- OTSeeker http://www.otseeker.com/

Figure 27.10 Some occupational therapy journals and Web sites.

may contain vital and specific information. Some organizations, such as the United Kingdom College of Occupational Therapists, London (http://www.cot.co.uk), have developed specialist libraries of gray literature that are available to review on request. The Internet significantly augmented the availability of gray literature. However, not all of this type information is electronically available.

Specific Content Web Sites

A number of Web sites are available that can provide access to various sources of information (including publications) related to a specific topic. One example is the Web site for Sensory Integration International (http://home.earthlink. net/~sensoryint/), a nonprofit corporation related to the sensory integration model of practice. The Web site lists publications relevant to sensory integration and provides a newsletter. Another example is the Model of Human Occupation (MOHO) Clearinghouse Web site (http://www.moho.uic. edu), which not only maintains an up-to-date bibliography of publications related to the model, but also has a search engine that can be used to identify published materials related to specific topics such as MOHO-based assessments and interventions in specific practice areas.

Conclusion

Skill in online searching is fundamental to information literacy, and a valuable asset for professional development and practice. Occupational therapists seeking to improve information literacy skills should begin by identifying a core set of useful occupational therapy information resources, and then concentrate on mastering the intricacies of the search tools or interfaces required to access their information content. Ultimately, the *only* way to improve online searching skills is by continuing

to actively perform and refine searches, and to evaluate information retrieval.

REFERENCES

Association of College and Research Libraries (ACRL). (2000). *Information literacy competency standards for higher education.* Retrieved August 9, 2004 from http://www.ala.org/ala/acrl/acrlstandards/informationliteracycompetency.htm

Bates, M. J. (1989). *The design of browsing and berrypicking techniques* Retrieved August 10, 2004 from http://www.gseis.ucla.edu/faculty/bates/berrypicking. html

Dalrymple, P. W. (2001). Bibliographic control, organization of information, and search strategies. In R. E. Bopp, & L. C. Smith (Eds.), *Reference and information services: An introduction* (3rd ed., pp. 69–96). Englewood, CO; Libraries Unlimited.

Guyatt, G., Rennie, D., Evidence-Based Medicine Working Group, & American Medical Association. (2002). *Users' guides to the medical literature: A manual for evidence-based clinical practice* (JAMA & archives journals) Chicago: AMA Press.

Jenson, J. D. (2004). It's the information age, so where's the information? *College Teaching, 52*(3), 107–112.

Kluegel, K. M. (2001). Electronic resources for reference. In R. E. Bopp & L. C. Smith (Eds.), *Reference and information services: An introduction* (3rd ed.). Englewood, Colorado: Libraries Unlimited.

Lyman, I., & Varian, H. R. (2003) *How much information? 2003 Executive summary* Retrieved August 10, 2004 from http://www.sims.berkeley.edu/research/projects/how-much-info-2003/execsum.html

National Library of Medicine. (2004). FAQ: Finding medical information in MEDLINE. Retrieved September 8, 2004 from http://www.nlm.nih.gov/services/usemedline.html

Rieh, S. Y. (2002). Judgment of information quality and cognitive authority in the web. *Journal of the American Society for Information Science and Technology, 53*(2), 145–161.

Saranto, K., & Hovenga, E. J. S. (2004). Information literacy—what it is about?: literature review of the concept and the context. *International Journal of Medical Informatics, 73*(6), 503–513.

Swanson, T. A. (2004). A radical step: Implementing a critical information literacy model. *Libraries and the Academy, 4*(2), 259–273.

Taylor, A. G. (2004). *The organization of information* (2nd ed.). Library and Information Science Text Series. Westport, CT: Libraries Unlimited.

CHAPTER 28

Generating Research Questions, Design, and Methods

Marian Arbesman • Hector W. H. Tsang

The research question is a statement of the specific knowledge that is being sought in the study. Generating this question is the most important step of the entire research process, as this directs the course of the subsequent study, particularly the design and methods of the investigation (Bordage & Dawson, 2003). Not surprisingly, generating the question, design, and methods is one of the most challenging aspects of the research process. In this chapter we examine key aspects of this process and discuss the role of creativity in developing sound research questions, design, and methods.

> Research problems are broadly defined gaps in knowledge, while research questions are narrow, focused, and specific questions intended to generate knowledge to help close the gap.

The Research Problem, Question, Purpose, Hypothesis, Design, and Methods

Investigators usually begin the research process by identifying their main area of interest. After this, they proceed to clarify a research problem, which is a gap in current knowledge within a specific topic area. Once the research problem is identified, it provides the groundwork for defining specific research questions that can be answered in the research study. Research problems are broadly defined gaps in knowledge, while research questions are narrow, focused, and specific questions intended to generate knowledge to help close the gap.

After delineating the research questions, one clarifies the research purpose. The statement of research purpose should be precise and concise. It describes what the study will accomplish and what will be the value of the study.

A research hypothesis states the expected results of quantitative study. Not all quantitative studies will have stated hypotheses. Most commonly, hypotheses are stated when the analysis will involve inferential statistics or when the study is comparing a dependent variable across two or more groups. More specific discussions of hypotheses are found in Chapters 7 and 17.

The research design and methods refers to the specific strategies that the investigator will use to answer the question or questions that guide the research (or to test a hypothesis where a hypothesis is included). Decisions about design and methods begin broad and become more detailed as the specific investigation is planned. Generally an investigator first decides whether a study will be quantitative or qualitative, or whether it will combine methods from these two approaches. Then the investigator makes a decision about the specific type of research design such as whether the study will be:

- A mailed survey to a national sample,
- A participant observational study of a specific setting,
- A single-subject design replicated across three clients,
- A series of focus groups with providers and consumers of service in a type of setting, or
- An experimental study with two independent variables composed of two different intervention approaches.

Once the decision is made about the study design, the investigator will proceed to more specific decisions and tasks such as selecting the data collection instruments, determining the sample for the study, planning the specific analysis and how it will be done, and determining logistical aspects of the study such as timing, costs, space, and equipment. Importantly these decisions are often iterative. That is, as one attempts to operationalize a research question into specific methods and design, new insights are gained that may lead to revision of the research question. Sometimes as one proceeds to plan the specific methods, it becomes apparent that the research design will not adequately answer the question or that another question needs to be added to the study. Thus, while an investigator generally proceeds from the question to the design and methods, it is not unusual to work back and forth between these tasks.

Uncovering the Research Problem and Question

There are many ways an investigator can uncover a research problem and question. Later in this chapter, we discuss a process for identifying the research question and translating it into a design and methods for the study. Below are some key sources of information that can help lead to identification of a research question.

Clinical Experience

Clinical experience is a good medium from which to identify a research problem and related questions. For instance, therapists often encounter problems such as not having an assessment for a specific purpose or not knowing which services will best help a given client group. Therapists routinely raise questions about clinical phenomena such as:

• Is an assessment reliable or valid?
• Is a treatment approach or modality effective?
• What accounts for different treatment outcomes within a defined population?
• Are there ways to improve the treatment outcome for a particular group?

These types of clinical questions can be tremendously helpful to uncover relevant research questions.

The following is an example of how a research question emerged from practice. Psychosocial skills training and a supported employment are two intervention approaches that have been typically used to improve vocational outcomes of individu-als with severe mental illness. As a practitioner-researcher, one of the authors had used both of these approaches separately. Thus, the question arose as to whether vocational outcomes would be better if these two interventions were combined. This led to an investigation that examined an integrated supported employment model that combined both approaches (Tsang, 2003).

Occupational Therapy Theory

A number of conceptual models or theoretical frameworks have been developed in occupational therapy. Their theory often serves as the basis for developing a research question. Theories explain phenomena and predict what things will happen given certain circumstances. Researchers can use theories to logically deduce expected observations or to make predictions. Research questions derived in this manner can be used to guide studies that test occupational therapy theory. An example of how theory directs research is provided later in the case illustrations.

Directions of Professional Organizations and Funding Agencies

Local, state, and national professional organizations (both for occupational therapy and for other fields) develop strategic plans that may incorporate short- and long-term research goals. By examining the goals and policy statements, whether or not they are related to research, one may discover an approach that can lead to a viable research problem and question.

For example, in recent years, the aging population of Hong Kong has increased. In response to this trend, the Hong Kong Occupational Therapy Association has put a great deal of emphasis on research and development of services for the elderly population. A study on psychosocial functioning of elderly people in Hong Kong was developed in response to this development (Tsang, Cheang, Tong, & Tse, 2004).

Another important consideration in the generation of research questions is consideration of funding priorities. As discussed in Chapter 30, funding agencies often have mission statements or indications of their overall funding priorities. Moreover, some funding agencies routinely generate requests for proposals that indicate research problems they would like to see addressed in grant proposals. Paying attention to what funding agencies consider as priorities for research can be helpful not only in generating ideas, but also in identifying research problems and questions for which there is likely to be funding support.

Literature Review

Reading the literature is key to developing any research question. There are many ways that one can find gaps in knowledge that will lead to a research question. For example, reviewing a study involving a specific population or context may trigger the question as to whether a described approach can be applied to different types of clients or in another setting. Or, one may recognize inconsistencies of findings across several studies that point out the need for further research efforts to account for these inconsistencies.

Narrowing Down the Research Focus

After identifying the general problem and question for the study, one must refine the question to become practical and manageable. As noted earlier, the research question will serve as a framework working out the design and methods of the study. Since the research question implies many elements of the actual study, one must think forward to these when developing the research question.

How one frames the research question will, first of all, determine whether a quantitative or qualitative approach is most appropriate to answer the research. As discussed in previous chapters these two traditions of research involve very different assumptions about the research process and include different approaches to assuring the dependability and validity of findings. Table 28.1 shows examples of research questions reflecting quantitative and qualitative approaches.

Similarly, every research question implies a research design best suited to answer it. For example, if the research question asks about the characteristics of a particular group, a descriptive research design will be appropriate. If the question asks about whether two groups experiencing different treatments would have different outcomes, an experimental design is required (Portney & Watkins, 2000).

Different research questions also require differing amounts and kinds of resources to answer them. Identifying available resources is important in designing your research. Questions should be formulated with an understanding of the kinds of funding, space, instruments, personnel, access to participants, and other resources that will be necessary to answer the question.

As discussed in Chapter 29, the consideration of participants' rights needs to be foremost in the development of any research protocol. Ethical issues and privacy regulations such as the Health Insurance Portability and Accountability Act in the U.S. (HIPAA, 2004) may constrain the kind of questions that can be asked.

The Role of Creativity in Developing Research Questions, Design, and Methods

The research process can appear to be the antithesis of creativity. Nonetheless, creativity can be a

Table 28.1 **Examples of Quantitative and Qualitative Research Questions**

Quantitative Research Questions	Qualitative Research Questions
Will children identified with tactile defensiveness assigned to 6 weeks of therapy based on sensory integration show greater reduction of their tactile defensiveness when compared to children assigned to receive play-oriented therapy?	What is the experience of children with tactile defensiveness when they participate in occupational therapy based on sensory integration principles?
Is higher confidence for returning to work related to an increase in job-seeking behavior among persons with AIDS?	What is the perspective on working among persons with AIDS whose work has been interrupted, and what are the range of concerns they express about returning to work?
Will persons living in nursing homes report fewer occupational roles than a matched samples of persons living in their homes?	What happens to the occupational roles of persons when they enter a nursing home?

The Creative Process and Brainstorming

Descriptions of the creative process fall into two camps. The first describes creative problem solving as taking place within the unconscious, involving incubation of an idea followed by sudden illumination that produces an "Aha!" or "Eureka!" (Simon, 1981). The second sees creativity as dependent on a conscious, systematic process and asks, "How can we develop strategies that enable us to come up with more creative and innovative research ideas?" In time, researchers may have their share of spontaneous inspirations but most of the creative process in research involves the conscious, systematic use of strategies that support creativity.

Definitions of Creativity

Ackoff and Vergara (1988) and Sternberg and Lubart (1999) point out that:

- Creativity is the process of producing something that is both original and valuable, and
- The development of a creative idea is a process that can be developed and enhanced, not just something that occurs by chance.

Creativity also involves two complementary divergent and convergent processes:

- Openness to new ideas combined with efforts to generate as many divergent ideas as possible (e.g., brainstorming), and

- Creativity incorporates a disciplined evaluation component to determine the utility of any idea and thus converge on the idea or ideas that have the greatest usefulness.

Brainstorming

The best known of the divergent tools is "brainstorming," a term coined by Osborn (1979). Brainstorming requires deferring judgment while striving for a large number of ideas including those that are free-wheeling and wild along with conservative ones. There are many ways to engage in brainstorming related to research. When doing individual brainstorming, the process of coming up with new ideas can be augmented by using the Forced Fitting tool (i.e., spending a minute or two looking at objects that have no obvious link to the problem that one is working on) (Isaksen et al., 2000). Brainstorming in groups can enable members to piggyback or build on the ideas of others. Evidence indicates that electronic brainstorming (i.e., requests for ideas sent out by email requests) can successfully generate new ideas (Dennis & Valacich, 1993). This process may be highly effective if one is working as part of a research team that is spread out geographically or when one wants to consult with international experts in a particular area.

---

powerful tool in developing the research question, design, and methods. There is a long history of creativity in the scientific and social science research literature (Bohn & Peat, 1987; Popper, 1959; Root-Bernstein, 1997)

The Creative Problem-Solving (CPS) Process

The Creative Problem-Solving Process (CPS) is a specific disciplined approach to creativity that can enhance one's ability to generate creative ideas and solutions (Noller, 1977). It is a way of looking at problems that combines:

- The generation of many new ideas, and
- The critical thinking needed to decide whether or not a given idea will work.

It also provides the tools to determine how a specific idea can be put into practice. In this section we examine how the CPS process can be applied to the task of generating a research question and selecting the research design and methods.

Components and Stages of the CPS Process

Originally developed by Osborn (1979), the CPS process has been refined into six stages that make up three main components (Figure 28.1) (Isaksen, Dorval, & Treffinger, 2000; Lewin & Reed, 1998). Each stage of the process incorporates tools that facilitate divergent or convergent thinking. Applied to the task of generating a research question, divergent thinking tools allow one to generate many ideas and to speculate about possibilities related to a given research topic. Convergent tools enable one to select from the ideas and possibilities generated and to formulate a focused research topic and generate an appropriate research question.

In the sections that follow, we apply the CPS process to the task of generating research questions and deciding on the methods for addressing the question or questions that are finally selected. The feature box on the next page titled "An Example of the Creative Problem-Solving Process" illustrates

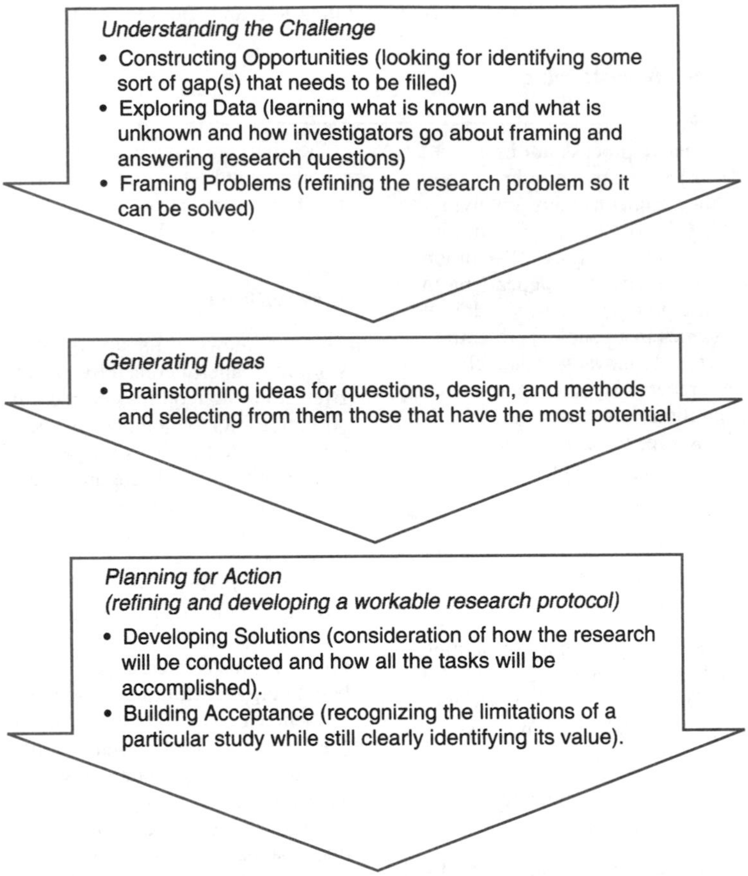

Figure 28.1 The creative problem solving process applied to generating a research questions and translating them into research plans.

An Example of the Creative Problem-Solving Process

The following is a hypothetical example of an occupational therapy researcher who is generally interested in the topic of head injury.

Understanding the Challenge

Constructing Opportunities

During this first phase, an occupational therapy researcher interested in head injury might:

- Read some key chapters in occupational therapy texts to identify what are the main types of services offered, and what theories guide services in this area;
- Identify one or more settings where occupational therapists are providing services to persons with head injury in order to observe and discuss intervention with therapists;
- Attend workshops in which experts discuss practice and research in the area, and/or
- Begin to read some studies related to occupational therapy and head injury in order to identify different approaches to research in this area.

By engaging in these activities, our hypothetical occupational therapy researcher may identify a particular interest in acute care and early rehabilitation services. It would also become apparent that the main services in this area are focused on cognitive–perceptual problems and on problems of motor coordination. Furthermore, input from practitioners and from reading would identify that there is a relatively new, motor control approach in this area for which there are not yet detailed assessment procedures or interventions. Thus, as a result of this phase, the researcher decides that the lack of assessments and intervention protocols related to motor control represents important gaps in knowledge.

Exploring Data
Having identified these potential gaps in knowledge, the investigator would next begin to gather systematic information by identifying and reviewing the major texts and research articles in the area of motor control. This review would identify, for instance, that most research in this area has

(continued)

An Example of the Creative Problem-Solving Process (continued)

focused on controlled laboratory experiments that examine theoretical ideas behind the motor control theory. For instance, these studies have shown that involving a person in a real life task produces different quality movements than having the person attempt to perform movements outside a meaningful task. It also reveals that there is very little research that has applied this approach to an actual clinical situation. Discussions with clinicians show that they are particularly interested in research that would demonstrate the impact of this approach on outcomes.

However, exploring data can also involve consulting experts (clinical and research) in the topic one is exploring.

Framing Problems

After considering the literature and feedback from practitioners, the researcher decides to frame the problem in the following statement:

Many practitioners use an approach to service based on concepts of motor control. Where there is substantial basic science evidence to support the theory underlying this approach, there is limited evidence about its impact on improving functional outcomes of persons with head injury. This study will aim to generate such knowledge.

Generating Ideas

At this stage, the investigator goes back to the literature. Since there are few studies of the motor control approach in practice, the investigator decides to examine ways that other researchers have studied the outcomes of other types of occupational therapy interventions. This literature identifies a number of group studies that examine the impact of different interventions on outcomes. Also the investigator finds some examples of single-subject designs that have been used to examine the impact of interventions. The investigator also contacts two investigators in the area of motor control via e-mail and exchanges ideas with them. Finally, the investigator engages in a brown bag discussion over lunch with a group of practitioners working in the area of head injury who use the motor control approach. As a result of this process, several alternative ideas for research are identified including an experimental study that compares the motor control approach to another more traditional approach

to research. However, several problems are identified related to this option. First of all, such a study is costly and given that there is little research in the area, it may be difficult to secure funding. Second, the motor control approach is based on "individualizing" the intervention for each client, which would make it challenging to define a single independent variable for the experimental group. For this reason the investigator begins to focus on the idea of using a single-subject design with a few clients. Consequently, the following first draft of the research question is formulated:

Will the introduction of motor control services demonstrate an improvement in a client's functional capacities?

Developing Solutions and Building Acceptance

Once the investigator has reached the tentative research question noted above, developing solutions to addressing the question would involve the following kinds of considerations:

- Where is a head injury service where one could undertake the research (i.e., where there would be administrative support and therapists' willingness to participate in the study)?
- What kind of single subject design is feasible in the specific head injury service?
- What single subject design would provide the most rigorous findings?
- Will the study design be replicated across several clients?
- What kind of functional measure could be used in the context of the study (i.e., a measure that could be easily administered several times since single-subject designs require repeated measures)?

As the answers to these and other detailed questions become apparent, the researcher would further refine both the study design and the question (and possibly a hypothesis) to operationalize the question in an experimental context. As these decisions are made to refine the study question and design, the investigator and others (e.g., practitioners) who may have been involved in earlier stages of planning the research will have to recognize and accept that the study is appropriate given context, resources, the state of existing knowledge, and other factors.

---

this process by using a hypothetical example of a researcher who is interested in occupational therapy for persons with head injury.

Understanding the Challenge. The initial component of the process, Understanding the Challenge, consists of three stages:

- Constructing Opportunities,
- Exploring Data, and
- Framing Problems.

Constructing Opportunities. The first stage, constructing opportunities, refers to the process of identifying potential areas where gaps in knowledge may exist. This stage may involve, for instance, talking to clinicians or researchers about a topic to identify potential areas where knowledge is needed. It can involve initial reading of the literature, attending lectures, workshops, or colloquia in the area where one is potentially interested. It may involve observing practice in the area of interest. At this stage one aims to identify a range of potentially fruitful avenues for research based on gaps in current knowledge (i.e., the potential research problem).

Exploring Data. Once one or more potential gaps in knowledge are identified, one needs to get a better handle on the nature and scope of problem that might be addressed. To do this one needs to gather systematic information regarding the problem one is considering. This stage is called exploring data. It is crucial to the development of a research question since it is here that one learns what is already known about the potential problem. Exploring the data always involves a review of the literature, which is discussed in more detail later. However, exploring data can also involve consulting experts (clinical and research) in the topic one is exploring. The aim of this step is to develop a comprehensive understanding of an area that focuses on:

• What knowledge is already available,
• How questions are ordinarily addressed and framed in this area of study,
• Where existing knowledge leaves off, and
• What gaps in knowledge are considered most important by those involved.

This step can often result in generating a number of possible problems that could be addressed in a study, as well as different approaches that might be taken to address them.

Framing Problems. The next step, framing problems, involves refining the issue that will be addressed in the study in such a way as to make clear exactly what the problem is that will be addressed. The process that results in this third stage is critical to planning any study, since it is impossible to come up with an effective solution to a research problem if the problem is not clearly identified and translated into a workable research question.

Generating Ideas. After a problem statement is selected, one moves on to the next CPS component (and stage) known as generating ideas. At this stage, investigators first seek to generate a range of ideas concerning how one might go about addressing the problem in a study. Once again, a review

of the research literature in a particular area is important. It will identify how other researchers are going about solving the problem (i.e., what types of questions they address, what design and methods they use in their investigations).

If the problem one has generated is an applied problem for which the investigation is likely to involve practitioners and clients and for which one expects the research results to have practical significance, it is important to discuss possible solutions with these stakeholders. Informal meetings and discussions or formal focus groups can be used to achieve this end.

After generating a range of ideas about how the research problem might be addressed (i.e., types of questions that might be asked and designs and methods that might be used to answer these questions), one must engage in a focusing phase. Focusing involves selecting ideas that have the most potential for solving the problem. At this stage, investigators will typically begin to draft a specific research question and outline the anticipated design and methods. These will be subject to refinement in the stages that follow.

Planning for Action: Developing Solutions and Building Acceptance. Once a potential research question has been identified to address the research problem, it is time to put energy into refining and developing a workable research protocol. This is the component of planning for action. There are two stages in this component:

• Developing Solutions, and
• Building Acceptance.

This step of developing solutions involves designing the actual research protocol. It involves consideration of how the research will be conducted (design and methods) and how the study will be implemented (logistics). The logistic factors include such details as:

• Establishing deadlines for all the necessary steps,
• Planning for how to compensate participants, and
• Determining how data will be entered into systems for data analysis.

Thinking through these details allows one to determine the feasibility of the study. It also allows one to make modifications in plans so the research will be feasible.

While the notion of building acceptance may not intuitively seem necessary for the process of planning research, it is an important step. Often researchers (individuals and research teams) begin with high aspirations for the research process that must be tempered in light of logistics, available resources, and the nature of the knowledge in the area. Inevitably, designing a study involves making compromises between the ideal study and the one that is possible given actual circumstances and resources. In part, acceptance means realizing the limits of the study one will undertake while still clearly identifying what will be valuable about the study. When a team is involved in the research, this process is important to generating "buy in" for the study.

Choosing the Best Research Question, Design, and Methods

Early in planning a study, one may be left with more ideas than one could complete in a typical lifetime. Consequently, one needs to select the idea or ideas that best fit a particular situation. Developing criteria helps one to clarify which research questions, design, and methods might be the best to pursue. These criteria may include whether the study question will be:

- Important,
- Answerable,
- Feasible based on skill, background, time, money, available participants, and additional resources,

- Have adequate support from mentors, collaborators, and institutions involved,
- Able to be completed, and
- A satisfying process for those involved.

Tools for Decision-Making

A variety of tools have been developed to systematize the kind of decision-making that underlies planning a study. One tool that uses criteria to make a systematic choice is the Evaluation Matrix (Isaksen et al., 2000; Lewin & Reed, 1998). The first step of the Evaluation Matrix is to make a grid with rows and columns. Along the columns, one would put all the criteria, and the potential choices would be put along the rows. Using a scale of 1 to 5, with 1 being poor to 5 being excellent, one then rates each option under consideration. By comparing each option across the criteria, one can better understand the implications of each choice. Table 28.2 illustrates a matrix that might facilitate the decision making when considering three different design options for studying outcomes of occupational therapy services based on motor control concepts in the area of head injury.

In using the Evaluation Matrix, it is important to evaluate each criterion across the choices. This is done to avoid a potential halo effect that could occur if one has a favorite option. When the grid is

Table 28.2 An Evaluation Matrix for Considering Different Design Options for a Study of Functional Outcomes of Occupational Therapy Services Based on Motor Control for Persons with Head Injury

	Survey of Therapists About Their Perceptions of the Value of Control Approaches	Two-Group Experiment Comparing Motor Control to Other Approaches	Single-subject Design to Examine Impact of Motor Control on Functional Outcomes Across Three Subjects
Can study be accomplished with a small seed grant (i.e., $5,000)?	4	1	5
Can study be completed in 12 months?	5	2	5
Will study contribute rigorous evidence about impact of motor control functional outcomes?	2	5	4
Can study be done on local rehabilitation unit with an average of 45 clients and 3 therapists?	1	3	5

Note: 1 = poor fit; 5 = excellent fit.

complete and all the criteria have been evaluated, one can have a general picture of the value of each choice.

A careful decision-making process can often leave one with few or no valuable potential choices. In this situation, another valuable tool is the Advantages, Limitations, and Overcome the Limitations (AL-O) process (Lewin & Reed, 1998). By taking each choice and generating its advantages and limitations, one has the ability to see the choice through new eyes. Through the generation of ideas to overcome the limitations to a given research question and design one can creatively problem solve how to make a given option more viable. In a sense, the AL-O process helps one to move directly to planning the research protocol since one is able to see what will support and what will be a barrier to a given research option.

The Literature Review

One should continuously review the literature as the research question, design, and methods are being developed. Understanding background information, past research, and theoretical concepts help to make sure that the correct research question is being formulated. While it may be relatively easy for the researcher to know where to begin the search for background information, it is often difficult to know that enough literature has been cov-

ered in terms of the quantity and quality of the literature.

Finding the Right Literature

There is no specific formula for how much literature review is necessary. The expectation for the depth and breadth of the review will vary based on the topic and the type of study one is planning. A review of the literature may be somewhat limited, for example, if the area is clearly defined and research on the topic is quite focused. On the other hand, if one is examining a new area or an area where extensive work has already been done, it may be necessary to do a very large literature review. In the former case, one may need to explore a number of related areas to the new area to generate ideas about how to approach the new area chosen for the study. In the latter case one would need to do a literature review of sufficient depth to make sure one is not asking a question for which there already is substantial evidence.

In all situations, beginning the search with a rather broad approach to the topic will allow the researcher to get a picture of how the topic is understood by other researchers. An example of this can be seen in the area of falls in the elderly. At the start of searching in this area one might broadly examine risk factors for all elderly persons. As one's understanding of the area deepens, one would be aware of the different risk factors

Table 28.3 Checklist of Things to Consider When Planning the Design and Methods of a Research Study.

Task	Dates for Task—Deadlines	Completed
Select appropriate research type (qualitative or quantitative).		
Select type of study design.		
Identify the study group.		
Formulate a plan to select study participants.		
Obtain approval to carry out research at organization, if necessary.		
Organize appropriate resources (money, support, time, knowledge) to carry out study.		
Apply for ethical approval of study.		
Complete thorough literature review that can demonstrate importance and need of proposed study.		
State research problem/hypothesis in format approved by department/research committee.		
Complete thorough description of methods section that can describe research process to research group and other readers.		
Develop timeline for study.		

among community-based falls, falls to hospitalized elderly, and falls that take place in a nursing home. With this framework in place, one may then limit further searching to a more specific area such as falls that take place in nursing homes.

Another factor that determines the type of literature review is one's own understanding of the research topic. The novice researcher will need to spend time uncovering background information to make sure that all areas are covered. While this process may involve following up on what appear to be many unimportant paths, it is necessary to keep digging a bit deeper to make sure that a strong web of understanding of the topic has developed. For the more seasoned researcher, the literature review will most likely focus on providing an update on the latest information. It will also serve to challenge experienced researchers to broaden and deepen their understanding of the research question/hypothesis so that he or she does not rely only on past comprehension of the topic.

It is important to examine literature from a variety of sources, and, in most instances, to examine references that span more than a single discipline. Following along on the example of falls in the elderly, one would find that the literature spans occupational therapy, physical therapy, social work, exercise physiology, public health, and nursing literature.

Finding the appropriate literature for a literature review involves a process of searching the literature. Using appropriate search strategies can ensure that one's literature review has sufficient breadth and depth. The process of searching the literature is described in depth in Chapter 27.

Synthesizing the Discovered Literature

Synthesizing the discovered literature requires two interdependent steps:

- Critically analyzing each article, book, or chapter found, and
- Figuring out how to present the information from the literature in a coherent and influential manner.

Staying focused on the task of refining the research question helps to focus and integrate these two steps. The evolving research question should drive the critical analysis and development of the framework for the presentation of the information.

Critical analysis of the literature involves:

- Assessing the quality of an article (e.g., comprehensiveness in a review article, or rigor in a research article), and

- Asking how appropriate a given source is to the selected topic.

The quality of an article, book, or chapter is based on many factors. For example, if an assessment tool is involved in a study, is the reliability and validity of the instrument discussed? If a study examines the effectiveness of a given intervention, are the reported results consistent with the type of study design? It is not possible to exhaustively list all the things one might consider in evaluating an article. Several sources of information in this text are helpful to this end. First of all, the chapters discussing various methods provide the rationale and the criteria for rigor in studies. Second, the discussions of evidence-based practice in Chapter 41 also discuss criteria that can be used to analyze research reports.

Deciding the relevance of each piece of literature to the research topic can be somewhat complicated by the fact that the research topic often changes in scope as the literature review process unfolds. For example, one might begin with a very broad topic, in which case a wide range of articles are relevant. As the literature is reviewed and the topic narrowed, a smaller subset of articles will be identified as relevant. In some instances, the research topic expands, necessitating that an initially narrow search be broadened.

When reviewing research literature, it is a good idea to characterize each article by:

- Summarizing the research question, and
- Describing key elements of the methods, results, conclusions, and implications.

Doing so not only clarifies the important points of an article, but also creates a record to which one can return when writing up the literature review.

There is no substitute for carefully examining each piece of literature included in the literature review. Reading and reviewing an article more than once may allow the reader to see more of the limitations and strengths of the article. It will also permit the researcher to more easily make the determination if an article fits the research question.

In some cases, writing the research question out and having it available when deciding if an article fits may be enough to move the process along. For some researchers, or for some types of research questions, it may be necessary to create a schematic or map of the research question. The map will look at relationships in the question, what is known and what is not known. It can also include the relationship to the theoretical framework. A schematic map allows the researcher to figure out what is needed and will enable the individual to understand the parameters of the research question and to easily answer the question "Does it fit or not?". Figure 28.2 is an example of a schematic map used for the development of a research question.

Another way to create a structure for information is to use a table format to summarize the results found in the most important supporting literature. This framework can then be used to write the literature review. Table 28.4 provides an example of how the articles to be included in a literature review can be summarized in tabular form. Whether the researcher is involved in quantitative or qualitative research, the two main goals of a literature review are to be accurate and to be persuasive. If one is accurate but not persuasive, one will be left with a literature review that is technically good but does not convince the reader that the topic has merit. If the review is fervent but without substance, the same readers will have the impression that the author was attempting to get by on his or her passion. A good literature review should lead one down a well-structured path that convinces the reader of both the completeness of one's examination of the literature and the merit of the research question. Finally, the literature review should lead naturally to the choice of research question, design, and methods.

Case Illustrations: Identifying the Research Question, Design, and Methods

Case One: Studying Attitudes Using Conjoint Analysis

Constructing Opportunities

The study of public attitudes toward disability, especially regarding people with severe mental illness, has been an important research topic in the occupational therapy and related literature. Researchers have been particularly interested in the attitudes of occupational therapy professionals and students toward people with disabilities. My personal experience as an occupational therapist and the findings of previous studies indicated that negative attitudes toward people with disabilities affect the successful rehabilitation, integration, and independence of people with disabilities (Antonak & Livneh, 1988).

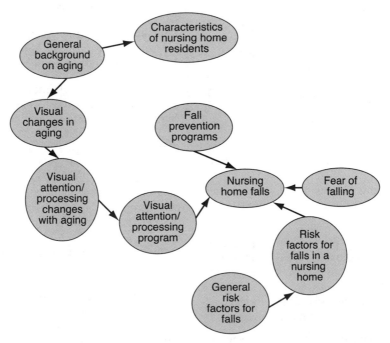

Figure 28.2 Schematic of literature review for research question: *Does participation in a visual attention/visual processing program reduce falls in nursing home residents?*

Table 28.4 Example of Table for Summarizing Articles to Be Used in a Literature Review

Author/Year/ Section of Literature Review	Study Objectives	Design/ Participants	Intervention and Measures Used	Results
Owsley & McGwin, 2004 Visual attention/ processing changes with aging	To examine the association between visual attention/ processing speed and mobility in older adults.	Cross-sectional 342 older adults (aged 55–85) living independently in the community. Recruited from primary eye care practices.	Survey as part of prospective study on mobility. Measured visual attention/processing speed, performance mobility, self-reported measures of falls, fall efficacy, mobility/ balance, and physical activity, demographics, health, and functional information.	Lower scores on visual attention/processing speed were significantly related to poorer scores on performance mobility, after adjustment for age, sex, race, education, number of chronic conditions, cognitive status, depressive symptoms, visual acuity, and contrast sensitivity (P =.04).
Becker et al., 2003 Fall prevention programs	To evaluate the effectiveness of a multi-faceted fall prevention program.	Randomized controlled trial (randomized by clusters) 1981 nursing home residents, 60 years of age and older.	Staff and resident education on fall prevention, advice on environmental adaptations, progressive balance and resistive training, and hip protectors. Number of falls and fractures.	The incidence density of falls for the intervention group was slightly more than half of that for the control group. There was no difference between both groups for number of fractures.

Exploring Data and Framing Problems

My personal interest in this area prompted me to systematically review the literature, which included Science Citation Index, Social Sciences Citation Index, CINAHL, and MEDLINE. Results show that many researchers have questioned the utility of using overt and obtrusive direct methods to measure attitudes using the traditional self-report and interview methods, especially when the targeted attitude referent is emotionally loaded and socially sensitive. The conscious or unconscious mechanisms of the respondent may interfere and alter his or her attitudes so as to conform to prevailing norms and socially sanctioned beliefs (Livneh & Antonak, 1994). These concerns are relevant in measuring public attitudes on issues related to the community integration of people with severe mental illness. While I was fully aware of the limitations of the current techniques of measuring attitudes, I did not have a strategy that could overcome this barrier.

Generating Ideas

My personal experience of having a breakthrough in research on several occasions has been to learn

from and collaborate with other disciplines. At one point, I discussed my concerns regarding the limitations of the traditional methods of studying attitudes with a professor from rehabilitation psychology at the University of Wisconsin–Madison who was interested in the study of public attitudes on individuals with mental illness. He introduced me to an indirect measure market research technique called "conjoint analysis." The virtue of conjoint analysis is that it asks the respondent to make choices in the same fashion as the consumer presumably does—by trading off features, one against another. Compared to the commonly used rating and ranking methods, the innovative conjoint analysis is less obtrusive, and its task design simulates real-life considerations more closely. It provides attitude/preference scores that are more realistic, less abstract, less declarative, and less tainted by social desirability (Shamir & Shamir, 1995). As an indirect method to evaluate attitudes as relative to the combinations of characteristics of persons with disabilities, conjoint analysis also has the advantage of being less affected by social desirability than the traditional methods of assessment. This enhances the validity of research results from well-educated healthcare professionals who were the subjects of interests in this study (Shamir & Shamir, 1995). Knowing its uniqueness and essential features, we brainstormed its potential uses in the field of rehabilitation. I had an intuition that it had great potential to be used to study attitudes of disabilities in occupational therapy. To use the terminology of CPS, I identified new ideas and developed a new way of framing the traditional problem.

Developing Solutions and Building Acceptance

With this creative idea in my mind, I performed a systematic literature review again to see if there were previous attempts to use this innovative approach to study public attitudes of disabilities, and I was delighted to see that there were no such studies. This confirmed that this new idea was original. My research question became: "Is conjoint analysis applicable to the study of public attitudes toward people with disabilities?"

To explore the application of conjoint analysis in occupational therapy research, we first identified the scope and objectives of the study. We planned to employ the conjoint analysis procedure to examine factors influencing occupational therapy students' context-specific attitudes toward people with disabilities. The relationships between sex of the occupational therapy students and their preferences for people with disabilities as well as the occupational therapy curricula effects on attitudes were also examined. Factors influencing context-specific attitudes of occupational therapy students toward persons with disabilities were examined by studying their preferences for placing a residential rehabilitation facility in their own neighborhood. This context was chosen as community integration of people with disabilities is still a controversial and sensitive issue in Hong Kong (Cheung, 1990).

A quantitative research design was employed for the study (Heppner, Kivlighan, & Wampold, 1999) as it included research strategies that enabled the investigator to describe the occurrence of variables, the underlying dimension in a set of variables, and the relationship between or among variables. Specifically, passive research designs (e.g., ex post facto designs and multiple regression) were considered to examine complex relationships among variables. In this study, conjoint analysis (a nonparametric multiple regression) was used to determine the effect of disability-specific and other demographic variables on attitudes toward people with disabilities and an ex post facto design was used to determine the sex and curricula effects on attitudes.

The next step was to transfer the above into a workable research protocol. The main considerations were the sample and sampling procedure, the instruments to be used, the procedure for data collection, and how the data should be analyzed to answer the research questions (Tsang, Chan, & Chan, 2004).

Case Two: Family Burdens of the Mentally Ill Offenders

Constructing Opportunities

Another illustration of the process of developing a research question involved the development of theoretical model using a qualitative research design. Based on my past clinical experiences and discussion with some experienced researchers in the field, it came to my notice that a number of research projects had been devoted to the study of needs, responsibilities, and intervention programs of families and caregivers of psychiatric clients because of the emphasis on deinstitutionalization and community integration. As I had worked as an occupational therapist in a forensic psychiatric setting for a number of years, I was fully aware that the responsibilities for families when looking after a client with a criminal history were even heavier and more complicated than for those without a criminal history.

Exploring Data

Studies on identifying family needs and responsibilities for mentally ill offenders have been very limited, however, and I recognized that this could be a new area of research. I first completed a comprehensive literature review on family stress and studies on family needs for psychiatric clients with a forensic history with particular emphasis on the methodological problems of available studies. Since research in this area was limited, I felt that building a theoretical model could act as a conceptual guide for subsequent studies to identify burdens of families of mentally ill offenders. Based on the literature review and my own experience, I postulated a model (Figure 28.3) suggesting that the core source of stress of families of the mentally ill offenders appeared to be the criminal offense itself. A secondary source of stress and burden were the events associated with the offense, including the court proceedings; dealing with the police and the media; and admission to a special hospital. The crime and the secondary events in turn add to the severity of the burdens to the families along the four classical dimensions (Tsang, Pearson, & Yuen, 2002).

Features of a Good Research Question

The following are elements of a good research question:

- The question should clearly state what is being described, compared, or contrasted in the study.
- The question should correspond to the type of research method and design that will be used (e.g., type of study, sample, planned analysis).

- The question should be operational, that is, it should not be too abstract and should refer to actual variables under investigation.

The table below illustrates research questions that conform or fail to conform to these elements.

Strong Research Questions	Weak Research Questions
Do therapists who use the Occupational Performance History Interview view it as providing information helpful to understanding the client, treatment planning, and discharge planning?	Is the Occupational Performance History Interview a good assessment?
Are lower scores on the Functional Index Measure at discharge related to type of discharge setting (home, nursing home, assisted living) in persons with cerebrovascular accident?	Does functional level determine where patients are discharged to?
Will young adults (18–30 years) diagnosed with bipolar disorder attending a monthly occupational therapy follow-up program following discharge have less rehospitalization rates in the 12 months post-discharge than a control group that does not attend this follow-up program?	Would an occupational therapy follow-up program reduce rehospitalization?
What factors do occupational therapy clients with AIDS enrolled in a vocational rehabilitation program find most helpful to their return to work?	How do clients with AIDS think occupational therapy helps them return to work?

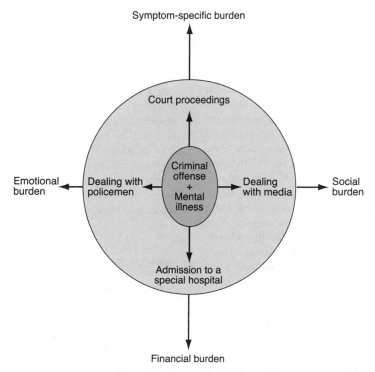

Figure 28.3 Stress and burden for families of forensic psychiatric clients.

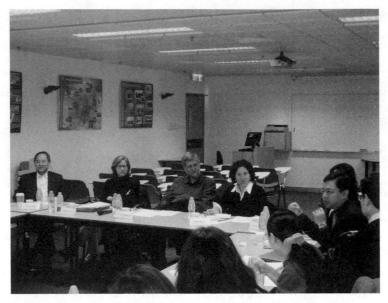

Figure 28.4 Dr. Tsang (right, holding the microphone) discusses a collaborator research with researchers of other disciplines from Chicago, Illinois and Beijing, China.

Framing Problems

With the theoretical model, we worked out the research questions. What were the experiences and needs of families of forensic psychiatric patients in Hong Kong with particular respect to their contact with the police, courts, media, and service providers? What suggestions for service provisions could be made after the needs of the families had been identified (Figure 28.4)?

Generating Ideas and Developing Solutions. My collaborators and I brainstormed the different methodologies that we might use in answering the above questions. Based on the fact that this would likely be a pioneering and exploratory study, we decided to use a qualitative approach. In-depth interviews were planned to be conducted among sufficient numbers of participants using a semi-structured interview schedule. Another problem we faced at that time was whether there was an appropriate assessment tool. The Relative Assessment Interview was found to be appropriate. However, modification was needed to include extra items related to the forensic nature of the patients. We therefore again read the literature on research methods involved in scale development and modification. We eventually developed the Chinese Relative Assessment Interview for our own purposes (Tsang & Pearson, 2001). The interviews were successfully completed among 23 partici-

pants and the results were published in a peer-reviewed journal (Pearson & Tsang, 2004).

Conclusion

This chapter discussed the process of generating a research question, and deciding design and methods. We emphasized the extent to which this is a creative, if disciplined, process. While there is no single pathway to developing a sound and doable research question and to designing rigorous research to answer it, one important rule of thumb is to employ the process of divergent and convergent thinking. The former is useful for generating opportunities, options, and ideas. The latter is necessary for choosing between these various elements in making good decisions that lead to a sound and valuable study.

REFERENCES

(2004). The Health Insurance Portability and Accountability Act.

Ackoff, R. L., & Vergara, E. (1988). Creativity in problem solving and planning. In R. L. Kuhn (Ed.),*Handbook for creative and innovative managers* (pp. 77–89). New York: McGraw-Hill.

Antonak, R., & Livneh, P. (1988). *The measurement of attitudes toward people with disabilities—Methods, psychometric and scales.* Springfield, IL: Charles C Thomas.

Bohn, D., & Peat, P. (1987). *Science, order and creativity*. Toronto: Bantam.

Bordage, G., & Dawson, B. (2003). Experimental study design and grant writing in eight steps and 28 questions. *Medical Education, 37*(4), 376–385.

Cheung, F. (1990). People against the mentally ill: Community opposition to residential treatment facilities. *Community Mental Health Journal, 26,* 205–212.

Dennis, A., & Valacich, J. (1993). Computer brainstorms: More heads are better than one. *Journal of Applied Psychology, 78*(4), 531–537.

Heppner, P. P., Kivlighan, D. M., & Wampold, B. E. (1999). *Research design in counseling*. Belmont, CA: Wadsworth.

Isaksen, S. K., Dorval, B., & Treffinger, D. (2000). *Creative approaches to problem solving*. Dubuque, IA: Kendall/Hunt.

Lewin, J., & Reed, C. (1998). *Creative problem solving in occupational therapy*. Philadelphia: Lippincott.

Livneh, H., & Antonak, R. (1994). Indirect methods of attitude measurement: Reply to Linkowski and Yuder. *Rehabilitation Education, 8,* 144–148.

Noller, R. (1977). *Scratching the surface of creative problem solving*. Buffalo, NY: DOK Publishers.

Osborn, A. (1979). *Applied imagination*. New York: Charles Scribner's Sons.

Pearson, V., & Tsang, H. (2004). Duty, burden, & ambivalence: Families of forensic psychiatric patients in Hong Kong. *International Journal of Law and Psychiatry, 27,* 361–374.

Popper, K. (1959). *The logic of scientific discovery*. New York: Harper & Row.

Portney, L., & Watkins, M. (2000). *Foundations of clinical research—Applications to practice*. Upper Saddle River, NJ: Prentice-Hall.

Root-Bernstein, R. (1997). *Discovering*. Cambridge, MA: Harvard University Press.

Shamir, M., & Shamir, J. (1995). Competing values in public opinion: A conjoint analysis. *Political Behavior, 17,* 107–133.

Simon, H. (1981). The psychology of scientific problem solving. In R. Tweney, M. Doherty & C. Mynatt (Eds.), *Scientific thinking*. New York: Columbia University Press.

Smalheiser, N., & Swanson, D. (1998). Using ARROW-SMITH: A computer-assisted approach to formulating and assessing scientific hypotheses. *Computer Methods and Programs in Biomedicine, 57,* 149–153.

Sternberg, R., & Lubart, T. (1996). Investing in creativity. *American Psychologist, 51,* 677–688.

Sternberg, R., & Lubart, T. (1999). The concept of creativity: Prospects and paradigms. In R. Sternberg (Ed.), *Handbook of creativity* (pp. 3–15). Cambridge, UK: Cambridge University Press.

Swanson, D., & Smalheiser, N. (1997). An interactive system for finding complementary literatures: A stimulus to scientific discovery. *Artificial Intelligence, 91,* 183–203.

Tsang, H. W. H. (2003). Augmenting vocational outcomes of supported employment with social skills training. *Journal of Rehabilitation, 69*(3), 25–30.

Tsang, H. W. H., Chan, F., & Chan, C. C. H. (2004). Factors influencing occupational therapy students' attitudes toward persons with disabilities: A conjoint analysis. *American Journal of Occupational Therapy, 58*(4), 426–434.

Tsang, H. W. H., Cheang, C. T. K., Tong, B. Y. M., & Tse, S. S. L. (2004). Psychosocial functioning of Chinese older people with chronic physical illness. *International Journal of Therapy and Rehabilitation, 11*(3), 99–105.

Tsang, H. W. H., & Pearson, V. (2001). A work-related social skills training for people with schizophrenia in Hong Kong. *Schizophrenia Bulletin, 27*(1), 139–148.

Tsang, H. V. H., Pearson, V., & Yuen, C. H. (2002). Family needs and burdens of the mentally ill offenders. *International Journal of Rehabilitation Research, 25*(1), 25–32.

RESOURCES

Computational Scientific Discovery

Computational scientific discovery (Swanson & Smalheiser, 1997) was developed specifically to facilitate the development of hypotheses across specialties that typically are not linked together. Arrowsmith (Smalheiser & Swanson, 1998), a form of computational scientific discovery, uses interactive software and database strategies to uncover potential links that had not been identified before. In a regular search, for example, one may find no references when combining two disparate areas. Through the use of Arrowsmith, one is able to retrieve the keyword terms that the two disparate areas have in common. By using the filters available through Arrowsmith, one can then reduce the number of potential choices for research. Arrowsmith is available on the Web at http://arrowsmith.psych.uic.edu/arrowsmith_uic/index.html

Creativity-Based Information Resources (CBIR)

Creativity Based Information Resources (CBIR) is a literature database maintained by the International Center for Studies in Creativity at Buffalo State College, State University of New York. The database contains more than 12,000 annotated references of works focusing on creativity, and includes articles on research related to creativity. CBIR is available on the Web at http://www.buffalostate.edu/orgs/cbir.

Creativity for Life

Creativity for Life.com is a Web site containing articles and links related to creativity and creative thinking. While not specifically dealing with the research process, the included links and articles contain information on enhancing writing and improving creativity. This Web site can be found at http://www.creativityforlife.com.

Innovation Tools

Innovation Tools is a catalog of creativity resources including tools, links, and articles. While this Web site is focused on business innovation, the tools that are discussed are directly transferable to the research process. Innovation Tools can be found on the Web at http://www.innovationtools.com.

CHAPTER 29

Integrity and Ethics in the Conduct of Human Subject Research

Don E. Workman • Gary Kielhofner

Overview of Issues of Integrity and Ethical Conduct Surrounding Research

This chapter summarizes issues related to research integrity and ethics. Conducting research in an ethical manner requires an investigator to develop knowledge beyond a common-sense understanding of moral issues. In this chapter, we cover the basic ethical principles that should guide the conduct of research.

Moreover, in much of the world today, investigators doing research that involves human subjects come under the jurisdiction of national principles and regulations that govern the ethical conduct of research. When discussing such governmental regulations[1] we focus mainly on the United States in this chapter. However, since these regulations reflect degrees of international consensus about research ethics, they will parallel many aspects of how ethical conduct of research is managed throughout much of the world. The structure of this chapter is partly based on an Office of Research Integrity publication entitled "Introduction to the Responsible Conduct of Research" (Steneck, 2004).

It is important to note at the outset of this chapter that the application of the general principles of

> Ethical conduct in research must go beyond compliance with the letter of the law and, instead, involve behavior consistent with a knowledgeable awareness of research ethics and an underlying spirit of integrity.

integrity and ethics are complex. There are situations when it is impossible to perform research without impinging upon one or more of the ethical principles, in which case the investigator may need to develop additional safeguards to protect the subjects of the research. For instance, one of the basic principles of research ethics requires that subjects be enrolled in research only when they have provided fully informed consent (this is included under the principle of *respect for persons*) (The National Commission for the Protection of Human Subjects of Biomedical and Behavioral Research, 1979). However, to answer important questions about clinical interventions, some occupational therapy research needs to be performed with persons whose impairments prevent them from fully understanding the research and who, therefore, have a limited capacity to give informed consent. In such cases, the investigator may be required to obtain permission on behalf of the patient from a spouse or other family member before enrolling the patient as a subject of research. In still other situations, it may simply not be ethically permissible to enroll the subjects at all (for instance, when the research represents more than minimal risk) (HHS Working Group on the NBAC Report, n.d.).

In the end, ethical research depends on the knowledge and integrity of the investigator. Everyone who undertakes an investigation assumes a moral responsibility to abide by commonly accepted ethical standards. In this chapter we discuss compliance with regulatory principles and procedures that enforce these ethical standards. However, it is important to underscore that ethical conduct in research must go beyond compliance with the letter of the law and, instead, involve behavior consistent with a knowledgeable

---

[1]In the United States, researchers who are not federally funded, or who conduct their research in institutions that have no federal funding, may not be obligated at the time this chapter is being written to learn and abide by these rules, but should be aware there is a movement underway at the federal level to require all research, regardless of whether there is federal funding involved, to abide by these same standards.

awareness of research ethics and an underlying spirit of integrity.

Regulation of Research Ethics and Integrity

To ensure that there is a reasonably objective review of the ethical issues related to human subject research, many institutions worldwide require that research plans be reviewed and approved by an ethical review board (known in the United States as an Institutional Review Board [IRB]) prior to the initiation of the research study. This requirement was codified in U.S. federal regulations in 1981 when 17 federal agencies agreed to a common set of rules to govern research on human subjects that they funded or over which they provided oversight (Office for Human Research Protection, 2001). It is also reflected in the national regulations of many countries throughout the world. The role and function of ethical review/IRB boards is discussed later in this chapter.

Occupational therapy research may fall under the jurisdiction of specific federal regulations or it may not be specifically governed by any regulations, depending on the institution or country where the research is conducted. Anyone conducting research is responsible to conduct the research ethically and with integrity, whether or not specific regulations pertain to the study. Moreover, when there are regulations they must be followed and it is the responsibility of the investigator to find out what the rules and procedures are.

Policies Governing Research Integrity

In the United States, the Office of Research Integrity (ORI) (see the feature box titled International Regulations Governing Research) is responsible for both the promotion of the responsible conduct of research (RCR) and the resolution of allegations of research misconduct. The Public Health Service has identified nine core areas that need to be addressed for investigators to know how to conduct research responsibly:

• Data acquisition, management, sharing and ownership,
• Conflict of interest and commitment,
• Human subjects,
• Animal welfare,
• Research misconduct,
• Publication practices and responsible authorship,
• Mentor/trainee responsibilities,
• Peer review, and
• Collaborative science.

ORI has and follows a number of federal policies for resolving allegations of misconduct. The following is their definition of misconduct:

Misconduct in Science means fabrication, falsification, plagiarism, or other practices that seriously deviate from those that are commonly accepted within the scientific community for proposing, conducting, or reporting research. It does not include honest error or honest differences in interpretations or judgments of data. [Cited from 42 CFR 50.102]

Definitions and examples of fabrication, falsification, and plagiarism are included in the feature box titled Fabrication, Falsification, and Plagiarism. These constitute the primary issues that fall under research misconduct, but it is important to note that the definition also includes other practices that seriously deviate from established scientific norms. Thus researchers in occupational therapy need to be familiar with established scientific norms, both within and outside the field of occupational therapy.

The Relationship Between Ethical Conduct and Regulatory Compliance or Noncompliance

Often an inherent tension arises concerning compliance and noncompliance with regulations. It is easy to feel offended when one is told that one has "broken a rule" (consider the average response to a policeman when someone has been pulled over for speeding). Higher stages of moral development, however, involve guiding one's behavior by ethical principles rather than rules. This allows one, at times, to understand that the morally right thing to do may indeed be inconsistent with an established rule.

In watching *Les Miserables*, one readily identifies with the hero who has been imprisoned for 20 years because he broke into a house and stole a loaf of bread for his sister's starving child. Nonetheless, one would also concede that laws against stealing are generally just and there should be consequences for individuals who break into houses and steal from others.

The regulations regarding research ethics and research integrity are not different. Knowing the regulations is helpful for understanding the broad parameters for acceptable conduct. Ethical research behavior is usually achieved by being compliant with those regulations. Nonetheless, as already noted, investigators should think beyond

There is growing international consensus conerning ethical principles that govern research. For instance, the Declaration of Helsinki (http://www.wma.net/e/policy/b3.htm) sets forth the principles regarding the ethical conduct of human subject research originally adopted by the World Medical Association in 1964. The current document, adopted in 2000, includes 32 principles and has two subsequent clarifications.

Nonetheless, most countries have their own specific guidelines or regulations that govern ethical conduct of research and investigators must be familiar and comply with them. Below is information on Australia, the United States, Canada, and the United Kingdom

Australia

National Statement on Ethical Conduct in Research Involving Humans (National Health and Medical Research Council, 1999) (available from: http://www.nhmrc.gov.au/issues/researchethics. htm) provides guidelines made in accordance with the National Health and Medical Research Council Act 1992, to which research involving humans must conform. This document:

• Sets out the ethical principles and values that should govern research involving humans,
• Provides guidance about how research should be designed and conducted so as to conform to these principles, and
• Outlines the procedures for consideration and approval of all such research by Human Research Ethics Committees (HRECs).

All research involving humans must be conducted in accordance with the principles contained in this statement.

United States

All research that is funded through the U.S. Public Health Service (PHS) falls under the jurisdiction of the Office for Research Integrity (http://ori.dhhs.gov/). PHS-funded research must be conducted in compliance with the federal regulations at Title 42 of the Code of Federal Regulations (CFR), Part 50 and Subpart A (http://ori.dhhs.gov/misconduct/reg_subpart_a. shtml). In addition, all research involving human subjects that is funded through the Department of Health and Human Services (HHS), which is part of the Public Health Service, is subject to the oversight of the Office for Human Subject Protections (OHRP) (http://www.hhs.gov/ohrp/). OHRP is responsible for ensuring that HHS-funded research is conducted in accordance with the federal regulations at Title 45, Part 46 of the Code of Federal Regulations (CFR). OHRP is the federal office that provides oversight over

the local IRBs just as the local IRB provides oversight of the human subject studies that are underway.

Canada

This Tri-Council Policy Statement: Ethical Conduct for Research Involving Humans describes the policies of the Medical Research Council (MRC), the Natural Sciences and Engineering Research Council (NSERC), and the Social Sciences and Humanities Research Council (SSHRC). The document replaces SSHRC's Ethics Guidelines for Research with Human Subjects, MRC's Guidelines on Research Involving Humans, and MRC's Guidelines for Research on Somatic Cell Gene Therapy in Humans. The Councils will consider funding (or continued funding) only to individuals and institutions that certify compliance with this policy regarding research involving human subjects.

This joint policy expresses the continuing commitment by the three Councils to the people of Canada, to promote the ethical conduct of research involving human subjects. This commitment was first expressed in the publication of guidelines in the late 1970s. Work on the joint policy was started by formation of the Tri-Council Working Group in 1994. The Councils published three documents prepared by the Working Group: an Issues Paper in November 1994, a Discussion Draft in May 1996, and its Final Report (Code of Ethical Conduct for Research Involving Humans) in July 1997. Each of these documents stimulated extensive discussion in the academic community. The present Policy Statement was prepared by the Councils by revision of the Working Group's Final Report in the light of consultations between mid-1997 and May 1998.

United Kingdom

In the United Kingdom, the Department of Health has produced a framework outlining the principles of all research within its remit that is undertaken in health and social care. The Research Governance Framework for Health and Social Care (2005, 2nd ed.) is available at: http://www.dh.gov.uk/Policy AndGuidance/ResearchAndDevelopment/Research And DevelopmentAZ/ResearchGovernance/fs/en

Research Governance, which applies to all those who undertake or participate in research, and sets out standards to improve research and safeguard the public. Requirements include:

• Independent review of research proposals to ensure ethical standards are met,
• Scientific review by independent experts,
• Informed consent and safeguards for patient data,
• Clear and accessible dissemination strategies, and
• Provision of a quality research culture.

regulations to a thorough consideration of ethical issues that inevitably arise in doing research. Moreover, investigators should seek to become as knowledgeable about ethical issues as they are in other aspects of the conduct of research.

The Benefits of Responsible Conduct

The benefits of responsible conduct of research go far beyond avoiding the negative consequences of noncompliance. Researchers usually are internally motivated to do things right, and a familiarity with the principles of the responsible conduct of research allows researchers to proceed with confidence that they are abiding by accepted standards of ethical conduct. Moreover the training of professionals and researchers in RCR will increase the common knowledge base and will contribute to the

furthering of a culture of compliance and respect among researchers.

Research Integrity

For the sake of summarizing the key elements of research integrity in this chapter, we present a summary of the basic tenets of research integrity as elucidated by Steneck (2004). These tenets are available for review or downloading on the Web site of the Office of Research Integrity (http://ori.dhhs.gov/documents/rcrintro.pdf). It is worth noting that in the introduction to this helpful booklet, the Director of the Office of Research Integrity (ORI) clearly indicates that the teaching and application of these principles will vary for different professions.

Fabrication, Falsification, and Plagiarism

The key aspects of scientific misconduct include fabrication, falsification, and plagiarism. Each is defined and exemplified below.

Fabrication: Fabrication is making up data or results and recording or reporting them. [*cited from 42 CFR 93.103 (a)*]. For example, an occupational therapy graduate student has been told by his or her advisor that a minimum of 30 subjects are required for a thesis project he or she is undertaking. The student obtained data on 29 subjects and is facing a deadline that would prevent graduation on time. Under the pressure of time, the student makes up a 30th subject, entering that subject into the database for analysis.

Falsification: Falsification is manipulating research materials, equipment, or processes, or changing or omitting data or results such that the research is not accurately represented in the research record [*cited from 42 CFR 93.103 (b)*]. Two occupational therapy researchers involved in a qualitative study have data providing support of a conceptual argument they have previously published in the literature. They are discussing the data in a research team meeting when a research assistant points out a number of instances in the fieldnotes that call into question their argument. Nonetheless, the investigators decide to complete an article based only on the data that support their argument. They not only ignore the contravening data but also do not mention its existence in the research report. This is an instance of falsification and it constitutes scientific misconduct.

Plagiarism: Plagiarism is the appropriation of another person's ideas, processes, results, or words without giving appropriate credit [*cited from 42 CFR 93.103 (b)*]. An occupational therapist has been working on a paper and discusses it with a colleague from nursing. This colleague points out that a paper addressing the issue has been published in the nursing literature and provides a copy. The occupational therapist used the fundamental ideas for and structures the occupational therapy paper much the same as the nursing paper. When the occupational therapy paper is published it has no reference to the nursing paper. This would be an example of plagiarism and it constitutes scientific misconduct.

In each of the three hypothetical instances of scientific misconduct given above, it is likely that those involved will have "good reasons" for their behavior. For instance, the student who fabricates a subject may reason that 1 subject out of 30 won't really change the findings. The qualitative investigators are convinced that their conceptual argument is mainly correct. They reason that mentioning contradictory data will only undermine others' confidence in what is basically a sound conceptual argument. The writer reasons that, since the original work was published in another field, it doesn't matter if the author is not cited. However, in each instance, the reasoning masks the fact that each of these hypothetical persons gained something from their misconduct. An investigator must always be careful to ask whether personal gain is influencing a decision that involves an ethical issue. Moreover, decisions should always be guided by the ethical principles involved and not by personal, logistic, political, or other considerations.

The Price of Irresponsible Conduct

When researchers receiving federal funding are investigated and judged to have engaged in research misconduct, they can bring significant penalties and consequences upon themselves and their host institutions. These can include:

- Requirements that federal funding be returned (paid back),
- Additional penalties and fines to the individual investigator and to the institution for not maintaining regulatory compliance,
- Institutional sanctions such as halting of all federal funding of research, or possibly even stopping all ongoing human subjects research (regardless of the source of funding) until the institution is "brought into compliance."

There are agencies that "blacklist" investigators so that they are prevented from participating in future research.

Data Acquisition, Management, Sharing, and Ownership

In the practice of science, data collection and storage are crucial activities. Given the advent of the personal computer, and the proliferation of easy ways to replicate, share, and store electronic copies of data (laptop computers, handheld storage devices, flash memory cards, and e-mail to name a few), there are many new mechanisms that can be used to facilitate the acquisition, management, and sharing of data. While these streamline many aspects of research, they also require additional care in how data are stored, managed, and shared.

In conducting research, one or many people may be collecting the data, but this does not necessarily infer rights of ownership over that data. There may be important limits to what one can ethically do with the data that are collected. For instance, when research is funded through a grant by the federal government, the research institution (e.g., university or hospital) is assigned ownership rights to the data gathered under that research. The research institution is held accountable for ensuring the integrity of the data that are collected. In this case neither the individual researcher nor the government have immediate ownership rights to the data—they belong primarily to the research institution that received the award (e.g., grant).

In other cases, the federal or state government may fund research through a contract, in which case the data are usually required to be "delivered" to the government which then retains ownership

interest. In the case of research that is sponsored (funded) by a private corporation, there is usually a contract that specifies the terms of the funding that is provided and that clarifies the ownership of data resides with the private corporation who retains this right in hopes of applying it for commercial use. Philanthropic organizations may also fund research, and they may either retain rights or give them away depending on their interests.

Finally, there are student research projects and clinician-initiated studies where the ownership interests in the data are not clearly articulated or understood. It is important for researchers to understand the nature of the agreements that provide funding for the research as well as any applicable policies in the settings where the research is conducted in order to know whether or not they have the right to publish those data.

Accepted Practices

For the results of research to be of value, it is essential that the data that are gathered are reliable. There is no one way to ensure the reliability of the data, but the responsible investigator will use acceptable standards within his or her field of research to ensure the careful collection of accurate information. In addition, the investigator must understand (or consult with others who understand) statistical methods adequately to ensure that they are using an appropriate strategy for the analysis of the data. Although this point is covered elsewhere in this text as an issue of scientific rigor, it is important to understand that following accepted scientific practice is also an ethical mandate.

The investigator must also understand what levels of authorization might be required to collect some forms of data. For instance, under the "Privacy Rule" (the rule many in the United States refer to by the legislation that required it—Health Information Privacy and Access Act or HIPAA), individuals who are collecting protected health information for research purposes in a setting such as a clinic or hospital will be required to obtain the written authorization of the patient/subject, or a data use agreement from the clinic or hospital, or a waiver of authorization from the IRB or Privacy Boar (Department of Health and Human Service, n.d.).

Finally, the investigator must ensure that data are properly protected so as to ensure the integrity of the data. This often means using appropriate filing strategies, including security measures such as locked file cabinets within locked offices, and password protected files on computer disks or other electronic storage devices. In many circumstances data must be retained for a number of years after they are published, or after the funding period is over. Specific data retention policies for the institution where data is gathered and stored should be consulted before data (or signed consent documents or authorizations) are destroyed.

Paper and Electronic Storage

Investigators frequently store their raw data on paper documents called case report forms. This information may subsequently be summarized in computer files for subsequent statistical analysis or for creating charts or graphs. The investigator should maintain the "source documents" as well as the computer files for some time after the results of the research are published or the grant or contract has ended.

Under HIPAA, in addition to the Privacy Rule there is also a Security Rule (Centers for Medicare and Medicaid Services, 2004) that requires that all electronically stored protected health information (e-PHI) be safeguarded according to acceptable standards. Each covered entity (e.g., clinic or hospital) is required to develop its own policies and procedures for ensuring the security of e-PHI. The researcher must be sure to comply with the applicable policies for his or her institution.

Mentor/Trainee Relationships

One of the most important, but least standardized mechanisms for training professional students in the proper conduct of research is the mentor–trainee relationship. Students are usually required to have a supervisor over their research activities, but the form and quality of the supervision will vary widely from mentor to mentor, and may be different with each trainee.

Mentors are required to invest time and resources in their trainees. Because of their experience base and relative power in the relationship, it is usually helpful for mentors to establish many of the ground rules for the mentoring relationship. These might include topics such as:

- How much time will the trainee be required to spend on the mentor's research?
- How much direct time will the mentor spend with the trainee providing individual or group supervision?
- What criteria will be used to evaluate the performance of the trainee?
- What are the authorship expectations for different research projects?
- What are the standard operating procedures regarding the conduct of the research, including the acquisition and storage of data?

- Who is entitled to access and use the data that are collected by the trainee?
- How will the data be stored, and by whom, after the trainee has completed his training?

It is helpful for a research laboratory to consider development of standard operating procedures governing the nature of the mentor/trainee relationship, and for standardizing authorship/publication practices.

The trainee also has responsibilities in the mentoring relationship. These include conscientious conduct that is consistent with research protocols, and other local institutional requirements. In the mentoring relationship, like in other aspects of academic training, trainees are responsible to understand the nature of their role and to seek out opportunities to learn from their teachers and mentors, who by virtue of their qualifications and experience should be in a position to be role models and resources for the trainee.

Many institutions or agencies funding research or research training require trainees to undergo formal training in the responsible conduct of research. This requirement has led to the development of a significant number of online resources that can be found in research institutions and on the ORI Web site. All persons who plan to collaborate in research or conduct research would be well advised to take advantage of these educational tools as well in order to consider ways they can maximize their benefit from the mentoring relationship.

Publication Practices and Responsible Authorship

The sharing of the results of research occurs in numerous contexts, and can easily be one of the more contentious issues related to research integrity. Early results from experiments are often shared in laboratory meetings, local research meetings, and clinical conferences, as well as scientific meetings. Later analysis of research results are frequently published in scholarly journals and books.

At a minimum, any communication of the results of research must be accurate and honest. Researchers should strive to accurately report their methods, the results obtained, and the conclusions they have drawn from the research. Scientific publication allows for the replication of methods, and the generalization of results from the study being reported. In human subject research, it allows for the generalization of the results from the experimental sample to others from a larger population. The publication of findings allows others to learn from the experiences and data collected during the conduct of the research.

Assignment of Due Credit

Authorship, or the assignment of names to a publication or presentation, is an important aspect of the responsible conduct of research. Persons who made substantive contributions to the research should be represented by inclusion in the authorship listing. This ordinarily can include:

• Persons who were instrumental in the initial conception and design of the study,
• Persons who were responsible for the collection and interpretation of the data, and
• Those who wrote up the results or substantively edited the presentation before publication.

Persons who play more minor roles are often acknowledged in the publication, but not given authorship credit. Individuals should not be given "honorary" authorship credit by virtue of their relationship to one or more of the authors, but included in the author listing only if they have made a substantive contribution. Open conversations between the parties conducting the research are essential regarding this topic as it is a frequent area of misunderstanding.

Within an organizational unit where members engage in research (e.g., a department or college), it is a good idea to develop policies that govern authorship. These policies should reflect:

• Consideration of ethical issues involved,
• Protection of less powerful individuals (e.g., students in relation to faculty members), and
• Local consensus about issues of fairness and responsibility.

Deciding authorship can be a challenging issue when students are involved with research under the supervision of faculty advisors or within the faculty member's research projects/teams. In such cases, it is useful to have departmental policies that guide decisions about authorship (see the feature box titled "Policies Governing Authorship," as an example). Finally, it should be noted that policies alone can never cover all contingencies, so open and honest communication combined with fair-minded negotiation is also important. This process should begin before the research commences and continue as persons shift responsibilities, contributions, and roles.

Repetitive and Fragmentary Publication

It is important that the same results not be published more than once without clear acknowledg-ment of the prior presentation or publication. This avoids wasting resources and keeps the research record clear. It is also important for readers to know whether one is reporting the same results again or an independent replication of the previous research (whether it is the same data being presented again or a new set of data). This is also important when researchers conduct meta-analyses (see Chapter 18), since it is essential that the "sample of samples" contain an accurate accounting and that research samples not be inadvertently repeated.

Citations

The appropriate and accurate citation of supporting evidence for one's own research is an important aspect of research integrity. When ideas, data, or conclusions are based on other published work, including prior publications of the author or co-authors, there must be appropriate attributions made through inclusion of a citation. As exemplified in the feature box titled "Fabrication, Falsification, and Plagiarism," not properly citing someone else's work can be cause for allegations of plagiarism (presenting someone else's work or ideas as if they were your own).

Conflicts of Interest or Commitment

There can be numerous conflicts of interest in the research enterprise. One of these is the desire to attain status and gratification from being the one to make new information available to others. However, it is important in research not to make public statements about the results of the research prematurely. When preliminary results are presented, this practice is usually limited to presentations at scientific meetings where the audience will understand and the presenter will clearly articulate the results as being preliminary and subject to additional analysis and the scrutiny of peer review before being published for more general scientific consumption.

In addition, there are circumstances when the results are not favorable, and when the reporting of those results might be harmful to the funding opportunity or career of the researcher. There are times when it would be a clear violation of principles of integrity to hide or suppress unexpected, contrary, or negative results for the sake of self-promotion or interest.

Conflict of commitment tends to address issues such as hours spent on an outside job or other income generation, which may prevent researchers from having their full energy and effort for their primary employment and, in particular, for dis-

Developing local policies of authorship that involve faculty–student collaboration should follow careful discussion that takes into consideration multiple factors including such things as ethical principles that guide the policy, the local organization culture, and how faculty and students ordinarily work together within the setting. Below is the policy published in the Student Handbook of the Department of Occupational Therapy at the University of Illinois (http://www.uic.edu/ahs/OT):

Policy on Joint Authorship

An important part of the recognized mission of the Department of Occupational Therapy and the University is the generation and dissemination of knowledge. Publication is the primary process through which knowledge is disseminated in a profession. Therefore, the Department expects its faculty to publish and encourage students to consider publication of their scholarly work. Although publication can never be a requirement for a student paper or thesis, student scholarship and research is often of a caliber to merit publication. In many cases the final product is the effort of several people including the student and joint-authorship will be a consideration.

Authorship connotes ownership of ideas, findings, conclusions, and so on. It is indicative of an individual's work and intellectual contribution to a final published product. It is both criteria by which individuals can be judged for such consequential processes as merit, tenure, and promotion. Moreover, it is something for which an individual may receive substantial recognition and career advancement. Thus, for these several reasons authorship should never be taken lightly.

The overriding principle that should always govern inclusion of an individual as an author is that the person has made a significant contribution to the scholarly piece and that this contribution was made with the explicit intention of sharing in the publication. Implied, then, is that authorship should be determined at the beginning of the process and not at the end. Also, since persons' roles in a particular scholarly process may change while it is underway, authorship should be subject to renegotiation if an individual's role becomes much greater or much less than originally intended. Because application of useful information is not only a privilege but also a responsibility, persons involved in a potentially publishable activity should always make provisions and plans for bringing the material to the jury process.

Not all authorship is equal. Generally the first author is recognized as the senior author—i.e., the person who had major responsibility for the published contents. Authorship can be diluted if the list of contributors is excessive; therefore, authorship should be limited to those with significant roles. Some activities that generally do not warrant authorship are: commentary on a draft of a paper, one or two consultations to a project, editorial assistance which focuses on grammar, punctuation, and composition, compensated data collection or limited voluntary data collection and compensated statistical analysis. Such contributions are generally noted in an acknowledgment. Authorship should never be used as a reward for limited assistance to a project; it should always be based on a negotiated significant role in the process.

The following are some guidelines that should be helpful in determining authorship:

1. The first author is someone who does all or many of the following: initiation of the idea, determination of the method to be used, making major decisions concerning variables and control of intervening variables, determining methods of data reduction, making interpretation of results, assumes a major role in writing the paper and assumes responsibility for communicating between authors, with the journal editor, and for any revisions following review and for submission of a flawless final manuscript and galley editing if it is used by the journal. (Note: In the event that two people equally shared this first level of responsibility, alphabetic order is the protocol for entry of names.)

2. The second author is someone who may do some of the things noted above and who typically assists in the development of ideas, method, and instrumentation and who assists in data reduction and analysis and in writing.

3. The third author may be someone who assists or carries out data collection of a significant portion of the data or who makes a substantial contribution to one or more phases of the project such as statistical analysis and interpretation. (Note: In the event that authors other than the first author have made equal contributions, alphabetic order is the protocol for order of entry of names.)

4. In the event that the original negotiated first author chooses not to assume his/her responsibility to pursue publication in good faith within 1 year of completion of the project, other persons who originally negotiated to be second or third authors may assume this responsibility. In any case the first author's name should be included in the publication, although first authorship may be renegotiated.

5. Everyone whose name appears on a published article should have the opportunity to view and approve the final draft unless he/she explicitly designates the responsibility to a coauthor(s).

charging research obligations. Local institutions are likely to have developed their own thresholds and definitions of when an activity constitutes a conflict of financial interest or commitment. Both the investigator and the research team members are responsible for complying with the institutional and federal requirements for disclosure and management of conflicts of interest and commitment.

Peer Review

One of the hallmarks of scholarly publication is the practice of peer review. This process involves a review of the planned publication by other scientists who are neutral in response to the publication and have sufficient expertise to provide a scientific critique and evaluation. Part of their evaluation includes judgments as to the potential value of the research to the current literature.

Peer review, like IRB review of human subject research, is intended to be an evaluative process through which quality scientific publications are vetted. The role of peer review then is one that requires honest appraisal and feedback. Journal and book editors rely on peer reviewers to provide them with expert opinions with regard to potential publication manuscripts. Granting agencies rely on peer review to make decisions about which research proposals should be funded. Therefore, it is important that the peer reviewer adopt a facilitative role. This requires putting aside personal disagreements with others in the discipline or deferring one's own ambitions to the sake of the scientific enterprise. Reviewers must also respect the confidentiality of the information with which they are provided.

Peer reviewers are usually selected in confidence by the editors of a journal or book. The reviewers usually are blind to the author of the manuscript under review, and the authors of the manuscript are not informed regarding the identity of the reviewers. Reviewers are not paid for their time and efforts, but are expected to provide timely and honest reviews in accordance with the format of feedback desired by the editors. Typically, editors will provide reviewers' comments back to the author, who will then revise the manuscript to address the issues raised. The editor may also notify the author that there is not support for the publication of that manuscript in their journal, in which case the author can consider submission of the manuscript to another journal for review. It is important to refrain from submitting a manuscript to more than one journal at a time.

Peer reviewers are obligated to provide honest feedback regarding the grants or manuscripts they are reviewing. It is not acceptable for a reviewer to allow someone else to assist him or her in performing the review, since this would be a breach of the confidentiality requirement. They also must not use ideas they find in grants or manuscripts until the information is publicly available. The manuscripts or grant applications that have been reviewed should be returned to the editors/granting agencies after the review is completed or they should be shredded or otherwise destroyed.

Collaborative Science

Scientific investigation is becoming increasingly interdisciplinary and inter-institutional. This has led to an increase in collaborative efforts between investigators and between scientific disciplines. It has also led to consortium arrangements whereby multiple institutions may share some common scientific resources. The responsible conduct of collaborative science entails attention to establishing clear roles and responsibilities, as well as written agreements that will satisfy institutional officials at the various institutions.

It is helpful to be able to establish the ground rules for conduct and reporting of the research early in the collaboration. Various co-investigators may share interest in common research aims, and so there should be some discussion of the proposed authorship arrangements in relation to the proposed conduct of and responsibility over the study.

Sharing of Materials and Data with External Collaborators

There may need to be contractual agreements, including material transfer agreements, that convey ownership rights to intellectual property or materials that will change hands during the course of the study. These agreements are usually negotiated through the grants and contracts office of a larger institution and by corporate counsel at a smaller institution.

Special Concerns Related to HIPAA. Following implementation of the HIPAA Privacy Rule, and more recently the Security Rule, it is prudent to consider the HIPAA-related issues early in the research development process to ensure adequate time to accrue the appropriate waivers, agreements, or approval for authorization agreements. It is important to remember that the institution where PHI is created has a primary responsibility for ensuring that there are appropriate mechanisms for accessing PHI for research, especially when PHI will be shared with co-investigators outside of the covered entity.

Protection of Human Subjects in Research

Of all the ethical considerations in research, the most compelling pertain to humans who will be subjects or participants in a study. Unfortunately, the impetus for contemporary ethical standards for the protection of human research subjects is grounded in previous abuses of humans under the guise of research. Two of the most well known instances are the Nazi doctors' trials and the Tuskegee experiment.

Nazi Doctors' Trials

In the Nazi doctors' trials following World War II, the tribunal identified numerous experiments that had been conducted in the interest of science, which represent horrific abuses of human beings. For instance, concentration camp prisoners were exposed to low atmospheric pressures, to simulate what might happen to pilots if they were exposed to atmospheric conditions at high altitudes. Individuals would lapse into coma, and sometimes died as the Nazi scientists established some of the limits of human endurance. In other experiments, prisoners were placed naked into tubs of icy water in order to establish limits for hypothermia. They were then often rescued using various techniques that sometimes produced scalding burns and even death. While these experiments provided the Nazi military with valuable information regarding the length of time human beings can survive in water at various temperatures, and information about effective methods for reviving soldiers who were partially frozen, those hapless prisoners were involuntarily exposed to experimental torture and even death. The experiments by the Nazi doctors were ethically reprehensible because they caused harm without regard for the well-being or for the informed consent of the subject. They also exposed individuals to unacceptably high levels of risk without regard for their pain and suffering, and in ways in which the risks were not reasonable in light of the benefit that might be gained from the information that was derived from the research.

Tuskegee Experiment

When an agency of the American Public Health Service began its study of syphilis in the African-American male, they selected a rural area in the south (Macon County, Alabama) with a high concentration of men who had the disease (Dunn and Chadwick, 2002). They intended to study the natural history of the disease for a period of 6 months, but then considered the research important enough that it was continued. They collected spinal fluid through nontherapeutic spinal taps, telling the unknowing research subjects that they were being provided with treatment for "bad blood."

In 1943, penicillin was recognized as an effective treatment for syphilis. In the eyes of the researchers from the Public Health Service (PHS), this made the cohort of patients in the Tuskegee trial even more precious as they might be one of the last cohorts of individuals with the disease who would be studied longitudinally (over a long period of time). For this reason, the PHS researchers made additional efforts to ensure that their research subjects remained under study. This meant preventing them from knowing they had a disease, and preventing them from obtaining medical treatment for syphilis. During World War II, the PHS investigators managed to convince the local draft board not to enlist any of the Tuskegee subjects into the armed forces because they would have been readily diagnosed and treated.

In retrospect, and from a perspective outside of the investigators, this is easily viewed as a morally repugnant study. Investigators deceived innocent and vulnerable men into thinking they were getting some form of treatment, when they were actually being denied information about a disease they had (and were sharing with others in their community), and were not provided with or actively prevented from receiving a treatment for their syphilis. This study was exposed by the media in 1972 and the study was finally halted in 1973. The public outcry led to the regulations and the IRB and federal oversight processes which make up today's human subject protection programs in the United States (Dunn & Chadwick, 2002).

Nuremberg Code

One of the earliest U.S. codes regarding the ethical conduct of research was written during the Nazi doctors' trials. Because the trials were conducted in Nuremberg, Germany, the 10 principles of ethical human subject research became known as the Nuremberg Code. Dunn and Chadwick (2002, p. 16) cite from the code the following protections:

- Informed consent of volunteers must be obtained without coercion in any form.
- Human experiments should be based upon prior animal experimentation.
- Anticipated scientific results should justify the experiment.
- Only qualified scientists should conduct medical research.

- Physical and mental suffering and injury should be avoided.
- There should be no expectation of death or disabling injury from the experiment.

The Principles of Belmont

In 1979, the U.S. National Commission for the Protection of Human Subjects of Biomedical and Behavioral Research published a document summarizing for the Department of Health, Education and Welfare (later to become the Department of Health and Human Services) the basic ethical principles for human subject research. In the paper, they distinguish between clinical practice and clinical research, and they set out three basic principles that are intended to apply to all research involving humans:

- Respect for persons,
- Beneficence, and
- Justice.

Respect for Persons

Respect for persons is the most basic of the three principles, and asserts that human persons must be respected in terms of their right to self-determination. Key to this principle is the notion of informed consent as a required prerequisite for most kinds of research, in particular when the research involves imposing some risks on the subjects.

The Belmont Report's principle of respect for persons emphasizes the importance of the individual to make choices whether or not to participate in a research study as an exercise of free will. Respect for persons assumes that the researcher can provide enough information, in a language the prospective subject can understand, for the individual to provide fully informed consent to be involved in the research. The report goes on to recognize that there are circumstances and populations that are not able to provide fully informed consent, and requires that additional protections be afforded to these vulnerable populations. Pregnant women and fetuses are considered to be a vulnerable population, as are prisoners and children.

Beneficence

Beneficence is the principle that requires that human subjects research minimize risk to the greatest extent possible and maximizes the potential for benefits to be gained from the research (either for the individuals participating in the research or from the knowledge that will be gained). Risks must be reasonable in relation to the potential for benefit to be derived from the research. This means that the risks are reasonable in light of the potential for benefit from participation (to the subjects themselves, or from the knowledge to be gained from their participation). The risks considered include reasonably anticipated physical and mental risks, as well as physical and mental discomforts. Beneficence also requires the use of sound research methodology, since no degree of risk is acceptable if the research design is inadequate. That is, there would be little likelihood for benefit from the knowledge to be gained if the study is not sound, and without any anticipated benefits no risk to subjects is justified.

Finally, beneficence also requires that risks must be minimized. This means that investigators should take every precaution and make every effort to anticipate and prevent or minimize physical or mental discomfort or harm that may accrue from participation in the study.

Maximizing Potential for Benefit. There are numerous ways in which the IRB and the investigator can design the study to maximize potential for benefit, both for the individual subjects and from the potential knowledge that may be gained from the research. For instance, a study might increase the potential for individual subjects to benefit by incorporating a crossover design rather than a placebo control. In the case of the placebo control, those subjects receive no therapy at all, while in the crossover design everyone has a period of time when they are receiving the new treatment. The IRB's insistence on sound research methodology is a way of ensuring that there is a maximum potential for benefit from the research in terms of its providing generalizable knowledge.

Justice

The principle of justice requires that the research impose the burden of risk and the potential for benefit upon the same groups of people. It is unacceptable from the perspective of the principle of justice for an investigator to take advantage of a vulnerable population, for instance the poor, in order for others to reap the benefits of the research. Consequently, ensuring justice typically involves examination of the composition of subjects who have been enrolled according to such categories as sex and race/ethnicity.

Informed Consent

The principle of informed consent requires that prospective research subjects be given enough information, before they choose to participate in a research study, that they can make an informed decision as to whether or not they want to participate. While there are some circumstances in which the requirement of prospective informed consent may be waived or altered, usually research involving human subjects requires they provide written informed consent (and possibly a HIPAA authorization for research use of protected health information) before they participate in the research.

Informed consent usually requires:

- That subjects be prospectively informed that they are being asked to participate in research,
- That their participation is voluntary, and
- That they may choose to discontinue their participation at any time.

Prospective subjects must also be informed of reasonably anticipated risks and discomforts from participation, as well as any benefits that may be expected to result from their participation or from the knowledge gained from the study. The IRB may waive or alter the required elements of informed consent under some circumstances.

The Process of Consent

A central component of informed consent is a well written informed consent document, and a process of obtaining consent that involves a careful review of the information in the document with ample opportunity for the prospective subject to have any questions answered. The process under which investigators inform prospective subjects about the research is even more important than the document that the subject signs. Consent conferences should reflect the information in the consent document, but also include questions to allow the person obtaining consent to be assured the potential subject understands the information that is being presented.

Consent usually is not a one-time event, but an ongoing process through a subject's participation in research. If a study goes for a prolonged period of time, it may be prudent to revisit the consent document, ask about willingness to continue in the research, and offer to answer questions about ongoing participation.

Assent and Surrogate Permission

Consent refers to the process whereby a competent adult gives permission for something to be done to his or her own person or information. One cannot give consent for something to be done to others. Therefore, in the case of children and adolescents, the regulations usually require a combination of parental permission and the active assent (not the failure to dissent) of the children and adolescents.

In the case of adults who may have cognitive impairments (e.g., psychotic episodes or dementia), the researcher will need to obtain the assent of such persons to the extent they are able to provide it and the permission of a surrogate. Ideally the surrogate is a legally authorized agent under the local laws. When such laws do not exist, it is important for the investigator who may be enrolling adult subjects who are cognitively impaired to consult with legal counsel to ensure that appropriate surrogate consent is being obtained.

Documentation of Consent

The documentation of consent refers to obtaining the appropriate signature on (an) IRB-approved consent or assent document(s). The original documents are very important to keep as any audit of the research study will require the investigator to produce them. Funding agencies require that these original documents be maintained for a number of years after the completion of the study. Investigators are usually required to provide a copy of the consent document to the subjects as an information sheet they can take with them. Under HIPAA, if an investigator is also obtaining an authorization for the research use of protected health information, the investigator is required to provide subjects with a copy of the signed consent document.

Informed consent is often a complex process that involves a number of considerations. These include, for instance:

- Making sure the prospective subject understands the study and the risks/benefits involved (this increasingly involves not only ensuring that the study will be explained in lay terms but indicating how the researcher will ascertain that the subject has understood what was explained),
- Consideration of whether prospective subjects have the ability to give consent,
- Balancing any incentives or reimbursement for participation to avoid coercion (e.g., giving financial incentives that would be difficult for some potential subjects to decline), and
- Assuring freedom of consent in situations where other obligations or roles might pressure individuals to consent.

It is important the investigators consider and make plans to deal with these and other considerations that may be unique to a particular study when developing informed consent procedures. The feature box titled "Informed Consent Procedures," illustrates an occupational therapy informed consent procedure and the forms used in association with it.

Ethics Committees or Institutional Review Boards

Most institutions that have research involvement have established committees that oversee issues of ethical conduct in research. In the international context these bodies are usually referred to as Ethics Committees. In the United States research institutions that receive federal funding for human subject research are required to have an Institutional Review Board (IRB) that will exercise oversight authority over the research (Steneck, 2004). In such institutions, an individual must be designated to oversee this process; that individual is usually given a title such as Research Integrity Officer. IRB/ethics committee review is established as a mechanism whereby a group of diverse individuals, with scientific and nonscientific interests review the research to ensure that the research plan is ethical.

The IRB is responsible for reviewing research proposals (including grant funding applications) to ensure there are adequate provisions to minimize risk and maximize the potential for benefit from the research (to the subjects or from the knowledge that will be gained). The IRB is also responsible for ensuring that adequate safeguards are in place, including the requirements for informed consent, so that the risks to subjects are minimized to the greatest extent possible.

The specific operations of the IRB and the application of the regulations (laws) will vary from one institution to another. They also may vary depending on the source of funding or the nature of the research. IRBs are responsible to make numerous determinations about the level of risk related to participation in the research, the adequacy of the informed consent documents or processes, the appropriateness of recruitment materials, as well as ensuring there are additional safeguards for protecting vulnerable subjects. The IRB process may involve several series of responses to questions, modifications of the research plan, recruitment materials, and informed consent documents before the project is approved to begin (Matthews-Lopez & Watson, 2004).

Informed Consent Procedures

The approval of Informed Consent procedures by an IRB requires the researcher to:

• Describe how subjects will be recruited,
• Describe the informed consent process, and
• Submit the informed consent letter that will be used for approval.

Below is the section from an Approved Protocol at the University of Illinois at Chicago for a Psychometric Study of the Child Occupational Self-Assessment.

Recruitment and Consent Procedure

The initial contact will be made by the Occupational Therapist.

When subjects are recruited under the UIC collection protocol, guardians of the subjects and subjects will be asked if they will be willing to participate in a research study to improve the Child's Occupational Self-Assessment (COSA).

It will be explained that:

Children are being asked to participate in a research study to improve the Child's Occupational Self-Assessment (COSA) and that the purpose of the assessment is to study how children perceive their strengths and weaknesses regarding performance of daily activities.

The guardians and children will be given the information sheet (that has been attached for IRB review) and will be asked to read the form (or have the form read to them) and to ask any questions they may have before agreeing to be in the research.

They will be told that:

• *As part of the research their child will be asked to complete a questionnaire and to discuss information obtained through the questionnaire.*
• *The child's name will not be used to identify them on the test form. They will not be identified in any way in any oral or written report of this study.*
• *There are no benefits or risks involved in participating in the study.*

Because this is a study involving children, both the children and their parents/legal guardians are explained the study and asked for consent. The procedure for asking parents/guardians is considered consent since the children are considered not yet able to give full consent on their own behalf. However, children's right to refuse participation is respected and thus they are explained the study; the procedure for asking children is referred to as assent. Below are the consent and assent letters used for the informed consent process in this study.

(continued)

University of Illinois at Chicago

**WRITTEN AND VERBAL ASSENT
TO PARTICIPATE IN RESEARCH
COSA STUDY**
(For children ages 8-17)

My name is Gary Kielhofner.

I am asking you to take part in a research study because we are trying to learn more about the lives of children who receive occupational therapy. We are trying to make a better questionnaire so that occupational therapists can have better information about the children they work with, especially how children think about their own strengths and weaknesses.

If you agree to be in this study, we will ask you to answer questions on a form.

Filling out the form will take place during your regular occupational therapy time.

There are no direct benefits to taking part in the study. However, your participation in the study will help to develop a questionnaire that may help other kids receive better occupational therapy.

Please talk this over with your parents before you decide whether or not you want to be in the study. We will ask your parents to give their permission for you to take part in this study. But even if your parents say "yes" you can still decide not to do this.

If you don't want to be in this study, you don't have to participate. Remember, being in this study is up to you and no one will be upset if you don't want to participate or even if you change your mind later and want to stop.

You can ask any questions that you have about the study. If you have a question later that you didn't think of now, you can call me, Gary Kielhofner, at 312-996-6901 or ask your occupational therapist.

Signing your name at the bottom means that you agree to be in this study. You and your parents will be given a copy of this form after you have signed it.

_____   _____

Name of Subject   Date

_____   ____   _____

Signature   Age   Grade in School

(continued)

University of Illinois at Chicago
Consent for Participation in Research
"Child Occupational Self Assessment"

Why am I being asked?
You are being asked if your child can participate in a research study to examine a self-rating evaluation form of occupational function. By using information obtained through this assessment, occupational therapists will be better able to provide therapy that is responsive to the individual needs of the child.

This study is conducted by Dr. Gary Kielhofner at the University of Illinois at Chicago. Your child has been asked to participate in the research because he/she has been referred to Occupational Therapy and may be eligible to participate. We ask that you read this form and ask any questions you may have before agreeing to be in the research.

You and your child's participation in this research is voluntary. Your decision whether or not to participate will not affect your current or future relations with the University. The occupational therapy your child receives will not be affected in any way by your decision to participate or not. If you decide to participate, you are free to withdraw at any time without affecting that relationship.

Why is this research being done?
Objectives: The objective of this project is to refine and determine the reliability of a self-rating form, the Child Occupational Self Assessment (COSA). The purpose of this research is to obtain information about a child's self perceptions of his /her occupational functioning.
Study Method: Data will be collected on a self rated form as part of the occupational therapy assessment procedure that your child would normally be involved in.
Risk/Benefits: There are no expected risks or benefits from participating in this research.

What is the purpose of this research?
The purpose of this research is to obtain information about a child's self perceptions of his /her occupational functioning. By using such an assessment, occupational therapists will be better able to provide therapy that is responsive to the individual needs of the child.

What procedures are involved?
If you agree to be in this research, we would ask your child to do the following things:

* Complete a self-assessment form and
* Take part in a subsequent discussion with an occupational therapist concerning his/her responses.

This form will be completed during his/her ordinary time for therapy or at a time scheduled for your own convenience. Your child's name will not be used to identify him/her on the test form and will not be identified in any way in any oral or written report of this study. Approximately 1,000 people may be involved in this research at the University of Illinois at Chicago.

What are the potential risks and discomforts?
There are no known risks associated with participation in this study beyond those that you would encounter in any supervised therapy session. Most of the questions are related to your child's ability to care for himself/herself. In the unlikely event that your child is injured while completing the assessment, the University of Illinois at Chicago will not be responsible for providing either medical care or compensation for such care as required by law.

Are there benefits to taking part in the research?
Although you will not directly benefit from participating in this study, your child's participation will help to develop an assessment that may be of benefit to children receiving therapy.

What about privacy and confidentiality?
The information that the research team receives will not have any information on it that will identify your child as a subject.

What if my child is injured as a result of my participation?
In the event of injury related to this research study, treatment will be made available through the University of Illinois at Chicago Hospital. However, you or your third-party payer, if any, will be responsible for payment of this treatment. There is no compensation and/or payment for such medical treatment from the University of Illinois at Chicago for such injury, except as may be required of the University by law. If you feel your child has been injured, you may contact the researcher, Gary Kielhofner, at (312) 996–6901.

What are the costs for participating in this research?
There are no additional research costs for which the subject would be responsible.

Will I be reimbursed for any of my expenses or paid for my child's participation in this research?
There will be no monetary compensation for participation in the research.

Can I withdraw or be removed from the study?
You can choose whether your child will be in this study or not. You may withdraw at any time without consequence. Your child may also refuse to answer any questions he/she doesn't want to answer and still remain in the study. The investigator may withdraw your child from this research if circumstances arise which warrant doing so.

Whom should I contact if I have questions?
The researcher conducting this study is Gary Kielhofner. You may ask any questions you have now. If you have questions later, you may contact the researchers at: (312) 996–6901.

What are my child's rights as a research subject?
If you have any questions about your rights as a research subject, you may call the Office for Protection of Research Subjects at (312) 996–1711.

Remember:
Your child's participation in this research is completely voluntary. Your decision whether or not to participate will not affect your current or future relations with the University. If you decide to participate, you are free to withdraw at any time without affecting that relationship.
You will be given a copy of this form for your information and to keep for your records.

Signature of Subject or Legally Authorized Representative

I have read (or someone has read to me) the above information. I have been given an opportunity to ask questions and my questions have been answered to my satisfaction. I agree to participate in this research. I have been given a copy of this form.

Signature   Date

Printed Name

Signature of Researcher   Date (must be same as subject's)

When research proposals are not approved, and even if they are disapproved by the IRB, the IRB is required to inform the investigator what changes to the research would make it approvable. After initial approval, IRBs are required to promptly receive and review information related to unanticipated problems involving risks to subjects or others, and to review and require changes or approve any planned modifications to the research before they are implemented (except when changes to the protocol would remove subjects from risk of immediate harm—in this case the changes can be implemented right away and the IRB should be notified and an amendment submitted as soon as possible). Finally, the IRB is responsible for substantive re-review of the research no less often than once every 365 days.

Institutions that have IRBs generally publish guidelines, procedures, and forms that are used to submit proposed research and research progress reports. Investigators are responsible to find out and comply with these procedures and necessary documentation. In some institutions, the Principal Investigator and others who are part of a research team are required to undergo training in research ethics before submitting research for approval.

The necessary documentation for a planned study is submitted to the IRB. This minimally includes:

- A basic description of the study design and methods,
- Justification for the research (including the general benefits expected to accrue from the study),
- The numbers of subjects/participants planned in the study and their characteristics including whether they represent vulnerable populations,
- A description of the planned procedures used to recruit (including inducements and reimbursements) and obtain informed consent from subjects (including consent forms that will be used),
- What subjects will be asked to do as participants in the study,
- What if any benefits will accrue to subjects from participation,
- What if any risks to subjects are involved and how these will be minimized,
- How confidentiality will be maintained (including how data will be stored and how long it will be retained), and
- Who will be the personnel in the study.

Increasingly, institutions provide forms or structured formats for submitting this information to the IRB for approval.

Until the IRB has approved the study, the investigator cannot proceed with the research. As noted earlier, approval sometimes involves several steps in which the IRB responds to the original or previous submission with questions and required changes. Investigators should find out deadlines for submission of IRB documentation and the schedule of IRB meetings, factoring these into overall deadlines and planning for a research project.

The Role of the Investigator and Research Team

The investigator and research team have the most direct responsibility for ensuring human subject protections are implemented and maintained as approved by the IRB. The Principal Investigator (i.e., the researcher in charge of the project) is ultimately responsible for ensuring that the required human subject protections are followed. The Principal Investigator may delegate some of the responsibilities for the conduct of the study, but may not delegate ultimate responsibility for the conduct of the research team. In addition, the Principal Investigator is responsible for reporting any unanticipated problems involving risks to subjects or others, and for abiding by the IRB approved protocol and consent document/process. Ultimately, it is the Principal Investigator who is held responsible for the conduct of the research, but each individual member of the research team is also responsible for his or her own conduct. When questions arise regarding research integrity or some aspect of the research conduct in light of regulations, it is the responsibility of the Principal Investigator and the research team to find a satisfactory answer.

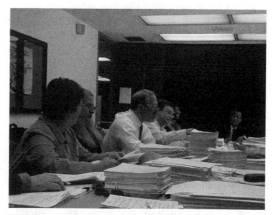

Figure 29.1 An Institutional Review Board (IRB) reviews a research proposal.

Research Misconduct

As noted earlier, misconduct in science refers to fabrication, falsification, plagiarism, or serious deviation from commonly accepted practice for proposing, conducting, or reporting research. Misconduct does not include honest error. Nor does it include honest differences in interpretations or judgments concerning research data. These criteria for research misconduct are from the U.S. regulations at Title 42 CFR 50.102. This regulation also establishes the criteria for allegations of research misconduct as well as for determinations made after a formal inquiry or investigation into the allegations. To qualify as misconduct, the behavior of the investigator or member of the research team must represent a significant deviation from commonly accepted practices, and it must be intentional, knowing, or reckless. In its view, Office of Research Integrity in the U.S. considers plagiarism to include outright theft and misappropriation of intellectual property, as well as the substantial unattributed textual copying of another's work. It does not include authorship or credit disputes (Office of Research Integrity, 2005). Finally, the allegations need to be proven by a preponderance of evidence for such a determination to be made. Thus, there are forms of misconduct that may not warrant sanctions, but that clearly breach ethical standards. Therefore, as we noted earlier, conduct in research is better guided by a concern for ethics and integrity than a concern to avoid sanction.

Mechanisms for Resolving Allegations

Research institutions usually develop policies for resolving allegations of misconduct in a timely manner and through a two-step process. Typically there is an inquiry phase during which the allegation is initially explored to determine whether it meets the institutional and federal definitions of misconduct, and whether there seems to be evidence of the alleged misconduct. If the allegation appears meritorious, then the matter is referred to a more comprehensive investigation phase, during which the allegations and the evidence are reviewed by a larger group. During the investigation, the institution is seeking to find out whether or not the allegation of misconduct is true. The institutional policy must also define a person with authority in the institution to act on the results of the investigation. That person can impose sanctions upon the individual if found guilty of misconduct or can vindicate the person if cleared of the allegation. Finally, the institutional policy makes provisions for reporting the findings to ORI.

Conclusion

There are many policies that govern the ethical conduct of research. These policies reflect a long history of efforts to correct past abuses of human right as well as efforts to identify and attain the highest standards of integrity in research. Researchers and students who participate in research are well advised to familiarize themselves with the basic requirements for the responsible conduct of research. This can be accomplished through online browsing and through continuing education sections at professional meetings and is often provided within research institutions. Some useful Web sites are noted at the end of this chapter in the Resources section.

In addition to the federal regulations, researchers need to be familiar with their own local policies and procedures. These local policies will often go into greater detail regarding how the researcher needs to conduct his or her research and stay in compliance. Many institutions have administrative offices that handle conflicts of interest, responsible conduct of research, and that coordinate grant and contract applications or ethical approval of research. Officials in those offices and their local Web sites are both likely to be rich sources of additional guidance.

In the end, the best way for investigators to ensure compliance with human subject protections is for the investigator to be well informed. Understanding the ethical principles and the regulatory requirements should increase a researcher's motivation to ensure that adequate protections are provided. A commitment to and thorough understanding of the ethical principles and the requirements for the responsible conduct of research are essential to conducting research with integrity.

REFERENCES

Centers for Medicare and Medicaid Services. (2004). *HIPAA Security and Electronic Signature Standards; Proposed Rule.* Retrieved at the time of publication from http://www.cms.hhs.gov/hipaa/hipaa2/regulations/security/default.asp.

Department of Health and Human Services. (n.d.). *Protecting personal health information in research: Understanding the HIPAA Privacy Rule.* Retrieved at the time of publication from http://privacyruleandresearch.nih.gov/pdf/HIPAA_Booklet_4-14-2003.pdf.

Dunn, C. M., & Chadwick, G. L. (2002). *Protecting study volunteers in research: A manual for investigative sites* (2nd ed.). Boston: Thomson.

HHS Working Group on the NBAC Report. (n.d.). *Research involving individuals with questionable capacity to consent: Points to consider* (Appendix C). Retrieved at the time of publication from http://aspe.hhs.gov/sp/nbac/appendixc.shtml.

Matthews-Lopez, J. L., & Watson, K. D. (2004). Navigating the review process for research involving human participants: An overview and practical guidelines [Electronic Version]. *Ohio Research and Clinical Review, 14*, 7–13. Retrieved at the time of publication from http://www.ohiocore.org/Research/documents/ORCR/ORCR_2004.pdf.

National Commission for the Protection of Human Subjects of Biomedical and Behavioral Research. (1979). *The Belmont Report.* Retrieved at the time of publication from http://www.hhs.gov/ohrp/humansubjects/guidance/belmont.htm.

Office for Human Research Protections. (2001). *Policy for the Protection of Human Subjects (Basic DHHS Policy for Protection of Human Research Subjects)*, Title 45 Public Welfare, Part 46, Protection Of Human Subjects, The Common Rule. Retrieved at the time of publication from http://www.hhs.gov/ohrp/humansubjects/guidance/45cfr46.htm.

Office of Research Integrity. (2005). *Policies: ORI provides working definition of plagiarism.* Retrieved at the time of publication from http://ori.dhhs.gov/policies/plagiarism.shtml.

Steneck, N. H. (2004). *ORI introduction to the responsible conduct of research.* Washington, DC: U.S. Department of Health and Human Services. Retrieved at the time of publication from http://ori.dhhs.gov/documents/rcrintro.pdf.

RESOURCES

U.S. Federal Research Integrity Policies

There are several U.S. federal research integrity policies posted on the Office of Research Integrity (ORI) Web site (including those from the Public Health Service and the National Science Foundation) (http://ori.dhhs.gov/). The federal regulations regarding the conduct of human subjects research that is funded by the Department of Health and Human Services, as well as guidance and online information resources is readily available at the OHRP Web site (http://www.hhs.gov/ohrp/) and the FDA Web site for regulating medical devices (http://www.fda.gov/cdrh/index.html). Many academic careers have ended with a finding of research misconduct, or have been impaired because of noncompliance with other regulations. In addition, institutions have faced very stiff fines or sanctions that have cost millions of dollars. The ORI Web site contains informative case summaries of closed cases and the sanctions that have been made (http://ori.dhhs.gov/misconduct/cases/index.shtml) The OHRP Web site includes access to determination letters regarding findings of noncompliance (http://www.hhs.gov/ohrp/compliance/letters/index.html). Reviewing these documents can be quite informative for the student and researcher alike as we all try to better understand how to conduct research responsibly.

The Belmont Report

In recognition of the 25th anniversary of the Belmont Report, and in tribute to its important contribution to our thinking about the ethical conduct of research, there is a special Web site with historical information pertaining to the report and the process of its development (http://www.hhs.gov/ohrp/belmontArchive.html).

The Declaration of Helsinki

Within the international context, the major document summarizing ethical principles for research is the Declaration of Helsinki. The World Medical Association initially adopted this statement of ethical principles in 1964, and last amended the document in 2000. It is available online at: http://www.wma.net/e/policy/b3.htm.

A study course is available to occupational therapists entitled: "Promoting Research Integrity in the Next Generation of Occupational Therapy Researchers." It was developed through a contract to the American Occupational Therapy Association and Foundation (AOTF/AOTA) from the Office of Research Integrity administered by the American Association of Medical Colleges. Information can be found at the AOTA Web site; www.aota.org.

CHAPTER 30

Obtaining Funding for Research

Renée R. Taylor • Yolanda Suarez-Balcazar • Geneviève Pépin • Elizabeth White

The most common mechanism for funding of research is a grant. A grant award is a specified amount of money given to an investigator or to the investigator's parent institution to undertake a specific research project. Grants may also include funding for development, educational, training, and/ or evaluation projects that often have a research component. A grant application is the document that an investigator prepares to request the funding. This chapter covers the nature of grant awards, what they fund, who provides them, and how to prepare a competitive grant application.

The Purpose of Grant Funding

The various agencies that provide grants do so to make possible a research project that might otherwise not occur. Thus, they often cover all or most of the expenses associated with the research study. Depending on the guidelines of the granting agency, grant funding may be used to cover:

- All or a certain percentage of team members' salaries,
- Tuition waivers and small monetary stipends to graduate research assistants,
- Supplies and equipment that is necessary for the conduction of the study (e.g., tests, mechanical devices for experiments, computers, printers, and relevant software),
- Incentives to participants, and
- The costs of ancillary needs such as telephone, postage, transportation, printing, and photocopy costs.

Some grants also cover indirect costs of doing the research, including, for example, space rental or maintenance, the cost of heating and air conditioning, and electricity.

Major Types of Grants

There are four major types of grants that may be obtained by occupational therapy researchers:

1. Research grants,
2. Demonstration grants,
3. Training, educational, and professional development grants, and
4. Center grants.

Research Grants

Research grants allow investigators to address scientific questions that will contribute to knowledge in a given topic area. There are numerous kinds of studies that research grants tend to fund, but they can generally be classified into two major groups:

1. Basic (bench) science studies, and
2. Applied science studies.

Basic science studies are typically narrow in focus. Rather than addressing a practical issue or clinical problem, basic science studies provide the necessary knowledge and background for later applied research. They are designed to generate knowledge about a particular theory or about a basic diagnostic, biological, behavioral, attitudinal, or emotional phenomenon. Basic science studies may include, but are not limited to, epidemiological studies, laboratory studies, and field observations.

Applied science studies aim to test the application of a particular theory to a practical life problem. Applied science studies may be used to develop new technologies or intervention approaches (e.g., rehabilitation strategies). Applied studies commonly involve evaluating the effectiveness of the application of one or more of these technologies or intervention approaches. A well-known example of an applied study is a clinical outcomes study (e.g., a randomized clinical trial) in which one or more technologies or intervention approaches are compared against a control condition to evaluate their efficacy in addressing a given clinical problem. Participatory research that seeks to empower individuals to transform their current skills or circumstances through education and social action is another example of applied research. More information about participatory research methods is provided in Chapters 38 to 40 of this text.

Alternative Mechanisms of Funding

Depending on the funding agency or sponsor, funding can be achieved through different mechanisms. For example, in the United States, the National Institutes of Health (NIH) uses three types of funding venues to support researchers: grants, contracts, and cooperative agreements. Grants differ from contracts and cooperative agreements in that the investigator has more influence in deciding the research topic to be designed or developed and the accompanying methodological approach. With contracts the government or private funder usually decides on and selects the research that fulfills the perceived need and then specifies detailed logistical or methodological requirements that an investigator is then asked to carry out. A cooperative agreement is similar to a grant, but the awarding institute or center and the researcher both have significant involvement together in carrying out the activities of the project. Because most funding agencies tend to utilize research grants as their primary funding source, this chapter focuses on describing the process of writing and applying for research grants. Information about contracts and cooperative agreements can be obtained from literature provided by individual funding agencies (see http://www.npguides. org/guide/index.html for resources).

Demonstration Grants

The aim of a demonstration grant is to allow investigators to develop, expand, and evaluate a specific set of healthcare services, a model program, or a particular methodological approach (Gitlin & Lyons, 2004). For example, some occupational therapy investigators use demonstration grants to develop new assessments, interventions, new ways to disseminate healthcare information, or assistive devices. Demonstration grants allow investigators to build on existing knowledge about the efficacy of a given approach to service or programming (Gitlin & Lyons, 2004). They typically involve some kind of program evaluation component that involves elements of research. These grants typically take place in settings seeking to expand or alter their services and those wanting to develop new programs that can serve as models for later replication in other settings. Demonstration grants may also be used to support the evaluation and modification of ongoing programs in clinical, industry, educational, and community settings.

Training, Educational, and Professional Development Grants

Training and educational grants are used to support professionals and students to develop or extend their knowledge or skills. These grants can be used to support professional activities that involve training and education (e.g., conferences or symposia). They can also be used to support the implementation of specialized academic programs. For example, a training grant can be issued to a university for the purpose of supporting first-generation undergraduate students from underserved groups who have a goal of pursuing graduate training in occupational therapy. Similarly, a professional development grant is used to enable an individual who is already employed in a professional capacity to begin a career in research or to further develop research-related skills and contributions.

Center Grants

Center grants are usually large grants; they are typically funded for about 5 years with the possibility of competitive renewal. Center grants generally involve several related projects that incorporate research, development, implementation, training, and dissemination activities. Center grants also involve identifying multiple partners and collaborators, which might include several researchers from across the country and/or multiple agencies who have access to potential participants or who want to participate in training and/or dissemination activities. Although center grants often involve multiple collaborators and disciplines, they are focused and theme-related. As such, all proposed research, development, or training activities are designed to make contributions to the advancement of knowledge, practice, and policies in a specific area. Overall, center grants are unique opportunities to develop state-of-the art innovations and engage in multidisciplinary research, dissemination, and training activities.

See the feature box on the next page for an example of a center grant.

Reasons to Apply for Grant Funding

In many academic settings, grant funding is vital to the daily operation and activities of the organization. Many clinics, clinical training programs, and academic departments would not exist in the

The University of Illinois at Chicago Center for Capacity Building for Minorities with Disabilities Research (CCBMDR)

This center grant was funded for 5 years for a total amount of $ 3 million by the National Institutes of Disability and Rehabilitation Research (see Balcazar & Suarez-Balcazar, 2004). The center was funded to increase the capacity of community-based organizations such as Centers for Independent Living, State Vocational Rehabilitation Agencies, and other agencies serving minorities with disabilities to identify services, improve their capacity to provide culturally competent services, and improve their capacity to evaluate the impact of services on the lives of participants. The center will also develop state-of-the-art scientific knowledge on issues related to cultural competence, adaptation and development of culturally appropriate vocational rehabilitation assessment tools, and the development of disability identity among minorities. The center grant also will undertake five research projects.

The center involves a principal investigator and a co-principal investigator from the University of Illinois at Chicago, nine research collaborators from five different states (California, Illinois, Massachusetts, Montana, and Texas), and a number of community partner agencies in each of the five states including Centers for Independent Living, other community-based organizations, and Vocational Rehabilitation agencies. These collaborators will be working together to conduct a national conference and then produce a state-of-the-science book and other forms of scholarship such as publications and professional presentations.

absence of grant funding. Within the field of occupational therapy, grants support the refinement, advancement, and empirical study of education, theory, assessments, technologies, and services. Grant funding is also an indirect source of reputation-building and publicity for an organization and the occupational therapists involved.

For all of these reasons, grant funding is often an expectation of occupational therapy faculty members working in top research universities. Likewise, occupational therapists working in practice settings may be involved in writing grants. Such grants enable advancing, maintaining, and/or evaluating programs of service.

Grants also provide individual benefits to the investigators who receive them. They allow an investigator to have the resources to conduct a study that otherwise would not be possible. Or, they allow a study to be larger in scope and greater in impact than would otherwise be possible. Moreover, grants allow an investigator to work with a funding agency to produce peer-reviewed research that serves public, legislative, and/or private interests. Grants also allow an investigator to advance his or her career and work collaboratively with a research team that mutually enriches and supports the efficiency, productivity, and professional development of all of its members.

How Grants Get Funded

In most cases, grant funding occurs as a result of a rigorous review process, discussed in a later section of this chapter. One thing is certain: Grant funding does not occur in a vacuum. It requires the involvement of a number of entities, including:

- One's sponsoring university, clinic, or home institution,
- Administrators within the funding agency (often referred to as project officers),
- Individuals charged to review the relevance and quality of the grant application (often referred to as peer reviewers or grant reviewers), and
- Individuals who take the feedback of project officers and reviewers and ultimately oversee the allocation of funds within a granting agency (e.g., agency trustees or a board of directors).

In addition to these individuals, investigators are wise to identify experienced colleagues, mentors, or hired reviewers to evaluate their ideas, methods, and eventual written grant proposal before it is submitted for formal review. When appropriate (e.g., when using research methodologies that emphasize consumer participation and representation), investigators should also involve and include prospective research participants in the grant writing and initial grant review and evaluation process.

The Process of Grant Writing and Application

Grant writing takes time and commitment as well as advance planning and preparation. In the grant writing and application process, one must justify and plan the research, write and package the proposal to meet the requirements of the funding agency, gather institutional support and necessary collaborators or consultants, submit the proposal to the funding agency, and follow up with the funding agency once the grant has been submitted. A successful grant includes a good idea, knowledge of hot topics and current funding initiatives and policies, sophisticated understanding of research design and methods, a good track record, and patience.

Grant writing encompasses the following steps:

* Developing an idea,
* Evaluating and negotiating with the sponsoring institution,
* Identifying and enlisting support from co-investigators, consultants, and other future personnel,
* Selecting the appropriate funding agency, funding institute, and funding avenue,
* Knowing regulations, policies, and guidelines,
* Working with funding agency administrators,
* Identifying a theoretical basis for the study,
* Demonstrating expert knowledge of the topic area,
* Demonstrating good scholarship,
* Conducting pilot research,
* Identifying specific aims,
* Developing hypotheses,
* Choosing an appropriate and rigorous design,
* Ensuring an ethical design and methodological approach,
* Addressing logistical issues and obstacles in data collection up front,
* Planning analyses,
* Developing a timeline and evaluation plan,
* Developing a reasonable budget request,
* Obtaining letters of support, and
* Determining where to send the grant.

Although these steps are presented and discussed below sequentially, in reality many of them are often performed simultaneously. Some steps will be left incomplete as others are initiated. The scramble to prepare a competitive application often requires substantial multitasking and cross-checking between all of the steps. Moreover, the order of the steps may vary depending on the funding source and the kind of competition to which one is applying. Nonetheless, in most cases, the steps discussed below will be required for preparing a grant proposal.

Developing an Idea:
The Importance of Impact

The most critical aspect of preparing a grant proposal is developing a research idea that is significant and innovative enough to warrant funding. Agencies want to utilize their money wisely and parsimoniously. They want to be sure that studies have the potential to be of high impact in terms of understanding, preventing, reversing, or alleviating certain health conditions. Developing a grant proposal idea with potential to be of high impact involves the following considerations:

* Defining impact,
* Taking into account policy documents and legislative initiatives,
* Matching your idea to the goals and priorities of the funding agency, and
* Building on existing contemporary scientific trends.

Often, one of the main challenges in evaluating one's idea in terms of impact involves knowing the ideology and funding priorities of the agency to which one is applying.

Defining Impact

Some agencies consider the severity, imminence, and potential for reversibility of a condition in determining their funding priorities and decisions. They may consider some diseases, chronic illnesses, or impairments to be more worthy of funding than others based on fatality rates or other characteristics of the disease or population. Other agencies may value certain methodological approaches over others. For example, an agency whose priority is to reduce and eradicate highly prevalent diseases with high mortality rates may be more inclined to fund medically innovative research that involves biomarkers and/or aspects of the human genome over research that focuses on improving the quality of life of individuals living with the condition. Conversely, a different agency may be more inclined to fund research that focuses on empowerment and capacity-building for individuals with existing impairments. An added priority for many agencies is reducing health disparities. Such agencies will tend to fund researchers that work with participants who do not have adequate economic resources, educational and employment opportunities, and access to healthcare. Knowing these priorities can help a researcher determine how reviewers might evaluate a proposal in terms of its overall significance and potential for impact.

Taking into Account Policy Documents and Legislative Initiatives

Being knowledgeable about politics, current events, and legislative initiatives can aid in determining whether a funding idea will be considered to be important and of high impact. Knowledge of legislative initiatives is particularly important when it comes to obtaining funding from federal agencies (Gitlin & Lyons, 2004). One can become familiar with legislative initiatives as they are reflected on funding agency Web sites, in government publications such as the *Federal Register* in the United States, and in funding announcements. At the broadest level, one can obtain knowledge about upcoming federal funding priorities by reading the daily newspaper and watching the news, and by watching and otherwise keeping current on issues in healthcare policy through other media outlets.

Matching One's Idea to the Goals and Priorities of the Funding Agency

One should always ensure that the research topic, population, and methodological approach reflect the goals and priorities of the funding agency to which one applies. A number of steps can be applied to effectively match one's research idea to the agenda of the funding agency:

- Consult relevant Web-based and other resources (many of which are discussed in this chapter) to develop a preliminary working list of possible funding agencies to approach,
- Periodically scan the Web and other resources for program announcements and/or funding agencies that reflect one's area of interest,
- Consult with respected peers, mentors, and program officers to receive feedback about the match of funding agencies to one's idea, and
- Refine and define one's proposal ideas to match chosen potential agencies based on the information gathered.

Building on Existing Contemporary Scientific Trends

Most funding agencies keep relatively current in terms of their knowledge of methodological approaches that are contemporary and/or on the cutting edge of science. In addition, certain scientific trends tend to develop and some gain a substantial amount of credibility and support within the research community. For example, recent trends within healthcare research include:

- A focus on participatory approaches to program development, service provision, and healthcare reform,
- Interdisciplinary research (e.g., research that draws upon the expertise of professionals from a wide range of disciplines), and
- Translational research (e.g., studies that incorporate a range of approaches that span the basic and applied concerns).

Evaluating and Negotiating with the Sponsoring Institution

Before deciding to write a grant, one must identify and evaluate existing resources within one's own institution. Sponsoring institutions often have internal rules and regulations that govern the grant submission process, many of which involve budgetary and resource issues. For example, some sponsoring institutions specify a minimum requirement for indirect cost support provided by a granting agency. Conversely, to award grant funding to an investigator, some funding agencies require a certain level of commitment of monetary or in-kind support (e.g., a certain percentage of cost-sharing or matching funds) from a sponsoring institution. It is important to clarify issues of resource allocation and administrative rules and regulations before a grant proposal is submitted so that all agreements are in place should a grant get funded.

Another important factor to consider during negotiations with one's sponsoring institution is that grant writing takes time and commitment. Applicants will need support in the form of time allocated to writing and preparing the grant proposal and other types of support such as access to secretarial, research assistant, and administrative support for such diverse things as conducting literature searches, gathering protocols and instruments, gathering letters of cooperation, preparing a budget, and making photocopies. The sponsoring institution should also be willing to release the applicant from other responsibilities (e.g., committee work, teaching) so he or she has the necessary time to construct a strong proposal.

Identifying and Enlisting Support from Co-Investigators, Consultants, and Other Future Personnel

Most grant evaluation criteria include an assessment of the strengths and credentials of the various members of the investigative team. Thus, selection of one's team members is critically important and requires thought and effort. Depending on the size of one's study, research team members can include:

- Co-investigators/subcontractors,
- Consultants (e.g., biostatisticians),
- Grant staff,
- Student research assistants, and
- Volunteers.

Co-investigators (commonly paid as subcontractors unless they are housed within the same institution) are research personnel critical to conducting the study. They:

• Share responsibility for the intellectual contributions made to the development of the study idea, design, and methods and analyses, and

• Collaborate with the principal investigator in interpreting the findings and in accessing avenues for dissemination.

Co-investigators are typically senior-level scientists with the knowledge base, technical skills, publication history, and a scientific reputation that support the central aims of the study and complement the credentials of the principal investigator and other collaborators. Increasingly agencies expect a research team reflecting diverse and complementary disciplines.

Consultants are of similar status and complete similar functions as co-investigators. However, their role is often more circumscribed and their contributions to the overall study are proportionally smaller than those of the co-investigators. Co-investigators and consultants are usually selected before a proposal is written and they are always identified in the grant proposal. Most funding agencies require that they provide curricula vitae and written letters of support. In many cases, a subcontract agreement will be in place that allows for formal budgetary relationships to be established.

Other members of the research team, including grant staff, student research assistants, and volunteers, can be named once the grant has been funded. However, some reviewers look more favorably upon grant applications that identify key grant staff because it leaves an impression that the investigator has a stable research team. However, it is often not possible to name the more junior-level or secondary contributors up front.

Selecting collaborators involves deciding what intellectual and physical resources are needed to complete a study and determining who might be available to meet those needs (Gitlin & Lyons, 2004). Selecting strong collaborators will not only increase the likelihood of a positive review, but also ensure the overall success of the study. Enlisting support from collaborators early in the grant writing process can be vital to idea development. In addition, collaborators may support activities such as grant writing, study implementation, and the write-up and dissemination of study findings.

Selecting the Appropriate Funding Agency, Funding Institute, and Funding Avenue

Being knowledgeable about the missions, values, and funding priorities of the different agencies that fund the kind of research one intends is vital.

Sometimes, funding decisions are made even before the review process begins because the investigator has selected the wrong agency, funding institute, or funding avenue for the proposed project. Some of the more widely utilized funding sources that may be accessed by occupational therapy researchers and their collaborators include:

• Grants awarded by professional organizations,
• Grants awarded by private foundations,
• Grants awarded by self-help organizations,
• Grants and grant competitions within university settings, and
• Grants awarded by the federal government.

Grants Awarded by Professional Organizations

Grants awarded by professional organizations are useful resources for individuals seeking to advance the profession. As such, their scope is limited to projects within the singular discipline of occupational therapy and typically funding is provided for tightly constructed, time-limited, and highly focused research studies, projects, or professional educational activities. Examples of organizations that award grants to occupational therapists are noted in the feature box titled "Professional Organizations Funding Occupational Therapy Research."

Grants Awarded by Private Foundations

Numerous private foundations support research, developmental, and educational activities. The mission and funding agenda of private foundations are as varied as the individual donors (e.g., Tiger Woods Foundation), families (e.g., Field Family Foundation of Illinois), and private industries (e.g., Procter & Gamble) that provide grants. Private foundation grants can range from small award amounts to awards in excess of US$1,000,000 for a single application. Topics for funding generally focus on, but are not limited to, community-based initiatives directed at improving communities, improving education, reducing conflict and violence, improving access and participation for individuals with disabilities, increasing job skills and employment for underserved, mentally ill, homeless, or adjudicated individuals, and reducing disease and disability and improving health outcomes for a wide range of populations and human conditions. The feature box titled "Private Foundations" discusses three foundations that fund research relevant to occupational therapy.

Occupational therapy professional associations are increasingly becoming sources of funding. Below information is contained on occupational therapy professional bodies form the United States, Canada, the United Kingdom, and the World Federation of Occupational Therapy. Occupational therapy researchers in countries other then those mentioned here are encouraged to identify additional possible sources of funding within their own national professional bodies.

American Occupational Therapy Foundation

The American Occupational Therapy Foundation (AOTF) is a nonprofit organization whose mission is to advance occupational therapy research specifically as it informs clinical practice. AOTF is also focused toward efforts that increase public understanding of occupational therapy services. In conjunction with ongoing support from the American Occupational Therapy Association (AOTA), AOTF has provided nearly $4,000,000 in support for research grants and projects. Currently, there are three types of research studies that AOTF and AOTA conjointly fund: innovation studies (US$8,000 maximum award amount per application), impact studies (US$30,000 maximum award amount per application), and student research grants (US$1,000 maximum award amount per application). A listing of 10 current occupational therapy research priorities of AOTF/AOTA can be found at http://www.aotf. org. Gillette (2000) has published a 20-year history of research funding in occupational therapy that describes the various activities and awards made by AOTF and AOTA. More information about grants funded by AOTF and AOTA can be found at http://www.aotf.org.

British Association/College of Occupational Therapists

In the United Kingdom, the professional body administers a range of grants for research, education, and professional development. These are available mainly on an annual basis, though some support is also available for low-cost courses that occur at short notice. In addition, travel bursaries are offered at three points in the year. Awards arise both from restricted funds held by the College of Occupational Therapists (COT) and grants made available from companies and charitable organiza-

tions. Details are advertised on the Web site at http://www.cot.org.uk.

Canadian Occupational Therapy Foundation

The Canadian Occupational Therapy Foundation (COTF) is a nonprofit professional organization that works in tandem with the Canadian Association of Occupational Therapists (CAOT) to develop mechanisms for granting awards to individuals and organizations for research, scholarship, and publication (COTF, 2005). COTF provides opportunities for occupational therapy researchers whose aim is to address the evolving needs of the occupational therapy community in Canada. COTF generates, receives, and maintains funds to support a broad range of research and scholarship in the field of occupational therapy.

With the support from CAOT and donations from individuals, corporations, organizations, and foundations, COTF has awarded a total of CAN$51,500 to occupational therapy researchers. COTF has three different grant programs: The Research Grants (CAN$28,000), the Scholarships Grants (CAN$22,000) and a third category, Other (CAN$1,500). Further details regarding each program, their policy, eligibility and reviewer criteria can be found at http://www. cotfcanada.org.

World Federation of Occupational Therapists

Every 2 years, the World Federation of Occupational Therapists (WFOT) reviews applications for the Thelma Cardwell Foundation Award for Research and Education. This award supports any project aiming to enhance the development of occupational therapy in any way. The award does not support research projects for which funds could be sought from governmental agencies or other grant-giving foundations. The budget is restricted to include only coverage for equipment, maintenance, or technical assistance for an already approved research project. Thus, WFOT funding is best used to supplement other types of funding provided for a given study. The Thelma Cardwell Foundation Award offers investigators a maximum amount of US$5,000 per application. More information about this grant award and evaluation criteria used to select applications can be found at http://www.wfot.org.

(continued)

Private Foundations

Below a few private foundations from thousands in existence around the world are described.

U.S. Foundations

The Robert Wood Johnson Foundation is the largest private philanthropy within the United States that is exclusively devoted to improving health and healthcare. This foundation has made basic science and applied research grant awards ranging from US$1,200 to US$50,000,000. Grants are announced through *calls for proposals* that are highly specific to the goals and agenda of the program that issues the call. Independent grants (i.e., unsolicited grant applications that reflect an investigator's unique ideas) can also be funded. Some of the foundation's interest areas are prevention and treatment of addictions, building human capital within the healthcare workforce, health disparities, quality healthcare, and pioneering research that promotes fundamental breakthroughs in health and healthcare. More information about funding through the Robert Wood Johnson Foundation can be found at http://www.rwjf.org/index.jsp.

The John D. and Catherine T. MacArthur foundation is a private, independent organization dedicated to promoting a lasting improvement in the human condition. The foundation awards large (i.e., over US$1,000,000) and small (i.e., under US$5,000) basic science and applied research. More information about funding from the MacArthur Foundation can be found at http://www.macarthur.org.

The Jacob and Valeria Langeloth Foundation is a private philanthropy that awards applied research grants in the area of healthcare (mainly to hospitals and other healthcare facilities). In 2004, Langeloth awarded 31 grants totaling to US$5,261,943. This averages to approximately US$169,740 per grant award. Langeloth's mission is to support effective and creative healthcare practices and policies related to recovery from illness, accident, and physical, social, or emotional trauma. For more information about funding from the Langeloth Foundation, readers may access the foundation's Web site at http://www.langeloth.org.

Canadian Foundations

In Canada, most grants for occupational therapy-based research come from private organizations, charities, and associations such as the Alzheimer Society of Canada, the Canadian Cystic Fibrosis Association, the Parkinson Society of Canada, the Canadian Mental Health Association, or the Royal Canadian Legion Fellowship in Gerontology. Other important sources of funding come from each province's own funding agencies. Regardless of whether they are governmental or private, each has specific research interests, a mission, and procedures for submitting a research project, and policies and criteria for funding. For example, in the province of Québec, the *Fonds de recherche en santé du Québec* (http://www.frsq.gpouc.qc.ca) funds specific rehabilitation programs, such as the *Reseau Provincial de recherche en Adaptation-Réadaptation*. The *Fonds de recherche sur la société et la culture du Québec* (http://www.fqrsc.gouv.ca) is another funding agency that opens doors for occupational therapists concerned with social inclusion, diversity, and adaptation.

United Kingdom Foundations (Charities)

In the United Kingdom, sources of grants for occupational therapists arise from a wide range of charities. For instance, the Wellcome Trust is an independent charity that funds research to improve human and animal health. Two of its funding streams of relevance to occupational therapists are Biomedical Science and Medical Humanities. The Wellcome Trust also funds 4-year PhD scholarships in Life Sciences. Further information is available from http://www.wellcome.ac.uk/funding. The Joseph Rowntree Charitable Trust was founded by Joseph Rowntree, a Quaker businessman, in 1904. This Trust makes available grants totaling some £4m each year. Information can be obtained from http://www.jrct.org.uk.

Grants Awarded by Self-Help Organizations

Grants awarded by self-help organizations largely serve the interests of clients who have experienced or are experiencing a specific illness, trauma, or impairment, their loved ones, and their specialist healthcare providers. As such, the scope of grants provided by self-help organizations is limited to projects that focus on a given condition or disease process. The size of grants awarded by self-help organizations is generally commensurate with the size of the membership and the amount of contributions made to a given organization. However, because self-help organizations are largely supported by small donations made by clients, their loved ones, and their healthcare providers, they tend to make smaller or more mid-sized grant awards. There are thousands of self-help organizations that fund grants throughout the world. The feature box titled "The Arthritis Foundation" highlights an organization that tends to fund a larger number of grants per annum than many others.

Grants and Grant Competitions Within University Settings

Two general types of grant competitions occur within university settings: limited internal competitions and seed grants. Limited internal competitions are made available to research-oriented universities by certain kinds of funding agencies (mostly federal agencies). These competitions involve two or more phases. The first phase occurs between faculty within the university to limit the number of applications from that university. Many limited internal competitions accept only one or two applications per university. The application that emerges as strongest and most relevant from the internal competition is the one that is selected.

Many university settings, particularly those with a research focus or emphasis, offer opportunities for faculty internal to the university to compete for small grants that are offered by the university itself. These grants are often referred to as seed grants. In large part, they are designed to provide funding (or other resources) to help an investigator collect pilot data for a later grant

The Arthritis Foundation

The Arthritis Foundation is a multifaceted national self-help organization that has funded more than 2,100 researchers with more than US$272,000,000 over the past 50 years. As the largest, private, nonprofit contributor to arthritis research in the world, the Arthritis Foundation funds a wide spectrum of large and small basic and applied research studies conducted by a broad range of disciplines that focuses on arthritis prevention, treatment, and cure. Clinical studies have been funded to test novel medical, rehabilitation, surgical, and psychoeducational treatments. Epidemiological studies and health services/quality of care research are also important funding priorities. In addition to studies of various forms of arthritis, the foundation also funds studies of related conditions, including systemic lupus, osteoporosis, Lyme disease, scleroderma, and fibromyalgia. The foundation funds investigator-initiated grants, career development and training programs, and special targeted research initiatives. More information about grant funding through the Arthritis Foundation can be located at http://www.arthritis.org/research.

application to be submitted elsewhere, or to initiate a new line of research that is perhaps too novel to receive funding in a competitive environment outside of the university setting. The amount of funding available for these grants tends to be small, and usually funding is limited to only a few proposals. Information about limited internal competitions and seed grants is generally provided through a university research office.

Grants Awarded by Governments

Each country, and often subjurisdictions such as states or provinces, have granting programs. These vary widely by country or jurisdiction. Major governmental funding bodies in the United States, Canada, and the United Kingdom are briefly reviewed in this chapter. Readers from other countries will want to investigate their national and local governmental sources of funding. Ordinarily, information is publicly available on Web sites and official government publications. Nonetheless, it often takes substantial time and effort to learn all the mechanisms, rules, regulations, deadlines and so on that are part of government funding. Before applying for a government grant, one should become as familiar as possible with this type of information.

Federal Grants in the United States. A number of federal granting agencies have programmatic interest areas relevant to occupational therapy researchers in the United States. This section will discuss those with the largest history of funding occupational therapy research. The National Institutes of Health (NIH) is the primary federal funding agency that supports medical research.

Most applications sent to NIH are investigator initiated. This means that the research idea (e.g., central aims of the research, topic area, study design, and methodology) is unsolicited and uniquely a product of the investigators' thinking. The investigator must be responsible for the planning, direction, and execution of the project. Despite the implicit intellectual liberties associated with this funding avenue, a caveat that many applicants forget is that their ideas still must incorporate ideas, aims, study populations, and methods that are considered of relevance to at least one of the various institutes or centers within NIH.

Opportunities for grant funding are announced in a number of ways. A Program Announcement (PA) is a formally prepared statement in writing that invites applications in a defined area of interest. A PA is not a guarantee that funds have been set aside to support the defined interest area, and applications are generally treated as being investigator initiated in all other respects. In a Request for Applications (RFA), NIH invites applications for a one-time competition in a specific topic area and describes an institute's initiative in a well-defined scientific area to stimulate research in an area of exceptionally high priority to the institute. In this case, the RFA does guarantee that a certain amount of funding has been set aside to support the defined interest area, and it specifies up front how many awards will be made. A Request for Proposals (RFP) is similar to an RFA except that an RFP involves a contractual relationship between the investigator and NIH, rather than a grant. RFAs and RFPs are dedicated mainly to problem-oriented research efforts that focus on disease-specific initiatives, particularly in the beginning stages of research.

NIH is comprised of a number of different institutes and centers, each dedicated to a specific health-related topic area and mission. Some examples of NIH institutes that may be of particular relevance to occupational therapy researchers include:

• The National Institute on Child Health and Human Development (NICHD), which also houses the National Center for Medical Rehabilitation Research,
• The National Institute on Aging (NIA),
• The National Institute on Alcohol Abuse and Alcoholism (NIAAA),
• The National Institute on Drug Abuse (NIDA),
• The National Institute of Arthritis and Musculoskeletal and Skin Diseases (NIAMS),
• The National Institute of Mental Health (NIMH), and
• The National Institute of Neurological Disorders and Stroke (NINDS), among several others (see http://www.nih.gov/icd for a complete listing).

Specific research topics that represent strong interest areas for the NIH can be searched regularly by accessing the *NIH Guide for Grants and Contracts*, which can be found at http://grants.nih.gov/grants/guide/index.html.

Table 30.1, which was composed from information in several tables provided on the NIH Web site (http://grants1.nih.gov/grants/funding/funding_program.htm), describes some of the different types of grants awarded through the NIH that are relevant to occupational therapy researchers.

Agency for Healthcare Research and Quality. The Agency for Healthcare Research and Quality (AHRQ) is a Federal funding source within the U.S. Department of Health and Human Services Public Health Service dedicated to funding research that enhances the quality, appropriateness, and effectiveness of healthcare services and service access. Topical areas of research cover the organization, financing, and delivery of healthcare services, disease prevention, and the improvement of clinical healthcare practices. Most of the large grants that AHRQ funds involve research projects, demonstration projects, program evaluations, and dissemination activities.

Because priorities are based on legislation, policies, and public need, areas of specific interest for AHRQ change regularly. AHRQ interest areas tend to be published in the form of Requests for Proposals (RFPs), program announcements (PAs), and notices. More information about current AHRQ funding opportunities can be accessed at http://www.ahrq.gov/fund/ongoing.htm. In addition, announcements can be searched regularly by accessing the *NIH Guide for Grants and Contracts*, which can be found at http://grants.nih.gov/grants/guide/index.html.

U.S. Department of Education. The U.S. Department of Education is comprised of nine principal offices (somewhat akin to NIH institutes). A full listing can be found at http://www.ed.gov. Among them, the Office of Special Education and Rehabilitation Services (OSERS) is one of the offices of highest relevance to the work of occupational therapy researchers working in educational, university, and clinical rehabilitation settings. Within the principal offices of the Department of Education, there are program offices. For example, the National Institute on Disability and Rehabilitation Research (NIDRR), the Office of Special Education Programs (OSEP), and the Rehabilitation Services Administration (RSA) are housed within OSERS. All of NIDRR's programmatic efforts are aimed at improving the lives of individuals with disabilities throughout the entire lifespan. Projects that are funded by NIDRR aim to maximize the full inclusion, independent living, employment, and economic self-sufficiency of individuals with disabilities. OSEP supports educational, technological, and developmental initiatives for infants, toddlers, children, and adolescents with disabilities. RSA focuses on funding efforts that enable individuals with disabilities to obtain employment and live more independently through supports such as counseling programs, medical and psychological services, job training, and other individualized services.

The U.S. Department of Education's name for what NIH calls an extramural grant is a discretionary grant. A discretionary grant is an award that the Department has chosen to make based on

Table 30.1 Selected* Funding Awards Made by NIH

Award Type*	Brief Definition
Research Grants	
NIH Research Project Grant Program (R01) http://grants1.nih.gov/grants/funding/r01.htm	An R01 is typically a larger research grant award made to support a very well-defined and highly specific research project. RO1s provide support to investigators for health-related research and development projects that coincide with the NIH mission. R01s can be funded for a period of 1–5 years and can total to more than US$2,000,000 for a full 5-year funding period.
NIH Small Grant Program (R03) http://grants1.nih.gov/grants/funding/r03.htm	An R03 is a research grant award that provides limited funding for a short period of time. It can be used to fund pilot or feasibility studies, secondary analysis of existing data, small, self-contained research studies, development of research methodology, or the development of a new technology.
NIH Academic Research Enhancement Award (AREA Grants) (R15) http://grants1.nih.gov/grants/funding/area.htm	AREA grants are small awards that support individual biomedical and behavioral-science research projects that are conducted collaboratively by faculty and students in undergraduate institutions that are housed in schools that have not been major recipients of other types of NIH research grant funding.
NIH Exploratory/Developmental Research Grant Award (R21) http://grants1.nih.gov/grants/funding/r21.htm	An R21 provides a limited amount of support for research projects, ideas, and methodologies that are exceptionally novel, potentially groundbreaking, or innovative.
NIH Clinical Trial Planning Grant Program (R34) http://grants1.nih.gov/grants/funding/r34.htm	The R34 is a 1-year grant award that supports the development of Phase III clinical trials.
NIH Research Career Development Awards	
Mentored Research Scientist Development Award (K01) http://grants1.nih.gov/grants/guide/pa-files/PA-00-019.html	The K01 supports 3–5 years of an intensive, supervised, career development experience for an investigator entering a new area of research in a biomedical, behavioral, or clinical science.
International Research Scientist Development Award (KO1–IRSDA) http://grants1.nih.gov/grants/guide/pa-files/PAR-04-058.html	The K01–IRSDA supports U.S. postdoctoral biomedical, social, and behavioral scientists in newer stages of their research careers to conduct research or extend their current research into developing countries.
Independent Scientist Award (K02) http://grants1.nih.gov/grants/guide/pa-files/PA-00-020.html	The K02 award provides up to 5 years of salary support for newly independent scientists that can demonstrate a need for a period of intensive research focus that will enable them to expand their potential to make significant contributions to their selected area of research.
Senior Scientist Award (K05) http://grants1.nih.gov/grants/guide/pa-files/PA-00-021.html	The K05 provides salary support for up to five years for scientists of outstanding caliber that have demonstrated sustained, high-level productivity and whose expertise, research accomplishments, and contributions to the field are critical to the mission of the particular NIH center or institute.
Mentored Clinical Scientists Development Award (K08) http://grants1.nih.gov/grants/guide/pa-files/PA-00-003.html	The K08 supports specialized study for individuals with a health professions doctorate that want to gain independence as a laboratory or field-based researcher.
Mentored Patient-Oriented Research Career Development Award (K23) http://grants1.nih.gov/grants/guide/pa-files/PA-00-004.html	The K23 was designed to increase the number of clinicians trained to conduct high-quality patient-oriented clinical research. This area covers mechanisms of human disease, therapeutic interventions, clinical trials, and the development of new technologies.

(continued)

Table 30.1 **Selected* Funding Awards Made by NIH** (continued)

Award Type*	Brief Definition
NIH Small Business Funding Opportunities	
NIH Small Business Innovation Research Program (SBIR) http://grants1.nih.gov/grants/funding/sbir.htm	The SBIR program is designed to encourage U.S.-based small businesses to engage in research and development activities that have an impact on health and a potential for commercialization.
NIH Small Business Technology Transfer Research Program (STTR) http://grants1.nih.gov/grants/funding/sbir.htm	The STTR is similar to the SBIR program in that both programs seek to increase the participation of smaller businesses in federal research and development and to increase subsequent commercialization of technologies developed by this program within the private sector. One difference is that STTR program applicants are required to formally collaborate with a research institution.

*Generally, the research awards (preceded by an "R") are designed to provide support for well-defined research and development projects. The research career development awards (preceded by a "K") provide support for new, mid-career, and senior scientists who are seeking to bring greater focus and/or knowledge. The small business awards promote the development and private commercialization of new technologies, and to promote collaboration between research scientists and small business owners.
A more comprehensive listing of the numerous types of grant awards offered by NIH can be found at http://grants1.nih.gov/grants/funding/funding_program.htm. Because the types of awards offered by NIH change periodically, readers are encouraged to access the Web site for the most updated information.

a competitive review process. Table 30.2, which was composed from information in several tables provided on the U.S. Department of Education Web site (http://www.ed.gov), describes some of the different types of grants that are awarded through the U.S. Department of Education.

United Kingdom. The purpose of funding for occupational therapy research in the United Kingdom is to both generate new knowledge and also to develop research capacity. Many research funders support interdisciplinary research, reflecting the team approach that is essential for effective health and social care interventions. Among the most prestigious funding sources for health and social care research in the United Kingdom are the government-funded research councils. The Medical Research Council (MRC) and the Economic and Social Research Council (ESRC) invest in funding for high-quality, world-class research.

The National Health Service is another highly regarded funding avenue within the United Kingdom. Three programmes of research are supported by funding from the National Health Service (NHS). First, the NHS Health Technology Assessment (HTA) Programme aims to provide research information relating to the costs, effectiveness, and impact of health technologies (i.e., any approach that is used to promote health, treat illness, and improve rehabilitation or long-term care). Further information on the HTA programme can be found at http://www.hta.nhsweb.nhs.uk/

aboutHTA. Second, the New and Emerging Technologies (NEAT) programme supports applied research in health and social care http://www.neat-programme.org.uk/. Third, the Service Delivery and Organisation (SDO) programme is a national research programme that develops the evidence base on the organization, management and delivery of healthcare services. Further detail on this programme is available from http://www.sdo.lshtm.ac.uk.

Within the United Kingdom, there has been recognition of the need to strengthen the research capacity of occupational therapists by supporting opportunities to undertake research and develop research careers (Creek and Ilott, 2002; Department of Health, 2000, 2005; Higher Education Funding Council for England, 2001; Ilott & White, 2001; Scottish Executive 2004). As a result, increased funding is available for occupational therapy through various government agencies. This funding supports not only specific research projects but also efforts to build research capacity.

Canada. Canada's major federal funding agency for health research is the Canadian Institute of Health Research (CIHR) (http://www.cihrirsc.gc.ca). The CIHR promotes research through an interdisciplinary structure made up of 13 institutes. Its philosophy rests on networks of researchers brought together to focus on specific and important health issues. Therefore, the Institute's structure encourages partnerships and

Table 30.2 **Selected Grant Awards Made by the US Department of Education Office of Special Education and Rehabilitation Services (OSERS)**

Name of Award	Program Office	Brief Description
Rehabilitation Engineering Research Centers (RERC)	National Institute on Disability and Rehabilitation Research (NIDRR)	Support efforts that lead to the development of methods, procedures, and devices that will benefit individuals with disabilities, particularly those with the most severe disabilities.
Research Fellowships Program	National Institute on Disability and Rehabilitation Research (NIDRR)	Enable individuals to build their research capacity. Individuals with 7 or more years of experience relevant to rehabilitation research are eligible for a distinguished fellowship award. Merit fellowships are awarded to individuals in earlier stages of rehabilitation research careers.
State Vocational Rehabilitation Unit In-Service Training	Rehabilitation Services Administration (RSA)	Promote the availability of skilled personnel to serve the needs of individuals with disabilities through vocational rehabilitation, supported employment, and independent living programs.
Field-Initiated Research Projects	National Institute on Disability and Rehabilitation Research (NIDRR)	Facilitate research and development activities that maximize the full inclusion, employment, independent living, and economic sufficiency of individuals with disabilities.

collaboration across sectors, disciplines, and regions. Some institutes of most relevance to occupational therapy include:

• Institute of Aging,
• Institute of Health Services and Policy Research,
• Institute of Human Development, Child and Youth Health,
• Institute of Musculoskeletal Health and Arthritis, and
• Institute of Neurosciences, Mental Health and Addiction.

Each Institute, while focusing on a specific area, is open to research initiatives that range from fundamental biomedical and clinical research to research that focuses on cultural dimensions of health and environmental variables that affect well-being.

Summary

This section provided a brief overview of different types of funding agencies. These agencies represent numerous opportunities available to occupational therapy researchers and practitioners working in a wide range of academic, private, educational, and community-based settings. These opportunities change continually in conjunction with federal and private foundation health agendas and funding priorities. Each year, new foundations emerge that fund research related to healthcare while at the same time others cease to offer funding opportunities related to healthcare research.

Many research-oriented universities have formal or informal research development services or offices, which are geared toward disseminating funding opportunities like these and others to faculty and staff. In addition to university research development services, prospective grant applicants can subscribe to a wide range of publications and Web-based resources that allow access to updated information about funding agencies and priorities. Some of these links and guidelines for accessing information about private funding opportunities were provided in the section of this chapter on private foundation funding sources. For federal resources within the United States, the Web site, http://www.grants.gov/Find, contains updated information about many types of funding announcements.

Knowing Regulations, Policies, and Guidelines

Because most funding agencies receive numerous applications for each funding cycle, and because grants involve (sometimes complex) financial arrangements between the agency and the applicant's home institution, all granting agencies rely heavily on policies and regulations that guide the application and award process and are generally uniformly upheld for all applicants.

Once an investigator is funded, many agencies have a number of requirements that must be met in order for the investigator to retain the funding award. Depending on the agency, examples may include providing periodic written progress reports that demonstrate that the research team is completing the work that they promised to complete within the expected time frame, and budget monitoring or occasional audits to ensure that the research team is not spending the award money inappropriately or purchasing items that have not been approved within the budgetary guidelines. Investigators must take great care to follow guidelines like these or an agency can and will discontinue funding. Grant writing and proposal preparation, administrative and budgetary maintenance, and the provision of periodic progress reports are not areas in which an investigator is permitted to cut corners or relax standards.

Working with Funding Agency Administrators

There are many different types of funding agency administrators. These may include, but are not limited to:

- Agency directors, advisory councils, and directorial boards (whose main job is to set agency funding priorities and provide ultimate oversight over the types of grants that receive funding),
- Referral officers (whose main job is to scan the titles and abstracts of grant applications and assign specific reviewers),
- Scientific review administrators (whose main job is to oversee the logistical, legal, and administrative aspects of the review process), and
- Project officers (whose main job is to guide applicants and grantees through the review and grant management processes).

The type of agency administrator with whom an investigator is likely to have the most contact is the project officer (or program officer). Project officers may be involved with a grant at all stages of its development and implementation. Generally, however, a project officer can educate an investigator about:

- The agency's funding priorities (i.e., the topic areas of most interest to the agency),

- The administrative aspects of applying for the grant (i.e., how to complete required forms and progress reports), and
- The review process (i.e., whether to resubmit an application and to what extent an investigator should respond to certain types of feedback from the reviewers).

More information about working with project officers in deciding whether to resubmit an application is provided later in this chapter.

Identifying a Theoretical Basis for the Study

High-quality research aims to evaluate the relevance of theory that underlies the research activities. In fact, one of the central reasons why many grant proposals receive poor scores from reviewers lies in the fact that the study is not well justified in terms of its relationship to a larger idea or system of ideas that support the central hypothesis. Theoretical justification is also a requirement for studies that focus on the development of an assessment, program, or other rehabilitation resource. Regardless of the nature of the study, a central theory must be closely linked and utilized to support the specific aims and methodology of the study.

For example, if one is designing a clinical trial that tests the efficacy of a given approach to rehabilitation, it would be expected that one would have based his or her approach to rehabilitation on an existing or emerging theory that defines the mechanisms that are expected to underlie the anticipated change.

Demonstrating Expert Knowledge of the Topic Area

For many granting agencies, one of the criteria by which a proposal is evaluated includes the estimated expertise of the principal investigator and the research team. Level of expertise is typically judged according to a number of variables, including:

- Number of peer-reviewed publications in the area under study,
- Quality of the journals in which the articles are published,
- History of prior grant funding in the area under study,
- Evidence of specialized training and research mentorship in the area under study, and
- An established area of focus and a tradition of research.

One of the most important determinates of an investigator's expertise is the number and quality of publications that the investigator and research team members have in the area under study.

Another variable that is commonly evaluated is whether the investigator and/or other team members have a history of prior grant funding and participation on experienced research teams. A history of prior grant funding coupled with a consistent stream of high-impact publications emerging from prior grants are reasonable indicators that the investigator has experience successfully managing the intellectual, managerial, budgetary, and logistical challenges involved in carrying out a grant-funded study.

One of the most basic indicators of expertise, particularly for emerging research professionals, is evidence of an area of focus and a tradition of research (Taylor, Fisher, & Kielhofner, 2005). This most basic indicator overlaps with all of the other criteria mentioned in this section because developing an area of focus and a tradition of research necessarily involves receiving good training and mentorship in research and building a portfolio of evidence of ongoing research involvement in the area. For those just starting out, more information about how to establish an area of focus within occupational therapy and build a tradition of research can be found in Kielhofner (2002), and Kielhofner, Borrell, and Tham (2002). Before submitting any application for research, Gitlin and Lyons (2004) recommend that conducting a self-evaluation to ensure one is ready to assume the role of principal investigator. The points that have been covered in this section can be used as a guide to this kind of self-evaluation.

One caveat is that it is important to recognize that the criteria used to evaluate an investigator's expertise are not uniformly applied within and across granting agencies. Some granting agencies issue classes of grant awards that are designed specifically to allow a new investigator or a clinician seeking to transition into a research role to develop his or her research skills in a given area. One contradiction to many of the criteria outlined in this section exists in some of the K-award funding (described in Table 30.3 later in this chapter) that is offered through the National Institutes of Health (NIH). As described earlier, the very purpose of the K-awards is to support the professional development of researchers and prospective researchers at varied points within their research careers. The Mentored Research Scientist Development Award (K01) is one example of a K-award that allows for newer researchers in a given area to receive funding for their research. The K01

requires a prospective investigator new to a given area of science to design a study and then obtain ongoing supervision and intensive training in his or her proposed area from an experienced researcher who serves as a career mentor for the investigator. The newer investigator is expected to accomplish the same research objectives as a more experienced researcher with the assistance of a mentor. In addition to professional development options offered by federal agencies, some private foundations and self-help organizations wanting to attract new investigators into an emerging or understudied area may place more value upon an investigator's demonstrated interest in the research agenda and funding priorities of the agency than upon the investigator's preestablished track record of research in that area. Seed funding is also offered within many university settings to assist newer investigators in establishing an area of focus, a tradition of research, and a publication record.

Demonstrating Good Scholarship

One often unspoken but critical criterion for successful grant writing is to demonstrate good scholarship in writing and assembling the grant proposal. Good scholarship is indicated by:

- Organizing the proposal so that it adequately responds to each of the proposal sections,
- Weaving a comprehensive and up-to-date literature review into various sections of the proposal;
- Including appropriate citations of prior, high-quality research in the area,
- Providing a well-reasoned and well-justified argument or rationale for the central aims and hypotheses,
- Presenting a meticulous and well-written document, and
- Obtaining mentorship, good advice, and peer reviews in advance of formal submission.

Because good scholarship is central to successful grant writing, the following section extends each of these points.

Organizing the Proposal So that It Adequately Responds to Each of the Proposal Sections

One of the most basic aspects of grant writing that differentiates it from other forms of academic writing is that administrators and reviewers usually demand that the proposal follow a highly structured and organized format that is presented in the application instructions package. In addition to providing a highly organized structure for the proposal, some funding agencies assist applicants even further by asking them to organize the proposal in sections that perfectly mirror each of the criteria by which the proposal will be evaluated. Some agencies even provide questions that frame each section of the proposal to which the applicant is asked to respond. Most grant applications must contain many or all of the following sections (Gitlin & Lyons, 2004):

- Title,
- Abstract,
- Introduction (including a literature review that reflects the background and significance of the problem, potential impact and feasibility of the study, theoretical foundation for the study, and general importance and relevance of the study to the scientific topic area),
- Specific aims (i.e., goals or objectives),
- Methods (including a research, evaluation, dissemination, and/or educational plan),
- Timeline and management plan (delineating roles and responsibilities of each research team member and timeframes in which the work will be expected),
- Biographical information (i.e., biographical sketches and/or curriculum vitae for each member of the research team illustrating credentials, level of expertise, and capacity to carry out the study),
- A summary of the resources and qualifications of the applicant's institution,
- A budget and budget narrative (justifying anticipated costs associated with the study),
- References (mirroring the citations provided in the text), and
- Appendices (containing consent forms, measures, treatment manuals and more detailed study protocols, fidelity rating scales, etc.).

Good scholars ensure that each of these sections is equally strong in terms of content and presentation.

Weaving a Comprehensive and Up-to-Date Literature Review into Various Sections of the Proposal

Within any scientific tradition, it is critical to convey knowledge of the empirical findings that form the background of one's decision to develop and/or test a given concept, assessment, or intervention. A literature review should be utilized to accomplish the following objectives:

- Establish the need for the project and the significance of the problem to be addressed. For example, epidemiological research may be cited to describe the nature, course, prevalence, incidence, and long-term impact of a given condition on functioning.
- Provide evidence of the potential impact of the study. This may be accomplished by citing established unknowns or contradictions within the literature that need resolution.
- Provide evidence of the reliability, validity, and feasibility of the proposed study methods. This may be accomplished by citing studies that support an applicant's plans and provisions for recruiting and retaining an adequate number of subjects, by citing studies that have utilized similar methods of data collection, and by citing studies that attest to the reliability and validity of the measures, data collection methods, and statistical analyses to be used.
- Describe, explain, and provide evidence for the chosen theoretical foundation for the study.

In sum, the literature review should reflect both wide-ranging and highly specialized knowledge about the topic area proposed for study. Grant proposals are typically criticized if the background information, theoretical ideas presented, and rationale for the study are not well supported by an abundance of accurate citations of prior studies.

For proposals that are written in highly complex or controversial areas, it is not sufficient to cite studies that support only one side of a scientific argument. In most cases it is essential to cite representatives of both sides of the argument, provide an accurate and respectful summary of the work on each side, and then justify why one plans to take one side over another or explain how one's work will attempt to resolve the controversy.

Including Appropriate Citations

Keeping updated and being knowledgeable about the work of important leaders and scientist-peers in one's area of research is an ongoing but important process. The literature review must include not only broad-based and highly specific studies that justify the problem and explain the study approach, but also the most updated and cutting-edge work of key scientist-peers working within one's area. In some cases, important, not-yet-published preliminary findings from researchers willing to share their work privately can and should be included in the literature review to reflect the applicant's knowledge of evolving findings within the area closest to his or her field of study. For example, when applying for a successful grant that aimed to estimate the rates of nonrecovery from acute infectious mononucleosis in adolescents, the first author included not-yet-published findings of adult rates of nonrecovery from a scientist-leader within the same field of study.

Findings presented by other scientists at recent conferences or scientific meetings may also be used to support or provide background for an applicant's proposed work. In some cases, personal communications regarding key methodological issues, study feasibility issues, or other evidence of communication with leaders working in the same topical area is regarded positively (though cited work is always best). Having knowledge about the evolving and cutting-edge work in one's area demonstrates that an applicant is careful to remain absolutely current.

Providing a Well-Reasoned and Well-Justified Argument or Rationale for the Central Aims and Hypotheses

Another critical step in demonstrating good scholarship involves ensuring that one's proposal builds a logical justification for the central aims and hypotheses of the study. This rationale and justification must be articulated clearly and concretely in the proposal so that the reviewers are able to view the study as relevant and important to the field and link the background literature review to the aims and methods of the study. Building a rationale for the study may, for example, involve an explicit description of gaps or questions within the existing knowledge base that the study seeks to answer.

Presenting a Meticulous and Well-Written Document

Each application cycle, funding agency administrators scan hundreds of proposals to determine whether they should be accepted for review. Subsequently, reviewers may be assigned to read or scan up to 20 to 30 proposals per meeting. For these reasons, it is important to write one's grant proposal in a clear, well-organized, and meticulous manner. Applicants must also ensure that their spelling is correct and that there are no careless typographical errors, formatting mistakes, or confusing and half-written sentences in the proposal. All of these errors can and do reflect poorly on the overall presentation of the proposal.

Obtaining Mentorship, Good Advice, and Peer Reviews in Advance of Formal Submission

Even if an applicant thinks he or she has made all possible provisions to ensure good scholarship in preparing a grant proposal, it is always wise to seek reviews or opinions from mentors or respected peers before formally submitting the proposal for review. The process of advice-seeking and opinion-gathering should be initiated in the early stages of idea formulation and sustained throughout the writing process.

Conducting Pilot Research

Many funding agencies require an investigative team to have conducted preliminary research studies or pilot research that provides evidence for the feasibility and likelihood of success of the proposed research. The extent of pilot research or preliminary studies necessary depends on the requirements of the funding agency, the size of the proposed study, the research question, and the extent to which the collection of pilot data is economically and logistically feasible in the absence of grant funding. Pilot research is traditionally defined as a trial application of some, many, or all of the methods that a researcher plans to utilize in a larger, anticipated study using a smaller sample size. It can also include collection of data that helps demonstrate the need or value of the proposed project.

Thus, in grant writing, pilot research may be used to:

- Provide evidence of need for the study or intervention,
- Identify unanticipated logistical roadblocks in data collection,
- Test aspects of the reliability or validity of administering a given measure with a new population,
- Assess the feasibility of planned strategies for subject recruitment and retention, and
- Determine the likelihood of finding anticipated results in the larger study.

Identifying Specific Aims

All grant proposals require applicants to identify specific aims. Specific aims are brief statements that accurately reflect the central outcomes that will result from the study (or program). Specific aims should cohere with any hypotheses or questions that the application seeks to answer. Often, specific aims are the first items within the proposal that administrators and reviewers read to get an overall sense of the direction and contents of the study. As such, the content and way in which specific aims are worded deserves careful attention and often a great deal of rewriting.

Generally, a single grant proposal contains between two and five specific aims. Some studies also have secondary aims. Specific aims should contain as much action-oriented language as possible. They should be realistic and not overly ambitious. They should be written clearly and concisely, and they should convey the expected outcomes of the study.

Developing Hypotheses

In tandem with the specific aims, the central hypotheses frame a research study and convey anticipated outcomes. They should be supported by theory and by the preceding literature review. As mentioned in the preceding section, hypotheses should correspond with the specific aims. In addition, hypotheses should be written in such a way that they may easily incorporate or reflect the study design and/or statistical approach that will be utilized to analyze the expected outcomes.

Choosing an Appropriate and Rigorous Design

Funding agencies and review groups vary widely in terms of what they consider to be appropriate and rigorous designs for research. Agencies that fund basic science studies and clinical research tend to value traditional experimental and quasi-experimental research designs, such as randomized controlled studies, epidemiological research, and prospective follow-up studies that utilize repeated measures designs.

Agencies that fund research on healthcare services and quality, innovative program development and program evaluation studies, and other forms of community-based research have a broader vision of what is considered to be an appropriate and rigorous design for a research study. In any case, it is important to ensure that the design chosen matches the central aims of the study, the resources (budget requested), and the sample size, and is likely to produce the expected data.

For example, participatory approaches to research and approaches that are descriptive have become widely utilized in community-based research. Qualitative research methodologies have also been incorporated. Over the past decade, occupational therapists and other medical and rehabilitation scientists have witnessed the incorporation of more of these designs into medical and rehabilitation research.

Ensuring an Ethical Design and Methodological Approach

A fundamental aspect of grant writing involves ensuring that the ethical guidelines established by one's home institution and the funding agency will be followed. All investigators are required to complete an Institutional Review Board (IRB) application to ensure that all ethical issues have been considered to protect to the fullest extent possible the rights of participants.

In selecting designs and methodologies for grant-funded research studies, applicants must balance the demands of methodological rigor with the necessity to treat research subjects in an ethical manner and protect their rights to confidentiality.

For example, Taylor (2004) conducted a randomized clinical trial that examined the effectiveness of a rehabilitation program on quality of life using a sample of adults with chronic fatigue syndrome. Half of the sample (the treatment group) was assigned to receive the program immediately following recruitment and the other half (delayed-treatment controls) was assigned to receive the program 1 year later. In a traditional randomized clinical trial, the investigator would not inform participants of their group assignment because expectancy effects might confound study findings. Specifically, delayed treatment controls would not be told they would be receiving the program 1 year later because their knowledge that they would eventually receive the program might bias their responses before, during, and after the program.

However, when the investigator developed the study in consultation with the ethics board it was determined that all participants should be informed of their group assignment so that those in the delayed treatment control group knew that they would eventually be receiving the treatment. This approach triggered criticism about the violation of traditional randomization when the investigator submitted the findings from the study for publication. However, in this case ethics demanded a less rigorous design in which all participants were informed of their group assignment.

When applicants are faced with ethical dilemmas in writing grant proposals, it is advisable to consult with ethics board representatives from the funding agency and from one's home institution (since both must approve the proposal before it is funded and conducted). In situations that are ambiguous or debatable, applicants should make it explicit within the grant proposal that alternative designs or methodologies were considered, and then justify why one approach was chosen over another. When complex situations arise, being explicit about ethical dilemmas demonstrates that an applicant has been thoughtful about these issues and opens the door for reviewers to support the selected approach or recommend alternatives. More detailed information and guidance about ethical considerations in occupational therapy research is provided in Chapter 29 of this text.

Addressing Logistical Issues and Obstacles in Data Collection

In addition to dilemmas involving competing ethical and methodological considerations, grant applicants often encounter dilemmas involving logistical and implementation issues. Expert reviewers are well aware that data collection that seeks to respond to a single research question can be approached from multiple methodological perspectives and it can be completed in a wide range of settings. In applications that involve complex research questions that have the potential to be approached using a variety of different measures, methods, and/or statistical approaches to analysis, reviewers often look for evidence that an applicant is aware of and has considered the entire range of choices.

For example, in a proposed study that aimed to examine outcomes of an occupational therapy program for persons with human immunodeficiency virus who were living in residential facilities, the investigators first considered a randomized clinical trial since it was ideally the most rigorous design for studying outcomes of an intervention. However, in the grant proposal the investigators, Kielhofner and Braveman (2001) made the following argument:

> Designing this study required us to deal with the following logistic constraints. Within a given facility, it would not be feasible to assign residents to different conditions. The model program will result in changes in the milieu of the facilities and cannot be implemented without contamination of control subjects in the same facility. Furthermore, once the intervention starts, it would be impossible for the facility to return to the control condition, for similar reasons. This rules out both a conventional randomized design at the level of the client and an interrupted times series design at the level of the facility.

The investigators then went on to propose their nonrandom control group design, describing statistical techniques that would be used to attenuate the effects of identified initial differences in the experimental and control groups. Since reviewers understood that the design proposed was the most rigorous design that could be implemented, given the circumstances of the study context, the grant was funded.

As in this case, a grant proposal should always:

• Make any study implementation dilemma explicit within the application and weigh the pros and cons of each approach or indicate why a more rigorous approach is not feasible, and
• Provide a rationale and justification for why the chosen approach was selected.

Planning Analyses

Most applications for research-related grants require investigators to specify how they plan to analyze the results and to describe in detail the statistical or qualitative methods that will be used. The data analysis plan is typically included in the methods section. In the case of quantitative studies, this section of the grant application is usually written by a statistical consultant or co-investigator with a high proficiency in mathematics and statistical methods. In many cases, it is expected that this plan will be accompanied by a power analysis. A power analysis (see Chapter 17) is typically completed by a statistical consultant or by an investigator that is experienced in the use of statistics. It is used to demonstrate that the proposed sample size will be large enough to detect any significant effects given the proposed experimental design.

For research studies that involve hypothesis testing, it is essential that all of the proposed statistical approaches represent an accurate and appropriate way to test the study hypotheses. In addition, each proposed statistical approach should correspond with each hypothesis listed. Each planned statistical approach should be described very clearly in lay terms in as much detail as possible. Any plans for the treatment of missing data and plans for troubleshooting other unanticipated complexities within the proposed dataset should also be accounted for in this section.

Qualitative data analysis plans should be as complete as possible. However, if some of the analysis will depend on the unfolding research process, it should be specified how decisions about analysis will be made. If software for analysis is to be used, it should be noted. The analysis should clearly reflect the study question, be embedded in the specific qualitative approach to analysis, and reflect thorough efforts to maintain trustworthiness of findings.

Developing a Timeline and Evaluation Plan

Most grant applications require a specific timeline of activities and when those activities are to be

Occupational therapy researchers throughout the world are increasingly receiving funding for research. This section contains examples of three funded research grants obtained by occupational therapy researchers in Scotland, Canada, and the United States, respectively. They illustrate a range of funding situations including a fellowship, interdisciplinary research, and research designed to test an occupational therapy intervention.

Developing a Research Career in the United Kingdom Through Fellowship Funding

After being awarded his PhD, an occupational therapist in the United Kingdom was looking for the next step in his research career. He was able to obtain a postdoctoral research Fellowship specifically designed for nurses, midwives, and allied health professionals in Scotland. The Fellowship, which is funded jointly by the Scottish National Health Service (Education for Scotland), the Scottish Executive Health Department, and the Health Foundation, provides an award of £65,000 for 2 years. It is designed to provide the highest possible quality of experience.

The Fellowship has three components:

1. Research development,
2. Research training, and
3. Leadership.

The award includes startup funds (£10,000) to cover setting up costs and the cost of pilot research studies. The aim of the fellowship is to provide the next generation of principal investigators, strengthen existing research collaborations, develop new ones, and allow focused research in Scotland to develop rapidly.

The application process was rigorous and competitive. The first stage entailed a detailed application and research proposal, developed in collaboration with an identified research unit where the Fellowship was proposed to occur. Following short listing, the applicant was informed that there would be an interview and a panel presentation of eminent academics from a range of collaborating Universities in Scotland.

Expected outcomes from the fellowship revolve around developing the applicant's capacity and capability as a lead occupational therapy researcher. In real terms, success will be judged by the number of publications and successful grants that he manages to secure during the 2-year period.

A Canadian Grant in Progress: The Effects of Early Intervention Programs for Children with Intellectual Disabilities

This multidisciplinary grant includes a Canadian occupational therapist. The grant evaluates programs offered to children newborn to 7 years old that present with global developmental delays in Rehabilitation centers in the province of Québec. This provincial study has been funded by the *Consortium National de Recherche sur l'Intégration Sociale* (CNRIS).

The CNRIS is a consensus-building organization whose goal is to energize and foster the development of research in the fields of intellectual disability and pervasive developmental disorders. Inspired by Quebec approaches to integration and social participation, the Consortium pursues the following main objectives:

- Foster networking amongst researchers and partners, as well as the development of research projects and programs in the areas targeted by its mission,
- Support orientations that deal with important social issues for users, parents, caregivers, and service managers,
- Foster the emergence of research that encourages or brings other sectors to invest in the development, adaptation, and improvement of services to persons with an intellectual disability or a pervasive developmental disorder,
- Encourage the dissemination of research results in various formats, and
- Collaborate with health and social service organizations in developing the ability to use research results in designing intervention programs and management methods.

The overarching goal of this provincial study is to develop knowledge about the current state of early intervention programs offered to children presenting a global developmental delay without a diagnosis of pervasive developmental disorder or autism age newborn to 7 years old. First, the study will explore the literature specific to the clientele and early intervention programs in Québec, but also throughout North America and around the world. This first step will paint the portrait of the situation from the point of view of the scientific community with regard to the object of the study. Then, a vast process of data collection will take place throughout the province of Québec in the different rehabilitation centers for children with intellectual disabilities. Healthcare professionals and other professionals involved with children ages from newborn to 7 years old will be met via focus groups to document in details the reality as it is in these rehabilitation centers. The second phase of the study will provide an empirical and detailed view of the situation. The results of these two phases will be compared and challenged to identify best practices and put forward promising trends in early intervention programs.

(continued)

Examples of Funded Projects (continued)

The team of researchers implementing this study is made up of occupational therapists, psychologists, and educators coming from three different universities located in the province of Québec. It is a 2-year project funded for CAN$100,000.

An American Study in Progress: Enabling Self Determination of People with AIDS

A project funded by the National Institute of Disability and Rehabilitation Research is studying an occupational therapy intervention for people with AIDS. In partnership with four supportive living facilities in Chicago, the investigators are implementing and studying an innovative model program of services based on the Model of Human Occupation and concepts from disability studies (Kielhofner & Braveman, 2001). The study design will compare outcomes of the program with a con-

trol group comprised of individuals who will receive basic educational services. Participatory research methods are also being used to identify potential obstacles and solutions to program implementation and efficacy, and to evaluate how the services impact upon and are viewed by the clients. Over the 3 years, the project, which is funded for U.S. $450,000.00, will:

* Implement and rigorously test an innovative model program designed to enable persons with AIDS to live and participate in the community and to become employed,
* Generate knowledge to refine the model program and describe best strategies for its implementation in supportive living contexts,
* Build capacity of four supportive living facilities to sustain this program, and
* Actively disseminate the model and evidence about its impact.

implemented, a detailed evaluation plan and a description of performance indicators. Proposals ordinarily include:

* A detailed listing of all grant activities (e.g., from recruiting participants and sites to data collection, data analysis and dissemination, etc.),
* When the specified activities will take place,
* Who will perform them, and
* The criteria by which they will be judged successfully competed (which is part of the evaluation plan as discussed below).

Grant reviewers appreciate seeing a table with these elements included across the duration of the grant.

The evaluation plan ordinarily must include two separate levels of evaluation:

* A formative evaluation of all the activities proposed in the timeline (according to criteria included for successful performance as noted earlier), and
* A summative evaluation of the impact of the research study, or training activity that the grant application has proposed.

Summative evaluation of the overall project usually involves specifying how one will determine the extent to which the aims and objectives proposed have been achieved and how they will be measured.

Many funders now require a project logic model to guide the evaluation process; it provides a visual representation of project goals, inputs,

outputs and outcomes (see Chapter 37 for a description of logic models). The logic model gives the researcher an overview of the outcomes of the project and also of the process of its implementation (or realization). Furthermore, it provides a framework that can serve as a reference point for the researcher to go back to and make sure that each step is achieved or that the proper adjustments are made.

Developing a Reasonable Budget Request

An important feature of any grant application is the budget request and budget narrative; together they justify the applicant's request for a certain amount of funding in each budget category. The budget narrative also provides the reviewers with a rough overview of the applicant's thinking about the logistical, timing, and implementation aspects of the study. In addition, the construction of the budget allows for the principal investigator and research team to anticipate and think through the personnel-related managerial and contractual aspects of the study.

Creating a budget upfront allows the team to anticipate the amount of salaried release time from other duties that will be required by each team member to implement the grant. In addition, it allows for subcontract agreements to be negotiated between the principal investigator's sponsoring (home) institution and any other institutions that house the co-investigators in which certain study duties will be carried out.

Most funding agencies provide detailed instructions regarding the level of detail and budgetary planning that is required for documentation in an application. For example, some budget narratives can be so detailed that they specify the estimated number of study-related phone calls that will be made by each member of the research team, the estimated length of each call, and the estimated charge for each call. Other agencies and reviewers may accept a more loosely written budget justification provided that the applicant is requesting what the reviewers and administrators consider to be a reasonable amount for each category. When possible, it always behooves an applicant to seek accounting consultation and assistance from an individual experienced in the assembly of a grant budget.

As outlined in an earlier section of this chapter (i.e., selecting an appropriate funding agency), funding agencies are highly diverse in terms of the amount of money they are willing to provide to support a single study or research group. The total amount for a grant award can range from $500 to well over $1,000,000 to support a single study. Despite this diversity, one characteristic that funding agencies have in common is that they all limit what they are willing to provide and they all have regulations on how money can be spent in a given category. Thus, it is always wise to consult with a program officer if there are any questions about how much money can be requested in a single category or if there are other ambiguities regarding the budget in the application instructions. Generally, grant budgets for health-related research may be broken down into the following categories:

- Personnel and fringe benefits,
- Tuition waivers and training stipends for students,
- Consultants,
- Travel,
- Equipment,
- Supplies,
- Inpatient or outpatient costs,
- Subcontractual costs,
- Construction costs, and
- Other costs.

The costs for each category are generally added together in different combinations using a formula that subdivides the total into the following three categories:

- Total direct costs: This is defined by the sum of all or a certain combination of the categories listed above. (For example, a granting agency

might define direct costs as the sum of all of the above categories excluding the costs of equipment and training stipends for students.)
- Indirect costs: Indirect costs cover basic infrastructure and operational costs involved in running a research study, such as office space, electricity, heating, and air conditioning.
- Total budget request: This is the sum total of the direct and indirect costs across all years of the study.

Each funding agency has a different formula that is applied in the calculation of direct versus indirect costs. Many agencies put a cap on the percentage of indirect cost funding that a sponsoring (home) institution can request in proportion to the total direct costs of a study. Some agencies do not allow a sponsoring institution to request any indirect costs because they expect an institution to provide the basic infrastructure support to operate the study. Under some circumstances the percentage of indirect costs that an institution is permitted to extract from a grant is negotiated between the funding agency and the sponsoring institution.

Obtaining Letters of Support

Many funding agencies require letters of support to be appended to the grant application. Letters of support are formal testimonials that describe a collaborator's level of experience working in the research area, overall enthusiasm about the idea and/or methodological approach of the study, and planned role or contribution to the study. Letters of support are obtained from collaborators who intend to participate directly as members of the research team; from consumers who intend to serve in advisory capacities; and from collaborating sites such as community organizations, practice sites, or other individuals who intend to support the study in a more peripheral way (e.g., practitioners who have agreed to refer their patients to participate as subjects in the study). Letters of support are typically obtained from co-investigators, consultants, subcontractors, referral sources, and advisory board members.

Determining Where to Send the Grant: Ensuring Appropriate Review

One of the most important steps in submitting a grant for review involves determining where and to whom to send the application. Each agency has its own unique policies and procedures for receiving grants and assigning them for review. It is always best to check with a reliable representative from an agency (usually a program officer or higher administrator) for first-hand information about the grant submission process.

After the Grant has been Submitted

The following section explains the critical processes and interactions that occur within the funding agency and between the program officers and the principal investigator after a grant has been submitted. It is important for investigators to have as much information about these processes as possible so that they better understand the details that contribute to a funding agency's decision to make a grant award. The three critical processes that will be discussed in this section include:

• Review process,
• Grant scores and funding decisions, and
• Feedback and resubmission.

Understanding the Review Process

For most funding agencies and competitive grant applications, the outcome of the review process is the most critical determinant of whether an investigator's grant proposal will receive funding. In many agencies, the review process can take from several months to nearly a year to complete. During the review process, one or more individuals serving as representatives for the funding agency carefully scrutinize each application to determine whether it meets a set of prespecified criteria for funding. Agencies differ in terms of these criteria. To a certain extent, these differences depend upon the overall mission, values, or objectives of the funding source. Knowing as much as possible about the review process, evaluation criteria, and the individuals serving as reviewers is important in preparing as competitive an application as possible (Gitlin & Lyons, 2004).

Agencies differ in terms of the number of grant applications they receive and in terms of the numbers and kinds of individuals that are assigned to review a given application. For example, the U.S. Public Health Service, which includes the National Institutes of Health (NIH) and the Agency for Healthcare Research and Quality (AHRQ), receives and reviews approximately 40,000 grant applications per year. Because few proposals relative to this overall number are actually funded, the application process is highly competitive. Similarly, certain offices within the U.S. Department of Education have been known to fund only the top 4% of discretionary grant applications for certain competitions.

Because the review procedures for U.S. federal granting agencies tend to be more complex than those for other granting agencies, this section focuses on describing the review procedures for federal agencies (i.e., NIH, AHRQ, and the U.S. Department of Education). Private industry and foundations use many of the evaluation criteria and review procedures that are employed by federal agencies. Thus, the general ideas provided herein should be somewhat transferable for applications to other funding sources. However, it is important to keep in mind that all agencies will differ between and within themselves in terms of the evaluation criteria they designate as most important for an investigator to address for any given type of grant. Following application instructions to the letter and tailoring the proposal to each and every aspect of the evaluation criteria is the most critical aspect of preparing any grant proposal.

Many funding agencies adhere to a peer review process in which reviewers are selected based upon their expertise in a scientific area that matches that of the grant proposals being reviewed. Peer reviewers are typically selected based on a history of exceptional scholarship and achievement in the given area. The designation of peer reviewer does not mean that the investigator knows or works with the reviewer. In fact, many agencies have strict conflict-of-interest regulations against dual relationships or research collaborations between peer reviewers and applicants.

Usually, at least three reviewers are designated to provide a detailed review of a grant application. These reviewers are sometimes referred to as first, second, and third reviewers, for example. For some agencies, an additional group of as many as 20 other reviewers that comprise a review panel may be asked to score and give input on a single application. Often, this larger group of reviewers will skim the applications and base their scores on the reports given by the primary review group and on the contents of the discussion that followed those reports.

Some funding agencies assemble review panels that consist of both peer (professional) reviewers and lay reviewers or consumers. Lay reviewers may be members of the same community or population from which participants in the research project will be drawn (e.g., individuals with chronic fatigue syndrome from a wide range of work or professional backgrounds). Alternatively, they may be individuals who represent the voice of an even broader group of individuals of which the prospective participants may be a part (e.g., individuals with disabilities). Lay reviewers will inevitably read the application through different lenses than peer reviewers. It is important to know upfront whether a lay reviewer will be reviewing the grant so that one will know whether his or her language and writing style should be tailored to a broader audience. Lay reviewers are usually charged with the same responsibilities and given as much power in the vote as peer reviewers regarding whether a given application should be funded.

If a grant received a fundable score as a result of the peer review process, some granting agencies employ a second tier of reviewers that are housed within the agency or closely linked to the agency (e.g., a board of directors) to make the final funding decision. For example, within NIH the National Advisory Council functions as an oversight board that consists of scientists and administrators. This board reviews each highly scored grant that has been recommended for funding to ensure that it provides adequate provisions for the protection of human subjects and that it is consistent with the overall policies, values, and vision of NIH. Similarly, the U.S. Department of Education has what is called a grants team that conducts an internal review of each highly scored grant to ensure that the reviewer's scoring sheets are correctly completed and to verify that the application meets all of the requirements of the program.

Criteria by which a grant application is judged vary widely. In many cases, evaluation criteria are provided in instructional format along with the initial grant application package. Some agencies have a rather rigid set of criteria by which an application is judged, whereas other agencies only offer general guidelines or do not offer much detail in the way of evaluation criteria. Examples of evaluation criteria set forth by the National Institutes of Health and the U.S. Department of Education are provided in Tables 30.3 and 30.4, respectively.

The evaluation criteria presented in Tables 30.3 and 30.4 are simply examples and they are not entirely comprehensive or exact. Even within a given agency, the evaluation criteria may change depending on the nature of the competition and the type of grant for which one is applying. Knowing and continually evaluating one's grant proposal against the published criteria for a given competition throughout the planning and writing process is fundamental to increasing the application's competitiveness. Just as evaluation criteria vary from agency to agency, so do approaches to scoring a grant proposal. More information about how applications are scored and how scores are typically interpreted is provided later in this chapter.

Interpreting Grant Scores in Light of Funding Decisions

Obtaining grant funding from most agencies is a highly competitive process. Agencies vary widely in their approaches to scoring grant applications. For example, the U.S. Department of Education scores applications such that high scores are given to the strongest applications and low scores to the weakest. Conversely, NIH scores applications such that low scores are given to the strongest applications and high scores are given to the weakest. Applications that score above the 50th percentile based on preliminary review are generally not forwarded for formal review and are not scored. Within NIH, this process is called *streamlining* because it is more time efficient and it facilitates the more detailed review of the stronger applications. Even though a review panel may assign a potentially fundable score to a grant application, it is not a guarantee that the application will be funded.

In conjunction with the requirement for additional evaluations of the overall relevance of the highly scored proposal to agency values and priorities, many agencies have cutoff points (often represented by percentile rankings) that determine which of the highly scored applications will be funded and which will not. For example, one agency may fund only the top 2% of applications for a given competition, whereas another agency may fund the top 15%. These cutoff points fluctuate depending upon accounting formulas that are developed by each agency. These formulas typically incorporate the number of applications received for each funding cycle and the amount of money available from cycle to cycle. Many program officers are willing to provide investigators with information regarding percentile funding cutoffs once it becomes available.

Evaluating Feedback and Determining Whether to Resubmit the Proposal

After having worked numerous hours to write and assemble a grant proposal, receiving critical or negative feedback is a challenging process for even the most experienced grant writer. When a grant application is not funded, it is not only difficult to read feedback from reviewers, but at times it is also difficult to interpret it and decide whether others consider the proposal worthy of revision and resubmission. Some agencies, such as the U.S. Department of Education and NIH, make the process of interpreting feedback somewhat easier by using a two-tier system. These agencies score

Table 30.3 Typical NIH Evaluation Criterion and Questions for Competing Research Applications*

Criterion	Types of Questions for Reviewers
Significance	• Is the scientific problem that the application addresses important? • Are the outcomes of the study likely to have a significant impact on existing scientific knowledge in this area? • How will this application advance existing knowledge, theoretical concepts, treatment approaches, or methodologies in this area?
Approach	• Is the study based on an overarching theory or conceptual framework? • Are the theory, design, methods, and statistical analyses cohesive and well developed? • Do they adequately reflect the specific aims and hypotheses of the study? • Is the proposed approach feasible and methodologically rigorous? • Does the investigator anticipate possible pitfalls or problems with the approach and does he or she provide alternative ways of addressing those problems should they occur?
Innovation	• Does the study introduce new theoretical concepts, approaches, or methodologies? • How does the project challenge existing paradigms or seek to revise or reformulate existing treatments or methodologies?
Investigator	• Are the investigator and his or her research team sufficiently knowledgeable, experienced, and adequately trained to carry out the work of the proposed project?
Environment	• Does the scientific environment in which the study will take place provide adequate resources and increase the likelihood that the study will be successful? • Does the project involve useful and relevant collaborations between agencies or organizations? • Does the study take advantage of unique resources or equipment within the investigator's home institution?
Inclusions, budget, and protections	• Are the plans to include both men and women in the project adequate? • Are there adequate provisions for the recruitment and retention of individuals from minority groups? • Is the proposed budget reasonable given the amount of professional effort put forth, logistical requirements, methods, and length of the proposed study? • Are there adequate provisions in place for the protection of subjects participating in the research?

*Based on evaluation guidelines for reviewers provided at http://grants.nih.gov/grants/guide/notice-files/ NOT-OD-05-002.html.

and comprehensively evaluate only the stronger applications. Written feedback from the reviewers is forwarded only to investigators who achieved the higher scores. If an applicant's proposal is rejected but he or she receives written feedback from an agency, it indicates that the reviewers considered the application worthy enough of a detailed discussion regarding its merits and weaknesses.

In many cases, federal agencies consider applications that are streamlined (or not scored) as not salvageable because they are limited by major flaws. Such flaws may include ideas that lack significance or do not reflect the objectives of the funding agency, flaws in the design and methods, absence of an adequate theoretical basis, confusing or inconsistent aims and hypotheses, poor overall scholarship, and ethical or logistic problems (Gitlin & Lyons, 2004).

Proposals worthy of revision and resubmission include those that are given scores near the percentile cutoff for funding. In many cases, feedback will indicate that the reviewers were enthusiastic about the application and would encourage revision and resubmission. Sometimes reviewers will provide the applicant with questions to answer in the revised proposal or suggestions about how to address the concerns that have been raised. The program officer can often speak to the general level of enthusiasm about an application and can assist an applicant in deciding whether to revise and resubmit the grant application.

Conclusion

This chapter provided an orientation to the main kinds of funding opportunities for occupational

**Table 30.4 Examples* of U.S. Department of Education General Evaluation
Criteria for Grant Reviews**

Criterion	Questions
Need for project	• Is the problem to be addressed of sufficient magnitude or severity? • How does the proposed project meet the need for services, identify gaps or weaknesses in existing services, and address those gaps? • How will the proposed project prepare personnel for fields in which shortages have been demonstrated?
Significance	• What is the national significance and likely impact of the proposed project in terms of improving employment? • How significant is the problem to be addressed by the project? • What is the potential contribution of the project to increased knowledge or understanding of rehabilitation or educational problems, issues, or effective strategies? • What is the likelihood that the project will result in system change or improvement? • How likely is the project to contribute to the development and advancement of theory, knowledge, and practices in the field of study? • How replicable will the program be in a variety of settings and how generalizable will the findings be? • To what extent will the proposed project yield findings or products that will be utilized by other agencies or organizations. • How likely will the proposed project build local capacity to provide, improve, or expand services? • Will the results be disseminated in ways that will enable others to use the information or strategies?
Quality of the project design	• To what extent are the goals, objectives and predicted outcomes clearly specified and measurable? • Is the project based upon a specific and rigorous research design? • Does the design reflect up-to-date knowledge from research and effective practice? • Is the design appropriate to the needs of the target population and is it likely to address those needs? • Is there a high-quality conceptual framework underlying the proposed research or demonstration activities? • Do the proposed activities add to a coherent and sustained program of research, training, or development in the field? • Do they add substantially to an ongoing line of inquiry? • Is the proposed design accompanied by a thorough, high-quality review of the literature, a quality plan for research activities/project implementation, and the use of appropriate theoretical and methodological tools to ensure successful achievement of the project objectives? • Will the design lead to replication of project activities or strategies? Are proposed development efforts accompanied by adequate quality controls and repeated testing of products? • Will the project build capacity and yield results that will extend beyond the funding period? • Does the proposed project represent an exceptional approach for meeting the priorities established for the competition and/or the statutory purposes and requirements? • To what extent will the project be coordinated with related efforts and establish linkages with appropriate community, state, and federal resources and organizations providing services to the target population? • Does the project encourage consumer involvement? • Are performance feedback and continuous improvement integral to the design of the project? • What is the quality of the methodology to be employed in this project?
Quality of Project services	• Are there strategies for ensuring equal access and treatment for eligible project participants that are members of groups that have traditionally been underrepresented based on race, color, national origin, sex, age, or disability? • Are the services to be provided by the project appropriate to the needs of the intended recipients or beneficiaries of those services? • Do entities that are to be served by any proposed technical assistance project demonstrate support for the project?

(continued)

511

Criterion	Questions
	• Do the services to be provided reflect up-to-date knowledge from research and effective practice?
	• What is the likely impact of the services to be provided on the intended recipients?
	• To what extent are training or professional development services to be provided by the proposed project of sufficient quality, intensity, and duration to lead to improvements in practice among recipients of those services?
	• Will the training or professional development services alleviate the personnel shortages that have been identified?
	• Will the project lead to improvements in the academic achievement of students as measured against rigorous standards?
	• Will the project lead to improvements in the skills necessary to gain employment or build capacity for independent living?
	• To what extent will the project involve the collaboration of appropriate partners for maximizing the effectiveness of services?
	• To what extent are the services to be provided focused on those with greatest needs?
Quality of project personnel	• Will the investigator encourage applications for project staff positions from persons who are members of groups that have traditionally been underrepresented based on race, color, national origin, sex, age, or disability?
	• How qualified, trained, and experienced are the investigators, key project personnel, consultants, and subcontractors?
Adequacy of resources	• Are the facilities, equipment, supplies, and other resources from the applicant organization adequate?
	• Has each partner demonstrated commitment to the implementation and success of the project?
	• Is the budget adequate to support the proposed project?
	• Are the proposed costs reasonable in relation to the objectives, design, potential significance and benefit, and number of persons to be served?
	• Is there potential for continued support of the project by appropriate entities after federal funding ends?
	• Is there a potential for the incorporation of project purposes, activities, or benefits into the ongoing program of the agency after the funding period?
Quality of the management plan	• Is the management plan adequate to achieve the objectives of the project on time and within the budget?
	• Does the management plan include clearly defined responsibilities, timelines, and milestones for accomplishing project tasks?
	• Are the procedures for ensuring feedback and continuous improvement in project operations adequate?
	• Are the mechanisms for ensuring high-quality products and services from the project adequate?
	• Are time commitments from the investigators and other project personnel adequate to meet the objectives?
	• How will the applicant ensure that a diversity of perspectives are brought to bear in the operation of the proposed project, including those of parents, teachers, the business community, other disciplines and consumers?
Quality of the project evaluation	• Are the methods of evaluation thorough, feasible, appropriate to the context within which the project operates, and appropriate to the goals, objectives, and outcomes of the project?
	• Do the methods of evaluation provide for examining the effectiveness of project implementation strategies?
	• Do the methods of evaluation include the use of objective performance measures that are clearly related to the intended outcomes of the project and will they produce quantitative and qualitative data to the greatest extent possible?
	• Will project evaluation methods provide timeline guidance for quality assurance?
	• Will the evaluation provide guidance about effective strategies suitable for replication or testing in other settings?

*Based on guidelines adapted from evaluation guidelines for reviewers provided by the Education Department General Administrative Regulations, Part 75, Subpart D at http://www.ed.gov/policy/fund/reg/edgarReg/edlite-part75d.html. A specific competition will typically use a subset of the types of questions listed on this table.

therapy researchers. The authors explained the steps involved in writing and applying for grants that fund research studies and other research-related programs and initiatives. Twenty steps that the authors considered necessary for the attainment of grant funding were reviewed. The authors explained elements of grant writing that ranged from idea development to ensuring an appropriate review once a grant has been submitted. The authors then described the review and evaluation process and explained how funding decisions are made. The chapter also provided information on how to revise and resubmit a grant proposal that was rejected. Explanations of international funding procedures and mechanisms available in the United Kingdom and Canada were provided and examples that described the process of obtaining different kinds of grant funding from different funding sources were provided.

REFERENCES

Balcazar, F., & Suarez-Balcazar, Y. (2004). *Center for capacity building for minorities with disabilities research*. The University of Illinois at Chicago, Department of Disability and Human Development and Department of Occupational Therapy. Grant proposal submitted to and funded by the National Institutes of Disability and Rehabilitation Research.

Canadian Occupational Therapy Foundation (2004). Opportunities for Researchers. Retrieved December 5, 2005, from http://www.cotfcanada.org/site_page.asp?pageid=672

Creek, J., & Ilott, I. (2002). *Scoping study of occupational therapy research and development activity in Scotland, Northern Ireland and Wales*. London: College of Occupational Therapists.

Department of Health (2000). *Meeting the Challenge: A strategy for the allied health professions*. London: Department of Health.

Department of Health (2005). *Research governance framework for health and social care (2nd ed.)*. London: Department of Health.

Gillette, N. (2000). A twenty-year history of research funding in occupational therapy. *The American Journal of Occupational Therapy, 54*(4), 441–442.

Gitlin, L. N., & Lyons, K. J. (2004). *Successful grant writing: Strategies for health and human service professionals*. New York: Springer.

Higher Education Funding Council for England (2001). *Research in nursing and allied health professions: Report of the Task Group 3 to HEFCE and the Department of Health*. Bristol: Higher Education Funding Council for England.

Ilott, I., & White, E. (2001). 2001 College of Occupational Therapists' research and development strategic vision and action plan. *British Journal of Occupational Therapy, 64*(6), 270–274.

Kielhofner, G. (2002). UIC's scholarship of practice. *OT Practice, 7*(1), 11–12.

Kielhofner, G., Borell, L., & Tham, K. (2002). Preparing scholars of practice around the world. *OT Practice, 7*(6), 13–14.

Kielhofner, G., & Braveman, B. (2001). *Enabling self determination for people living with AIDS*. Department of Occupational Therapy, University of Illinois at Chicago. Grant proposal submitted to and funded by the National Institute of Disability and Rehabilitation Research, U.S. Department of Education (H133G020217-3).

Scottish Executive (2004). *Allied Health Professions Research and Development Action Plan*. Edinburgh: Scottish Executive.

Taylor, R. R. (2004). Quality of life and symptom severity for individuals with chronic fatigue syndrome: Findings from a randomized clinical trial. *American Journal of Occupational Therapy, 58*, 35–43.

Taylor, R. R., Fisher, G., & Kielhofner, G. (2005). Synthesizing research, education, and practice according to the scholarship of practice model: Two faculty Examples. *Occupational Therapy and Health Care, 19*, 107–122.

RESOURCES

For Grant Writing

Gitlin, L. N., & Lyons, K. J. (2004). *Successful grant writing: Strategies for health and human service professionals*. New York: Springer.

Additional resources can be found at (http://.www.npguides.org/guide/index.html and http://www.cpb.org/grants/grantwriting.html).

To find a potential match between a private source of funding and an idea/project:

United States

• The Foundation Center: A nonprofit information clearinghouse and library that collects and disseminates information on more than 80,000 private foundations for organizations and individuals seeking information about grants. It is one of the most widely accessed search engines used by research development personnel to inform investigators of available funding opportunities and competitions. The Foundation Center can be accessed at http://www.fdncenter.org.

• Foundations On-Line: A foundation directory and search tool that can be accessed at http://www.foundations.org

• FundingSearch.com: Provides grant funding resource services for nonprofit organizations, consultants, and proposal writers.

• GrantsWeb: Provides links to grant resources, funding opportunities and a grants database.

Additional links and resources to granting agencies, funding announcements, and grant writing tips:

• http://www.npguides.org/guide/index.html. Nonprofit guides is a grant writing resource with tools and links for funding for nonprofit organizations.

• http://www.foundations.org. The Doundation Center is a great resource for finding private and public foundations, the foundation directory, and matching of topics and foundations.

• http://fconline.fdncenter.org/ The foundation center online has a comprehensive directory of private, community, and corporate grant makers.

United Kingdom

In the United Kingdom, information on many funding opportunities for health-related research can be obtained from the web-based resource RDInfo (http://www.rdinfo.org.uk). Support for new researchers is a recent addition to the information provided, while a special edition devoted to funding opportunities for allied health professionals, produced in 2003, can also be downloaded.

Information About the Grant Review Process

Most funding agencies will have information on their grant review process posted on their Web sites. Detailed information about the review process within NIH can be found at http://grants1.nih.gov/grants/peer/peer.htm

CHAPTER 31

Securing Samples for Effective Research Across Research Designs

Anne E. Dickerson

Selecting a Sample

The research process has clearly defined steps. One of the most critical of these is securing the study sample. An adequate, carefully selected sample, suitable to the research design, is essential to rigorous research. Whether undertaking quantitative or qualitative research, there is a process for determining who should participate in the study.

Selecting a sample determines who is studied. However, it is intimately tied to what is studied. It is important to delimit the specified group of individuals who will be studied according to the phenomena, or conceptual idea under investigation. For example, if an investigation is examining the use of a training technique for increased mobility in clients who experienced a cerebrovascular accident (CVA), it may be very important to limit the scope of the research to clients who had either a right or left CVA, since training may affect differently depending on the location of the CVA. On the other hand, if the research question is on the effectiveness of the Canadian Occupational Performance Measure (Law et al., 1998), CVA clients with both right and left CVA should be included, but persons with expressive aphasia would not be appropriate subjects, since they could not participate in the assessment.

Issues Affecting Selection of Subjects

The term *subject pool* refers to those who are identified as eligible to participate in the study. How a subject pool is selected depends on several issues. First, as mentioned previously, the subject pool clearly depends on the study question. For example, if a study question asks about the efficacy of sensory integrative (SI) therapy for children, the subject pool would be children who have SI problems. If the question pertained to SI effectiveness with children who have tactile defensiveness, then the subject pool would be further narrowed to those children with this particular SI problem. Thus, the specific nature of the research question directly impacts the selection of subjects.

The research approach also affects sampling. For example, a quantitative study of the efficacy of sensory integration would compare a group of children randomly assigned to receive sensory integrative treatment to a group randomly assigned to a control group. In this instance, there would be concern to have a sufficiently large sample size in order to achieve statistical significance. In contrast, a qualitative researcher examining efficacy would be likely to select a small number of children who could be interviewed and observed in great depth. In this instance, the investigator might systematically select children who are better able to articulate their experience.

A researcher may address the research question using a single-system design as discussed in Chapter 11. Such an inquiry would require only one subject. Alternatively, a narrative history design could involve an in-depth interview with a child, members of his/her family, and the therapist providing the SI therapy. As these examples illustrate, a third issue that affects sampling is the research design.

Finally, the practical considerations such as access to the populations under interest influence the selection of subjects. In many cases, these logistic issues have a major impact on a researcher's sampling plan. For example, if a study focuses on a population that has limited numbers (e.g., people with amyotrophic lateral sclerosis), the sample size will be limited by access. More commonly, the limitations of budget, time, and space lead the researcher to limit the sample size or diversity. Often, sampling limitations undermine the integrity of a study, jeopardizing its usefulness. Unfortunately, many studies are ultimately not published because the sample size or sampling approach was inadequate to provide the necessary rigor. While practical considerations are necessary, an investigator will need to be prepared to explain and defend the sample and sampling strategy at the conclusion of the study. In the end, the researcher has to balance the research question, the approach to inquiry, the research design, and pragmatic considerations, to achieve an optimal sample.

What to Call Individuals Participating in a Study

What should the individual who participates in the study be called? Traditionally in quantitative research, the term *subject* is used. This term denotes the ideal of objectivity and the often passive nature of participating in a quantitative study. On the other hand, qualitative research often stresses the researcher's joining with those studied in their everyday lives. Thus, the term *participant* is more typically used to refer to those whose lives are studied. *Informant* is also used in qualitative studies to designate the person who gives the researcher valuable information about the phenomena under study. In survey research, the term *respondent* is most frequently used to refer to the individual answering the survey. In participatory research where the investigation is designed to affect the lives of those under study, the term *stakeholder* is common. Each term reflects a different way the individual participates in the study and it is the researcher who selects which term accurately portrays the role that the individual plays in the study.

Gender and Race/Ethnicity Issues

Historically, large-scale studies funded by national grant funding focused on majority male subjects. Government task force reports on women's health indicated there was an absence of research data on women (Schroeder & Snowe, 1994). Similar observations were made concerning the lack of research on minorities. As a consequence, the government mandated that women and minorities must be included in clinical research studies. Now the National Institute of Health Revitalization Act of 1993 ensures that there is representation of women and minorities, unless there is a clear and compelling rationale that their inclusion is inappropriate for the purpose of the study or health of the subjects (Hayunga & Pinn, 2002). Although the National Institute of Health has required awardees of grants to furnish enrollment data by sex and race/ethnic group and substantial numbers of women and minorities have been included as research subjects, more emphasis on identifying potential differences between men and women and individuals of diversity is still needed (Hayunga & Pinn, 2002).

As with any research question, it is important to consider if gender or race factors will impact the study. For example, in a study of persons with spinal cord injury, Tzonichaki and Kleftara (2002) found that males had a higher level of self-esteem than females. In another example, Kizony and Katz (2002) found in a study of persons with stroke that significantly more women than men scored above the cutoff point of the process scale of the Assessment of Motor and Process Skills. As these examples illustrate, gender can make a difference in occupational performance and volition.

Relevant to occupational therapy, there is evidence that Latinos and African-Americans with disabilities in the United States are more likely to receive fewer comprehensive services, and less culturally relevant services compared to white families (Belgrave & Walker, 1991; Moritsugu & Sue, 1983; Wells & Black, 2000; Zea, Quezada, & Belgrave, 1994).

Decisions about sampling should always, therefore, give careful consideration to issues of gender and race/ethnicity. Including diverse samples and analyzing data within these subcategories can also have important implications for sample size. This is addressed later.

Steps to Sampling

The first step in the sampling process is defining the population of interest (Figure 31.1). This is ordinarily done through a literature review. A thorough examination of completed research in the area of concern, will define the parameters of the

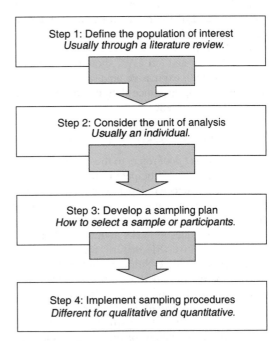

Figure 31.1 Steps to sampling.

population that will be important for a given study. Knowing the population of interest is the first step in defining the sample.

The next step is to consider the unit of analysis. What is analyzed in the study, will determine the unit. In most occupational therapy research, the unit of analysis is an individual (e.g., the client). However, the unit of analysis can be settings (e.g., comparing long-term care facilities with rehabilitation centers), families, caregivers, or couples, geographical areas, or other elements. For example, in comparing the efficacy of sensory integration by evaluating performance of children, the unit of analysis would be individual children because each child's scores would be used in the data analysis. However, if the goal is to determine the efficacy of one private pediatric setting using sensory integration against another setting, the unit of analysis would not be the settings and groups of clients as a whole. If the goal of the study was to examine the impact of therapy on families with a disabled child, the unit of analysis could be the family.

Once the population and the unit of analysis have been identified, the third step is developing a sampling plan. This plan outlines how the investigator will select the sample. In quantitative research, researchers should use theoretically defined methods of sampling that are required for making inferences about the population of interest and that are assumed by more powerful parametric, and even some of the non-parametric statistics. As part of the plan, the researcher determines the sample size or how many individuals are needed for the study. The rigor of a quantitative study depends on a well planned sampling plan that is strictly followed.

In qualitative studies, sampling is designed to be less rigid, but it is not any less important. A key distinction of the qualitative design is that, although the qualitative researcher does outline a sampling plan, the sample can be changed during the study including the number, type, and description of the subjects to be studied. In some cases it is critical to the rigor of the study to change the boundaries of the sample.

The last step is to implement the sampling procedures. The next sections elaborate on these critical steps for quantitative and qualitative research separately.

Sampling in Quantitative Research

In quantitative research, the specifications of the subjects are set before the study begins. As noted earlier, defining the population is the starting point in sampling. The population of the study includes all the individuals that share the defined characteristics of interest. Sometimes the population is the key element of the research question. For example, consider an investigator who wants to find out the most appropriate assessment for determining if the client with head injury is ready to return to work. The population for the study would be individuals with brain injuries who are of working age.

In contrast, if a researcher wants to validate an assessment, the actual focus or question of the research is the construct validity or the predictive validity of the assessment tool. In this case, the population could be very broad (i.e., all persons who could potentially be assessed with the instrument). The population is still important since the assessment should be shown to have validity for the entire population for whom it is intended. Depending on the assessment, the population may be defined either broadly (e.g., any disabled clients) or narrowly (e.g., clients with chronic mental illness). Whatever the research question, the researcher must clearly define the characteristics of the population about whom conclusions will be drawn from the study.

The target population is the population to which the researcher wants to generalize his or her intended findings. For example, if the study's target population is defined as individuals with schizophrenia, it would include all individuals who have this diagnosis. The researcher selects a subset of that target population for the sample. The sample will be the subjects whom the researcher uses in his or her research study. The degree to which the selected sample represents the target population is the degree to which the results can be generalized to the population.

The researcher wants to ensure that the sample is representative of the population in order that the results of the study are valid for the population whom the sample was chosen to represent. For instance, if a researcher wants to investigate an

> The degree to which the selected sample represents the target population is the degree to which the results can be generalized to the population.

occupational therapy intervention for CVA clients, the sample must represent all CVA clients who are candidates for occupational therapy. If the study was done in a regional hospital in a specific state, the researcher would need to defend how CVA clients admitted to this hospital are typical of the population. Just as importantly, the investigator will need to define how the individuals in the study sample were actually selected from this hospital to maximize their representativeness of the target population. The main purpose of sampling in quantitative research is to be able to accurately draw conclusions about the population by studying the sample.

The investigator defines the parameters of the target population by specifying the inclusion and exclusion criteria. The inclusion criteria are the traits that the researcher has identified as characterizing the population. They serve as the criteria that qualify someone as a subject or participant in the study. For example, an inclusion criterion for the earlier example would be a diagnosis of CVA. The exclusion criteria are the characteristics that will prohibit the subject from being an appropriate candidate for the study. These are typically factors that could potentially confound the results of the study (Portney & Watkins, 2000). In other words, the subject may have characteristics that would interfere with the interpretation of the results of a study, and thus need to be excluded from the study. For example, if the investigation sought to examine the impact of an intervention on persons with CVA it might produce different outcomes of the person with CVA who also had a major mental illness. In such a case co-morbid mental illness might be an exclusion criterion. In some instances, clients are excluded because they are unable to participate in the study. For example, if the intervention and the outcome measure require a participant or subject to speak a given language, those who do not speak the language would be excluded.

The sample pool must possess the inclusion criteria, not possess the exclusion criteria, and be available for selection. Good inclusion and exclusion criteria are specific and clearly identified. For example, Mathiowetz (2003) had the following specific inclusion criteria for his study of the Fatigue Impact Scale for persons with multiple sclerosis:

- A diagnosis of multiple sclerosis,
- Age of 18 years or older,
- Functional literacy,
- A Fatigue Severity Scale score of four or greater (i.e., moderate to high fatigue severity),
- Living in the community, and

- Functionally independent in the majority of self-care and daily activities.

In this same study participants were excluded if they:

- Did not attend at least five support group and energy conservation sessions,
- Had an exacerbation of symptoms,
- Changed fatigue medication, or
- Had other major illnesses, hospitalizations, or rehabilitation during the course of the study.

In quantitative research, the specification of the number of persons in the sample is established after the design is determined. For example, if the research study calls for a pretest/posttest comparison group design, the researcher can know that two groups of subjects are required. The number of subjects necessary will depend on the desired power as discussed in Chapter 7 and later in this chapter.

External Validity

The purpose of getting a representative sample is to increase the generalizability of the study. A worthwhile study is one whose results can be generalized to a broader population or similar populations. External validity relates to this generalizability (i.e., a study whose sample allows generalization to the broader population, has greater external validity). Validity refers to the "approximate truth of propositions, inferences, or conclusions" so external validity refers to the "approximate truth of conclusions that involve generalizations" (Trochim, 2002, p. 1).

To make generalizations, the researcher must be able to assume the characteristics of the sample members will represent the target population. Unfortunately, sampling bias occurs when individuals are selected who overrepresent or underrepresent certain population characteristics (Portney & Watkins, 2000). A bias can be deliberate when an investigator purposefully includes certain kinds of subjects. However, even when bias is unplanned, it can jeopardize a study's external validity.

The three major threats to external validity are people, place, or time (Trochim, 2002). A potential criticism of any study is that the study's results occurred because there was an "unusual" group of subjects in the study. For example, if the sample for an intervention study included individuals who volunteered for the study and were highly invested in results, these volunteers may "work" beyond what the non-volunteer or average individual would choose to do. Thus, their outcome from the intervention may not generalize to all others who might receive the intervention.

Another threat to external validity is the place or location of the study. For example, if an outcomes study occurred in an area of a city where the average income is well above average, affluence may influence the results. Other areas with fewer resources or more environmental stressors linked to poverty may not achieve the same benefits from an intervention because there may not be any follow through or resources to meet the basic requirements of an intervention (i.e., no resources to pay for assistive devices).

There is the element of time in a study (i.e., when data are collected from the sample). For example, a study on the incidence of depression could be affected if the study occurs immediately after the holidays when more people report depression. Thus, the researcher must evaluate these factors prior to starting any study in order to limit threats to external validity with sampling or sampling bias.

Kinds of Sampling and Sampling Error

In quantitative research, there are two kinds of sampling:

• Probability, and
• Nonprobability.

Probability or random sampling is based on probability theory that is addressed later in this chapter. Random sampling means that each member or element of the population can theoretically have an equal chance of being selected for the sample. For example, consider a study in which the population consists of all the voters in a particular state. If an investigator could obtain a complete voters list, then a sampling design could be developed that ensures that each voter will have an equal chance of being selected for the sample.

If the population parameters are known, the sampling error can be calculated. Sampling error represents the difference between the values obtained by the sample and the actual values that exist in the population. However, it is very unusual to have this information. Therefore, calculating the exact sampling error is usually not possible. In this case, an estimated sampling error can be calculated. Since sampling error represents the degree to which the sample is representative of the population, the larger the sample error, the less representative the sample is to the population and the lower the external validity.

Sampling error is due to:

• Random error, or
• Systematic error.

Random errors are those that happen by chance. For example, suppose 50 subjects for a study on normal grip strength were randomly selected in a geographic area. If one of these subjects happened to be an Olympic shot putter, his grip strength will skew the mean higher than the true average since there is not 1 Olympian for every 50 persons in the population. This type of random error is expected, but cannot be predicted. For this reason larger numbers of subjects are preferred since they reduce random error. For example, if 500 subjects had been selected for the study of grip strength, it is highly improbable another Olympian would have been selected in which case the effect of the 1 Olympian on skewing the mean grip strength would be much less.

Systematic error is a serious problem for a study. It represents a flaw in the sampling process, which results in the subjects differing from the population systematically. For example, if the investigator studying grip strength recruited subjects at a men's gym, the resulting sample would include individuals who are likely to have greater grip strength than average.

The major sources of systematic error are:

• Using volunteers (because those who volunteer for any study are likely to be different from those who refuse), and
• Using groups that are available and convenient (but likely to share some common characteristic that makes them different than the intended population).

Avoiding these two sources of error often creates a dilemma for researchers. For example, consider an occupational therapist who wants to study the efficacy of sensory integration for learning disabled children. If the researcher seeks volunteers from a clinic that evaluates and treats children using sensory integration techniques, which parents are most likely to volunteer? Those who volunteer will tend to be motivated parents who want any kind of information that might help to address their child's issues.

Since the children with the most motivated parents are not "typical" of all learning disabled children, systematic error will have been introduced into the selection of subjects.

Methods of Probability Sampling and Assignment

Randomization is considered to be the cornerstone of quantitative research. It balances both the measured and unmeasured characteristics that affect the outcomes of a study, allows for masking, and

**Selected Examples of Quantitative Studies in Occupational Therapy
Illustrating Sampling Bias Identified by the Investigators**

- The sample was composed of college students in an introductory psychology class who got credit for participation in the study. Although it was possible that there were students with varying degrees of health, the sample was biased toward healthy college students. "The extent to which the participant sample of college students might be representative of other participant samples is unknown. This leaves some uncertainty about the generalizability of the results of the study" (p. 55). Additional research comparing healthy individuals with those of varying degrees of illness would need to be conducted to enhance the validity of this particular study (Reich & Williams, 2003).
- Participants were recruited from the "students, faculty, and staff at the university, friends, and family" (p. 101). Older adults were recruited from a research registry developed at the university. The participants all lived in the Midwest and most in urban areas. Findings may not be generalized to those who reside in other parts of the country and other settings. In addition, the sample of older adults was highly educated. "A more diverse representation of education levels in future work is needed" (Pohl, Dunn, & Brown, 2003, p. 105).
- The response rate from the survey was 52%. "This response rate indicates a self-selected sample (volunteers) that may be biased in their views about *AJOT* and the usefulness of research. Consequently, study results may not accurately reflect general leadership views" (Philibert, Snyder, Judd, & Windsor, 2003, p. 457).
- The participants were kindergarten students from one school district. "The participants did not effectively represent a heterogeneous population of kindergarten students as a random sample would have" (Daly, Kelley, & Krauss, 2003, p. 462).
- The participants were kindergarten students from one school district. "Only typically developing students were assessed; thus, the research has no implications for learning disabled students" (Daly, Kelley, & Krauss, 2003, p. 462).
- One hundred and twenty-nine volunteers were recruited. There was no effect for gender on the reaction time to the visual stimulus. "However, it should be remarked that the relatively small number of female participants (28) did not reflect the actual gender distribution of older drivers" (Lee, Lee, & Cammeron, 2003, p. 327).
- 129 volunteers were recruited. "The participants who volunteered for this study cannot be taken as representative of the target population because the sample was not randomly selected but only came from some sectors of the community" (Lee, Lee, & Cammeron, 2003, p. 327).

provides a basis for inference (Berger & Bears, 2003). In other words, it is the best method of removing selection bias (Torgerson & Roberts, 1999). As will be discussed, randomization can be used both for subject selection (sampling) and subject assignment (allocation to different experimental groups).

When the population is known, methods of probability sampling can be relatively simple and unbiased. With simple random sampling, all the individuals in a defined target population have an equal and independent chance of being selected for a sample. Simple random sampling is also known as sampling without replacement (Portney & Watkins, 2000); once a person is selected, he or she is out of the pool and has no further chance of being selected. Often a table of random numbers or a computer-generated list of random numbers is used to select the sample from the list of the target population.

In addition to using random sampling to choose a subject pool from a population, investigators who are studying groups of subjects use random assignment to allocate subjects to groups. The principle of random assignment is the same as for sampling. However, instead of eliminating bias that makes the sample unrepresentative of the population, random assignment seeks to eliminate bias due to differences in the groups being compared. Thus, by randomly assigning subjects into the groups that make up a study, an investigator achieves groups that, according to probability theory, are likely to be equivalent.

True randomization is often difficult or prohibitive in occupational therapy studies owing to the structure of the practice environment. Fortunately, randomization is also considered as referring "... to a broad collection of allocation methods" (Berger & Bears, 2003, p. 468). For example, Berger and Bears argue that, in studies in which groups are compared, strict allocation (assignment) methods can eliminate selection bias as effectively as randomization. If the terms of allocation are identified before identification (or screening) of subjects, selection bias is controlled. However, if terms of allocation are done after the identification of subjects, then direct selection bias is introduced. In other words, if it is determined how subjects will be assigned to particular groups prior to the start of the study, then it can be argued the bias is eliminated (e.g., every other subject will be assigned to the control group). If subjects are identified and *then* assigned to groups, direct selection bias is likely (e.g., the more willing subjects might be assigned to the treatment group).

Bias can also be introduced if the investigator has discretion to approve or deny enrollment in the study or has advanced knowledge of the groups. In addition, if alternation of assignment of subjects (e.g., every other identified subject is assigned to a particular group) is used instead of randomly assigning groups, the sequence becomes predictable and problematic (Berger & Bears, 2003).

Stratified Random Sampling

If a study requires that certain groups be represented equally, a stratified random sample may be more appropriate. Stratified sampling is similar to a simple random sample, but the selection is from identified subgroups in the population. For example, if a study about the occupational therapy profession was undertaken, the researcher may want to ensure that both the professional and technical levels of the profession are represented. Therefore, a stratified random sample of the professional level therapists and the occupational therapy assistant population would be separated and the appropriate number from each group selected randomly. It is important to ensure that representation from the stratified categories is proportional to that category's proportion of the whole population. For example, if there were two occupational therapists for every assistant in the profession then the resulting sample should reflect that proportion.

Systematic Sampling

Systematic sampling is considered equivalent to random sampling as long as there is no reoccurring pattern or order in the listing (Portney & Watkins, 2000). The number of subjects for the sample is known and divided into the number of the population. Then, individuals are selected from the list by taking every "k"th name. For example, if a list of licensed occupational therapists from Pennsylvania includes 1,500 occupational therapists and the researcher has decided to survey 300 therapists, the research would select every fifth individual from the comprehensive list to survey.

Cluster Sampling

Another common probability sampling method is cluster sampling. In cluster sampling individuals are not randomly selected. Rather, groups or programs are selected and every member of that group or program is invited to participate in the study. For example, cluster sampling may be used to determine the usefulness of an evaluation in outpatient rehabilitations centers. Centers in certain states or counties may be selected and all therapists in the centers asked to participate.

Nonprobability Sampling Methods

When the parameters of a population are not known or when it is not feasible to do some type of probability sample, nonprobability sampling is used in quantitative research. In this instance, it is very important to try to attain the greatest degree of representation for the sample. When nonprobability sampling is used, the investigator must:

• Clearly define the process of the sampling,
• Acknowledge the limitations of the sampling procedure, and
• Justify why the sampling limitations do not jeopardize the research question being answered.

The sample characteristics still need to be defined clearly in terms of inclusion and exclusion criteria.

Convenience Sampling

Convenience sampling method is the most problematic, yet widely used nonprobability method to obtain subjects. Convenience sampling is the use of volunteers or easily available subjects such as a group of students in a program or clientele in a clinic. In a convenience sample, subjects are enrolled as they agree to enter the study, until the desired number is reached. While a convenience sample is always the weakest sampling method, the degree of appropriateness of using a convenience sample depends on the research question. For example, if the research question asked about normal grip strength for female college students, selecting the women in an occupational therapy class, on the face of it, does not appear to enter a large amount of bias. However, if the research question asked about average knowledge of health issues among college students, an occupational therapy class might be very biased in terms of such knowledge. In the latter case, using the class as a convenience sample is much less defensible.

Purposive Sampling

Purposive sampling is the deliberate selection of individuals by the researcher based on certain predetermined criteria (usually stated as inclusion and exclusion criteria) (Portney & Watkins, 2000). For example, if a study sought to understand the impact of being involved in a wellness group on health behaviors among women, an investigator might seek subjects from a wellness group at a local women's center.

Snowball or Network Sampling

Snowball or network sampling is a method in which initially identified subjects provide names of others who may meet the study criteria. Snowball sampling is used when potential subjects are difficult or impractical to obtain and when the intended subjects are likely to be aware of others who share their characteristics. For example, consider a researcher who wants a sample of mothers of children with spina bifida. If the researcher has some initial contacts, such mothers usually know other members of the same group through support groups and other means. They can, thus, be useful in recruiting additional subjects. However, with the snowball method, the sampling pool can become biased and the researcher has no control over who is nominated for the study.

Quota Sampling

Quota sampling is used when different proportions of subject types are needed so that there is appropriate representation in the sample that may not be attainable with purposive or convenience sampling. For instance, an investigator who wanted to compare male to female occupational therapists might use quota sampling to attain equal numbers of subjects in both groups.

Determining Sample Size

It is important to determine the right sample size for every study. The sample size will influence many factors in the design and implementation of a study, especially the costs and time involved in a study. A general rule of thumb is that one should obtain the largest sample possible. Larger samples make a study more challenging to complete and require more resources. On the other hand, if there are too few subjects, a study is not worth undertaking since any findings would be suspect.

Researchers have agreed on a minimum number of cases needed for specific research designs. For example, in correlational research, it is traditional to use a minimum of 30 subjects (Gall, Borg, & Gall, 1996). Survey research requires a minimum of 100 in each major subgroup and 20 to 50 in each minor subgroup whose responses will be analyzed (Gall, Borg, & Gall, 1996). In causal–comparative or experimental research, there should be at least 15 subjects in each group. However, within this category, there are variations of appropriate numbers of subjects. For example, in crossover two-period designs, the same subjects are used in the treatment and control groups. The subjects are their own controls and therefore sample sizes for this can be substantially smaller than the parallel groups (Albert & Borkowf, 2002).

Statistical Power and Sample Size

It has become good research practice to base decisions about sample size on statistical power. Statistical power refers to the likelihood of finding a significant difference between groups or association between variables when one exists (Albert & Borkowf, 2002). The number of subjects is directly related to the *statistical power* of a study. As discussed in Chapter 7 and this chapter, investigators can determine before a study is undertaken how many subjects are needed.

To determine the number of subjects necessary to have sufficient statistical power, four interrelated components need to be considered:

1. Sample size,
2. Effect size,
3. Alpha level or level of significance, and
4. The power or the odds of observing a treatment effect when it occurs (Trochim, 2002).

If the values of three of these components are known, computation of the fourth factor is possible. Thus, the number of subjects needed can be determined based on reasonable estimates of the other factors. The goal is to balance these components so that maximum level of power is available to detect an effect if one exists, given constraints on the other components (Trochim, 2002).

Effect Size

Effect size is the "effect of differences between two means or the degree of relationship between two variables in the results of a study" (Stein & Cutler, 2000, p. 502). The smaller the effect size, the more subjects a study will need. For example, consider a study about the changes in handwriting for children who were enrolled in a 6- month long sensory processing program. Such a study would compare

Selected Examples of Quantitative Studies in Occupational Therapy Using Specific Types of Sampling Strategies

Randomly Assigned

- Subjects needing bathing devices were chosen from inpatient and outpatient services from one hospital in Hong Kong. The subjects were randomly assigned to the intervention group or a control group (Chiu & Man, 2003).
- Subjects were randomly assigned to test administrators and either of the two treatment groups or control group. "Environments and treatment schedules for both groups were matched" (Shaffer, Jacokes, Cassily, Greenspan, Tuchman, & Stemmer, 2001, p. 157).

Stratified Random Sampling

- Stratified random sampling was used in order for the total sample to have "…equal numbers of boys ($n = 20$) and girls ($n = 20$), 6- and 7-year olds ($n = 20$ each), and to allow for equal numbers of right-handed ($n = 32$) and left-handed ($n = 8$) children in each group" (Smith-Zuzovsky & Exner, 2004, p. 383).
- Adolescents 12 to 18 years were recruited from a target population of 110,000. "The use of a sample stratified by age allowed for exploration of the potential differences to emerge during adolescent development…" (Passmore, 2004, p. 66).
- The investigators selected five states from various parts of the country based on their geographic location and variety of occupational therapy programs. AOTA member mailing lists were ordered. Faculty members, students, and occupational therapy assistants were eliminated from the mailing lists. The proportion of AOTA members in each state was determined and based on proportions, and the surveys were mailed to randomly selected AOTA members from the five states (Philibert, Snyder, Judd, & Windsor, 2003).

Purposive

- "Participants were identified by their occupational therapist, school psychologist, or special education teacher according to predetermined criteria including having a learning disability as defined by the State of Washington" (Handley-More, Deitz, Billingsley,& Coggins, 2003, p. 141).
- The sample of low-income older adults was purposely selected if they met inclusion criteria of reporting impairments in one or more areas of the Functional Independence Measure motor subscale and indicated a need for environmental modifications to their home to increase performance capacity (Stark, 2004).

Convenience

- The sample was 140 participants who were selected from four groups with different levels of neurological impairment and community participation. There was a limitation in that the levels of education were not equal among the four groups. Education was used and controlled for as a covariate in the statistical analysis to compensate (Goverover & Josman, 2004).
- Participants were recruited through day programs located in one large metropolitan area and postings at two mental health centers. Participants received a small monetary honorarium. Sampling bias may be present since more motivated and socially oriented individuals may have volunteered (Laliberte-Rudman, Hoffman, Scott, & Renwick, 2004).
- Volunteers were recruited by the investigator at the acute psychiatric hospital where she was employed (McNulty & Fisher, 2001).

Snowball or Network

- "All were recruited via word-of-mouth" (Niemeyer, Aronow, & Kasman, 2004, p. 589).
- Use of posters and brochures were used to recruit subjects. "Word of mouth and personal contacts were also used" (Clemson, Manor, & Fitzgerald, 2003, p. 109).
- Participants were recruited from several settings including "a health club, a school employee retirement community, a folk dancing group, a student group, and a military base community" (Dickerson & Fisher, 1997, p. 248).

---

handwriting proficiency in children who received the sensory processing programming to a group of children who did not receive the program. The size of the expected difference in handwriting proficiency between the two groups (the effect) would need to be estimated. Several considerations might enter into this estimate. For instance, the investigator might consider the sensitivity of the measure of handwriting used, any pilot data or previous studies that give an indication of how much change could be expected as a result of the intervention, and how much change might occur naturally in the control group as a result of maturation or learning.

Level of Significance

The level of significance or "alpha" is typically set at .05 in occupational therapy studies. This means that investigators are willing to accept a 5% chance that they will find an effect by chance when there really is no true effect. This is known as a type I error (we mistakenly accept the alternative hypothesis when the null hypothesis is in fact correct and should be accepted). Decreasing alpha (e.g., to .01), decreases the chances of making a Type I error; however, it also decreases the "power" or the chances of rejecting the null when the alternative hypothesis is true. "Power is the probability of rejecting the null hypothesis when the alternative hypothesis is true. Power equals 1 minus the probability of making a Type II error" (Albert & Borkowf, 2002, p. 179).

Calculating Sample Size

Using expected effect size, alpha level, and power, an appropriate sample size can be established. Traditionally, occupational therapy studies use .05 as the alpha level and .80 for statistical power. The following are points that need to be considered in calculating a necessary sample size:

- As the sample size increases, the power increases.
- If variation in outcome decreases, the power increases.
- If variation in outcome increases, the sample size needs to increase,
- The power increases as the effect size increases, and
- If the effect size decreases, the sample size needs to increase.

Researchers often consult with a statistician to perform analyses that determine the right number of subjects based on a power estimate.

Other Factors Affecting Sample Size

In addition to the statistical power analysis, several other factors affect the determination of sample size including subgroup analysis, expected attrition, and reliability of measures (Gall, Borg, & Gall, 1996). In group comparison studies, there is often a need to compare subgroups after the primary analysis is complete. For example, there may be a need to compare right-handers and left-handers within the experimental and control group. If the subgroups do not have enough subjects, the analysis may not yield any significant results. Thus, it is important to plan for any subgroup analysis prior to the start of the study in order to plan for enough subjects.

Selected Examples of Quantitative Studies in Occupational Therapy Illustrating Sample Size Issues

- "The sample size precluded investigators from conducting a factor analysis to further establish validity" (Laliberte-Rudman, Hoffman, Scott, & Renwick, 2004, p. 20).
- With this pilot study's small sample size, the study was able to identify one significant difference in self-care performance between the control and experimental groups. However, "...further research, with a greater number of participants over longer duration, is recommended in order to detect other differences that may exist" (Gange & Hoppes, 2003, p. 218).
- To help determine what sample size was needed for this study, the investigators looked at similar studies and found that two in which a sample size of 20 was needed to achieve a power of .91 at .05 with an effect size around 31. However, in this study, the investigators wanted to compare males and females, thus requiring a larger sample. "Therefore, in order to achieve a power of .80 at .05 with an affect size of .68, a sample size of 56 was needed" (Dudek-Shriber, 2004, p. 511).

Attrition (or subject dropout) is an issue that needs to be considered. Especially for studies that involve considerable time and effort on the part of the subjects, the projected sample size should take into account the possibility of attrition. Finally, if the measure used has a low reliability, the power of tests of statistical significance is decreased and an increase in the number of subjects is justified (Gall, Borg, & Gall, 1996).

Sampling in Qualitative Studies

Morse and Field (1995) identify two principles that guide qualitative sampling:

- Appropriateness, and
- Adequacy.

Appropriateness is the identification of participants who will best inform the researcher about the phenomena under inquiry. In qualitative research, although the sample size is often small, the amount of data can be substantial and expensive to collect. Therefore, research must be efficient and effective (Meadows, 2003). The researcher must interview participants who are in a position to offer the most information.

Since randomization would not serve this end, random selection is not considered an effective sampling strategy for qualitative research. The researcher theoretically should know who would be the best participant based on the needs of the study. Moreover, the *number* of participants or informants is not as important as their amount of exposure to and knowledge of the phenomena to be studied.

Adequacy of the data means that enough data will be available to provide a rich description of the phenomena of interest (Meadows, 2003). The goal is saturation, meaning that after continued interviewing and/or observation, no additional information is gained.

Depending on the study, participants may be obtained from the community or formal or informal groups. Frequently, volunteers are sought to participate and those who usually volunteer tend to be more receptive to the interviewer and readily offer information (Meadows, 2003). However, it is important not to select informants based just on convenience, but on what that person can offer in terms of illuminating a particular concept, experience, or cultural context.

In some organizations or groups, there will be informants who are in key positions or have information that will be more insightful than other individuals in the organization. It is important to identify those key informants and include them as participants. Key informants are selected on the basis of their role, knowledge or insights, and the type of relationship they have with others in the query. However, it can be valuable to also pay attention to the quiet, less verbally expressive individuals (Meadows, 2003). These individuals may have a different perspective and offer insight that would otherwise be ignored.

Douglas (1976) has identified four types of individuals in any setting that are useful to the qualitative researcher:

- The "social gadflies" are the well-liked and lively individuals who mix and talk to everyone in the group,
- The "constant observers" are the individuals who are the longer, well-established members of the group who will freely speak of the details of past events,
- The "everyday philosophers" who think a great deal about the setting, can give insights to what is going on, but who are not as forthcoming, and

- The "marginal people" are the individuals who do not feel like they really belong to the group or feel ambivalent about the group. Because they do not have strong loyalty, they will often talk to outsiders and be able to give valuable insights about the group. Using marginal participants requires caution lest the researcher be seen as aligned with a member whom the others believe to be the least trust worthy.

Most participants can only give part of the picture or have only one perspective on a setting that includes many perspectives. It is therefore critically important to make sure that all perspectives are represented in the collection and verification of the data. Sometimes the researcher does not know who are the best participants. In this case, Morse (1991) recommends that the researcher use secondary selection. This means that the researcher conducts many interviews. If a participant does not have the information that is needed or does not meet the qualities of a good interviewee, the researcher does not use the interview in the analysis. Such data is set aside for possible use in the future if it turns out to have some validity.

A necessary factor in acquiring good participants for qualitative research is the amount of rapport and trust established between the participants and researcher. This element is paramount to the success of the study. If the key participants are not receptive to the researcher or the project, they may give shallow or partial information, not disclose their true feelings, or provide invalid information on the topic.

As with all research studies, the sampling methods are determined by the nature of the study. The fluid nature of the qualitative study process is also reflected in how participants are selected. This process is inductive and dynamic and may change as the study evolves. In fact, it is common for new participants to be sought out as a study progresses.

> Two principles guide qualitative sampling—appropriateness and adequacy.

Unit of Analysis

The unit of analysis for qualitative studies tends to be either people-focused or structure-focused (Patton, 2002). In people-focused studies, the researcher examines individuals and small informal groups such as friends, gangs, or families. Structure-focused units include projects, programs, organizations, or units within organizations (Patton, 2002).

Some of the most common factors that are considered when determining participants for a qualitative study are:

- Culture,
- Geographic or organizational location,
- Time or event-related experience, and
- Personal experience of a unique condition.

One of the most common considerations in qualitative research is the culture of the participants. For example, Bazyk, Stalnaker, Llerena, Ekelman, and Bazyk's (2003) study on use of play with Mayan children; in this study, how culture influenced play was a major concern. Another example is a study of two undocumented immigrants and their child's participation in an early intervention program (Alvarado, 2004). As these two examples illustrate, qualitative studies often focus on individuals who represent unique cultural experiences.

Geographic location or membership in an organizational group can be used to initially define the participants for a study. Ward's (2003) study of the clinical reasoning of occupational therapists working in community mental health is an example of such a study. Other factors leading to sample selection may be time or event-related. For example, qualitative studies often focus on experiences during events such as the Depression, 9/11, or the Vietnam War era (DePoy & Gitlin, 1998; Patton, 2002).

Personal experiences are frequently a focus of qualitative studies, particularly phenomenological studies. Neville-Jan's (2003) study of chronic pain and Kinnealey, Oliver, and Wilbarger's (1995) study of the experience of being an adult with sensory defensiveness are both examples of this type of research focus. In such studies, investigators seek out participants who experience the phenomena under study.

Strategies for Selecting Participants

Selecting participants in qualitative research is always purposeful. That is to say, the researcher strategically determines who would make the best participants. Obviously, the best participants are those who have the knowledge and are willing and able to share the knowledge in enough depth so as to be understandable and useful to the researcher.

Nevertheless, there are specific strategies for selecting informants. One of the most commonly used strategies is maximum variation. Maximum variation involves seeking individuals who have extremely different experiences of the phenomenon being studied. In this strategy, the researcher

is seeking to find the broadest range of experiences, information, and/or perspectives possible. Homogeneous selection is the opposite. In this instance, the investigator seeks informants who have the same experience. The researcher wants to simplify the number of experiences, characteristics, and/or conceptual domains under investigation. This strategy is used for exploring a particular phenomenon in-depth, rather than examining all the variations of which it is an instance.

Theory-based selection is when the researcher selects only individuals who exemplify a particular theoretical construct for the purpose of expanding the current understanding of a theory. This strategy focuses on a particular concept and seeks to explore its meaning in-depth.

Yet another strategy involves finding confirming or disconfirming cases. In this instance, the investigator looks purposefully for the informant who will support or challenge an emerging interpretation. This is a useful strategy in the later stages of the qualitative study, when the researcher begins to feel confident that the data are leading the investigation in a specific direction. Finding informants who can confirm or disconfirm that direction is critical for increasing the confidence of the analysis and expanding the understanding of the phenomenon.

Finally, the researcher can select cases on the criteria that they represent an extreme example of a phenomenon or that they represent the average case. In each of these instances, the design or purpose of the study determines what the most useful strategy is.

Determining the Number of Participants

In qualitative research, there are no standards or set rules for determining the "right" number of subjects or informants. In fact, the number of participants is less important than selecting participants who can ensure richness of information and depth of understanding. In some instances, exploring the experiences of a very few subjects in depth, may be sufficient to thoroughly exhaust a topic. In other instances, an investigator may need to continue selecting participants to gather necessary information on all elements of the question.

In the end, the quality of the data obtained in relation to the study question drives the sampling process. When the researcher wants to explore a phenomenon, explain diversity, or understand variation, then a larger sample is needed (Patton, 2002). Lincoln and Guba (1985) recommend that the appropriate sample size be determined by the information gathered. When no new information

Selected Examples of Qualitative Studies in Occupational Therapy Using Specific Types of Sampling

Purposefully Selected Settings

- The study's aim was to investigate the use of occupation with individuals with life threatening illnesses. A hospice attached to a hospital was selected (Lyons, Orozovic, Davis, & Newman, 2002).
- The study was limited to physical rehabilitation settings because of the variability of occupational therapy settings and physical rehabilitation represents one of the largest areas of practice (Scheirton, Mu, & Lohman, 2003).

Purposefully Selected Participants

- Participants were recruited from local Parkinson's disease support groups. The criteria included individuals who would be able to hear and respond verbally in a face-to-face interview. "Purposive sampling (Lincoln & Guba, 1985) was used to select four participants from the pool of seven people who indicated interest" (Doyle Lyons & Tickle-Degnen, 2003, p. 28).
- "I used purposive sampling to select three children with physical disabilities." (Richardson, 2002, p. 298).

Purposefully Selected Process

- Participants were adults with acute hand injuries who were receiving outpatient therapy. "Usual treatment protocols are followed because the intent is to document the adaptation process as it naturally occurs" (Chan & Spencer, 2004, p. 129).

Maximum Variation

- Participants interviewed were from many different sites, varied in years of experience, and used the income for a variety of purposes. The participant craft workers used a variety of media processes (Dickie, 2003).

Homogenous

- All the participants were Caucasian females who graduated from the same occupational therapy program at the same university (Scheerer, 2003).

Convenience

- The participants were recruited through support groups associated with the local chapters of the National Multiple Sclerosis Society. Interested individuals contacted the study office and were screened to determine eligibility (Finlayson, 2004).

Snowball or Network

- Seven participants were selected from known contacts and an additional participant was suggested by one of the original participants (Egan & Swedersky, 2003).
- Participants were chosen based on their reputation as expert occupational therapists in community mental health as well as their ability to communicate and reflect on their practice (Ward, 2003).

---

on the study question is forthcoming from new subjects, then the "right" number of subjects has been achieved. Patton (2002) recommends that the design specify minimum samples based on the expected description of the phenomena. As with all other aspects of qualitative study, the sample size will need to be flexible, fluid, and subject to change.

Depth Versus Breadth

Before and during the data collection process, a qualitative investigator must be acutely aware of the implications of the participant selection choices and be prepared to define why all participants were selected, interviewed, and/or observed. There is generally a trade-off between breadth and depth. The researcher needs to decide whether to explore specific experiences of a large number of

individuals (seeking breadth) or a greater range of experiences from a smaller number of individuals (depth) (Patton, 2002).

Gaining Access

Gaining access is the entry point into a qualitative inquiry and affects the selection of subjects. Frequently the investigator enters the setting through the gatekeeper or the person in charge of the setting or organization. Winning the trust of the gatekeeper through a straightforward approach or through contacts in the organization impacts the ability to freely select participants.

Domain Analysis

The researcher makes ongoing judgments on who to interview and/or observe based on the unfolding research question(s) and how well the questions are being answered. Usually the researcher starts with broad sampling. As the research progresses, the question (and thus sampling) becomes more focused and narrowed. Domain analysis is the critical process of selecting and adding pieces of information through interview and observation and analyzing it for further discovery. The subject selection process is strategically guided by the aim of achieving rich data for discovery.

Conclusion

This chapter overviewed the process of securing samples in order to do effective research. Issues affecting the selection of subjects include the study question, research approach and design, and pragmatic considerations. The steps to sampling include defining the population through a literature review, considering the unit of analysis, and developing a sampling plan.

In quantitative research the main concern of sampling is whether the sample represents the target population, whether compared groups are equivalent, and whether sample size is large enough to achieve statistically significant results. In qualitative studies, the investigator seeks participants who will best inform the researcher about the topic under inquiry and purposefully samples until the topic is saturated. The number of participants is not as critical as selecting participants who can ensure the richness of information and depth of understanding.

Careful sampling is essential to a rigorous study. Good sampling takes planning, effort, and resources. In the end, it is the foundation for having confidence in the study findings.

REFERENCES

Albert, P. S. & Borkowf, C. B. (2002). An introduction to biostatistics: Randomizations, hypothesis testing, and sample size. In J. Gallin (Ed.), *Principles and practice of clinical research* (pp. 163–185). San Diego: Academic Press.

Alvarado, M.I. (2004). Mucho camino: The experience of two undocumented Mexican mothers participating in their child's early intervention program. *American Journal of Occupational Therapy, 58,* 521–530.

Bazyk, S., Stalnaker, D., Llerena, M., Ekelman, B., & Bazyk, J. (2003). Play in Mayan children. *American Journal of Occupational Therapy, 57,* 273–283.

Belgrave, F. Z., & Walker, S. (1991). Differences in rehabilitation service utilization patterns of African Americans and White Americans with disabilities. In S. Walker, F. Z. Belgrave, R. Nicholls, & K. Turner (Eds.), *Future frontiers in the employment of minority persons with disabilities.* Washington, DC; Howard University Research and Training Center.

Berger, V.W. & Bears, J.D. (2003). When can a clinical trial be called 'randomized'? *Vaccine, 21,* 468–472.

Chan, J., & Spencer, J. (2004). Adaptation to hand injury: An evolving experience. *American Journal of Occupational Therapy, 58,* 128–139.

Chiu, C., & Man, D. (2003). The effect of training older adults with stroke to use home-based assistive devices. *Occupational Therapy Journal of Research, 24,* 113–120.

Clemson, L., Manor, D., & Fitzgerald, M. (2003). Behavioral factors contributing to older adults falling in public places. *Occupational Therapy Journal of Research, 23,* 107–117.

Daly, C. J., Kelley, G. T., & Krauss, A. (2003). Brief report-Relationship between visual-motor integration and handwriting skills of children in kindergarten: A modified replication study. *American Journal of Occupational Therapy, 57,* 459–462.

DePoy, E. & Gitlin, L. N. (1998). *Introduction to research: Understanding applying multiple strategies.* St. Louis: C. V. Mosby.

Dickerson, A. E. & Fisher, A. G. (1997). *Psychology and Aging, 12,* 247–254.

Dickie, V. A. (2003). Establishing worker identity: A study of people in craft work. *American Journal of Occupational Therapy, 57,* 250–261.

Doyle Lyons, K., & Tickle-Degnen, L. (2003). Dramaturgical challenges of Parkinson's disease. *Occupational Therapy Journal of Research, 23,* 27–34.

Douglas, J.D. (1976). *Investigative social research: Individual and team research.* London: SAGE Publications.

Dudek-Shriber, L. (2004). Parent stress in the neonatal intensive care unit and the influence of parent and infant characteristics. *American Journal of Occupational Therapy, 58,* 509–520.

Egan, M., & Swedersky, J. (2003). Spirituality as experienced by occupational therapists in practice. *American Journal of Occupational Therapy, 57,* 525–533.

Finlayson, M. (2004). Concerns about the future among older adults with Multiple Sclerosis. *American Journal of Occupational Therapy, 58,* 54–63.

Gall, M. D., Borg, W. R., & Gall, J. P. (1996). *Educational Research,* (6th ed.). White Plains, NY: Longman.

Gange, D. E., & Hoppes, S. (2003). Brief report—the effects of collaborative goal-focused occupational therapy on self-care skills: A pilot study. *American Journal of Occupational Therapy, 57,* 215–219.

Goverover, Y, & Josman, N. (2004). Everyday problem solving among four groups of individuals with cognitive impairments: Examination of the discriminant validity of the observed tasks of daily living-revised. *Occupational Therapy Journal of Research, 24,* 103–112.

Handley-More, D., Deitz, J., Billingsley, F. F., & Coggins, T. E. (2003). Facilitating written work using computer word processing and word prediction. *American Journal of Occupational Therapy, 57,* 139–151.

Hayunga, E. G., & Pinn, V.W. (2002). NIH policy on the inclusion of women and minorities as subjects in clinical research. In J. Gallin (Ed.), *Principles and practice of clinical research* (pp. 145–160). San Diego: Academic Press.

Kinnealey, M., Oliver, B., & Wilbarger, P. (1995). A phenomenological study of sensory defensiveness in adults. *American Journal of Occupational Therapy, 49,* 444–451.

Kizony, R. & Katz, N. (2002). Relationships between cognitive abilities and the process scale and skills of the assessment of motor and process skills (AMPS) in patients with stroke. *Occupational Therapy Journal of Research, 22,* 82–92.

Laliberte-Rudman, D., Hoffman, L., Scott, E., & Renwick,R. (2004). Quality of life for individuals with schizophrenia: Validating an assessment that addresses client concerns and occupational issues. *Occupational Therapy Journal of Research, 24,*13–21.

Law, M., Baptiste, S., McColl, M. A., Polatajko, H., & Pollock, N. (1998). *Canadian Occupational Performance Measure* (3rd ed.). Ottawa, Ontario: Canadian Association of Occupational Therapists Publications ACE.

Lee, H. C., Lee, A. H., & Cammeron, D. (2003). Validation of driving simulator by measuring the visual attention skill of older adult drivers. *American Journal of Occupational Therapy, 57,* 324–328.

Lincoln, W. S. & Guba, E. G. (1985). *Naturalistic inquiry.* Beverly Hills, CA: SAGE Publications.

Lyons, M., Orozovic, N., Davis, J., & Newman, J. (2002). Doing-being-becoming: Occupational experiences of persons with life-threatening illnesses. *American Journal of Occupational Therapy, 56,* 285–295.

Mathiowetz, V. (2003). Test-retest and convergent validity of the Fatigue Impact Scale for persons with multiple sclerosis. *American Journal of Occupational Therapy, 57,* 463–467.

McNulty, M. C., & Fisher, A. G. (2001). Validity of using the Assessment of Motor and Process Skills to estimate overall home safety in persons with psychiatric conditions. *American Journal of Occupational Therapy, 55,* 649–655.

Meadows, K. A. (2003). So you want to do research? 4: An introduction to quantitative methods. *British Journal of Community Nursing, 8,* 519–526.

Moritsugu, J., & Sue, S. (1983). Minority status as a stressor. In R. D. Felner, L. A. Jason, J. Moritsugu, & S. S. Farber (Eds.), *Preventive psychology: Theory, research, and practice* (pp. 162–174). New York: Pergamon.

Morse, J. M. (1991). Strategies for sampling. In J. D. Morse (Ed.). *Qualitative nursing research: A contemporary dialogue* (rev. ed., pp. 127–145). Newbury Park, CA: SAGE Publications.

Morse, J. & Field, P. (1995). *Qualitative research methods for health professionals.* Thousand Oaks: SAGE Publications.

Neville-Jan, A. (2003). Encounters in a world of pain: An autoenthography. *American Journal of Occupational Therapy, 57,* 88–98.

Niemeyer, L. O., Aronow, H. U., & Kasman, G. S. (2004). Brief report—A pilot study to investigate shoulder muscle fatigue during a sustained isometric wheelchair-propulsion effort using surface EMG. *American Journal of Occupational Therapy, 58,* 587–593.

Passmore, A. (2004). A measure of perceptions of generalized self-efficacy adapted for adolescents. *Occupational Therapy Journal of Research, 24,* 64–71.

Patton, M. Q. (2002). *Qualitative research and evaluation methods.* Thousand Oaks, CA: SAGE Publications.

Philibert, D. B., Snyder, P., Judd, D., & Windsor, M. M. (2003). Practitioners' reading patterns, attitudes, and use of research reported in occupational therapy journals. *American Journal of Occupational Therapy, 57,* 450–458.

Pohl, P., Dunn, W., & Brown, C. (2003). The role of sensory processing in the everyday lives of older adults. *Occupational Therapy Journal of Research, 23,* 99–106.

Portney, L. & Watkins, M. (2000). *Foundations of clinical research: Applications to practice* (2nd ed.). Upper Saddle River, NJ: Prentice-Hall Health.

Reich, J., & Williams, J. (2003). Exploring the properties of habits and routines in daily life. *Occupational Therapy Journal of Research, 23,* 48–55.

Richardson, P. K. (2002). The school as social context: Social interaction patterns of children with physical disabilities. *American Journal of Occupational Therapy, 56,* 296–304.

Scheerer, C. R. (2003). Perceptions of effective professional behavior feedback: Occupational therapy student voices. *American Journal of Occupational Therapy, 57,* 205–214.

Scheirton, L., Mu, K., & Lohman, H. (2003). Occupational therapists' responses to practice errors in physical rehabilitation settings. *American Journal of Occupational Therapy, 57,* 307–314.

Schroeder, P. & Snowe, O. (1994). The politics of women's health. In C. Costello & A. J. Stone (Eds.), *The American woman 1994–95.* New York: W. W. Norton .

Shaffer, R. J., Jacokes, L. E., Cassily, J. F., Greenspan, S. I., Tuchman, R. F., & Stemmer, P. J. (2001). Effect of Interactive Metronome training on children with ADHD. *American Journal of Occupational Therapy, 55,* 155–162.

Smith-Zuzovsky, N., & Exner, C. E. (2004). The effect of seated positioning quality on typical 6- and 7-year old children's object manipulation skills. *American Journal of Occupational Therapy, 58,* 380–388.

Stark, S. (2004). Removing environmental barriers in the homes of older adults with disabilities improves occupational performance. *Occupational Therapy Journal of Research, 24,* 32–39.

Stein, F. & Cutler, S. K. (2000). *Clinical research in occupational therapy* (4th ed.). San Diego: Singular Publishing Group.

Torgerson, D. J. & Roberts, C. (1999). Randomization methods: Concealment. *British Medical Journal, 319,* 375–376.

Trochim, W. M. (2002). *Research methods knowledge base* (2nd ed.). Retrieved May 19, 2005 from http://www. socialresearchmethods.net/kb/external.htm.

Tzonichaki, I. & Kleftara, G. (2002). Paraplegia from spinal cord injury: Self esteem, loneliness, and life satisfaction. *OTJR: Occupation, Participation, and Health, 22,* 96–103.

Ward, J. D. (2003). The nature of clinical reasoning with groups: A phenomenological study of an occupational therapist in community mental health. *American Journal of Occupational Therapy, 57,* 625–634.

Wells, S. A., & Black, R. M. (2000). Cultural competency for health professionals. Rockville, MD: American Occupational Therapy Association.

Zea, M. C.; Quezada, T., & Belgrave F. Z. (1994). Latino cultural value and their role in adjustment to disability. *Journal of Social Behavior and Personality, 9*(2), 185–200.

RESOURCES

Additional Readings Beyond References

Fink, A. (1995). *How to sample in surveys.* Thousand Oaks, CA: SAGE Publications.

Trochim, W. (2000). *The research methods knowledge base (2nd ed.). Cincinnati, OH: Atomic Dog Publishing.*

CHAPTER 32

Collecting Data

Renée R. Taylor • Gary Kielhofner

All research depends on data. Data are pieces of information that have been gathered according to specified rules and procedures to answer questions under investigation in a study (Crotty, 1998; DePoy & Gitlin, 1998; Neuman, 1994; Portney & Watkins, 2000). Answering the research questions requires that information be gathered on the phenomena or variables under study. In the end, the dependability of the research findings are all linked to whether the data collected are reliable and valid.

The purpose of this chapter is to discuss the process of data collection within a research study. It begins with a brief review of how issues of data reliability are approached in the quantitative and qualitative traditions. Then, approaches to data collection are discussed. Next, the steps involved in research data collection are identified and discussed. The chapter concludes with a discussion of professional and ethical issues that involve the treatment of research participants during data collection.

Qualitative and Quantitative Data

Data can be either quantitative (i.e., numeric) or qualitative (e.g., narrative) in nature. How investigators think about and ensure the dependability (i.e., reliability and validity) of data depend on whether the data are being collected within the quantitative and/or qualitative traditions (Neuman, 1994). Each tradition is briefly considered below.

Quantitative Data Collection

Quantitative approaches to data collection are basically concerned with judgments of category or amount (Portney & Watkins, 2000). In quantitative data collection, variables of interest are assigned a numeric value that reflects the category or amount of that variable. Numeric quantities of one variable

can then be examined in isolation or compared to those of other variables.

Levels of Data

As discussed in Chapters 12 and 15, quantitative data can be:

- Nominal or categorical, in which case numeric labels are assigned to designate specific categories of a given variable (e.g., determining whether a research participant belongs to a category pertaining to sex, race, religion, or political affiliation),
- Ordinal, which determines the rank order of a variable (e.g., the rating, 1 = never, 2 = sometimes, 3 = frequently, 4 = always, is a rank order of frequency),
- Interval (also described as continuous), which is characterized by the assignment of numbers along a continuum of less to more of a variable divided into equal intervals,
- Ratio (also described as continuous), which differ from interval data only in that there is a true zero point at which none of what is being measured exists.

Approach to Data Collection

Ordinarily, in quantitative research the same data will be collected from all subjects, or there will be a specific plan for more in-depth data collection depending on subjects' responses or scores from the first phase of data collection. For example, a study may be structured so that only clients who report or demonstrate the presence of a trait will be asked to engage in more in-depth data collection. In quantitative research, investigators will also undertake data collection so as to minimize the amount of missing data, since statistical analyses are most rigorous when there are no or few missing data points.

Quantitative data collection that focuses on human behavior, thought, attitude, or emotions pri-

> In the end, the dependability of the research findings is linked to whether the data collected are reliable and valid.

A Note on Terminology

Considerable differences in terminology are used in the research literature to refer to different approaches and tools for data collection. In this chapter, the term *data collection procedures* is used to refer to any form of data collection regardless of whether it is quantitative or qualitative. When discussing quantitative procedures for data collection, we use the generic term *instruments*, and when referring to more specific kinds of instruments, we use the terms most often associated with them (e.g., questionnaires, checklists, rating scales, measures). When discussing qualitative procedures for data collection we refer to them as strategies. Unlike the quantitative researchers who employ preselected instruments to collect data, qualitative researchers use approaches that are at least in part strategically designed to fit the research context. These strategic approaches are used within qualitative research to generate optimal data given the natural conditions encountered in the setting and to respond to emerging research questions that develop as the research unfolds. It is recognized that qualitative researchers also use tools that may be referred to as instruments. However, for purposes of clarity in this chapter, the term *strategies* is used to refer to all qualitative data collection procedures.

marily uses structured methods of collecting data such as observational rating scales, self-report questionnaires, structured interviews, and standardized tests. Within occupational therapy, quantitative research also involves the use of functional performance data collection procedures (e.g., motor coordination, self-care, driver safety, and work capacity). These data collection procedures ordinarily require equipment or standardized tests for collecting data. Finally, quantitative research also can involve biometric data collection, which ranges from procedures such as measuring the kinematics of movement to imaging techniques that capture brain activity.

Methodological Rigor and Dependability of Quantitative Data

In quantitative research, investigators carefully choose and justify their data collection procedures when planning the research. Researchers either:

• Choose instruments that have previously been developed and investigated, or
• Spend substantial time prior to or in the early stages of the research developing instruments

and refining and documenting the reliability and validity of those instruments.

While it is sometimes necessary to construct instruments for research, a wide array of suitable instruments is increasingly available that had been previously developed and studied.

When it is necessary to create a new instrument for a study, the development of that instrument is, of itself, a substantial research undertaking. Chapters 12 and 13 provide an introduction to the issues and procedures involved in developing and assessing a valid and reliable data collection instrument. Moreover, in many research institutions there are centers or laboratories that provide technical assistance to investigators who need to develop new data collection instruments. Investigators often seek the resources of such entities when developing an instrument.

Concerns with the dependability of quantitative data are centered on reliability and validity (Benson & Schell, 1997). Reliability of data seeks to ensure that the accuracy of information collected was not unduly affected by any extraneous circumstances surrounding data collection. Reliability is typically concerned with how accuracy may be affected by circumstances of data collection (i.e., who collects it, what kind of instrument is used to collect it, and how and when it was collected).

Validity concerns in quantitative data collection basically ask whether the data collected actually represent the variable under study. Empirical assessment of validity focuses on such factors as the extent to which items used to quantify a variable coalesce together and whether the instrument's scores converge with measures of variables that are theoretically related to the variable the instrument intends to measure.

When collecting quantitative data for a study, investigators who wish to ensure the reliability and validity of their data ordinarily:

• Select data collection methods for which there are published reliability and validity findings relevant to the intended study population, and/or
• Test the reliability and validity of the data collection procedure in their own investigation.

There is reason to question the reliability and validity of data collection procedures when:

• There is not sufficient previous research on the reliability and validity of the instrument,
• The sample under study differs from those on which the instrument has been studied,
• An aspect of how the instrument will be used varies from its standard use or how it has been used in previous research, and

• A new data collection procedure has been developed specifically for the study, for which reliability and validity are unknown.

In these cases, investigators will ordinarily:

• Test the reliability and/or validity prior to using an instrument to collect data in the study, or
• Collect data within the study that simultaneously provide evidence pertinent to the reliability or validity of the instrument.

For example, consider a data collection procedure (e.g., administering a self-report measure by telephone) that has been shown to be reliable and valid with an adult sample. An investigator who wishes to use it in a study of adolescents must consider two questions:

• Will the self-report measure provide valid measures for an adolescent sample?
• Does administering the measure by telephone still yield reliable data in an adolescent sample or is there something unique about adolescents that would make telephone administration an unreliable data collection procedure in a given study?

Under these circumstances, an investigator may do a pilot study to investigate:

• Whether adolescents give stable responses (e.g., test–retest reliability), or
• Whether obtained measures correlate with another means of collecting the same information (i.e., concurrent validity).

As the example illustrates, rigor in quantitative data collection emphasizes determining the dependability of data collection procedures before or at the beginning of the research process.

Methodological Rigor and Trustworthiness of Qualitative Data

Within the qualitative tradition, data collection tends to be strategic and emergent (Glaser & Strauss, 1967; Lincoln & Guba, 1985; Pelto & Pelto, 1978; Strauss & Corbin, 1990). That is, the investigator ordinarily begins collecting data with the overall research question in mind and a general plan of data collection. Then, as data are collected and the questions and preliminary findings emerge, the investigator tailors and refines the data collection process accordingly.

Another important influence on data collection is the ongoing discovery of who, when, and where are the best sources of data. Data collection often

proceeds in an iterative fashion going back and forth between analysis and data collection. In this instance, the data collection process is guided by the need for data that elaborates and looks for counter instances of emerging findings.

Qualitative research is basically concerned with understanding and reporting on human behavior and experience while at the same time being faithful to how subjects experience their own behavior. In this instance the concerns for data dependability are whether they faithfully represent circumstances as they are experienced by those under study (Glaser & Strauss, 1967; Lincoln & Guba, 1985; Pelto & Pelto, 1978; Strauss & Corbin, 1990). This is often referred to as the trustworthiness of data. Consequently, the concerns for reliability and validity of qualitative data ordinarily center on:

• Do the data faithfully represent the phenomena as experienced by the participants?
• Do the participants believe that the findings accurately portray their problem, experience, or situation?
• Are the data comprehensive such that all existing perspectives on the given problem, experience, or situation are represented?
• Do the data accurately and completely reflect the problem/experience/situation as it exists within a given environmental context?

These questions are best answered in the unfolding context of the qualitative study. Thus qualitative researchers ordinarily monitor, choose, and modify their data collection strategies as the research process unfolds.

As discussed in Chapter 20, there are a number of ways that qualitative researchers seek to ensure the reliability and validity of qualitative data. These include but are not limited to:

• Engagement over time,
• Reflexivity,
• Triangulation, and
• Member checking.

Most qualitative research involves an extended period of engagement in the field of study. This not only allows the investigator to develop trust with participants but also helps ensure the investigator gains an insider perspective. In addition, prolonged engagement allows the researcher to judge when data collection has saturated a question (i.e., when little or no new information or insights are forthcoming).

Reflexivity is a systematic process of self-reflection that examines insights as well as emotions and reactions to people and events that occur during data collection. In many instances the personal reactions of the researcher also become data. Triangulation means using two or more strategies to collect data on the same phenomena (e.g., combining observation with interviewing). Triangulation can also include using two or more data gatherers who independently collect data on the same phenomenon. Triangulation increases the likelihood that data capture all relevant features of the phenomena under study. Member checking is a process whereby the investigator returns to the study participants to ask whether representations of the data accurately and adequately represent their experience and understanding of the phenomena. It is a means of ensuring that the investigator's data adequately reflect an insider view. Unlike quantitative investigators that seek to ensure the reliability and validity of data collection procedures a priori, qualitative researchers seek to ensure these characteristics of data collection in situ (i.e., as part of the ongoing process of data collection). All of these approaches and others are typically used in qualitative research to ensure the trustworthiness of data. Within a particular study, the combination of approaches for ensuring trustworthiness will depend on the study question, the sample, and other contextual factors.

Approaches to Data Collection

Data can be collected in a wide variety of ways. The most common forms of data collection are:

- Observation,
- Interviews,
- Self-report measures,
- Standardized tests and performance measures,
- Contextual/environmental assessment,
- Focus groups and town hall meetings,
- Biometric measures, and
- Document/records review.

While many of these methods are used in both quantitative and qualitative research, some are more or less exclusively used in one approach or the other.

Observation

Observational approaches to data collection are suited to both qualitative and quantitative studies. When the aim of research is to answer questions related to performance or behavior, observation is frequently the data collection method of choice. Observational data also provide a richer under-

The Importance of Multiple Sources of Data in Research

It is becoming increasingly important to gather data on multiple independent and/or dependent variables and to collect data at multiple time points to enhance the explanatory power of research. For example, a study designed to help clients achieve employment may collect data on work status, activity level, and quality of life over three time points following the intervention in order to demonstrate the broad effects of the intervention and to illustrate that they are sustained over time. Similarly, an intervention designed to improve participants' use of assistive devices to maximize independent functioning might document the individual and combined effects of initial training and ongoing support on improving overall quality of life, job functioning, social contacts, and physical activity level.

Moreover, research increasingly emphasizes the collection of functional, psychological, and social data along with biological data in order to study the interaction of factors across the biopsychosocial continuum. For example, an occupational therapy researcher investigating an intervention to improve feeding behavior in children with severe developmental delays may aim to demonstrate that intervention improves the participants' emotional well-being and nutritional status while reducing family caregiving burden.

standing of an unfolding or ongoing behavior, process, or other situation in real-time. Observation is most straightforward when there is tangible physical evidence, outcomes, or products that can be seen or heard.

In some circumstances, observational methods are used to corroborate data that have been collected through other assessment methods, such as interviews or self-report measures. In other cases, observational methods are used when subjects lack insight or self-evaluation skills or are not able to participate in an interview or provide an accurate self-report (e.g., infants or individuals with severe cognitive limitations).

Observational data collection methods are also useful in providing direct information about a variable under study that is not filtered through the perceptual lens of the person under observation. For example, in occupational therapy, home visits to assess features of an individual's physical environment is a more reliable and valid means of assessing the risk for falls than gathering this information through self-report (Clemson, Fitzgerald, Heard, & Cumming, 1999).

Types of Information Gathered Through Observation

The information typically sought through observation includes:

- Subjects' characteristics or affective states (e.g., whether a person is sad, anxious, agitated, calm),
- Behavior (e.g., what a person does in a given situation, how a person performs a task, level of endurance to activity, or whether a person shows signs of restlessness, inattention, hyperactivity, fatigue, etc.),
- Communication (e.g., what a person says to others, how a person acts toward others, or what a person expresses to others through gestures, facial expressions), and
- Environmental circumstances (e.g., objects and their arrangement in space, social conditions, safety, task demands).

The observer ordinarily watches and/or listens to participants, recording the information. Methods of recording information include:

- Observational guides (i.e., highly structured printed forms or booklets that provide probes or codes for various topic areas and corresponding space to record observations). These can be used for both qualitative and quantitative research.
- Structured checklists (i.e., paper-and-pencil forms used primarily to indicate the presence versus absence or frequency of certain states, behaviors, or communication). These yield categorical data most often used in quantitative research.
- Quantitative rating scales (i.e., forms that assign ordinal numerical scores to a number of items designed to represent the variable under study). The most common is the Likert or Likert-type scale, which uses an ordinal rating technique in which qualitative statements are used to differentiate positions along a continuum (e.g., frequently = 1, sometimes = 2, never = 3).
- Semistructured or unstructured note taking (field notes). This involves taking notes based on broad topics or thematic areas (semistructured) or based on spontaneous observations (unstructured). This approach is most common to qualitative research, although it is used in quantitative research to provide supportive anecdotal data.
- Electronic/digital recording of data: Data can be collected using audiotape or videotape recording. Recording can occur in any stage of the research depending on the aims and nature of the study. For example, recording can be used as an investigator's "third eye" to gather observational data

that involve interaction between the subject(s) and the investigator.

Another advantage of recording is that playbacks can allow the researcher to view the data at any speed and as many times as he or she desires. Thus it is best used in circumstances where the question under study must be rated in a very detailed manner and a given behavior must be slowed down or replayed to ensure that the researcher has observed and understood all aspects of the behavior correctly.

Forms of Observation

There are two widely known types of observation, *passive observation* and *participant observation*. The first and most commonly utilized form of observation in quantitative research is passive observation. Passive observation involves observing subjects and recording data on the variables of interest with little to no interaction with the subjects, in the interest of maintaining objectivity and minimizing any biasing influence on what is being observed.

The second general form of observation is participant observation; it is commonly utilized in qualitative research. When using participant observation, the investigator joins the subjects and participates in the same discussion or activities as the subjects. The aim of the participatory process is for the investigator to gain understanding of the phenomena under study as experienced by the participants (Rice & Ezzy, 1999).

Role of the Observer

In general, the observer's role is to capture certain details about the subject, discern important from unimportant observational data, interpret the observed data accurately and in light of the environmental context, and validate observations over time. In studies that utilize observation, the role of the observer also depends largely on whether the study is quantitative or qualitative. In quantitative research, the aim of the data collection is ordinarily for the observer to:

- Remain as objective as possible in gathering/recording the data to prevent any biases in data interpretation or other personal expectations imposed on the data by the observer.
- Prevent artificiality or other changes in subjects' behavior due to the presence of the observer. In circumstances where the question under study does not involve interaction with the investigator, the investigator is to remain as unobtrusive and

uninvolved as possible so as to avoid contaminating the observational context or influencing the behavior of the subjects. In some cases, this involves observing through a one-way mirror or from a location that is outside of a subject's vision or awareness.

- Take precautionary measures to ensure the reliability and validity involved in recording the data, particularly if the nature of the observation involves subtle changes in behavior, rapidly changing behavior, or some other highly detailed or nuanced aspect of behavior. Precautionary measures include audio taping, videotaping, and/or corroborative rating checks by an independent rater.

In qualitative research, the role of the observer usually involves a sustained level of interaction with participants over an extended period, during which time the researcher(s) become increasingly familiar with the phenomena under study. As previously noted, prolonged involvement allows for building trust with participants and developing a more accurate, insider understanding of the group's perceptions and experience. Alternatively, a qualitative researcher may observe without being a direct participant in or member of the population under study. For example, such investigators may sit in on a weekly support group or they may follow a group of subjects around in the field observing activities and asking questions without engaging in the same activities as the subjects.

In large part, the comfort level of the subjects will depend on the interpersonal skills of the researcher and the research questions under study. The interpersonal skills of researchers may be reflected in the roles they take within the group, the kinds of questions they ask, the tone of voice and body language used, the comments they make in response to obtaining information, and the nature and phrasing of the questions to which they seek answers.

Observational Context

Observation can take place in a number of contexts including:

- Natural contexts,
- Semistructured (e.g., clinical) contexts, and
- Standardized or laboratory contexts.

In its purest form, qualitative research takes place within the natural environment or context in which subjects live and function. Natural contexts may include, but are not limited to, a subject's home, workplace, neighborhood, and/or general community environment (e.g., in a grocery store or on public transportation).

In the field of occupational therapy, observational data are often collected in semistructured settings, such as within an inpatient or outpatient clinical setting. Unlike a subject's natural environment, a semistructured setting introduces the following structures:

- Time (i.e., length of therapy session),
- Space (i.e., size and configuration of the therapy space),
- Objects (i.e., therapeutic equipment, assessment tools, assistive technologies, arts and crafts, and other objects within the clinical setting),
- Sensory variation (i.e., different lighting, sounds, smells), and
- People (i.e., therapists, support staff, administrators, other clients) that are artificial to a subject's natural environment.

Standardized or laboratory contexts offer the highest degree of control over confounding factors. Within occupational therapy research, a standardized context is typically created within a staged or highly structured treatment room in a clinical setting or within a standardized laboratory space. Depending on the research question, any variety of characteristics of these settings can be controlled, including room temperature, lighting, sound, contents, and space configuration. In addition, standardized or laboratory contexts allow use of specialized measurement devices or test situations.

Advantages and Disadvantages of Different Observational Contexts

The primary advantage of collecting data within a natural environment is the ability to gather data that are authentic and ecologically valid. Natural environments do not introduce extraneous variables that might otherwise be imposed by an artificial laboratory or clinical environment. Semistructured and structured settings can raise questions of ecological validity. However, unlike a highly structured laboratory setting, a semistructured clinical context may be construed in such a way as to simulate enough of a subject's natural environment to increase ecological validity. For example, a researcher seeking to answer an observational research question pertaining to environmental impact on attentional problems in persons with schizophrenia might compare the subject's attention within three semistructured clinical contexts that simulate aspects of everyday settings. First the researcher might take the subject into the dining room of the hospital during lunchtime and test the subject's ability to follow a conversation in a highly stimulating environment. Then the researcher might take the subject into the waiting room of the outpatient rehabilitation clinic to test the subject's ability to follow a conversation in a moderately stimulating environment. Finally, the research might test the subject's ability to follow a conversation in a private therapy room.

Distinct from variation that would be inherent in observing subjects in their natural settings, semistructured settings can be applied uniformly across subjects. However, in contrast to a laboratory setting in which even more control can be imposed over the level of environmental stimulation, semistructured environments still introduce certain risks for confounding the research question. The obvious advantage of standardization is that it allows the researcher to control the environment across subjects. The disadvantages include limitations to the generalizability to the subject's natural environment and elicitation of responses to the artificiality of the environment.

In deciding the level of control over observational context, a researcher must consider a number of variables. These include, but are not limited to, the nature of the research question and the vulnerability of the research subjects to the influence of environmental variation on their behavior. Finally, the researcher must consider the feasibility of conducting the observation within different types of environments.

Interviews (Structured and Semistructured)

Interviews typically allow a researcher to collect information that leads to a broader, more holistic, or more integrative view of a subject's impairment or life situation. In occupational therapy research, interviews are most commonly utilized to obtain the following types of information:

• Sociodemographic and sociocultural information about subjects (e.g., age, ethnic identification, educational status, annual income, and extent to which culturally diverse clients identify with and practice health-related beliefs and behaviors that are related to their culture of origin),
• Historical information (e.g., health history, history of events leading up to the impairment),
• Information about a subject's experience of his or her current impairment and its functional consequences (this may include information about a subject's volition, habits, roles, and performance capacity),
• Psychosocial information (e.g., available social support, other resources and coping abilities, available sources of assistance within a subject's social network, sources of stress or conflict within a subject's social network),
• Information about a subject's physical living environment (e.g., safety and accessibility within home, work, and community environments), and
• Employment information (e.g., work history, current work status, work performance issues, need for and access to reasonable accommodation).

Methods of Recording Interview Data

There are three general methods of interviewing:

• Structured interviews,
• Semistructured interviews, and
• Unstructured interviews.

Structured interviews are comprised of a set of preestablished questions that follow strict administration and scoring rules. They are used in quantitative research and mostly gather ordinal and nominal data. In many cases, the scoring of structured interviews follows a very rigid and well-defined set of rules or template. In many instances these interviews ask subjects to select from among responses provided by the interviewer. Questions that ask interviewees to give an open-ended response are generally focused and the interview either records or codes the response using a standard coding scheme. Structured interviews may contain skip patterns within it that tell an interviewer that he or she may skip certain questions based on a subject's responses to prior questions. They also may contain allowable probing questions or explanations that interviewers can use when subjects do not respond accurately or fully or when they do not understand a question.

The high level of structure is designed to minimize interviewer bias. The structured interview also helps eliminate inaccuracies in scoring or subjective interpretation of responses on the part of the interviewer. Other advantages of structured interviews include their ease of administration (particularly for beginning therapists or researchers), their time-limited nature, and their ease in scoring.

Semistructured interviews may be used in quantitative research to generate data that is later coded or categorized. They are also used to generate more narrative accounts for qualitative research. These interviews use a preestablished schedule of open-ended questions, but allow considerable flexibility in how they are administered. Semistructured interviews typically also allow interviewers to tailor questions and probes in order to obtain more in depth and trustworthy information. When administering a semistructured interview, an interviewer may pursue questioning in a related area to obtain a different perspective or to shed light on the subject's responses to the interview questions at hand. Semistructured interviews require a higher level of clinical judgment, interpersonal skill, knowledge, and expertise on the part of the interviewer. Because scoring or coding rules are much less rigid and, in qualitative research not predefined, interviewers must decide:

- Whether a respondent's answer to each item is accurate, detailed, and comprehensive enough,
- What additional information is needed,
- What kinds of questions are required to probe for that information, and
- How to limit tangential or overly lengthy responses.

The advantages of semistructured interviews are that they allow for better rapport-building and more detailed and in-depth understanding of the variables of interest. The disadvantages can include length of administration and greater vulnerability to interviewer bias.

Unstructured interviews are used in qualitative research. These interviews may be guided by only a general topic or short list of topics that the interviewer pursues. Alternatively, the content of the interview may depend on an issue that is raised by a participant or a recent observation. While investigators conducting this type of interview are usually guided by a broad study question, they remain open to new topics that may emerge in the interview itself.

Unstructured interviews have the advantage of being able to discover new information and establish a sense of trust (that the investigator really wants to understand and hear the participant's perspective). They require substantial time, interviewing skill, and contextual knowledge. Since, however, unstructured interviews ordinarily take place as part of an ongoing qualitative study in which the investigator is also a participant observer, they benefit from the background knowledge of the interviewer.

Sources of Interview Data

In every interview, there are three possible sources of data:

- Verbal data provided by the subject/respondent,
- Behavioral data, and
- Proxy verbal data provided by significant others, family, friends, and coworkers.

When interviews are used in occupational therapy, the most common source of interview data is the subject him/herself. During an interview, a subject is required to respond to questions based on some degree of reflection about his or her experience and/or needs. All interviews require subjects to have the ability to reflect honestly upon their impairments and experiences with a reasonable level of accuracy. Depending on the variables of interest in a research study, participating in an interview may require varying degrees of self-awareness or insight.

Depending on the nature of the interview and the variables under study, behavioral information may also be generated during an interview. In some cases, it may be factored into the overall outcome or score of the interview. Nonverbal information may include subjects' behavioral and affective responses to interview questions, their facility in processing auditory information, and communication/interpersonal skills.

In many circumstances, a researcher may wish to obtain information about a subject through reports from significant others, family, friends, or coworkers. Data provided on behalf of a subject by others who are close to the subject may be used to corroborate information provided by a subject or to fill in informational gaps within the subject's self-report. In some cases, it is not possible to obtain self-reported interview information from a subject directly owing to impairment-related issues. Under these circumstances, interview data from proxy sources may be helpful.

Role of the Interviewer

Establishing rapport is fundamental to every interview. Depending on the preferences and reactions of the subject, achieving rapport can be a relatively straightforward process, or it can be rather lengthy and complex. Some individuals will respond well to a brief period of introductions and small talk before an explanation of interview procedures is provided. Others will prefer that the researcher assume a more professional stance and explain the procedures upfront without preliminary chatter. The interviewer's first role is to make his or her best estimate of the interpersonal preferences of any given subject and act accordingly.

Because there is a potential for the researcher to be viewed as an authority figure in any interview situation, it is important to know or predict how the subject might respond given the automatic power differential involved in an interview situation. Some subjects will feel uncomfortable providing difficult or intimate information to a relative stranger. In such circumstances the researcher must do everything possible to ensure confidentiality and to create an atmosphere of unconditional acceptance and positive regard.

Although the role of an interviewer is clear with respect to the nature of the task, the need to establish rapport, and the power differential involved, interviewers can differ in significant ways in terms of their more nuanced behavior and roles. For example, an interviewer's role may vary according to whether the research is quantitative or qualitative. During an interview that seeks to obtain quantitative data, an interviewer may assume a more formal role. The interviewer may ask the subject to select an answer among a limited number of options, set more limits on side conversations, and/or discourage the interviewee from providing unnecessary details or extraneous information when answering open-ended questions. Qualitative interviews require the researcher to assume a less structured role.

Self-Report Measures

Self-report measures are written instruments on which subjects are asked to record information. They typically ask the subject to self-reflect on his or her experience or needs and select the best option from a finite number of categories or to provide an open-ended explanation as a response. Self-report measures are typically self-administered by subjects and responses are usually provided in writing. However, under certain circumstances (e.g., subjects that require accommodations) subjects may provide verbal responses that the researcher records.

When asking for factual information, self-reports may ask a subject to:

- Report demographic characteristics (e.g., age, sex, race),
- Rate the severity or frequency of certain symptoms or impairments (e.g., "I am able to walk a flight of stairs with no pain" never, sometimes, frequently, always),
- Respond to open-ended questions (e.g., what one typically does at a specific time of the day, or what types of difficulties one has performing a given task), or
- Respond to dichotomous questions (e.g., yes–no questions as to whether one can or does perform a given task).

Self-Rating Scales

Some self-reports involve completing self-rating scales. Self-rating scales are used to capture con-

structs such as personality characteristics (e.g., degree of assertiveness in relationships), attitudes (e.g., how much value one attaches to leisure or work), emotional states (whether one is depressed or anxious), and behavior patterns (to what extent exercise is part of an individual's daily routine).

They can also ask an individual to evaluate him- or herself more directly in terms of his or her performance capacity (e.g., how competent one is at performing a task). The most common form of a unidimensional rating scale is the Likert scale. It most frequently uses a five-category ordinal rating technique in which qualitative statements are used to differentiate positions on a continuum. One example of a commonly utilized self-report measure in occupational therapy research that utilizes Likert scaling is the Medical Outcomes Survey Short-Form 36 (SF-36). The eight subscales of this measure each contain Likert scale items that are designed to assess self-reported health-related quality of life and functional impairment. In addition to instruments that utilize Likert scales, another type of self-report instrument is the semantic differential (Polit & Hungler, 1999).

Semantic Differential, Q-Sort, and Visual Analogue Scales

The semantic differential asks the respondent to rate a given concept on a series of bipolar adjectives that are used to characterize one's reaction or feelings (e.g., free versus constrained, dull versus exciting). The Q-sort is a self-report method that encourages respondents to organize data into visual categories (e.g., adjectives written on index cards are sorted into piles). During the Q-sort procedure, respondents are expected to sort the visual data into piles that represent meaningful categories. Visual analogue scales employ a straight line with labels to anchor each end. Subjects are then asked to mark the point on the line that corresponds most closely to their experience. Visual analogue scales typically employ a line that is 100 mm in length so that scoring can be accomplished with use of a standard ruler (Polit & Hungler, 1999). Semantic differentials, Q-sorts, and visual analogue scales are typically used in the assessment of subjective experiences or less tangible phenomena that are sometimes difficult to describe verbally, such as pain or fatigue.

Unstandardized Questionnaires

No data exist on the reliability and validity of unstandardized questionnaires. They are typically created by investigators for their own use in preliminary studies to gather wide-ranging information about a novel variable or to gather information about a novel population. Researchers are more likely to use unstandardized questionnaires when existing measures do not address the variables of interest and a new measure must be generated. For example, an occupational therapy researcher interested in gathering general information about practitioners' attitudes and knowledge about treating a new type of disability in practice might wish to administer a preliminary questionnaire that contains items that assess a broad range of variables.

The benefit of unstandardized questionnaires includes their potential to provide rough preliminary information about a wide range of variables. Because of the need for standardized instruments to contain items that cohere with one another and reflect a general construct or constructs, reliable and valid questionnaires tend to be more limited in their breadth and scope. Despite this, unstandardized questionnaires carry a number of limitations. Generally, their accepted use in research is limited to descriptive studies that are preliminary in nature and aim to report general information about a single sample. They are less frequently used in experimental and clinical outcome studies.

Administration of Self-Reports

The most common method of administration of a self-report measure is to provide individuals with a written form. Forms may be given to a subject to be filled out in the presence of the investigator or to be completed at the respondent's discretion and returned later. In addition, forms may be mailed to individuals for responses. Instructions for completing the form may be given verbally or provided in writing on the form itself. When self-reports are mailed to respondents, the instructions are typically provided in writing.

Increasingly, self-reports are being administered using computer-based technologies. For example, researchers who work with relatively large samples of subjects are increasingly posting and administering self-report measures online via the World Wide Web. An advantage to online administration is that it can be organized so that subjects' responses are automatically downloaded and scored using a data entry and scoring program. Depending on sample size, online administration may save costs that would otherwise be incurred through printing and postage. However, one must weigh the overall cost of the computer software and programming required to develop, post, protect, and manage the survey and the data records of each of the respondents. This approach requires that subjects in the study have computer access

and computer aptitude. There are also a number of considerations regarding the confidentiality and overall security of the data that must be taken into account.

Portable approaches to computer-based administration can be used to gather repeated, self-report measurement. Subjects are typically provided with a handheld personal computer or a small data recording device. They can be programmed to cue (e.g., beep) an individual to provide his or her self-report at various times throughout the day, week, or month. Studies that aim to measure an outcome variable that is subject to change periodically throughout the day typically use this approach. For example, if an investigator wished to measure the effects of overall activity levels on the subjective experience of pain, subjects might be provided with a handheld device that would cue the person periodically (e.g., at fixed or random time points) throughout the day to answer questions about what the subject is currently doing and to rate pain level on a visual analogue scale.

Standardized Tests and Performance Measures

Standardized tests involve contrived cognitive or motor tasks that are administered and scored under strictly standardized conditions and typically generate norm-referenced or criterion-referenced scores. Examples of standardized tests include intelligence and aptitude tests, tests of motor proficiency, and cognitive performance tests. A substantial amount of research goes into developing these tests.

Performance measures commonly involve everyday tasks (although they may be somewhat standardized) that are observed to allow researchers to measure performance in the task. For example, the Assessment of Motor and Process Skills (Fisher, 1993) is used to observe clients in selected activities of daily living (ADLs) and instrumental activities of daily living (IADLs). It measures the quality of an individual's performance (i.e., motor and process skills).

One advantage of standardized tests and performance measures is that they are widely used and widely accepted as rigorous measures of outcomes. Because they are widely used, they facilitate comparison of any investigator's findings from a given study with those of another investigator from a different study. Disadvantages of standardized tests and performance measures are that they are sometimes too general or broad to answer the more detailed questions that a researcher may have. In addition, not all are cross-cultural in nature and may not be relevant to all sociodemographic and sociocultural groups.

Administration of Standardized Tests and Performance Measures

Standardized tests are typically administered under standardized conditions that are consistent with those that were set when the test was initially developed. Depending on the nature of the test, these conditions might involve having a subject sit at a desk within a research office to respond to a written questionnaire or having a subject perform certain behaviors or tasks in a laboratory or clinical area using standard equipment.

Contextual/Environmental Assessment

In occupational therapy, contextual and environmental assessments typically measure aspects of physical, social, educational, or work-related settings in which subjects perform daily life occupations. An example of a contextual assessment that measures the extent to which an individual's physical environment facilitates or thwarts his or her occupational adaptation is The School Setting Interview (Hoffman, Hemmingsson, & Kielhofner, 2005), a semistructured interview that measures the extent to which all of a child's educational environments support engagement and participation in learning activities. Similarly, the Work Environment Impact Scale (WEIS) (Moore-Corner, Kielhofner, & Olson, 1998) is a semistructured interview scale that evaluates features of an individual's work environment as they support or interfere with job functioning.

Occupational therapy researchers who incorporate qualitative strategies may focus on the social and cultural aspects of a subject's occupational context. For example, a researcher interested in the daily routines of homeless individuals with mental illness might observe and document the effects of a number of contextual and environmental variables.

Focus Groups and Town Hall Meetings

A focus group is a group discussion conducted by an investigator who serves as a moderator, guiding the discussion by introducing questions, usually from a written set of questions or topics. Ordinarily, data are recorded in the form of:

• Audiotapes that are then transcribed, and
• Notes taken by the moderator or another investigator whose role is to record information.

Focus groups ordinarily include between 5 and 15 participants; the aim of the group size is to achieve a balance between ensuring that all members have an opportunity to share their views while including enough members to represent the diversity of existing viewpoints (Krueger & Casey, 2000). Focus groups are used to explore people's perceptions and attitudes regarding topics in which the participants have some investment or stake (Bernard, 1994; Krueger & Casey, 2000; Morgan & Spanish, 1984; Nabors, Ramos, & Weist, 2001).

The advantages of focus groups are that data can be collected from several people at once and that the interaction between members can stimulate data that the investigator might not otherwise have gained. One of the main reasons for using focus groups is to obtain the kind of data that emerge when participants interact with and modify each other's responses. One disadvantage is that some persons, especially those with minority opinions, might be discouraged from sharing their views. Therefore the researcher aims to create a milieu that encourages participants to share their perceptions and views without the need for overall group consensus (Krueger & Casey, 2000).

Within a single study, researchers may replicate the focus group with different sets of participants who represent a particular constituency. Replication of focus groups representing a particular constituency can reveal common themes, trends, and patterns (Krueger & Casey, 2000). Investigators will also sometimes conduct different focus groups composed of persons who represent different constituencies in a setting (e.g., a focus group composed of staff and a focus group composed of clients in a healthcare setting). In this instance the focus groups are designed to emphasize differences in the perceptions of different constituencies.

Focus groups are increasingly used as a method of data collection in both qualitative and quantitative research. In quantitative research, focus groups often serve as a first stage of research or as a pilot study to ensure that later data collection procedures will focus on relevant questions, reflect the perspectives, and be understandable to subjects. In qualitative research focus groups can be the only or a primary means of data collection.

Focus groups are increasingly used to develop and evaluate health-related interventions and programs (Heary & Hennessy, 2002; Hildebrandt, 1999). The following is an example. Ivanoff (2002) used focus groups to develop an occupation-based health education program for adults with macular degeneration. Focus groups were conducted to gain an insider perspective on how vision problems affected their daily lives. The focus group revealed both these elders' insecurities regarding their daily occupations and the strategies they employed to be able to perform their occupations. Findings generated from the focus groups informed the development of the intervention. Post-intervention focus groups were used to evaluate the program and to generate ideas for further program development.

Biometry/Physiological Measures

Biometry and physiological measures are objective means of assessing any range of variables that involve physical, biological, or physiological functioning. Examples of biometric measures of physical functioning that are commonly used by occupational therapy researchers include measures of grip strength (e.g., dynamometer), endurance (e.g., how long an individual can sustain a motor movement), and range of motion (e.g., joint range of motion specific to seating). Increasingly, occupational therapy researchers are beginning to conduct interdisciplinary and translational studies in which they collaborate with researchers from other disciplines to measure relationships between occupationally based variables and other biological or physiological variables, such as immune function, physical fitness, and/or cardiovascular functioning.

Document/Records Review

In many cases an important source of research data is preexisting documents or records. In health care, an important source of information is the medical record. Medical records can be used to extract a wide range of information that might be important to a researcher, including, but not limited to:

• Sociodemographic information,
• Medical and psychiatric diagnoses,
• Access to health insurance,
• Number, reason, and nature of contacts with medical care providers,
• Prior treatment plans,
• Treatments prescribed, provided, or recommended, and
• Treatment follow-through and outcomes.

In addition to medical records, qualitative researchers often use a range of documents as sources of data. These may include written communication (memos, notices, letters); artwork; diaries that contain information about daily activities, symptoms, or other information relevant to occupational performance; brochures; policy and procedure documents; educational records; legal records; insurance records; or job performance records maintained by an individual's employer. Within health care, access to historical information of this nature, particularly without direct consent from the subject, is becoming increasingly difficult because of the necessity to protect the confidentiality and rights of the subjects on whom the documentation or records are based.

Planning and Implementing Data Collection

The next section of this chapter reviews three steps generally taken by researchers to plan and implement data collection. These include:

• Selecting instruments and procedures for data collection,
• Developing a data collection plan, and
• Selecting and preparing personnel for data collection.

Each of these steps is discussed in detail below. The feature box titled "A Checklist for Preparing for Data Collection" contains a checklist that can be used by researchers to facilitate self-evaluation of their selected approach to data collection.

Selecting Instruments and Strategies for Data Collection

One of the most important steps in the data collection process involves choosing the appropriate instrument and/or strategy for data collection. This choice has implications for the ease and efficiency of data collection and the quality of the data that are ultimately collected.

Generally, identification of data collection procedures requires careful and sometimes extensive investigation. Some useful strategies are:

• Examining the research literature and attending conference presentations to identify strategies and instruments being used by other investigators in one's topic area.
• Corresponding with other researchers about the state-of-the art strategies and instruments being used in a given topic area. This allows one to have a more extensive dialogue about the strengths, limitations, and receptivity of a given procedure or instrument. It also allows an investigator to ask other researchers about details such as logistical considerations in administration, preferred approaches to scoring, and issues involving the instrument's sensitivity to change.

A Checklist for Preparing for Data Collection

I) Has the appropriate data collection procedure been selected? _____
(Check off only if criteria A–E are endorsed.)

A) Is the information gathered relevant and sufficient to answer the study question? ____

B) Is the data collection approach methodologically rigorous enough to adequately address the study question? ____

C) Have all relevant logistical variables related to the overall study design, available resources, and subject characteristics been accounted for? ____

D) Are norms or other criteria for interpreting the instrument needed and available? ____

E) Is the type of data that the instrument yields appropriate for the study question and will it need to be normalized or transformed? ____

II) Has a data collection plan or protocol been developed? ____
(Check only if all of the following questions have been answered.)

• What data are to be collected?

• Who will obtain the necessary equipment, exam space, and instruments for data collection and by when will they be obtained?

• Who will be collecting which types of data? Who will be administering each of the instruments?

• What training and qualifications will data collectors need and by when will they be expected to have completed this training?

• At what time point in the study will data collection be initiated for each instrument or type of data that will need to be collected?

• What are the deadlines for completion of data collection for each data collection time point, instrument, or procedure?

• How will data be identified and coded for data entry? Who will enter the data, how will it be entered, and by when will it be entered? What program will be used for data entry?

• Who will analyze the data and how will they be analyzed?

• How will data be disseminated? To what audiences?

III) Are the personnel involved in data collection adequately trained and prepared? ____

IV) Have all relevant professional and ethical considerations been met? ____

• Consulting Web-based and published compilations of assessments (see Resources at end of chapter).

When a tradition of research exists on a topic, there are often one or more quantitative instruments that are considered gold standards for collecting data on certain variables. For example, in rehabilitation-related outcome studies of health-related quality of life, the Medical Outcomes Study Short-Form Survey (SF-36) (Ware & Sherbourne, 1992) is frequently the measure of choice, but the Quality of Life Index (Ferrans & Powers, 1992) is an equally valid and reliable instrument that measures somewhat distinct dimensions of health-related quality of life.

Criteria for Selecting Instruments and Strategies

In choosing one instrument or strategy over another, the following considerations have been identified as important in guiding the selection of one's means of data collection (Depoy & Gitlin, 1998):

• Relevance and sufficiency of the information gathered to answer the study question,

• Extent to which the instrument or strategy conforms to standards of methodological rigor,

• Logistical considerations related to the overall study design, available resources, and subject characteristics,

• Availability of norms or criteria for interpreting the information gathered, and

• Type of data the instrument or strategy yields.

Relevance and Sufficiency of Data. In selecting an overall approach to data collection, the first consideration involves whether the approach is relevant to the research question on which the study is based. For example, an observational approach to data collection should be used when one is studying a question that involves a concretely observable phenomenon or behavior. If the research question involves a variable that is highly complex or difficult to observe self-report or interview may be the correct approach. In the case of a complex research question or variable, a self-report approach may be combined with an observational approach to triangulate measurement.

A second important consideration when selecting an approach to data collection is whether the instrument or strategy represents an accurate reflection of the research question. Consider, for example, investigators studying the outcomes of an occupational therapy program designed to improve fine-motor skills in children or one designed to improve communication/interaction skills in adults. These investigators should select sound instruments that specifically measure the dependent variables (i.e., fine motor skills and communication/interaction skills) identified in the research questions.

In addition to these considerations, the way in which an investigator approaches the questions of relevance and sufficiency of data collection approaches depends on the methodology of the study. In quantitative studies, the primary focus of relevance is whether the method of data collection provides accurate data that reflect the variable(s) under investigation and is suitable to the anticipated sample. In qualitative studies, one must ensure that the method of data collection is likely to generate the right kind of data of sufficient quality, quantity, and detail to address the central question under study. As noted earlier, this process of planning the data collection strategy begins when the study is being planned but generally continues through its implementation in qualitative research.

Methodological Rigor. The methodological rigor of data collection depends on whether there is evidence in the literature that a quantitative instrument is valid and reliable or that a qualitative strategy is trustworthy. Researchers should ask themselves four questions in evaluating whether a given instrument or strategy to data collection is indicated.

- What does this evidence say about the reliability and validity of the instrument or about the trustworthiness of a strategy?
- Does research evidence of reliability, validity, or trustworthiness of the instrument/strategy have relevance for the proposed study sample? Are there any reasons to expect this sample may respond differently to the procedure than those with which the procedure has been studied?
- If there is not sufficient evidence for dependability of the procedure with the proposed study sample, then is there some precedent in the literature for successful use of the instrument or strategy with the proposed study population?
- Are there any logistical aspects of the study that would preclude recommended administration of an instrument or strategy?

One should examine what strategies or instruments have been successfully used by other researchers studying the same or similar research questions or populations. Consideration should be given to what strategies or instruments are most likely to give reliable and valid data given the particular phenomena to be studied and who the study participants will be. Sometimes preliminary pilot testing of strategies or instruments can give useful information about what are likely to be the best data collection strategies in a given context.

Logistical Considerations. In selecting appropriate instruments and strategies for data collection, researchers must also consider logistical elements of the study. The first logistical consideration is what the planned strategies and/or instruments require of participants in terms of their mental and physical performance capacity, personal time, and level of effort. One should also consider the impact of any strategies or instruments on their health and well-being. Participants should be asked to do only what is within their capacity and absolutely necessary to obtain necessary data. For ethical reasons, any inconvenience, stress, or risk involved in data collection must be clearly outweighed by the importance of the research question.

A second logistical consideration involves the resources that a given data collection procedure would require. Human resources (i.e., time and effort of the investigator or other study personnel) required by data collection procedures is the first major resource that must be considered. The anticipated number and length of different collection instruments or strategies should be examined in light of sample constraints (e.g., the schedules, locations, and availability of participants).

Economic resources are also important when selecting an appropriate data collection procedure. Considerations include the level of education or specialized training data collectors need since they have salary and cost implications. Moreover, the availability or cost of instruments, test kits and forms, scoring and data management and analysis software packages, necessary space, computers, telephones, and other equipment should be considered. If a study will involve data collection within the field, transportation resources and costs must also be considered.

A final logistical consideration in data collection involves the appropriateness of the data collection procedures for any unique characteristics of the sample and the subject burden posed by the data collection procedures. A particular concern in occupational therapy research is whether the intended participants have impairments that affect their ability to participate in any of the data collection methods to be utilized in the study. In some cases, the investigator may resolve this issue by removing barriers (e.g., providing a sign language interpreter or a written instrument in interview format, on audiotape, or in Braille). In other cases the investigator will select a data collection method that does not require skills affected by the impairment.

Subject burden refers to the effort, inconvenience, pain, risk, and other factors that affect what will be required for or may be a consequence of data collection procedures. Subject burden increases with the time involved in data collection, the number of data collection instruments utilized, and the negative effects of any data collection procedure on a participant's emotional or physical well-being.

If subject burden is unduly high in a study, it will lead to low participation rates and high dropout rates. In turn, this will limit sample size and introduce sampling bias, which limits the degree to which the sample is representative of all individuals in the population under study. Researchers must constantly balance the need to obtain adequate, detailed, and comprehensive information against human and other costs involved in actually obtaining that information.

Availability of Norms or Criteria for Interpretation. A consideration in selecting an appropriate quantitative instrument for data collection involves whether norm-referenced scores are available for a given instrument. For many research questions, the availability of norms for a particular instrument may not be required. For example, if a researcher wishes to examine attitudes among occupational therapists regarding the importance of therapeutic use of self to occupational therapy outcomes, he or she does not need to utilize an instrument with norm-referenced scores. Alternatively, if the same researcher wishes to examine the extent of impairment in physical functioning among adults with cardiovascular disease over time, he or she may wish to compare subjects' baseline physical functioning scores against the instrument's available norms for individuals with cardiovascular disease on the physical functioning domain. This would yield added information about the comparability of the baseline physical functioning of the sample against national norms. If physical functioning findings are comparable, findings from the researcher's study are more likely to have greater generalizability to the larger population of individuals with cardiovascular disease.

In other instances investigators may wish to use instruments that are criterion referenced. As discussed in Chapters 12 and 13, there are different approaches to criterion referencing. In some cases there will be cutoff points assigned to scores that may indicate the presence of a problem or the point beyond which a person will be incapable of some criterion (e.g., independent living). Instruments based on item response theory have built-in criteria as the items serve to represent a hierarchy of capacities, skills, attributes, etc. For example, the Volitional Questionnaire (de las Heras, Geist, Kielhofner, & Li, 2003) measures motivation for occupation and it can indicate the level of motivation as indexed by items that range from low to high motivation. A person at a basic exploratory level shows interest but does not seek out challenges. The highest level of interest would be labeled achievement motivation behavior. A person's score on this instrument indicates, then, which of the items on the instrument are below and which are above the person's level of motivation. This kind of criterion referencing is very helpful in interpreting a score.

In qualitative research, norms and criterion referencing are not specific considerations. However, investigators will be interested to know what information has been generated on the phenomena under study so that the data that emerge from their data collection strategies can be assessed in terms of whether it is new information or contradicts or confirms previously reported findings.

Type of Data the Instrument Yields. The final consideration in selecting an approach to data collection involves examining the type of data that an instrument or strategy yields. By definition, quantitative instruments yield numeric data and qualitative instruments typically yield written descriptive data that can later be coded or otherwise categorized. In quantitative studies, researchers need to consider whether the type of numeric output is sufficient for the kinds of analyses that will be needed to answer the research question (e.g., scale of measurement, sensitivity of the instrument so that its scores will detect change). Quantitative researchers also need to consider whether the type of numeric output yielded by a given instrument will require transformation to make it consistent with the numeric output yielded by other instruments used in the study.

Qualitative investigators will be concerned with whether strategies are likely to provide comprehensive data that will lead to saturation. For example, if an investigator is interested in how children experience certain types of sensory problems, observation alone would likely be insufficient to answer the question. Thus, interviews with the children would also be required. Moreover, since children may not be as articulate as desired in discussing the details of experience, the investigator might want to video the child, select certain scenes to view with the child, and then discuss in order to obtain richer data. Or, the researcher may decide to do interviewing as the child is engaged in motor behavior to discuss the experience as it occurs.

Developing a Data Collection Plan or Protocol

After evaluating all of the considerations involved in selecting the appropriate procedures and instruments for data collection, a researcher must develop a data collection plan or protocol. This can often be incorporated into an overall study timeline. This plan should answer the following questions:

- What data are to be collected?
- Who will obtain the necessary equipment, exam space, and instruments for data collection and by when will they be obtained?
- Who will be collecting which types of data? Who will be administering each of the instruments?
- What training and qualifications will data collectors need and by when will they be expected to have completed this training?
- At what time point in the study will data collection be initiated for each instrument or type of data that will need to be collected?
- What are the deadlines for completion of data collection for each data collection time point, instrument, or procedure?
- How will data be identified and coded for data entry? Who will enter the data, how will it be entered, and by when will it be entered? What program will be used for data entry?
- Who will analyze the data and how will it be analyzed?
- How will data be disseminated? To what audiences?

To the greatest extent possible, all of these questions should be answered prior to initiating data collection. In qualitative research, the data collection plan typically evolves with the study. Nonetheless, it is equally important to begin with a clear initial plan for data collection. Then, the investigator or research team should periodically revisit and revise the plan of data collection. This may entail decisions about where to seek data, what type of data to seek, and from whom. It may also involve multiple revisions of semistructured interviews, observational guides or checklists, and other instruments that are commonly used in qualitative research.

Selecting and Preparing Personnel for Data Collection

In selecting and preparing personnel for data collection, a number of considerations need to be taken into account. For example, in some studies the quality of data collection is higher when data collectors share as many characteristics in common with study participants as possible. Depending on the research question and the degree of interpersonal interaction required in a given study, similarities in language, age, racial or ethnic background, and disability status can facilitate rapport and trust during data collection procedures. Other characteristics that will enhance data collection are good clinical judgment, interpersonal skills, observational skills, and the ability to grasp and understand the theoretical foundations for the data collection procedures.

In addition to these more fundamental qualities, data collectors should have adequate training and experience required for the data collection procedure. This may include generic training and more specialized training associated with the particular procedure. In most instances study-specific training and ongoing supervision of data collectors will be necessary. These measures help ensure that the particular approach to data collection is fully understood and implemented correctly. They also are useful to ensure that data collectors can relate well with the study population.

Professional and Ethical Considerations in Data Collection

Professional and ethical considerations ensure the safe and humane treatment of research participants. In addition to the required steps for obtaining ethical approval and complying with ethical procedures (e.g., informed consent and risk management), researchers need to take special precautions to limit subject burden. Although most institutions out of which research is conducted have internal review boards that ensure appropriate treatment of research participants, a number of more subtle issues must be considered during data collection.

Before beginning any data collection procedure, adequate rapport with subjects must be established. It is also the data collector's responsibility to maintain rapport throughout the procedure to the extent that it does not distract the participant or interfere with or confound the quality and effi-

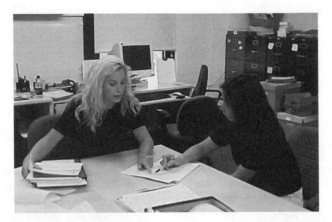

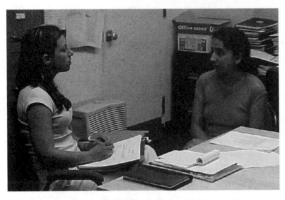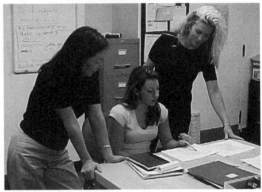

Figure 32.1 Dr. Taylor (top picture, left) and her research team make sure data collection procedures and responsibilities are well defined before initiating data collection.

ciency of the data collection procedures. Rapport can be maintained during data collection by responding humanely and empathically to any uncomfortable circumstances or difficult disclosures made by the subject during data collection. Empathic responding involves:

• Naming, witnessing, and/or verbally acknowledging a difficult circumstance,
• Questioning the participant about his or her emotional or physical well-being, and
• Following through with any necessary actions to ensure the participant's safety and/or physical and emotional well-being.

Maintaining professional boundaries during data collection is equally important for the protection of research subjects. This means that researchers should avoid nonprofessional relationships with participants. Researchers should avoid unplanned disclosure of highly personal information to participants, and they should not accept personal gifts or money from participants. Researchers must ensure that participants are clear in

their understanding of the limits to the researcher's role and availability in their care.

Conclusion

This chapter reviewed the process of data collection. It began with an overview of how data collection is viewed and approached within the quantitative and qualitative methodological traditions. It defined and evaluated a wide range of procedures and approaches used for data collection within these traditions. This was followed by a review of the three steps involved in the actual implementation of data collection within an investigation. We concluded with a discussion of professional and ethical issues that involve the treatment of research participants during data collection. While this chapter overviewed the major considerations involved in selecting and using data collection procedures, readers who are planning data collection for a study should also refer to other chapters in the text that discuss qualitative data collection and quantitative instruments in more detail.

REFERENCES

Benson, J., & Schell, B. A. (1997). Measurement Theory: Application to Occupational and Physical Therapy. In J. Van Deusen & D. Brunt (Eds.), *Assessment in occupational therapy and physical therapy* (pp. 3–24). Philadelphia, PA: W. B. Saunders.

Bernard, H. R. (1994). *Research methods in anthropology: Qualitative and quantitative approaches*. Thousand Oaks, CA: SAGE Publications.

Clemson, L., Fitzgerald, M. H., Heard, R., & Cumming, R. G. (1999). Inter-rater reliability of a home fall hazards assessment tool. *Occupational Therapy Journal of Research, 19*, 83–100.

Crotty, M. (1998). *The foundations of social research: Meaning and perspective in the research process*. Crows Nest, Australia: Allen & Unwin.

de las Heras, C. G., Geist, R., Kielhofner, G., & Li, Y. (2003). *The Volitional Questionnaire*. Chicago, Illinois: University of Illinois at Chicago.

DePoy, E., & Gitlin, L. N. (1998). *Introduction to research: Understanding and applying multiple strategies* (2nd ed.). St. Louis: C. V. Mosby.

Ferrans, C. E., & Powers, M. J. (1992). Psychometric assessment of the Quality of Life Index. *Research in Nursing and Health, 15*, 29–38.

Fisher, A. G. (1993). The assessment if IADL motor skills: An application of many faceted Rasch analysis. *American Journal of Occupational Therapy, 47*, 319–329.

Glaser, B., & Strauss, A. (1967). *The discovery of grounded theory*. New York: Aldine.

Heary, C. M., & Hennessy, E. (2002). The use of focus group interviews in pediatric health care research. *Journal of Pediatric Psychology, 27* (1), 47–57.

Hildebrandt, E. (1999). Focus groups and vulnerable populations: Insights into client strengths and needs in complex community health care environments. *Nursing and Health Care Perspectives, 20* (5), 256–259.

Hoffman, O. R., Hemmingsson, H., & Kielhofner, G. (2005). The School Setting Interview (Version 3.0). Nacka, Sweden: The Swedish Association of Occupational Therapists

Ivanoff, S. D. (2002). Focus group discussions as a tool for developing a health education programme for elderly persons with visual impairment. *Scandinavian Journal of Occupational Therapy, 9* (1), 3–9.

Krueger, R. A., & Casey, M. A. (2000). *Focus groups: A practical guide for applied research* (3rd ed.). Thousand Oaks: SAGE Publications.

Lincoln, Y. S., & Guba, E. G. (1985). *Naturalistic inquiry*. California: SAGE Publications.

Moore-Corner, R. A., Kielhofner, G., & Olson, L. (1998). *Work Environment Impact Scale*. Model of Human Occupation Clearinghouse. Chicago: Department of Occupational Therapy, College of Applied Health Sciences, University of Illinois at Chicago.

Morgan, D. L., & Spanish, M. T. (1984). Focus groups: A new tool for qualitative research. *Qualitative Sociology, 7*, 253–270.

Nabors, L. A., Ramos, V., & Weist, M. D. (2001). Use of focus groups as a tool for evaluating programs for children and families. *Journal of Educational and Psychological Consultation, 12* (3), 243–256.

Neuman, W. L. (1994). *Social research methods: Qualitative and quantitative approaches*. Needham Heights, MA: Allyn and Bacon.

Pelto, P., & Pelto, G. (1978). *Anthropological research: The structure of inquiry*. New York: Cambridge University Press.

Polit, D. F., & Hungler, B. P. (1999). *Nursing research: Principles and methods*. Philadelphia: Lippincott.

Portney, L. G., & Watkins, M. P. (2000). *Foundations of clinical research: Applications to practice* (2nd ed.). Upper Saddle River, NJ: Prentice-Hall.

Rice, P. L., & Ezzy, D. (1999). *Qualitative research methods, a health focus*. Melbourne: Oxford University Press.

Strauss, A., & Corbin, J. (1990). *Basics of qualitative research*. California: SAGE Publications.

Ware, J. J., & Sherbourne, C. D. (1992). The MOS 36-item short-form health survey (SF-36). Conceptual framework and item selection. *Medical Care, 30*, 473–483.

RESOURCES

There are useful publications that identify and review occupational therapy and related instruments for data collection. The following are two examples:

* Law, M., Baum, C. & Dunn, W (2001) *Measuring occupational performance*. Thoroughfare, NJ: Slack. This book covers a wide range of measures that capture data on such aspects of occupational performance as play, work, activities of daily living, occupational role, and time use. There is also a discussion of qualitative procedures for obtaining data on occupational performance. This text includes information about studies of reliability and validity. Readers should be careful to search for additional publications beyond the publication date of this text.
* *Buros mental measurements yearbook*, published by the Buros Institute of Mental Measurements, the University of Nebraska-Lincoln, provides descriptive information, references, and critical reviews of tests in the areas of personality, achievement, behavior assessment, education, and science.

There are also useful Web sites for identifying instruments and research on their reliability and validity.

* One such occupational therapy sight is located at: moho.uic.edu. It contains information on a number of instruments related to the Model of Human Occupation. Visitors to the site can learn about the available instruments, view copies of forms, and use a search engine to identify publications on reliability and validity.
* Health and Psychosocial Instruments (HAPI) is a searchable online database that contains research on published and unpublished information-gathering tools that are utilized in health and psychosocial research studies. Information on questionnaires, interview schedules, tests, checklists, rating and other scales, coding schemes, and projective techniques is available from 1985 onward. The database pertains to any medical or medically related condition or treatment outcome. It contains citations to actual test documents, bibliographic citations to journal articles that contain information about specific instruments, and a catalog of commercial test publishers and their available test instruments.

CHAPTER 33

Data Management

Marcia Finlayson • **Toni Van Denend**

The ultimate goal of any research is to produce findings that others can trust and use. This goal is the same regardless of whether the study is quantitative, and the findings will be judged on their reliability, validity, objectivity, and generalizability, or whether the study is qualitative, and the findings will be judged on their dependability, credibility, neutrality, and transferability (Krefting, 1991). Occupational therapy researchers should always strive to do rigorous work that will contribute to the advancement of our theories and clinical practices (Kielhofner, Hammel, Finlayson, Helfrich, & Taylor, 2004).

Earlier chapters discussed many different factors that can threaten the quality of the research. Unfortunately, even the best designed study can fail if the research team does not plan for and address issues of data management. Despite many publications and the wealth of knowledge about how integral data management is to rigorous investigation, its importance is still sometimes underestimated. Many researchers learn about data management by watching their mentors, talking to other researchers, picking up ideas at conferences, and learning from their own mistakes.

The chapter provides a framework for thinking about and planning data management processes and infrastructure. We also share some of our own experiences from investigations that we have planned and implemented, and provide tools and resources that can be used and modified for other studies.

Basic Definitions

For the purposes of this chapter, data management is defined as the logistical, reflective, and behind-the-scenes processes and infrastructure that allow a researcher to:

• Produce high-quality information to address the study questions, and
• Describe how and what has been done during a study accurately and comprehensively.

In the context of data management, data refer to all of the pieces of information that are collected from research participants to address a study's questions, as well as all of the information that is gathered to monitor and manage study progress. A few examples of this latter type of information include:

• Recruitment processes and outcomes,
• Progress on data collection, coding, entry and cleaning,
• Status of data storage and security, and
• Documentation of decisions that will make it easier for the investigator to describe what he or she has done during the course of the study when it is time to disseminate the study findings.

For simplicity and clarity, the term *data* is used to refer to the information collected from participants, and *project information* is used to refer to the other types of information that a data management system must track.

> In the context of data management, data refer to all of the pieces of information that are collected from research participants to address a study's questions, as well as all of the information that is gathered to monitor and manage study progress.

The Context of Data Management

To begin, it is important to understand the overall context of data management and how it fits within the research process. Figure 33.1 depicts the relationship between data management and research design, and illustrates that the ultimate goal of data management is to support the production of findings that are trustworthy and are useful to others. The figure also illustrates that data management is done in conjunction with design. In other words, designs that are truly rigorous must include planning for data management as part of the process, and strong data management systems must take into account the research design (McFadden, LoPresti, Bailey, Clarke, & Wilkins, 1995). These two processes are inseparable in the production of good quality data (Nyiendo, Attwood, Llyod, Ganger, & Haas, 2002).

Finally, the figure emphasizes that good quality data does not automatically mean trustworthy findings that others can use. Selecting the correct analytic techniques for the data that are available, and using these techniques appropriately will determine the value of a study's findings. Using techniques appropriately means that a researcher must understand the type of data needed for a given analytic strategy, understand the assumptions of the technique and how these can be determined, and interpret results correctly.

> The ultimate goal of data management is to support the production of findings that are trustworthy and are useful to others.

- How and where information about new recruits is to be documented, and
- How calculations on response rates are to be summarized.

Documenting the steps and processes of a project makes it easier for all parties involved to be consistent during the course of a research study, regardless of the project's size or the type of research being conducted (e.g., ethnographic, experimental, survey, etc.) (Antonakos, Miller, & Caruso, 2002; Gassman, Owen, Kuntz, Martin, & Amoroso, 1995).

Using consistent processes and procedures throughout a project will reduce the likelihood of making errors in the course of data collection and/or its entry into analytic software systems. Minimizing errors at the beginning and throughout a study will reduce problems later in the process that could negatively influence the speed or accuracy of data analysis, limit the types of analyses that are possible, or increase the challenges of preparing the research report (Hosking, Newhouse,

Importance of Data Management

The larger the project, the more sophisticated the data management plan will be, but all investigators need to plan for and implement a basic system, regardless of the size of their study. The reasons data management is important are summarized in the feature box on the next page and explained in Figure 33.2.

At the most basic level, a data management plan will facilitate and support communication about the research study across members of a project team, as well as between the team and external parties (e.g., participants, funders, colleagues, editors). The plan will offer guidance about how to carry out and document all research-related procedures and their consequences. For example, a data management plan should identify:

- Which members of the research team are responsible for identifying and contacting potential participants,
- What forms are to be used in this process,

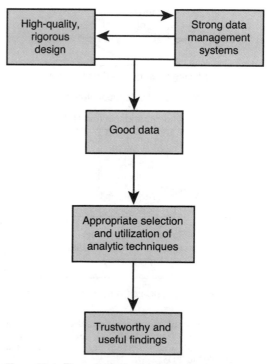

Figure 33.1 The context of data management.

Data Management is important for:

- Supporting a culture of consistent communication,
- Minimizing data collection and entry errors,
- Facilitating data analysis and interpretation of findings,
- Maximizing data quality by promoting internal validity (credibility) and reliability (dependability) of data,
- Ensuring data security and confidentiality,
- Ensuring compliance with relevant laws,
- Facilitating the preparation of the research report, including the identification of study strengths and limitations, and
- Facilitating data archiving and sharing.

Bagniewska, & Hawkins, 1995; Pogash, Boehmer, Forand, Dyer, & Kunselman, 2001). For example, one of the data management processes used in the *Aging with MS: Unmet Needs in the Great Lakes Region Study*[1] was a regular team meeting to dis-

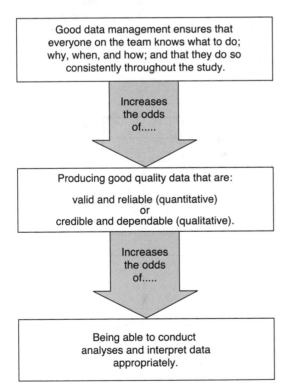

Figure 33.2 Importance of data management.

cuss problems encountered in coding unusual participant responses. During these meetings, the interviewing team and principal investigator discussed the problem, made a coding decision, and then documented that decision for inclusion in the policy and procedure manual. In this way, everyone on the team had access to the decision, and was able to code the data in a consistent way if and when the problem occurred again. Without this process it is likely that unusual responses would not have been consistently coded and would have caused problems later in the analysis phase.

Documentation of policies (rules) and procedures (explanations about how to implement the rules) is a major aspect of a data management plan (Gassman et al., 1995). Documentation for a study should explain:

- How to track what member of the research team has collected what data from which participants,
- When the data were collected,
- If any additional information needs to be collected,
- What the status of the data currently is (e.g., entered or not, where), and
- What data are missing and why (Antonakos et al., 2002).

By having all of this information at hand, a data management system facilitates the preparation of a comprehensive and detailed methods section of research and technical reports, as well as other forms of dissemination (see Chapter 34). Methods that are well documented will be transparent and therefore will be viewed as supporting the internal validity (credibility) and reliability (dependability) of the study.

A strong data management system also ensures that a research team is able to maintain the security of the data collected from participants and demonstrate that guidelines for the protection of human subjects have been followed. It also ensures that the research is in compliance with any other laws that are relevant to the conduct of the research (e.g., Health Insurance Portability and Accountability Act[2] (HIPAA), professional licensing when delivering an intervention, etc.) (Hosking et al., 1995; McFadden et al., 1995). It is important to remember that the human subjects committee that approves a study is free to audit the research for compliance at any time. Failing to follow regulations regarding human subjects or other relevant

---

[1]This project is based on a contract awarded to Dr. Marcia Finlayson by the National Multiple Sclerosis Society through a Health Care Delivery and Policy Research Contract, 2002 to 2005.

[2]HIPAA is specific to the United States, but other countries and jurisdictions have similar laws. The focus of HIPAA is on the protection of personal health information.

guidelines or laws could result in a project being closed.

Finally, data management will facilitate study and data archiving that will, in turn, make it easier for a research team to:

• Compare its findings to other similar studies,
• Provide data to students for thesis or dissertation work based on secondary analyses, and
• Share data with other researchers who seek to build on the work that has already occurred.

Being able to explain to others what was done, and how and why will facilitate later data analyses by members of the team or others who have an interest in the topic.

Failing to address data management in a comprehensive, methodical, and consistent way will result in inconsistencies within and across staff or over time, limit the quality or detail of the methods description in a published article, jeopardize data quality and confidentiality, or even worse, raise questions about the internal validity or credibility of an entire study. Consequently, data management needs to be included during the initial proposal preparation stages of any research study (see Figure 33.1). The system needs to be updated as the project evolves so that new issues are addressed and new decisions are documented.

It should be clear at this point that developing a strong data management system involves more than just recording participants' responses to the study questions and measures. It is an administrative process that supports rigorous research and involves:

• Documenting how all forms of data and project information will be collected, handled, stored, and prepared for use,
• Developing tools and systems to operationalize the documentation, and
• Following through on the use of these tools and systems, refining and adding to them as the project evolves over time.

Components of Data Management

Translating the knowledge of why data and project information should be tracked to the actual creation of a data management system is often not that straightforward. The process can be significantly complicated by the breadth and depth of what must be monitored, and will clearly be influenced by the size and scope of the research project,

the number of staff involved, and the presence of more than one research site (Gassman et al., 1995; McFadden et al., 1995). Therefore, it can be helpful to think about the components or parts of a data management system when beginning the process.

Figure 33.3 illustrates that a strong data management system, including both participant data and project information, includes processes and infrastructure related to staff, and a clearly defined set of policies and procedures. Furthermore, these components are premised on a foundation of a culture of consistent communication. In the context of data management, consistent communication includes (Gassman et al., 1995; McFadden et al., 1995):

• Verbal and written communication *among* members of the team (e.g., principal investigator, co-investigators, research assistants, analysts) via team meetings, e-mails, memos, etc., and
• Documentation of individual work and decisions (e.g., maintenance of study notebooks, lab books).

Written documentation enables the team and others (e.g., funders, collaborators, people using the data for secondary analyses) to track decisions about different aspects of the project easily, and to clearly understand the logic behind these decisions. As a project unfolds, documentation will facilitate consistency in how data management problems are resolved (e.g., coding unusual participant responses) (Gassman et al., 1995).

Ultimately, without consistent communication, any data management system is at risk of crumbling and therefore compromising both the quality of the data produced, and the ability to support the production of trustworthy and useful findings.

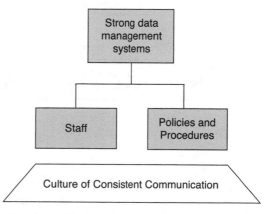

Figure 33.3 Key components of a data management system.

Later sections of this chapter elaborate on some of the specific tools and strategies that can be used to support the production of good quality data. We will also point out specific strategies that promote consistent communication.

To summarize this discussion on the components of data management, it is important to think of a data management system as both a product as well as a dynamic process. When done well, it is the infrastructure that allows the research study to be carried out as planned. When there are problems with data management, even the best designed and funded study can fail to address its intended objectives.

Data Management Issues to Consider and When to Consider Them

Before discussing some of the specific tools that can facilitate data management, we will identify a number of issues that need to be considered when developing a data management system. We have already alluded to some of these issues in our discussions of the importance and components of data management, for example, specifying the roles and responsibilities of team members, documenting activities, tracking respondents, etc. To highlight key issues we have taken Figure 33.3 and expanded it in Figure 33.4.

This figure illustrates the different types of issues that an investigator needs to consider under both the staff component (e.g., selection of team members) and the policies and procedures component (e.g., data access and security, documentation) of the data management system. Clearly, this figure is not all-inclusive, given the variability across projects, research designs, populations being studied, and the size of different studies. Nevertheless, experience suggests that addressing each of the seven issues included in Figure 33.4 is key to increasing the likelihood of high-quality data management.

The specific tasks that need to be completed to address each of the data management issues identified in Figure 33.4 are outlined in Table 33.1. In addition, the importance of doing each of these tasks and when to do them is provided in Table 33.1. A quick scan of the final column of Table 33.1 shows that most of the issues for data management need to be considered during the initial proposal development. This timing is critical because human and financial resources are often required to manage data and project information

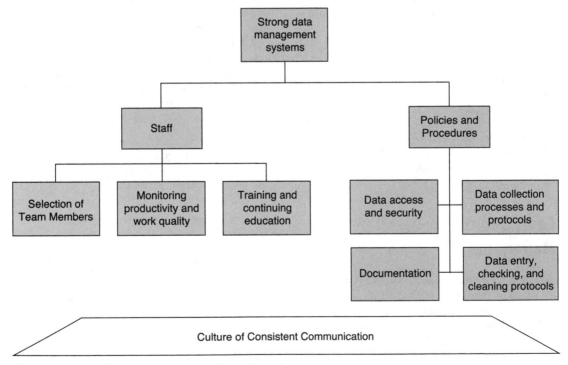

Figure 33.4 Specific issues to be considered in a data management system.

Table 33.1 Data Management Issues, Tasks, Importance, and Timing

Issues to Consider (from Figure 33.4)	Specific Tasks	Importance	Timing
	• Determine what skills are needed across the members of the team (e.g., administering specific assessments, delivering interventions, creating data files, entering data, conducting analyses). • Determine the qualifications of individuals who can fulfill these skill requirements.	• Ensures all aspects of project are being addressed across the members of the team. • Enables the principal investigator to put together a team that can meet all of the needs within a project.	• Consider during proposal development. • Reconsider and refine at time of project initiation.
Selection of team members	• Clarify the roles, responsibilities, and performance expectations associated with specific jobs on a research team. • Outline reporting and accountability lines, which are important for staff monitoring. • Develop job descriptions. • Use job descriptions to recruit potential team members. • Screen qualifications of potential team members. • Select individuals who have the necessary skills and experience to meet the project needs. • Ensure that members of the research team understand their job descriptions.		
Monitoring productivity and work quality	• Track whether staff members are doing the tasks they are assigned, in the way that they were trained. • Monitor staff for ongoing continuing education needs. • Provide opportunities for team members to identify potential problems that may later influence data quality, and solve them before it is too late. • Create and implement systems to address problems in productivity and work quality.	• Ensures that the principal investigator can maintain the rigor of the project.	• Consider during proposal development. • Begin and maintain after project is started and staff is hired. • Update as required during project.
Training and continuing education	• Identify project specific training needs for staff members as a group, as well as individually (e.g., roles and responsibilities, specific job duties, lines of authority and accountability). • Prepare and deliver staff training and continuing education materials. • Develop a system to keep staff up-to-date on the latest developments in the field that may impact a project.	• Enables the principal investigator to contribute to the maturation and sophistication of a team over time.	• Consider during proposal development. • Begin and maintain after project is started and staff is hired. • Update as required during project.

Staff

(continued)

Table 33.1 Data Management Issues, Tasks, Importance, and Timing (continued)

Issues to Consider (from Figure 33.4)	Specific Tasks	Importance	Timing
Data access and security	• Design and implement a system for assigning ID codes. • Identify who has access to what information (e.g., budgets, participant information, specific data files). • Provide team members with explicit guidelines for: • How and where data and project information are to be stored, • What information is to be password protected (e.g., participant contact information), and • What data needs to be separated (e.g., consent forms from data sheets). • Design and implement a system for conducting data and file backups.	• Ensures compliance with relevant laws, rules and regulations. • Protects participant confidentiality.	• Consider at proposal development. • Refine upon human subjects review submission. • Follow upon project initiation. • Modify as required during project.
Documentation	• Identify what project information must to be documented (e.g., recruitment responses, participant attrition and reasons). • Identify where project information is to be documented (e.g., specific files and their locations). • Determine when project information is to be documented (e.g., frequency). • Explain to members of the team the rationale for the documentation.	• Facilitates consistent decision-making. • Supports all other aspects of the data collection system. • Facilitates report preparation. • Ensures compliance with relevant laws, rules and regulations.	• Consider at proposal development. • Begin at project initiation. • Refine and update throughout project.
Data collection processes and protocols	• Explain each of the specific steps to be taken during the data collection, including: • Prepare necessary scripts. • Prepare any anticipated protocols for addressing participants with cognitive impairments, use of proxy respondents, etc. • Prepare any resource materials data collectors will require (e.g., list of relevant phone numbers such as abuse or suicide hot lines). • Specify tasks and responsibilities for each member of the team during data collection. • Educate team members about how to consistently address challenging situations that may arise during the data collection process (e.g., dealing with participants who disclose abuse; uncovering cognitive impairment that may compromise informed consent).	• Ensures consistency in data collection, and therefore maximizes data quality. • Ensures compliance with relevant laws, rules, and regulations.	• Consider at proposal development. • Reconsider and refine upon project initiation. • Update and refine as new challenges emerge.
Data entry, checking and cleaning protocols	• Identify each step of the data entry and cleaning process, including: • Who is responsible, • What specific tasks must be completed at what time, • What processes are to be used to confirm data entry, and • How data entry errors are to be documented and resolved. • Develop and maintain a code book. • Identify timing for data checking and cleaning.	• Ensures quality data for analysis. • Saves time at end of project by maintaining data files throughout project.	• Consider at proposal development. • Begin at project initiation, in conjunction with decisions about data collection. • Refine during data collection, but before data are being entered.

Policies and Procedures

well (McFadden et al., 1995). Often, new investigators do not fully appreciate the amount of time that is required to manage the everyday administrative aspects of a study, and fail to incorporate adequate staff time in their project budget. By thinking through data management, and carefully analyzing the requirements of the project from beginning to end, an investigator will be in a better position to plan the necessary resources to support project infrastructure (McFadden et al., 1995).

Specific Tools and Resources to Facilitate Data Management

Good data management involves a range of tools and processes that allow the researcher to:

- Track what has been done,
- Track what is still needs to be done, and
- Ensure that the final research report and findings will be recognized as products of a rigorous and believable process.

This section includes specific examples of tools that can be used in the process of managing data. Table 33.2 presents the linkages between the tools and resources that are presented in this section, and the data management issues from Figure 33.4 and Table 33.1.

These tools and resources are ones we have found to be particularly helpful; their use is also supported in the existing literature on data management. What is presented here represents only a sampling of what is possible, and does not include all of the different tools that can be used to facilitate data management. The tools described are intended to offer a starting point for those with little or no experience in developing data management systems. Not everything that is presented over the next few pages will be relevant to every project.

Management Plan and Project Timeline

The management plan and project timeline is typically prepared as part of the research proposal. A

Table 33.2 Examples of Data Management Tools and Their Correspondence with Specific Data Management Issues

Tool, Resource or Strategy	Data Management Issue Influenced by Tool, Resource or Strategy	
	Staff	Policies and Procedures
Management plan and project timeline	• Monitoring productivity and work quality	• Documentation
Job descriptions	• Selection of team members • Monitoring productivity and work quality	• Data access and security • Data collection processes and protocols • Data entry, checking, and cleaning protocols
Systems to track participants and their data including: • Participant identifiers • Master file • ID sheets	• Training • Monitoring productivity and work quality	• Data access and security • Documentation • Data collection processes and protocols
Systems for data entry and confirmation: • Protocols for data coding, checking, and cleaning • Codebooks • Development of data collection forms	• Training • Selection of team members • Training • Monitoring productivity and work quality	• Data collection processes and protocols • Data entry and checking processes and protocols • Documentation
Team meetings	• Training • Monitoring productivity and work quality	• Documentation
Backup protocol	• Training	• Documentation • Data access and security

brief example is provided in Table 33.3. As a data management tool, a management plan and project timeline is helpful in the identifying the specific tasks that will need to be done over the course of an entire project and when these tasks need to be completed. Having this information will facilitate the process of identifying the skills and knowledge that will be required of the research team, which will aid in their selection. Later on in the project, the management plan and project timeline will provide guidance for monitoring the productivity and work quality of team members, and help in setting goals for data collection and for monitoring its progress.

Job Descriptions

For a research project to operate smoothly, the principal investigator must ensure that the people who are performing the various tasks within the project have the necessary skills and expertise to do so. Specifying these tasks and identifying the necessary qualifications of the individuals who will be performing these tasks are the first steps in developing job descriptions. In large projects when staff members are hired into a specific role, job descriptions facilitate a culture of consistent communication by clearly identifying the roles and responsibilities of each team member. For small projects in which one or two people play multiple roles, job descriptions can ensure that all tasks are addressed and assigned, and that each person understands his or her responsibilities. Typical areas to include in a job description are:

- Job title,
- Name and title of direct supervisor,
- Summary of job character and purpose of the position,
- Qualifications and/or specific skills required, and
- Specific list of job duties.

Systems to Track Participants and Their Data

To obtain good quality data, it is critical that an investigator can track participants throughout the course of a study (Nyiendo et al., 2002; Pogash et al., 2001). This information ensures that all information is collected from participants at the right times, that the data gathered from each participant are handled correctly, and that everyone can be accounted for at the end of the study, including the individuals who were recruited but never actually participated, those who dropped out, or those who were lost to the study (e.g., moved, died, etc.).

In the study, *Addressing Concerns about Falling Among Older Adults with Multiple Sclerosis,*[3] we explained in detail the process of tracking participants and their data in our policy and procedure manual, including who is responsible to

[3]This project is based on a grant awarded to Dr. Marcia Finlayson and Ms. Elizabeth Peterson by the Retirement Research Foundation, 2004 to 2007.

Table 33.3 **Sample of a Part of a Management Plan and Project Timeline**

Specific Project Tasks	Time Frame	People Responsible	Measure of Task Completion
Activity no. 2: Conduct focus groups with key informants			
2.1. Work with collaborators to select dates, times and locations for focus groups	July to August, 2002	PC and RA	Dates and times set
2.2. Work with collaborators and Advisory Group members to identify potential participants for focus groups	July to August, 2002	PI, PC, AG, and RA	Potential participants identified
2.3. Set up office systems to manage focus group documents and data (e.g., master file, logistics task lists, transcription processes, etc.)	July to August, 2002	PI, PC, and RA	Office systems completed
2.4. Contact potential participants to invite participation and provide basic information about the focus group	August to September, 2002	PI, PC, possibly AG	No. of participants contacted

AG = members of advisory group; PC = project coordinator; PI = Principal investigator; RA = research assistant.
Excerpted from the data management plan for the study: "Aging with MS: Unmet needs in the Great Lakes Region," Finlayson, principal investigator. Funded by the National Multiple Sclerosis Society, July 2002–June 2005, Contract no. HC0049.

complete which parts of the process, when, and where. Figure 33.5 summarizes the process used showing the connections between the initial recruitment of a participant and the final data file for analysis.

Figure 33.5 illustrates how a system for tracking participants and their data involves a series of individual tools, all of which are used in concert to achieve the goal of good quality data. The specific tools and processes within these systems that will be discussed in more detail in this section include:

• Developing and assigning participant identifiers,
• Creating and maintaining a master file, and
• Developing and using participant ID sheets.

Developing and Assigning Participant Identifiers

To be able to track participants and their data, it is necessary to be able to link individual data items to the people from whom the data were collected.

A participant identifier is a tool critical to this process. A participant identifier is a numeric or alphanumeric code (e.g., A-001) that is used in place of the participant's name on all documents pertaining to that individual. In terms of data management, assigning identifiers is more than simply ensuring that participant names are kept confidential, although that is a major reason for using identifiers. The actual process of assigning identifiers can facilitate the data collection and management process by providing a consistent variable that can be used to link files across the study (e.g., master participant list, data file, follow-up files, etc.).

To illustrate how the assignment of identifiers can facilitate data collection, consider the example of the study *Addressing Concerns about Falling Among Older Adults with Multiple Sclerosis* that is provided in the feature box on the next page. In this project, a national sample was used for telephone interviews. To facilitate the interviewing process, and reduce the risk that participants would be called at inappropriate times of the day

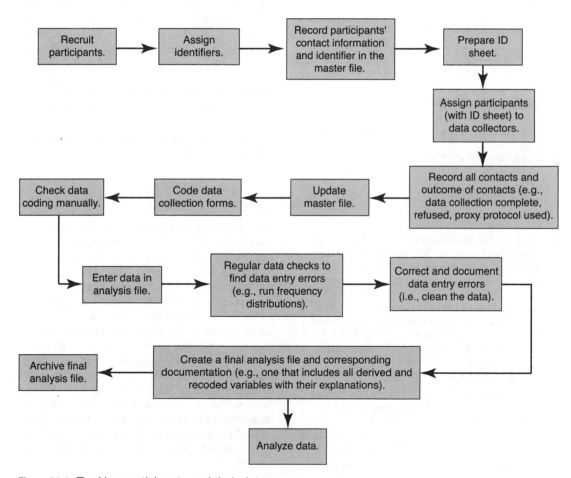

Figure 33.5 Tracking participants and their data.

(as a result of differences in time zones), information about the participant's time zone was embedded into the identifier. In addition, because participants were divided into two age groups for sampling, age group was also embedded in the identifier to make it easier to identify how many interviews had been completed in each group.

Identifier information should be maintained in a password-protected file. When working in larger multisite studies, assigning identifiers must be considered carefully so that when the final data are merged, there is no possibility that identifiers are duplicated. For example, one site may be assigned to use alphanumeric codes starting with the letter "A," while the second site may be assigned identifiers starting with the letter "B."

For therapists who are conducting research as part of their regular clinical duties, assigning identifiers must be done carefully to ensure that the research data and clinical data cannot be confused and inadvertently mixed together. Research data must be kept separate from the medical record, and under separate identifiers.

Assigning Identifiers—Sample Explanation

The Senior Research Assistant will be responsible for intake, entry, and assigning ID no.'s to all eligible respondents.

- ID numbers will be assigned based on time zone and age group.
- Time zone will be the first two digits in the ID code:
  - Eastern Time = ET
  - Central Time = CT
  - Mountain Time = MT
  - Pacific Time = PT
  - Alaska = AT
  - Hawaii = HT
- There are two age groups of interest in this study, 55–64 and 65+. The age groups will be designated as 01 (55–64) and 02 (65+). These will be the second two digits in the ID code.
- The remaining part of the ID code will be the sequential number of the respondent, e.g., 001, 002, 003, etc. Each age group is to have its own sequential numbering starting with 001. Time zone will not be considered in the sequential numbering—only age group.
- A sample ID would therefore be: MT-02-005.

Excerpted from the Policy and Procedure Manual from the study: "Addressing Concerns about Falling Among People Aging with MS" (Finlayson & Peterson, 2004–2007, with funding from the Retirement Research Foundation).

Creating and Maintaining a Master File

When tracking participants and using forms and files to do so, it is important to note that documents containing both the participant's name and identifier should be kept to a minimum because of the sensitivity and confidentiality of these materials. Nevertheless, it is important in most studies to be able to link a participant identifier to information such as name, address, and/or telephone or other means of contact. A master file is one tool to address this data management need.

A basic master file typically contains participant identifying information (e.g., name, contact information) together with the participant identifier code. Because of the sensitivity of this information, this file must be password protected and access to the file should be restricted to key members of the research team. Master files are usually electronic spreadsheet files. As new participants are recruited into a study, a participant identifier is assigned, and then the master file is updated (see Figure 33.5). Depending on the project, the master file may also include process related information such as how many contacts were attempted with a participant, whether baseline or outcomes measures have been administered, or when follow-up appointments are to be scheduled. It is important to note that this type of information is not data for analysis, but rather data to track the progress of a participant through the study. Data that will be used for analysis is maintained in the analysis file. Personal contact information should never be kept in the analysis file.

Developing and Using Participant ID Sheets

After recruiting participants, assigning identifiers, and adding individuals to the master file, it is very important to do everything possible to maintain participant confidentiality. This typically means that only minimally necessary information about the participant is recorded on other data collection forms. In fact, actual data collection forms should never include the participant's name, but rather only the participant identifier. A key challenge of occupational therapy research is that data collectors usually need both the participant identifier as well as contact information, particularly if an intervention or interview is involved, and if the data collector must go out to the participant's home or workplace. Balancing the need to have this information and keeping it confidential can be challenging.

A Participant ID sheet is one data management tool that can be used to address this dilemma and ensure that data collectors have the pieces of information they need to maintain their records, and at the same time minimize the number of places where the participant's name and identifier appear together. A sample Participant ID sheet is provided in Figure 33.6. A major advantage of an ID sheet is that it can easily be removed from the participants' files when the information it contains is not germane to the activities of the research team. Maintaining clear protocols about how to handle the ID sheet, where it is to be stored, who can have access to it, and when it is to be destroyed is very important. Often, the human subjects' ethics committee will have guidelines about these issues.

Systems for Data Entry and Confirmation

While data collection is often a major focus during the process of planning a study, it is equally important to consider how to enter and confirm these data after the collection is completed. The issues of data coding, checking, and cleaning are most often discussed in relation to data management, and other authors have described these processes in detail (see Aday, 1989; Hosking et al., 1995; Hulley, Cummings, Browner, Grady, Hearst, & Newman, 2001; McFadden et al., 1995; Pogash et al., 2001; Portney & Watkins, 2000). Given that data coding, checking and cleaning are process-oriented tasks, most investigators develop protocols to manage them. Therefore, the data management tools are the protocols themselves. In addition to these protocols, other related data management tools and strategies include codebooks and how data collection forms are developed.

Protocols for Data Coding, Checking, and Cleaning

In quantitative research, data coding involves translating participant responses into numerical values to facilitate statistical analysis. For variables that are continuous in nature (e.g., age, years since diagnosis), responses are already numerical so coding simply involves entering a participant's value into the analysis file. For variables that are nominal or ordinal in nature, responses must be assigned a numerical value. For example, consider a survey question that asks participants to reflect on how they are managing today compared to a year ago. Response options might be either "about the same," "worse," or "better." To be able to use

Aging with Multiple Sclerosis Study	

ID Form for Interviewers

Date reply form received:	
Date interview assigned:	
Participant name:	
Participant ID #:	
Participant telephone #:	
# of calls to obtain interview:	
# of calls to complete interview:	
Date interview completed:	
Contact log: Please note when contacts were made with participant (date, time, outcome of contact).	

CONFIDENTIAL

Figure 33.6 Participant ID sheet.

these responses statistically, the answers must be translated into numbers, for example, "about the same" equals 1, "worse" equals 2, and so on. This process is called data coding. In qualitative research, data coding involves applying labels to sections of text. Details on qualitative data coding are provided in Chapter 21.

Once data are coded, and the values for each response for each participant is entered into the analysis file, the investigator or a designate (e.g., research assistant, statistician) must do the data checking. The term *data checking* primarily relates to quantitative data. Data checking involves running frequency distributions and measures of central tendency and variability on each of the individual variables in the analysis file to check for missing or out of range values. If such values are found, it may indicate a data entry error. Potential errors can be checked against raw data, and if necessary, corrected. The process of correcting data entry errors is referred to as data cleaning. A sample protocol for data coding and checking is pro-

vided in the feature box titled "Sample Protocol for Data Coding and Checking," and one for data cleaning is provided in the feature box titled "Sample Protocol for Data Cleaning."

Codebooks

There can be many variables in a project, and keeping track of each of them is critical. Codebooks are one data management tool that can address this need. Codebooks are relevant to both qualitative and quantitative research (MacQueen, McLellan, Kay, & Milstein, 1998; Nyiendo et al., 2002; Shi, 1997). A codebook can be considered the dictionary for the data set generated by the study. The key contents of a quantitative codebook include the list of variables, their names and labels, and the coding for the different responses. Information in a qualitative codebook can include the list of codes, a definition of each code, and a description of when and how to use it.

In quantitative research, a codebook often con-

Sample Protocol for Data Coding and Checking

1. During any of the interviews, record information directly on the form being used—*do not use the coding boxes to record information as it is being collected.*
2. All interviews should be coded by the interviewer in BLUE INK.
3. All interviews should be coded within 24 hours of the completion of the interview.
4. Initial and date the interview guide to indicate when the interview was completed, and when it was coded. Mark initials and date on the bottom.
5. Each interviewer's first 25 interviews should be checked by the project coordinator for accuracy of coding. The Principal Investigator will check the project coordinator's coding accuracy. After these checks, the principal investigator or project coordinator will complete random coding checks at regularly scheduled intervals, unless otherwise assigned. These random checks will be made of 5% to 10% of the participants from the data files. Random numbers will be applied to the ID codes to select the interviews for checking.
6. If an error is made during the initial coding process, the error is to be stroked out with a SINGLE LINE. Corrections are to be marked BESIDE the initial code and initialed by the team member assigned to data cleaning.
7. Any coding corrections that are made by the team member assigned to complete the data checking are to be done in RED INK, and are to

follow the same procedure (i.e., single line, correction beside).
8. Special Codes:
   - 777—Skip
   - 880—Person with MS is deceased
   - 888—Don't know. If the participant is unable to decide between two categories, code the response as **888** "Don't know".
   - 899—Skipped due to the use of the cognitive impairment[4] protocol
   - 990—Skipped due to the use of the proxy protocol
   - 997—Not applicable (e.g., in nursing home, don't ever do stairs, apartment complex mows yard and does yard work)
   - 998—Refusal. If the participant refuses to answer a question or a series of questions.
   - 999—Interviewer error

Excerpted from the Policy and Procedure Manual from the study: "Aging with MS: Umet Needs in the Great Lakes Region" (Finlayson, 2002–2005, with funding from the National Multiple Sclerosis Society, Contract no. HC0049).

[4]Depending on the nature of the participants who may be recruited into a study, sometimes it is necessary to develop protocols for dealing with participants with certain characteristics. In our work, we sometimes come across individuals with cognitive impairment or individuals who need assistance to complete an interview (i.e., proxy). To ensure consistency across interviewers, we have specific protocols on how to proceed with these interviews.

Sample Protocol for Data Cleaning

---

1. Interview data will be entered into SPSS' Data Builder program. For this project, use the Data Builder on computer D.

2. The research assistants will take responsibility for entering the interview data into Data Builder. As each interview is entered, initial and date the form in black ink to indicate that it was entered. Mark initials and date on the appropriate line on the bottom of the form.

3. The co-principal investigator will be responsible for exporting the data file from Data Builder on the <u>first Monday of the month.</u>

4. The co-principal investigator will complete frequency distributions on the full exported file to check for data entry errors, specifically out of range values and missing values.

5. The co-principal investigator will give the senior research assistant any identified errors to check against raw data and correct as necessary.

6. The co-principal investigator and senior research assistant will maintain a log of identified errors and the corrections made. The principal investigator has final authority for making decisions about how to handle data corrections that are not obvious (i.e., not simply a matter of missed entry).

Excerpted from the Policy and Procedure Manual from the study: "Addressing Concerns about Falling Among People Aging with MS" (Finlayson & Peterson, 2004–2007, with funding from the Retirement Research Foundation).

---

tains information on the origins of items, instructions on how to complete the coding, how to code unusual responses, where individual data files are kept (raw data as well as electronic), who maintains the passwords for the files, and how derived variables were developed. A derived variable is one that is computed using other variables that already exist in the analysis file. An example of a derived variable would be "number of ADL limitations," which could be derived by counting the number of individual ADL items with which each participant identifies requiring assistance.

Development of Data Collection Forms

The key to coding, checking, and cleaning is forethought, careful documentation, and attention to detail. Forms and files need to be linkable, and many models exist for achieving linkage (e.g., relational databases, interface files, etc.) (Hulley et al., 2001). A key strategy that can be employed to facilitate linkage and data entry and cleaning is the format and preparation of the data collection forms (Antonakos et al., 2002; Nyiendo et al., 2002; Shi, 1997). For example, all of our interview guides include the data coding for each of the response options (e.g., stable = 1, improving = 2, etc.) for each question right on the data collection form, as illustrated in the feature box titled "Examples of Items from an Interview Guide." In addition, the variable label that is used in the analysis file for the question is included on the data collection form. In this feature box, the variable labels are "Msstatus" and "Ablechg." These labels are the ones that appear in the analysis file. The variable labels and codes on the data collection form match the ones in the electronic data file (e.g., SPSS, SAS). Being able to link files and forms together facilitates data management by ensuring that data can be cross-checked, confirmed, and, if necessary, corrected or updated as errors or omissions are found.

In addition, we also include the participant's identifier on each page of each document that is connected to that person. Doing so facilitates data management by ensuring that data collection forms that are unintentionally separated during the data collection process can be reconnected.

Team Meetings

Throughout this chapter, the importance of consistent communication across members of the research team has been emphasized to ensure that data are managed well. One important strategy for facilitating communication is the team meeting, to which we have previously alluded. Team meetings are an opportunity for everyone involved in the project to come together to discuss progress, address problems and make decisions to solve them, share achievements, and to make joint decisions that influence the project.

To facilitate a culture of consistent communication, everyone on the research team should be included in a team meeting, even if it appears on the surface that the discussion is not directly relevant to his or her duties. Team meetings provide an opportunity for all staff members to see how their own activities and decisions influence the work of others.

Taking minutes during team meetings is advised, particularly if decisions are made regarding data collection processes, changes to data coding protocols, etc. In addition, having team meeting minutes can make it easier for an investigator to summarize technical decisions at the end of a project.

Examples of Items from an Interview Guide that Include the Coding for Each Response, and the Variable Names that Will Be Used in the Data File

Survey Items and Response Options	Explanation
Would you say that your MS is within the last year (*read all but don't know option*): _____ Stable (1) Msstatus_____ _____ Improving (2) _____ Deteriorating (3) _____ Variable (4) _____ Don't know (888) Thinking about your symptoms and your ability to do everyday activities, how do you think you manage now compared to one year ago? (*read all but don't know option*) _____ About the same (1) Ablechg_____ _____ Worse (2) _____ Better (3) _____ Don't know (888)	Both of the survey items that are shown to the left include the response options and the coding for each option (the number in the bracket behind the response). "Msstatus" and "Ablechg" are the variable names that will be used in the data file. The line to the right of these names in the interview guide is used for "coding" after the interview is complete. For example, if a participant responded that in the past year, his or her MS had been "stable," a "1" would be recorded in the line beside "Msstatus." "1" would also be recorded in the data file for that respondent for this variable.

Fear of Falling study

ID code:_____   Interview completed: Data entered: _____

Backup Protocols

Nowadays, most of the information investigators retain for a research study is done so electronically. For this reason, developing and implementing backup protocols as part of a data management system is essential. There are two basic rules of backups: do them regularly and frequently (McFadden et al., 1995). One never knows when a file will become corrupted, fall victim to a computer virus or worm, or when the computer hardware might fail. Therefore, planning for and doing backups of all files is an absolute necessity.

In addition to actually planning for and doing the backups, the protocol should include directions about where the backup files are to be stored (in another location is always best, in case of fire), as well as instructions on how backups can be retrieved if that becomes necessary.

Final Thoughts on Data Management

So far this chapter has described the components of data management, explained why it is important, outlined issues to consider, and described some of the tools and strategies used to address these issues. This last section provides some general tips on data management, including what things to do at different points in the planning

process. This latter information will elaborate on the information provided in the last column of Table 33.1, presented earlier in this chapter. The feature box titled "General Tips on Setting Up Data Files" summarizes some of these tips.

Considerations During Proposal Development

As noted earlier, a good data management system will be initiated during the process of preparing a study proposal. At the time of proposal writing, decisions about staffing, project activities and timelines, computers and software, and storage needs (e.g., locking filing cabinets) must be made so that a realistic budget can be developed. Realistic budgets support good data management by providing the necessary financial resources to a project. At the time of project planning, the following data management tools and resources will need to be decided upon, developed, or at least initiated:

• Management plan and project timelines,
• Job descriptions,
• Equipment and supply needs (e.g., locking filing cabinets and data management and analysis software), and
• Submissions for human subjects protection (ethics review) and, if necessary, submissions related to the use and protection of personal health information (In the USA, HIPAA).

General Tips on Setting Up Data Files

Tip 1: Remember to include variables on your data collection forms and in your data files that will help you describe your study later (e.g., start and end times so you can calculate interview length).

Tip 2: Avoid using a single code to describe all "missing" data. Instead, use specific codes to detail the specifics of why data are missing— e.g., interviewer error, refused, skip, not asked—proxy, etc. These details can assist the statistician when making decisions about the analysis.

Tip 3: Remember: Detail is good. Categories can always be collapsed later, during analysis.

Tip 4: When setting up your files, consider whether you may need to link the new file to another one at some point in the future. Include variables that will facilitate these linkages, and determine if any variable names need to be the same between the files.

Tip 5: Maintain a file documenting all of your data files, where they are located, and their passwords (if electronic).

Issues During Project Initiation

The startup phase of any project can be hectic, as many different tasks must be completed. In relation to data management, an investigator needs to review all of the data management-related materials developed during the proposal phase of the project, and adjust as necessary. In addition, he or she must:

• Recruit and hire[5] individuals who meet the qualifications of the positions available,

• Train or arrange training for staff on protection of human subjects, use and protection of personal health information (if necessary), and all necessary aspects of their job,

• Decide what policies and procedures will be needed, and work with staff to prepare a policy and procedure manual,

• Set up staff monitoring procedures that can be reasonably followed (e.g., weekly team meetings),

• Develop systems to track participant recruitment and outcomes, including how ID numbers will be assigned,

[5]In clinical research, the principal investigator may not be hiring staff, but rather involving therapists or others who will be engaged in the data collection as part of their daily duties. Even in these types of situations, investigators must ensure that the individuals involved in the project have the qualifications necessary to conduct the duties related to the study.

• Review data collection tools and ensure that their design will facilitate accurate data entry,

• Test data entry systems, including data export protocols, and

• Set up and test data storage, security, and backup protocols.

Issues During Data Collection

Many data management problems will first emerge during the actual data collection phase. Some of them will be unexpected while others may have been overlooked in the original planning. During this phase, most of the data management involves following the protocols that were previously set, refining or adding to them as necessary, and documenting all decisions that are made. Specifically, the investigator will need to:

• Document methods and responses to each recruitment strategy,

• Document the outcome for each potential participant—who is in and who is out, and why an individual does not participate or complete the study,

• Update policies and procedures as new situations emerge,

• Maintain and adjust (as necessary) staff monitoring procedures, and

• Document as decisions are made (e.g., how to code unusual responses).

Issues During Data Preparation and Analysis

Once the data collection is completed, data entry will need to begin. For some studies, data entry can and will occur simultaneously with the data collection process. Either way, during the time period

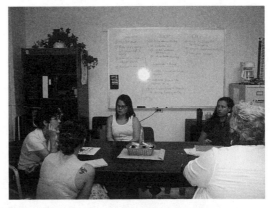

Figure 33.7 Dr. Finlayson and team members review a policy and procedure manual.

in which the data are being prepared for analysis, data management protocols will be in the forefront. The investigator will need to:

- Implement the data checking and cleaning protocols,
- Document corrections made to the data files,
- Document the construction of derived variables,
- Document the process of recoding variables,
- Apply weights to the data, if necessary, and document this process,
- Transfer, if necessary, the data to the analyst, and
- Ensure that all files are archived for later use and sharing.

Conclusion

This chapter emphasized the critical nature of data management and how it influences the quality of the data that a project produces. It also emphasized that data management involves both the information gathered from participants as well as the project information that facilitates overall study management. Data management is a complex set of tasks and processes. The key to doing it well is to be logical and methodical, and plan for problems before they emerge.

REFERENCES

Aday, L. (1989). *Designing and conducting health surveys.* San Francisco, CA: Jossey-Bass.

Antonakas, C. L., Miller, J. M., & Caruso, C. C. (2002). Critical elements of documentation in data-based research. *Western Journal of Nursing Research, 24* (1), 87–100.

Gassman, J. J., Owen, W. W., Kuntz, T. E., Martin, J. P., & Amoroso, W. P. (1995). Data quality assurance, monitoring and reporting. *Controlled Clinical Trials, 16,* 104S–136S.

Hosking, J. D., Newhouse, M. M., Bagniewska, A., & Hawkins, B. S. (1995). Data collection and transcription. *Controlled Clinical Trials, 16,* 66S–103S.

Hulley, S. B., Cummings, S. R., Browner, W. S., Grady, D., Hearst, N., & Newman, T. B. (2001). *Designing clinical research* (2nd ed.). Philadelphia, PA: Lippincott Williams & Wilkins.

Kielhofner, G., Hammel, J., Finlayson, M., Helfrich, C., & Taylor, R. R. (2004). Documenting outcomes of occupational therapy: The Center for Outcomes Research and Education. *American Journal of Occupational Therapy, 58* (1), 15–23.

Krefting, L. (1991). Rigor in qualitative research: An assessment of trustworthiness. *American Journal of Occupational Therapy, 45,* 214–222.

MacQueen, K. M., McLellan, E., Kay, K., & Milstein, B. (1998). Codebook development for team based qualitative analysis. *Cultural Anthropology Methods, 10* (2), 31–36.

McFadden, E. T., LoPresti, F., Bailey, L. R., Clarke, E., & Wilkins, P. C. (1995). Approaches to data management. *Controlled Clinical Trials, 16,* 30S–65S.

Nyiendo, J., Attwood, M., Llyod, C., Ganger, B., & Haas, M. (2002). Data management in practice-based research. *Journal of Manipulative and Physiological Therapeutics, 25* (1), 49–57.

Pogash, R. M., Boehmer, S. J., Forand, P. E., Dyer, A., & Kunselman, S. J. (2001). Data management procedures in the asthma clinical research network. *Controlled Clinical Trials, 22,* 168S–180S.

Portney, L., & Watkins, M. P. (2000). *Foundations of clinical research: Applications to practice* (2nd ed.). Upper Saddle River, NJ: Prentice-Hall.

Shi, L. (1997). *Health services research methods.* Clifton Park, NY: Delmar.

Disseminating Research

Gary Kielhofner • Ellie Fossey • Renée R. Taylor

Research that is not publicly shared is incomplete. Dissemination is a key step in the research process and, thus, before any investigation is undertaken, the researcher should plan ahead for how and when it will be shared. This chapter discusses the rationale, process, and range of mechanisms for disseminating research.

Research is undertaken for the larger benefit of the scientific community and the public. Research dissemination communicates new knowledge to these constituencies. Moreover, when disseminating research, the investigator describes the research process so that peer scholars are able to evaluate its rigor and to replicate or build upon the study to advance science. Finally, dissemination shares knowledge with stakeholders so it can be used for practical ends (Mercier, Bordeleau, Caron, Garcia, & Latimer, 2004).

There is a growing emphasis in many sectors on assuring the utilization of research results. As a result, researchers are combining traditional concerns for scientific rigor with "new outcomes planning and performance measurement requirements which focus on the effects and utilization of findings" (Campbell & Schutz, 2004, p. 7). This growing emphasis on ensuring the practical impact of findings has underscored the importance of a comprehensive approach to dissemination. Such an approach helps ensure that the information generated through the research reaches the right audiences in a format that allows them to effectively use it to change and enhance their behavior and practices.

The Nature and Role of Dissemination

Dissemination refers to the processes by which researchers inform others within and beyond the scholarly community about their research process and what they have learned from it. As we will see, there are multiple ways that research can be disseminated. Each of these is suited to a particular audience and purpose.

In occupational therapy, the dissemination of research addresses the following aims:

• Making new information available to members of the profession in order to build and support evidence-based practice,
• Making information available to scholars in related disciplines who are doing research in the same or related areas so that they can incorporate and build upon one's methods and findings,
• Permitting criticism and replication, each of which is necessary to the refinement and further development of professional knowledge,
• Making information available to consumers, and
• Making information available to entities and persons who fund and/or make decisions and policy that impact the availability and delivery of occupational therapy services.

In planning and implementing a particular form of dissemination, one should always consider its purposes. Below, we briefly discuss each of the aims to which dissemination can be directed. It should be kept in mind that any particular act of dissemination has the potential to address more than one of these aims.

> In planning and in reporting research, investigators should consider how their research can contribute to practice.

Making New Information Available to Members of the Profession

As discussed in Chapter 41 there is a professional obligation to base practice on evidence. Many different forms of evidence can inform practice; however, the most rigorous is generated through research. Most research conducted by occupational therapy researchers will have either direct or indirect implications for practice. By making their findings available, researchers are supporting their practitioner peers to provide services in line with evidence. In planning and in reporting research, investigators should consider how their research can contribute to practice. Thus, a critical part of research dissemination is to discuss the practice implications of the findings.

Making Information Available to Scholars in Related Disciplines

Occupational therapy researchers conduct their investigations within an interdisciplinary context. First, occupational therapists mostly use research methods that were developed in other fields. Second, occupational therapy researchers are often investigating topics on which there is also interdisciplinary research. Further, even when therapists are investigating topics of specific interest to the profession, it is likely that their findings will have some relevance to members of other professions and disciplines.

Making one's research available to an interdisciplinary audience is an important way of participating in the discourse that advances research in a particular area. Reporting findings in an interdisciplinary context allows others to incorporate and build upon one's methods and findings. It is a way of returning something to the larger scientific community, from which the profession benefits. Moreover, the reputation of occupational therapists is enhanced when others encounter quality research conducted by them. Finally, disseminating findings in the interdisciplinary context informs others of the profession's particular perspective and concepts.

Permitting Criticism and Replication

One of the most demanding aspects of research is submitting to public scrutiny. Anyone who has submitted for review or published research is aware that such efforts almost assuredly generate feedback concerning the limitations and flaws of the research and its presentation. After one has worked hard for months or years to plan and implement research, it is not easy to hear others criticize it.

Nonetheless, this critique is an essential aspect of all research. By explicating how findings were generated, dissemination allows others to judge how much confidence they wish to place in the findings, given the limits and flaws in the particular research process. No investigation is ever perfect and it is important that others can objectively critique and learn from it.

Dissemination is also important so that others can understand and replicate one's research. Replications are conducted to confirm whether similar results are obtained when studies are repeated by others, and to test the generalizability of findings to different samples and situations. Subsequent research that fails to reproduce the earlier study's findings can help to illuminate flaws that were not apparent in the original research, or to distinguish the context-specific elements of the findings from those that are common across settings. When research findings are replicated by others, the scientific community places more confidence in them.

Making Information Available to Consumers and/or Participants

Consumers include persons who themselves or whose family members are receiving or may receive occupational therapy services. Consumers also include advocacy and lobby groups, who represent the interests of people in the community for whom the research has relevance. Research should be shared with consumers whenever it can enable them to make informed decisions about the need for and likely outcomes of services. This means that researchers should be willing to share research findings in ways that are accessible to consumers. Moreover, investigators are ethically obligated to provide information about research findings to agencies and/or individuals who participate in the research (Sieber, 1992).

Making Information Available to Funding and Decision-Making Entities

Research can serve as a means of demonstrating the value of occupational therapy services. Such research has the potential of influencing persons to make affirmative decisions concerning reimbursing and making available occupational therapy services.

Typical Venues for Dissemination

Dissemination can be thought of as falling into two broad audience categories: professional/scientific and stakeholders. We will discuss the various forms of dissemination for each of these audiences.

Professional/Scientific Audiences

The most common ways of disseminating research to professional and scientific peers occurs in the form of presentations and posters at conferences and journal publications. These venues can be either peer-reviewed or non-peer-reviewed. Peer-reviewed venues are more common for the presentation of the research methodology and findings. Non-peer-reviewed professional publications are generally more appropriate for emphasizing the significance of research findings for practice.

Peer-Reviewed Dissemination

In most professional and virtually all scientific venues, one must submit the proposed poster, presentation, or journal article for peer review. The review process is used to ensure the quality of information disseminated, and its suitability for the particular conference audience or journal readership.

The Purpose of Reviews. Review procedures are intended to maintain the quality and standard of conferences and academic journals. For conference presentations and posters, this review process focuses on the quality and suitability of submitted abstracts (i.e., brief summaries of proposed presentations/posters), and is typically undertaken by an expert panel/committee responsible for selection of the program content.

In contrast, the review process for journal publication involves review of full-length research papers (also referred to as manuscripts) written and submitted to the journal by the researchers, which are then reviewed by designated members of the journal's editorial board or team of referees. For occupational therapy journals, peer review also ensures that published papers reflect, and

Choosing Venues for Dissemination

> Dissemination mechanisms should be chosen to ensure that research findings are effectively communicated and utilized (Patton, 1997). Thus, it is important to consider:
>
> • Who should know about the outcomes of this research?
> • What information will be of most relevance to each of these various audiences (e.g., individuals, agencies, policymakers)?
> • What will be the most effective mechanisms for sharing this information with them?

build on current thinking and developments within the field of occupational therapy.

Each journal has its own requirements for the format of papers, how many copies must be submitted, whether electronic copies are required/permitted, and so forth. These requirements are noted in the guide to authors, which can generally be found on the journal's Web site (if it has one) and/or in a copy of the journal itself. Journals ordinarily do not have deadlines. An exception is when a special issue of a journal is announced. Generally special issues of a journal focus on a given research topic, or method, and may involve one or more guest editors. These special issues are usually announced though a call for papers with a specified submission deadline.

Referees, the people who undertake reviews of papers submitted to journals, usually have experience in writing for publication, and represent the broad range of professional backgrounds relevant to the journal's particular field. In occupational therapy, this means referees are likely to be occupational therapists and scholars in the field of occupational therapy and related fields, who have the necessary publishing experience and expertise in particular practice areas and/or inquiry method to review and constructively evaluate the types of work submitted for publication in occupational therapy journals.

Blind Review. Many, but not all, scientific/professional journals utilize blind review. Blind review means that the review procedure is undertaken by the referee(s) without the author(s) of a manuscript being identified to the referee(s). Blind review procedures are intended to foster fair evaluation of the quality and standard of the manuscript on its merits, by minimizing the extent to which knowledge of the authorship might influence opinions expressed by the referee about the work, or bias the referee's judgment.

Consumer Review. Although less common than review by scientific/professional peers, consumer review is increasingly considered important and included for some dissemination venues. Consumer reviews offer the perspective of persons who participated in the study, or those for whom the research is intended. Consumer review is intended to evaluate the relevance and applicability of research and its presentation for consumer audiences.

> Dissemination can be thought as falling into two broad audience categories: professional/scientific and stakeholders.

The American Journal of Occupational Therapy® *(AJOT)* is the official peer-reviewed journal of the American Occupational Therapy Association. We welcome the submission of manuscripts that are relevant to the study of occupation and the practice of occupational therapy. Categories of peer-reviewed articles include feature-length articles, case reports, brief reports, and issue papers. The journal also publishes book reviews, the Evidence-Based Practice Forum, Technology and Occupation, Letters to the Editor, and the official archival material of the Association.

AJOT uses the fifth edition of the *Publication Manual of the American Psychological Association* (APA) as the style guide. Consult this manual for style questions unless specified otherwise in this Author's Guide.

One original and three copies of all manuscripts should be sent to Mary A. Corcoran, PhD, OTR/L, FAOTA, Editor, 2901 Oak Shadow Drive, Oak Hill, VA 20171, USA; ajoteditor@aol.com.

Manuscripts must be submitted with the authors' explicit written assurance that they are not simultaneously under consideration by any other publication. The journal cannot assume responsibility for the loss of manuscripts.

1. Authors' Responsibility

Signatures. Before publication of any accepted manuscript, all authors must provide original signatures for the statement of authorship responsibility, the statement of financial disclosure, and the statement of copyright release. Signed statements of authorship responsibility and financial disclosure must be included with the manuscript submission (see form at end of this guide). The form containing the copyright release statement will be mailed to the corresponding author on acceptance of the manuscript (after peer review).

The statement of authorship responsibility is certification that each author has made substantial contributions to (a) the conception and design, acquisition of data, or analysis and interpretation of data; (b) drafting and revising the article; *and* (c) approval of the final version. Further, each author takes public responsibility for the work.

Author order. The order of authors in the byline follows APA guidelines. The principle contributor appears first, and subsequent names are in order of decreasing contribution.

2. Categories of Articles

Feature-length article. Feature-length articles (18 to 20 pages) include (a) original research reports that focus on philosophical, theoretical, educational, or practice topics and (b) critical reviews (including meta-analyses) that offer the systematic review and critical analysis of a body of literature as related to occupation and occupational therapy.

Brief Report. A Brief Report (8 to 10 pages) is a short report of original research that is of a pilot or exploratory nature or that addresses a very discrete research question and lacks broad implications. References are abbreviated (10 to 15).

Case Report. A Case Report (8 to 10 pages) is a short report of original work that focuses on a case example of a clinical situation. The focus can be on a patient or client, a family, an institution, or any other defined unit. The case should represent elements of practice that are not already represented in the literature. References are abbreviated (10–15).

The Issue Is. Papers submitted for The Issue Is (8 to 10 pages) department are those that address timely issues, policies, or professional trends or that express opinion that is supported by cogent argument. Papers for The Issue Is have no abstract; references are abbreviated (10–15).

Letters to the Editor. Letters discussing a recent *AJOT* article or other broad issues relative to the journal are welcome. Letters should ordinarily not exceed two double-spaced typed pages. Submission may be via e-mail or hard copy. If using e-mail, the letter should be pasted in the e-mail message; do not send as an attachment.

Manuscripts for all categories above, except Letters to the Editor, are peer reviewed.

Evidence-Based Practice Forum and Technology and Occupation. Authors interested in submitting manuscripts for these departments should contact the appropriate associate editor before submission to discuss topics and manuscript preparation guidelines. Linda Tickle-Degnen is the associate editor for *Evidence-Based Practice* (Tickle@bu.edu), and Roger O. Smith is the associate editor for *Technology and Occupation* (smithro@uwm.edu).

3. Manuscript Preparation

For format and reference style, consult the APA style manual and recent issues of *AJOT*. Careful attention to style details will expedite the peer-review process.

Double-space the entire manuscript, including abstract, text, quotations, acknowledgments, tables, figure legends, and references. Leave 1-inch margins on all sides, and keep the right side unjustified. Number all pages, starting with the abstract page. Use only standard 12-point font size. Do not copy pages back to back.

Title page. The title should be short and reflect the primary focus of the paper. List three key words or phrases (not already in the title). List full names, degrees, titles, and affiliations of all authors. Designate corresponding author and give full address, telephone number, fax number, and e-mail address.

(continued)

Abstract page. A 150-word abstract is required for all full-length feature articles, Brief Reports, and Case Reports. Abstracts may be structured (organized with subheadings Objective, Method, Results, and Conclusion) or unstructured (narrative description of the focus and key content of the paper). The abstract is page 1 of the manuscript.

Acknowledgments page. The acknowledgments page follows the last page of the text and precedes the reference list. Brief acknowledgments may include names of persons who contributed to the research or paper but who are not authors (e.g., statistician) followed by acknowledgments of grant support. Prior presentation of the paper at a meeting should be briefly described last.

References. Follow the APA style manual for referencing, listing references in alphabetical order starting on the page after the acknowledgments and inserting authors' surnames and year of publication for in-text citations. Personal communications or other nonretrievable citations are described in the text only with name and date for a person and name, date, and address for an organization. *Authors are solely responsible for the accuracy and completeness of their references and for correct text citation.* The following are examples of commonly used reference listings:

Journal article:

Abreu, B. C., Peloquin, S. M., & Ottenbacher, K. (1998). Competence in scientific inquiry and research. *American Journal of Occupational Therapy, 52,* 751–759.

Book with corporate author and author as publisher:

American Psychiatric Association. (1994). *Diagnostic and statistical manual of mental disorders* (4th ed.). Washington, DC: Author.

Book with author(s):

Frank, G. (2000). *Venus on wheels: Two decades of dialogue on disability, biography, and being female in America.* Los Angeles: University of California Press.

Edited book:

Law, M. (Ed.). (1998). *Client-centered occupational therapy.* Thorofare, NJ: Slack.

For instructions on citing electronic references, see the following APA Web page: www.apa.org/journals/webref.html.

Tables. Provide full titles and put each table on separate pages following the references. Number the tables consecutively as they appear in the text. Data appearing in tables should supplement, not duplicate, the text.

Figures and illustrations. Submit one original and three copies of all figures or illustrations. Number figures in order of mention in the text.

Affix a label with name of first author, figure number, and arrow indicating "top" on the back of the figure. Figures may be submitted as high-quality laser printouts, black-and-white glossy prints, or digitized electronic files. Provide a caption for each figure. List all captions on one page, double-spaced. Place the figure caption page after the tables and before the figures.

Abbreviations. Do not use abbreviations in the title or abstract of the paper; the use of abbreviations in the text should be minimal.

4. Permissions

Authors who wish to reprint tables, figures, or lengthy quotations are responsible for obtaining permission from the original copyright holder. Letters of permission with original signatures must be submitted to the editor. AOTA does not reimburse authors for any expense incurred when obtaining permission to reprint. The need for permission applies to adapted tables and figures as well as exact copies.

Signed statements of permission to publish must accompany all photographs of identifiable persons.

Authors must submit signed statements of permission from persons cited for personal communications.

5. Manuscript Review

Manuscripts and reviews are confidential materials. The existence of a manuscript under review is not revealed to anyone beyond the editorial staff. All submitted manuscripts are initially reviewed by the editor for suitability for the journal. Suitable manuscripts are then sent to editorial board members or guest reviewers for peer review. The identities of the reviewers and of the authors are kept confidential. Initial review takes approximately 3 months; subsequent review of revisions takes less time.

Authors are responsible for ensuring that a blind review process can take place. Except for the title page, manuscripts should contain no identifying names of specific persons or places.

All accepted manuscripts are subject to copyediting. Authors will receive a photocopy of the edited manuscript for review and final approval, as well as reprint order forms, before publication. The author(s) assumes final responsibility for the content of the manuscript, including copyediting.

6. Copyright and Patent

On acceptance of the manuscript, authors are required to convey copyright ownership to AOTA. Manuscripts published in the journal are copyrighted by AOTA and may not be published elsewhere without permission. Permission to reprint

(continued)

AJOT Author Guidelines (continued)

---

journal material for commercial or other purposes must be secured in writing from the director of AOTA's Publications Department.

Any device, piece of equipment, splint, or other item described with explicit directions for construction in an article submitted to *AJOT* for publication is not protected by AOTA copyright and can be produced for commercial purposes and patented by others, unless the item was already patented or its patent is pending, at the time the article is submitted.

Checklist for Authors

_____ Original and three copies of manuscript and figures

_____ Cover letter

_____ Signed authorship responsibility and financial disclosure forms

_____ All references checked for accuracy and completeness and for exact match between list and text

_____ Manuscript contains no identifying names of specific persons and places within the text

_____ Pages numbered starting with abstract on page 1

_____ Written permissions obtained as needed (photographs, personal communications, publishers of copyrighted material)

_____ Labels on back of all figures

_____ All material double-spaced (including abstract, references, quotations, figure captions)

_____ On title page—name, full address, telephone and fax numbers, and e-mail address of corresponding author as well as three key words or phrases

Note. Do not send a diskette with the initial submission of a manuscript. A diskette will be requested if the manuscript is accepted for publication.

The Review Process. The process of review for conference presentations or posters begins with a call for abstracts with a deadline. Calls for papers and posters generally occur several months in advance of the conference. Authors are notified of the decision about whether their paper/poster is accepted well in advance of the conference. Each conference has its own rules for the length and content of an abstract. Some conferences publish abstracts of papers and posters that are selected for inclusion in a conference proceeding. Historically, abstracts were submitted on paper. Many conferences today use electronic formats, such as submission via a Web site.

Peer review for journal articles requires submission of a full manuscript that is intended for publication. The manuscript will be forwarded to two to three reviewers whose expertise overlaps with the methodological and/or substantive content of the manuscript. Reviewers ordinarily are provided with detailed guidelines and forms for completing the review process and making recommendations about the disposition of the manuscript. Generally reviewers are asked to make one of the following recommendations:

• Rejection,
• Invitation to make major revision and submit for re-review (in which case the revised manuscript is ordinarily re-reviewed by one or more of the original reviewers), or
• Acceptance pending minor or no revisions.

In addition to recommending disposition of the manuscript, reviewers generally provide detailed feedback, which provides the rationale for the recommendation and, when revisions are asked for, guidance to the author(s) of the manuscript as to the kind of revisions required.

The journal editor considers the reviewers' feedback, decides on a course of action, and then communicates to the author(s) whether the paper is rejected, invited to be resubmitted with revisions, or accepted with minor or no revisions. The editor ordinarily shares the outcome in a detailed letter, which provides the rationale and spells out any requested revisions.

Different journals have differing standards for and rates of manuscript acceptance. For extremely competitive journals, the majority of manuscripts submitted will be rejected. Authors who have had articles rejected from these top tier journals often find their manuscripts accepted by less competitive journals. Experienced investigators choose the level of journal to which they originally submit papers based on their assessment of the quality and sophistication of their study as determined by such factors as design rigor, sample size, and degree of innovation.

In the case of papers that are accepted for publication, the most common experience of authors is to make fairly substantial revisions, which are then re-examined by reviewers and/or the editor. Anyone who wishes to publish research must be prepared to accept criticism and have a full measure of patience. After submitting a manuscript, one ordinarily waits 3 to 6 months for initial feedback. If revisions are required, a similar period after submission of the revised manuscript lapses before the

An Example of a Research Abstract for a Conference

Title: Attending to Clients' Stories: Use of the Occupational Performance History Interview (OPHI-II)

    Author(s): Ellie Fossey, Karen Roberts, and Melanie Gray

    Abstract accepted for paper presentation at the OT AUSTRALIA 20th National Conference, Canberra 1999.

    Abstract: Attending to clients' life stories is an essential part of developing positive relationships with clients, and gaining an understanding of their illness experiences, as well as their life goals, and the part that therapy could play in enabling clients to achieve these goals. Ultimately, our success in designing therapeutic interventions that are meaningful and relevant to our clients depends on our ability to develop such relationships and understanding.

    The Occupational Performance History Interview (OPHI-II) (Kielhofner et al., 2004) is a revised version of the OPHI currently being developed through an international collaboration, to which the authors are contributors. This interview gathers information about a person's occupational identity (self-understanding), perceived competence in occupational performance, and his/her environment, as well as providing a framework to explore the direction, and important events in the person's life story.

    This paper will briefly describe the OPHI-II, then present occupational narratives (stories), obtained using OPHI-II, to illustrate the richness of information and understanding of clients' lives that may be gained with this tool. Stories from people in Australian rehabilitation and community settings will be included to discuss their therapeutic implications, and illustrate some potential uses for the OPHI-II in occupational therapy practice.

author(s) receive the second round of feedback. Often at this stage the author must make additional (usually more minor) edits and submit a manuscript, which is then copyedited in most instances. Some months later, and prior to publication, the author ordinarily receives a galley proof (i.e., a facsimile of the article as it will appear in the journal), which must be checked for accuracy and returned with any corrections to the journal. A minimum of 6 months can be expected to elapse from the time of submission until publication, and more often the process takes upwards of a year.

Oral Presentations and Posters at Conferences. Professional and scientific conferences provide

opportunities for investigators to share the process and results of recent research on a shorter timeline than publication. Conferences also provide a unique opportunity for members of the scientific/professional community to meet each other, discuss research informally, make connections, and share information that can benefit future research, as well as to interact with other stakeholders. The feedback that presenters receive can be helpful to preparation of a manuscript for publication. For these reasons, investigators frequently seek to present the results of their research first at conferences and later in published format.

Presentations. Presentations of scientific papers are usually brief (i.e., 10 to 30 minutes). Some time is ordinarily scheduled following presentations for brief public discussion. Verbal presentations are primarily an oral medium so they rely on both the content of the presentation and its delivery by the presenter(s).

A good presentation is characterized by clarity, conciseness, and attention to the target audience. Generally, the quality of a presentation depends not only on the verbal content, but also on the graphic representation of the research. PowerPoint presentations are typical in modern conferences and they may be supplemented with audience handouts. The use of these elements allows the presenter to emphasize major points, to supplement verbal presentation with visual illustration, and provide attendees with information that goes beyond what can be presented within the time limit of the presentation (Figure 34.1).

Scientific Posters. Poster presentations are ordinarily exhibited in a large room or hall that accommodates a number of posters simultaneously. Conference attendees view and select those they wish to read in detail. The authors are expected to be present during scheduled poster sessions, so they can further explain the content of their posters in response to questions. Posters may also be available for viewing outside the scheduled poster session, depending on the conference rules.

The essential feature of a good poster is that the message is clear and understandable without the presenter, and that it achieves a balance between words and graphics. A range of visual techniques can assist in presenting information in interesting and informative ways. These include, for instance: photographs; diagrams; tables; graphs; and layout methods, such as flow charts and dot points.

Conference organizers typically provide specific guidelines about poster content, format, and size requirements. Familiarity with these requirements and attention to production design,

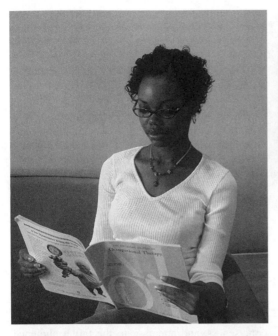

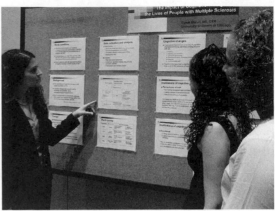

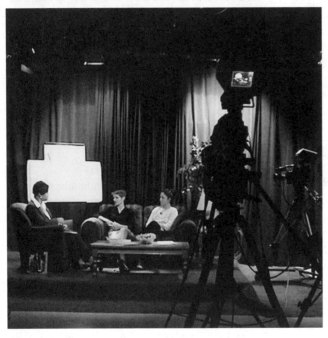

Figure 34.1 Researchers disseminate results in a variety of ways, including poster presentations at national professional conferences such as the annual meeting of the American Occupational Therapy Association, through publications in journals such as American Journal of Occupational Therapy, and through local media such as local news programs.

clarity of content, colors, layout, and finishing are important to maximize effectiveness. It is important to be selective—that is, to include the key information to make the research understandable to the reader, but not to overload the poster with details.

Choosing a Poster or Verbal Format for Presentation. Choosing whether to orally present a paper or to present a poster at a conference involves several considerations. Generally, oral presentations are more competitive than posters, so depending on the overall level of acceptance rates for papers at a conference, one may consider the likelihood of having a verbal presentation versus a poster accepted. Poster sessions are also more likely to accept presentations of preliminary findings and research in process.

Posters are primarily a visual medium for sharing information. Poster presentations provide graphic and textual means to illustrate studies and their outcomes. They are particularly valuable for information that is best presented using schematic diagrams and flow charts. The fact that a poster can be viewed at one's own pace and discretion may make it possible for others to better absorb the information than from verbal presentation. Since conference poster sessions involve face-to-face interaction, they tend to facilitate networking with others interested in related research.

Verbally presenting a paper allows one to share information with an audience in real time. For many investigators, it is the only time one shares research face to face with members of the scientific and professional community. Since much of research can involve long hours of private writing and interaction with others through written means, the verbal presentation is something many researchers value. Presentations are usually competitively selected, so the fact of presenting research gives it an air of authority. All in all, presentations are a time for researchers to engage in the most public aspect of the scientific process.

Summary: The Importance of Peer-Reviewed Dissemination. Dissemination through peer-reviewed channels is essential to all research. Its importance is linked to the fact that the peer review process provides quality control. Presentations, posters, and published articles that have gone through a review process have been scrutinized. The peer review process assures that investigators have fully described their methods to allow evaluation of rigor and replication. It also serves to ensure that the claims about discovered knowledge made by the author(s) are warranted and that adequate attention is paid to the limitations of the study. Thus peer review often improves the quality of the information presented about both the research process and findings to better serve those listening to, or reading, that information.

Non-Peer-Reviewed Presentations and Publications

Non-peer-reviewed venues for dissemination also serve important roles. These venues include:

• Invited presentations,
• Continuing education,
• Books,
• Professional publications and newsletters,
• Nonprint materials containing information about research findings and their implications.

Each of these venues is described briefly below.

Invited Presentations. Conference organizers and academic and practice organizations and associations often invite outside speakers to present information generated from research. While the specific content of these presentations is not peer reviewed, it is ordinarily the case that speakers (and sometimes their topics) are chosen because of the positive reputation of the quality of the speaker (and the research presented). Some invited presentations are associated with awards or honors and the choice of speakers and topics is highly selective. Other venues, such as a routine research colloquium or "brown bag" lunch presentations offered in an academic department, have open invitations for persons of varying levels of research accomplishment to present their work and obtain feedback. All of these venues from the most prestigious to the routine can be important opportunities for sharing information about research.

Continuing Education. Continuing education provides an important means of ensuring that professionals and researchers remain current in their knowledge and skills. The typical vehicle for continuing education is a workshop (ranging from a few hours to several days). Typically one or more persons, who are recognized experts, will organize a program of sequential topics in a specific area of interest. Such workshops may provide opportunities for related studies to be presented and synthesized. Workshops are also an excellent venue for discussions of the practical challenges of doing research, and the practice implications of findings.

Books. In some fields, it is common to report the results of research in a full book. It is not commonplace in occupational therapy. However, books do often describe, summarize, and synthesize research. For example, occupational therapy textbooks often make reference to research findings in discussing practice. In addition, books that present theoretical models typically describe the kinds of research that has been conducted to develop, apply, and test those models.

Professional Publications and Newsletters. A variety of professional magazines and newsletters can be useful resources for sharing research findings and its implications. *OT Practice*, published by the American Occupational Therapy Association, is one example of such a professional magazine. While it does not feature the more technical discussions of research that appear in refereed journals, it can be an appropriate venue to discussing how research findings can be integrated into practice.

Newsletters are another appropriate vehicle for discussing the applied relevance of research. Some large institutional research programs and federal agencies that fund research also produce publications that share research findings. Finally, there are agencies whose purpose is to disseminate research. They produce a variety of publications that share research. Most of these venues secure articles by inviting authors to write, accepting contributed articles, and using in-house writers to compose articles. If there are not published guidelines for accepting contributed papers, this information can usually be obtained from the editor. In most cases, it is up to the editor of the publication to decide whether or not to include a particular topic or paper.

Nonprint Materials Containing Information About Research Findings and Their Implications. With the growth of the Internet, a wide range of electronic sources now contain information related to research. These include sites specific to areas of research, or even specific to individual research projects. Often Web-based dissemination can serve both professional and other stakeholder audiences. Information can also be made available in different formats to suit these constituencies.

Stakeholder Audiences

Historically, the focus on research dissemination was to the scientific and professional communities through the kinds of means discussed above. There is increasing emphasis today on sharing research with various stakeholder audiences. Stakeholders refer to anyone outside the scientific and professional community who may be informed or influenced by the research findings either in their personal lives or in the exercise of their responsibilities. These include but are not limited to:

- Individuals and agencies who participate in the research,
- Consumers of health services for whom the research has relevance,
- Officials and agencies who make decisions and policy that might be informed by the research,
- Entities who address needs and/or fund services related to the research, and
- The general public whose attitudes or behavior might be influenced by the research findings.

The avenues for disseminating research to these audiences are multiple. Major ones include:

- Procedures for sharing findings with the study participants;
- Public presentations to consumer and community groups and collaborating organizations;
- Reports to government and private agencies, legislative bodies, and public officials;
- Web sites, targeted brochures, and other media for laypersons; and
- Releases to the popular press and media.

Each of these means offers opportunities to disseminate research to audiences beyond scholarly and professional communities. They are discussed below.

Sharing Information with Research Participants

There is an ethical responsibility to disseminate information about research findings and outcomes with research participants (Sieber, 1992). This responsibility is ordinarily not fulfilled by publication of results. Therefore, other dissemination mechanisms should be considered. One such mechanism for disseminating information to research participants is to prepare and send a written summary of the research findings to all participants and participating agencies. This approach has the advantages of being both low cost and time efficient, so it is particularly well suited to studies with large numbers of participants. Limitations of this approach are that it does not promote discussion about the potential uses of the research findings, nor does it enable participants to give feedback to the researchers.

The use of technologies, such as e-mail, Web sites, and Internet discussion groups, have the potential to both efficiently disseminate research findings and enhance dialogue among researchers, participants, and relevant community groups about research. For this approach to be effective, use of these technologies must be widespread among the relevant stakeholder groups. Face-to-face meetings with participants, participating agencies, and community groups provide more targeted opportunities to discuss findings with relevant audiences and to gain feedback from them (McConnell & Kerbs, 1993).

Individually tailored feedback is labor intensive, but particularly useful in research involving performance-based assessments and disempowered or marginalized groups (Fossey, Epstein, Findlay, Plant, & Harvey, 2002). For example, in an Australian study involving participants with psychiatric disabilities, Fossey et al. (2002) developed and evaluated a process for sharing individual feed-back with the participants about their occupational performance, based on results of the Assessment of Motor and Process Skills (AMPS) (Fisher, 2003). The investigators prepared written information for each participant, adopting a strengths-based approach, in which the person's occupational performance strengths were described, and some ways in which these strengths could be used to overcome areas of difficulty were suggested. This written information was shared face to face, accompanied by verbal explanation. Participants reported that the focus of the feedback on strengths was helpful, while the verbal explanation was seen as essential to enabling their understanding and use of the written information.

Different research traditions have approached the issue of dissemination to stakeholders in different ways. For example, in the quantitative tradition, research tends to be viewed as the researcher's expertise, product, and property. Thus providing feedback is usually viewed as a didactic process, in which the researcher gives information to stakeholders (Fossey et al., 2002). In contrast, qualitative research traditions, and particularly participatory inquiry approaches, view knowledge production as a shared process and findings as shared property. Feedback then is considered integral to the research process, being a mechanism for ensuring validity and sharing power in the research relationship (Fossey et al., 2002; Guba & Lincoln, 1989; Patton, 1997). In participatory research, information sharing tends to be iterative, rather than unidirectional. Thus, sharing information with the research participants is an essential part of the research process.

Choosing an Approach to Dissemination

Choosing one's approach to dissemination with participants depends on the nature of the research process, the kind of information generated, and the audience being addressed. The following questions are helpful to consider in developing mechanisms for sharing information about research in these forums:

- What information from this research project could be helpful, or useful to the research participants?
- What methods of information sharing are likely to facilitate respectful and sensitive communication with the research participants?
- What methods of information sharing are most likely to facilitate the research participants' understanding of this research?

- What methods of information sharing are likely to empower the research participants to engage with the material and identify its potential uses/implications for them?
- What resources are available for sharing the findings?

Public Presentations to Consumer and Community Groups, Collaborating Organizations

Research findings may be shared with consumer groups through a variety of channels. One commonly utilized channel for presentation-based dissemination to consumers includes conferences and conventions hosted or co-hosted by consumer interest groups, or by professional organizations that cater to consumer interest groups. For example, the National Fibromyalgia Awareness Campaign and Whole Health co-hosted a conference in Chicago that featured the research findings of medical and rehabilitation professionals who treat individuals with fibromyalgia. Similarly, a biannual, international conference sponsored by the American Association for Chronic Fatigue Syndrome offers a "patient conference day" during which research-based presentations are distinctly tailored to consumers attending the conference. Presentations are selected based on their relevance to patients and clinical utility. Similarly, the International Association of Psychosocial Rehabilitation Services (IAPSRS) in the USA and The Mental Health Services of Australia and New Zealand (The MHS) respectively run integrated conferences that foster mutual dissemination and learning opportunities for consumers, care givers, and professional groups in the mental health field.

A second common means by which research findings may be disseminated to consumers is through more informal, direct presentations to consumers within their own organizational contexts. For example, a researcher might give a presentation at a self-help group meeting, weekly staff meeting, or board meeting of a consumer organization with whom he or she is collaborating. Alternatively, if the consumer group is not a research collaborator, research findings may be shared in a public presentation to inform the consumer/lobby group about findings that have relevant implications (e.g., for quality of life or service delivered). Such presentations may also serve to forge new collaborative relationships with lobby groups and organizations. Recent advances of computer-based tele-health and tele-rehabilitation technologies also allow for public presentations of research findings to be disseminated through online broadcasting and DVDs.

Reports to Government and Private Agencies, Legislative Bodies, and Public Officials

It is not unusual for governmental agencies or bodies to ask for reports of research findings to use in their deliberations as they set policies and make laws. For example, the Office of the Surgeon General may request a report on the prevalence of a given health condition so that appropriate resources can be allocated to prevent. In addition, researchers can offer to make such reports available, even when they are not requested, as a means of facilitating public awareness about a key issue, or in an effort to advocate for increased support and funding for continued research and resources to address a given issue.

The following is an example of dissemination to a government body. The National Institutes for Disability and Rehabilitation Research funded a study to examine the impact of an alternative financing program for disabled persons to obtain loans to finance needed assistive technology. Under this study, two occupational therapy investigators, Hammel and Finlayson, developed a Web-based data management and outcomes system (Hammel, Finlayson, & Lastowski, 2003; Finlayson & Hammel, 2003) to study the impact of the program. They produced annual reports to inform U.S. congressional policymakers about the outcomes of their federal appropriations. The evidence they shared with Congress was used to justify sustaining and expanding the program funding from $3.8 million in 2000 to $35.8 million allocation in 2003. As with this example, dissemination to governmental agencies can have a significant impact in directly influencing policymaking and systems change.

Web Sites, Targeted Brochures, and Other Media for Laypersons

Research that leads to consumer-relevant information and products, such as educational curricula, resource directories, treatment tips, prevention guidelines, and frequently answered questions, can be made available to the public through linkable Web sites, printed brochures or booklets, and computer media. Printed materials are the most easily accessed by individuals capable of reading print, but they are also one of the most expensive and time-consuming to produce and distribute. Computer disks, or CDs, are inexpensive and easy to work with but documents must be converted to universally acceptable formats (e.g., converting files to text-only formats, or using an Adobe file). They offer the advantage of being readily convertible to accessible formats for persons with some kinds of disabilities (e.g., audio-translation by computer software for people with visual impairment). However, they are not yet as appropriate for mass distribution as printed material because they require consumers to have access to computers and computer proficiency.

Web sites are a common means of disseminating research-based information to consumers. Though development of a Web site, or Web page, requires training and knowledge in Web site design and construction, once developed, Web sites are relatively easy to maintain and update. All consumer-based Web sites need to be approved so that they are automatically accessible to individuals with visual and auditory impairments. The "Bobby-approval" is perhaps the most stringent of many available means of evaluating a Web site to ensure that barriers to accessibility are eliminated. Examples of Web site barriers to accessibility include audio messages displayed in the absence of a written transcript (for hearing impairment), or pictures without written descriptions that can be broadcast through an audio device that describes the contents of that picture (for visual impairment). Bobby approval can be accomplished by submitting the Web site address to the following Web site for approval: http://bobby.watchfire.com/bobby/html/en/index.jsp.

Web sites or Web pages that are well designed and easy to navigate are easily accessible by any individual with access to a computer. They also offer the research a greater degree of visibility. One example of a Web site that was designed for accessibility by individuals with chronic fatigue syndrome was developed by the third author: http://www.ahs.uic.edu/ahs/files/ot/bookler/CFS_Website/index.htm.

This Web site is a product of a field-initiated research and demonstration program for individuals with chronic fatigue syndrome funded by the National Institute on Disability and Rehabilitation Research. The Web site contains educational information about chronic fatigue syndrome, a copy of the curriculum used as the basis for the group phase of the rehabilitation program, and a copy of the resource directory that contains information about referrals to medical and legal professionals and other essential information necessary for consumer rights and access to employment, transportation, food, and housing. Both the curriculum and resource directory were co-developed by research staff and participants.

Releases to the Popular Press and Media

Everyone has read, heard on the radio, or seen on television reports of recent research findings considered to have importance for the general public. A number of strategies can be used to foster coverage of occupational therapy research in the popular media. Most medical centers, colleges, and universities have marketing or "public relations" departments whose personnel are responsible for communicating with the press. Working with these communications personnel is typically the best strategy for getting media coverage of research. Nonetheless, individual researchers can directly contact local TV or newspaper health writers to inform them of newsworthy research findings. Sometimes an investigator can foster the potential for media coverage by being responsive to lay requests for information. The following is an example.

Research that led to the development and investigation of a program designed to reduce fear of falling among community-dwelling seniors (Tennstedt et al., 1998) was the subject of a National Public Radio (NPR) broadcast of a story on fear of falling after one of the occupational therapy researchers associated with that program responded to questions posed by a woman who was concerned about her mother. Following the telephone conversation, that woman, who happened to be a health correspondent for NPR, pitched the idea of a story on fear of falling to her editor.

Conclusion

This chapter covered the nature and role of dissemination in research, reviewing a range of options for disseminating research. As stated at the outset, dissemination is an essential component of any inquiry. In this age of information, the options for sharing research are myriad. When the investigator takes seriously the obligation to disseminate

to the various constituencies, who have a right to know about and who could potentially benefit from awareness of the research, it is clear that substantial energy and time must be devoted to dissemination. Without this expenditure of effort, research will not realize its potential value and impact.

REFERENCES

Campbell, M. L., & Schutz, W. V. (2004). *The Research Exchange* (Vol. 9, No. 2). Austin, TX: National Center for the Dissemination of Disability Research, Southwest Educational Development Laboratory.

Finlayson, M., & Hammel, J. (2003). Providing alternative financing for assistive technology: Outcomes over 20 months. *Journal of Disability Policy Studies, 14*(2), 109–118.

Fisher, A. G. (2003). *AMPS Assessment of Motor and Process Skills, Volume 1: Development, standardization and administration manual* (5th ed.). Fort Collins, CO: Three Star Press.

Fossey, E., Epstein, M., Findlay, R., Plant, G., & Harvey, C. (2002). Creating a positive experience of research for people with psychiatric disabilities by sharing feedback. *Psychiatric Rehabilitation Journal, 25*(4), 369–378.

Guba, E. G., & Lincoln, Y. S. (1989). *Fourth generation evaluation.* Newbury Park, CA: SAGE Publications.

Hammel J., Finlayson M., & Lastowski, S. (2003). Using participatory action research to create a shared assistive technology alternative financing outcomes database and to effect social action systems change. *Journal of Disability Policy Studies, 14*(2), 98–108.

Kielhofner, G., Mallinson, T., Crawford, C., Nowak, M., Rigby, M., Henry, A., & Walens, D. (2004). *The Occupational Performance History Interview-II* (version 2.1). Model of Human Occupation Clearinghouse, Department of Occupational Therapy, College of Applied Health Sciences, University of Illinois at Chicago.

McConnell, W. A., & Kerbs, J. J. (1993). Providing feedback in research with human subjects. *Professional Psychology: Research and Practice, 24*(3), 266–270.

Mercier, C., Bordeleau, M., Caron, J., Garcia, A., & Latimer, E. (2004). Conditions facilitating knowledge exchange between rehabilitation and research teams—a study. *Psychiatric Rehabilitation Journal, 28*(1), 55–62.

Patton, M. (1997). *Utilization-focused evaluation.* Beverly Hills, CA: SAGE Publications.

Sieber, J. E. (1992). *Planning ethically responsible research: A guide for students and internal review boards.* Newbury Park, CA: SAGE Publications.

Tennstedt, S., Howland, J., Lachman, M., Peterson, E., Kasten, L., & Jette, A. (1998). A randomized, controlled trial of a group intervention to reduce fear of falling and associated activity restriction in older adults. *Journals of Gerontology Series B-Psychological Sciences & Social Sciences, 53*(6), 384–392.

CHAPTER 35

Writing a Research Report

Gary Kielhofner • Ellie Fossey • Renée R. Taylor

This chapter discusses the process of writing a research report. As noted in Chapter 34, research can be documented in many different formats. Most common is the research article intended for publication in a refereed scientific/professional journal. Consequently, this chapter is organized around creating such a paper. At the same time, the discussion will be useful to the writer who is preparing another type of document such as a research proposal, thesis, or dissertation.[1]

In addition to discussing the content of a research paper, we also address the underlying task of writing. Writing is absolutely necessary for research. Without it, one cannot garner the necessary approval and resources for research. More importantly, without writing, research is not shared with the scientific and professional community. For all practical purposes, an unpublished study never took place. Therefore, anyone who wishes to do research must commit to the task of writing.

Investigators have a wide range of reactions to the obligation of writing. Nonetheless, writing a research report can be a satisfying culmination to the process of inquiry. It is, after all, an opportunity to share one's discovery.

When to Begin Writing

The process of writing a research report should begin when the research is first conceived and continue throughout the investigation. This is a wise approach to writing since the content of a research report mainly follows the sequence of action that is necessary to carry out a study. By writing up a study as one proceeds through it, one not only doc-

uments the unfolding logic and procedures of the study, but also creates material that is eventually integrated into one or more research reports that flow from it.

Structure and Format of a Research Paper

Research papers, or reports, are typically written according to a well-known and defined structure, which includes the following components:

• Abstract,
• Introduction, purpose, and significance,
• Literature review,
• Statement of the research problem,
• Statement of the research question and/or hypotheses,
• Methods (design, sample, procedures),
• Results (findings),
• Discussion, and
• Conclusion.

We briefly discuss each below. While all of these components are similar across topics and methods, there is variability in the style of research papers. Thus, while these components are generally part of a paper reporting research findings, how they are sequenced and integrated into the paper can differ with the discipline, research method of the study, or the journal.

One should seek to identify both the targeted journal or other venue for publication and the intended audience for a paper as soon as possible. Identifying the journal will provide technical information (e.g., page limit, manuscript preparation format) necessary for preparing a final manuscript. Identifying the audience means becoming familiar with:

• Who is likely to read the manuscript,
• What their level and type of knowledge is likely to be, and
• What perspectives they are likely to bring to reading the paper.

This information is essential not only to writing a paper that will be understood by its intended

---

[1]Some graduate programs traditionally required lengthier theses, but it is increasingly recognized that these are not the standard formats in which career researchers report their work. Consequently, more and more programs require the master's thesis presented in the standard format and length of a research paper. Some programs are also following a model for doctoral dissertation work in which the dissertation is composed of "chapters" that are each, in effect, a stand-alone, publishable research report. These reports are either derived from a series of studies that make up the dissertation research, or represent several papers reporting different aspects of the research.

Every journal follows a particular referencing and formatting guideline, often termed an editorial style. Editorial style refers to the set of rules that are followed to ensure that material published in a particular journal is presented consistently.

The most common one used by occupational therapy and related social and behavioral science journals is the American Psychological Association's APA Style. Details about its Publication Manual (American Psychological Association, 2001), as well as information about self-teaching materials for learning APA Style, and guidelines for citing electronic media and creating effective visual materials can be found online at the Web site http://www.apastyle.org/.

Before submitting a manuscript to a journal, one must become knowledgeable about the editorial style required by the journal and ensure that the manuscript submitted adheres to the format in all its details.

audience, but also to its being considered appropriate for publication by the chosen journal.

It is invaluable to read research papers from the journal in which one intends to publish and papers on the same research topic and using the same methods as one is using. When reading, one should pay attention to how each of the components of the research paper is written. This will help one become familiar with subtle but important stylistic and technical differences that characterize different types of research papers. Finally, reading research papers will provide examples of how the components, discussed below, are best organized and incorporated into the paper one plans to write.

The Abstract

An abstract is a summary of the key features of the paper. Arguably, it is the most important part of the paper since its purpose is to enable the reader to decide whether to read the entire paper (Brown, 1996; Hocking & Wallen, 1999). In the end, more people will read an abstract than will go on to read the entire paper.

Abstracts should be written to stand alone, that is, to be understandable without a reading of the entire paper. Moreover, the abstract should convey the main messages of the paper. A good abstract does more than provide readers with an overview of the contents (Brown, 1996). Using phrases such as "the results are described" and "the implications are discussed" is insufficient. Rather, one should succinctly characterize the actual results and their main implications.

An informative abstract will describe the following elements:

* Why the study was conducted/the importance of the research topic,
* What was done in the study,
* Who the subjects/participants were,
* What the main results/findings were, and
* What the implications are for practice, theory, and/or future research (Brown, 1996; Hocking & Wallen, 1999).

When these elements are all included, the abstract will be informative to readers and make it clear what the benefit of reading the entire paper would be (Brown, 1996).

Introduction, Statement of Purpose, Significance

The introduction to a research paper provides the context for what follows in the rest of the paper. In other words, it sets the scene by outlining:

* The area and topic to which the study belongs,
* The nature of the problem or issue being addressed by the study, and
* The relevance of the study to the professional and/or scientific community that is assumed to be the audience for the paper.

The introduction section typically serves to frame the research topic. As such, it may define and discuss key concepts/theory pivotal to understanding the research topic.

The purpose of the paper is generally outlined at the end of the introduction. This statement of purpose may be quite closely related to the aim of the research. However, it should communicate the aim of the paper, rather than that of the overall study, unless the two are exactly the same. Often, however, a research paper will report only one aspect of a larger study. The author(s) will have decided why to present the particular set of findings that will be reported in the paper. It is this rationale that constitutes the aim of the paper, and which will be more specific than the aim of the overall study.

The introduction will also often include a statement of the significance of the study, although this element can also be included as part of the conclusion of a literature review. Wherever the significance is noted, it should address the question of why the study needed to be done. Thomas (2000) suggests that a significance statement should be phrased along the following lines: "The problem I am studying affects lots of people in a particularly unfortunate way and/or costs a lot of money"

Abstracts, like entire research reports, can vary in their format according to the methods used in the study. Below are two examples of abstracts. The first is from a quantitative study and the second is from a qualitative study.

Abstract by Roche and Taylor (2005)

Existing studies have shown that individuals with chronic fatigue syndrome (CFS) demonstrate functional impairment in a number of domains related to occupational participation. Researchers have not yet explored whether coping styles may be associated with occupational participation in individuals with this condition. The aim of this study was to examine the effects of coping styles on occupational participation among adults with CFS. We hypothesized that occupational participation would be associated with coping strategies oriented toward information seeking and maintaining activity, and that this relationship would endure despite individual differences in illness severity. The study used a cross-sectional design to describe the associations between coping and occupational participation for 47 individuals diagnosed with CFS. Findings from linear regression analysis revealed that the coping style of maintaining activity was positively associated with occupational participation whereas accommodating to the illness was negatively associated. Implications of the findings for continued research and clinical practice in occupational therapy are discussed.

Abstract by Farnworth, Nitikin, and Fossey (2004)

Institutional environments are challenging settings in which to provide rehabilitation. This study describes the time use of a group of inpatients, the majority diagnosed with schizophrenia, in a secure forensic psychiatric unit in Australia. Time diaries, interviews, and field notes were collected over 5 weeks. Eight participants completed time diaries for 2 consecutive days, of whom five were also interviewed using the Occupational Performance History Interview-II.

Participants' time use was dominated by personal care and leisure occupations. In general, participants were dissatisfied with their time use, describing themselves as "bored" or "killing time." Many perceived that the environment created barriers to their participation in valued occupations, yet some also found occupations that provided solace, challenge, or connection with the outside world.

The findings indicate the importance of understanding individuals' unique occupational histories, interests, and skills to create opportunities to engage them in relevant occupations that utilize personal resources, as part of forensic rehabilitation programs, and the utility of the Occupational Performance History Interview-II in this context. Further research exploring patient and staff perspectives on the challenges of occupational programming in forensic settings and the longitudinal impact of such programming on inpatients' occupational functioning, health, and well-being is recommended.

(p. 35). In essence, then, the significance of a study is the underlying reason that it was important to undertake the study.

Literature Review

A literature review is a critical evaluation of existing literature relevant to the topic under study (DePoy & Gitlin, 1993). A good literature review informs, evaluates, and integrates relevant existing literature (Thomas, 2000). If the literature review is done well, it will make apparent to the reader how the research was a logical next step in building knowledge and/or how the research fills a critical gap in an area of knowledge (DePoy & Gitlin, 1993). Thus, in writing the literature review for a research paper, it is important to make sure that it is organized so as to tell a story, or provide an

argument that leads directly to the research question and study. A literature review that simply reports previous research is inadequate.

Before one begins a study, a review of the literature is undertaken to identify what is already known about a topic and the methods with which it is typically studied. The purpose of that initial literature review is formative—that is, it helps shape the development of the research plan. Generally, much of the literature reviewed initially will be incorporated into the literature review written for the research report. If the report presents a subset of the study findings relevant to a narrower topic than the overall study topic, then the review will also tend to be more narrowly focused than the original literature review.

Before preparing the literature review for a research paper, the investigator should update the original literature review with any newly published relevant research and/or theory. If one is preparing to report an aspect of the findings from a large study, the nature of particular findings may need to be framed with different literature than that originally reviewed in planning the study. Such a review is undertaken to appropriately context the particular findings that will be reported in the paper. This kind of review typically is related to the initial literature review, but may focus in one area in more depth, or it may pursue a topic related to the initial literature review that was not originally examined. Both quantitative and qualitative research may produce results/findings that require the investigator to review a new body of literature to prepare a report.

The major tasks in preparing and writing a literature review, therefore, are to locate, critically appraise, and then summarize the previous research relevant to the topic. One should address the issues and controversies that are raised in the literature, and identify the gaps in the current knowledge base that provide the rationale for the research and its design. Brown (1996) poses seven questions that should be answered in writing a review of literature for a research paper:

• Why is this topic important?
• What is known about the topic?
• What is unknown about this topic?
• Why are some things unknown?
• Why should the gaps be filled?
• Which gaps does one propose to fill and has one chosen them?
• How does one propose to fill them?

In the literature review section of a research paper, it will not be possible to discuss the full scope and volume of literature on the research topic. The aim of a literature review is not to demonstrate the breadth and depth of the investigator's knowledge of the literature. Rather the aim is to address the above questions and, in so doing, to make apparent the underlying logic for undertaking the study.

Both accurate representation and critical appraisal of the literature are important to an effective literature review. Critical appraisal will:

• Identify the current trends and ways of thinking about the topic and how to research it,
• Identify the boundaries of the literature (e.g., what particular populations, settings, and perspectives were studied in the previous research?),
• Illuminate the gaps in the current knowledge base and the way in which it has developed,

• Evaluate the strengths and weakness of existing research approaches to studying the topic, and
• Make an argument for why any conflicting or differing research findings exist (if they exist).

DePoy and Gitlin (1993) suggest the following structure for organizing a literature review:

• Introduction, defining the focus and scope of the review,
• Discussion of each specific concept, principle, or theory in the current literature on the topic,
• Brief overview of key studies, compared in parallel rather than serially to achieve a critical appraisal of the current research,
• Integration of the work reviewed, identifying the relationships, inconsistencies among findings across studies, controversies, and gaps in the literature,
• Identification of the niche in the current knowledge base that your research fills, and
• Justification/rationale for the study and its design.

These components are typical of many literature reviews, but it should be remembered that the review is designed to characterize the content of literature that is relevant to the topic, and that makes sense of the chosen question and research methods. Thus, there are instances in which the state of the literature, or the nature of the research question, may dictate a somewhat different structure. For example, if a study examines something for which little or no previous research is reported, the literature review may focus on providing the rationale for the importance of the topic area or extrapolate from literature that is only partly related to the research question. Also, some journals have formats that require literature to be succinctly reviewed as part of the introduction, rather than as a separate section. In these cases, the review may be structured differently, but still needs to appraise the key literature of relevance.

Statement of Research/Scholarly Problem

An explicit statement of the nature of problem being addressed by the study tells the reader why this research is important. In other words, it lets readers know why they should care about the research reported in the paper. For this reason, the statement of the research problem is best located early in the paper, generally in the introduction. In journal formats that allow separate introduction and literature review sections, the problem area may be more broadly outlined in the introduction, and the specific nature of problem more narrowly defined in the conclusion of the literature review.

Statement of Research/Scholarly Aim, Questions, and/or Hypotheses

All research inquiry is guided by its aim and the specific research question(s) or hypotheses being addressed. Hence, a statement of the research aim accompanied by the question(s) and/or hypotheses allows the reader to understand the researcher's intentions behind designing a study in a particular way. In research papers, this statement is typically contained in the conclusion of the literature review since it is supported by the reader's conclusions from appraising the literature. In some journal formats, however, it is expected that the research question(s) or hypotheses are stated as part of the study design.

Methods: Design, Procedure of Study, Sample, and Analysis

The methods section of a research paper contains a succinct description of the research design. The aim of this section is to provide adequate detail to enable the reader to understand what was done and how. This part of the paper allows the reader to determine the degree of rigor in the study procedures, and provides information that is essential for replicating the study.

This section of the paper is often challenging to write since the limits on page length in journals generally allow only the most key elements of the research to be described. The following elements are typically included in the methods section:

- A description of the fundamental design of the study,
- A statement of the ethical approval and procedures (for studies involving human subjects),
- A description of the sampling procedure (whose participation was sought and how),
- A statement of the number of participants and depiction of their salient characteristics (in some types of studies, this element is reported in the results/findings section),
- A description of any experimental procedures and equipment used,
- A description of the methods for data collection and how they were used (e.g., tests, interviews, observations), along with a discussion of their suitability for the study and evidence of their adequacy (validity and reliability), and
- An explanation of the data analysis procedures.

How these elements are described in a particular research paper will depend on the actual methods used. For example, when an investigator has used a well-known quantitative design and common statistical analyses, it may be sufficient simply to name the design and analysis technique with minimal details about its use in the study. On the other hand, a qualitative study in which the methods were constructed as the study unfolded, or a study with a more unconventional or innovative research element, may require much more explication for the reader to grasp what was actually done.

Results or Findings

This section of a research paper informs the reader about the most salient discoveries of the study. Whether one uses the term results or findings depends to an extent on the type of study done as well as the journal preference. As a rule, the term results is more typically used with quantitative studies and findings in reporting qualitative findings. How the results/findings are presented also depends to a large extent on the method of the study.

Quantitative study results are generally presented through a combination of text, statistics, summary tables, and figures. Quantitative figures provide visual representation of data such as histograms, plots, and charts. They are generally organized according to the questions or hypotheses posed.

Qualitative findings are generally text-based. They usually incorporate depictions of themes or a narrative depiction of the nature of the finding, supplemented with evidence from the study, such as quotes from interviewees or observations from fieldnotes. The use of these data serves to illustrate a theme or demonstrating a concept in such as way as to deepen the reader's appreciation or understanding. Qualitative reports may also include tables, which usually contain textual information, or figures to illustrate a finding.

Tables and figures that are used to present results/findings should be self-contained and complementary to the text. In some cases, they contain information that is not specifically stated in the text. In other cases, they amplify or serve as another way of representing findings that are discussed in the text. Tables and figures are used when they are more efficient and succinct in presenting results/findings and when they are likely to add to the reader's comprehension of the results/findings.

The interpretation of results/findings also depends on the nature of the study being presented. A rule of thumb for quantitative results is that interpretation should not extend beyond what the data indicate. So, interpretation serves to clarify the findings. It should not evaluate the data. In qualitative research, interpretation is much more interwoven into the presentation of the findings because the author(s) of the study are serving as guides to allow the reader to comprehend the reality of the phenomena studied.

Discussion and Conclusion

The discussion and conclusion may be two separate sections offered in sequence at the end of the paper, or they may be presented as a single section that covers all the elements discussed below. The purpose of the discussion in a research paper is to consider the meaning and significance of the results/findings. This means both:

- Examining the findings in relation to the study question(s) and its purpose advanced in the literature review, and
- Considering the findings in light of the results of previously published studies.

The discussion section does not recount the results themselves. However, it serves to interpret or further explain the meaning or implications of the findings. Moreover the discussion will typically offer evaluative statements about the findings/results, noting the strength of the evidence or how compelling it is. The discussion may also draw together or synthesize different aspects of the findings. Finally, the discussion should draw the reader's attention to the salient similarities and differences between the reported results and those from previous studies and to the factors. It should seek to account for these similarities and differences.

A research paper is usually concluded with some discussion of the theoretical and practice implications of the results, the limitations of the research, and recommended avenues for further research. When it is well written, this section can highlight the key lessons to be learned from the research for the reader, guide the reader in weighing the strengths and limitations of the research, and suggest an agenda and directions for further research to the reader. In other words, its impor-

tance lies in providing the researcher with an opportunity to explicitly tell readers how they might use the information gained from this research for themselves in practice, or in further research (Brown, 1994).

Summary

The previous sections discussed the main elements that ordinarily make up a research report. As noted at the outset and highlighted throughout the discussion, these elements can be woven into a research report in a variety of ways. What is emphasized and how it is organized in a paper depends on the type of research being reported, the methods used, and, to an extent, the topic of the research. As stressed earlier, there is no substitution for becoming familiar with how articles on the research topic, using similar methods and/or published in the intended journal are composed, as preparation for writing one's own research report.

Selecting a Venue for Publication

Writing for publication is essentially a task of communication with a specific audience.

Therefore, as already emphasized, knowing one's expected audience is crucial to effective communication of one's research in written form. Academic and professional scholarly journals target different readerships, and so it is important to identify one or two suitable journals at an early stage. One, then, writes so as to speak to the journal's readers.

Selecting the wrong journal can result in the rejection of a paper (see Chapter 34 for a discussion of the review process) that would otherwise be acceptable for another journal. Moreover, if one does not pay attention to the guidelines of a journal or the way in which articles are typically written for that journal, the likelihood of having to make major revisions to an article is greater.

> Writing for publication is essentially a task of communication with a specific audience.

Criteria for Selecting a Journal

Journals differ according to their level of rigor, their subject matter and/or intended audience, and sometimes their preference for methodology.

There is no magic formula for selecting an appropriate journal. Overall, the strategy should consider two main factors. The first is whom the author wishes to be the audience. For instance, if a study has a strong applied focus and the author wishes it to have an impact on practice, then a professional journal is probably a wise choice. If communicating with interdisciplinary colleagues might make more impact on practice, then an interdisciplinary journal might be a good choice. On the other hand, if the study contributes new knowledge to understanding the nature of a specific problem or diagnosis, then the author may wish to consider a journal that focuses on that problem or diagnosis.

The second factor that needs to be considered is the fit between one's study and the anticipated paper with the characteristics of the journal. To assess this fit, it can help to ask the following questions:

- Is the rigor of the study being reported consistent with the level expected for this journal?
- Does this journal typically publish articles on the topic of this study?
- Does this journal publish studies with the kind of sample in this study (as defined by such factors as age or disability)?
- Does this journal publish studies that use the kind of methods employed in this study?
- Does this journal emphasize applied, basic, or participatory research and, if so, how does this emphasis fit with the study?
- Does this journal have restrictions on article length that will affect how well the study can be presented?

These questions can be answered by examining the journal's statement of mission, editorial statements that indicate the special focus or emphasis of the journal, and guidelines for manuscript submission. It is equally helpful to examine the typical content of articles in the journal. If in reading a selection of recent articles in that journal, one finds articles of a similar nature to the planned paper, then the journal is probably a good choice.

The Writing Process

Writing research papers is a skill that can be learned and maintained through deliberate and regular practice.

This section describes strategies that can be used to become and remain an effective writer. While writing is a creative process, it requires deliberate and disciplined management of several interrelated tasks (Brown, 1994). Figure 35.1 illustrates some of the range of tasks to be managed by the writer.

People often try to manage writing from the bottom up, that is, by focusing on the least complex tasks of writing shown at the bottom of Figure 35.1, such as grammar, language use, punctuation, and so forth. However, it is more effective to take a top down approach to writing, attending to the more complex tasks earlier in the writing process. Doing so will tend to lead to a more coherent, readable, and engaging writing style.

Writing Strategies

The following are key strategies for anyone who wishes to become an effective research writer:

- Setting aside and structuring time for writing,
- Discovering and developing one's own writing style and habits,
- Writing for a particular audience,
- Clarifying one's focus,
- Drafting, sequencing, and rewriting, and
- Seeking and using feedback.

Each of these strategies is briefly discussed below.

Setting Aside and Structuring Time

Writing takes time. Most writers find that they require large blocks of time to focus on writing. Hence, there is no substitute for structuring one's schedule to include regular writing time. These blocks of time should be periods when one is alert and able to attend to the writing task. Scheduling writing in one's spare time, when one is tired or easily distracted, will only invite frustration. It can also be helpful to allocate less optimal or smaller blocks of time for the more mundane or concrete aspects of writing (i.e., those tasks nearer the bottom of Figure 35.1).

Discovering and Developing One's Own Writing Style and Habits

While some things are essential to all writing, it is also a highly personal process. Individuals who are experienced and successful writers have paid

> Writing research papers is a skill that can be learned and maintained through deliberate and regular practice.

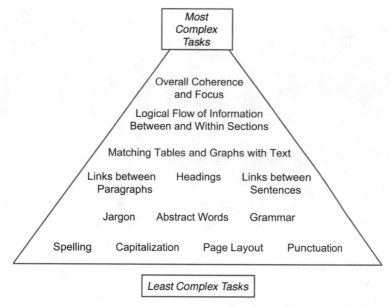

Figure 35.1 The hierarchy of tasks that writers need to master in managing the writing process. (Adapted from Brown [1994, p. 4].)

attention to and developed their own writing style and habits. This includes consideration of such factors as what are optimal times and contexts for writing, and what is the best way to organize resource materials.

Writing requires discipline. Anyone who has done substantial writing will admit that a key element is following through on planned time and making oneself focus during scheduled writing time. In scheduling writing times and tasks, one should take into consideration what times of the day/week are best for one to concentrate on the writing task and how long one can effectively write. Some people write better earlier in the day, whereas others prefer late at night. Some persons can write at a variety of times.

One should assess how long one can write optimally. Some people can write for only an hour or two. Others can write for an entire day. Some persons require frequent breaks, whereas others want to stay focused throughout the writing. Knowing and respecting one's own writing patterns is vital. It is important to pay attention to when one gets the most writing done and when one has difficulty writing, and then to plan one's schedule accordingly.

It is also useful to structure one's writing time. Some people find it helpful to set short-terms goals for the next hour or day such as writing so many pages or finishing a particular section of a paper. Some people find it best to write for a period and then review what was written, revise, and go on to the next task. Once again, it is important to identify and use what works best.

An often underestimated element is finding the right context for writing. Scientific writing conjures up images of some quiet corner in a library, but such a context does not work for everyone. Some persons need quiet space; others write effectively with background noise or music. In the end, if a writer discovers ways to make the writing process enjoyable and fulfilling, it will require less effort to motivate oneself to write and the routine of writing will be easier to sustain.

Most of the time, we write with resources that have been accumulated over time. These materials include such things as articles accumulated for a literature review, notes taken from reading, and boilerplates (i.e., previously written materials that are edited and incorporated into papers). Organizing these materials in ways that optimize one's writing style will facilitate efficient writing. For instance, one of the authors of this chapter prefers to take notes in a laptop computer while reading and then uses those notes later when composing a chapter. This author tends to begin writing while reading. This author also typically works on several articles or chapters at a time and maintains a folder for each work in process in the computer. That way, notes, references, and other materials can be inserted in the folder whenever new information or new thoughts about a work in progress arise. When writing, the author takes all these resources and weaves them together into an

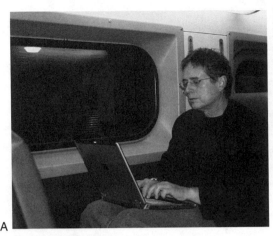

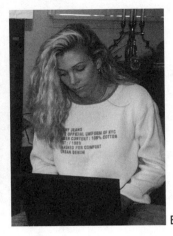

A

B

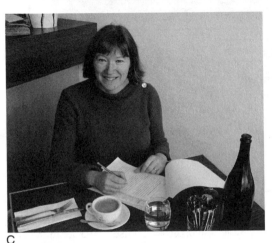

C

Figure 35.2 (A) Gary writes effectively in a variety of places and times. One of his most productive times for writing is during the daily commute to and from Chicago on the train. It provides over 2 hours a day of time away from interruptions. For him, the background noise helps him concentrate since he is unable to write in silence. (B) Renée writes best in a comfortable and quiet environment with large chunks of time. She needs relatively frequent short breaks. Writing in front of the fireplace in winter and in a sunny spot in the yard during summer works well for her. (C) Ellie writes drafts on computer at home or work, but prefers to rework the structure of material, or to edit it on paper. Her favorite venues for editing are her local neighborhood cafes in Melbourne with the music and activity of the café going on around her.

"organic" document that generally gets revised multiple times, often quite dramatically as it evolves into the final written manuscript.

Another of the authors prefers to first read, surrounded by hard copies of the readings, highlighting aspects of the readings that are important. Then, the author outlines the plan of the manuscript and proceeds to write the paper progressively from beginning to end, thinking carefully about each section of the manuscript as it is being written and doing most of the rewriting along the way. Once finished with a paper or manuscript, the author seeks feedback and then generally completes one overall rewrite before the paper is finished.

These differences in writing are matters of personal style that a new writer must discover through experimentation. Of course, writing style will also vary somewhat according to what one is writing, how familiar the topic is, and how tight a deadline one is facing. Respect for one's style, tempered with practical considerations of getting the task done, is a wise course.

When collaborating on papers, it is a good idea to discuss writing styles and figure out how they can be meshed over the course of working together. For example, one of us has found discussion, written comments, electronic editing, and time spent working together on the computer to each be effective at different stages in the process of writing collaboratively with colleagues. Sometimes, of course, this is not possible. For instance, this chapter was written without any face-to-face discussion among the authors. Each person took turns working on the manuscript, which was shared by e-mail.

Writing for a Particular Audience

No scientific article will be readily understood or interesting to everyone. Readers bring to a written piece their own training and knowledge and their sense of what is important. The sole purpose of writing is to communicate with readers. This may seem obvious, but it requires one to read one's writing from the imagined perspective of the reader. Writers, of course, understand their own writing since it is an outpouring of what they know. Readers, however, do not know what the writer knows and, thus, the paper needs to be written and edited with the reader's perspective in mind.

Thus, the writing and rewriting process begins with a sense of one's audience, including their knowledge base, interests, and expectations. Writers who do not consider their intended audience will inevitably be frustrated with rejected papers or requests for substantial rewriting. Hence, as previously noted, one should identify who one's audience is at the outset. Having done so, it is important to read one's own writing and rewriting from the perspective of that intended audience (Brown, 1994).

It takes some practice to develop this skill of reading your own work from another's perspective. Nonetheless, it is a skill worth cultivating. It can help to think of three or four specific people who are potential readers of your work, and to write and read your work with them in mind. It may also be useful to seek someone who represents that audience to give feedback, as a way of getting a sense of how the intended audience will approach your writing. In doing so, one should pay careful attention not only to the implications for a given paper, but also to how the person approaches the paper. This helps one develop the sense of what it means to pay attention to an audience.

Clarifying One's Focus

Clarifying the main message of an intended paper will:

- Make the writing task more efficient, and
- Result in a paper that is easier for readers to understand (Brown, Rogers, & Pressland, 1993, 1994).

This advice sounds deceptively simple. Typically researchers find themselves with much more information then they can include in a single research report. Thus, they must make challenging decisions about what to include in their papers, what to leave out, and how to organize the information reported. Lack of clarity about the focus of a paper can create difficulty in making these decisions.

Mind-Mapping and Abstracting

Based on their experiences of running workshops for researchers about how to write papers, Brown and his colleagues (1993, 1994) recommend two strategies that are helpful in creating a clear focus:

- Mind-mapping to distill the main message, and
- Developing a working abstract as a framework for the first draft of a paper.

Mind-mapping and similar techniques, such as concept-mapping, involve generating and refining a visual representation of the ideas to be contained in a paper (Bihl-Hulme, 1985; Brown et al., 1994; Buzan & Buzan, 2000).

The process begins with laying out on paper a detailed free-form diagram of all the facts, ideas, thoughts, questions, and linkages that could go into a paper. One then identifies the most important parts of the mind-map by assigning priorities to the information contained in it (Brown et al., 1994). This process allows one to more readily see the relationships or connections between materials, and to identify the material of most importance to the topic. Mind-mapping also helps to define the boundaries of a paper, letting one decide what not to include (Brown et al., 1994).

To further clarify the main message it is often helpful to generate a brief (approximately 25-word) working abstract from the mind-map. The discipline of this word limit is useful to creating a clear focus! This abstract should not be confused with the abstract that is written for publication. Rather, it is a mission statement that guides one's writing process. The contents may, indeed, go into the final abstract in some form, but the purpose of writing an abstract as part of this process is to make sure one has clear in one's own mind what is being written.

The use of outlines is often recommended as a tool for structuring written papers and organizing the material within them, but they can be difficult to create when one is not clear what the paper is going to be about. Clarifying the main message and creating a working abstract can provide the foundation for creating an outline. The priorities identified in the mind-map often yield the section headings and subheadings for an outline.

Finding One's Story

Mind-mapping will not work for all writers and it probably works better for visual thinkers. Other writers may find it more helpful to think about the paper as a story. A research paper basically involves telling the story of how one came up with the research question and went about answering it in the research process, and then revealing the answers obtained.

In this case, one needs to identify the basic plot of the story. The plot involves a beginning, middle, and end that flow together into a whole. Each part of the writing contributes to the unfolding of the story.

Inspiration

Most writers will publicly say they don't believe in inspiration, pointing out rightly that writing simply takes hard work. However, almost every writer will have at least one good story about the time he or she was stumped and couldn't figure out how to pull together a paper or present a particular argument. Then, suddenly in the middle of the night, in the midst of taking a shower, or while driving home, the solution came in a flash. The writer could suddenly see how to put it all together.

We have heard enough such stories (and have some of our own) to assert that inspiration can definitely be a part of writing. The problem with inspiration is that one can't will it. However, there are some things a writer can do to enhance the possibility of getting the sudden vision that makes everything clearer:

Do your homework: Inspiration does not come to those who don't do the basics first. If inspiration is anything, it's the synthesis of many elements or pieces of information into a higher order whole. However, if you have not fully immersed yourself in the various informational components, the synthesis will never come. Reading thoroughly and carefully in order to become knowledgeable and organizing concepts and information in some fashion are necessary foundations.

Take a break at critical times: Writing tempts many of us to take frequent breaks. Nothing inspires us to check out the weather, see if we have anything in our e-mail inbox, or even clean out the refrigerator more than staring at a blank computer screen or an empty piece of paper. However, that's not the type of break we are suggesting. When writers have spent effort over an extended time organizing volumes of materials and writing different pieces of a paper, they have a difficult time seeing the proverbial forest for the trees. At such times, it can sometimes be useful to step away form the writing for a short period (from a day or two to perhaps a week or so). One should not leave the writing so long as to let memory fade about the contents or it will take additional work to get restarted. However, stepping back from the immediate writing task to reflect on the paper and let thoughts percolate as they occur can sometimes be the catalyst for a new insight or inspiration.

There are also ways of way of taking a break without losing momentum. One way is to work on some of the less intellectually demanding tasks of writing such as double checking one's references or updating a literature search. Another way is to switch to writing another paper. Many investigators who are working on more than a single investigation or paper find that when they hit a wall writing one paper, it can be productive to switch to another.

Seek someone's opinion: Talking to someone about one's paper is often a very helpful strategy. Sometimes inspiration comes in the form of some solid advice. Other times, the act of discussing one's writing and, in particular, the problem one is trying to resolve, helps to clarify what one is really having difficulty with and that, in turn, leads to identification of a solution to the writing puzzle.

To use this approach, one should write out the story in as few words as possible. In a sense, it's like creating the abstract. However, it is a good idea to create the story for a layperson. One can imagine, for instance, how one would explain to one's mother or to a friend what the paper is about. This requires one to pare down everything to a fairly simple story line.

Once one is able to articulate the story in straightforward terms, deciding what to include and leave out is facilitated. Moreover, determining the best way to chunk the successive parts of the story and link them together becomes easier. As with the mind-mapping technique, one can create a more effective and integrated outline once one is clear about the underlying story.

Drafting, Sequencing, and Revising

For most authors, writing typically involves a substantial number of drafts to refine the content, to enhance the synthesis of ideas in a paper, and improve the organization of information to communicate effectively with readers. This is because writing is itself a learning process and the more one learns about the topic, the more effectively one can write about it. Successive drafts tend to get better because one is more knowledgeable.

The process of writing is also not linear. The typical structure of research papers as outlined earlier may constitute a sequential series of writing tasks. However, one does not necessarily begin at the beginning when writing a research paper.

For instance, working first on sections that are more straightforward can help one make more effective progress. The methods section is typically one of the more straightforward to write, followed by results section. This is because in these sections one is describing what one has done and found, these being the most familiar parts of the story one is telling.

The introduction and discussion require a greater degree of abstraction and interpretation to frame the story of one's research for the reader.

Consequently, these sections may be easier to write at a later stage, once the main body of the paper is complete. The introduction, in particular, is more straightforward to write once one is clear about what is being introduced

Although there are different styles of writing and rewriting, redrafting sections in parallel, rather than sequentially, often helps to achieve better structural and conceptual integration. It also helps to ensure consistency in writing style and language use through the paper. Every paper should be read at least once as a whole with an eye toward editing it to be a more integrated piece.

Seeking and Using Feedback

Seeking feedback by having others read and comment on drafts of a paper can be very helpful. Writers always know more about what they want to say than do their readers. Consequently, when rereading one's own work, it is easy to make mental assumptions and linkages that are not in the paper or apparent to the reader. Constructive feedback from someone else can help to identify assumed knowledge, missing links, and unanswered questions that a reader may have. Such feedback is extremely helpful for redrafting a paper.

There are different ways to get feedback on a paper. The following are some examples:

• Coaching from an experienced writer in one's discipline/area of research (someone who knows the topic, the intended audience and journal). This type of reviewer may provide feedback paragraph by paragraph on technical aspects of the writing, as well as on larger issues central to research, such as how to articulate the rationale or methods.
• Participating in writing groups with peers. This process is helpful for developing overall writing skills since one not only receives feedback but also learns from reading and critiquing others' writing. Also, by mutually agreeing on deadlines for writing part or all of a manuscript, writers can help each other maintain discipline in writing.
• Asking for feedback from colleagues with differing disciplines or professional backgrounds who reflect the targeted audience. This type of feedback can be valuable in helping one step outside of familiar ways of presenting things and point out when papers are too full of jargon or insider perspectives. This type of feedback is especially useful when one is aiming for publication in an interdisciplinary journal.

An important form of feedback also comes as part of the review process following submission of a paper for consideration for publication. Written comments prepared by referees for authors are intended to provide constructive feedback about the content, structure, and presentation of the manuscript, and to guide the authors in subsequent revision of their manuscripts. Revisions are almost always required, so being asked to make some revisions should not be taken by authors as an indication that a manuscript is of poor quality. Authors are well advised to pay careful attention to the referees' comments and recommendations in revising a manuscript.

If a journal decides not to accept a manuscript for publication, one should carefully examine the feedback. Rejection may mean the paper does not rise to the level of quality necessary for publication. It may mean that one needs to submit the paper to another journal. Generally, it is necessary also to revise the manuscript to address the new journal's style and format requirements, to ensure the writing "speaks" to the new readership, and to improve the manuscript on the basis of feedback from the previous submission. Attending carefully to the referees' feedback and seeking advice, or coaching, from colleagues with publishing experience can often be helpful at this stage.

Conclusion

This chapter presented the process of writing a report of research. It discussed both the usual content that goes into such a paper and the process of writing itself. As noted at the outset, many investigators thoroughly enjoy the writing process. Even those who find it very enjoyable know that good writing takes time and effort, and requires personal discipline, persistence, and an openness to criticism and feedback.

REFERENCES

American Psychological Association (2001). *Publication manual of the American Psychological Association* (5th ed.). Washington, DC: Author.

Bihl-Hulme, J. (1985). Creative thinking in problem-based learning. In D. Bond (Ed.), *Problem-based learning in education for the professions* (pp. 177–183). Sydney, Australia: HERDSA.

Brown, R. (1994). The "big picture" about managing writing. In O. Zuber-Skerritt & Y. Ryan (Eds.), *Quality in postgraduate education—Issues and processes* (pp. 90–109). London: Kogan Page.

Brown, R. (1996). *Key skills for writing and publishing research* (3rd ed.). Brisbane, Australia: WriteWay Consulting.

Brown, R. F., Rogers, D. J., & Pressland, A. J. (1993). Righting scientific writing: Focus on your main message! *Rangelands Journal, 15*(2), 183–189.

Brown, R. F., Rogers, D. J., & Pressland, A. J. (1994). Create a clear focus: the 'big picture' about writing better research articles. *American Entomologist, 40,* 144–145.

Buzan, T., & Buzan, B. (2000). *The mind map book* (3rd ed.). London: BBC Worldwide.

DePoy, E., & Gitlin, L. N. (1993). *Introduction to research: Multiple strategies for health and human services*. St. Louis: C. V. Mosby.

Farnworth, L., Nitikin, L. & Fossey, E. (2004). Being in a secure forensic psychiatry unit: Every day's the same, killing time or making the most of it. *British Journal of Occupational Therapy, 67*(10), 430–438.

Hocking, C & Wallen, M (1999). *Australian Occupational Therapy Journal Manual for referees: Guidelines to assist referees and authors review manuscripts.* Melbourne, Australia: OT AUSTRALIA.

Roche, R., & Taylor, R. R. (2005) Coping and occupational participation in chronic fatigue syndrome. *Occupational Therapy Journal of Research 25,* 75–83.

Thomas, S. A. (2000). *How to write health sciences papers, dissertations and theses*. Edinburgh: Churchill Livingston

RESOURCES

Brown, R. (1996). *Key skills for writing and publishing research* (3rd ed.). Brisbane, Australia: WriteWay Consulting.

Hayes, R. L. (1996). Writing for publication: solutions to common problems. *Australian Occupational Therapy Journal, 43,* 24–29.

Thomas, S. A. (2000). *How to write health sciences papers, dissertations and theses*. Edinburgh: Churchill Livingston

C H A P T E R   3 6

Assessing Need for Services

Marcia Finlayson

Every day, occupational therapists are faced with determining if an individual client has a problem or set of problems that could be remediated through occupational therapy services and, if so, which intervention would be the most appropriate to apply. Consequently, practitioners are well versed in how to assess the needs of individual clients, translate these needs into intervention goals, assess progress toward goals, and determine when discharge should occur. Equally important is the process of identifying the needs of broader groups of people in order to develop or modify services, programs, and policies and their respective goals. This process is a requirement for occupational therapists who are:

- Developing new areas of practice,
- Expanding services within existing settings,
- Examining ways to allocate limited resources to best meet the needs of a particular client base, or
- Trying to advocate for policy changes that will affect entire populations.

To succeed in these broader types of activities, occupational therapy practitioners and researchers must have a basic but solid grounding in the theories and methods of needs assessment. This foundation must include the knowledge and skills that are necessary to conduct high-quality needs assessments, and the ability to work with others to translate findings into action. Therefore, the objectives of this chapter are to:

- Provide a theoretical overview of the concept of need,
- Examine the processes and dimensions of a needs assessment,
- Describe and compare models and approaches to needs assessment,
- Evaluate methods commonly used in needs assessments, and
- Outline how needs can be translated into actions for solutions.

What Is a Needs Assessment?

The term *needs assessment* is commonly used and seemingly easy to understand. At the most basic level, it refers to the process of determining what a group of individuals, an organization, a community, or a population requires to achieve some basic standard or to improve its current situation. Reviere, Berkowitz, Carter, and Ferguson (1996) describe a needs assessment as "a systematic and ongoing process of providing useable and useful information about the needs of the target population – to those who can and will utilize it to make judgments about policy and programs" (p. 6). Consequently, a needs assessment is simultaneously a form of applied research and a political process (Hancock & Minkler, 1997; Martí-Costa & Serano-García, 1983). Needs assessments vary across four dimensions: the sophistication of the project design, the level of involvement of the stakeholders, its political orientation, and the scope of the issue being addressed (see Figure 36.1).

Dimension 1: Sophistication of the Project Design

As a form of applied research, needs assessments range in quality and rigor, just like any other form of research. This variability is reflected in the first dimension of a needs assessment: the sophistication of the project design. To accurately inform judgments about policies and programs, and ultimately the allocation of resources, the ideal needs assessment is one that is rigorously designed. This means that it takes into account all of the key components of a high-quality study—clearly defined questions that are grounded in theory, appropriate sampling, psychometrically sound data collection tools and processes, and correctly applied analytic strategies. As previous authors have noted, needs assessments should be:

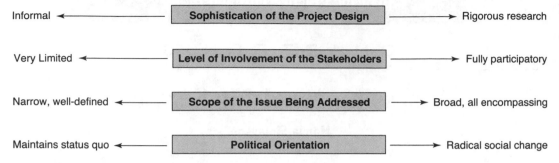

Figure 36.1 Dimensions of a needs assessment.

• Systematic,
• Empirically based,
• Outcome oriented, and
• Focused on solving real-world problems through the application of a variety of research methodologies and methods (Reviere et al., 1996; Witkin & Altschuld, 1995).

Often, though, the term *needs assessment* is used loosely for projects that are little more than informal questioning of convenient individuals with little to no rigor or possibility of replication.

As a political process, needs assessments are value laden, focus on collectives rather than individuals, and raise awareness of everyday problems and their causes. They seek to mobilize communities into action in order to influence and inform policymaking, infrastructure changes, and human and financial resource management and distribution (Martí-Costa & Serano-García, 1983). Through these processes, the ultimate goal of a needs assessment is to gather meaningful data to inform actions that build on community strengths and remediate any problems that are uncovered (Kretzmann & McKnight, 1997; Witkin & Altschuld, 1995). As such, two additional dimensions of a needs assessment are the level of involvement of stakeholders and its political orientation.

Dimension 2: Level of Involvement of Stakeholders

Stakeholders are the individuals, organizations, and policymakers who have a role in defining the issues and/or addressing the concerns that arise from the needs assessment process. Witkin and Altschuld (1995) conceptualize stakeholders at three levels—individuals who are receiving services, the providers of services, and organizations as a whole. An example of these different levels may include older adults who have experienced a stroke, the occupational therapists who provide

services to these individuals, and the hospital that employs the therapists. It is important to realize that stakeholders can also include individuals and organizations associated with the individuals in each of these three levels. For example, additional stakeholders could include families, friends, other professionals providing services (e.g., physical therapy, social work), organizations to which clients are referred on discharge (e.g., home care, stroke support group), and insurance companies.

A needs assessment that is fully participatory would seek input and direction from all three levels of stakeholders at all points during the assessment process (e.g., setting the question, determining the methods, collecting data, etc.). This type of needs assessment would draw on the principles of community building (Minkler, 1997) and participatory action research (Reason & Bradbury, 2001). (See Chapters 38–40.)

Involvement of stakeholders in the needs assessment process is critical to increase the odds of results uptake and utilization of the findings (Green & Mercer, 2001). At the opposite end of the continuum are the needs assessments that do not actively involve stakeholders. In these types of needs assessments, an external needs assessor is brought in to act as an expert consultant who designs and implements the project, analyzes the findings, and presents recommendations to the contracting group.

Dimension 3: Political Orientation

The political orientation of a needs assessment will to a large extent depend on who initiated the process. Some needs assessments are initiated by organizations in order to maintain the status quo, or alternatively, justify a decision that has already been made (Martí-Costa & Serano-García, 1983; Witkin & Altschuld, 1995). For example, hospital administrators may conduct a needs assessment that recommends a new computerized documentation system or a different staffing configuration on the rehabilitation units in order to improve patient care. While these infrastructure changes may benefit patients indirectly, they often do not emerge from the issues and concerns of patients themselves.

At the opposite end of the continuum are needs assessments that are initiated for the purposes of raising awareness of the issues within a community, and for promoting community building and social change. For example, a needs assessment of older adults who have experienced a stroke and are being discharged back to the community may uncover issues and concerns related to housing accessibility, lack of social support, and inadequate outpatient follow-up. By documenting these issues and sharing findings with the community, a needs assessment team can provide empirical data to support social change efforts such as mobilizing community volunteers, changing discharge policies, or developing a fund to subsidize home modifications for older adults who require home modifications after a catastrophic health event.

> Defining and operationalizing need is critical to conducting a needs assessment that is rigorous and can produce findings that have utility for informing political action.

Dimension 4: The Scope of the Issue Being Addressed

A final dimension of a needs assessment reflects the scope of the issue or problem being addressed. Many needs assessments are narrow and well defined in their orientation, for example, determining the recreational needs of teenage members of a specific community center. Other needs assessments are much broader in their orientation, for example, determining the needs of individuals in the United States who are newly diagnosed with multiple sclerosis.

What Is It that We Are Assessing?

At the heart of the needs assessment process is the concept of need. It is a vague term that is poorly understood and rarely defined in the research literature. Nevertheless, defining and operationalizing need is critical to conducting a needs assessment that is rigorous and can produce findings that have utility for informing political action. Within many disciplines, need is essentially viewed as a discrepancy between what an individual's or group's present situation or status is and what is desired (Reviere et al., 1996; Witkin & Altschud, 1995). But the definition raises two key questions: What is desirable? Who defines desirable?

Trying to answer these questions illustrates the complexity of defining and then trying to assess need. Authors from the disciplines of psychology, sociology, philosophy, and political science (Bradshaw, 1972; Dill, 1983; Doyal & Gough, 1991; Maslow, 1954; Thomson, 1987) suggest that the concept of need is complex because of the different ways the term is used (noun as well as verb), the extent to which need is value laden, and because of its links to ideas about what is moral and good. For example, the term *need* itself is used to describe basic physiological drives, goals that are sought after (ends), as well as the strategies to achieve those goals (solutions) (Dill, 1983; Doyal & Gough, 1991). Furthermore, need can be conceptualized at both an individual level as well as a collective one. These ideas are explored below.

Need as a Physiological Drive

As a basic physiological drive, need is a "motivational force instigated by a state of disequilibrium or tension set up in an organism because of a particular lack" (Thomson, 1987, p. 13). Defining needs as drives is illustrated in the classic hierarchy described by Maslow (1954), which suggests that humans are motivated to first address physiological needs for food and water, then safety and security, and finally to belong, to develop self-esteem, and to seek self-actualization. Examples of needs as drives can be illustrated in the following statements: "I need a glass of water," "I need a house," or "I need to participate in a meaningful activity." Note that in all of these statements the term *need* is used as a verb, and "points to what is required or desired to fill the discrepancy – solutions, a means to an end" (Witkin & Altschud, 1995, p. 9). Yet, the discrepancy itself is not explicit, nor is the specific end (e.g., becoming hydrated, having shelter, being engaged in an occupation).

Need as a Solution

While needs as drives is not the perspective used for the majority of needs assessments that are conducted by occupational therapists, using the term *need* as a verb and conceptualizing need as a solution is very common. Take for example the situation of a community mental health agency that is examining life skills programming for its clients. Staff members set off to conduct a needs assessment to help its Board of Directors determine if clients need more occupational therapists within the scope of the agency's service package. What is missing in this scenario is an explicit indication of what the actual goal might be, and a willingness to explore solutions other than more occupational therapists.

Presumably, the goal of this needs assessment would be improved ability of the agency's clients to manage in the community independently. Unfortunately, by framing the needs assessment from a solution orientation (i.e., do clients need more occupational therapists?), it is unlikely that other options to achieve this goal will be identified. If alternatives are not identified, the Board of Trustees cannot consider them in their decision-making and resource allocation decisions.

For this reason, Altschuld and Witkin (2000) argue against conceptualizing needs as solutions because such an approach fails to identify the underlying issues and concerns, thereby limiting the opportunity to explore and examine a range of possible solutions. Yet, many needs assessments completed within health and social services conceptualize need in this way. A classic example of this type of needs assessment is the survey that provides respondents with a list of services, and then asks them to review the list and check off what they "need". Such an approach risks the possibility of identifying "needs" that do not address the underlying issue.

Need as Relative to the Assessor

In addition to conceptualizing need as either goals or solutions, it is also possible to consider needs relative to the assessor and the method of determining the need. The classic typology presented by Bradshaw (1972) is an example of conceptualizing needs from these perspectives. Bradshaw discusses four types of needs: normative, felt, expressed, and comparative. Table 36.1 provides definitions and examples of these types of needs, as well as related terms that have been used by other authors.

Normative Need

Normative need is defined by professionals and experts rather than by members of the community themselves. Consequently, a needs assessment that uses a normative needs perspective would have little to no involvement of the stakeholders. In addition, defining needs using this approach is highly subject to the cultural and value biases of the expert and can vary greatly across experts. For example, when asked to identify the needs of young men in a homeless shelter, an occupational therapist may identify needs related to their roles and habits. For the same group of young men, a social worker may identify needs related to communication and social interactions. A drug and alcohol counselor may identify the primary need of these young men as substance abuse rehabilitation. As a result, using a normative perspective means that the needs assessor must be vigilant about the reliability of the data collection tools and processes so that the findings can be replicated.

Expressed and Felt Need

In comparison, individuals themselves determine expressed need and felt need. Felt need refers to want, with or without actions to obtain that which

Table 36.1 **Bradshaw's Categories of Need**

Bradshaw's Need Categories	Explanation/Illustration
Normative need	Expert definitions
Expressed need	Refers to demand for a service as measured by actual use as well as requests for services (i.e. waiting lists).
Felt need	Want
Comparative need	Need based on comparisons to and equity with others. For example, Group A receives a service, but Group B does not even though the groups are equivalent on key characteristics. Therefore, Group B is determined to be in need of the service.

is wanted. Expressed need refers to demand for a service, either through current use or waiting lists. The problem with both felt and expressed need is twofold. First, both frame needs in terms of solutions—a problem that has already been discussed earlier in this section. Second, these ways of defining need cannot account for people who do not know about a service—one cannot want something of which one is unaware. Expressed need is further problematic because there are often individuals who want a service, but who do not request it because they know it is not physically or financially accessible, or because they are simply tired of fighting the system. Consider for example individuals who have been consistently refused third-party funding for assistive technology and simply give up asking for it. Both felt and expressed need focus on the solution, and not necessarily the underlying issue or concern.

Comparative Need

Conceptualizing need from a comparative perspective is relatively common in public health, and the health and social services. Consider the situation in which a group of older adults living in one seniors' apartment complex (baseline group) is compared to a group of older adults living in another complex (comparison group). If the comparison group does not have the same programs and services as the baseline group, they are determined to have need. Through this approach, need is framed in terms of solutions (i.e., the programs and services provided), which is problematic because it carries with it important assumptions that are often difficult to test. Specifically, taking a comparative need approach assumes that the baseline group actually needs the programs and services that their complex provides, and that they are receiving them in the correct amount. It further assumes that all of the baseline group's needs are actually being met and that the programs that are being provided are the best solution to the underlying problem.

Identifying Needs as a Political Process

At the beginning of this chapter, needs assessment was described as both a form of applied research and as a political process. Regardless of whether need is viewed as a goal or a solution, it is value laden and culturally influenced. As such, it is affected by sociopolitical factors that are operating within the organization, community, or region in which the needs assessment is being conducted. Sociopolitical factors encompass basic beliefs about what is moral or good, overriding political philosophies, and the nature and operations of systems that are either leading the needs assessment efforts, or will respond to the findings (Dill, 1983; Doyal & Gough, 1991; Shi & Singh, 2001). As such, the process, measures, outcomes, and actions of a given needs assessment are fundamentally linked to either the principles and values of the marketplace (e.g., a needs assessment to determine whether to expand a private practice rehabilitation clinic) or to a commitment to the social good (e.g., a needs assessment to determine the accessibility of public housing in an urban center) (Shi & Singh, 2001).

While the majority of needs assessments will have a primary link to one of these positions, it may also have secondary goals and objectives in the other. For example, a health management organization may conduct a needs assessment in a rural area to determine the demand for an assistive technology clinic and the economic viability of developing one. This needs assessment would be linked primarily to the principles and values of the marketplace, and the organization's need to be economically successful. Nevertheless, it may also be linked to a secondary understanding that access to assistive technologies is not equitably distributed between rural and urban areas, and that the health and quality of life of individuals with a wide range of disabilities may be negatively influenced by the lack of such a program.

Needs Assessment Grounded in a Marketplace Philosophy

Needs assessments that are grounded in a marketplace philosophy equate need with demand, and define needs in terms of solutions. In other words, they take both a felt needs and an expressed needs conceptualization that focuses primarily on the individuals. Individual preferences and autonomy are viewed as key to determining need (Shi & Singh, 2001). While there is room within a marketplace philosophy of needs assessments for expert definitions of needs (i.e., normative needs), it could be argued that this approach would focus more on the needs of the organization that would deliver the service rather than the individual receiving it.

Using the marketplace philosophy, needs can best be met through the free market and through a conservative approach to the development and maintenance of health and social service policies. Services that are provided as a result of the needs assessment are viewed as an economic good and are distributed based on people's ability to pay, either independently or through various types of insurance (Shi & Singh, 2001).

Needs Assessment Grounded in a Philosophy of the Social Good

Alternatively, needs assessments that are grounded in a philosophy of the social good equate need with disparities across groups and inequities of service supply and access, and focuses on the collective rather than the individual (Shi & Singh, 2001). As such, needs assessments grounded in this way have the potential to address underlying problems and issues, as well as identify potential solutions. Two types of need are key to this perspective: normative need and comparative need. From the perspective of the social good, the purpose of conducting needs assessments is to identify areas that need to be remediated in order to improve the standard of living and/or quality of life of the collective and to determine how to allocate services fairly.

> Ultimately, the results of needs assessments allow decision makers to justify expenditures to develop new services, or to refocus, modify, or eliminate existing services.

The provision of services to address the identified needs is seen as a social good (if one person is better off, everyone is better off), and generally involves governmental intervention whether at the community, county, state, regional, or national level. The products of these types of needs assessments guide actions that emphasize equity and ensure that some basic set of standards is met. Actions to remediate these needs are more likely to be met through liberal or democratic policies, and social advocacy and action movements (Shi & Singh, 2001). Consequently, needs assessments grounded in this philosophy are more consistent with ones that are participatory in orientation, and are directed at social change (see Figure 36.1).

Summary

These discussions suggest that need is ultimately "created" by the people and organizations that are conducting needs assessments, particularly when needs are conceptualized as solutions. The question then becomes: Why try to measure need? As a number of authors have pointed out, needs assessment is one of many potential tools in the processes of strategic and ongoing planning, quality improvement, and outcomes management. Ultimately, the results of needs assessments allow decision makers to justify expenditures to develop new services, or to refocus, modify, or eliminate existing services.

In summary, the concept of need is complex and multilayered. The term need is used in different ways, and these ways influence the processes and outcomes of a needs assessment. In addition, the conceptualization of needs is influenced by values, culture, politics, and ideas about what is moral and good. While the idea of "needs assessment" is seemingly easy to understand, this theoretical overview suggests that it is much more complex than many people realize. It would be easy to become mired in these theoretical perspectives, and be unable to move forward to assess the needs of a group of individuals, an organization, a community, or a population. Instead, the intention of this overview is to highlight the importance of being clear on what is being assessed and to provide potential frameworks within which current or future needs assessors can consider their work.

Models for Approaching Needs Assessments

While the definitions of need are multifold, and the philosophical basis for doing needs assessments varies, the actual process of needs assessment is systematic. Over the years, a number of models or approaches to needs assessments have been presented in the literature. Five important approaches include:

- Logic models,
- Three-phase model,
- Concerns report method,
- Community building, and
- Participatory approaches.

The key features of these models are summarized in Table 36.2.

Table 36.2 Comparison of Key Features of Different Models and Approaches to Needs Assessment

	Logic Model	Three-Phase	Concerns Report Method	Participatory Approach	Community Building
Is there a clearly defined philosophical or theoretical stance?	No	No	Yes	Yes	Yes
Is it apparent what research approach fits with this model (i.e. qualitative, quantitative, or mixed)?	No	No	Yes	Yes	No
Are the specific research methods fitting with this model defined?	No	No	Yes	No	No
Is it clear within this model what tasks are done in what order, by whom, etc.? In other words, does it have a defined structure?	Somewhat	Yes	Somewhat	No	No
Is it clear how a needs assessor would move through the process of a needs assessment based on this model?	Somewhat	Yes	Yes	Yes	Somewhat
Would the use of this model be resource intensive?	No	Maybe—depends on the issues and the community	Maybe—depends on the issues and the community	Yes	Yes
What is the expected outcome of a needs assessment using this model?	Planning tool	Action plans	Task forces that develop solutions to community concerns	Stronger community with ownership over issues	Stronger community with ownership over issues

Logic Models

Logic models were originally developed as a tool to facilitate program planning and evaluation. While logic models continue to be primarily used for these purposes, they also have great utility for the process of planning a needs assessment (Rush & Ogborne, 1991). Figure 36.2 presents a logic model that was developed by a group of students at the University of Illinois at Chicago for a needs assessment they conducted for a local suburban department of public health. Although a logic model does not identify the philosophical stance of the needs assessment, nor points to particular types of methods, it does offer a concrete way of communicating the work of a needs assessment team to people outside of the immediate group. It is also an excellent tool to keep a needs assessment focused on the long-term goal of the project, and how the information that is being gathered will be used.

Three-Phase Model

The three-phase model is another tool that can be used to facilitate the planning of a needs assessment. This model is described in detail by Witkin and Altschuld (1995), and fundamentally operates as a checklist of steps and activities that must be achieved over the different stages of a needs assessment. The first phase of this model is the preassessment, during which:

• A planning group is established,
• The purpose of the needs assessment is defined, and
• Preliminary data gathering is completed to contextualize the main needs assessment.

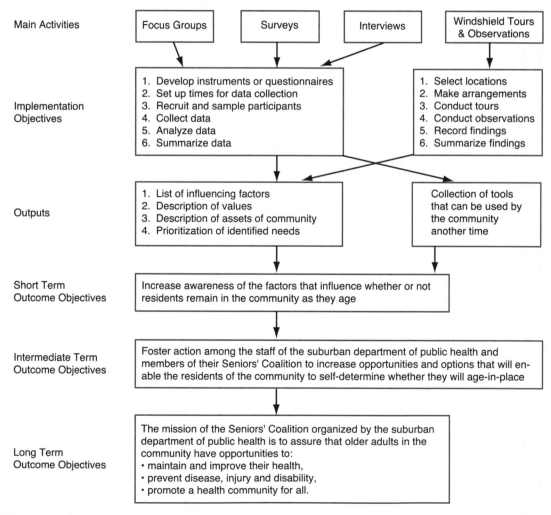

Figure 36.2 Sample logic model.

The preassessment phase is an opportunity for the needs assessment team to learn about the community and its social and political context.

The second phase of this model is called the assessment phase. Using information obtained during the preassessment, the needs assessment team determines the scope of their work, plans the data collection, and determines time lines, budgets, and necessary resources. It is also during this phase that the needs assessment team actually gathers data and analyzes findings.

The final phase of this model is the postassessment phase, during which needs are translated into priorities for action, potential solutions are identified and compared, the needs assessment process is evaluated, and results are communicated. Like the logic model, the three-phase model is a structural and planning tool that does not have a clear philosophical or theoretical stance, nor does it identify particular methods of data collection.

Concerns Report Method

In comparison to the logic model and the three-phase model, the Concerns Report Method has a clear grounding in theories of empowerment, self-help, and community development (Ludwig-Beymer, Blankemeier, Casa-Boyots & Suarez-Balcazar, 1996; Schriner & Fawcett, 1988). This grounding leads to a participatory action research approach to needs assessments that use this model. Methodologically, the Concerns Report Method draws on focus groups, survey research, and analytic strategies that originate in discrepancy modeling (Ludwig-Beymer et al., 1996). Through the use of the Concerns Report Method, communities work with the needs assessment team to identify community strengths as well as issues and concerns. Strengths are then built upon to address the issues and concerns. The basic steps of the Concerns Report Method are as follows:

- Focus groups are conducted to identify community values, concerns, and priorities,
- Findings from the focus groups are used to develop a structured survey in which each item has an importance dimension and a satisfaction dimension,
- The survey is administered to members of the community,
- Data are analyzed,
- Results are shared with the community through public meetings,
- During the public meetings, community members discuss ways to preserve and enhance community strengths and address issues and concerns,

- Action committees are established, and
- A final report is disseminated throughout the community.

One of the interesting and unique features of the Concerns Report Method is the survey, and how the way it is structured produces a prioritization of community needs. The feature box on the next page provides examples of statements from a Concerns Report Method survey that focused on identifying older adults issues and concerns related to food acquisition and preparation. From the results of these surveys, a needs index is calculated for each statement as follows:

- The proportion of respondents who state that an item is very important is calculated,
- The proportion of respondents who state that they are very satisfied with the item is calculated, and
- Need index = proportion very important – proportion very satisfied.

Through this strategy, the needs assessment team is able to provide the community with a list of issues in order of priority. The range of scores on the need index can range from +100, which

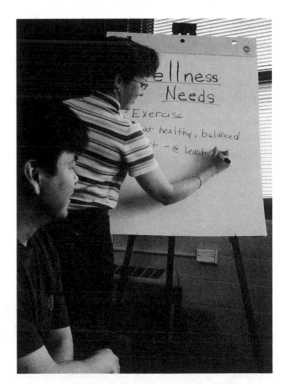

Figure 36.3 Dr. Finlayson conducts a focus group in order to identify student wellness needs.

Sample Statements from a Concerns Report Method Survey

I have access to transportation for shopping.
How important is this to you personally?
Very important _____ Somewhat important _____ Not important _____
How satisfied are you with your own situation?
Very satisfied _____ Somewhat satisfied_____ Not satisfied _____

I am able to shop independently.
How important is this to you personally?
Very important _____ Somewhat important _____ Not important _____
How satisfied are you with your own situation?
Very satisfied _____ Somewhat satisfied _____ Not satisfied _____

I am able to prepare nutritious meals independently.
How important is this to you personally?
Very important _____ Somewhat important _____ Not important _____
How satisfied are you with your own situation?
Very satisfied _____ Somewhat satisfied _____ Not satisfied _____

I am aware of community programs that provide nutritious meals.
How important is this to you personally?
Very important _____ Somewhat important _____ Not important _____
How satisfied are you with your own situation?
Very satisfied _____ Somewhat satisfied _____ Not satisfied _____

indicates a very high need (i.e., the issue is very important to everyone, but no one is very satisfied), to −100, which indicates a very low need or alternatively, a community strength (i.e., the issue is very important, yet everyone is very satisfied). A score of zero on this score range indicates that needs are being addressed (i.e., there is a balance).

Community Building and Participatory Approaches

Both community building and participatory approaches to needs assessment focus on social change, and draw from practices of community development and participatory action research. Both approaches are based in critical social theory, and therefore focus on the critical examination of rules, habits, traditions, and beliefs about an issue and how these factors impact social relationships and structures (Lindsey & McGuinness, 1998; Lindsay, Shields, & Stajduhar 1999; Wallerstein & Duran, 2003). In both of these approaches to needs assessment, the key is community involvement and community ownership over the entire process.

In participatory approaches to needs assessment, the underlying assumption is that knowledge is power, and that knowledge development within a community will lead to social action (Lindsay et al., 1999; Lindsey & McGuinness, 1998; Wallerstein & Duran, 2003). Therefore, participatory approaches to needs assessment link social science to social activism, and link research, action, and education into a single project. For the purposes of a needs assessment, participatory approaches provide significant theoretical guidance in terms of process. For example, using a participatory approach will require active involvement of the stakeholders in all aspects of the research process and associated decision-making. Developing effective partnerships will be key, and the primary needs assessor will take the role of facilitator and technician. Beyond these theoretical and process guides, taking a participatory approach does not dictate the use of specific methods during the needs assessment process.

In community building approaches to needs assessment, the focus is on the community and on fostering development of a collective to promote social change. Raising critical consciousness and promoting reflection are key to the use of a community building approach to needs assessment. There are four aspects or components to this model of needs assessment, and they include citizen action, voluntary participation and collaborative problem solving, empowerment, and holistic community-wide outcomes (Wallerstein & Duran, 2003). Like the participatory approach to needs assessment, the community building approach provides strong theoretical and process guidance, but does not dictate the use of particular methods.

Summary

Through this review of models and approaches to needs assessment, it should be apparent that this

Table 36.3 Advantages and Disadvantages of the Different Models and Approaches to Needs Assessment

	Advantages of Using this Model	Disadvantages of Using this Model
Logic model	• Tool that can assist with planning. • Promotes communication among stakeholders. • Keeps the project focused on the long-term outcome.	• Provides no theoretical guidance. • Provides no guidance about methods.
Three-phase model	• Clearly defined, step-by-step process. • Good for novices who need checklist formats to guide them through the needs assessment process. • Emphasizes use of a needs assessment advisory committee.	• Provides no theoretical guidance. • Provides no guidance about methods.
Concerns report method	• Clearly defined, step-by-step process. • Clearly defined guiding theory. • Clearly defined methods. • Role of community explicit.	• May be time and resource intensive depending on the community.
Participatory approach	• Clearly defined guiding theory. • Role of community explicit. • Community controls process. • Involving community members in research process increases likelihood of ownership over findings.	• Time and resource intensive. • Provides no guidance about methods. • May require needs assessor to train community members in research processes.
Community building approach	• Clearly defined guiding theory. • Role of community explicit. • Community controls process. • Typically involves multiple constituencies (e.g., business, social services, government, etc.).	• Time and resource intensive. • Provides no guidance about methods. • Involvement of multiple constituencies is likely to require specialized and experienced facilitators to negotiate multiple viewpoints.

is an area of research that requires further methodological and conceptual clarity. Each of these models and approaches offers advantages and disadvantages, and these are summarized in Table 36.3. Logic models and the three-phase models are really structural and organizational in nature, providing guidance for process but little else. Community building and participatory approaches provide theoretical guidance, and therefore a philosophical stance to guide the needs assessment process. They do not provide guidance for the step-by-step activities of a needs assessment, nor the methods that can and should be used. The Concerns Report Method falls in between these two extremes. It has a clear structure, and a step-by-step process about what activities to complete in which order. It also has a clear theoretical orientation that can guide the process conceptually. Ultimately, mixing and matching these models and approaches may have the greatest utility for a needs assessment team. For example, using the

three-phase model together with a community building approach would provide guidance to a needs assessment team in terms of theory as well as step-by-step activities.

Common Data Collection Methods for Needs Assessment

Up to this point in the chapter, variability in needs assessments and how they are designed has been the message. Yet, one factor that high-quality needs assessments have in common is that multiple and mixed methods are used to collect the data (Müllersdorf & Söderback, 1998). In fact, both Witkin and Altschuld (1995) and Reviere et al. (1996) caution against using a single method to inform a needs assessment process. It is this feature of needs assessment—multiple and mixed methods—that make this form of applied research unique as well as exciting and challenging. Using multiple methods means that the research team often must be larger and more diverse to ensure that adequate expertise is available for designing and analyzing the data from each method. It also means that preparing the findings and making recommendations may become more complicated, particularly when trying to integrate qualitative and quantitative data, and data from different methods that may contradict each other. These challenges can often be overcome by revisiting the stakeholders, refocusing on the values of the community, and being clear about the scope and purpose of what is and can be addressed.

> Using multiple methods means that the research team often must be larger and more diverse to ensure that adequate expertise is available for designing and analyzing the data from each method.

Table 36.4 summarizes the most commonly used methods in needs assessments, as well as their advantages and disadvantages. Since many of these methods are discussed in other chapters in this book, they are not discussed here. Instead, Table 36.4 provides a cross-reference to other chapters that address the method. In addition, references are provided at the end of the chapter for readers who wish to learn more about the particular methods described in the table.

Preparing Needs Assessment Findings, Developing Recommendations, and Taking Action

Early in this chapter, needs assessment was described as both applied research and a political process. Although early needs assessments were often simply a list of problems, modern needs assessments do not stop there (Reviere et al., 1996). Needs assessors have a responsibility to translate their findings into recommendations that the community can consider for action. Typically, recommendations to address the identified needs fall into one of three categories (Carter, 1996):

> To prepare recommendations that a community can use, it is critical that the needs assessor understands his or her audience.

- Development of a new policy or program,
- Modification of an existing policy or program, or
- Modification to the delivery processes of an existing program or policy (e.g., eligibility criteria, staffing, funding, etc.).

To prepare recommendations that a community can use, it is critical that the needs assessor understands his or her audience. This understanding includes issues such as what they want to know, what they value and think is important, what they have the ability to change/influence, and how they prefer to acquire information. Needs assessors that engage the community members in their work should be able to develop a strong sense of the audience for the needs assessment findings and recommendations. Developing recommendations that can be used by the community can be facilitated in a number of ways.

Developing Recommendations

First, the needs assessor can draft and share findings as the needs assessment is being conducted, and seek feedback and interpretation from key stakeholders as the project proceeds. Taking this action has a number of benefits. First, it provides these individuals with the opportunity to become familiar with the findings, and begin to think about possible solutions to the issues being addressed. It may make it easier for some individuals and organizations to be open to radical changes if they have an opportunity to contemplate the findings well before the final report is disseminated.

Engaging stakeholders in the process of determining priorities for action can also facilitate the development of recommendations. Most needs assessments uncover more problems and concerns than can be reasonably addressed. Therefore, setting priorities for action is critical. Many strategies can be used to set priorities, for example, simple rank ordering based on the frequency with which a need was identified during the data collection process (e.g., results of a

Table 36.4 Commonly Used Methods in Needs Assessments

	Advantages	Disadvantages	Chapters in Which Method Is Discussed
Self-administered surveys (mail or in-person)	• Can be longer (people can be interrupted and return later). • Nonthreatening for sensitive information. • Don't have to hire or train interviewers. • Potential for broader coverage of population. • Medium length of data collection period.	• Low response rates generally, particularly for mail-outs. • Biased against people with low literacy levels or visual impairments. • Usually have to do a lot of data cleaning and editing. • Don't know who really filled out survey. • Questions must be simple (e.g., generally avoid skip patterns).	8
Interviewer-administered surveys (telephone or face-to-face)	• Consistent data across all subjects. • Enables statistical analysis. • Relatively quick method, generally speaking.	• Must train interviewers extensively for good reliability. • Don't get participant's own words. • Choices may not fit participant's experiences.	8, 20
Semistructured and open-ended interviews (including key informant interviews)	• Good when the researcher knows little about the topic. • Allows the researcher to obtain "natural wording." • Provides the participant with the opportunity for self-expression. • Enables the researcher to identify relevant variables from the participant's perspective.	• Quality of data is dependent on the quality of the interviewer. • Interviewer ability to listen and probe. • Interviewer ability to guide the discussion without controlling it. • Interviewer ability to cover all topics. • Sensitive topics are difficult to address, risk of obtaining socially acceptable responses only. • Time consuming. • Challenging to analyze.	20
Focus groups	• Provide data from a group of people more quickly and less expensively than one-on-one interviews. • Researcher can directly interact with participants. • Allows for clarification, follow-up questions, nonverbal cues. • Obtain respondents' own words. • Allows respondents to react and build on the responses of other people. • Can be used with children. • Can be used with people with low literacy levels.	• Need to think carefully about sampling and focus group member mix. • Responses of participants are not independent of one another. • Results can be biased by a dominant or opinionated member. • Summarization of results can be challenging if the group members have very divergent opinions. • Moderator can bias results.	20

(continued)

Table 36.4 Commonly Used Methods in Needs Assessments (continued)

	Advantages	Disadvantages	Chapters in Which Method Is Discussed
Delphi technique	• Does not require participants to meet. • Accommodates stakeholders with different levels of power in the same group. • Allows researcher to identify and use the experience of experts.	• Can be very time consuming, depending on the number of iterations.	24
Nominal group technique	• Focuses on identifying priorities quickly. • Accommodates stakeholders with different levels of power in the same group. • Good for setting priorities for action.	• Not a brainstorming technique, so issues become very focused very quickly. • Must get participants together.	24
Secondary data (e.g., administrative records, census figures, social indicators)	• Provides a broader perspective and larger sample sizes. • Can provide contextual information that other methods cannot. • Good for determining the size and scope of a problem.	• Often requires sophisticated statistical knowledge. • Access can sometimes be problematic (e.g., HIPPA, cost to buy data). • Quality of findings dependent on quality of original data collection procedures.	9, 20
Observation, including windshield tours	• See community in its natural form. • Permits descriptions of people, behaviors, settings and person–environment fit. • Can be qualitative or quantitative. • Can accommodate different levels of participation.	• Requires good training and data management. • Analysis can be challenging. • Researchers who are external to the environment may have inadequate knowledge to interpret observations accurately.	20

Concerns Report Survey) or Sork's approach (Witkin & Altschuld, 1995).

Sork's approach is based on two criteria for setting priorities: importance and feasibility. The importance of a need can be considered in a number of ways, as outlined by Witkin and Altschuld (1995). Important needs are ones that:

• Are experienced by greater numbers of people,
• If addressed, would contribute to the mission and goals of the community,
• Are immediate in nature, and cannot be resolved by time, and
• If resolved, would have additional benefits in other areas.

Feasibility addresses the extent to which addressing the identified needs is possible. Factors that play a role in feasibility include current knowledge, the availability of human and financial resources, and the commitment of the stakeholders to make changes to their operations (e.g., change policies, develop programs, change resource allocations). For occupational therapists, evidence-based practice plays a large role in determining feasibility—what evidence exists that the needs can be addressed effectively?

To evaluate the importance and feasibility of a list of needs identified through the needs assessment data collection, one can use the Q-sort methodology or other methods to rank order items (Chinnis, Paulson & Davis, 2001; McKeown & Thomas, 1998). Ultimately, the goal is to identify those needs which are both high importance and highly feasible to address. For these needs, one then moves to consider potential solutions. As already noted, recommending solutions to the identified needs may take the form of suggesting modifications to existing programs or policies, or the development of new ones.

The key to these final steps of the needs assessment process is to engage the community and listen to what they value. It is also critical to be open to a range of possible solutions, and to work with the community to explore what might be possible. Various brainstorming techniques such as townhall meetings and the nominal group technique

The key to these final steps of the needs assessment process is to engage the community and listen to what they value. It is also critical to be open to a range of possible solutions, and to work with the community to explore what might be possible.

(Delbecq, Van deVen & Gustafson, 1975/1986) can all be used to facilitate the discussion of possible solutions. Townhall meetings in particular are useful for obtaining commitment from stakeholders to take action on the findings of the project, and to engage community members in the process of enacting solutions.

Conclusion

The objectives of this chapter were to provide a theoretical overview of the concept of need, examine the processes and dimensions of a needs assessment, describe and compare models and approaches to needs assessment, evaluate methods commonly used in needs assessments, and outline how needs can be translated into actions for solutions. The foundation presented here, in addition to some extra reading on methods, should give readers a better and stronger understanding of the needs assessment process and its importance in occupational therapy research and practice. To close this chapter and summarize its important points, here is a list of proposed criteria for a good quality needs assessment:

• Develop a clear conceptualization of need, focusing on the underlying issue rather than the potential solution,
• Ground the needs assessment in a clear philosophical and theoretical stance,
• Actively involve stakeholders,
• Design a rigorous project,
• Use multiple data collection methods,
• Make recommendations based on empirical evidence, and
• Ensure that plans are put in place to address the needs that are uncovered.

REFERENCES

Altschuld, J. W., & Witkin, B. R. (2000). Setting needs-based priorities. In: *From needs assessment to action: Transforming needs into solution strategies* (pp. 99–132). Thousand Oaks, CA: SAGE Publications.

Bradshaw, J. L. (1972). A taxonomy of social need. In G. McLachlan (Ed.), *Problems and progress in medical* care: Essays on current research (pp. 71–82). London: Oxford University Press.

Carter, C. (1996). Using and communicating findings. In: R. Reviere, S. Berkowitz, C.C. Carter, and C.G. Ferguson (Eds.), *Needs assessment: A creative and practical guide for social scientists* (pp. 185–201). Washington, DC: Taylor & Francis.

Chinnis, A. S., Paulson, D. J., & Davis, S. M. (2001). Using Q methodology to assess the needs of emergency medicine support staff employees. *Journal of Emergency Medicine, 20*(2), 197–203.

Delbecq, A. L., Van de Ven, A. H., & Gustafson, D. H. (1975/1986). *Group techniques for program planning: A guide to nominal group and Delphi processes.* Middleton, WI: Green Briar Press.

Dill, A. (1983). Defining needs, defining systems: A critical analysis. *The Gerontologist, 33*(4), 453–460.

Doyal, L., & Gough, I. (1991). *A theory of human need.* New York: Guilford Press.

Green, L. W., & Mercer, S. L. (2001). Can public health researchers and agencies reconcile the push from funding bodies and the pull from communities? *American Journal of Public Health, 91*(12),1926–1929.

Hancock, T., & Minkler, M. (1997). Community health assessment or healthy community assessment – Whose community? Whose health? Whose assessment? In M. Minkler (Ed.), *Community organizing and community building for health* (pp. 139–156). New Brunswick, NJ: Rutgers University Press.

Kretzmann, J., & McKnight, J. (1997). *Building communities from the inside out: A path toward finding and mobilizing a community's assets.* Chicago, IL: ACTA Publications.

Lindsey, E., & McGuinness, L. (1998). Significant elements of community involvement in participatory action research: Evidence from a community project. *Journal of Advanced Nursing, 28*(5), 1106–1114.

Lindsey, E., Shields, L., & Stajduhar, K. (1999). Creating effective nursing partnerships: Relating community development to participatory action research. *Journal of Advanced Nursing, 29*(5), 1238–1245.

Lugwig-Beymer, P., Blankemeier, J. R., Casas-Byots, C., & Suarez-Balcazar, Y. (1996). Community assessment in a suburban Hispanic community: A description of method. *Journal of Transcultural Nursing, 8*(1), 19–27.

Martí-Costa, S., & Serrano-García, I. (1983). Needs assessment and community development: An ideological perspective. *Prevention in Human Services, 2*(4), 75–88.

Maslow, A. H. (1954). *Motivation and personality.* New York: Harper & Row.

McKeown, B., & Thomas, D. (1998). *Q-methodology.* Thousand Oaks, CA: SAGE Publications.

Minkler, M. (Ed.). (1997). *Community organizing and community building for health.* New Brunswick, NJ: Rutgers University Press.

Müllersdorf, M., & Söderback, I. (1998). Needs assess-

ment methods in healthcare and rehabilitation. *Critical Reviews in Physical & Rehabilitation Medicine, 10,* 57–73.

Reason, P., & Bradbury, H. (Eds.). (2001). *Handbook of action research: Participatory inquiry and practice.* Thousand Oaks, CA: SAGE Publications.

Reviere, R., Berkowitz, S., Carter, C. C., & Ferguson, C. G. (1996). *Needs assessment: A creative and practical guide for social scientists.* Washington, DC: Taylor & Francis.

Rush, B., & Ogborne, A. (1991). Program logic models: Expanding their role and structure for program planning and evaluation. *The Canadian Journal of Program Evaluation, 6*(2), 95–106.

Schriner, K. F., & Fawcett, S. B. (1988). Development and validation of the community concerns report method. *Journal of Community Psychology, 16*, 306–316.

Shi, L., & Singh, D. (2001). *Delivering health care in America: A systems approach* (2nd ed.), Gaithersburg, MD: Aspen.

Thomson, G. (1987). *Needs.* London: Routledge & Kegan Paul.

Wallerstein, N., & Duran, B. (2003). The conceptual, historical and practice roots of community based participatory research and related participatory traditions. In M. Minkler & N. Wallerstein (Eds.), *Community based participatory research for health* (pp. 27–52). San Fransisco, CA: Jossey Bass.

Witkin, B. R., & Altschuld, J. W. (1995). *Planning and conducting needs assessments: A practical guide.* Thousand Oaks: SAGE Pubications.

METHODS RESOURCES

Allen, S. M., Mor, V., Raveis, V., & Houts, P. (1993). Measurement of need for assistance with daily activities: Quantifying the influence of gender roles. *Journal of Gerontology: Social Sciences, 48*, S204–S211.

Bowling, A. (1997). Questionnaire design. In A. Bowling (Ed.), *Research methods in health: Investigating health and health services* (pp. 242–271). Buckingham, UK: Oxford University Press.

Fowler, F.J. Jr. (2002). *Survey research methods* (3rd ed.). Thousand Oaks, CA: SAGE Publications.

Gubrium, J. F., & Holstein, J. A. (Eds.). (2002). *Handbook of interview research.* Thousand Oaks, CA: SAGE Publications.

Krueger, R. A., & Casey, M. A. (2000). *Focus groups: A practical guide for applied research* (3rd ed.). Thousand Oaks, CA: SAGE Publications.

Morse, J. M., & Field, P. A. (1995). *Qualitative research methods for health professionals* (2nd ed.). Thousand Oaks, CA: SAGE Publications.

Weiss, R. S. (1994). *Learning from strangers: The arts and method of qualitative interview studies.* New York: The Free Press.

Using Research to Develop and Evaluate Programs of Service

Brent Braveman • Yolanda Suarez-Balcazar • Gary Kielhofner • Renée R. Taylor

This chapter explores the integration between research and the development and evaluation of occupational therapy programs. Examples are presented throughout this chapter to illustrate this integration and to highlight the relationship between the research methodologies presented in this book, evidence based on research, and the processes of developing and evaluating programs of service.

Program Development

Program development is the systematic design, planning, and implementation of new services, innovations, or initiatives. It can range from relatively simple ventures such as implementing a standard approach to care in a given setting to complex endeavors such as the creating interventions for populations facing new conditions and significant challenges. For example, program development occurs when the administrator of a rehabilitation center decides to develop and introduce a new approach (e.g., sensory integration) into an existing program of occupational therapy pediatric services. Another example of program development would include an occupational therapist who collaborates with a local YWCA to design services for women and children who have self-identified as being victims of domestic violence.

Regardless of the level of complexity, the integration of research methods into the program development process can foster success. Integrating research methods into program development can:

- Provide formative data that shape what services are provided and how they are delivered,
- Provide evidence about the effectiveness of services,
- Increase the likelihood that services will be used, sustained over time, and designed to meet the needs of participants, and
- Provide evidence about the effectiveness of underlying theory being tested.

Program Evaluation

Program evaluation is a process documenting the impact of a newly developed or existing intervention or program of services. Impact can be assessed using process and/or data on outcomes (indicators of change). Similar to program development, approaches to program evaluation can range in complexity. They may involve evaluation of a single aspect of an intervention or program with a limited number of clients or evaluation of multiple related interventions with a large population in order to establish their effectiveness.

Relationships Among Program Development and Evaluation, Theory, and Research

In some circumstances, program development and program evaluation are taken on as separate activities in isolation of one another. For example, this might occur when an evaluation of outcomes is requested of a program of occupational therapy services that has been in existence for a long period of time. Other circumstances might call for the development of a new program or intervention. In these cases, program development is often accompanied by formative evaluation (ongoing evaluation and refinement of the process of service implementation) and followed by a summative evaluation (evaluation of the ultimate outcomes or effectiveness of the program). In this chapter, program development and program evaluation are treated as coexisting along a continuum that includes program development, formative evaluation, and summative evaluation. This approach of undertaking program development and program evaluation simultaneously is widely supported as the preferred approach by different fields including the health and social sciences.

A Scholarship of Practice

Regardless of how familiar or complex an intervention is, the process of developing and evaluating a program of service can be made easier if it is guided by sound principles that connect theory and research (both methods and the resulting evidence) to practice. The relationship between theory, research, and practice has been described as a scholarship of practice (Crist & Kielhofner, 2005; Hammel, Finlayson, Kielhofner, Helfrich, & Peterson, 2002; Kielhofner, 2005).The scholarship of practice envisions a process in which theoretical and empirical knowledge is brought to bear on the practice problems and practice raises questions to be addressed through scholarship. Maintaining a discourse between theory, practice and research is an ideal framework for program development, since programs translate theory into services and research can guide the process and demonstrate its impact.

For example, Braveman and Kielhofner (2006) describe the use of theory and research evidence to develop occupational therapy programming focused on preparing persons living with human immunodeficiency virus/acquired immunodeficiency syndrome (HIV/AIDS) to return to employment in a community-based setting in which occupational therapy previously had not been provided. Similarly, Fisher and Braveman (2006) describe the use of methods commonly used in research such as interviews and focus groups to collect and organize data, information, and other forms of evidence to help with the processes of needs assessment, program planning, and program evaluation.

As noted earlier, the range of program development efforts and the resulting need to evaluate services can vary widely in complexity. While less complex efforts may require less sophisticated evaluation approaches, the amount and usefulness of the resulting evidence are also limited. Naturally, more complex program development efforts require more sophisticated evaluation approaches and these approaches may result in a greater amount of evidence with broader applications.

In research as well as in program development and evaluation there is always a trade-off between the investment of time and effort and the value of the results. Figure 37.1 represents a continuum of research and evaluation approaches and the advantages and disadvantages that come with expending less or more time and effort. The key is to match the approach and level of effort with the desired outcome and the needs of your situation. The left side of the figure represents "low-complexity programs" such as the implementation of an established approach to care in a familiar setting to a limited population (e.g., developing a cardiac rehabilitation protocol for a new cardiology program in a general hospital). The right side of the figure represents "high-complexity programs" such as a two-site randomized control trial that examined the efficacy of an energy conservation education program for people with multiple sclerosis (Mathiowetz, Finlayson, Matuska, Chen, & Lou, 2005).

Using Research to Guide Program Development

The primary tenets of both evidence-based practice and of a scholarship of practice are that the most effective programs are designed using the best available evidence. While other forms of evidence such as the testimony of experts, clinical guidelines provided from professional groups, information from Internet sites, and even one's own clinical experience are valid and sometimes the only evidence available, the strongest evidence is obtained through the application of sound research strategies, tools, and methodologies. Such strategies, tools, and methodologies are described throughout the other chapters of this book. While these approaches are used to carry out research to develop or validate the theories that guide programming, many of the same strategies, tools, and methodologies may also be used to collect and synthesize data, information, and other forms of evidence *during* the program development process. In other words, rather than associating a strategy, tool, or methodology just with the generation of knowledge one should realize that they also assist with the application of knowledge.

The process of program development may be conceptualized as a series of four steps that include:

- Needs assessment,
- Program planning,

> The process of developing and evaluating a program of service can be made easier if it is guided by sound principles that connect theory and research.

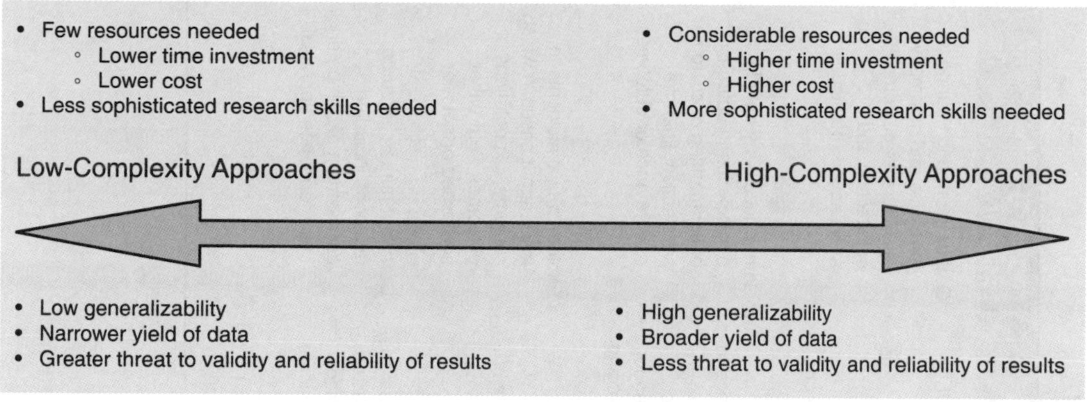

- Few resources needed
  - Lower time investment
  - Lower cost
- Less sophisticated research skills needed

- Considerable resources needed
  - Higher time investment
  - Higher cost
- More sophisticated research skills needed

Low-Complexity Approaches

High-Complexity Approaches

- Low generalizability
- Narrower yield of data
- Greater threat to validity and reliability of results

- High generalizability
- Broader yield of data
- Less threat to validity and reliability of results

Figure 37.1 A continuum of research and evaluation approaches.

- Program implementation, and
- Program evaluation (Braveman, 2001; Braveman, Kielhofner, Belanger, Llerena, & de las Heras, 2002; Braveman, Sen, & Kielhofner, 2001).

Table 37.1 lists each of these four steps across the top of the table. In addition, common research strategies, tools, and methodologies are listed along the left side of the table. Each cell of the table provides an example of how the strategy, tool, or methodology could be applied in the process of developing a new program or service. The strategies, tools, and methods presented in Table 37.1 are not an exhaustive list, but rather represent a sampling of such approaches. Next, each of the fours steps of program development is described in more depth and additional examples of the use of research strategies, tools, and methodology in the program development process are provided.

Needs Assessment

The first step in developing a program of service is to determine the needs of the target population that the program addresses. Needs assessment is a systematic set of procedures undertaken to make decisions about program improvements (Witkin & Altschuld, 1995). As noted in Chapter 36, it is a process of determining what a group of persons, a community, or a population requires in order to achieve some basic standard or to improve their current situation. The needs assessment process can range from simple to complex depending on the characteristics of those who will receive services and the scope of planned services. In more complicated examples, determining the needs of a target population may in fact be the *focus* of a research effort (Witkin, 1991; Witkin & Altschuld, 1995). In most cases of program development however, previous research is combined with the

results of a needs assessment to guide the choice of conceptual practice models and other elements of an intervention designed to respond to identified needs.

Strategies for needs assessment should be chosen based on ease of use, resources available, and the results they produce. Research strategies and tools such as questionnaires, surveys, or reviews of records may help you obtain specific information about the needs of a target population such as demographic characteristics and services already utilized. For example, an occupational therapist interested in developing occupational therapy services for a client population not yet served (e.g., adults with sensory impairment who reside in an underserved urban neighborhood) might begin by initiating a relatively simple needs assessment. This needs assessment might involve reviewing existing information on the prevalence of individuals with sensory impairment in the neighborhood served by the medical center and information about sensory impairment services offered by other medical centers or community-based organizations within the same neighborhood.

Other situations might require a more systematic approach to needs assessment. For example, once preliminary data are obtained, the same administrator might gain access to the clients with sensory impairment and survey them directly to assess the likelihood that they would use occupational therapy services. Such quantitative strategies can assist one to begin to understand how the target population may be similar or different to previously researched populations. Interviews or focus groups may generate deeper insights on the needs of the target population such as perceived barriers to accessing services or desired outcomes of services. Qualitative strategies such as focus groups can also be useful.

Table 37.1 Sample Applications of Research Strategies, Tools, and Methodologies Within the Steps of Program Development

Research Strategy, Tool or Methodology	Needs Assessment	Program Planning	Program Implementation	Program Evaluation
Questionnaires and surveys	Identify desires and needs of target populations and customers internal and external to an organization.	Determine customer preferences, validate perception of needs, and gather data to plan for personnel, equipment, and other programmatic needs.	Monitor and improve staff satisfaction, identify opportunities for continuous quality improvement efforts, facilitate communication with key stakeholders.	Gather information during formative and summative evaluation of customer satisfaction and assessment of outcomes.
Record reviews	Gather demographic data, rates of incidence, prevalence, and service utilization.	Establish baseline benchmarks for productivity and financial monitoring as well as assessment of outcomes.	Determine levels of productivity, compliance to accreditation or other standards, and collect trend data to help plan for financial management and budgeting.	Gather necessary data for participation in database benchmarking of customer satisfaction, financial performance or outcomes.
Interviews or focus groups	Identify needs and desires of stakeholders internal and external to the organization.	Garner support of key stakeholders, identify roadblocks to success, validate the focus of your product or service, and collect information on program competitors.	Plan and conduct human resource functions including performance appraisal and staff development.	Explore critical incidents to learn about cases in which customer expectations or outcomes were either surpassed or not met.
Observation	Visit existing programs to learn about space needs and space design, work flow, and customer expectations.	Ensure compliance with accreditation and safety standards and gather information to help plan continuous quality improvement and other evaluation systems.	Become more familiar with the challenges and obstacles faced by staff in service delivery and communicate a desire for open communication.	Carry out human resource functions including assessment of competency or performance appraisal.

Program Planning

The same strategies (and sometimes the same tools or assessments) used to assess the needs of a target population can be adapted and used to guide program planning. Program planning involves:

• Determining the type of service to be provided,
• Enumerating resources needed to provide the services,
• Characterizing the population, and
• Identifying how the services/program will be delivered.

Continuing with the example of using an evidence-based approach to plan a new program of services for adults with sensory impairment, program planning would follow the comprehensive needs assessment described in the preceding section. Following the needs assessment, the act of program planning might involve creating a spreadsheet in which the collected information about the needs of the population and the information about other existing services within the community would be analyzed, compared, and discussed. In addition, findings from a literature review of any existing outcomes research on the efficacy of various approaches to occupational therapy with individuals with various types of sensory impairment would be summarized, added to the spreadsheet, and compared in order to guide the development of a conceptual model of care.

Many resources are available to help occupational therapy practitioners become skilled at finding, evaluating, and integrating evidence into their practice (Braveman, 2006; Law, 2002). Questionnaires or surveys may assess how potential users view planned services and the extent to which they intend to use a service if it is offered. Quantitative data gained during these efforts can also help with planning for personnel, equipment, and space needs as they may provide information related to potential volume and intensity of service utilization.

Qualitative methods including interviews, focus groups, and observations can assist with planning a program by uncovering potential roadblocks to the program's success. Such strategies may also be useful in learning information about existing services or competitors and why members of your target population might choose to use your service rather than another option. As one approaches the step of program implementation, these strategies also assist with planning management and human resource functions such as systems for continuous quality improvement, the assessment of competencies, and the development of job descriptions.

Program Implementation

Program implementation involves the actual delivery of the program or services. Data collection is used during program implementation to document:

• When the service was provided,
• How many hours of services were provided,
• Who provided the service,
• What type of service was provided, and
• How many clients were provided with services.

Maintaining an activity log will help the occupational therapist generate a record of program implementation. Both quantitative and qualitative approaches can be used to collect and analyze data, information, and other forms of evidence from various sources for ongoing program evaluation. The output of these efforts may be used for functions such as monitoring and improving customer and staff satisfaction, planning and conducting human resource functions such as performance appraisals and staff development, or in continuous quality improvement efforts.

Unfortunately, once program implementation begins the evidence-based strategies used in program planning often lapse. However, the relationship between research and the development, implementation, and evaluation of programs of service should be both reciprocal and continuous. Practitioners should continuously raise questions that may be answered by researchers. Researchers should continuously provide new evidence that should be evaluated by practitioners to improve programs of service.

> The relationship between research and the development, implementation, and evaluation of programs of service is both reciprocal and continuous.

Program Evaluation

The fourth step of the program development process is program evaluation. While listed last, program evaluation is actually a continuous process that is integrated throughout the planning and implementation of a program of service. In this section, the different types of program evaluation, the different methodological strategies used to evaluate occupational therapy interventions, and a framework that includes practical steps to conduct program evaluation are introduced.

Program evaluation is the use of tools, methods, and skills to determine if a human service or program is meeting the needs of participants, if the program is offered as planned, and if it is having the desired impact on the lives of participants (Posavac & Carey, 2003; Stufflebeam, 2001). Program evaluation implies a process that contributes to the provision of quality services (Posavac & Carey, 2003) and to decisions about improving a program or intervention (Fawcett et al., 1996; Suarez-Balcazar & Harper, 2003).

The need for program evaluation has grown quite rapidly during the last 10 years (Posavac & Carey, 2003). The demand for community-based services has come with an increased demand from funders for agencies and organizations to conduct evaluations of their interventions and programs, especially in times of budget cuts. Philanthropic entities as well as private and public sources of funding are requesting program evaluations. It is now a common practice among funding agencies to make financial support of community programs and services contingent on evaluation of such initiatives. Program evaluation provides information about human services and interventions in ways that such information can be used to improve services, policies, or practices (Posavac & Carey, 2003).

Human services staff and professionals deem the evaluation of their initiatives both as a necessity and as a challenge (Connell & Kubisch, 1998; Cousins, Donohue & Bloom, 1996). Finding the appropriate measurement tools and specifying the right indicators can be challenging (Flora & Grosso, 1999; Suarez-Balcazar, Orellana-Damacela, Portillo, Sharma, & Lanum, 2003). Nevertheless, professionals are now under pressure to engage in practice supported by evidence.

Program evaluation supports evidence-based practice. By documenting the impact of occupational therapy interventions, practitioners will be engaging in practice supported by evidence. Evaluation theory is rooted in outcomes-based evidence models, which have gained much attention in Occupational Therapy literature and have major implications for research and practice (Dysart & Tomlin, 2002; Holm, 2000; Kielhofner, Hammel, Finlayson, Helfrich & Taylor, 2004; Law & Baum,

1998; Ottenbacher, Tickle-Degnen, & Hasselkus, 2002).

General Approaches to Program Evaluation: Formative and Summative

Most generally, evaluation can be summarized under two broad categories: formative and summative. Formative evaluation occurs during the initial steps of planning and implementing a program and reports *process* information. It is used to assess the extent to which actual programming matches that which was planned and the extent to which programming and services address the identified needs of the target population. Formative evaluation often focuses on the process of documenting the delivering of services. The evaluation of process is designed to examine how a program or intervention is being implemented; it helps verify program implementation (Linney & Wandersman, 1996). Therefore, by using process information, the evaluation can improve not only the plan for services but also the implementation and delivery of programs. When information is gathered to document the implementation and delivery of a program, the purpose of the evaluation is then formative evaluation.

More specifically, formative evaluation, or the evaluation of process answers questions about the program such as, Is the program or intervention being implemented as planned? For instance, an occupational therapy intervention designed to teach self-advocacy skills to family members of children with disabilities may ask the following questions to respond to process evaluation: Does the parents' need for advocacy training match what they are being taught? How is the intervention being implemented? How many parents have been trained? What specific advocacy training strategies and topics are being covered? Is the training going as planned?

Keeping detailed records of program implementation allows for the documentation of process. Often the information collected is reported in terms of outputs about program descriptors such as:

- How many training sessions were implemented?
- How many parents were trained?
- What do parents say about the program?

Monitoring the implementation of a program is also a part of formative evaluation. This is the most common practice in terms of evaluation. For the most part, all human services document their programs by maintaining records of the services they provide and participants served. In fact, before conducting an outcomes evaluation, monitoring the program allows for an actual record of the program itself and of the population being served.

Another example of formative evaluation involves conducting weekly staff meetings to determine whether a given program of services is being delivered as it was originally designed and intended. Meetings might determine whether the intended content of services is being delivered, whether services are being delivered at the anticipated rate, whether the anticipated number of clients are utilizing the services, and how staff are experiencing the process of service delivery. Asking clients to complete weekly "feedback forms" that reflect how they are experiencing the occupational therapy services offered is another example of a type of formative evaluation. One uses process information to report on a formative evaluation.

> Evaluation of outcomes documents the impact the program or intervention is having on participants' attitudes, knowledge, skills, abilities/competencies, and/or conditions.

Summative evaluation is also an ongoing process but typically focuses on the outcomes or effectiveness of service delivery. Summative evaluation provides information about the extent to which a program achieves the objectives for which it was developed. As with the other steps described, both quantitative and qualitative data and information may be gathered using strategies, tools, or methodologies that match the evaluation question and the resources available for evaluation. One example of a summative evaluation involves collecting data from clients with hand injuries on functional outcomes following a course of therapy. Evaluation of outcomes documents the impact the program or intervention is having on participants' attitudes, knowledge, skills, abilities/competencies, and/or conditions. The data collected through summative evaluation should help assess the merit of a program or select among interventions.

Outcome evaluation answers questions such as:

- Which intervention is most effective in producing changes in participants' skills (when comparing more than one intervention)?
- Did the attitudes of participants change as a result of the program?
- Did participants' behaviors or skills/competencies change as a result of the intervention?

- Did participants' knowledge change as a result of the intervention?
- Which intervention produced the most impact on participants?
- Did participants' conditions change as a result of the intervention?

Researchers have also classified outcomes in terms of short-term outcomes, intermediate outcomes, and long-term outcomes (Fawcett et al., 1996; United Way, 2003). Short-term outcomes speak for changes in participant's knowledge and/or attitudes, intermediate outcomes speak for changes in behavior, and long-term outcomes speak for changes in an individual's skills/competencies and/or condition. For instance, an occupational therapy intervention designed to increase job related-skills and employment status of individuals with disabilities may document the following:

- Short-term outcomes: Did participants' knowledge of employment resources change as a function of the training?
- Intermediate outcomes: Did participants' job-seeking skills (e.g., writing a resume, preparing for an interview) change as a function of the intervention?
- Long-term outcomes: How many participants found jobs and maintained them at 3 months? Six months? And 12 months after training?

To evaluate the impact of an intervention, researchers need to rely on scientific methods of inquiry. The next section provides an overview of research methods used in evaluation, from the least sophisticated design to the most sophisticated design.

Scientific Research Strategies in Program Evaluation

The type of strategy used to assess the outcome of an intervention and the success of the program depends on many factors, including the evaluation information needs of different stakeholders, resources available for the evaluation, timeline, and deadlines imposed by stakeholders, type of program being evaluated, and the timing of the evaluation (Gabor & Grinnell, 1994). The evaluation of outcomes may go from the least sophisticated design, such as single group evaluation design, to the most complex, such as experimental group evaluation design.

This section only briefly overviews designs that can be used for program evaluation. See Chapter 7 for a detailed discussion of group comparison designs that can be used in program evaluation. Table 37.2 displays a summary of the characteristics, advantages and disadvantages of each of the designs and methodological strategies available for evaluating occupational therapy programs and interventions.

Single-Group Evaluation Design

According to Posavac and Carey (2003), the simplest form of outcome evaluation is the single-group design, which includes one observation after the intervention has taken place. For instance, in the example of a job training program for people with disabilities, the single-group evaluation design may answer the following question: How many individuals with disabilities who completed training are employed at 6 months after training? Or in the example of family members learning advocacy skills, outcome evaluation may answer how many individuals acquire advocacy skills?

Although this design might be an easy way for human service professionals to evaluate the program, it does not answer the questions of whether participants' knowledge or skill would have changed if no intervention was provided. Also, the degree of change cannot be assessed because of the lack of a premeasure or baseline.

Pretest–Posttest design

This design implies an observation before and after the intervention has taken place. This design will help answer the question of whether participants improved or changed while receiving the intervention. For instance, in the example of advocacy skills training program for families of children with disabilities, the occupational therapist could assess the level of advocacy skills and knowledge of disability rights using a validated instrument before and after training. Posavac and Carey (2003) advise that when there are clear standards for the outcome of a human service program and no participants drop out of the program that the pretest–posttest design is an alternative that is inexpensive, simple, and might provide enough information for human service staff.

Quasi-experimental Approaches to Evaluation

Quasi-experimental and experimental designs according to Posavac and Carey (2003) allow for establishing cause–effect relationships and answering the following questions:

• Does the cause precede the effect?
• Does the cause covary with the effect?

These designs also allow alternative explanations of the observed effects to be ruled out. Within quasi-experimental designs, one might use a time-series design in which data are collected several times across a period of time. This design allows for control of some alterative explanations for the observed effects such as maturation (Campbell & Stanley, 1963). Another potential design is the nonequivalent control group design. In this design, more than one comparable group is observed, at least one of which does not receive the intervention. Another possibility is to combine designs such as the time-series and the nonequivalent control design.

Experimental Designs

Experimental designs include by definition the use of random assignment to groups. In this case, a group of similar participants is assigned to different treatment and nontreatment groups randomly. Although this is an optimal design in terms of responding to questions of causation, the reality is that human services and occupational therapy interventions maybe not necessarily need or have the resources or support for a more sophisticated type of evaluation to learn if their programs are having an impact. Experimental designs, for the most part, are more costly and time consuming.

Qualitative Strategies in Program Evaluation

Evaluators often rely on the use of qualitative research strategies as a compliment or an alternative to quantitative methods. Qualitative research methods may be the most appropriate program evaluation methods when:

• The program has complex and multifaceted goals,
• Using empowerment and/or participatory strategies,
• There is a strong need to be culturally sensitive to participants, and

Table 37.2 Program Evaluation Designs: From the Least Sophisticated to the Most Sophisticated

Design	Characteristics	Advantages	Disadvantages
Qualitative strategies	Examples: Focus groups, interviews, public forums, participant observation	- Rich narrative information from the perspective of participants based on their personal experience. - Helps to understand the intervention. - Helps to interpret quantitative data. - Culturally sensitive to some populations.	- Difficult to identify outcome indicators. - Difficult to generalize to other similar populations. - Difficult to establish cause–effect relationships.
Post-measure design only	One systematic observation/assessment after the intervention	- Simplest form of evaluation. - Useful to follow-up on simple, discrete behaviors (e.g., how many people have jobs after 6 months of completing training).	- Does not show change over time. - Difficult to generalize to other similar populations (threats to external validity). - Difficult to establish cause–effect relationships. (threats to internal validity).
Pre–post measure	An observation/assessment is done before and after the intervention	- Simple form of evaluation, appropriate for simple, inexpensive, and standard interventions. - Identifies change over time.	- Difficult to generalize to other similar populations (threats to external validity). - Difficult to establish cause –effect relationships (threats to internal validity).
Quasi-experimental designs Time series	Collection of data across several time intervals on a single unit of behavior	- Controls for some internal validity threats (maturation). - Use by behavior analysts.	- Not appropriate for complex behaviors.
Nonequivalent comparison group	Comparison of two groups that have not been selected randomly and are nonequivalent but somehow similar	- Allows for comparing the target group with a nontreated control group.	- Groups are nonequivalent, which threatens external validity.
Experimental design	Participants are selected randomly and assigned to control and experimental group	- Allows for cause–effect relationships. - Control for treats to internal and external validity.	- Is expensive and complex. - Random assignment to groups is not that feasible in applied settings.

• There may be different desires or conflicts of interest among key stakeholders (Posavac & Carey, 2003; Suarez-Balcazar et al., 2003).

Qualitative strategies include observational methods such as participant observation and direct observation, and other strategies such as interviews with key stakeholders, focus groups, and public forums. Qualitative strategies, for the most part, provide rich narrative information from the perspective of those who experience the program or intervention. Program evaluators recommend combining strategies, qualitative and quantitative, and using multiple informants. Different stakeholders (e.g., participants, significant others, and program staff) can provide useful and relevant information about a program.

Planning and Conducting an Evaluation

The following framework for conducting a program evaluation includes the following four phases:

• Planning the evaluation,
• Developing a program logic model,
• Selecting the methodology and data collection procedures, and
• Reporting research findings and utilizing findings (Suarez-Balcazar et al., 2003). See Figure 37.2 for phases of an evaluation.

Phase I: Planning the Evaluation

The planning of the evaluation should begin at the same time that the program is being developed and planned. This is critical because the use of some evaluation designs imply collecting information about participants and about the program at the onset of the program. During this phase, the evaluation team needs to clarify the following:

• The program/intervention to be evaluated,
• Stakeholders who need to be involved,
• Information needs of different stakeholders,
• Timeline for the evaluation, and
• Resources needed.

It is also important to discuss roles and expectations and to identify evaluation questions of interest to different stakeholders as well as how the data gathered are going to be utilized.

Phase II: Developing an Outcomes Logic Model

A program logic model is a visual representation of the link between program goals, resources and activities, outputs, outcomes, and impact (United Way, 1996). A program logic model is usually developed in an outcomes brainstorming session that fosters critical thinking and self-determination about the program or service (Fetterman, Kaftarian, & Wandersman, 1996).

A number of outcomes models, also referred to as program logic models, have been proposed in the evaluation of human service programs and interventions. Among these frameworks are: the United Way of America (1996) Outcomes Measurement Model; Milstein & Chapel (2002) Model of Change; Linney and Wandersman (1996) Prevention Plus Model; and Connell and Kubisch (1998) and Weiss (1995) Theory of Change Approach.

The outcomes model proposed by United Way of America (1996) highlights the connection between program goals, inputs, activities, outputs, and outcomes. Within this model, program goals are specific statements of who the target population is and what the program is intended to achieve; inputs are defined as program resources and context. Activities and outputs include the pro-

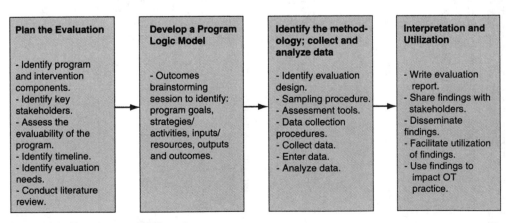

Figure 37.2 Program evaluation phases.

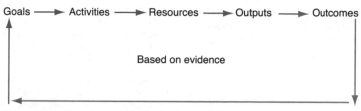

Figure 37.3 Development of a logic model.

gram components and strategies that take place, while outcome evaluation involves measuring changes in participants' knowledge, skills and behaviors, and/or attitudes; or changes in community conditions (Figure 37.3).

Phase III: Identifying the Methodology and Data Collection

During this phase, one must select the evaluation design that is most suitable to the problem and intervention being evaluated. In addition, important decisions about sampling, assessment tools, and methods to measure relevant outcome indicators need to be considered. These important decisions are followed by data collection and data analysis. Most commonly, the sampling, assessment tools, and data collection strategies depend on the design selected. In this decision making process, one needs to keep in mind what is feasible, measurable, realistic, objective, and reliable.

Evaluation experts have called for the use of multiple levels of analysis and multiple measures in the evaluation of human services. Those supporting a more participatory and empowering approach to evaluation have also recommended using both qualitative and quantitative strategies (Fetterman et al., 1996) and that the unit of analysis include the individual and community conditions (Hollister & Hill, 1995).

The selection of a methodology is dependent on the program to be evaluated and the population being served. It is critical that tools and methods selected be culturally sensitive to the population of interest (Marín, 1993). For instance, researchers have asserted that ethnic minority individuals—African-Americans and Hispanics—are more likely to respond to one-on-one interviews and focus groups than to mail surveys (Suarez-Balcazar et al., 2003). Similar strategies have been reported as successful ways to collect information from people with disabilities.

Phase IV: Reporting and Utilizing Findings

During this phase, a report needs to be produced based on the data analysis conducted. Once an evaluation report is developed, the findings are disseminated among different stakeholders. The findings must be interpreted carefully as decisions are likely to be made based on the evaluation findings. The use of an experimental design calls for stronger recommendations, however, while a nonexperimental design may yield weak results about key outcome indicators. Qualitative methods may yield interesting and rich subjective comments from participants about the program.

Dalton, Elias, and Wandersman (2001) consider effective communication of findings imperative, given its potential impact on community members and agencies' subsequent actions in their communities. However, working together with agency staff, other health professionals and diverse stakeholders in interpreting and reporting findings can minimize the challenges (Harper & Salina, 2000).

Maximizing the use of evaluation information is a crucial component of any evaluation effort. Currently, there is an emphasis in the evaluation field on assessing the impact of the evaluation process on the agencies (Cousins, Donohue & Bloom, 1996). This is a reaction to the fact that evaluation results have sometimes been ignored by stakeholders (Mayer, 1996; Weiss, 1995). Several authors have reported that participatory and empowerment approaches to evaluation increase the likelihood of the stakeholders using the information generated by the evaluation. This increase occurs due to:

- A sense of ownership of the evaluation,
- Credibility and trust in the process, and
- A more thorough cognitive processing of the information (Cousins & Earl, 1995; Suarez-Balcazar & Harper, 2003; Wandersman et al., 2004).

Utilization should be a focus of the evaluation throughout the entire process. At the beginning of the evaluation process, all stakeholders invested in the evaluation should be asked to consider ways in which they would use the evaluation information. During the planning and data collection phase, stakeholders should be included in the decision making process and should be kept informed of the preliminary information to ensure utilization. Evaluation utilization should be prompted through a thorough discussion of findings.

Conclusion

This chapter described general approaches to developing and evaluating occupational therapy programs of service. A four-step process for program development was described and the step of program evaluation was explored in further detail. Throughout the chapter, the value of integrating research strategies, methodologies, and findings into program development and program evaluation (e.g., an evidence-based approach) was emphasized. Examples of the types of services that might be developed, implemented, and evaluated by occupational therapy personnel were provided to reinforce that these efforts may occur across a continuum of complexity and effort. Regardless of the level of complexity, the tools, methodologies, and approaches covered in other chapters of this book may be utilized to foster success in program development and evaluation endeavors.

REFERENCES

Braveman, B. (2001). Development of a community-based return to work program for people living with AIDS. In B. P. Velde & P. P. Wittman (Eds.), *Community occupational therapy education and practice* (pp. 113–132). New York, NY: The Haworth Press.

Braveman, B. (2006). *Leading and managing occupational therapy services: An evidence-based approach.* Philadelphia: F. A. Davis.

Braveman, B., & Kielhofner, G. (2006). Developing evidence-based occupational therapy programming. In B. Braveman (Ed.), *Leading and managing occupational therapy services: An evidence-based approach* (pp. 215–244). Philadelphia: F. A. Davis.

Braveman, B., Kielhofner, G., Belanger, R., Llerena, V., & de las Heras, C. G. (2002). Program development. In G. Kielhofner (Ed.), *The model of human occupation: Theory and application* (3rd ed., pp. 491–519). Baltimore, MD: Williams & Wilkins.

Braveman, B., Sen, S., & Kielhofner, G. (2001). Community-based vocational rehabilitation programs. In M. Scaffa (Ed.), *Occupational therapy in community-based practice settings* (pp. 139–161). Philadelphia: F. A. Davis.

Campbell, D. T., & Stanley, J. C. (1963). *Experimental and quasi-experimental designs for research.* Chicago: Rand-McNally.

Connell, J., & Kubisch, A. C. (1998). Applying a theory of change approach to the evaluation of comprehensive community initiatives: Progress, prospects, and problems. In K. Fulbright-Anderson, A. C. Kubisch, & J. P. Connell (Eds.), *New approaches to evaluating community initiatives* (pp. 15–44). New York: Aspen Institute.

Cousins, J. B., Donohue, J. J., & Bloom, G. A. (1996). Collaborative evaluation in North America: Evaluators'

self-reported opinions, practices and consequences. *Evaluation Practice, 17,* 207–226.

Cousins, J. B., & Earl, L. M. (1995). The case for participatory evaluation: Theory, research, practices. In J. B. Cousins & L. Earl (Eds.), *Participatory evaluation in education: Studies in evaluation use and organizational learning* (pp. 3–17). London: Falmer.

Crist, P., & Kielhofner, G. (2005) *The Scholarship of Practice: Academic and practice collaborations for promoting occupational therapy.* Binghamton, NY: Hayworth Press.

Dalton, J. H., Elias, M. J., & Wandersman, A. (2001). *Community psychology: Linking individuals and communities.* Belmont, CA: Wadsworth/Thomson Learning.

Dysart, A. M., & Tomlin, G. S. (2002). Factors related to evidence-based practice among U.S. occupational therapy clinicians. *American Journal of Occupational Therapy, 56,* 275–284.

Fawcett, S. B., Paine-Andrews, A., Francisco, V. T., Schultz, J. A., Richter, K. P., Lewis, R. K., et al. (1996). Empowering community health initiatives through evaluation. In D. Fetterman, S. Kaftarian, & A. Wandersman (Eds.), *Empowerment evaluation: Knowledge and tools for self-assessment and accountability* (pp. 256–276). Thousand Oaks, CA: SAGE Publications.

Fetterman, D. M., Kaftarian, S., & Wandersman, A. (Eds.). (1996). *Empowerment evaluation: Knowledge and tools for self-assessment and accountability.* Thousand Oaks, CA: SAGE Publications.

Fisher, G. S., & Braveman, B. (2006). Understanding health systems. In B. Braveman (Ed.), *Leading and managing occupational therapy services: An evidence-based approach* (pp. 23–52). Philadelphia: F. A. Davis.

Flora, C., & Grosso, C. (1999). Mapping work and outcomes: Participatory evaluation of the farm preservation advocacy network. *Sociological Practice: A Journal of Clinical and Applied Sociology, 1*(2), 133–155.

Gabor, P. A., & Grinnell, R. M., Jr. (1994). *Evaluation and quality improvement in the human services.* Boston: Allyn & Bacon.

Hammel, J., Finlayson, M., Kielhofner, G., Helfrich, C., & Peterson, E. (2002). Educating scholars of practice: An approach to preparing tomorrow's researchers. *Occupational Therapy in Health Care, 15,* 157–176.

Harper, G. W., & Salina, D. (2000). Building collaborative partnerships to improve community-based HIV prevention research: The university-CBO collaborative (UCCP) model. *Journal of Prevention and Intervention in the Community, 19,* 1–20.

Hollister, R. G., & Hill, J. (1995). Problems in the evaluation of community-wide initiatives. In J. Connell, A. C. Kubisch. L. B. Schorr, & C. H. Weiss (Eds.), *New approaches to evaluating community initiatives: Concepts, methods, & contexts* (pp. 127–172). Washington DC: Aspen Institute.

Holm, M. B. (2000). Our mandate for the new millennium: Evidence-based practice, 2000 Eleanor Clarke Slagle lecture. *American Journal of Occupational Therapy, 54,* 575–585.

Kielhofner, G. (2005). Scholarship and Practice: Bridging the Divide. *American Journal of Occupational Therapy, 59,* 231–239.

Kielhofner, G., Hammel, J., Finlayson, M., Helfrich, C., & Taylor, R. R. (2004). Documenting outcomes of occupational therapy: The center for outcomes research and education. *American Journal of Occupational Therapy, 58*(1), 15–23.

Law, M. (2002). *Evidence-based rehabilitation: A guide to practice.* Thorofare, NJ: Slack.

Law, M., & Baum, C. (1998). Evidence-based occupational therapy. *Canadian Journal of Occupational Therapy, 65,* 131–135.

Linney, J. A., & Wandersman, A. (1996). Empowering community groups with evaluation skills: The prevention plus III model. In D. Fetterman, S. Kaftarian & A. Wandersman (Eds.), *Empowerment evaluation: Knowledge and tools for self-assessment and accountability* (pp. 256–276). Thousand Oaks, CA: SAGE Publications.

Marin, G. (1993). Defining culturally appropriate community interventions: Latinos/as as a case study. *Journal of Community Psychology, 21,* 149–161.

Mathiowetz, V., Finlayson, M., Matuska, K., Chen, H. Y., & Lou, P. (2005). Randomized controlled trial of an energy conservation course for persons with multiple sclerosis. *Multiple Sclerosis 11*(5), 592–601.

Mayer, S. E. (1996). Building community capacity with evaluation activities that empower. In D. Fetterman, S. Kaftarian, & A. Wandersman (Eds.), *Empowerment evaluation: Knowledge and tools for self-assessment and accountability* (pp. 256–276). Thousand Oaks, CA: SAGE Publications.

Milstein, B., & Chapel, T. (2002). Developing a logic model or theory of change. *Community tool box* (Chapter 2, section 7). Retrieved April 25, 2004, from http://ctb.ku.edu/tools/EN/chapter_1002.htm.

Ottenbacher, K. J., Tickle-Degnen, L., & Hasselkus, B. R. (2002). Therapists awake! The challenge of evidence-based occupational therapy. *The American Journal of Occupational Therapy, 56*(3), 247–249.

Posavac, E. J., & Carey, G. (2003). *Program evaluation: Methods and case studies.* Englewood Cliffs, NJ: Prentice-Hall.

Stufflebeam, D. L. (2001). Evaluation models. *New directions for program evaluation*(no. 89). San Francisco, CA: Jossey-Bass.

Suarez-Balcazar, Y., & Harper, G. W. (Eds.) (2003). *Empowerment and participatory evaluation of community interventions: Multiple benefits.* New York: The Haworth Press.

Suarez-Balcazar, Y., Orellana-Damacela, L., Portillo, N., Sharma, A., & Lanum, M. (2003). Implementing an outcomes model in the participatory evaluation of community initiatives. In Y. Suarez-Balcazar & G. W. Harper (Eds.), *Empowerment and participatory evaluation of community interventions: Multiple benefits* (pp. 5–20). New York: The Haworth Press.

United Way of America (1996). *Outcome and measurement resource network.* Retrieved April 25, 2004, from http://national.unitedway.org/outcomes/.

United Way of America (2003). *Outcome measurement resource network.* Retrieved April 25, 2004, from http://national.unitedway.org/outcomes/.

Wandersman, A., Keener, D., Snell-Johns, J., Miller, R., Flaspohler, P., Livet-Dye, M., Mendez, J., Behrens, T., Bolson, B., & Robinson, L. (2004). Empowerment evaluation: Principles and action. In L. Jason, K. Keys, Y. Suarez-Balcazar, R. Taylor, M. Davis, J. Durlak, & D. Isenberg (Eds.), *Participatory community research: Theories and methods in action* (pp. 139–156). Washington, DC: American Psychological Association.

Weiss, C.H. (1995). Nothing as practical as good theory: Exploring theory-based evaluation for comprehensive community initiatives for children and families. In J. P. Connell, A. Kubisch, L. Schorr, & C. H. Weiss (Eds.), *New Approaches to evaluating community initiatives: Concepts, methods, and contexts* (pp. 65–92). Washington, DC: Aspen Institute.

Witkin, B. R. (1991).Setting priorities: Needs Assessment in a time of change. In R. V. Carlson & G. Awkerman (Eds.), *Education planning: Concepts, strategies, and practices* (pp. 241–266). White Plains, NY: Longman.

Witkin, B. R., & Altschuld, J. W. (1995). *Planning and conducting needs assessments: A practical guide.* Thousand Oaks, CA: SAGE Publications.

RESOURCES

American Evaluation Association: Information about evaluation practices, methods, and uses through application and exploration of program evaluation. http://www.eval.org/

Getting to Outcomes: Methods and Tools for Planning, self-evaluation and accountability: A manual that works through 10 questions that incorporate the basic elements of program planning, implementation, evaluation and sustainability. http://www.stanford.edu~davidf/empowermentevaluation.html#GTO

Enhancing program Performance with Logic Models: Step by step development of a logic model. http://www.uwex.edu/ces/lmcourse/#

Electronic Resources for Evaluators: This site contains many different links to program evaluation resources. www.itrs.usu.edu/AEA

The Promising Practice Network: Practical programmatic and practice information to help increase the effectiveness and positive impact of work with children, families and communities. http://www.promisingpractice.net/

W. K .Kellogg Foundation Evaluation Handbook: You can get a free copy of their evaluation manual and logic model development guide. www.wkkf.org/documents/wkkfevaluationhandbook/evalhanbook.pdf

Occupational Therapy Evidence-Based Practice Internet Resources

OTSeeker http://www.otseeker.com/

Occupational Therapy Critically Appraised topics http://www.otcats.com

AOTA Evidence-based practice project http://www.aota.org

Center for Evidence-based Rehabilitation at McMaster University http://www.fhs.mcmaster.ca/rehab/centre.htm

Participatory Research in Occupational Therapy

Renée R. Taylor • Yolanda Suarez-Balcazar • Kirsty Forsyth • Gary Kielhofner

Participatory approaches to research have been applied by investigators to address a number of health issues ranging from macro-level community needs to specific needs of disabled clients for resource acquisition and empowerment (Balcazar, Taylor, et al., 2004). Recently, participatory approaches have been discussed and used in occupational therapy (Boyce & Lysack, 2000; Cockburn & Trentham, 2002; Hammel, Finlayson, & Lastowski, 2003; Letts, 2003; Redick, McClain, & Brown, 1999; Townsend, Birch, Langley, & Langile, 2000). This chapter overviews participatory research and discusses its rationale, principles, procedures, and steps. In addition, it illustrates how participatory research can be used within occupational therapy.

> Ultimately, the difficulties of applying research in practice can be linked to the fact that practitioners ordinarily have little influence over what gets studied and how it is studied.

The Need for Participatory Research in Occupational Therapy

The need for participatory research in occupational therapy is indicated by two important circumstances. The first is the gap that often exists between research and practice in occupational therapy. The second is the growing call for clients' voices in shaping the aims and content of occupational therapy services they receive.

The Research–Practice Gap

There can be a significant gap between what research suggests and what actually occurs in professional practice (Kielhofner, 2005a). While many factors contribute to this gap, a key factor is how the knowledge that is supposed to guide practice is created (Schon, 1983). Traditionally, academics who create theory and evidence for practice are isolated from practice settings and practitioners (Peloquin & Abreu, 1996; Thompson, 2001). As a result, they may not be aware of important circumstances and constraints faced by the practitioners who are expected to use that research (Higgs & Titchen, 2001). Even when conducting applied research studies in occupational therapy, academics have largely conceived and executed the research, with practitioners mostly filling secondary roles as consultants, advisors, service providers, or data collectors.

Not surprisingly, practitioners have expressed concerns that research findings lack relevance to clinical situations, address irrelevant topics, and fail to present findings so as to facilitate application (Creek & Ilott, 2002; Dubouloz, Egan, Vallerand, & Von Zweck, 1999; Dysart & Tomlin, 2002; Metcalfe et al., 2001; Sudsawad, 2003). Even when practitioners indicate that they believe that research holds value for practice, they report substantial difficulty integrating it into their practice (Dubouloz et al., 1999; McCluskey, 2003; McCluskey & Cusick, 2002). Ultimately, the difficulties of applying research in practice can be linked to the fact that practitioners ordinarily have little influence over what gets studied and how it is studied.

The Need for Consumer Voice

Within occupational therapy, the concept of client-centered practice makes the important point that individual clients should have a voice in determining their services (Law, 1998). However, outside the field, disability scholars and activists are calling for more. They argue that the disability community should have a voice in the development and validation of services they receive (Fawcett, Seekins, Whang-Ramos, Muiu, & Suarez-Balcazar, 1987). This call suggests that occupational therapy needs to go beyond client-centered practice to embrace a disability community-centered practice that is informed by the collective experiences and perspectives of disabled consumers of our services (Kielhofner, 2005b).

Scholars from disability studies argue that the experience of living with a disability is, in part, a function of social oppression, discrimination, and exclusion, and that individuals with disabilities have been exploited, oppressed, ridiculed, excluded, and disadvantaged by society (Fine & Asch, 1990; Hahn, 1990; Katz, Hass, & Bailey, 1988; Meyerson, 1990; Oliver, 1990). Moreover, they argue that rehabilitation services, including occupational therapy, have the potential to be oppressive, stigmatizing, and largely irrelevant to the needs of individuals with disabilities (Kielhofner, 2005b). This situation exists, in part, because of the lack of control given to the consumer in deciding what services are needed and how they should be provided (Charlton, 1998). Frequently, disabled consumers observe that their individual and collective voices are missing from how occupational therapy construes disability and how to improve such services (Kielhofner, 2004).

> Frequently, disabled consumers observe that their individual and collective voices are missing from how occupational therapy construes disability and how to improve such services.

The Promise of Participatory Research in Addressing These Needs

Participatory research is predicated on the belief that research should be committed to solving practical problems, and to that end, should involve stakeholders as equal partners in the research process. In occupational therapy, stakeholders are the therapists who deliver, the clients who receive, and the communities or groups that are affected by occupational therapy services. Hence, participatory research is well suited to address the need for greater practitioner and client voice in developing and studying occupational therapy service. As such, it promises to contribute knowledge that practitioners can readily use and that consumers will find relevant to their needs.

Definitions and Approach of Participatory Research

Participatory research is an approach to doing research that embraces certain values, perspectives, principles, and processes outlined in this chapter. Many researchers integrate qualitative research methods into participatory research. However, participatory research is also compatible with rigorous experimental designs (Taylor, Braveman, & Hammel, 2004). Participatory research often uses a combination of quantitative and qualitative strategies. For example, data collection in a study may combine standardized measures along with interviewing key informants and conducting focus groups and public forums. Moreover, participatory research is compatible not only with exploratory and case study designs but also with quasi-experimental and experimental designs.

Participatory research can take many forms but the following are four key characteristics:

* Participatory research is conducted in the setting or type of setting where the knowledge to be generated is expected to have relevance. In occupational therapy this means that participatory research takes place in practice contexts,
* Participatory research involves innovation and experimentation that allows inquiry to generate new or modified services and examine how they work. Consequently, participatory research typically combines an ongoing and reflective process of initial investigation, ongoing input from the stakeholders, changes and modifications in the services, and examination of the impact of those changes. This process is used to continuously improve services in concert with gathering evidence about their impact (Reason & Bradbury, 2001),
* Participatory research seeks to empower stakeholders by allowing them to shape the research agenda so that their needs remain the focus of the research process. By definition, participatory research aims to achieve practical outcomes as they are defined by therapists, clients, and other stakeholders, rather than simply to address problems conceptualized by the researcher (Freire, 1970, 1993; Park, 1999). In participatory research, stakeholders engage in many or all aspects of the research process (Park, 1999), and
* Participatory research brings stakeholders into a mutual dialogue and cooperation with investigators to address issues of relevance to those involved. The researcher's role in participatory research is to become an intimate knower and

facilitator of the research process (Balcazar, Garate-Serafini, & Keys, 2004).

General Principles for Implementing Participatory Research in Occupational Therapy

Because participatory research takes place in practice settings and must be responsive to the circumstance of those settings and to the stakeholders who are involved, it requires considerable flexibility on the part of the researcher. Consequently, there is no single or fixed way to conduct participatory research. Nonetheless, scholars have suggested general principles for this type of inquiry (Balcazar, Keys, Kaplan, Suarez-Balcazar, 1998; Nyden, Figert, Shibley & Burrows, 1997; Selener, 1997). Building on their recommendations we offer the following key principles that should shape participatory research in occupational therapy.

Stakeholders Must Be Recognized as Having the Capacity to Participate Fully in the Research Process

In participatory research, researchers must recognize stakeholders' capacity to be involved in research. This recognition begins with acknowledging the kind of expertise that stakeholders bring to the research process. For instance, practitioners bring their accumulated experience in day-to-day practice as well as their local knowledge of the context under study. Consumers bring their intimate knowledge of the problems they face in everyday life as well as their own desires and aims for improving their lives. Ultimately, in participatory research, stakeholders must be viewed as co-researchers working in partnership with the investigators.

Participatory Research Should Empower Everyone Involved

Everyone involved in participatory research has their own agenda. Researchers typically want to create new knowledge, generate publications, meet the expectations of funders, and provide practical and research opportunities for students. Practitioners typically want to increase their skills, provide better services, and have evidence to support what they do. Consumers want to improve their quality of life and have more control over their own lives. Participatory research is most successful when all partners are empowered to address their agendas as much as possible. Moreover, when there are conflicting agendas a process of negotiation must occur and result in a fair compromise.

Elden and Levin (1991) argue that participatory research empowers those involved in three ways: First, specific insights, new understandings, and new possibilities for addressing issues are generated, empowering those involved in the process of discovery. Second, those who engage in participatory research learn how to learn. This aspect is especially beneficial to practitioners or consumers who may feel insecure about themselves and their own knowledge. Third, participatory research is empowering because it often leads those involved to change their own circumstances. True empowerment occurs when stakeholders are increasingly able to sustain what they learned to do through the research process in order to address new needs and barriers that occur in the future.

Participatory Research Should Involve a Dialogical Process Among Constituents that Leads to Critical Awareness

Dialogue gives researchers a more accurate understanding and appreciation of practice settings and consumers' lives. Conversely, it gives practitioners and clients an understanding of how inquiry works and can address practical problems with which they are concerned. Beyond the learning that occurs with the exchange of information, dialogue can also lead those involved to reflect on their own assumptions, attitudes, knowledge, and behavior in a critical way that leads to new awareness.

The dialogue between practitioners, consumers, and researchers is facilitated by using strategies such as listening sessions, focus groups, public forums, and constant ongoing team meetings in which all stakeholders are involved. When implemented in this way, participatory research can be a transformative and liberating process of mutual discovery.

The Research Agenda Is Shaped by the Researchers, Practitioners, and Consumers and It Aims to Address Local Social Issues

Participatory research works best when the agendas of all those involved are openly discussed and addressed. Participatory research means that stakeholders other than the researchers are involved to some significant extent in helping to identify what gets studied, how questions are formulated, what kinds of data will be collected, and how data will be analyzed, shared, and used to make change. Involving practitioners and clients in these decisions often requires a great deal of discussion and negotiation between the stakeholders and the researchers. In traditional occupational therapy scholarship, the research agenda is formulated by the researchers based on personal research agendas (i.e., the desire to prove or disprove an existing theory). In participatory research, the researcher's agenda is important but it must be balanced with the agendas of stakeholders such as the therapists or consumers.

Participatory Research Generates Knowledge that is Intended to be Used

Utilization of findings to either inform or shape services, practices, and policies is a key feature of participatory research. Moreover, participatory research often involves an ongoing cycle of research informing practice and practice informing research. Thus, scientific knowledge and practical knowledge mutually inform each other.

In participatory research, practical real-world utility is considered, along with empirical rigor, as a hallmark of good research (Higgs & Titchen, 2001). Participatory research recognizes that genuine knowledge arises out of efforts to achieve desired changes or solve problems in a particular context (Bradbury & Reason, 2001; David, Zakus, & Lysack, 1998). Participatory research projects are interested in practical outcomes at the local level. In the case of occupational therapy, they ask such questions as: What are the specific changes in practice and its impact resulting from the research process?

Inserting Stakeholders' Voices into the Research Process

As we have noted, participatory research aims to give stakeholders a genuine role in the research process so that their perspectives and needs are addressed. A key challenge of participatory research is to find ways in which practitioners and consumers have a true voice in shaping the questions, methods and outcomes of the research process (Boyce & Lysack, 2000; Suarez-Balcazar, Harper & Lewis, 2005; Taylor et al., 2004). The appropriate approach to involving stakeholders in the research process depends on many factors.

Creating a Genuine Dialogue

Because participatory research involves bringing together people with quite different backgrounds and perspectives, interactions can readily involve mistrust and misunderstanding. A productive dialogue requires finding common ground between what are often the disparate perspectives of researchers and practitioners. Genuine dialogue requires:

- Hearing others' perspectives in a nonjudgmental way,
- Sharing one's knowledge and perspectives openly with others,
- Willingness to change one's own perspective,
- Working toward a common language with others,
- Confronting legitimate disagreements over what is most important,
- Negotiating and compromising,
- A two-way communication style,
- An attitude of being as ready to learn as to teach,
- Recognizing that others have important knowledge to contribute, and
- Being ready to acknowledge diversity of opinions.

These factors include:

- The aims and scope of the research,
- Organizational and contextual policies,
- The culture of those involved,
- Available resources,
- The level of readiness and desire of stakeholders for participation, and
- The collaborative attitude and approach taken by the researchers.

Approaches to Practitioner and Consumer Participation in Research

The particular form that the participatory research process actually takes depends on the context of the research. An important factor to consider is the degree of power or control that the stakeholders have over the research process. Danley and Langer-Ellison (1999) suggest that we can think of a continuum of power held by stakeholders that spans from little power to full power or control. At the low end of the spectrum are advisory committees, which are sometimes called participatory. The reality in such research is that stakeholders

> In participatory research, the researcher's agenda is important but it must be balanced with the agendas of stakeholders such as the therapists or consumers.

have some involvement but ultimately very little power or authority over the research project.

On the other end of the continuum are projects in which participants have full control over the research process, including hiring and firing authority over the professional researchers. Midpoints on the continuum include hybrid projects in which stakeholders have high degree of control over the research process, but researchers are responsible to outside funding agencies and thus retain decision-making authority over some areas. For example, Whyte's (1991) approach involves stakeholders in the research process "from the initial design of the project through data gathering and analysis, to the final conclusions and actions arising out of the research" (p. 7). In this approach, stakeholders become actively involved in the quest for information and ideas to guide their future actions.

Table 38.1 was derived from a schema proposed by Danley and Langer-Ellison (1999) and revised by Balcazar, Taylor, et al. (2004). This version, which is an adaptation to occupational therapy research, provides a means of conceptualizing the extent of stakeholder involvement in the clinical research process. Practitioners' and consumers' roles are classified on the basis of three criteria: the degree of control that participants have over the research process (Litvak, Frieden, Dresden, & Doe, 1997), the extent of collaborative decision-making between stakeholder participants and professional researchers (Turnbull & Friesen, 1997), and the levels of input from and commitment of participants with the research process (Gordon, 1997).

This schema can be useful in evaluating how "participatory" a research project is. It is important to note that one end of the continuum is not automatically superior to the other. Rather, the continuum should be seen as a structure for thinking about the amount of stakeholder involvement the researcher is willing to negotiate, is good for the project, and is allowed by funders and other organizational constituencies who affect the research resources and implementation.

Knowledge-Creation and Evaluation in Participatory Research

Within participatory research, knowledge is redefined and judged in ways that go beyond the traditional focus on propositional, rationally deduced forms of knowledge and the processes for ensuring rigor of such knowledge. There is a new emphasis

Sharing Power

Participatory research often challenges investigators to share power in unaccustomed ways. Conversely, it asks therapists and clients to take on responsibilities for and control over matters for which they ordinarily have little or no involvement or influence. As a result, all those involved in participatory research have to constantly reflect on their own attitudes and behaviors with reference to issues of power. This is not necessarily an easy task, as often researchers are the ones who come in with the resources and funding and the aura of expertise of research and therapists and/or clients can be readily intimidated. Among other things, true power sharing requires:

- Shared responsibility, voice, and decision-making about all aspects of the investigation,
- Respect and acknowledgement of the unique expertise and insights of all those involved,
- Willingness to step outside their usual roles and responsibilities,
- Identification and remediation of sources of power imbalance such as money and access to technology, and
- Sharing resources (e.g., paying for a staff time to devote to the project, providing participants with stipends).

on alternative epistemologies that recognize, for example, the importance of experiential and procedural knowledge (Bradbury & Reason, 2001; Maxwell, 1992). This means that participatory research values the kind of knowledge that is generated among the participants in the study (i.e., what they have experienced and what they have learned to do). In this same vein, Selener (1997) suggests that feeling and acting are ways of knowing that should also emerge from research. He argues that traditional scientific methods rely exclusively on cognitive activities as a source of knowledge. Participatory researchers typically embrace the idea that reflection and action are important to the research process.

Participatory research also values the stakeholders' knowledge and experiences as important resources. Such subjective knowledge is viewed as a necessary part of the process of understanding any situation Elden and Levin (1991) argue that those inside a particular context get to know more about it and have more ways of making sense of their world than would be possible for any outsider to appreciate. The best way to access such knowledge is through dialogue, allowing individuals to share their views in a free and supportive

Table 38.1 **The Continuum of Stakeholder Involvement in Participatory Research Implementation**

Level of Participation	Degree of Control Influence	Typical Amount/ type of Collaboration	Degree of Commitment/ Ownership
Nonparticipatory	Practitioners and clients have no control or influence on the research process.	Serve as implementers or recipients of services studied or as participants in the study.	None
Low	Practitioner and/or client opinions and feedback are considered and used by researchers at the latter's discretion.	Serve as advisors to the research project. Provide feedback in pilot studies or discuss implications of findings at advisory board meeting.	Minimal commitment and ownership
Medium	Practitioners and/or clients, and/or representatives of consumer groups participate in research meetings and in aspects of the research implementation.	Provide ongoing advice, review, and consultation. Participate in discussions leading to decisions about the research.	Multiple commitments to and partial ownership of the research process
High	Practitioners, clients, and/or representatives of consumer groups function as equal partners with researchers in making all decisions about the research.	Full partners in making key research decision.	Full commitment to and equal ownership of the research process with the researchers
Very high	Practitioners, clients, and/or consumers groups lead the research with researchers assisting them.	Research leaders.	Full commitment and complete ownership of the research process

process. In this way, stakeholders' perspectives can define:

- What issues are important,
- How problems can be framed and defined,
- What strategies work in the community, and
- What are local challenges and barriers to change.

This kind of local knowledge is critical to the success of participatory research and is included whether the primary research design is qualitative or quantitative. In qualitative participatory studies, the subjective experiences of stakeholders are used throughout. In quantitative participatory studies, subjective knowledge and experiences may be used at critical points (e.g., when deciding on the content of services to be studied or when interpreting the findings).

A Framework for Knowledge Generation in Participatory Research

One challenge of participatory research is how to balance traditional concerns for developing rigor-

ous generalizable knowledge with concerns of solving real-world problems and empowering stakeholders in the research context (Kielhofner, 2005a). According to Elden and Levin (1991), participatory research involves coming to understand a particular situation by working with those within it to develop, test, and enhance knowledge that improve people's lives. In this approach, researchers are interested in generating knowledge that helps people learn how to better control their circumstances. This approach implies a cycle of knowledge generation in which theory shapes practice and practice shapes theory. Theory that is generated or enriched through participatory research builds on knowledge that accumulates as people work together to improve understanding of a particular situation (Park, 1993).

Senge and Scharmer (2001) express a similar view of participatory research, proposing that it involves "a knowledge-creating system." We have adapted their ideas to discuss a general model of participatory research for occupational therapy. In our model, researchers, practitioners, and con-

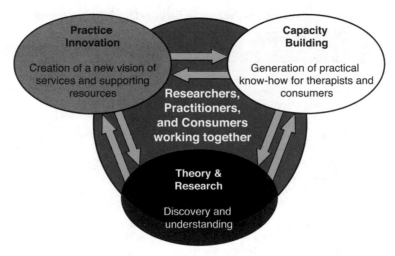

Figure 38.1 A knowledge-creating system.

sumers work together as part of what Senge and Scharmer (2001) call a "continuing cycle of creating theory, tools and practical know-how" (p. 238). They further engage in three interacting domains of activity:

- Discovery and understanding of concepts and data whose relevance transcends the particular situation—that is, knowledge that is generalizable. This knowledge is generally the primary objective of the researcher.
- Creation of practical knowledge and capacity-building, which enhances practitioners' and clients' awareness and capabilities. Practical knowledge emphasizes utilization and usefulness of the knowledge generated in addressing social issues of importance to consumers. Capacity building is also critical in this model because it speaks for one of the essences of participatory research and that is increasing skills, knowledge, and capabilities of participants to address their own concerns. This kind of knowledge is local and personal since it involves such things as enhancing the practical know-how of occupational therapy practitioners and empowering clients with knowledge of how to manage their circumstances.
- Practice innovation, which involves creating new possibilities and means for achieving them. Such knowledge can involve rethinking practice aims or methods. It involves creating or improving practical tools and approaches that work out in a particular situation but that are irrelevant to other similar situations. Practice innovation often aims at creating tools that not only work in the situation at hand, but that can also be used in other practice situations.

These three components of knowledge creation are collectively addressed within a single community of people working together. As a result, concepts, evidence, and practice innovations are created at the same time that practitioners' knowledge of and use of these resources is increased.

In this knowledge-creating system, practitioners and clients are centrally involved along with researchers in the process of creating knowledge. Conversely researchers join practitioners and consumers in solving practice problems and innovating in practice. Furthermore, in a knowledge-creating system there is no artificial division between creating and assessing knowledge on the one hand and applying it on the other. Finally, all stakeholders are involved in co-generative learning in which their initial perspectives are altered or replaced through dialogue and co-discovery (Elden & Levin, 1991).

The Steps of Participatory Research in Occupational Therapy

Discussions of the process of participatory research have been offered in the literature (Balcazar, Keys, & Suarez-Balcazar, 2001; Fawcett et al., 2003; Selener, 1997; Suarez-Balcazar & Harper, 2003; Taylor et al., 2004). Based on these ideas, we propose here a framework for the process of participatory research in occupational therapy. According to this framework, participatory research involves six steps as depicted in Figure 38.2. These steps, discussed next, are part of an ongoing cycle of discovery, change-making, and evaluation of change. Although the research ordinarily begins with the first step, it can begin at any stage and may involve implementing elements of different stages simultaneously. Furthermore, it is important to recognize that before participatory research begins and throughout its implementation, there is a process of entry and building trust wherein the researcher establishes and maintains a true partnership with the stakeholders.

Phase 1: Delineating the Problem Through Critical Reflection and Analysis

In traditional research, problems to be investigated in the research are most often identified from careful study of the literature. In participatory research, delineating the problem to be studied also involves careful attention to how stakeholders define the problem locally and to the larger context that may be influencing the problem. Moreover, the problem to be addressed will emerge out of the practice context. In this phase it is important to ask the following questions:

- How does the literature shed light on the problem?
- How do different stakeholders view the problem?
- What are contextual and environmental factors affecting the problem?
- When all these dimensions are considered together how do they frame the problem?

In participatory research, researchers and stakeholders engage in ongoing reflection aimed at achieving a critical awareness of the problem. Without critical reflection, research can move forward to solve a problem before it is fully defined and its multiple dimensions are fully understood. Participatory research seeks to confront and address the full complexity of any problem rather than trying to isolate and study only one aspect. In this way, participatory research is more likely to generate solutions that actually work in the real-life situation. Often, given the cyclical nature of participatory research, the problem may be redefined as the research unfolds.

Phase 2: Analysis and Planning of the Participatory Research

Careful and critical analysis of the problem sets a foundation for the next step of the process, planning the research. This step involves selecting the research questions or hypotheses that will be answered or tested in the research. Because of the previous step, the research questions or hypotheses will not be grounded only in preexisting empirical and theoretical knowledge. They will also reflect key stakeholders' perspectives on what they need to understand or know. In this phase, it is important to consider the following kinds of questions:

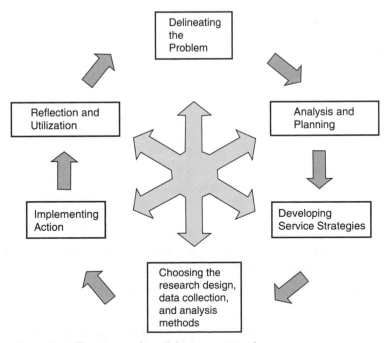

Figure 38.2 The steps of participatory research.

• Given the dimensions of the problem, what do we need to know to understand or address the problem?
• What kinds of information do we want to generate about the problem and how the solutions work?
• How would the information that is generated be used?

Since stakeholders are involved along with researchers, the questions generated will have not only theoretical but also utilitarian ends. Information is sought not only to create understanding of what is being studied but also to achieve workable solutions to local problems.

Phase 3: Developing Service Strategies

The third phase involves an analysis of potential service strategies that can be implemented to understand and address the problem and its dimensions. In occupational therapy these strategies can include such diverse things as modifying or generating a new assessment or intervention, developing a program to meet an unmet need, promoting organizational change that affects healthcare delivery for a client group, or engaging in advocacy efforts to change insurance legislation to affect a consumer group. Depending on the context, choosing or implementing a solution may require systematic deliberations, complex negotiations, and even struggles between different perspectives or with existing power structures.

In this phase it is important to consider the following questions:

• What are potential strategies to address the problem?
• Are the strategies appropriate given the situation and perspectives of the stakeholders involved?
• What are the anticipated likely consequences of applying the proposed strategies or ways of addressing the problem?

In answering these questions, the researchers and stakeholders work together to integrate existing scientific knowledge with local knowledge.

Phase 4: Choosing the Research Design and Data Collection and Analysis Methods

After strategies for addressing the problem have been chosen, the researcher and stakeholders engage in choosing the research design and the approach to data collection and analysis. Once again, these methods must fit the interests of stakeholders and available resources (Fawcett et al, 2003; Park, 1999). In participatory research, investigators and stakeholders often participate equally in data collection, data analysis, and in decisions as to how the success of a given strategy will be judged. By shaping such data analysis, stakeholders have an important role in determining what conclusions will be drawn from the research. In this phase, it is important to consider the following questions:

• Are the design, the methods for gathering data, and the kind of data collected appropriate for evaluating the strategies?
• Are the design, the methods for gathering data, and the kind of data collected appropriate to the context and the concerns of stakeholders?
• Will the design, data collection, and analysis provide information that is both credible in the scientific community and relevant to making future decisions in the research setting?

> Information is sought not only to create understanding of what is being studied but also to achieve workable solutions to local problems.

This phase requires achieving an important balance between scientific and practical concerns. The design and data will not only address concerns of a larger scholarly community but also provide information about whether a local problem has been effectively addressed.

Phase 5: Implementing Action

A key element of participatory research is that it involves action. Participatory research in occupational therapy will involve implementing the strategies that have been designed to address the problem. As noted earlier, these strategies can range from fairly minor modifications of services to new programs of services to large-scale changes in service delivery. Whatever the action being implemented, a key feature is that this action is undertaken in a reflective way. This means that the following kinds of questions are typically asked:

• Are the service strategies working as anticipated?
• What unexpected problems or barriers have emerged?
• Have efforts to implement the innovations in service been successful? Have they created new complications?

Depending on the design of the research, answers to these types of questions may be used to modify the services on an ongoing basis or they will be used to provide critical information about how the service strategies work.

Phase 6: Reflection and Utilization

In this phase, researchers and stakeholders reflect on the strategies implemented in the research and the results they have achieved as indicated by the data collected and by their experiences in the process. During this phase, questions such as the following are asked.

- What do the findings mean?
- What are their implications for future action in this setting?
- How can we use the results to improve services, programs, and practice in general?
- How can the knowledge be disseminated to others?
- What new questions or problems have emerged from taking action?

By addressing such questions, the research team is accountable for ensuring that the research findings can be used locally and broadly with the profession to improve occupational therapy practice.

Implementing the Six Phases of Participatory Research

As illustrated in Figure 38.2, the phases of participatory research are not linear. In fact, they are interactive and mutually informing. Often, stages will be combined and implemented simultaneously or iterated in small cycles. For example, it is common that phase 5 and phase 6 are interwoven. When this is the case, the research involves a reflection–action–reflection cycle (Freire, 1970, 1993) in which ongoing understanding of new problems and action to address those problems continues as knowledge is generated in the research process (Park, 1999).

Challenges of Conducting Participatory Research

Like all forms of research, participatory research has its own unique challenges. Two of the most challenging aspects of participatory research are creating a dialogue and sharing power. Participatory research inevitably involves the following elements (Balcazar et al., 2001; Prilleltensky & Nelson, 2002; Riger, 2001; Suarez-Balcazar et al., 2004):

- Working together with others who share different views,
- Taking on nontraditional roles,
- "Thinking outside the box" of traditional, discipline-defined research,
- Balancing power, control and resources, and
- Breaking from traditional researcher–participant relationships.

For this reason, participatory research can be, at its extremes, both frustrating and exhilarating. It requires a serious commitment to the underlying vision of why participatory research is important for the field, and careful attention to the guidelines and procedures we have outlined in this chapter. Chapters 39 and 40 discuss the challenges of participatory research further and provide strategies and examples of how they can be effectively addressed.

Conclusion

This chapter overviewed the rationale and need for participatory research in the context of occupational therapy and discussed its underlying epistemological assumptions. It also suggested ways to think about the extent of participation by stakeholders, it offered principles, and it offered a model to guide participatory research. In addition, this chapter noted some of the challenges involved in participatory research.

Participatory research protects the voice of consumers and clients and provides a venue for researchers and practitioners to work together and advance both scholarship and practice. Moreover, its emphasis on innovation and reflection makes it particularly suited to achieve creative new approaches to service. Consequently, participatory research has a unique role in advancing occupational therapy practice.

REFERENCES

Balcazar, F. E., Keys, C. B., Kaplan, D. L., & Suarez-Balcazar, Y. (1998). Participatory action research and people with disabilities: Principles and challenges. *Canadian Journal of Rehabilitation, 12*, 105–112.

Balcazar, F. E., Keys, C. B., & Suarez-Balcazar, Y. (2001). Empowering Latinos with disabilities to address issues of independent living and disability rights: A capacity-building approach. *Journal of Prevention and Intervention in the Community, 21*(2), 53–70.

Balcazar, F. E., Garate-Serafini, T. J., & Keys, C. B. (2004). The need for action when conducting intervention research: The multiple roles of community psychologists. *American Journal of Community Psychology, 33*(3–4), 243–252.

Balcazar, F. E., Taylor, R. R., Kielhofner, G. W., Tamley, K., Benziger, T., Carlin, N., & Johnson, S. (2004). Participatory action research: General principles and a study with a chronic health condition. In L.A. Jason, C.B. Keys, et al. (Eds.), *Participatory community research: Theories and methods in action* (pp. 17–35). Washington, DC: American Psychological Association.

Boyce, W., & Lysack, C. (2000). Community participation: Uncovering its meanings in CBR. In M. Thomas, & M.J. Thomas, *Selected readings in community based rehabilitation: CBR in transition (Series 1)*. Bangalore: Asia Pacific Disability Rehabilitation Journal.

Bradbury, H., & Reason, P. (2001). Conclusion: Broadening the bandwidth of validity: Issues and choice-points for improving the quality of action research. In P. Reason & Bradbury, H. (Eds.). *Handbook of action research: Participative inquiry and practice*. London: SAGE Publications.

Charlton, J. I. (1998). *Nothing about us without us*. Los Angeles: University of California Press.

Cockburn, L., & Trentham, B. (2002). Participatory action research: Integrating community occupational therapy practice and research. *Canadian Journal of Occupational Therapy, 69*, 20–30.

Creek J., & Ilott I. (2002) Scoping study of occupational therapy research and development activity in Scotland, Northern Ireland and Wales. Executive Summary, College of Occupational Therapists, London.

Danley, K., & Langer Ellison, M. (1999). *A handbook for participatory action researchers*. Boston: Center for Psychiatric Rehabilitation, Boston University.

David, J., Zakus, L., & Lysack, C. L. (1998). Revisiting community participation. *Health Policy and Planning, 13*(1), 1–12.

Dubouloz, C., Egan, M., Vallerand, J., & VonZweck, C. (1999). Occupational therapists' perceptions of evidence based practice. *American Journal of Occupational Therapy, 53*, 445–453.

Dysart, A. M., & Tomlin, G. S. (2002). Factors related to evidence-based practice among US occupational therapy clinicians. *American Journal of Occupational Therapy, 56*(3), 275–284.

Elden, M., & Levin, M. (1991). Cogenerative learning: Bringing participation into action research. In W. F. Whyte (Ed), *Participatory action research*. Newbury Park, CA: SAGE Publications.

Fawcett, S., Boothroyd, R., Schultz, J., Franciasco, V. T., Carson, V., & Bremby, R. (2003). Building capacity for participatory evaluation within community initiatives. *Journal of Prevention and Intervention in the Community, 26*, 21–36.

Fawcett, S. B., Seekins, T., Whang-Ramos, P., Muiu, C. & Suarez-Balcazar, Y. (1987). Involving consumers in decision-making. *Social Policy, 13*(6), 36–41.

Fine, M., & Asch, A. (1990). Disability beyond stigma: Social interaction, discrimination, and activism. In M. Nagler (Ed.), *Perspectives on disability* (pp. 61–74). Palo Alto, CA: Health Markets Research.

Freire, P. (1970). *Pedagogy of the oppressed*. New York: Continuum..

Freire, P. (1993). *Pedagogy of the oppressed*. New York: Herder and Herder.

Gordon, W. A. (1997). PAR: A realistic strategy for medical rehabilitation Research? In B. Phillips-Tewey, (Ed.). *Building participatory action research partner-*ships in disability and rehabilitation research*. Washington, DC: U.S. Department of Education, National Institute on Disability and Rehabilitation Research.

Hahn, H. (1990). The politics of physical difference: Disability and discrimination. In M. Nagler (Ed.), *Perspectives on disability* (pp. 118–123). Palo Alto, CA: Health Markets Research.

Hammel, J., Finlayson, M., & Lastowski, S. (2003). Using participatory action research to create a shared assistive technology alternative financing outcomes database and to effect social action systems change. *Journal of Disability Policy Studies, 14*(2), 109–118.

Higgs, J., & Titchen, A. (2001). Rethinking the practice-knowledge interface in an uncertain world: A model for practice development. *British Journal of Occupational Therapy, 64*, 526–533.

Katz, I., Hass, L., & Bailey, J. (1988). Attributional ambivalence and behavior toward people with disabilities. In H. Yuker (Ed.), *Attitudes toward persons with disabilities* (pp. 47-57). New York: Springer.

Kielhofner, G. (2004). *Conceptual foundations of occupational therapy* (3rd ed.), Philadelphia: F. A. Davis.

Kielhofner, G. (2005a). Scholarship and practice: Bridging the divide. *American Journal of Occupational Therapy, 59*, 231–239.

Kielhofner, G. (2005b). Rethinking disability and what to do about it: Disability studies and their implications for occupational therapy. *American Journal of Occupational Therapy, 59*, 487–496.

Law, M. (Ed). (1998). *Client-centered occupational therapy*. Thorofare, NJ:Slack.

Letts, L. (2003). Occupational therapy and participatory research: A partnership worth pursuing. *American Journal of Occupational Therapy, 57*, 77–87.

Litvak, S., Frieden, L., Dresden, C., Doe, T. (1997). Empowerment, independent living research and participatory action research. In B. Phillips-Tewey, (Ed.), *Building participatory action research partnerships in disability and rehabilitation research*. Washington, DC: U.S. Department of Education, National Institute on Disability and Rehabilitation Research.

Maxwell, N. (1992). What kind of inquiry can best help us create a good world? *Science, Technology, & Human Values, 17*, 205–227.

McCluskey, A. (2003). Occupational therapists report a low level of knowledge, skill and involvement in evidence-based practice. *Australian Occupational Therapy Journal, 50*(1), 3–12.

McCluskey, A., & Cusick, A. (2002). Strategies for introducing evidence-based practice and changing clinical behavior: A manager's toolbox. *Australian Occupational Therapy Journal, 49*(2), 63–70.

Metcalfe, C., Lewin, R., Wisher, S., Perry, S., Bannigan, K., & Moffett, J. K. (2001). Barriers to implementing the evidence base in four NHS therapies: Dietitians, occupational therapists, physiotherapists, speech and language therapists. *Physiotherapy, 87*, Part 8, 433–441.

Meyerson, L. (1990). The social psychology of physical disability: 1948–1988. In M. Nagler (Ed.), *Perspectives on disability* (pp. 13–23). Palo Alto, CA: Health Markets Research.

Nyden, P., Figert, A., Shibley, M., & Burrows, D. (1997). *Building community: Social science in action*. Thousand Oaks: Pine Forge.

Oliver, M. (1990). *The politics of disablement*. London: Macmillian.

Park, P. (1993). What is participatory research? A theoretical and methodological perspective. In P. Park, M. Brydon-Miller, B. Hall, & T. Jackson (Eds.) *Voices of change: Participatory research in the United States and Canada* (pp. 1–19). Westport, CT: Bergin & Garvey.

Park, P. (1999). People, knowledge, and change in participatory research. *Management Learning, 30,* 141–157.

Peloquin, S. M., & Abreu, B. C. (1996). The academia and clinical worlds: Shall we make meaningful connections? *American Journal of Occupational Therapy, 50*(7), 588–591.

Prilleltensky, I., & Nelson, G. (2002). *Doing psychology critically: Making a difference in diverse settings.* Basingstroke, UK: Palgrave, MacMillan.

Reason, P. & Bradbury, H. (2001). *Handbook of action research: Participative inquiry and practice.* London: SAGE Publications.

Redick, A. G., McClain, L., & Brown, C. (1999). Consumer empowerment through occupational therapy: The Americans with Disabilities Act Title III. *The American Journal of Occupational Therapy, 54,* 207–213.

Riger, S. (2001). Working together: Challenges in collaborative research. In M. Sullivan & J. G. Kelly (Eds.), *Collaborative research: University and community partnerships* (pp. 25–44). Washington, DC: APHA.

Schon, D. A. (1983). *The reflective practitioner.* New York, Basic Books.

Selener, D. (1997). *Participatory action research and social change.* Ithaca, NY: Cornell Participatory Action Research Network, Cornell University.

Senge, P., & Scharmer, O. (2001). Community action research: Learning as a community of practitioners, consultants, and researchers. In P. Reason & Bradbury, H. (Eds.), *Handbook of action research: Participative inquiry and practice.* London: SAGE Publications.

Suarez-Balcazar, Y., Davis, M., Ferrari, J., Nyden, P.,

Olson, B., Alvarez, J., et al. (2004). University-community partnerships: A framework & case study. In L. Jason, C. Keys, et al. (Eds.), *Participatory community research: Theory and methods in action* (pp. 105–120). Washington, DC: American Psychological Association.

Suarez-Balcazar, Y., & Harper, G. (Eds.). (2003). *Participatory and empowerment evaluation: Multiple benefits.* New York: The Haworth Press.

Suarez-Balcazar, Y., Harper, G., & Lewis, R. (2005). An interactive and contextual model of Community-University partnerships. *Health Education & Behavior, 32*(1), 84–101.

Sudsawad, P. (2003). Rehabilitation practitioners' perspectives on research utilization for evidence-based practice. Paper presented at the American Congress of Rehabilitation Medicine conference, October 24, Tucson, Arizona.

Taylor, R. R., Braveman, B., & Hammel, J. (2004). Developing and Evaluating Community Services through Participatory Action Research: Two Case Examples. *American Journal of Occupational Therapy, 58,* 73–82.

Thompson, N. (2001). *Theory and practice in human services.* Maidenhead: Open University Press.

Townsend, E., Birch, D. E., Langley, J., & Langille, L. (2000). Participatory research in a mental health clubhouse. *Occupational Therapy Journal of Research, 20,* 18–44.

Turnbull, A. P., & Friesen, B. J. (1997). Forging collaborative partnerships with families in the study of disability. In B. Phillips-Tewey (Ed.), *Building participatory action research partnerships in disability and rehabilitation research.* Washington, D. C.: U.S. Department of Education, National Institute on Disability and Rehabilitation Research.

Whyte, W. F. (1991). *Participatory action research.* Newbury Park, CA: SAGE Publications.

CHAPTER 39

Building Culturally Competent Community–University Partnerships for Occupational Therapy Scholarship

Yolanda Suarez-Balcazar • Jaime Phillip Muñoz • Gail Fisher

Occupational therapy researchers increasingly recognize the need for and benefits of building partnerships with community settings to support scholarship (Braveman, Helfrich, & Fisher 2001; Cockburn & Trentharn, 2002; Suarez-Balcazar, Hammel, Helfrich, Thomas, Head-Ball, & Wilson, 2005a). These multipurpose partnerships often combine research, student training and development, and implementation and evaluation of service delivery (Braveman et al., 2001). This chapter examines factors that contribute to effective partnerships with community settings. It offers key principles and a framework of cultural competence to guide community–university partnerships.

Factors such as the mental health movement, deinstitutionalization, and consumer self-help initiatives, combined with declining healthcare access, governmental services, and family support, have contributed to the growth of community agencies. There are many types of community settings; examples include:

- Grass-roots advocacy organizations,
- Shelters,
- Jails,
- Social service agencies,
- Community mental health programs, and
- Public health clinics.

These types of agencies provide a wide range of services, often to marginalized populations (e.g., low-income families, people with AIDS, refugees, survivors of domestic violence, the elderly, at-risk youth, individuals with disabilities) (Suarez-Balcazar, Harper, & Lewis, 2005b).

Community–University Partnerships

Community–university partnerships are mutually beneficial collaborative relationships that bring individuals from academia and the community together to work on common goals. Moreover, participants typically share the risks, responsibilities, resources, and rewards of their collaborative efforts (Suarez-Balcazar et al., 2004). Community–university partnerships are critical for research that aims to:

> Community–university partnerships are mutually beneficial collaborative relationships that bring individuals from academia and the community together to work on common goals.

- Apply theoretical and research-related constructs in a real-life setting,
- Study varied populations and cultural contexts, and
- Impact the health and life satisfaction of disenfranchised populations.

Benefits to the community partner can include:

- Access to the skills of a researcher for identifying and addressing unmet needs,
- Assistance with grant writing and accreditation, and
- Support for program development and evaluation.

Table 39.1 **Benefits of Community–University Partnerships**

Benefits to the Community	Benefits to the University
• Capacity building	• Opportunities to advance scholarship
• Improving the success of programs	• Access to research participants and sites
• Documentation of impact to inform decision makers and funders	• Stronger grant applications
• New perspectives for needs assessment and strategic planning	• Staff service as advisory board members for research proposals and studies
• Assistance in planning, implementing, and evaluating programs and services	• Capacity building to be more culturally competent
• Assistance in understanding problems and collecting data	• Opportunity to participate in a social change process
• Access to researchers with the skills to examine complex interventions	• Opportunities to engage in learning by doing
• Assistance in providing best services to clients	• Possibility to conduct applied and participatory action research
• Shared ownership over products and materials developed	• Opportunity to gain knowledge about the culture of the community including social norms and community values
• Adoption of innovations that are developed	• Entrée into a network of community health coalitions with legitimate power and leadership
• Practice and services based on evidence	• Collaboration with practitioners
	• Publications based on applied research

Thus community–university alliances can bring benefits to all those involved. Table 39.1 provides a summary of such benefits.

Key Principles of University–Community Partnerships

Previous literature has identified characteristics and models of successful community–university partnerships (Braveman et al., 2001; Harper & Salina, 2000; Suarez-Balcazar et al., 2004; Suarez-Balcazar et al., 2005a,b) and articulated methodological strategies for Participatory Action Research with community agencies (Balcazar, Keys, Kaplan, & Suarez-Balcazar, 1998; Taylor, Braveman, & Hammel, 2004). Building on this work, we argue that the key principles of community–university partnerships belong to two overarching characteristics of successful partnerships:

• Shared commitment, and
• Joint responsibility.

Table 39.2 illustrates these key principles which are discussed.

Shared Commitment

Successful community–university partnerships occur when both parties share commitment to:

• Address complex social problems,
• Achieve mutuality,
• Create learning communities,
• Use a participatory approach to research, and
• Advance scholarship and practice together.

Commitment to Address Complex Social Problems

Society today faces difficult problems such as domestic and school violence, AIDS, hunger, homelessness, unemployment, rising rates of incarceration, and addiction. Solutions to these problems are likely to be as complex and interdependent as the factors that give rise to them. Most

Table 39.2 **Framework of Key Principles for Successful Partnerships**

Shared Commitments	Joint Responsibility
• To address complex social problems	• For communication
• To mutuality	• For recognizing, utilizing, and exchanging resources
• To create learning communities	• For addressing challenges and assimilating change
• To participatory approach to research	• For sustainability
• To advance the Scholarship of Practice	

efforts to address these issues occur at the community level.

Occupational therapists in community-based settings are beginning to demonstrate how complex societal problems can be addressed from an occupational perspective (Daunhauer & Jacobs, 2003; Fazio, 2001; Muñoz, Reichenbach, & Witchger Hansen, 2005). Occupational therapy concepts are being used to address human problems that have their origins in complex social conditions (Abelenda, Kielhofner, Suarez-Balcazar, & Kielhofner, 2005; Kielhofner, 2002; Townsend, 1997). Thus, occupational therapists are increasingly able to bring their disciplinary perspectives to bear on research that addresses social problems.

Commitment to Mutuality

Mutuality is facilitated by:

* Making time to get to know a setting and its different stakeholders,
* Building a common vision,
* Mutually setting expectations/ground rules,
* Establishing common goals, and
* Sharing frameworks and ways of thinking about issues of importance to all involved.

In research involving community–university partnerships, a common agenda and clarification of shared values needs to be pursued from the very beginning. Mutuality requires the development of reciprocal trust and respect for each other's differences (Foster-Fishman, Berkowitz, Lounsbury, Jacobson & Allen, 2001; Mattessich & Monsey, 1992).

Decisions must be made collaboratively. Partnerships call for flexibility when working with multiple layers of decision-makers (Mattessich & Monsey, 1992). Moreover, community organizations typically have a number of stakeholders who must be involved in decision-making. These stakeholders range from executive directors and staff members, to community members and leaders. Moreover, in many agencies, staff turnover and work overload may mean that one's primary partner(s) change throughout the partnership (Suarez-Balcazar, Orellana-Damacela, Portillo, Sharma, & Lanum, 2003). Therefore, mutuality is served well by establishing relationships with a range of community members and leaders (Braveman et al., 2001).

> Researchers must move from seeing a community as a research site to seeing a community as a research partner.

Commitment to Create Learning Communities

Investigators should come to a partnership ready to learn, as well as to guide. It is useful for all to maintain a constant exchange of perspectives and flexible teacher–learner roles. Collaborative partnerships for occupational therapy research recognize that expert knowledge resides not only within the profession but also in the community. Moreover, an interactive building of knowledge is important.

Researchers must move from seeing a community as a research site to seeing a community as a partner. This means appreciating that the community is a repository of rich cultural and practical knowledge. For example, community partners are typically aware of important political and organizational relationships in a community. Further, they usually hold informed perspectives on the needs and strengths of the community, the prevailing issues, and the key players. Community partners often have legitimate power and authority in the community that is grounded in a sustained commitment to addressing the needs of the community as grassroots organizers or front-line service providers. Researchers who at best have limited experience and exposure as intermittent participant-observers in the community do well to rely on the information, expertise, and authority of their community partners.

Commitment to a Participatory Approach to Research

Participatory research emphasizes the inclusion of community partners in the earliest stages of defining research questions, setting research priorities, and designing research studies (Suarez-Balcazar et al., 2004; Taylor et al., 2004). In fact, in some cases it is the community who calls upon the researcher to be part of the partnership team. In participatory research, investigations are guided by the needs of the community rather than the intellectual interests of the researcher (Braveman et al., 2001; Suarez-Balcazar, 2005).

Successful community–university partnerships recognize that social issues originate in the community and are better understood, analyzed, and solved when members of the community are intimately involved (Balcazar et al., 1998; Balcazar,

Keys, & Suarez-Balcazar, 2001; Selener, 1997). Successful partnerships also require that researchers and community partners engage in joint reflection and analysis. Finally, successful partnerships occur when those involved use findings to support genuine change that addresses local problems.

Commitment to Advance a Scholarship of Practice

Community–university partnerships represent an opportunity for researchers to embrace a scholarship of engagement (Boyer, 1996) that both serves and develops a deeper understanding of the community (Jackson & Reddick, 1999; Sanstad, Stall, Goldstein, Everett, & Brousseau, 1999). Within occupational therapy, engaged scholarship has been referred to as a Scholarship of Practice. This perspective argues for occupational therapy research that addresses and solves practice problems in real-life contexts (Braveman et al., 2001; Crist & Kielhofner, 2005; Kielhofner, 2005). The Scholarship of Practice framework also emphasizes using occupational therapy theories to enhance service delivery and using the real life challenges and circumstances of service delivery to further develop theoretical constructs.

When scholars are immersed in the lived experience of community members, they tend to develop a greater sense of social responsibility that leads to participating in advocacy and social change efforts. In truly collaborative community–university research partnerships, researchers work together with community leaders, service providers, and consumers to create knowledge not only for the profession but also for solving local problems.

Joint Responsibility

Successful community–university partnerships are strong alliances where not only mutual benefit but also mutual responsibility occurs. Partners must assume equal responsibility for:

* Developing adequate communication,
* Recognizing, utilizing, and exchanging resources,
* Addressing challenges to assimilating change, and
* Ensuring sustainability of any change that is implemented.

Responsibility for Communication

Establishing a good communication system is at the heart of authentic and successful partnerships. A communication system is concerned with:

* What is communicated,
* How it is communicated, and
* The communication style and language used.

Communication is facilitated when goals and expected roles and outcomes are discussed and agreed upon and when hidden agendas or power plays are absent (Connors & Seifer, 2000; Panet-Raymond, 1992). Of course, goals and expectations may change throughout the process, but they need to be openly discussed and negotiated. Sensitivity to the communication mode and style of the setting is critical. Modes refer to such communication channels as formal memos, regularly scheduled meetings, e-mail messages, phone calls, and one-on-one visits (Suarez-Balcazar et al., 2004). Community settings can vary in their preferences or modes, and different modes can also symbolize such things as power, trust, and respect. Often researchers have to adjust to the communication style of the community setting.

For a relationship to be successful, it is essential to establish open and frequent communication by providing updates, discussing issues openly, and sharing all information with one another as well as the broader community membership (Mattessich & Monsey, 1992). Partners must establish regular ways of communicating in order to discuss how the partnership is unfolding, to quickly identify any issues, and to strategize how to address them.

Community–University Partnership Example of Shared Commitment

Faculty at Duquesne University built a partnership with a community nonprofit organization that has been dedicated to providing shelter and supportive services to homeless men and women for over two decades (Muñoz et al., 2005). This community–university partnership grew from a shared vision between the executive director of the agency and an occupational therapy faculty who envisioned a strong, reciprocal partnership that would address the comprehensive health and wellness needs of the consumers at agency with holistic, innovative programming. In addition to the Executive and Program Directors, faculty built relationships with others whose support has ensured the success of the partnership. These include administrators of the homelessness and hunger programs, directors of other programs serving homeless and incarcerated populations who might utilize services at the agency, and funders who were supporting programming at the shelter. Projects are chosen in collaboration with the agency staff and all partners share a commitment to scholarship and practice.

Researchers will be most successful at developing and sustaining an authentic relationship when using a nonhierarchical communication style (Suarez-Balcazar et al., 2005a; Harper et al., 2004). This means avoiding using academic language and jargon to impress the community. If community members feel they are being treated in condescending and paternalistic ways, their trust is impeded and they are more likely to develop resentment toward the researcher or the study (Gills, Butler, Rose, & Bivens, 2001). Effective communication is grounded in mutual respect for diverse viewpoints and ideas regardless of one's education or title.

Responsibility for Recognizing, Utilizing, and Exchanging Resources

Each of the partners brings into the relationship resources and strengths that need to be recognized and valued (Connors & Seifer, 2000; Mattessich & Monsey, 1992). Most typically, investigators bring access to resources (e.g., grant funding), knowledge of research design and methods, theoretical knowledge, and fresh perspectives. Community partners bring knowledge of the specific area or population of interest, legitimate power and leadership within the community, political savvy, experiential information of the issues involved, and awareness of the cultural and contextual characteristics of the setting and community (Braveman et al., 2001; Suarez-Balcazar et al., 2005b).

Moreover, resources might be differently perceived and available in academia and the community. For instance, not all members of a community organization may have their own computers or access to the Internet. For many people with disabilities, access to accommodations such as transportation, personal assistance, interpreting, and captioning are critical to their active participation in research. Communities with limited resources may perceive research as a low priority when other more fundamental needs are not being met. Many organizations in urban areas are struggling to attract resources and are cautious about how many resources (e.g., time and effort) they spend on research. Investigators must make a direct link between their research and meeting needs of the community and be sensitive to the resource flow that any investigation creates. In this regard, assisting agency partners in grant writing activities or bringing grant-related or university-based resources to a community agency can be very helpful.

Time frames might also be different. Researchers often operate within longer frameworks (such as a 3- to 5-year grant period), while community agencies often have briefer temporal horizons and operate around events shaped by a variety of factors such as cultural holidays, fund raising cycles, budget, or academic calendars. Unique features of sites may also influence issues of timing. For example, sites serving individuals without family connections may be able to provide more access

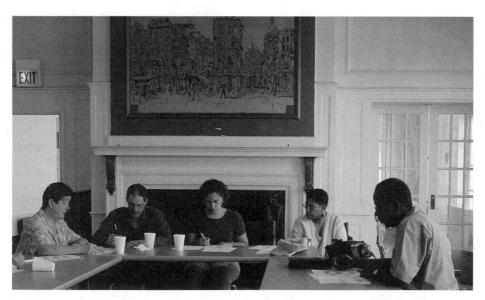

Figure 39.1 University researchers and members of a community organization meet to discuss the "next steps" related to findings from a previous project, resolve any concerns related to the current research project, and identify areas for future collaboration.

to potential research subjects over the holidays because they are providing expanded programming. Consequently, community–university partners need to talk about time frames and negotiate when certain activities and products are expected.

Responsibility for Addressing Challenges and Assimilating Change

An omnipresent feature in community–university partnerships is change and the challenges that come with it. Changes in personnel, governmental regulations, and funding priorities or levels, are but a few of the challenges that either partner may face. The challenges of partnerships have been discussed extensively in the literature (see, Connors & Seifer, 2000; Mattessich & Monsey, 1992; Riger, 2001; Suarez-Balcazar et al., 2004). Some of these challenges include:

- Managing conflicts of interest and differences in perspectives,
- Sustaining activities after termination of funding,
- Changing roles and redefining boundaries,
- Developing common ground, and
- Managing different external pressures.

Partnerships call for flexibility and tolerance. Challenges should be acknowledged up front, openly discussed, and addressed. Changes in personnel, funding, or timing may force a partnership to change. A key strategy for assimilating such change is to stay grounded in the central mission and vision that drew the partners together initially. When a clear and unified vision permeates thinking and planning, partners can adjust to changes without fracturing their mutual commitment.

Responsibility for Sustainability

Sustainability refers to the capacity for the partnership to maintain itself over time. Partnerships with community settings for research are not built overnight. They take time, a positive attitude from all those involved, and a strong commitment to make it work (Suarez-Balcazar et al., 2004). From the earliest stages of collaboration, partners should address sustainability with an open and frank discussion.

Research partnerships with a community setting minimally need to last the duration of an ongoing project. Longer-term commitments can be developed based on common interest and success in obtaining ongoing funding. Getting to know the program well, its constituents, the setting's mission, goals, constituents, and overall context well is part of the responsibility of the researchers who wish to develop a long-term relationship. They should also be prepared to volunteer time and talent to the agency (e.g., serving on the board of directors or providing technical and professional advice when needed).

Developing Cultural Competence for University–Community Partnerships for Occupational Therapy Scholarship and Practice

Community–university partnerships for research almost always involve managing diversity. Thus, respecting and celebrating diversity is essential to the relationship. Importantly, it requires researchers to building cultural competence (Prilleltensky, 2001; Suarez-Balcazar, Durlak, & Smith, 1994; Velde, Wittman, & Bamberg, 2003).

There are compelling reasons for occupational therapy researchers to become culturally competent. Recent U.S. census figures suggest that ethnic and racial minorities are becoming numerical majorities in parts of our pluralistic society (U.S. Census Bureau, 2000). Race, ethnicity, and socioeconomic status are consistent factors in studies of health disparities. A growing body of research is demonstrating that levels of health care, healthcare outcomes, and general health status are typically poorer for racial and ethnic minorities and economically disadvantaged populations (Institute of Medicine, 2002; Mayberry et al., 1999). Researchers need to address these entrenched disparities, study disadvantaged populations in their own environment, and advance the limited body of knowledge on the impact of occupational therapy with minority populations.

According to Papadopoulos and Lees (2002), the development of culturally competent researchers is important because:

- Research and most services tend to come from a unicultural perspective,
- There is growing recognition from funders, educators and health policy makers alike of the need to manage diversity and address inequalities in research knowledge and service development to minority and disadvantaged populations,
- Research with minority populations is often not integrated into subsequent research, practice and mainstream policy, and
- Culturally incompetent research may lead to inappropriate policies, services and programs.

Community–University Partnership Example of Joint Responsibility

A long-term relationship has developed between the University of Illinois at Chicago and an agency in Chicago that provides employment, life enrichment, advocacy, and residential services to primarily Hispanic adults with intellectual disabilities. Taking joint responsibility for the ongoing development of this relationship has provided the agency, clients, faculty members, students, and the occupational therapy academic program with multiple benefits. The relationship began with the agency requesting a clinical service contract, and expanded to include the agency's involvement in several research grants, a yearly commitment from the agency to host community practicum students, and collaboration on a number of master's projects. These projects, which embody the Scholarship of Practice framework, have addressed unmet needs expressed by the agency representative to the contact faculty member. For example, two students worked with a faculty member to develop a new assessment for the agency's group residences, which has provided the agency with strategies to improve their homes to promote occupational role development within the constraints of limited dollars and staff resources. A second project resulted in a staff development training model, with the students serving as coaches to the staff to develop skills areas that the staff member had identified. Both projects are now being used in research projects by the contact faculty member and other occupational therapy scholars (Taylor, Fisher, & Kielhofner, 2005). These new research grants will provide resources to the agency while the community site provides access to clients for the studies.

Both the faculty member and the community agency take responsibility to build the partnership by sharing resources, time, and expertise. They each have become familiar with the culture of the other's environment, and have both learned about celebrations, traditions, and priorities. The contact faculty member serves on the agency's strategic planning committee and has assisted with the development of a proposal for a new building. The community agency representative serves on the advisory board for the faculty member's allied health grant, assists with subject recruitment for research studies, and participates as a panelist for graduate courses. Both the contact faculty member and the community agency representative are committed to the sustainability of this relationship, letting it evolve over time to address emerging needs.

There is no universally accepted definition of cultural competence (Bonder, Martin, & Miracle, 2002). Several models of cultural competence have been proposed in the psychological (Cross, Bazron, Dennis & Issacs, 1989; Sue, Arredondo, & McDavis, 1992), nursing (Campinha-Bacote, 2001; Leininger, 2000; Purnell & Paulanka, 2002), and health professions literature (Bonder et al., 2002). Collectively, these models hypothesize that cultural competence is a multidimensional process. It involves a tripartite mix of cognitive, behavioral, and affective components. This tripartite conceptualization of cultural competence is not new. In cultural psychology, Sue et al., (1992) organized their framework of cultural competency around the domains of knowledge, skills, and awareness (Arredondo et al., 1996; Sodowsky, Taff, Cutkin, & Wise, 1997). In nursing, Sawyer et al., (1995) identified knowledge, sensitivity, and collaboration as the three key characteristics of cultural competence. While these models have been developed to describe competencies needed by the practitioner, they are relevant for the researcher as well.

In occupational therapy, Muñoz (2002) has proposed a process-oriented model of culturally responsive caring that also defines three distinct dimensions of cultural competence: *knowing, doing, and becoming*. This process-oriented conceptualization of culturally responsive caring is critical to the success of community–university partnerships in occupational therapy and is discussed below.

Knowing: Generating Cultural Knowledge and Building Cultural Awareness for Successful Partnerships

Culturally responsive researchers generate cultural knowledge when they develop a broad knowledge base that helps them understand the worldviews of people living in diverse communities. Sue and colleagues (1998) have argued that to be culturally competent, one needs to possess specific information and knowledge about particular social groups with whom one is working. Sawyer and colleagues (1995) defined cultural knowledge as the understanding of integrated systems of learned behavior patterns in a cultural group, including how members of a group talk, think, and behave and their feelings, attitudes, and values.

Knowing involves:

• Viewing partner communities as inherently multicultural,

• Cultivating a perspective on culture that encompasses attributes beyond race and ethnicity, and
• Acknowledging the differences that exist within any community.

Generating cultural knowledge entails "reaching and obtaining a sound educational foundation about the worldviews of different cultures" (Campinha-Bacote, 2001, p. 256). Sue and Zane (1987) have described this type of knowledge as cultural literacy. Cultural literacy is reflected in the way that a researcher studies the culture of a community. Culturally responsive researchers:

• Generate culture-specific knowledge about the people and social groups with whom they partner,
• Acknowledge within-group variations in the community, and
• Make conscious efforts to determine whether culture-specific information is applicable to community partners.

This approach to reasoning has been described by Sue (1998) as dynamic sizing.

Culturally responsive researchers also build cultural awareness of themselves as multicultural individuals. Awareness is enhanced by exploring their cultural heritage (Tervalon & Murray-Garcia, 1998). This self-knowledge is essential for researchers to recognize how their own cultural lenses may influence their analyses of data. Active reflection directed at understanding self and others as cultural beings is a key aspect of building cultural awareness. Researchers can also build cultural awareness through a conscious process of examining their own biases and their capacities and limitations for research with culturally diverse populations. This willingness to examine one's own prejudices and to remain open to the experience of diversity and multiculturalism has been described by Tervalon and Murray-Garcia (1998) as cultural humility.

Doing: Applying Cultural Skills and Engaging Culturally Diverse Others in Partnerships for Research

Doing is conceptualized as a behavioral component of culturally responsive research. It refers to demonstrable skills in communication and relationship building, advocacy, data gathering, data analysis, and collaborative dissemination of results and products. One of the primary ways that cultural responsiveness skills are manifest is in the interpersonal interactions that researchers employ to forge interpersonal connections with community partners. Researchers can establish a sense of mutuality with community partners by:

• Maintaining an open and welcoming stance,
• Reading and respectfully responding to the dynamics of each encounter, and
• Engaging each partner with a purposeful intent to identify and honor the cultural lifeways of the community.

Every partnership is a cross-cultural encounter. The researcher approaches the partnership with a knowledge base and social norms that reflect the academic culture while the community partners are seeped in a culture and knowledge base of their own. These cultural crossings sometimes compliment and sometimes clash. Culturally responsive researchers often serve as cultural brokers between the community partner and the wider university community.

Culturally responsive researchers must apply advocacy skills. Being an advocate or collaborating with community partners on self-advocacy recognizes the influence that socioeconomic and environmental conditions have on health status and the way that political, legal, and language barriers compound these situations. Rorie, Paine, and Barger (1996) suggested that skills in advocacy involve moving beyond recognition that racism and ethnocentrism influence health care to doing something to address this situation.

Researchers also apply cultural skills when they design data collection methods that respect the community partner's cultural practices and perspectives. These skills can entail the intentional consideration of culture when designing evaluation tools or intervention procedures.

To develop the skills of a culturally responsive researcher one must engage culturally diverse others (Campinha-Bacote, 2001). A researcher can develop skills through direct encounters with culturally diverse populations. Such encounters provide a context for researchers to test the depths and recognize the limits of their cultural knowledge and to practice skills for connecting and responding. Encounters are not always harmonious and friction is often rooted in a clash of cultural values. However, cultural missteps provide opportunities to generate cultural knowledge and build skills. This type of learning is supported by reflective processing of cultural encounters.

Spence (2001) has argued that cross-cultural encounters "have meaning prior to, in the moment, and on reflection" (p. 102). Lockhart and Resnick (1997) posit that the process of cultural competence begins with self-reflection. In partnerships the researcher will engage in several cultural exchanges that are likely to help shape his *knowing* and *doing* in becoming more culturally competent.

Culturally responsive research requires the integration of knowing and doing. A researcher must not only possess cultural knowledge and an intentional respect for varied cultural perspectives, but she must also develop skills and use them effectively in cross cultural encounters (Brach & Fraser, 2000).

Becoming: Exploring Cultural Competence in the Context of Partnerships

Becoming is a reflective process whereby researchers demonstrate an intentional drive to continually broaden their cultural understanding. Exploring multiculturalism is a purposeful act grounded in a commitment to address culture in the research context. Padilla & Brown (1999) have characterized the process of becoming culturally competent as a journey and lifelong process. Becoming culturally responsive is an intentional endeavor. Campinha-Bacote (2001) uses the term *cultural desire* to convey this sense of drive and commitment to exploring multiculturalism. The term *exploring* is used intentionally to capture a sense of discovery and intense reflexivity.

Becoming is a commitment toward multicultur-alism. It manifests in a desire and obligation to learn and experience cultural diversity while being humbled by the vastness of human multiculturalism (Tervalon & Murray-Garcia, 1998). Framing culturally responsiveness as exploration underscores the idea that cultural competency is a process not a state (Campinha-Bacote, 2001). It requires an openness to cultural understanding where one is informed but not-knowing (Laird, 1998). Not-knowing is manifest in an interpersonal approach that includes:

- Active listening,
- Intentional respect, and
- Questioning processes that conscientiously recognize persons as experts of their own experience (Anderson & Goolishian, 1992). Table 39.3 lists strategies that facilitate developing cultural competence in the context of community–university partnerships.

Conclusions

Community–university partnerships are increasingly important to scholarship. Through mutual

Table 39.3 Strategies for Developing Cultural Competence for Partnerships

Knowing	Doing	Becoming
• Be aware of one's own cultural heritage, cultural values, attitudes, ethnic experiences, and biases that can influence partnership processes.	• Identify educational and training opportunities that support the development of culturally responsive practice.	• Enact a personal commitment to social justice and multiculturalism.
• Develop understanding of health care disparities and factors that prevent effective care of marginalized groups.	• Seek opportunities for encounters with culturally diverse groups outside professional settings.	• Practice acceptance of ambiguity.
• Become aware of the effect of racism, discrimination, and oppression on the lived experience of marginalized groups.	• Use a variety of interpersonal strategies that recognize and respect cultural differences in communication styles.	• Remain flexible to accept differences and change.
	• Develop data collection methods that reflect preferred interaction styles of the cultural group.	• Recognize the limits of your cultural competencies and expertise.
• Learn the culture of the community, its population, and resources.	• Adapt services, research endeavors, and practice to meet the needs of diverse populations as defined from within those communities.	• Develop a high level of comfort with a broad array of cultural difference (race, ethnicity, religion, lifestyle preferences, etc.).
• Appreciate a variety of cultures and subcultures (e.g., disability culture).	• Challenge bias, stereotypes, and discriminatory practices.	• Be vigilant toward the dynamics that result from cultural differences.
• Learn the culture of the agency (e.g., traditions, ways of communicating).	• Participate in the traditions of the agency.	• Maintain a "not-knowing" posture that intentionally respects the beliefs, values, and knowledge base of the community.
	• Listen to the experiences of others and share experiences.	
	• Appreciate differences and recognize similarities.	

collaborative relationships, individuals from academia and the community come together to work on a common goals. In these partnerships, knowledge and practice innovations are produced in such a way that both occupational therapy theory and occupational therapy practice benefit.

Community–university partnerships require researchers to let go of traditional power relationships and to share commitment and responsibility. Researchers must work to achieve trust, mutual respect, and open communication, combined with clear expectations and shared goals. Finally, investigators who want to engage in such partnerships must value participatory research and commit to an ongoing process of becoming culturally competent.

REFERENCES

Abelenda, J., Kielhofner, G., Suarez-Balcazar, Y., & Kielhofner, K. (2005). The Model of Human Occupation as a Conceptual Tool for Understanding and Addressing Occupational Apartheid. In F. Kronenberg, S. Simo Algado, & N. Pollard (Eds.), *Occupational therapy without borders* (pp. 183–196). Edinburgh: Churchill Livingstone.

Anderson, H., & Goolishian, H. (1992). The client is the expert: A not-knowing approach to therapy. In S. McNamee & K. Gergen, (Eds.), *Therapy as social construction* (pp. 25–39). Newbury Park, CA: SAGE Publications.

Arredondo, P., Toropek, R., Brown, S. P., Jones, J., Locke, D. C., Sanchez, J., & Stadler, H. (1996). Operationalization of the multicultural counseling competencies. *Journal of Multicultural Counseling and Development, 24*, 42–78.

Balcazar, F., Keys, C., Kaplan, M. A., & Suarez-Balcazar, Y. (1998). Participatory action research and people with disabilities: Principles and challenges. *Canadian Journal of Rehabilitation, 12*, 105–112.

Balcazar, F., Keys, C., & Suarez-Balcazar, Y. (2001). Empowering Latinos with disabilities to address issues of independent living and disability rights: A capacity-building approach. *Journal of Prevention and Intervention in the Community, 21*, 53–70.

Bonder, B. R., Martin, L., & Miracle, A. (2002). *Cultural threads in clinical contexts.* Thorofare, NJ: Slack.

Boyer, E. L. (1996). The scholarship of engagement. *Journal of Public Service and Outreach, 1*(1), 11–20.

Brach, C., & Fraser, I. (2000). Can cultural competency reduce racial and ethnic health disparities? A review and conceptual model. *Medical Care Research and Review, 57*, 181–217.

Braveman, B., Helfrich, C., & Fisher, G. S. (2001). Developing and maintaining community partnerships within a 'scholarship of practice. *Occupational Therapy in Health Care, 15*(1/2), 109–125.

Campinha-Bacote, J. (2001). A model of practice to address cultural competence in rehabilitation nursing. *Rehabilitation Nursing, 26*(1), 8–11.

Cockburn, L., & Trentharn, B. (2002). Participatory action research: Integrating community occupational therapy practice and research. *Canadian Journal of Occupational Therapy, 69*(1), 20–30.

Connors, K., & Seifer, S. D. (2000). *Partnership perspectives, 1*(2). San Francisco, CA: Community–Campus Partnerships for Health.

Crist, P., & Kielhofner, G. (2005). *The Scholarship of Practice: Academic and practice collaborations for promoting occupational therapy.* Binghamton, NY: Hayworth Press.

Cross, T., Bazron, B. J., Dennis, K. W., & Issacs, M. R. (1989). *Towards a culturally competent system of care. Vol. I: Monograph on effective services for minority children who are severely emotionally disturbed.* Washington: Georgetown University Child Development Center, CASSP Technical Assistance Center.

Daunhauer, L., & Jacobs, K. (2003). *Occupational therapy's role in preventing youth violence.* Retrieved on February 4, 2004, from http://www.aota.org/members/area7/links/link18.asp?PLACE=/members/area7/links/link18.as

Fazio, L. S. (2001). Programming to support meaningful occupation and balance for the disenfranchised and homeless. In L. S. Fazio (Ed.), *Developing occupation centered programs for the community: A workbook for students and professionals* (pp. 256–274). Upper Saddle River, NJ: Prentice Hall.

Foster-Fishman, P., Berkowitz, S., Lounsbury, D., Jacobson, S., & Allen, N. (2001). Building collaborative capacity in community coalitions: A review and integrative framework. *American Journal of Community Psychology, 29*, 241–261.

Gills, D. C., Butler, M., Rose, A., & Bivens, S. (2001). Collaborative research and action in communities: Partnership building in the Chicago empowerment zone. In M. Sullivan & J. G. Kelly (Eds.), *Collaborative research: University and community partnership* (pp. 25–44). Washington, DC: APHA.

Harper, G. W., Lardon, C., Rappaport, J., Bangi, A. K., Contreras, R., & Pedraza, A. (2004). Community narratives: The use of narrative ethnography in participatory community research. In L. Jason, C. Keys, Y. Suarez-Balcazar, R. R. Taylor, M. Davis, J. Durlak, & D. Isenberg (Eds.), *Participatory community research: theories and methods in action* (pp. 199–217). Washington, DC: American Psychological Association.

Harper, G. W., & Salina, D. (2000). Building collaborative partnerships to improve community-based HIV prevention research: The university-CBO collaborative (UCCP) model. *Journal of Prevention and Intervention in the Community, 19*, 1–20.

Institute of Medicine (2002). *Unequal treatment: Confronting racial and ethnic disparities in health care.* Retrieved on April 1, 2004, from http://books.nap.edu/books/030908265X/html/

Jackson, R. S., & Reddick, B. (1999). The African American church and university partnerships: Establishing lasting collaborations. *Health Education and Behavior, 26*, 663–674.

Kielhofner, G. (2002). *Model of human occupation* (3rd ed.). Philadelphia: Lippincott, Williams & Wilkins.

Kielhofner, G. (2005). Scholarship and Practice: Bridging the divide. *American Journal of Occupational Therapy, 59*, 231–239

Laird, J. (1998). Theorizing culture: Narrative ideas and practice principles. In M. McGoldrick (Ed.), *Revisioning family therapy: Race, culture, and gender in clinical practice* (pp. 20–36). New York: Guilford Press.

Leininger, M. (2000). *Transcultural nursing: Concepts, theories, research & practices* (3rd ed.). New York: McGraw-Hill.

Lockhart, J. S., & Resnick, L. K. (1997). Teaching cultural competence: The value of experiential learning and community resources. *Nurse Educator, 22*(3), 27–31.

Mattessich, P., & Monsey, B. (1992). *Collaboration: What makes it work.* St. Paul, MN: Amherst Wilder Foundation.

Mayberry, R. M., Mili, F., Vaid, L., Samandi, E., Ofili, M. S., McNeil, M. S., Griffith, P. A., & LaBrie, G. (1999). *Racial and ethnic differences in access to medical care: A synthesis of the literature.* Menlo Park, CA: The Henry J. Kaiser Family Foundation.

Muñoz, J. (2002). *Culturally responsive caring in occupational therapy: A grounded theory.* Unpublished doctoral dissertation, University of Pittsburgh, Pittsburgh.

Muñoz, J. P., Reichenbach, D., & Witchger Hansen, A. (2005) Project Employ: Engineering hope and breaking down barriers to homelessness. WORK - A *Journal of Prevention, Assessment and Rehabilitation, 25(3),* 241–252.

Padilla, R. & Brown, K. (1999). Culture and patient education: Challenges and opportunities. *Physical Therapy Education, 13*(3), 23–33.

Papadopoulos, I., & Lees, S. (2002). Developing culturally competent researchers. *Journal of Advanced Nursing, 37*(3), 258–264.

Panet-Raymond, J. (1992). Partnership: Myth or reality? *Community Development Journal, 27,* 156–165.

Prilleltensky, I. (2001). Value-based praxis in community psychology: Moving toward social justice and social action. *American Journal of Community Psychology, 29,* 747–778.

Purnell, L. D., & Paulanka, B. J. (2002). *Transcultural health care: A culturally competent approach.* Philadelphia: F. A. Davis.

Riger, S. (2001). Working together: challenges in collaborative research. In M. Sullivan & J.G. Kelly (Eds.), *Collaborative research: University and community partnership* (pp. 25–44). Washington, DC: APHA.

Rorie, J. L., Paine, L. L., & Barger, M. K. (1996). Primary care for women: cultural competence in primary care services. *Journal of Nurse-Midwifery, 41,* 92–100.

Sanstad, K. H., Stall, R., Goldstein, E., Everett, W., & Brousseau, R. (1999). Collaborative community research consortium: A model for HIV prevention. *Health Education and Behavior, 26*(2), 171–184.

Sawyer L., Regev, H., Protor, S., Nelson, M., Messias, D., Barnes, D., & Meleis, A. I. (1995). Matching versus cultural competence in research: Methodological considerations. *Research in Nursing and Health, 18,* 556–567.

Selener, D. (1997). *Participatory action research and social change.* Ithaca, NY: The Cornell Participatory Action Research Network.

Sodowsky, G. R., Taff, R. C., Cutkin, T. B., & Wise, S. L. (1997). Development of multicultural counseling inventory: A self-report measure of multicultural competencies. *Journal of Counseling Psychology, 41*(2), 137–148.

Spence, D. G. (2001). Prejudice, paradox, and possibility: Nursing people from cultures other than one's own. *Journal of Transcultural Nursing, 12*(2), 100-106.

Suarez-Balcazar, Y. (2005). Empowerment and participatory evaluation of a community health Intervention: Implications for occupational therapy. *Occupational Therapy Journal of Research: Occupation, Participation, and Health, 25*(4), 133–142.

Suarez- Balcazar, Y., Davis, M. I., Ferrari, J., Nyden, P., Olson, B., Alvarez, J., Molloy, P., & Toro, P. (2004).

University–community partnerships: A framework and an exemplar. In L. A. Jason, C. B. Keys, Y. Suarez-Balcazar, R. R. Taylor, & M. I. Davis (Eds.), *Participatory community research* (pp. 105–120). Washington, DC: American Psychological Association.

Suarez-Balcazar, Y., Durlak, J. A., & Smith, C. (1994). Multicultural training practices in community psychology programs. *American Journal of Community Psychology, 22,* 785–798.

Suarez-Balcazar, Y., Hammel, J., Helfrich, C., Thomas, J., Head-Ball, D., & Wilson, T. (2005a). A model of university–community partnerships for occupational therapy scholarship and practice. *Occupational Therapy and Health Care, 19*(1/2), 47–70.

Suarez-Balcazar, Y., Harper, G., & Lewis, R. (2005b). An interactive and contextual model of Community–university partnerships. *Health Education & Behavior, 32,* 84–101.

Suarez-Balcazar, Y., Orellana-Damacela, L., Portillo, N., Sharma, A., & Lanum, M. (2003). Implementing an outcomes model in the participatory evaluation of community initiatives. *Journal of Prevention and Intervention in the Community, 26*(2), 5–25.

Sue, D. W., Arredondo, P., & McDavis, R. (1992). Multicultural counseling competencies and standards: A call to the profession. *Journal of Counseling and Development, 70,* 477–486.

Sue, D. W, Carter, R. T., Casas, J. M., Fouad, N. A., Ivey, A. E., Jensen, M., La Fromboise, T., Manese, J. E., Ponterotto, J. G., & Vasquez-Nuttal, E. (1998). *Multicultural counseling competencies: Individual and organizational development.* Thousand Oaks: SAGE Publications.

Sue, S. (1998). In search of cultural competence in psychotherapy and counseling. *American Psychologist, 53*(4), 440–448.

Sue, S., & Zane, N. (1987). The role of culture and cultural techniques in psychotherapy: A critique and reformulation. *American Psychologist, 42,* 37–45.

Taylor, R. R., Braveman, B., & Hammel. J. (2004). Developing and evaluating community-based services through participatory action research: Two case examples. *American Journal of Occupational Therapy, 58*(1), 73–82.

Taylor, R. R., Fisher, G., & Kielhofner, G. (2005). Synthesizing research, education, and practice according to the Scholarship of Practice model: Two faculty examples. *Occupational Therapy and Health Care, 19,* 107–122.

Tervalon, M., & Murray-Garcia, J. (1998). Cultural humility versus cultural competence: A critical distinction in defining physician training outcomes in multicultural education. *Journal of Health Care for the Poor and Underserved, 9*(2), 117–25.

Townsend, E. (1997). *Enabling occupation: A Canadian perspective.* Ottawa, ON: CAOT Publications ACE.

U.S. Census Bureau (2000, January 13). *Projections of the resident population by race, Hispanic origin, and nativity: Middle Series, 2025–2045.* Washington, DC: Author. Retrieved April 20, 2004, from Population Projections Program, Population Division database on the World Wide Web: http://www.census.gov/population/projections/nation/summary/np-t5-c.pdf

Velde, B., Wittman, P., & Bamberg, R. (2003). Cultural competence of faculty and students in a school of allied health. *Journal of Allied Health, 32*(3), 189–195.

CHAPTER 40

Participatory Research for the Development and Evaluation of Occupational Therapy: Researcher–Practitioner Collaboration

Gary Kielhofner • Lisa Castle • Claire-Jehanne Dubouloz

Mary Egan • Kirsty Forsyth • Jane Melton • Sue Parkinson • Mick Robson

Lynn Summerfield-Mann • Renée R. Taylor • Suzie Willis

This chapter discusses researcher–practitioner collaboration in the context of participatory research. The authors include both practitioners and researchers who have been participated in investigations that used a participatory approach. Thus, this chapter reflects not only the literature, but also first-hand experiences in implementing participatory research. The chapter covers:

- The importance of participatory research for occupational therapy,
- Principles that should underlie participatory research involving practitioners, and
- Guidelines for meeting the challenges of implementing participatory research.

Finally, the chapter ends with three examples that illustrate participatory research projects in which therapists and researchers collaborated to develop and investigate practice.

The Importance of Participatory Research

The majority of occupational therapists agree that it is a good thing to base practice on research (Dysart & Tomlin, 2002). However, practitioners sometimes:

- Question the relevance of the questions addressed and findings generated by research (Dubouloz, Egan, von Zweck, & Vallerand, 1999; Sudsawad, 2003),
- Express concern that research reflects occupational therapy conducted under ideal conditions or with resources not readily available in practice (McCluskey, 2003; McCluskey & Cusick, 2002), and

- Feel that research evidence does not fit with their perception of the practical situation or a particular client's needs (Dubouloz et al., 1999; Dysart & Tomlin, 2002).

As a result, it is not uncommon that experienced occupational therapists use a wide range of techniques that "appear to work rather than appraising the research evidence" (Creek, 2003, p. 27).

The disconnection between research and practice exists partly because generating knowledge and using knowledge are considered distinct and separate enterprises (Barnett, 1997; Higgs & Titchen, 2001; Schon, 1983). Researchers based in academic settings conduct most occupational therapy research. Moreover, since academics generally have the most advanced training for research, it is generally accepted that conducting investigation is their responsibility and prerogative.

In their quest for rigor, university-based investigators can be prone to overlook the circumstances of practice for which they aim to generate evidence (Peloquin, 2002; Peloquin & Abreu, 1996). Research is infrequently grounded in or guided by practice. Even when occupational therapists are involved in research, these practitioners serve mainly as consultants, advisors, service providers, or data collectors. Characteristically, the researcher ultimately controls the process of investigation.

These circumstances are beginning to change. There is an increasing recognition that the process of integrating research into practice should begin long before the research is completed. Investigators in occupational therapy are looking for ways to more clearly ground their research in practice contexts. An emerging form of participatory research in occupational therapy involves investigators and practitioners working together as partners to advance practice knowledge.

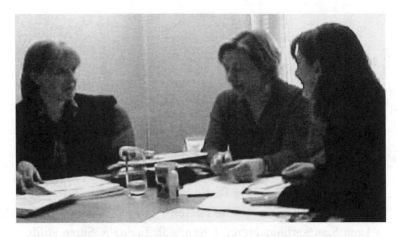

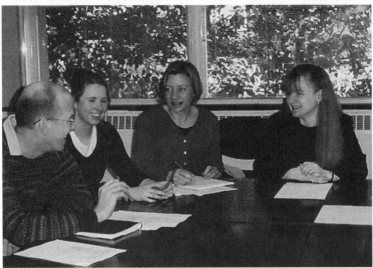

Figure 40.1 (A) Kirsty Forsyth, Suzie Willis and Lynn Summerfield Mann (L-R) discuss plans for academic–practitioner collaboration as part of the United Kingdom Center for Outcomes Research (UKCORE) that fosters participatory research in England and Scotland. (B) Clinicians Mick Robson, Janet Woodhouse, Suzie Willis, and Kirsty Forsyth (L-R), with Central and North West London Mental Health NHS Trust, present their experiences with practice innovation as part of the UKCORE effort.

Principles of Participatory Research for Examining Occupational Therapy

The idea of researcher–practitioner partnerships is a natural application of participatory research, as discussed in Chapter 38. Participatory research is an empowerment-oriented approach that involves researchers and stakeholders working together to shape the research questions and methods and to conduct the research (Bradbury & Reason, 2001;

Stringer, 1996; Taylor, Braveman, & Hammel, 2004). The following three principles are fundamental to participatory research in occupational therapy when the stakeholders are occupational therapists who will use the results of the research to shape their practice.

1. Therapists who ultimately use knowledge should be involved as equal partners in helping to generate and refine that knowledge.

This principle means that practitioners should be involved in research as true collaborators with the investigators, not merely as consultants, data collectors, or implementers of intervention. It could be further advocated that this principle expresses the belief that practitioners can also become the driving force behind clinical investigations. For example, practitioners are in an excellent position to identify areas of need for research as well as relevant research questions.

In participatory research, practitioners participate in making decisions about such critical research issues as the questions to be asked and the methods to be used. Experience indicates that, when practitioners shape research, it yields resources and evidence that is responsive to occupational therapists' perspectives, work styles, and practice realities.

> An emerging form of participatory research in occupational therapy involves investigators and practitioners working together as partners to advance practice knowledge.

2. Knowledge development should be grounded in real-life practice contexts.

For findings to be usable in practice, research must reflect actual practice. The surest way to reflect practice is to conduct research in practice settings. When grounded in practice settings, the outcomes of that research are relevant to the actual circumstances and demands of practice.

3. Knowledge development should be innovative and reflective.

Investigators and practitioners undertake participatory research to improve upon existing practice. This means that practitioners and researchers typically work together to create practice innovations and to examine how these innovations work. A reflective process in which researchers and practitioners share their ongoing insights and perspectives as the research unfolds is important to support practice innovation.

Meeting the Challenges in Participatory Research: Achieving Effective Researcher–Practitioner Partnerships

Participatory research that examines occupational therapy practice can be challenging to undertake for two primary reasons. First of all, participatory research involves interfacing issues of rigor that emphasize control and order with practice settings that are often changing and difficult to control. Enhancing both rigor and relevance requires a constant balancing act.

Second, participatory research involves the interface of two different perspectives. These practice and academic perspectives are each characterized by different concerns, values, time frames, and procedures. For researchers and practitioners to effectively collaborate, dialogue, compromise, and goodwill are required.

The following section considers typical challenges that emerge in participatory research where researchers and practitioners collaborate. It discusses how and why these challenges arise. Finally, it examines ways these challenges can be overcome. Importantly, these challenges can be surmounted as will be illustrated. Nonetheless, participatory research will be more successful when parties enter into the collaboration aware of the types of challenges that can arise. The authors of this chapter have found participatory research to be an exciting and productive form of inquiry as well as one that has its own unique challenges.

The Challenge of Knowledge and Power Differentials

As noted in Chapter 38, participatory research requires sharing power between investigators and stakeholders. However, this power sharing requires careful attention to subtle knowledge and status differentials between researchers and therapists. The scientific knowledge of researchers is typically considered a more privileged and prestigious form of knowledge. This discrepancy is heightened when the overall purpose of collaboration is to conduct research. Practitioners can feel that they don't have skills comparable to the researcher's, leading to an unequal initial footing. Since participatory research usually involves examination of some aspect of occupational therapy services, practitioners can also perceive that their own practice is being judged.

Challenges can arise around issues of who should control what aspects of the participatory research process. Researchers have more training and experience in research methods and feel responsible for the rigor of their investigations.

The following are examples of knowledge and power issues in participatory research. In one project involving some of the authors, the overall aim was to implement and investigate theory-based practice. At the beginning of the project, existing practice was characterized by a lack of clearly articulated theoretical rationale and by the use of nonstandard "home-grown" assessments. It was agreed that therapists in the setting would work to articulate and implement a common theory and begin to use standardized assessments that would also be used to generate data about intervention outcomes.

As part of the process of examining how the theory was being put into practice, the researchers suggested that practitioners would present cases so that there could be a public discussion of how the theory was working in practice. This process seemed relatively straightforward and benign to the researchers, who were accustomed to public discussion and criticism. After all, at the basis of research is the assumption that knowledge is always incomplete and tentative and, therefore, must be questioned, debated, and changed.

However, the prospect of having their cases discussed and critiqued was very threatening to practitioners who were not accustomed to having their practice publicly examined. They felt that it was important that they had confidence in their knowledge since it was being applied with real consequences. The idea of uncertainty and ever-changing knowledge appeared contradictory to the daily requirement to make decisions that impacted clients. In this same study, some practitioners spoke about feeling "brainwashed." As one practitioner put it, she "did not want to practice the same way as everyone else" or be "taken over" by researchers. Moreover, she saw the innovations as implying that her previous knowledge and practice were inadequate. As can be readily seen, these issues required some direct attention and negotiation.

Thus, researchers can be reluctant to relinquish control over decisions about research methodology that affects scientific rigor. On the other hand, practitioners may feel that their experience gives them a right to make the decisions about the practice issues that are addressed in the research process.

The Challenge of Different Agendas and Priorities

Practitioners and researchers sometimes have different agendas and expectations for the outcomes of their research efforts. For example, researchers who wish to make an objective study of the effec-

tiveness of an intervention may advocate a research design in which not all subjects receive the intervention. In such a situation, practitioners may have misgivings about withholding a form of treatment they believe their clients need. In such a case both perspectives have merit, although each emphasizes a different aspect of the situation (i.e., creating more certain knowledge that can improve services versus providing a group of clients with every possible form of service).

Differences in perspective can also affect the collaborative research process. For example, researchers whose job expectations include publishing often have higher priorities and tight timelines for writing up the results of studies. Practitioners who face other kinds of time demands and work expectations may not share this same sense of urgency for publishing.

Challenges Due to Differences in Work Styles and Settings

Researchers typically function in an entrepreneurial fashion, pursuing lines of inquiry that they are passionate about, securing funding, and publishing in a particular area of expertise. Researchers often have substantial discretion over their everyday use of time, but they also must deal with deadlines and timelines imposed by funding agencies, conferences, publishers, and the tenure and promotion timetable.

Some practitioners have highly structured workdays involving constant demands of client interventions with the ongoing necessity of getting documentation and billing done. Others are constantly responding to crises and must reprioritize their work on a daily basis. When researchers and practitioners collaborate, these differences in work demands and work styles can result in legitimate disagreements about priorities.

Research is a foreign activity in most practice contexts. While researchers experience the various tasks involved in designing and implementing participatory research to be natural, they are not part of the practitioner's accustomed routine. Thus, practitioners can experience research as increasing their workload. Even practitioners who are initially enthusiastic can grow weary of the extra work involved in doing research (Egan et al., 2004).

Many times, even when there are negotiated practitioner responsibilities for research, the demands of practice simply override research needs. Consider, for instance, the practitioner faced with the choice between covering clients who are part of a sick or vacationing colleague's caseload versus collecting data for research. These and other circumstances can leave clinicians feeling overwhelmed by the demands of research tasks and researchers frustrated with the lack of progress in an investigation.

A final challenge of collaborating across practice and academic work settings is the practical matter of physical distance. Sometimes the challenge is that academic and clinical sites are separate; other times the challenge is coordinating practitioners and academics across multiple settings. Thus, the usual challenges of communication are further complicated by the fact that some of this communication inevitably takes place in non face-to-face formats (e.g., Web-based communication).

Overcoming the Challenges of Practitioner–Researcher Collaboration in Participatory Research

Resolving differences of power, perspectives, and work style are among the major challenges of participatory research. True power sharing in participatory research means that all participants have a degree of responsibility, voice, and decision-making about all aspects of the research. This means that both researchers and practitioners must also commit to sharing what they know and to learning what the other knows. Each must respect the expertise and insights of the other. Above all, there must be ongoing dialogue to maintain understanding and trust.

True dialogue means more than simply talking together. Researchers and practitioners function in different worlds with different sets of concerns, and different constituencies to whom they are accountable. Dialogue requires that the parties discover their different values and perspectives and find common ground between them. Productive dialogue requires:

- Acknowledging and respecting expertise,
- Clarifying the purpose of participatory research,
- Communicating honestly with sensitivity,
- Suspending judgment while striving to understand the perspectives of others, and
- Negotiating and reformulating plans.

Acknowledging and Respecting Expertise

In participatory research that examines practice, it is important to underscore that the research requires two types of expertise:

- Practice expertise, and
- Research expertise.

Acknowledging the value of both these forms of expertise is essential to a successful participatory research project. While practitioners and investigators are likely to differ on the extent of expertise they have in these two areas at the outset, the participatory research process provides opportunity for learning from one another. Investigators become more knowledgeable about practice circumstances and practitioners learn more about the research process. Also, researchers and practitioners alike often discover that their counterparts have a mixture of both types of expertise. That is, researchers generate clinical insights while practitioners come up with useful research strategies.

Clarifying the Purpose of Participatory Research

As noted in Chapter 38, practitioners and investigators involved in participatory research share a common concern for addressing practice challenges in a particular situation and for generating knowledge that can be generated in the field as a whole. Practitioners who are involved in participatory research must open up their practice to inspection. Given this circumstance, it is critical for all to acknowledge that the purpose of research is to examine the field's knowledge, not therapists' personal knowledge.

Participatory research that examines practice is designed to determine how the field's prevailing knowledge works in a particular practice context. Moreover, it provides opportunity to generate new concepts and practice innovations that can become part of the field's knowledge base. While this knowledge is expressed in how individual practitioners go about doing their work, the focus should always remain on the concepts that inform, and the particular characteristics of, successful therapeutic strategies. For example, discussing how participatory research will improve practice can trigger practitioners to worry that their practice is inadequate. Framing such discussions as improving the knowledge available to therapists for their practice can help avoid such misgivings.

Communicating Honestly with Sensitivity

Everyone can readily see that dialogue works best when all parties honestly share perspectives. However, honest communication can have unintended consequences if not carefully enacted. For instance, direct statements of perspective have the potential to make those whose perspectives are different feel undervalued or dismissed. Similarly, honest feedback can exacerbate an individual's or group's vulnerabilities.

Experience teaches that it is generally easier to have the honest discussion among one's research or practitioner peers than it is to share perspectives or feedback with those from another group. Persons from another group are more likely to misunderstand or fail to appreciate what one is saying. There is a natural tendency to avoid potentially sensitive discussions. However, avoiding such discussions only ensures that gaps in perspective or beliefs will be perpetuated. Consequently, all parties need to put effort into recognizing the potential for information to be emotionally charged and to consider how it is best shared. Consistent, honest sharing of information with careful consideration to its impact on the receiving parties is always helpful.

For example, in one participatory research project, the primary aim was to make changes in practice. While most practitioners in the study setting had expressed a desire to achieve this change, one working group particularly struggled with practice innovation. Moreover, initial minor critiques of their work caused tension among the team members, indicating that their practitioners' confidence was low.

Consequently, the investigators avoided providing feedback that the group was falling behind others in the setting. Instead, they provided gentle but persistent nurturing and communicated suggestions for further development in the context of positive feedback concerning what had already been accomplished. In time, this group did generate successful innovations in their practice. Moreover, they felt empowered and grew in confidence. Importantly, these practitioners, who were initially wary of the researchers, came to trust them.

As noted earlier, participatory research often requires communication to take place through Web-based systems. While virtual communication allows collaboration across wide distances and thus makes possible participatory research that would otherwise not be possible, the lack of constant face-to-face encounters requires extra attention and effort.

Suspending Judgment While Striving to Understand the Perspectives of Others

Because they come from different work cultures, practitioners and researchers can sometimes misconstrue each other's knowledge, motives, and behaviors. Productive dialogue always begins with an openness to leave behind preconceptions or judgments about others. It further requires that col-

laborators actively question and carefully listen in order to generate understanding of another's knowledge, perspectives, and concerns. As Peloquin and Abreu (1996) note, it is important to find common ground between the thought processes that typically separate scholars and practitioners.

The following is an example of how a group of practitioners and researchers found such common ground. Some of the authors have been working for years to create, study, and publish standardized assessments. When they began a project to instate standardized assessments for documenting occupational therapy treatment outcomes, there were frustrated to learn that practitioners were using these standardized assessments in nonstandard ways. The investigators first decided to remedy the situation by providing the therapists with more training, reasoning that these practitioners lacked understanding of the importance and use of standardized tools.

Unexpectedly, these efforts initially frustrated practitioners who felt that the needs and demands of practice were being overlooked. Ensuing discussions underscored that the researchers' concerns about assessment centered on scientific evidence concerning validity and reliability while the practitioners' concerns centered on ease of administration, usefulness for treatment, and whether the interdisciplinary team valued the information they yielded. Moreover, both groups were convinced that their concerns were the ones that really mattered.

In ongoing discussions, both constituencies considered together how both sets of concerns might be integrated. This discussion led to a new way of thinking about assessments, upon which they all agreed. That is, they all wanted a practical way to dependably generate critical information for understanding clients' needs that the interdisciplinary team would understand, respect and support. With this new common ground, they were able work together on research that aimed to improve the assessment process.

Finding such common ground involves not only educating each other, but also pausing to consider other ways of thinking about things. The left-hand side of Table 40.1 illustrates some the assumptions that practitioners and researchers sometimes hold about each other. Through the kind of openness, dialogue, and reflection espoused here, common perspectives (shown on the right-hand side) can be generated. The unification of practitioner perspectives and academic perspectives is reflected in a term that collaborators have found helpful, namely, practitioner-scholars. When therapists and researchers work together in participatory research, they all become, in effect, practitioner-scholars.

Ongoing Negotiation and Reformulation of Plans

Participatory research, by definition, is not as linear or neatly controlled. Because it occurs in real-life settings and is designed to be responsive to the realities of those settings, participatory research often requires changes in aims, plans, and deadlines. The following is an example.

One of the authors was involved in a federally funded investigation of model occupational therapy services provided to clients living in residential facilities. The original plan of the study involved testing an intervention with a three-group design. According to this plan, the model intervention was to be implemented in the residential settings by occupational therapists who were part of a funded research team (the model program group) and

> When therapists and researchers work together in participatory research, they all become, in effect, practitioner-scholars.

compared to a control group. Following this, it was planned that the project team would train occupational therapists and interdisciplinary personnel indigenous to the settings to carry out the intervention.

This plan was initially agreed on by the facilities that were part of the study. Nonetheless, early in the project, it became apparent that the indigenous staff in the facilities wanted to be part of the program and help in its delivery. Moreover, the facilities' managers wanted all services in their facility to be integrated as a whole. Thus, the original plan to implement the model program separately from other services and service personnel was deemed infeasible.

Since this project was government funded, the investigators had to discuss the changes with the funding agency and secure its approval. Moreover, subject recruitment and implementation plans had to be redrawn and new timelines developed. Although not every participatory research project will involve such a

Table 40.1 The Transformation from Conflicting to Collaborative, Practitioner-Scholar, Perspectives and Attributions

Typical Conflicting Perspectives and Attributions of Researchers and Practitioners		New Collaborative Practitioner–Scholar Perspective
Researchers	Practitioners	
Research is essential to good practice—i.e., it helps therapists to understand the client and know what kinds of intervention to implement to achieve the best results.	Research is often out of touch with the "real world."	Scientific knowledge and practical experience can be complementary:
Practitioners undervalue theory and research and don't make the time to learn new approaches that contemporary evidence suggests would constitute best practice.	Experience is the best way to figure out what works in a given context.	• Practitioners' experience and expertise can inform and shape the researcher.
	Client-centered practice and building rapport with clients requires flexibility that can by stifled be the "standardization" of practice suggested by theory and research.	• Research can address practical issues and shed light on practical questions.
	Academics are out of touch with the real world of practice and don't understand its demands and constraints.	Practice can be systematic and evidence-based while also being client-centered.
		Practitioners and researchers can learn and create practice together, share accountability, and work toward improving and demonstrating the outcomes of practice.
		Researchers' and practitioners' differences *and* similarities can be assimilated into unique shared dialogue to create better visions for practice.

major change as altering the basic design of the study, minor changes are par for the course.

Participatory research results in practice innovations. Changing practice patterns means that therapists must justify what they are doing to the multidisciplinary team and convince them to accept the changes. Sometimes managers have to be convinced to allow therapists to change intervention protocols or to take time to develop new skills. Often, resistance by these constituencies can cause delays, necessitate changes in plans, or require extended negotiations and compromise.

For example, in one setting, where some of the authors are involved in ongoing research, a team of occupational therapists began to make practice modifications in anticipation of eventually studying outcomes. These changes involved more clearly basing practice on occupational therapy theory and doing client documentation in ways that reflected that theory. Initially, the physicians working on the service demanded that the occupational therapist revert back to their old form of documentation, complaining that they did not understand the new approach and language used by the therapists. A great deal of tact was required to educate the physicians as to the reasons for the changes and to achieve their support. The resulting reporting style accommodated concerns of physicians while preserving what therapists believed was important to document about their practice.

A comprehensive strategy that seeks to anticipate problems and reactions of others, and to inform and educate those impacted by innovation is often helpful. Nonetheless, comprehensive planning and action can never avoid the emergence of unforeseen problems. When these occur, flexibility is required.

Summary

The previous sections discussed some of the challenges that can arise in participatory research. It also highlighted strategies that can effectively manage these challenges. What follows are three cases that illustrate the principles and processes discussed in this chapter.

Case 1: Engaging in Participatory Research to Modify an Assessment Process

During a participatory research project involving some of the authors, new legislation mandated that clients with mental illness receive an evaluation of

vocational potential when they came into contact with the service system. Occupational therapists within a regional health organization felt that they had the expertise to assume this role and successfully negotiated with senior management to take on vocational evaluation. Therefore, they needed a validated assessment appropriate to capture the clients' motivation and potential for work. Researchers recommended the Worker Role Interview (WRI) (Velozo, Kielhofner, & Fisher, 1998).

When practitioners tested the WRI, which was originally designed for persons with acute physical impairments, they discovered that it was not well suited to clients with chronic disabilities and negligible work histories. At first the practitioners felt that the investigators lacked information about their client group and were simply advancing a favored instrument. In a meeting between the investigators and practitioners, both groups listened carefully to the concerns and perspectives of each. As a result of this discussion, a decision was made to modify the WRI so that it was more suitable to psychiatric clients, and then to test the psychometric properties of this modified assessment. This was done in two steps.

First, the practitioners in the setting worked with one researcher to develop, pilot, and refine an alternative interview format suitable to the person with limited work history. At the same time, other researchers collaborated with the practitioners to revise the rating scale of the WRI so that it was relevant to both acutely and chronically impaired clients. The result was a new and more flexible version of this standardized assessment (Braveman et al., 2003). The feature box that follows provides the perspectives of a practitioner and an investigator involved in this project.

A second innovation emerged from practitioners' observations. Implementing the WRI with clients took away from time that could be used to explore other aspects of a client's occupational functioning, which were important. Therapists in this setting previously used the Occupational Circumstances Assessment-Interview and Rating Scale (OCAIRS) (Forsyth et al., 2004). The OCAIRS is a generic assessment of occupational performance and participation. Doing both the OCAIRS and the WRI simply took too much time. Discussion between researchers and therapists resulted in the following innovation. Since the content of the OCAIRS and the WRI somewhat overlap, it was decided to develop a single interview format that combined the content of both the WRI and the OCAIRS. After doing the combined interview, therapists would complete the rating and

Engaging in Participatory Research to Modify an Assessment Process

The Practitioner's Account

In 2002, I was invited to collaborate on the redevelopment of the Worker Role Interview to make it more suitable for people with long-standing illness or disability. The original version was designed for people with an acute injury. Most of my clients have not worked for many years and have long term illness, so the suggested questions and rating scale just didn't work in my clinical practice.

I have plenty of experience of adapting assessments to suit my purposes, but this has always been done for pragmatic reasons without specific reference to any theoretical or research considerations. I like to work in an iterative way with assessments, slowly getting the feel for what information I need and adjusting them accordingly. I anticipated that working with an academic researcher was going to bring this way of working to an abrupt halt. Orderliness and precise, clear thinking would be the order of the day.

My actual experience was quite different. We worked very much in an equal partnership. I brought my day to day clinical and practical experience to the work with all its inherent ambiguities. My academic colleague brought her academic expertise (and of course her own extensive clinical experience).

We agreed on a timetable for achieving each stage of the initial development process over a 4-month period, meeting monthly and communicating in between by e-mail and phone. It seemed, in retrospect, somewhat like taking a course of study with no lessons to attend, but regular assignments to submit, each one building on what had already been achieved. This approach may sound rather rigid, but I found that it gave me a great opportunity to put my ideas down in writing within a structure designed to achieve very clear goals. My academic colleague worked with the material that I provided, returning it with her ideas and suggestions so that we worked our way step by step toward a mutually agreed-upon end product.

During this process, I had a clear sense that nothing was being taken for granted with regard to the eventual outcome, and that my input was as crucial to the success of the project as that of anybody else. I felt able to ask "dumb questions," knowing that I would either get an illuminating answer or that the question would highlight an issue in need of further thought and consideration by the team. In turn, I was encouraged to consider why I was seeing things a certain way and challenge my own assumptions and prejudices. As a personal benefit, this allowed me to reflect on my professional experience and relate my "gut feelings" to a theoretical framework. This process has helped me to validate my experience but also to extend my thinking and, I hope, understand my clients better.

Once we had agreed on the revised assessment—following a period of testing by therapists in London and Chicago—the final stage of collaboration involved a wider group of people communicating by e-mail to agree on the contents of the new manual. This was not simply a matter of proofreading, because it allowed everyone to contribute to mini-debates on the final content of the manual. I think these debates highlighted the importance of being able to challenge each others' assumptions and to put forward a different perspective on the situation. I am sure that they helped to improve the final version of the manual so that it will satisfy important academic requirements without forgetting the more pragmatic concerns of therapists.

The Researcher's Account:

When I first met my practitioner colleague, he was very skeptical of academics. He expected that the researchers would simply defend the existing standardized assessment in the first meeting. Instead, the researchers said in effect, "OK, you're right! Let's work towards making it better." That's when I saw his attitude change. His frustration turned into action. We met and communicated routinely over several months. I discussed the needs of measurement. But most of our discussions were around clinical cases—debating them, dissecting them, and applying the assessment to find out if it would embrace the complexity of the clients' situations. He took responsibility for the working up of the document with me and reviewing it routinely between meetings. I made sure the measurement aspects of building the new scale would be consistent with measurement principles. He was very engaged in the process, and he said he was surprised by my clinical knowledge.

---

reporting forms for both the OCAIRS and the WRI, thus saving substantial time.

In both cases, innovations arose from practice dilemmas. A local problem was solved, and, at the same time, new resources for other therapists in similar situations were developed and empirically studied. At the time of this writing, the two assessments are routinely used and data are being collected that will allow evidence to be generated about the assessments' reliability and validity as well as their practical utility in clinical decision-making.

Case 2: An Online Participatory Action Research Project

A Canadian-based project aimed to allow practicing occupational therapists to develop strategies for enhancing their use of research findings in practice. The main premise of this project was the belief that practitioners, through their own experience and knowledge, are skilled at reflecting, analyzing, and identifying solutions grounded in real-life practice contexts. During a 13-month Web-mediated action research project (Egan et al., 2004), 51 occupational therapists from eight Canadian provinces met online, using Stringer's three-step action research approach to problem resolution. The three steps of this approach are:

• Naming the problem of research utilization,
• Looking for an understanding of the use of research, and
• Acting on practical strategies to be tested (Stringer, 1996).

This process of inquiry structured the online communication and research activity.

Four virtual groups of approximately 12 occupational therapists each were assembled according to four clinical interests: adult institution-based care, adult community-based care, adult mental health care, and child health. Four academics coordinated the project. One of the debates among the research team, prior to the initiation of online exploration, concerned how much group leaders should instruct practitioners about the process of evidence-based practice. Academics anticipated that the practitioners would look to them for how they should go about finding and synthesizing research evidence. However, in previous research projects, instruction to healthcare providers on evidence-based practice methods had met with limited success. Thus, the investigators were interested to see the practitioners develop innovative solutions and procedures on their own. Thus, having academics instruct practitioners on how to go about evidence-based practice was seen as potentially stifling such creativity.

The solution to this dilemma was twofold. First, the investigators decided to stay in the background during the exploration of research utilization. Four post-professional graduate students were assigned to be at the forefront of communications, each one facilitating one of the four groups of practitioners. It was expected that this would be a practical method to prevent the tendency of the researchers to teach and control and to remove the temptation for practitioners to seek quick answers. Not only did the graduate students not have the same urge to provide answers, but they were also seen as credible to the participants since as recent practitioners they were aware of the clinical reality. In addition, these graduate students were asked not to provide instruction to participants on evidence-based practice methods.

Once the recruitment of the participants and the process of grouping participants were completed, the exploration began. Participants were keen to start their reflection and to follow the inquiry process. Each phase of the process was facilitated by the graduate student facilitator, keeping in mind the intention to empower the therapist participants. Practitioners successfully shared on-line reflections on their perceptions and experiences. At the end of the first phase (i.e., naming the issue), practitioners easily completed a collective account, accepted by all members of their group, that described the difficulties of using research in practice.

The second phase of the research process, understanding the issue, was felt by some practitioners to be a bit more complex, but still manageable. Although more time was required, the second phase was completed. Each group created an interpretative account to explain the problems under investigation.

At the beginning of the third, action, phase, challenges to creating new strategies in the work place were articulated. Practitioners were beginning to express the need for more direction from the researchers as the complexity of the task was increasing. It was challenging to empower practitioners as they started to feel reticent and somewhat inadequate to the task. They did not see creating a solution as entirely within their rights. They did not trust their own judgments and were not sufficiently reassured by the group process.

In each of the two groups that were most successful in identifying new strategies for using research evidence in practice, a group member emerged to take over leadership from the group facilitator. In one case, the group became frustrated with the software used in the project and formed alternate communication channels. While this decreased the researchers' access to communication between the group members, it was ultimately taken as a sign of the group's maturity and ability to work toward its goals. Successful internal leadership did not emerge in the two less successful groups. For example, in one group, discussions became rather circular without consensus and, thus, the group's work stalled.

While leadership and a sense of ownership were crucial factors in whether groups were able to create solutions to the problem of bringing research findings into practice, other factors were also involved. These other factors included lack of confidence, the challenge of using a new technology (i.e., asynchronous online communication), the unexpected amounts of extra time required for participation, and the real difficulty in moving from collecting information to critiquing and synthesizing it in order to form a plan of action.

Despite the different levels of success across groups, almost all the practitioners reported valuing the experience of being linked to other occupational therapists working in similar areas and struggling to determine the best care for their clients. Approximately half of the original practitioner participants completed the project. They reported beginning to consistently use evidence-based methods in their work, often applying skills learned in an academic setting within their workplaces for the first time. This practitioner–academic collaboration appeared to create an important bridge for them in applying skills, such as searching the literature and identifying a guiding theoretical model. This type of collaboration appears quite promising, particularly when leadership of the group can be shifted to the practitioners who then look to the academics for support rather than direction.

Case 3: Engaging in Participatory Action Research to Create a New Screening Tool

A group of practitioners in the United Kingdom who had reviewed a number of standardized assessments decided that none were routinely usable in the fast paced and often chaotic context of acute mental health care. Consequently, they began to develop their own assessment. These practitioners sought out academic involvement after they had piloted an initial version of their new assessment. In the spirit of participatory research, the investigators did not take over the development of the assessment, but rather they joined the practitioners as partners.

For nearly 5 years so far, researchers and practitioners have worked together to refine and study the resulting instrument, the Model of Human Occupation Screening Tool (MOHOST) (Parkinson, Forsyth, & Kielhofner, 2004). This collaboration required a constant process of educating each other about practice or research perspectives and concerns. It also required substantial compromise and negotiation about how to proceed. Importantly, neither those with academic roles, nor the practitioners, ultimately controlled the process. Rather, it unfolded with a degree of healthy tension and ebb and flow of whose agenda prevailed at critical junctures in decision-making about the developing instrument. The process of creating the MOHOST was less linear than previous projects in which researchers where clearly in charge. However, in the end, our power sharing resulted in an assessment that satisfied both academic and practical sets of concerns. Interestingly, the story does not end here. The feature box on the next page illustrates both a practitioner and a researcher perspective on this collaboration.

Practitioners in another setting began to use this instrument with the dual intention of incorporating it as part of client documentation and collecting data for a validation study. These practitioners used an electronic medical record and found it cumbersome to go from the paper-and-pencil instrument to creating a report in the electronic medical record. One practitioner requested to have a copy of the electronic file so he could create his own templates for reporting in the electronic medical record for all to be able to access. They went through many different versions based on the unit's need, user friendliness, and also based on other team members' feedback—in terms of the content and look of the report (too long, too much info on the page, etc.).

During meetings involving both investigators and practitioners, the idea emerged to develop a software package that incorporated the assessment, allowed it to be scored electronically, and particularly automated the process of writing a narrative note. Over time, with joint discussions between researchers and practitioners, the software was designed to include treatment goals, interventions, and documentation of goal attainment so that it could serve as a database for research. The software continues to be refined, adding both more practitioner-friendly features and enhancing its value as a database for investigating practice.

It is important to note that the creation of the software came out of a discussion of daily practice challenges rather than a long-term vision or plan. This highlights the importance of how having a dialogue about our daily practice challenges as part of participatory research can lead to innovations that no one could have predicted.

Engaging in Participatory Action Research to Create a New Screening Tool

The Practitioner's Account

In 1992, I read Creek's book, *Occupational Therapy in Mental Health* (1990), and found myself identifying with her assertion that, "vague and inaccurate assessment leads to vague and imprecise treatment" (p. 82). I determined that a new therapist-rated outcome measure was needed for use in acute mental health settings and I took the first steps toward creating an assessment that is now known as the Model of Human Occupation Screening Tool (MOHOST). The first drafts were rudimentary, and it was with some trepidation that I decided to share my early work with university-based researchers. I was concerned that "home-grown assessments" would be frowned upon, but I was also convinced that some locally devised tools could meet the specific needs of practitioners better than many generalized tools. To my delight, I discovered that new ideas were warmly welcomed, and that academics in two institutions wanted to support practitioners by matching the art of practice with the science of standardization.

The resulting collaboration to create a new assessment led to my becoming involved in a participatory research process—that is, research leading to concrete solutions for a recognized problem. This kind of collaborative research

> *differs from solo work because it is accomplished, not first in one person's mind, and then in the other's, but on the loom between them, ... The richness ... lies in effectively acknowledging, and where appropriate, resolving differences between the partners"* (Donaldson & Sanderson, 1996, p. 44).

In participatory action research all participants must be involved throughout the process as equal partners blending the insights of the practitioner and the expertise of the researcher. Throughout the research, the academics involved demonstrated respect for my experiential learning and this meant that I felt encouraged to maintain my own convictions and assert my knowledge of the needs of my clients and my colleagues. Their openness allowed us to work together to produce something that would be familiar and relevant to practitioners, and, as a consequence, the MOHOST has led to tangible results that have made a real difference to my practice and to other services.

The Researcher's Account

My role was ensuring that the theory was correctly reflected in the assessment and that we were following measurement rules. The most concerning issue for me about this assessment was the clinical request to have multiple data-gathering methods. I could see that such an approach would make it more usable in clinical practice and allow it to be reflective of how practitioners normally work. However, from a measurement point of view, this flexibility could be a serious source of error. Consequently, there were tense times, but our commitment to the field and to producing something useful that would engage practitioners took priority over any disagreements. We now get a kick out of practitioners saying how usable the tool is in practice. It makes all the hard work worthwhile.

Conclusion

This chapter examined the rationale and principles underlying participatory research that involves researchers and practitioners together. The challenges of doing this type of research and strategies for managing these challenges were discussed. As our three case examples illustrate, the unique potential of participatory research to create and test practice innovations far outweighs its challenges.

The following underscores this point. Earlier, this chapter illustrated an instance in which therapists were threatened by

the prospect of having their cases publicly discussed and critiqued. Investigators worked hard to assure therapists that the purpose of this discussion was not to critique their personal knowledge or expertise and, instead, to think together about how to best do theoretically driven and evidence-based practice. When such discussions took place, therapists were pleasantly surprised to learn that the researchers affirmed their own observations and recognized their expertise. Moreover, there was opportunity to creatively discuss and arrive at decisions about further innovations. Later in the research process, practitioners

> When researchers and practitioners work together in participatory research, they are transformed and empowered by the research process.

collaborated with researchers to submit abstracts and present at a national conference. Some of the clinician's cases were later incorporated into published materials. Recently, there was an opportunity in the ongoing research to have another public discussion of how therapists were using theory and standardized assessments. There were so many therapists who wanted to present their practice that all of them could not be accommodated!

This example highlights what is, perhaps, one of the most unique things about participatory research. Collaborators have opportunity not only to work together to create and examine practice innovations, but also to learn and grow professionally. When researchers and practitioners work together in participatory research, they are transformed and empowered by the research process. The old discrepancies between practitioners and scholars are broken down and all involved come to work together as practitioner-scholars.

REFERENCES

Barnett, R. (1997). *Higher education: A critical business.* Bristol: Open University Press.

Bradbury, H., & Reason, P. (2001). Conclusion: Broadening the bandwidth of validity: Issues and choice-points for improving the quality of action research. In P. Reason & Bradbury, H. (Eds.), *Handbook of action research: Participative inquiry and practice* (pp. 447–455). London: SAGE Publications.

Braveman, B., Robson, M., Velozo, C., Kielhofner, G., Fisher, G., Forsyth, K., & Kerschbaum, J. (2003). *Worker Role Interview (WRI) (version 10.0).* Model of Human Occupation Clearinghouse, Department of Occupational Therapy, College of Applied Health Sciences, University of Illinois at Chicago, Chicago, IL.

Creek, J. (1990) *Occupational therapy and mental health: Principles, skills and practice.* Edinburgh: Churchill Livingstone.

Creek, J. (2003). Occupational therapy defined as a complex intervention, London, College of Occupational Therapists.

Donaldson, G. A., & Sanderson, D. A. (1996) *Working together in schools. A guide for educators.* Thousand Oaks, CA: Corwin Press.

Dubouloz, C. J., Egan, M., von Zweck, C., & Vallerand, J. (1999). Occupational therapists' perceptions of evidence-based practice. *American Journal of Occupational Therapy, 53,* 445–453.

Dysart, A. M., & Tomlin, G. S. (2002). Factors related to evidence-based practice among U.S. Occupational therapy clinicians. *American Journal of Occupational Therapy, 56*(3), 275–284.

Egan, M., Dubouloz, C. J., Rappolt, S., Polatajko, H., King, J., Vallerand, J., Craik, J., Davis, J. A., &

Graham, I. D. (2004). Enhancing research use through on-line action research. *Canadian Journal of Occupational Therapy, 71,* 230–237.

Forsyth, K., Deshpande, S., Kielhofner, G., Henriksson, C., Haglund, L., Olson, L., Skinner, S., & Kulkarni, S. (2004). *User's manual for the Occupational Circumstances Assessment and Interview Rating Scale (OCAIRS) (version 4.0).* Model of Human Occupation Clearinghouse, Department of Occupational Therapy, College of Applied Health Sciences, University of Illinois at Chicago, Chicago, IL.

Higgs, J., & Titchen, A. (Eds.) (2001). *Practice knowledge and expertise in the health professions.* London: Butterworth Heinemann.

McCluskey, A. (2003). Occupational therapists report a low level of knowledge, skill and involvement in evidence-based practice. *Australian Occupational Therapy Journal, 50,* 3–12.

McCluskey, A., & Cusick, A. (2002). Strategies for introducing evidence-based practice and changing clinical behaviour: A manager's toolbox. *Australian Occupational Therapy Journal, 49,* 63–70.

Parkinson, S., Forsyth, K., & Kielhofner, G. (2004). *User's manual for the Model of Human Occupation Screening Tool (MOHOST) (version 1.1).* London: UK CORE.

Peloquin, S. M. (2002). Confluence: Moving forward with affective strength. *American Journal of Occupational Therapy, 56*(1), 69–77.

Peloquin, S. M., & Abreu, B. C. (1996). The academia and clinical worlds; Shall we make meaningful connections? *American Journal of Occupational Therapy, 50* (7), 588–591.

Schon, D. A. (1983). *The reflective practitioner: How professionals think in action.* New York: Basic Books.

Stringer, E. T. (1996). *Action research.* Thousand Oaks, CA: SAGE Publications.

Sudsawad, P. (2003). Rehabilitation practitioners' perspectives on research utilization for evidence-based practice. Paper presented at the American Congress of Rehabilitation Medicine conference, October 24, Tucson, AZ.

Taylor, R. R., Braveman, B., & Hammel, J. (2004). Developing and evaluating community-based services through participatory action research: Two case examples *American Journal of Occupational Therapy, 58,* 73–82.

Velozo, C., Kielhofner, G., & Fisher, G. (1998). *A user's guide to the Worker Role Interview (version 9).* Department of Occupational Therapy, University of Illinois at Chicago.

RECOMMENDED READINGS

Crist, P., & Kielhofner, G. (2005) *The Scholarship of Practice: Academic and practice collaborations for promoting occupational therapy.* Binghamton, NY: Hayworth Press.

Harrison, M., & Forsyth, K. (2005) Developing a vision for therapists working within child and adolescent mental health services: Poised or paused for action? *British Journal of Occupational Therapy, 68,* 1–5.

CHAPTER 41

Definition, Evolution, and Implementation of Evidence-Based Practice in Occupational Therapy

Pimjai Sudsawad

Definitions of Evidence-Based Practice

Evidence-based practice (EBP) is a practice approach developed based on the concept of evidence-based medicine (EBM). There are many definitions of EBP by several authors. However, the most widely cited definition is that by Sackett, Rosenberg, Gray, Haynes, and Richardson (1996) who defined evidence-based (medicine) practice as the conscientious, explicit, and judicious use of current best evidence in making decisions about the care of individual patients.

According to Sackett and colleagues (1996), evidence-based practice is an *integration of individual clinical expertise* with the *best available external clinical evidence* from systematic research. Clinical expertise refers to the proficiency and judgment that the individual practitioners acquire through experience. Best available external clinical evidence means client-centered research that is useful for informing practice.

It is clear from this definition that evidence-based practice relies on practitioners' clinical expertise when applying research evidence to practice. Sackett et al. (1996) stated that neither clinical expertise nor the best available external evidence alone is enough for evidence-based practice. They believed that external clinical evidence can inform but can never replace individual clinical expertise, and it is the clinical expertise that decides whether the external evidence applies to the individual patient (i.e., whether and how it matches the client's clinical state, predicaments, and preferences).

> Evidence-based practice relies on practitioners' clinical expertise when applying research evidence to practice.

More recently, Sackett, Straus, Richardson, Rosenberg, and Haynes (2000) described EBP as the integration of *best research evidence* with *clinical expertise and patient values*. With this updated version, the patient values are acknowledged as an equally important and necessary ingredient in the practice of EBP as research evidence and clinical expertise.

In another widely cited definition, Gray (1997) described evidence-based practice as an approach to decision-making in which the clinician uses the best evidence available in consultation with the patient to decide upon the option that best suits the patient. This definition stresses that the relationship between clinician and patient is centrally important in clinical decision-making.

According to Gray (1997), a clinical decision occurs based on three factors:

- Evidence,
- Values, and
- Resources.

He characterized current healthcare decisions that are based principally on values and resources as "opinion based decision-making." Gray further predicted that, as the pressure on resources increases, decisions will have to be made explicitly and publicly to justify the use of the resources. Therefore, those who make decisions will need to be able to produce and describe the evidence that informed each decision.

A third definition comes from the Canadian Association of Occupational Therapists' position statement on evidence-based occupational therapy (Canadian Association of Occupational Therapists,

Association of Canadian Occupational Therapy University Programs, Association of Canadian Occupational Therapy Regulatory Organizations, & the Presidents' Advisory Committee, 1999). It defines evidence-based occupational therapy as the client-centered enablement of occupation, based on client information and a critical review of relevant research, expert consensus, and experience. This definition of evidence-based occupational therapy recognizes the range of sources and scope of evidence available to occupational therapists (Zimolag, French, & Paterson, 2002) including:

- Research evidence,
- Information provided by the client for determining occupational priorities and capacities, and
- The knowledge that occupational therapists have gained from past experience.

Based upon those definitions, the essence of EBP may be summarized as follows:

- Evidence-based practice involves more than just the use of research evidence.
- Clinical expertise is as important to evidence-based practice as research evidence.
- Client input is vital to the decision-making process in evidence-based practice.
- Healthcare decisions are also influenced by available resources.

Evolution of Evidence-Based Practice in Occupational Therapy

Evidence-based practice (EBP) evolved from the principles of evidence-based medicine (EBM), a concept that originated in the 1980s at McMaster University in Canada (Taylor, 1997). EBP emerged within healthcare and health education in the 1990s (Turner, 2001). The need for increased accountability, in conjunction with the spending restraints in healthcare, has accelerated interest in the use of research evidence as the basis for occupational therapy practice (Law & Baum, 1998).

> The need for increased accountability in conjunction with the spending restraints in Healthcare has accelerated the interest in the use of research evidence as the basis for occupational therapy practice.

Discussions of Evidence-Based Practice in Occupational Therapy

Since the introduction of EBP in occupational therapy, there continues to be discussion about its implementation. There is an increasing recognition that the implementation of evidence-based practice is a complex process that may need some adaptations to ensure its applicability to occupational therapy.

To implement EBP in occupational therapy, the synthesis of the available evidence with clinical expertise and judgment, and knowledge of the values and preferences of the clients is viewed as critical (Gates & Atherton, 2001; Lee & Miller, 2003; Lloyd, King, & Bassett, 2002; Rappolt, 2003). Different authors have argued that the direct adoption of evidence-based medicine (EBM) and its established prescriptive guidelines may not adequately reflect the philosophical beliefs and the highly contextualized and dynamic nature of occupational therapy (Lee & Miller, 2003; Tse, Blackwood, & Penman, 2001; Welch, 2002).

Occupational therapy authors have also questioned the strict use of the Level of Evidence model (also based on EBM). According to this model, the strength of research evidence is ranked based upon predetermined criteria related to the study's designs and characteristics (with meta-analyses of randomized controlled trials usually considered the strongest and best evidence). The rationale for questioning this model is that the best evidence for each circumstance may differ depending on the type of clinical questions asked, and whether the questions relate to patterns and possibility or causality (Tickle-Degnen & Bedell, 2003; Tse et al., 2001).

Some authors have suggested qualitative research methods as one of the appropriate tools to identify and address clients' priorities. They argued that qualitative methods may enable occupational therapists to explore the complexities of clinical practice and of living with a disability, thereby informing a client-centered, evidence-based practice perspec-

International Developments in Evidence-Based Practice

Since the introduction of EBP, there have been several international developments for its support in the field of occupational therapy. EBP has been the main subject of prestigious lectures by several prominent scholars in different countries such as the Casson Memorial Lecture at the annual conference of the College of Occupational Therapists in the United Kingdom (Eakin, 1997), the Eleanor Clarke Slagle Lecture at the annual conference of the American Occupational Therapy Association (Holm, 2000), and the Silvia Docker Lecture at the annual conference of the Australian Association of Occupational Therapists (Cusick, 2001).

The American Journal of Occupational Therapy (AJOT) established the Evidence-Based Practice Forum as a regular department in 1999 (Tickle-Degnen, 1999). Numerous articles have been published in this department, providing information on different aspects of EBP. A new department in the journal now highlights clinical scholarship to enhance the links between research and practice (Kielhofner, 2005). There is also an increased drive for manuscripts that report applied research findings (Corcoran, 2003).

EBP has also been incorporated into educational requirements and professional conduct in occupational therapy. In the United States, educational standards require that occupational therapy graduates be able to "provide evidence-based effective therapeutic intervention related to performance areas" (Accreditation Council for Occupational Therapy Education, 1998, requirement 5.3, Section B). In addition, the occupational therapy code of ethics (American Occupational Therapy Association, 2005), Principle 4 E. states that "occupational therapy practitioners shall critically examine available evidence so they may perform their duties on the basis of current information." Similarly, the Code of ethics of the British College of Occupational Therapists Principle 5.4 states "Occupational therapists shall be personally responsible for actively maintaining and developing their personal development and professional competence," (College of Occupational Therapists, 2005) with a specific requirement that "Occupational therapy personnel shall be accountable for the quality of their work and base this on current guidance, research, reasoning, and the best available evidence."

To address the clinicians' and researchers' need for easily available research-grounded evidence documenting the value of therapeutic interventions, the American Occupational Therapy Association (AOTA) initiated a project to develop a series of evidence-based literature reviews of occupational therapy's effectiveness with health conditions addressed in AOTA's practice guidelines series (Lieberman & Scheer, 2002). The overarching goal of this project is to be part of the international effort to promote an outcome-based orientation among occupational therapists (Lieberman & Scheer, 2002). Several articles based on the evidence-based literature reviews have been published in AJOT (Baker & Tickle-Degnen, 2001; Ma & Trombly, 2002; Murphy & Tickle-Degnen, 2001; Trombly & Ma, 2002). There is also a plan to disseminate the reviews through submissions to the National Guideline Clearinghouse which is sponsored by the Agency for Healthcare Research and Quality, the American Medical Association, and the American Association of Health Plans so that the reviews will be part of the larger resources for evidence-based practice contributed by several other practice communities (Lieberman & Scheer, 2002).

In addition, AOTA has also made the evidence-based resource directory and Evidence Briefs Series available to its members through its Web site. The evidence-based resource directory includes links to many Web sites providing information in many areas related to evidence-based practice. The Evidence Briefs Series provides easy-to-read summaries of articles selected from scientific literature and indexed by topic area.

Most recently, AOTA, in collaboration with the American Occupational Therapy Foundation (AOTF), received a grant from the Agency for Healthcare Research and Quality to host a conference on evidence based practice. The conference served as an international forum to determine the state-of-the-art evidence-based occupational therapy practice and support the development of knowledge into the field including a set of consensus guidelines for evaluating and reporting research evidence, as well as a specific series of outcomes to be accomplished internationally (AOTF, 2003). The conference took place in July of 2004, and the final report of this international conference is available for AOTA members through the AOTA Web site and through a published article in AJOT (Coster, 2005).

A Web-based evidence resource containing abstracts of occupational therapy-relevant randomized controlled trials and systematic reviews, OTSeeker, has recently been established in Australia (Bennett et al., 2003). The OTSeeker database currently contains over 3500 abstracts (updated 12/20/05) and is expected to increase over time. The database was developed by a team of occupational therapists at that University of Queensland and University of Western Sydney with support from OT Australia, the Motor Accident Authority of New South Wales, and a Center for Evidence-Based Physiotherapy, Australia.

tive of occupational therapy (Gates & Atherton, 2001; Hammell, 2001).

There are also discussions about ethical issues related to EBP for both occupational therapy practitioners and researchers. An ethical dilemma can occur when the client's preference is contradicted by evidence (Roberts & Barber, 2001). Christensen and Lou (2001) suggested ethical considerations for occupational therapy researchers such as:

* Involving consumers in making research-related decisions,
* Ensuring that there is no conflict of interest in conducting a study due to sponsoring,
* Ensuring that disciplinary loyalty does not introduce potential bias into trials involving interventions associated with a given profession,

* Ensuring that informed consent was obtained in conducting a research study (despite the pressure to create research evidence to justify existing practice), and
* Being careful of biases in selection of research participants.

Hayes (2000) suggested that the best use of resources for research should be achieved through:

* Conducting a limited number of large, strategically designed, significant research projects rather than smaller, less consequential projects,
* Replicating existing studies to confirm their findings, and
* Conveying research findings in ways that practitioners are able to understand, critically interpret, and apply them to clinical practice.

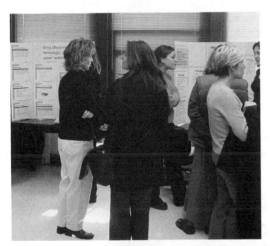
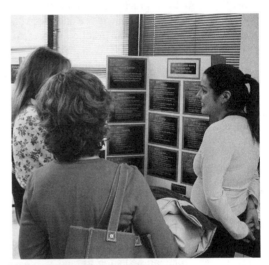
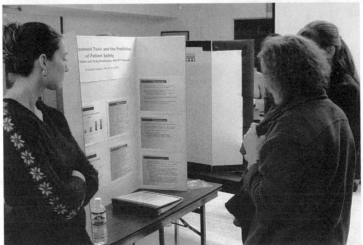

Figure 41.1 An evidence-based practice poster session is held annually at the University of Illinois at Chicago. Posters summarize and analyze evidence that addresses practice questions from Chicago area clinicians.

Implementation Status of Evidence-Based Practice

In general, occupational therapy practitioners have expressed positive attitudes toward an evidence-based practice approach (Bennett, Tooth et al., 2003; Curtin & Jaramazovic, 2001; Humphris, Littlejohn, Victor, O'Halloran, & Peacock, 2000; Upton & Lewis, 1998). However, the implementation of EBP in actual practice settings seems to face several barriers (Closs & Lewin, 1998; Bennett, Tooth et al., 2003; Curtin & Jaramazovic, 2001; Dysart & Tomlin, 2002; Humphris et al., 2000; McCluskey, 2003; Metcalfe et al., 2001; Philbert, Snyder, Judd, & Windsor, 2003; Sudsawad, 2004; Sweetland & Craik, 2001; Upton & Lewis, 1998). From the results of these studies, occupational therapy practitioners indicated that they still lacked adequate knowledge and the skills necessary for evidence-based practice at present. For example, they lacked:

- Information technology skills,
- The ability to undertake computer literature searches,
- Knowledge about electronic databases,
- Sufficient evidence appraisal skills, and
- Adequate understanding of statistics.

Problems with the logistics of EBP implementation were also apparent such as:

- The lack of time to read research and implement findings due to workload pressure,
- High staff turn over combined with staff shortages,
- The lack of organizational support, and
- Difficulty accessing research evidence since the literature is not available in one place.

Finally, the characteristics of research evidence can be another barrier to the implementation of evidence-based practice. Practitioners find that research evidence can be difficult to use due to such things as:

- Conflicting results,
- Methodological problems,
- Poor generalizability,
- Implications for practice not being made clear, and
- Lack of clinical relevance of findings.

These barriers are likely explanations for the slow adoption of EBP in occupational therapy. In addition, there seems to be evidence that occupational therapy practitioners continue to favor the use of clinical experience, information from continuing education, and colleagues to make clinical decisions, over the use of research evidence (Bennett et al., 2003; Dubouloz, Egan, Vallerand, & von Zweck, 1999; Sudsawad, 2004; Sweetland & Craik, 2001).

Several strategies have been proposed to alleviate barriers and help to facilitate the adoption of EBP. One strategy called for occupational therapy managers to find ways to provide time and support for EBP in a cost-effective manner (Closs & Lewin, 1998), and to create organizational conditions that promote the use of evidence-based practice (Humphris et al., 2000). Another strategy involved creating initiatives to assist the implementation of EBP (Curtin & Jaramazovic, 2001). There is also a call for occupational therapy programs to place more emphasis on reading and interpreting research and systematic reviews to help therapists overcome the obstacle of not being able to interpret research (Gervais, Poirier, Van Iterson, & Egan, 2002). Furthermore, there is a suggestion for occupational therapy researchers to create research evidence that is more usable for practice (Sudsawad, 2005).

There is a need to investigate the usability and the effectiveness of these strategies in addressing the barriers stated above, and it is likely that concurrent strategies will be necessary to help move the implementation of evidence-based practice in occupational therapy forward. Chapters 43 and 44 discuss strategies that are likely to support the change process that is necessary for the implementation of evidence-based practice.

Conclusion

Evidence-based practice is an approach that requires the integration of several factors in decision-making including research evidence, the practitioner's clinical expertise, the client's values and preferences, and available resources. From the EBP literature in occupational therapy, it seems apparent that the use of evidence-based practice continues to evolve as shown by the several debates and discussions on different aspects of the conceptual foundation of EBP, and the appropriate ways to interpret and use EBP in occupational therapy. The adoption of EBP is still limited, possibly due to the numerous barriers as indicated by practitioners, and there is a need to find effective strategies to alleviate those barriers in order for the implementation of EBP to move forward. Subsequent chapters in this section provide resources for the practitioner, and discuss factors that can enhance evidence-based practice and the usability of research in practice.

REFERENCES

The Commission on Standards and Ethics of the American Occupational Therapy Association (2005). Occupational therapy code of ethics. *The American Journal of Occupational Therapy, 59*, 639–642.

The American Occupational Therapy Foundation (2003). AHRQ funds international conference on evidence-based occupational therapy. *AOTF Connection, 10*(2), 1, 5.

Baker, N. A., & Tickle-Degnen, L. (2001). The effectiveness of physical, psychological, and functional interventions in treating clients with multiple sclerosis: A meta-analysis. *The American Journal of Occupational Therapy, 55*, 324–331.

Bennett, S., Hoffmann, T., McCluskey, A., McKenna, K., Strong, J., & Tooth, L. (2003). Introducing OTseeker (Occupational Therapy Systematic Evaluation of Evidence). A new evidence database for occupational therapists. *The American Journal of Occupational Therapy, 57*, 635–638.

Bennett, S., Tooth, L., McKenna, K., Rodger, S., Strong, J., Ziviani, J., Mickan, S., & Gibson, L. (2003). Perceptions of evidence based practice: A survey of Australian occupational therapists. *Australian Occupational Therapy Journal, 50*, 13–22.

Canadian Association of Occupational Therapists, Association of Canadian Occupational Therapy University Programs, Association of Canadian Occupational Therapy Regulatory Organizations, & the Presidents' Advisory Committee (1999). Joint Position Statement on Evidence-Based Occupational Therapy. *Canadian Journal of Occupational Therapy, 66*, 267–269.

Christensen, C., & Lou, J. (2001). Evidence-based practice forum. Ethical considerations related to evidence-based practice. *The American Journal of Occupational Therapy, 55*, 345–349.

Closs, S. J., & Lewin, B. (1998). Perceived barriers to research utilization: A survey of four therapies. *British Journal of Therapy and Rehabilitation, 5*, 151–155.

College of Occupational Therapists (2005). *Code of ethics and professional conduct.* London: Author.

Corcoran, M. A. (2003). A glance back and a glimpse ahead. *The American Journal of Occupational Therapy, 57*, 367–368.

Coster, W. (2005). International conference on evidence-based practice: A collaborative effort of the American Occupational Therapy Association, the American Occupational Therapy Foundation, and the Agency for Health Research and Quality. *The American Journal of Occupational Therapy, 59*, 356-358.

Curtin, M., & Jaramazovic, E. (2001). Occupational therapists' views and perceptions of evidence-based practice. *British Journal of Occupational Therapy, 64*, 214–222.

Cusick, A. (2001). OZ OT EBP 21C: Australian occupational therapy, evidence-based practice and the 21st century. *Australian Occupational Therapy Journal, 48*, 102–117.

Dubouloz, C-J., Egan, M., Vallerand, J., & von Zweck, C. (1999). Occupational therapists' perceptions of evidence-based practice. *American Journal of Occupational Therapy, 53*, 445–453.

Dysart, A. M., & Tomlin, G. S. (2002). Factors related to evidence-based practice among US occupational therapy clinicians. *The American Journal of Occupational Therapy, 56*, 275–284.

Eakin, P. (1997). The Casson Memorial Lecture 1997: Shifting the balance—Evidence-based practice. *British Journal of Occupational Therapy, 60*, 290–294.

Gates, B., & Atherton, H. (2001). The challenge of evidence-based practice for learning disabilities. *Learning Disability Nursing, 10*, 517–522.

Gervais, I. S., Poirier, A., Van Iterson, L. & Egan, M. (2002). Attempting to use a Cochrane review: Experience of three occupational therapists. *The American Journal of Occupational Therapy, 56*, 110–113.

Gray, J. A. M. (1997). *Evidence based healthcare: How to make health policy and management decisions.* New York: Churchill Livingstone.

Hammell, K. W. (2001). Using qualitative research to inform the client-centred evidence-based practice of occupational therapy. *British Journal of Occupational Therapy, 64*, 228–234.

Hayes, R. L. (2000). Evidence-based occupational therapy needs strategically targeted quality research now. *Australian Occupational Therapy Journal, 47*, 186–190.

Holm, M. B. (2000). The 2000 Eleanor Clarke Slagle Lecture. Our mandate for the new millennium: Evidence-based practice. *The American Journal of Occupational Therapy, 54*, 575–585.

Humphris, D., Littlejohn, P., Victor, C. O'Halloran, P., & Peacock, J. (2000). Implementing evidence-based practice: Factors that influence the use of research evidence by occupational therapists. *British Journal of Occupational Therapy, 63*, 516–522.

Kielhofner, G. (2005). Scholarship and Practice: Bridging the divide. *American Journal of Occupational Therapy, 59*, 231–239

Law, M., & Baum, C. (1998). Evidence-based practice occupational therapy. *Canadian Journal of Occupational Therapy, 65*, 131–135.

Lee, C. J., & Miller, L. T. (2003). The process of evidence-based clinical decision making in occupational therapy. *The American Journal of Occupational Therapy, 57*, 473–477.

Lieberman, D., & Scheer, J. (2002). AOTA's evidence-based literature review project: an overview. *The American Journal of Occupational Therapy, 56*, 344–349.

Lloyd, C., King, R., & Bassett, H. (2002). Evidence-based practice in occupational therapy—why the jury is still out. *New Zealand Journal of Occupational Therapy, 49*, 10–14.

Ma, H., & Trombly, C. A. (2002). A synthesis of the effects of occupational therapy for persons with stroke, part II: Remediation of impairments. *The American Journal of Occupational Therapy, 56*, 260–274.

McCluskey, A. (2003). Occupational therapists report a low level of knowledge, skill and involvement in evidence-based practice. *Australian Occupational Therapy Journal, 50*, 3–12.

Metcalfe, C., Lewin, R., Wisher, S., Perry, S., Bannigan, K., & Moffett, J. K. (2001). Barriers to implementing the evidence based in for NHS therapies. *Physiotherapy, 11*, 433–441.

Murphy, S., & Tickle-Degnen, L. (2001). The effectiveness of occupational therapy-related treatments for persons with Parkinson's disease: A meta-analytic review. *The American Journal of Occupational Therapy, 55*, 385–392.

Philbert, D. B., Snyder, P., Judd, D., & Windsor, M-M. (2003). Practitioners' reading patterns, attitudes, and use of research reported in occupational therapy journals. *The American Journal of Occupational Therapy,* *57*, 450–458.

Rappolt, S. (2003). The role of professional expertise in evidence-based occupational therapy. *The American Journal of Occupational Therapy, 57*, 589–593.

Roberts, A. E. K., & Barber, G. (2001). Applying research evidence to practice. *British Journal of Occupational Therapy, 64*, 223–227.

Sackett, D. L., Straus, S. E., Richardson, W. S, Rosenberg, W. M. C., & Haynes, R. (2000). *Evidence-based Medicine: How to practice and teach EBM* (2nd ed.). Edinburgh; New York: Churchill Livingstone.

Sackett, D. L., Rosenberg, W. M. C., Gray, J. A. M., Haynes, R., & Richardson, W. S. (1996). Evidence based medicine: What it is and what it isn't. *British Medical Journal, 312*, 71–72.

Sudsawad, P. (2004). *Developing a social validation model for effective utilization of disability and rehabilitation research*. Project summary. Submitted to the National Institute of Disability and Rehabilitation Research, US Department of Education, Grant no. H133F020023.

Sudsawad, P. (2005). A conceptual framework to increase usability of outcome research for evidence-based practice. *The American Journal of Occupational Therapy, 59*, 351–355.

Sweetland, J., & Craik, C. (2001). The use of evidence-based practice by occupational therapists who treat adult stroke patients. *British Journal of Occupational Therapy, 64*, 256–261.

Taylor, M. C. (1997). What is evidence-based practice? *British Journal of Occupational Therapy, 60*, 470–474.

Tickle-Degnen, L. (1999). Evidence-based practice forum—Organizing, evaluating, and using evidence in occupational therapy practice. *The American Journal of Occupational Therapy, 53,* 537–539.

Tickle-Degnen, L., & Bedell, G. (2003). Heterarchy and hierarchy: A critical appraisal of the "levels of evidence" as a tool for clinical decision-making. *The American Journal of Occupational Therapy, 57*, 234–237.

Trombly, C. A., & Ma, H. (2002). A synthesis of the effects of occupational therapy for persons with stroke, part I: Restoration of roles, tasks, and activities. *The American Journal of Occupational Therapy, 56*, 250–259.

Tse, S., Blackwood, K., & Penman, M. (2001). From rhetoric to reality: Use of randomised controlled trials in evidence-based occupational therapy. *Australian Occupational Therapy Journal, 47*, 181–185.

Turner, P. (2001). Evidence-based practice and physiotherapy in the 1990s. *Physiotherapy Theory and Practice, 17*, 107–121.

Upton, D., & Lewis, B. (1998). Clinical effectiveness and EBP: design of a questionnaire. *British Journal of Therapy and Rehabilitation, 5*, 647–650.

Welch, A. (2002). The challenge of evidence-based practice to occupational therapy: A literature review. *The Journal of Clinical Governance, 10*, 169–176.

Zimolag, U., French, N., & Paterson, M (2002). Developing expert practice. Striving for professional excellence: The role of evidence-based practice and professional artistry. *Occupational Therapy Now, 4* (6), 8–10.

RESOURCES

American Occupational Therapy Association: http://www.aota.org

American Occupational Therapy Foundation: www.aotf.org

Agency for Healthcare Research and Quality: www.ahrq.gov

National Guideline Clearinghouse: www.guideline.gov

OTSeeker: http://www.otseeker.com

CHAPTER 42

Analyzing Evidence for Practice

Nancy A. Baker

The emergence of consumer-driven health care and the advent of managed care has led to a movement toward evidence-based practice (Tickle-Degnen, 1998). In evidence-based practice, healthcare practitioners access and evaluate research to identify:

- The effectiveness of interventions,
- The accuracy of evaluations, and
- The expected prognosis of a disorder.

This information is then used to determine the best practice for different health conditions. Sackett and Richardson (1996) defined evidence-based practice as "the conscientious, explicit, and judicious use of current best-evidence in making decisions about the care of individual patients." (p. 71). The bottom line of evidence-based practice is that it provides practitioners with objective evidence that an intervention can improve a client's health and well-being.

Occupational therapy practitioners are mandated by the ethics of their practice (American Occupational Therapy Association, 2000) to demonstrate that the intervention they provide not only does no harm, but also helps their client. Nonetheless, many practitioners feel that the acquisition and development of the skills necessary to be evidence-based practitioners is a formidable task (Dubouloz, Egan, Vallerand, & von-Zweck, 1999; Straus & McAlister, 2000). While evidence-based practice may appear complex, some simple methods can be used to identify, access, and critically appraise evidence for making intervention decisions. This chapter provides a method to:

> The bottom line of evidence-based practice is that it provides practitioners with objective evidence that an intervention can improve a client's health and well-being.

- Develop an answerable question,
- Find the evidence,
- Do a critical appraisal of the evidence, and
- Calculate effect sizes to understand how an intervention affects outcomes.

Developing a Question

Many practitioners do not know how to start the process of evidence-based practice. The first step of evidence-based practice is to develop a clear, specific, answerable question (Law, 2002b; Sackett, Straus, Richardson, Rosenberg, & Haynes, 2000; Straus & McAlister, 2000). A well-developed clinical question serves several purposes:

- It helps clearly define and refine what is relevant to both the practitioners' knowledge needs and their clients' care needs,
- It suggests specific criteria to use for search strategies, and
- It provides a useful format for communicating the information to others (Sackett et al., 2000).

The key to asking a clinical question is to clearly specify what information is needed. For instance, practitioners working with clients with spasticity of the hand might want to establish the effectiveness of splinting for these clients. Their initial question might be:

- *Is splinting useful for clients with spasticity of the hand?*

While this is definitely a question, it is not specific. What kind of "splinting"? What is meant by "useful," and useful for what? Even the type of client is not clear. In what type of "spasticity" is the practitioner interested? A well-written clinical question contains specific information designed to assist a practitioner to specify the clinical problem (Richardson, Wilson, Nishikawa, & Hayward, 1995).

Questions in evidence-based practice can be divided into two types:

- Background questions, and
- Foreground questions (Sackett et al., 2000).

Each type of question is useful for gathering different types of knowledge. Generally novice practitioners ask more background questions and more experienced therapists ask more foreground questions as they are familiar with the disorder and are trying to develop interventions to address different deficits associated with the disorder (Sackett et al., 2000). Each type of question asks for certain types of information.

Background Questions

Background questions provide groundwork information about general aspects of the disorder such as the population involved, modes of evaluation, types of intervention, or overall prognosis. They have two essential components:

- A question root such as who, what, where, how, or why combined with a verb, and
- A disorder or aspect of a disorder (see Table 42.1).

While these questions do not answer a specific intervention question, they provide a practitioner with a general sense of what the disorder may look like, act like, or what kind of general implications the disorder may have.

Foreground Questions

Many times practitioners seek evidence to support an intervention for a specific client, or for a population of clients whom they see routinely. The foreground question focuses on specific knowledge about managing the care of clients with a specific aspect of a disorder. Foreground questions are often called PICO questions because this acronym spells out the key components of a specific clinical question:

- P—The patient or problem of interest,
- I—The intervention being considered,
- C—The comparison intervention (if any), and
- O—The anticipated clinical outcome (Sackett et al., 2000)

Specifying the PICO Question

P—The Patient or Problem. The P defines the criteria of the patient or population of interest and should include client information that may affect the outcome of the intervention. While a P should specify the patient, too many qualifiers will make it too hard to find any evidence at all. The P defines the criteria used to determine if the sample described in an article can be used with the clinician's clients.

For example, a question for splinting should specify clients potentially seen with this problem, such as clients post-CVA who have moderate to severe spasticity. The resulting P might read: *In clients 3 months post-CVA with moderate to severe spasticity…*

I—The Intervention. The I specifies a particular intervention method, or may identify different intervention options. The I should identify the key criteria of the intervention. This may include not only the type of intervention, but also how the intervention will be applied, and the frequency and duration of the intervention. One of the key aspects of naming an intervention is to use the most common terminology or description so that the evidence will be easy to access. Sometimes more than one name needs to be used in a search to track down the best evidence.

For the intervention for the clients with hand spasticity the intervention might be specified as a dorsal splint with digit abductors. The I portion of the PICO question about work might read: *…does the application of a dorsal splint with digit abductors…* or it can be further refined by including the duration or intensity of the intervention: *…does the application of a dorsal splint with digit abductors at night time for 5 days a week …*

C—The Comparison Intervention. Experimental research usually compares two different forms of intervention; one is the intervention of interest (the treatment group or experimental group) and one is an alternate, mock, or no intervention condition (the control group). The C specifies the alternate care. Defining a "control" intervention in the clinical question will focus on whether the intervention will be compared to an existing intervention or to receiving no intervention. In some studies there is no specific comparison and thus the comparison intervention can be omitted. For the splinting question, splinting will be compared to daily PROM: *…as compared to daily PROM…*

O—The Outcome. O specifies what outcomes the intervention will affect, and how the intervention will affect them. Outcome improvements can be in activity performance, such as activities of daily living; in impairments, such as speed, strength, flexibility, or endurance; or in less tangible outcomes, such as improvements in emotion, cognition, or social ability. The O for the question could be: *…cause a reduction in tone and increased use of the hand as a stabilizer?*

Table 42.1 Background and Foreground Question Formats

Background Question	
Question Root and Verb	Disorder or Aspect of the Disorder
• What causes...	• ...Guillain-Barré syndrome?
• What is...	• ...the incidence of chronic low back pain?
• What are...	• ...the characteristics of spastic quadriplegia?

Foreground Questions (PICO)			
P Problem or patient	I Intervention	C Comparison	O Outcome
• In workers with low back pain of at least 3 months duration...	• ...does work rehabilitation or functional rehab lasting 5 days a week and at least 4 hours a day...	• ...as compared to three times a week individualized occupational therapy...	• ... cause a reduction in sick days and improve strength and endurance?
• For a 30- to 50-year-old client with severe MS and associated tremors ...	• ...will a cold suit worn for 10 minutes prior to therapeutic intervention...	• ...as compared to no intervention...	• significantly increase dexterity?
• For a middle school boy with poor handwriting	• ...will 6 months of daily shape copying for 10 minutes...	• ...compared to 6 months of daily 10 minutes of handwriting practice...	• significantly improve handwriting?

Based on the points just made, the splitting question has become quite specific:

In clients 3 months post-CVA with moderate to severe spasticity, does the application of a dorsal splint with digit abductors at night time for 5 days a week as compared to daily PROM cause a reduction in tone and increased use of the hand as a stabilizer?

It defines the client, intervention, and outcome in a manner that allows a ready benchmark to match any accessed literature. Table 42.1 provides examples of some other PICO questions.

Searching the Literature

Once an answerable question is developed, the next step is to access the evidence. Chapter 27 in this book provides a discussion of how to find literature and there have been several excellent articles and chapters written on the process of searching the literature and accessing the articles (See Resources at the end of the chapter).

Critical Appraisal of the Evidence

After completing the search and retrieval, each resulting article's overall quality should be critically appraised to determine if the research methodology used is adequate to support using the results to guide treatment. Critical appraisal helps to identify the strength of the evidence for guiding practice. For example, if the question is about the effectiveness of an intervention, the highest quality research is that which accurately supports a causal association between the intervention and the outcome of interest.

It is difficult to show a causal association, particularly when there are complex interactions between biological, psychological and socioeconomic factors (Hulley et al., 2001; Newman, Browner, & Hulley, 2001; Rosenthal & Rosnow, 1991). To support a causal association between an intervention and an outcome, all other plausible alternate explanations must be ruled out. The presence of plausible alternate explanations for the effects

> ...critical appraisal helps to identify if potential threats to internal validity have been controlled through experimental design, thus preventing an artificial inflation or reduction of treatment effect.

seen in an article is often referred to as threats to internal validity. Thus, when reviewing intervention studies, critical appraisal helps to identify if potential threats to internal validity have been controlled through experimental design, thus preventing an artificial inflation or reduction of treatment effect (Moher et al., 1998). The feature box on the next page provides additional information about threats to internal validity.

There are many different methods to appraise an intervention study article quality (Ajetunmobi, 2002; GRADE Working Group, 2004; Law, 2002a), but all appraisal methods are designed to provide a level of confidence that the estimate of the effect is accurate (GRADE Working Group, 2004). For this chapter, the appraisal criteria described by Sackett et al. (2000) are used, but other authors provide variations on these criteria (see Resources for other critical appraisal methods). Also, when appraising other types of evidence (e.g., evidence about the psychometric soundness of an assessment, or diagnostic ability) other criteria relevant to that type of research should be used. This chapter does not provide in-depth information about article quality for articles other than those focused on intervention effects. For further information on appraising articles on diagnostic tests, instrument psychometrics, and prognosis, see the Resources.

The most basic critical appraisal is to identify the research design used for the study. The design most likely to prevent threats to internal validity for intervention studies is a randomized clinical trial (RCT). The RCT is considered better than a quasi-experimental study, which in turn is considered better than a case-control or cohort study, which are in turn considered to be better than a correlational study (see Table 42.2 for more information about different research design characteristics). One hierarchy used to assess intervention studies as described by Moore, McQuay, and Gray (1995) is detailed in Table 42.2, although there are many different variations of these basic hierarchal levels. These hierarchies can be used to assign a rating to different intervention articles to help ascertain the overall quality of any given article based on its design type.

This kind of hierarchy of evidence is widely accepted in medicine when examining the effectiveness of an intervention. However, as noted in Chapter 41, some occupational therapists have called for a more flexible approach to what is considered "best" evidence depending on the type of question being answered.

Methodological Considerations for Appraisal

The following sections will discuss major considerations for critical appraisal of intervention studies.

The Control Group

One of the most effective methods to control for plausible alternate explanations is a control group (Portney & Watkins, 2000). A control group is a set of subjects who are equivalent to the treatment group for all variables except they receive a "control" treatment, such as usual care. Often, in therapeutic research studies, the control group is made up of participants who are on a wait list; in this instance they receive no control intervention. This study design is somewhat weaker because the improvement in outcomes seen in the treatment group may be the result of the additional attention experimental subjects receive, not the actual intervention.

After the intervention is completed, the control group is compared to the treatment group statistically. If the control group has changed significantly less than the treatment group on the outcomes being measured, it is reasonable—within limits of the design rigor—to attribute any changes in the outcome to the intervention rather than some other reason.

An important aspect to consider is whether random allocation was used to assign subjects to the treatment and control groups. Random allocation is the best way to ensure that the treatment and control group are equivalent, as it is important to avoid the confounding of group differences with treatment effects (Ajetunmobi, 2002). In addition, the investigator determining if a person meets eligibility requirements for the study should do so without prior knowledge of what group the subject will be assigned. Concealed allocation ensures that subjects are retained or excluded from the study without conscious or unconscious bias (Altman & Schulz, 2001) which helps to prevent an inflation of results (Moher et al., 1998).

Even when there is random assignment, the treatment and control groups may be significantly different on some measure such as age, ethnicity, or a baseline outcome score. In this case investigators will often control for these differences through the statistical analyses, and should mention this in their description of the statistical analyses.

Intention to Treat Analysis

Another safeguard of internal validity is a method of statistical analysis called "intention to treat"

Threats to Internal Validity

In 1979, Cook and Campbell (1979) described some threats to internal validity that could occur during the process of a study. Others have elaborated on these threats to internal validity. The following table provides a review of some of these threats as well as a description of how they can be controlled.

Threats to Internal Validity

Threat	Definition	Control	Example
History*	Observed effect may be due to events that take place between baseline and follow-up.	Control group Random assignment Isolation	A single group (pre–post study) study examined the effect of exercise on reducing depression in individuals with fibromyalgia. During the course of the study a brand new drug was released that reduced depression in those with fibromyalgia. More than half the sample was placed on the drug. At the end of the study there was a big, significant difference in baseline and follow-up measures of depression.
Maturation*	Observed effect may be due to changes occurring simply as a function of the passage of time.	Control group Random assignment	A 2-year single group (pre/post study) study examined the effect of fine motor coordination training on improving handwriting skills in 7-year-olds. Subjects received weekly treatment. At the end of 2 years there was a big, significant difference between the 7-year-old (baseline) and 9-year-old (follow-up) scores.
Attrition (Mortality)*	Observed effect may be due to the differential loss of subjects between groups.	Make treatment easy Make visits easy Make measurements painless Encourage subjects to remain Find lost subjects Intention to treat analysis	A study examined the effect of OT on the health of the well-elderly. They recruited 300 well-elderly and initiated a 6-month program of OT with 150 of them. The other 150 received no treatment. At the end of the study, 75 had dropped out of the no treatment group (attrition rate 50%) and 30 out of the treatment group (20% attrition rate). There was a big, significant difference between the treatment and control group.
Testing*	Observed effect may be due to repeated testing causing improvements in the test due to familiarity/learning.	Control group Random assignment Vary tests Limit retests	A single group (pre–post study) study examined the effect of strength training on dexterity tested 10 subjects with the 9-hole-peg test, then initiated a daily strengthening program. At the end of each session, the subjects were retested with the 9-hole peg test. At the end of 10 sessions there was a big, significant difference between baseline and follow-up scores on the 9-hole peg test.
Instrumentation*	Observed effect may be due to changes in the instrument from baseline to follow-up. Instruments may be improperly calibrated and/or insensitive particularly at the extremes of measurement.	Control group Blinding Frequent instrument calibration Training/certifying raters Repeating measures Choose sensitive instruments	A single group (pre/post study) study examined the effect of a home program in Thera-putty® on hand strength. Unbeknownst to the raters, the dynamometer used to measure strength was dropped on the floor just prior to follow-up testing. All subjects showed at least a 10-lb difference in strength at follow-up which was significantly different from baseline score.

(continued)

Threat	Definition	Control	Example
	Raters may be unreliable and/or biased.		
Regression to the Mean*	Observed effect may be due to the tendency of extreme scores to retest nearer to the point of central tendency (mean).	Control group Random assignment Multiple measurement methods Reliable tests	A single group (pre–post study) study examined the effect of tai chi on balance by recruiting 40 individuals who scored below the 2nd standard deviation on the Berg Balance Scale. They participated in a 6-week program of tai chi. At follow-up, all subjects have improved to within at least one standard deviation of the mean. There was a big, significant difference between baseline and follow-up tests.
Selection*	Observed effect may be due to the difference in the type of people in each experimental group.	Random assignment Assess differences between groups pre intervention. Control in statistical analysis	A study examined the effect of night splinting on work related carpal tunnel syndrome. Those subjects who come in the morning were assigned to the control group, those in the afternoon were assigned to the treatment group. After the study was completed, an examination of the demographic data suggests that more of the people in the treatment group were currently at work, while those in the control group were off of work. There was no significant difference between the groups.
Diffusion/ imitation of treatment*	Treatment effect is eliminated if treatment involves informational programs and the treatment group shares information with the control group.	Blinding Limit contact between groups Reinforce need not to share information. Let both groups know information will be shared post-study.	A study examined the effect of training in patient handling techniques on reports of back pain. One unit in a hospital was the treatment group, another was the control. During the study the investigator finds the treatment group handouts in the lunch room used by both groups. There were no significant differences between groups on reports of pain at follow-up.
Compensatory equalization of treatment*	Treatment effect is eliminated if group receiving "less desirable" treatment receives additional services/ help by those aware of this "inequality".	Blinding Let all know that control group will receive treatment after study.	A study examined the effect of group Sensory Integration (SI) on reading in 7-year-olds. Children with SI problems were randomly assigned to receive SI intervention or no intervention. After 4 weeks of treatment the investigator found out that the teacher was assigning those in the control group to extra reading practice during the times when the treatment group was receiving SI. At the end of the study there was no significant difference between those receiving SI and the control group.

(continued)

Threats to Internal Validity (continued)

Threat	Definition	Control	Example
Compensatory rvalry[*]	Treatment effect is eliminated if members of group receiving "less desirable" treatment are motivated to work harder than usual ("John Henry effect").	Blinding Let all know that control group will receive treatment after study.	A study examined the effect of modeled work training on the productivity of individuals in sheltered workshops. One group in a facility was assigned to the treatment group, the other to the control group. At the end of a year, the productivity of the control group is 25% greater than any previous years' productivity. There was no significant difference between the two groups.
Resentful demoral-ization[*]	Observed effect may be due to the negative reaction of the group receiving "less desirable" treatment who may reduce their level of effort.	Blinding Let all know that control group will receive treatment after study.	A study examined the effect of weekend adventure camp on short term memory of individuals with TBI. The treatment group traveled to the camp while the control group remained in the group home over the weekend. At follow-up 1 week later, the control group's mean memory has decreased significantly from its mean baseline score. There was a significant difference between the two groups on short-term memory.
Placebo effect[**]	Observed effect may be due to the subjects expectation that the treatment will cause a change.	Control group Blinding	A study examined the effect of ultrasound on wrist tendonitis pain. The treatment group received the clinical protocol ultrasound treatment, the control received a sham treatment with the machine turned off. There was no significant difference between the treatment and control groups.
Hawthorne effect[**]	Observed effect may be due to the attention inherent in the research process, not the treatment itself.	Control group Sham treatment Blinding	A study examined the effect of playing gin rummy on memory and pain in elderly individuals in a SNF. Each individual in the treatment group played gin rummy three times a week one on one with the researcher, the control received no treatment. At the end of 4 weeks the treatment group shows significant improvements in both memory and pain.
Halo effect[**]	Observed effect may be due to researchers' expectations about the performance of their subjects which may bias their judgment or cause them to interact differently with subjects depending upon group assignment.	Blinding experi-menter	A study examined the effect of a new form of dressing training on individuals with CVA. The investigator developed the new training and plans to market it once the research proves it is better than the traditional method. Sixty subjects were randomly assigned to one of two groups, one received the new treatment and one received the traditional treatment. All evaluations were carried out by the investigator who was aware of what group each subject was assigned to. The outcome measures were along the five level continuum of dependent to independent. By the end of 2 weeks, all subjects in the treatment group were rated as basically independent by the evaluator, while only one third of the control group received a score of independent. There was a significant difference between the two groups.

[*]Cook and Campbell (1979); [**]Berg and Latin (1994)

Table 42.2 **Hierarchy of Levels of Evidence by Research Design**

Level	Research Design	
I	Systematic review of research studies (randomized clinical trial [RCT])	• In a systematic review, many articles about the topic are analyzed and synthesized together to develop an overview of the intervention based on many different sources. Systematic reviews are considered to be the strongest evidence because they combine the overall conclusion of all evidence.
II	Randomized clinical trial (RCT)	• An RCT research design includes at least one control group as well as the intervention group. It has random allocation of subjects to each group. All other variables are held constant except for the intervention which the researcher manipulates by group.
III	Quasi-experimental, pre–post, cohort, and case control studies	• A quasi-experimental study is similar to an RCT except subjects are not randomly assigned to the treatment and control groups. • A pre–post study has a single group of subjects assessed at baseline and at intervals. • A cohort study follows a group of subjects who do not yet have the outcome of interest over time to see who develops the disorder. The investigators then examine variables gathered at baseline to see which ones are associated with those who develop the disorder. Unlike an RCT, the investigator does not manipulate an intervention within the groups. • A case control study selects a group of subjects (cases) who have the outcome of interest and matches it to a group of subjects without the outcome (controls). The investigator looks in all the subjects' pasts to see what variables are associated with the outcome of interest.
IV	Correlational studies of multiple sites	• A correlational study has a group of subjects. The investigators look for associations between variables and the outcome of interest. To be a level IV, the subjects must be gathered from multiple sites.
V	Correlational studies, qualitative studies; expert opinion	• Qualitative studies examine thoughts and ideas by conducting in-depth interviews of subjects and analyzing these interviews for common themes. • Expert opinion is a idea or belief developed by someone with experience, but that idea does not have research to support the conclusions.

Adapted from: Moore, McQuay, & Gray (1995).

analysis (Hollis & Campbell, 1999). In this type of analysis, each subject is analyzed in the group to which he or she was assigned, regardless of whether the individual received the intervention. This qualification of analysis groups is important as some subjects switch groups or dropout during a research study. This is not an intuitive safeguard as it would appear to make more sense to analyze subjects' data as part of the group they attended, not to which they were assigned. However, factors such as attrition may seriously bias the results, destroying the random allocation and the equivalency of the groups (Sackett et al., 2000). The easiest way to be sure an intention to treat analysis was used is to look in the data analysis section for the term "intention to treat," although older articles may not list that this was done (Hollis & Campbell, 1999).

Length of Follow-Up

Investigators must allow sufficient time for the outcomes of interest to develop fully (Sackett et al., 2000). In some interventions the outcome will be immediately evident. For example, applying splints to improve coordination can be tested almost immediately. Other times, the follow-up period may need to be weeks or months. For example, many stroke studies follow subjects for at least 6 months to make sure the stroke has resolved fully in order to understand the implications of the intervention over the full span of the rehabilitation and healing process.

Blinding

Blinding, in which the client, investigator, assessor, or other important study personnel is unaware of who is and who is not receiving the intervention, is an important method of preventing bias (Schulz & Grimes, 2002). Subjects' knowledge of their treatment status or investigators' expectations can consciously or unconsciously influence outcomes, or the recording of outcomes. Blinding can include hiding the intervention status from:

• The subjects,
• Those who provide the intervention or measure outcomes, and
• Those who analyze the data.

These various levels of blinding are called single-blinding, double-blinding, and triple-blinding, respectively. Blinding is not always feasible, particularly where therapeutic interventions are involved as it may be impossible to hide from a subject or provider whether he or she is receiving or implementing an intervention (Schulz & Grimes, 2002).

Attrition

In studies that last for more than a few days, some of the research subjects may drop out or be lost before the final outcome measures are taken, called attrition. In general, if a study loses more than 20% of its sample before follow-up, there is a possibility of serious bias (Sackett et al., 2000). For example, if a large number of the less healthy subjects enter a nursing home and are not measured at follow-up, the research will be unable to describe the effect of the intervention on those with poorer health. Their loss may skew the results toward healthier subjects.

Critical Appraisal

The above criteria or criteria described in other critical rating systems (see Resources) should be used to critically appraise any evidence to determine if the article is worth further assessment and use in practice. Evidence-based practice is based on the premise that the "best available evidence" should be used (Sackett & Richardson, 1996). If the research design has serious design flaws (i.e. lacking several of the above criteria) the article

may not be worth further assessment if better evidence is available. When there is no other available evidence, the findings should be considered in light of the design weaknesses. Studies with serious design flaws tend to systematically either inflate or deflate the size of the effect on outcomes (Rosenthal & Rosnow, 1991), and therefore may suggest that an intervention has very large effects, when in reality, the true effect is negligible. In determining whether to use the results of a study, practitioners should consider:

• The type of intervention described,
• Whether the theory supporting its use is sound, and
• Whether it has been used routinely in clinical practice, or is a new, "innovative" technique.

In cases where weaker evidence is used to support practice, practitioners should continue to search the literature in the future for new evidence.

Effect Size Calculation

In clinical research, investigators measure the outcomes that are considered most important. For example, an investigator examining the effect of occupational therapy on function might choose an outcome measure that captures some aspect of functional ability. Investigators analyze data on these outcomes with inferential statistics (see Chapter 17), obtaining a p-value to determine if the results are significantly different. By convention, a p-value of less than .05 is considered statistically significant (Ajetunmobi, 2002; Portney & Watkins, 2000). Significance, however, does not refer to the size or magnitude of the observed effect. Statistically significant differences can occur in situations where there is only a very small clinical effect.

For example, Table 42.3 shows a hypothetical study examining the effect of Thera-putty® on grip strength. It reports the following after 6 months of daily Thera-putty®. There is a significant difference between the treatment and control group for right and left grip strength, as represented by the

Table 42.3 Hypothetical Results of a Study Examining the Effect of Thera-putty® on Hand Strength

	Treatment Group Mean		Control Group Mean		p-Value
	Pre-intervention	Post-intervention	Pre-intervention	Post-intervention	
Grip strength right	34 lbs	37 lbs	34 lbs	35 lbs	.03
Grip strength left	23 lbs	26 lbs	23 lbs	24 lbs	.04

p-values of less than 0.05. This finding suggests that the Thera-putty® intervention caused a change in the grip strength of the treatment group. However, a closer examination shows that the hypothetical treatment group's bilateral grip increased by only 3 pounds. This is not a clinically large effect, particularly for 6 months of daily therapy.

Significance, therefore, does not indicate the magnitude of the effect of the intervention. As discussed in Chapter 16, an effect size refers to the magnitude of differences found between the outcomes of persons in a treatment group and those in a control group (Tickle-Degnen, 1998). Increasingly, studies will report effect size. This section provides information on how to quickly calculate effect size (when it is not provided) from available information in an article. It also discusses how to interpret an effect size.

Outcomes usually come in one of two forms, frequencies and means. Frequencies are a count of the number of individuals who have had a particular result in each group, and are usually reported as percentages. Dichotomous data assume an all or nothing outcome frequency (e.g., the subjects stay at home or are placed in nursing homes; subjects find jobs or remain unemployed). In other cases results are measured as continuous data (e.g., grip strength or an ordinal scale such as the FIM scores of 0 to 7). Results in these studies are often reported as means and standard deviations.

The Number Needed to Treat (NNT) is one method for determining an effect size for dichotomous data, while statistics such as *d, r,* and *BESD* can be used to determine an effect size for continuous data.

In Table 42.1 one of the PICO questions was focused on work rehabilitation. A search of the literature found an article by Jousset et al. (2004) that had adequate article quality (see critically appraised paper [CAP] in Table 42.4). This study compared the effect of an intervention called functional restoration, which included daily occupational therapy as part of a comprehensive program, to a physical therapy intervention on reducing sick days and increasing fitness for clients with chronic low back pain. In the study, 84 patients were randomly assigned either to treatment (functional restoration for 6 hours a day for 5 weeks, *n* = 43) or control (3 hours a week of physical therapy for 5 weeks, *n* = 41). The investigators examined the effect of each type of intervention, functional restoration or physical therapy on several types of outcomes: some frequency data and some continuous measures. In the following sections, the magnitude of the differences between these two interventions on some of these outcomes will be examined using NNT, *d, r,* and *BESD*.

Calculating and Interpreting Number Needed to Treat (NNT)

Calculating NNT

Number Needed to Treat (NNT) compares the number of treatment group subjects (those receiving the intervention under study) who had a successful outcome to the number of people in the control group who had a successful outcome without that intervention. As illustrated on Table 42.5, to calculate NNT (Bandolier, 2003; Sackett et al., 2000) one must:

- Change the number of people who received the intervention and improved into a percentage by dividing this number by the number of people allocated to the treatment group at the beginning of the study. This is the Treatment Event Rate (TER).
- Change the number of people who did not receive the intervention and improved into a percentage by dividing this number by the number of people allocated to the control group at the beginning of the study. This is the Control Event Rate (CER).
- Take the absolute value of TER subtracted from CER. This is the Absolute Rate Reduction (ARR).
- Divide 1 by the ARR.
- Round the resulting number up to the next highest whole number. This is the Number Needed to Treat (NNT).

In the Jousset et al. (2004) article, the investigators evaluated several dichotomous outcomes including:

- The number of clients who subjectively rated their ability to work positively,
- The number of clients who subjectively rated that their physical condition was improved, and
- The number of clients who reported that they increased their participation in sports and leisure activities.

In all cases, the percentage of subjects in the treatment group who had positive outcomes was greater than the percentage of subjects in the control group who had positive outcomes. However, the treatment group was significantly better than the control group only for the number of clients who participated in more sports and leisure activities (see *p*-values in Table 42.5). To determine the magnitude of the clinical effect on these outcomes NNT must be calculated. Table 42.5 provides the calculations and the NNT for each of these outcomes.

Table 42.4 Critically Appraised Paper (CAP) Format for Jousset et al. (2004)

Clinical Bottom Line: Clients with low back pain show significant improvements in impairment and activity/ participation restrictions if they participate in any structured program (either functional rehabilitation or 3 times a week physical therapy). However, functional rehabilitation is more effective for impairment level outcomes (strength, endurance, and flexibility) and demonstrates a trend toward being more effective and having a larger effect size than 3 times a week physical therapy for most outcomes.

Finding the Article

Clinical population: Employed clients with chronic low back pain

Four-part question: (PICO)

In workers with low back pain of at least 3 months duration does work rehabilitation or functional rehabilitation lasting 5 days a week and at least 4 hours a day as compared to three times a week physical therapy cause a reduction in sick days and improve strength and endurance?

Study

Citation

Jousset, N., Fanello, S., Bontoux, L., Dubus, V., Billabert, C., Vielle, B., Roquelaure, Y., Penneau-Fontbonne, D., & Richard, I. (2004). Effects of functional restoration versus 3 hours per week physical therapy: A randomized controlled study. *Spine, 29*, 487–494.

Critical Appraisal

Threats to internal validity	Present (Yes/No)	Comments
Random allocation....?	Yes	
Concealed allocation...?	?	Not clear—person assigning subjects not specified.
Intention to treat analysis...?	?	Not specified; however, statistical *n* matches baseline *n*.
Long enough treatment/follow-up.?	Yes	5 weeks of treatment, 6 months follow-up.
Blinding...?	No	Researchers felt standardized testing and close communication reduced possibility of bias.
Groups equal at baseline...?	No	Significantly more workers in the treatment group had surgery, otherwise the groups were equal.
Attrition less than 20%...?	Yes	
Other threats?		

Evidence Level? II (based on Moore et al. (1995) hierarchy)

Subjects

Treatment group characteristics (*n* = 43): Age—41; Sex—male = 70%; on sick leave—47%; Previous surgery—35%; Previous depression—35%; Smokers—37%

Control group characteristics (*n* = 41): Age—39; Sex—male = 63%; on sick leave—51%; Previous surgery—15%; Previous depression—24%; Smokers—42%

Intervention/Method

Treatment group—Functional Restoration Program (FRP): Place: two different rehab centers. Duration: Six hours per day, for 5 weeks. Consisted of group treatment including warm-up/stretching, strengthening, aerobic activities, occupational therapy, endurance training, balneotherapy, individual interventions.

Control group—Active Individual Therapy (AIT): Place: Private physiotherapist practice. Duration: 1 hour per day, 3 times a week, for 5 weeks contact with therapist combined with a daily 50-minute home exercise program. First 2 weeks focused on flexibility, range of motion, and pain coping strategies. Strengthening and functional training were then added. Cardiopulmonary was achieved through sports activities.

(continued)

Table 42.4 **Critically Appraised Paper (CAP) Format for Jousset et al. (2004)** (continued)

Results: FRP group demonstrated significant, large improvements in participation in sports and leisure activities (NNT = 5), trunk strength (r = .24), and endurance (r = .29). There were no significant differences for any other outcome, although there was a trend for those in the FRP to show more improvement than the physical therapy group. A comparison of baseline and follow-up scores suggested that both interventions had significant effects on both impairments and activity/participation, but the FRP generally showed a larger effect. Selected r include: sick leave—FRP 0.50, AIT 0.41; flexibility—FRP 0.50, AIT 0.22; lifting—FRP 0.30, AIT 0.29; endurance—FRP 0.25, AIT 0.01; pain intensity—FRP 0.38, AIT 0.12; Activity/participation (Quebec scale)—FRP 0.37, AIT 0.25.

Additional Comments

This study was completed in France. The system for injured workers is different than for USA.

Date of Completion—September 26, 2004

Interpreting NNT

The NNT is the number of clients who would have to be treated with the intervention studied for benefit to occur in one additional client who otherwise would have had an unsuccessful outcome (Katz, 2001; Moore & McQuay, 2001; Sackett et al., 2000). The smaller a NNT the better the intervention works. In the case of the Jousset et al. (2004) article, the NNT can be interpreted in the following fashion:

- Thirteen clients would have to participate in functional restoration therapy in order for one additional client to report improved ability to work,
- Seventeen clients would have to participate in functional restoration therapy in order for one additional client to report improved physical condition, and

- Five clients would have to participate in functional restoration therapy in order for one additional client to participate in more sports and leisure activities.

Although the NNT for the first two outcomes, ability to work and physical conditioning, are included, the results of these outcomes are nonsignificant, suggesting that they might not apply to any subjects except those in the study itself. Calculating an effect size for a nonsignificant outcome has the benefit of identifying outcomes that may have a large effect (i.e., a small NNT), but had an insufficient number of subjects to obtain power. For those nonsignificant results that have a large effect, the practitioner may calculate the 95% confidence interval to better understand the range of possible effect sizes associated with that outcome

Table 42.5 **Calculation of NNT from Selected Outcomes from the Jousset et al. (2004)**

Outcome	Follow-up n		Event rate		ARR	NNT	p^*
	Control Group (baseline n = 41)	Treatment group (baseline n = 43)	Control (CER) $\frac{n_{follow-cont}}{n_{base-cont}}$	Treatment (TER) $\frac{n_{follow-tx}}{n_{base-tx}}$	$\lvert CER - TER \rvert = ARR$	$\frac{1}{ARR}$	
Improved ability to work	33	38	$\frac{33}{41}$=.805	$\frac{38}{43}$= .884	$\lvert .805-.884 \rvert$ =.079	$\frac{1}{.079}$ = 13	0.20
Improved physical condition	28	32	$\frac{28}{41}$=.683	$\frac{32}{43}$=.744	$\lvert .683-.744 \rvert$ =.061	$\frac{1}{.061}$ = 17	0.42
Sports and leisure activities	21	32	$\frac{21}{41}$=.512	$\frac{32}{43}$=.744	$\lvert .512-.744 \rvert$ =.232	$\frac{1}{.232}$ = 5	0.02

*Reported in the article.

How Precise Are the Effect Sizes Calculated from the Study—the 95% Confidence Interval?

In most research, the study effect size is considered to be an estimate of the magnitude of the effect of the intervention on the actual population. However, the study effect size actually represents an approximation of the population effect size. In many cases, the study effect size can vary greatly from the population effect size. The 95% confidence interval (95% CI) provides the range of population effect size values (Sackett et al., 2000; Sim & Reid, 1999), which can express the degree of uncertainty in relationship to that value representing the actual population effect size. This number is invaluable in providing the range of possible effect sizes and identifying the precision of the effect size that was obtained from the study.

To calculate a 95% CI around a NNT, first calculate the standard error for the ARR. (The table in this box provides the formula for the standard error of ARR). This is multiplied by 1.96, and the resulting number is both added and subtracted from the ARR calculated for the study. The resulting two numbers represent the range of possible NNT that might be obtained if this study was repeated again.

Calculation of the 95% Confidence Intervals (95% CI) Around NNT Calculated from Selected outcomes from Jousset et al. (2004)

Outcome	Event Rate		Standard Error (SE)			$\pm$ 95% CI ARR $\pm$ 1.96(SE)		NNT (95% CI)
	Control	Treatment				+95% CI	−95% CI	
	(CER)	(TER)	$SE_{NNT} =$	$\sqrt{\dfrac{TER(1-TER)}{n_t}}$	$+ \dfrac{CER(1-CER)}{n_C}$	ARR+	ARR−	
	(n = 41)	(n = 43)				1.96(SE)	1.96(SE)	
Improved ability to work	.81	.88	$.069 =$	$\sqrt{\dfrac{.90(1-.90)}{43}}$	$+ \dfrac{.88(1-.88)}{41}$	0.21	−0.06	11 (5 − ∞)
Improved physical condition	.68	.74	$.099 =$	$\sqrt{\dfrac{.74(1-.74)}{43}}$	$+ \dfrac{.68(1-.68)}{41}$	0.26	−0.13	17 (4 − ∞)
Sports and leisure activities	.51	.74	$.103 =$	$\sqrt{\dfrac{.74(1-.74)}{43}}$	$+ \dfrac{.51(1-.51)}{41}$	0.44	0.03	5 (3 − 34)

If the 95% CI of the ARR has a zero in the range, the overall result is considered to be nonsignificant. Thus, when the NNT is calculated from a negative ARR, the range of possible results is reported as being from the lower range of the 95% CI (calculated from the positive 95% CI) to infinity.

A 95% CI can also be calculated around an *r*. As an *r* has a skewed distribution, it must be translated to an *r* with a normal distribution, a Fisher *r*. A standard error (SE) is calculated from the Fisher *r* using the following formula $SE_r = \sqrt{\dfrac{1}{n_{tot} - 3}}$ where n equals the total *n* of the sample. As with the SE derived for the NNT, the SE derived for the *r* is multiplied by 1.96 and added to and subtracted from the Fisher *r*. The resulting numbers, as well as the original Fisher *r* are translated back into a regular *r*.

to help determine if the intervention may be useful to implement. In general, however, if a result is nonsignificant, the evidence-based practitioner will not calculate an effect size.

What constitutes a "low enough" NNT to justify using the intervention? Unfortunately, there is no absolute answer (Herbert, 2000). If an intervention improves the life of a client in a way that was not possible before, then an intervention with a "high" NNT may be of use. For example, consider an OT intervention that allowed 1 out of every 10 young adults with psychosis to stay in the community and out of a nursing home. If there was no alternative intervention, then this intervention would still be considered worth applying both because it addresses an important aim (i.e., preventing institutionalization) and it avoids the cost of a nursing home. However, if the intervention is one of many possible interventions to achieve this aim, then an NNT of 10 may be too high. To put the NNT in perspective, practitioners have to draw upon their clinical expertise and consider such issues as:

- Treatment alternatives,
- Resource availability for the intervention,
- Resource consequences of the intervention, and
- Their clients' values and needs.

Calculating and Interpreting Continuous Data Effect Sizes—d, r, BESD

The d statistic is essentially a standardized or z-score, or the difference between two scores in standard deviation units (Portney & Watkins, 2000). It is discussed in detail in Chapters 16 and 17. The d can be transformed into a r, which is a partial correlation coefficient that indicates the degree of association between receiving the intervention and having a successful outcome (Tickle-Degnen, 1998). An r of 1 indicates that everyone in the treatment group had a successful outcome while no one in the control group had a successful outcome. Conversely, an r of 0 indicates that there was absolutely no difference in successful outcomes between the treatment and control groups. In most studies, r lies somewhere between 0 and 1.

Both r and d can be interpreted in a clinically useful manner, however, Rosenthal and Rubin (1982) have created a method of translating r into a paired statistic called the Binomial Effect Size

Display (BESD), which appears to be most easily understood by both clinicians and clients. The BESD provides intervention success rates which compare the percentage of subjects who benefited with the intervention (treatment group) to the percentage of subjects who benefited without the intervention (the control group) (Tickle-Degnen, 1998). All three of these statistics are discussed below.

Calculating $\underline{d}$

To calculate an effect size d, subtract the mean of the control group (M_c) from the mean of the treatment group (M_T) (Rosenthal, 1994). This difference score is divided by the average of the standard deviations for the two groups (pooled standard deviation) (see Table 42.6 for d formula).

A d can be either a positive or a negative number. Whether a positive number indicates a higher success rate for the treatment or control group is dependent upon the direction of the outcome measure. For some outcome measures a higher score indicates a more positive outcome; for instance, strength and range-of-motion (ROM) are both such measures. On the other hand, for some outcome measures a smaller score indicates a more positive outcome. For example, in most pain measures a lower score usually indicates less pain; thus a lower score is better.

Since the control mean is subtracted from the treatment mean, a positive outcome indicates that the treatment group did better than the control group when a higher score indicates success. For an outcome where a lower score indicates suc-

Table 42.6 Mean, Standard Deviation, d Calculations, d, and p-Values for Selected Outcomes from Jousset et al. (2004)

	Treatment		Control		$\dfrac{M_T - M_c}{SD_{POOLED}}$		
	M	SD	M	SD		d	P**
No. of sick days*	28.7	44.6	48.3	66.0	$\dfrac{28.7 - 48.3}{55.3}$	−0.35	0.12
Lifting capacity (PILE)	35.1	12.6	33.7	12.7	$\dfrac{35.1 - 33.7}{12.7}$	0.11	0.65
Endurance (kJ)	92.7	49.3	66.3	36.7	$\dfrac{92.7 - 66.3}{43.0}$	0.61	0.01

*An outcome in which a lower score indicates a more successful outcome.
** = p-value reported in article.
PILE = Progressive isoinertial lifting evaluation.

Table 42.7 **Interpreting the Negative and Positive Signs Associated with** *d*

	The higher the score the more successful the outcome.	The lower the score the more successful the outcome.
d is positive.	Treatment did better on the outcome.	Control did better on the outcome.
d is negative.	Control did better on the outcome.	Treatment did better on the outcome.

cess a negative score indicates that the treatment did better than the control. Table 42.7 provides a brief summary of interpreting a positive or negative *d*.

Jousset et al. (2004) reported on several outcome measures that were interval scales, and the results were provided as means and standard deviations. Table 42.6 provides the measures, the means, standard deviations, and calculates the *d* for each outcome.

Interpreting *d*

The effect size *d* provides the size of the difference between the means in standard deviation units. An effect size *d* of 0.50 means the difference between the means is 1/2 standard deviation unit (Tickle-Degnen, 2001). An effect size *d* of 1 means that there is one standard deviation unit between the means. Cohen (1988) has provided an interpretative guideline for the *d* effect size that is shown in Table 42.8.

For the Jousset et al. (2004) (see Table 42.6), the functional restoration therapy in comparison to physical therapy had:

• A negligible effect on the subjects' lifting ability (PILE),
• A small effect on the number of sick days, and
• A moderate effect on the subjects' endurance.

In all cases the functional restoration group did better on each outcome than the physical therapy group. The results were significant only for the

Table 42.8 **Interpreting the Effect Sizes *d* and *r***

Interpretation	*d*	*r*
Negligible effect	0–0.19	0–0.09
Small effect	0.20–0.49	0.10–0.23
Moderate effect	0.50–0.79	0.24–0.37
Large effect	0.80–0.99	≥ 0.38
Very large effect	≥ 1.00	–

From Cohen (1988).

endurance outcome, suggesting that the magnitude of the difference for the other outcomes might be quite different if the study was repeated with other samples. It is also possible that the magnitude of effect would be different if compared to no treatment. The feature box titled "Comparing Baseline and Follow-up Results" discusses the changes in the magnitude of effect when comparing a new treatment to no treatment. A *d* can also be calculated from the difference between pretest and posttest scores. This method is described in the feature box titled "Calculating Effect Sizes from a Difference Score."

Calculating *r*

It can be useful to translate the effect size *d* to the effect size *r*. While the *d* examines the difference between the scores, the *r* looks at the association between a more positive outcome and participation in treatment (Tickle-Degnen, 2001). Table 42.9 provides the equation for calculating an *r* from a *d* (take the square root of *d* squared divided by *d* squared plus 4) and changes the *d's* calculated from the Jousset (2004) article into *r's* (Rosenthal, 1994).

Interpreting *r*

The effect size *r* is a partial correlation coefficient; it indicates the degree to which the independent measure (treatment vs. control) is associated with the outcome scores. Since it is a coefficient, *r* can range from -1 to +1. A negative *r* indicates that the control group was more successful than the treatment group. Since the *r* calculation always produces a positive *value*, the sign of an *r* must be assigned once the calculation is completed using the *d* as a guideline (i.e., if *d* indicated that the experimental group had a better outcome, then *r* should be assigned a positive value; if *d* indicated the control group had a better outcomes, then *r* should be assigned a negative value). The *r* can be interpreted something like a percent score (Tickle-Degnen, 1998). An *r* of .25, suggests that the treatment group was 25% more successful than the control.

Comparing Baseline and Follow-up Results from Jousset et al. (2004)

Although the effect sizes reported here appear to show that functional restoration intervention is not very effective, this is a misperception. Although the effect sizes for functional restoration appear low, it is because they were compared to another effective intervention, physical therapy. The table in this box provides an example of the effectiveness of both functional restoration and physical therapy in improving function for clients with chronic low back pain by calculating the effect sizes based on the differences between baseline and follow-up scores rather than the differences between the treatment and control group. The effect sizes are generally moderate to large (see table in this box). From these effect sizes, it appears that both physical therapy and functional restoration are effective interventions for some outcomes related to chronic low back pain, though functional restoration is more effective, particularly for endurance. What the example points out is that in interpreting an effect size, one must always take into consideration the nature of the control condition. When an experimental intervention is being compared to a control condition that has little or no benefit for subjects, it is easier to show a larger effect size. If the same intervention is compared to a control condition that also has a positive impact on the outcome variable(s), the effect size will appear smaller.

Effect Size r Comparing Functional Restoration Therapy and Physical Therapy Baseline and Follow-Up Scores for Selected Outcomes from Jousset et al. (2004)

		Baseline		Follow-up		
		M	SD	M	SD	r
No. of sick	Functional	101.3	79.1	28.7	44.6	0.50
days	Physical	109.8	70.4	48.3	66.0	0.41
Lifting capacity	Functional	27.5	13.3	35.5	12.5	0.30
(PILE)	Physical	27.5	11.6	35.0	13.0	0.29
Endurance	Functional	70.2	39.0	92.7	49.3	0.25
(kJ)	Physical	65.6	37.3	66.5	37.3	0.01

Calculating Effect Sizes from a Difference Score

Some articles do not provide mean scores, but difference scores. The difference score is most often the difference between the score at baseline and at follow-up. Difference scores can be treated like a mean to calculate the effect size d (see table in this box). Subtract the control difference score from the intervention difference score and divide by the pooled standard deviation of the difference score. This effect size is often more representative of the true effect because it controls for the differences between the intervention and control group at baseline.

A difference score can be created from information available in most articles. Simply subtract the baseline score from the follow-up score for both the treatment and control group. Divide this score by either the baseline or follow-up pooled standard deviation.

Calculating the Effect Size d from a Difference Score for Joussett et al. (2004)

	Treatment				Control				$\dfrac{M_T - M_c}{SD_{POOLED}}$	d
	M_{base}	M_{foll}	M_{diff}	SD_{base}	M_{base}	M_{foll}	M_{diff}	SD_{base}		
Lifting capacity (PILE)	27.5	35.1	7.6	13.3	27.5	33.7	6.2	11.6	$\dfrac{7.6-6.2}{12.5}$	0.11
Endurance (kJ)	70.2	92.7	22.5	39.0	67.2	66.3	−0.9	37.3	$\dfrac{22.5-(-.09)}{38.2}$	0.59

In the case of Jousset et al. (2004), the results of calculating an effect size from the difference score are no different than calculating an effect size from the follow-up score. This indicates that randomization worked well in this study to achieve experimental and control groups that were equivalent.

Table 42.9 **Transforming the Effect Size d to the Effect Size r for Selected Outcomes from Jousset et al. (2004)**

	d	$\sqrt{\dfrac{d^2}{d^2+4}}$	r	p^{**}
No. of sick days*	−0.35	$\sqrt{\dfrac{-.35^2}{-.35^2+4}}$	0.17	0.12
Lifting capacity (PILE)	0.11	$\sqrt{\dfrac{.11^2}{.11^2+4}}$	0.05	0.65
Endurance (kJ)	0.61	$\sqrt{\dfrac{.61^2}{.61^2+4}}$	0.29	0.01

*An outcome in which a lower score indicates a more successful outcome.
**p-value reported in article.
PILE = Progressive isoinertial lifting evaluation.

Like the d the r can also be classified as small, moderate, or large (Cohen, 1988) (see Table 42.8). For the Jousset et al. (2004) outcomes the functional rehabilitation intervention was:

- 17% more successful than physical therapy (a small effect) in decreasing the number of sick days,
- 5% more successful than physical therapy (a negligible effect) in increasing lifting capacity, and
- 29% more successful than physical therapy (a moderate effect) in increasing endurance.

If there is a negligible or small (although significant) effect, the case for implementing an intervention is weak since the client will do almost as well without the intervention. With a moderate or large significant effect, the intervention is probably worth implementing if the client or target population is similar to the treatment group and the outcome is relevant.

Calculating the Binomial Effect Size Display (BESD)

The BESD provides a result that is most readily understood by many clients and helps both client and therapist to decide if the intervention should be implemented (Tickle-Degnen, 1998). In the BESD, the r is used to develop success rates for both the treatment and control interventions, which can then be compared (See Table 42.10).

The treatment and control BESD can be compared when presenting the results. In considering the Jousset et al. (2004) article the following statements can be made:

- Number of sick days: 58.5% of clients improved with functional restoration while only 41.5% of the clients improved with physical therapy.
- Lifting capacity: 50.03% of clients improved with functional restoration while only 49.98% of the clients improved with physical therapy.

Table 42.10 **Calculating the BESD from r for Selected Outcomes from Jousset et al. (2004)**

Outcome	r	Treatment formula $50+\dfrac{(r\times100)}{2}$	Control formula $50-\dfrac{(r\times100)}{2}$	$\text{BESD}_{treatment}$	$\text{BESD}_{control}$
No. of sick days	0.17	$50+\dfrac{(.17\times100)}{2}$	$50-\dfrac{(.17\times100)}{2}$	58.5	41.5
Lifting capacity (PILE)	0.05	$50+\dfrac{(.05\times100)}{2}$	$50-\dfrac{(.05\times100)}{2}$	50.03	49.98
Endurance	0.29	$50+\dfrac{(.29\times100)}{2}$	$50-\dfrac{(.29\times100)}{2}$	64.5	35.5

PILE = Progressive isoinertial lifting evaluation.

- Endurance: 64.5% of clients improved with functional restoration while only 35.5% of the clients improved with physical therapy.

The BESD defines the relative effectiveness of both the treatment and control groups. The control group, whether it has no intervention or some standard intervention, will almost always show some improvement on most outcomes. The BESD allows the reader to make a determination of how successful both the treatment and control were, and determine if the success rate warrants using the intervention. Using the Jousset et al. (2004) research results to guide practice, a clinician might choose functional restoration for clients who are concerned about their endurance level, but would be less likely to implement the intervention for clients who are concerned about lifting ability. Since functional restoration is considerably more intensive (6 hours a day, 5 days a week compared to 3 hours a week total), the cost of the functional restoration therapy in time, manpower, and money is considerably larger than that for the three times a week physical therapy intervention. Therapists and clients must determine if the extra cost is warranted by the expected benefit to the client.

The effect size also provides an understanding of the overall strengths and weaknesses of the intervention. Compare the interpretability of these effect sizes with the means, standard deviations, and *p*-values provided in Table 42.6. Since the means are on different scales, it is impossible to compare and contrast the relative effectiveness of the intervention for different types of outcomes. Once effect sizes are calculated, the means are standardized, and it is possible to compare the results to each other and to other articles. The relative effectiveness of the intervention for improving each type of outcome becomes clear, whether the impairment involves attributes such as flexibility or endurance, or a function, such as lifting.

Putting It All Together: Building Evidence into Practice

Documenting the Evidence

Collecting and assessing evidence should be an ongoing part of effective practice (Law, 2002c;

Sackett, Haynes, Guyatt, & Tugwell, 1991; Sackett et al., 2000).

The evidence-based practitioner should work with other practitioners, both in their clinics and within their therapeutic communities, to access and assess relevant articles. The evidence developed in this process should be saved in a clinically useful manner so that it can be used to guide practice. One method is to summarize the information about the article in a critically appraised paper (CAP), also referred to as a critically appraised topic (CAT) (Suave et al., 1995). The following are standard elements of a CAP that should be used when documenting the results of the process of finding, selecting, and appraising the evidence (Law, 2002b):

- The date of completion: Evidence related to intervention can change rapidly. The date that review was completed helps determine if the information is still relevant.
- The clinical question: The PICO or background question that was originally used to find the article helps structure why the literature was accessed and how it was used.
- The clinical bottom line: The meat of the review, what the evidence suggests concerning the question of interest. The clinical bottom line summarizes the results of the critical appraisal, reports pertinent outcomes (e.g., effect sizes), and reports possible clinical applications of the evidence.
- The article citation: A citation of the article(s) used to develop the CAP. When possible a copy of the original article should be kept with the CAP.
- Comments: This section provides information on important aspects of the evidence that might otherwise not fit in else where.

Table 42.4 is an example of a CAP prepared for the Jousset et al. (2004) article and provides the basic format of a CAP.

Applying the Evidence

The final step in evidence-based practice is applying the evidence. There are numerous ways that critically appraised evidence can be used in practice. Evidence can be used to:

- Develop practice guidelines (Sackett et al., 2000; Tickle-Degnen, 2002),

> Collecting and assessing evidence should be an ongoing part of effective practice.

• Develop economic analyses of different intervention options (Tickle-Degnen, 2002),
• Evaluate clinical performance (Sackett et al., 1991),
• Inform consumers of the effectiveness of an intervention, and
• Shape clinicians' choices of the most appropriate intervention.

Evidence-based practice is not a cookie-cutter guide to intervention (Sackett & Richardson, 1996). Current available best evidence must be used judiciously by skilled practitioners in combination with their knowledge of treatment principles and their overall therapeutic skills. Part of this skill is matching potential evidence-based interventions with the needs and values of their clients. The ability to understand the needs of clients and present evidence so clients can make informed decisions about their treatment is an important part of evidence-based practice. In addition, practitioners should remember that there are "consumers" other than clients who are interested in the evidence about an intervention. For example, funders and managers will also be concerned about intervention options and choices (Tickle-Degnen, 2002). Practitioners can use evidence to justify their choices to these groups as well. Clinicians should be able to present the results to all three groups, using different language and focus for each. Tickle-Degnen (2002) suggests that when communicating the results of evidence, practitioners should:

• Use simple, concrete, nontechnical, culturally neutral language,
• Keep the information brief,
• Check frequently for confusion or lack of comprehension, and
• Suggest concrete actions related to the information (p. 229).

For example, a client has had several acute episodes of low back pain that he states has led to decreased participation in work, play, and home activities. After assessment it is clear that the client has low flexibility, endurance, and reports high levels of pain. He has had several courses of physical therapy, but continues to have problems. The client states that he would like to miss less work, improve his ability to play with his children, and improve his overall fitness level. The practitioner working with the client believes that a course of intensive work related occupational therapy will benefit the client, and provides him with the following information to help him make his decision.

Mr. X, you have had chronic low back pain for 1 year now. Your physical therapy has helped some, but you continue to have trouble with home activities, and you feel that you overall fitness level is low. I would like to suggest a course of therapy in which you attend daily therapy lasting 6 hours a day. The therapy is designed to improve your flexibility, endurance, strength, and work ability. A recent study reported that this type of therapy was superior to a three times a week physical therapy program in decreasing sick days, improving flexibility, endurance, and assisting people to getting back to leisure and sports activities. For example, there was a 17% greater decrease in sick days for those people who received this type of therapy, a 29% increase in endurance, and a 17% decrease in pain. In addition, one in five clients in this type of intervention report improved ability to participate in sports and leisure activities.

This type of statement provides the client with information that will help him to make an informed decision as to whether the additional time and effort required to attend the more intensive program is worth it.

Conclusion

This chapter provides an overview of some basic methods of applying evidence-based practice to treatment interventions. Using information from this chapter should help practitioners to use the literature to identify, assess, and implement treatment evidence in their own practice. Importantly, this chapter has not addressed how to use evidence to evaluate the literature relating to diagnosis, prognosis, or economic factors which are other topics of evidence-based practice that can be incorporated into treatment. There are several excellent texts that cover these important topics (Ajetunmobi, 2002; Law, 2002c; Sackett et al., 1991, 2000) and the reader is urged to explore the topic of evidence-based practice more fully through these texts and other resources. Moreover, this chapter did not address how to use evidence from research other than studies that involve a control and intervention group. While controlled studies represent some of the most valuable sources of information for evidence-based practice, many other forms of research are also valuable. These include:

- Psychometric studies that provide information about the dependability and utility of assessments,
- Qualitative studies that examine client experiences in intervention,
- Needs assessment studies that point toward unmet needs and/or desirable service outcomes, and
- Participatory studies that involve consumers and/or practitioners in identifying needs and in developing and/or evaluating services to meet those needs.

These and other approaches to research that provide evidence useful to practice are discussed throughout this text.

REFERENCES

Ajetunmobi, O. (2002). Making sense of critical appraisal. London: Arnold.

Altman, D. G., & Schulz, K. F. (2001). Concealing treatment allocation in randomised trials. *British Medical Journal, 323,* 446–447.

American Occupational Therapy Association (2000). Occupational therapy code of ethics. *American Journal of Occupational Therapy, 54,* 614–616.

Bandolier (2003). Calculating and using NNTs. Retrieved May 26, 2004, from the World Wide Web: http://www.ebandolier.com

Berg, K. E., & Latin, R. W. (1994). *Essentials of research methods in health, physical education, exercise science, and recreation* (2nd ed.). Philadelphia: Lippincott Williams & Wilkins.

Cohen, J. (1988). *Statistical power analysis for the behavioral sciences* (2nd ed.). Hillsdale, NJ: Lawrence Erlbaum.

Cook, T. D., & Campbell, D. T. (1979). *Quasi-experimentation: Design & analysis issues for field settings.* Boston: Houghton Mifflin.

Dubouloz, C. J., Egan, M., Vallerand, J., & vonZweck, C. (1999). Occupational therapists' perception of evidence-based practice. *American Journal of Occupational Therapy, 53,* 445–453.

GRADE Working Group. (2004). Grading quality of evidence and strength of recommendation. *British Medical Journal.* Retrieved September 26, 2004, from http://www.bmj.com

Herbert, R. D. (2000). How to estimate treatment effects from reports of clinical trials. II. Dichotomous outcomes. *Australian Journal of Physiotherapy, 46,* 309–313.

Hollis, S., & Campbell, F. (1999). What is meant by intention to treat analysis? Survey of published randomised controlled trials. *British Medical Journal, 319,* 670–674.

Hulley, S. B., Cummings, S. R., Browner, W. S., Grady, D., Hearst, N., & Newman, T. B. (2001). *Designing clinical research* (2nd ed.). Philadelphia: Lippincott, Williams & Wilkins.

Jousset, N., Fanello, S., Bontoux, L., Dubus, V., Billabert, C., Vielle, B., Roquelaure, Y., Penneau-Fontbonne, D., & Richard, I. (2004). Effects of functional restoration versus 3 hours per week physical therapy: A randomized controlled study. *Spine, 29,* 487–494.

Katz, D. L. (2001). *Clinical epidemiology & evidence-based medicine.* Thousand Oaks, CA: SAGE Publications.

Law, M. (2002a). Appendix C: Critical review form for quantitative studies. In M. Law (Ed.), *Evidence-based rehabilitation* (pp. 305–308). Thorofare, NJ: Slack.

Law, M. (2002b). Building evidence in practice. In M. Law (Ed.), *Evidence-based rehabilitation* (pp. 185–220). Thorofare, NJ: Slack.

Law, M. (2002c). *Evidence-based rehabilitation: A guide to practice.* Thorofare: NJ: Slack.

Moher, D., Pham, B., Jones, A., Cook, D. J., Jadad, A. R., Moher, M., Tugwell, P., & Klassen, T. P. (1998). Does quality of reports of randomised trials affect estimates of intervention efficacy reported in meta-analysis? *The Lancet, 352,* 609–613.

Moore, A., & McQuay, H. J. (2001). *What is an NNT?* Hayward Medical Group. Retrieved, 2004, from the World Wide Web: http://www.evidence-based-medicine.co.uk

Moore, A., McQuay, H., & Gray, J. A. M. (1995). Evidence-based everything. *Bandolier, 1* (12), 1.

Newman, T. B., Browner, W. S., & Hulley, S. B. (2001). Enhancing causal inferences in observational studies. In S. B. Hulley, S. R. Cummings, W. S. Browner, D. Grady, N. Hearst, & T. B. Newman (Eds.), *Designing clinical research* (2nd ed., pp. 125–142). Philadephia, PA: Lippincott, Williams, & Wilkins.

Portney, L. G., & Watkins, M. P. (2000). *Foundations of clinical research: Applications to practice* (2nd ed.). Upper Saddle River, NJ: Prentice-Hall Health.

Richardson, W. S., Wilson, M. C., Nishikawa, J., & Hayward, R. S. (1995). The well-built clinical question: A key to evidence-based decisions. *ACP Journal Club, 123,* A-12.

Rosenthal, R. (1994). Parametric measures of effect size. In H. Cooper & L. V. Hedges (Eds.), *The handbook of research synthesis* (pp. 231–260). New York: Russell Sage Foundation.

Rosenthal, R., & Rosnow, R. L. (1991). *Essentials of behavioral research: Methods and data analysis* (2nd ed.). New York: McGraw-Hill.

Rosenthal, R., & Rubin, D. B. (1982). A simple general purpose display of magnitude of experimental effect. *Journal of Educational Psychology, 74,* 166–169.

Sackett, D. L., Haynes, R. B., Guyatt, G. H., & Tugwell, P. (1991). *Clinical epidemiology* (2nd ed.). Boston: Little, Brown and Company.

Sackett, D. L., & Richardson, W. S. (1996). Evidence-based medicine: What its and what it isn't. *British Medical Journal, 312,* 71–72.

Sackett, D. L., Straus, S. E., Richardson, W. S., Rosenberg, W., & Haynes, R. B. (2000). *Evidence-based medicine* (2nd ed.). New York: Churchill Livingstone.

Schulz, K. F., & Grimes, D. A. (2002). Blinding in randomised trials: Hiding who got what. *The Lancet, 359,* 696–700.

Sim, J., & Reid, N. (1999). Statistical inference by confidence intervals: Issues of interpretation and utilization. *Physical Therapy, 79,* 186–195.

Straus, S. E., & McAlister, F. A. (2000). Evidence-based medicine: A commentary on common criticisms. *Canadian Medical Association Journal, 163,* 837–841.

Suave, S., Lee, H. N., Meade, M. O., Lang, J. B., Faroukh, M., Cook, D. J., et al. (1995). The critically appraised topic: A practical approach to learning critical appraisal. *Annals of the Royal College of Physicians and Surgeons of Canada, 28*, 396–398.

Tickle-Degnen, L. (1998). Communicating with clients about treatment outcomes: The use of meta-analytic evidence in collaborative treatment planning. *The American Journal of Occupational Therapy, 52*, 526–530.

Tickle-Degnen, L. (2001). From the general to the specific: Using meta-analytic reports in clinical decision making. *Evaluation and the Health Professions, 24*, 308–326.

Tickle-Degnen, L. (2002). Communicating evidence to clients, managers, and funders. In M. Law (Ed.), *Evidence-based rehabilitation* (pp. 221–254). Thorofare, NJ: Slack.

RESOURCES

General Evidence-Based Practice Resources

Agency for Healthcare Research and Quality (AHRQ) (http://www.ahcpr.gov/)—part of the Department of Health and Human Services, this site provides information about evidence-based treatment as well as clinical guidelines for healthcare professionals.

Ajetunmobi, O. (2002). *Making sense of critical appraisal.* London: Arnold.

Bandolier (http://www.jr2.ox.ac.uk/bandolier/)— Independent journal about evidence-based health care.

British Medical Journal (BMJ)—(http://www.bmj.com/)

Centre for Evidence-Based Medicine (http://www.cebm. net/)—Describes methods of finding, evaluating and using evidence.

Cochrane Collaboration (http://www.cochrane.org/ index0.htm)—A subscription-based organization that produces and disseminates systematic reviews of healthcare interventions.

OTseeker (www.otseeker.com)—An occupational therapy systematic evaluation of evidence.

PEDro (http://www.pedro.fhs.usyd.edu.au/index.html) — The Physiotherapy Evidence Database—a physical therapy systematic evaluation of the evidence.

Sackett, D. L., Straus, S. E., Richardson, W. S., Rosenberg, W., & Haynes, R. B. (2000). *Evidence-based medicine* (2nd ed.). New York: Churchill Livingstone.

Sackett, D. L., Haynes, R. B., Guyatt, G. H., & Tugwell, P. (1991). *Clinical epidemiology* (2nd ed.). Boston: Little, Brown and Company.

Search Methods

Coster, W., & Vergara, E. (2004). Finding the resources to support EBP. *OT Practice*, March 8, 2004, 10–15.

Katz, D. L. (2001). Appendix A. In *Clinical epidemiology & evidence-based medicine*. Thousand Oaks, CA: SAGE Publications.

Lou, J. (2002). Searching for the evidence. In M. Law (ed.) *Evidence-based rehabilitation* (pp. 71–96). Thorofare, NJ: Slack.

Oxford Centre for Evidence-based Medicine (2001). Searching for the best evidence in clinical journals. Retrieved January 10, 2002, from the World Wide Web: http://www.cebm.net/searching.asp

White, H. D. (1994). Scientific communication and literature retrieval. In H. Cooper & L. V. Hedges (Eds.), *The handbook of research synthesis* (pp. 41–56). New York: Russell Sage Foundation.

Hierarchies of Research Design

Baker, N. A., & Tickle-Degnen, L. (2001). The effectiveness of physical, psychological, and functional interventions in treating clients with multiple sclerosis: A meta-analysis. *American Journal of Occupational Therapy, 55*, 324–331.

Centre for Evidence-Based Medicine (2001). *Levels of evidence and grades of recommendation.* Retrieved January 10, 2002, from the World Wide Web: http://www.cebm.net/levels_of_ evidence.asp

GRADE Working Group. (2004). Grading quality of evidence and strength or recommendation. British Medical Journal, 328, 1–8. Retrieved September 26, 2004 from the World Wide Web: http://www. bmj.com

Critically Appraising the Evidence

Hill, A., & Spittlehouse, C. (2001). What is critical appraisal? Hayward Medical Group. Retrieved, 2004, from the World Wide Web: http://www.evidence-based-medicine.co.uk

Khan, K. S., ter Riet, G., Popay, J., Nixon, J., & Kleijnen, J. (2001). *Study quality assessment.* Retrieved February 6, 2004, from the World Wide Web: http://www.york.ac.uk/inst/crd/pdf/crd4_ph5.pdf

Law, M. (2002). Appendix C: Critical review form for quantitative studies. *Evidence-based rehabilitation: A guide to practice* (pp. 305–308). Thorofare, NJ: Slack.

Maher, C. G., Sherrington, C., Herbert, R. D., Moseley, A. M., & Elkins, M. (2003). Reliability of the PEDro Scale for rating quality of randomized controlled trials. *Physical Therapy, 83*, 713–721.

Verhagen A. P., de Vet H. C., de Bie R. A., Kessels A. G., Boers M., Bouter L. M., & Knipschild P. G. (1998). The Delphi list: a criteria list for quality assessment of randomized clinical trials for conducting systematic reviews developed by Delphi consensus. *Journal of Clinical Epidemiology*, 51, 1235–1241.

Calculating Effect Sizes

Bandolier. (2003). Calculating and using NNTs. Retrieved, May 26, 2004, from the World Wide Web: www. ebandolier.com

Guyatt G. H., Sackett D. L., & Cook D. J. (1993). User's guide to the medical literature: II. How to use an article about therapy or prevention: B. What were the results and will they help me in caring for my patients? *Journal of the American Medical Association, 271*, 59–63.

Herbert, R. D. (2000a). How to estimate treatment effects from reports of clinical trials. I: Continuous outcomes. *Australian Journal of Physiotherapy, 46*, 229–235.

Herbert, R. D. (2000b). How to estimate treatment effects from reports of clinical trials. II Dichotomous outcomes. *Australian Journal of Physiotherapy, 46*, 309–313.

Rosenthal, R. (1994). Parametric measures of effect size. In H. Cooper & L. V. Hedges (Eds.), *The handbook of research synthesis* (pp. 231–260). New York: Russell Sage Foundation.

Disseminating the Evidence

Centre for Evidence-Based Medicine (n.d.). The CATbank. Retrieved September 26, 2004 from the World Wide Web: http://www.cebm.net/cats.asp

Holm, M. B. (2001). Our mandate for the new millennium: Evidence-based practice. *OT Practice, July 2001*, CE-1-CE-14.

Tickle-Degnen, L. (1998). Communicating with clients about treatment outcomes: The use of meta-analytic evidence in collaborative treatment planning. *The American Journal of Occupational Therapy, 52*, 526–530.

Tickle-Degnen, L. (2001). From the general to the specific: Using meta-analytic reports in clinical decision making. *Evaluation and the Health Professions, 24*, 308–326.

Tickle-Degnen, L. (2002). Communicating evidence to clients, managers, and funders. In M. Law (Ed.), *Evidence-based rehabilitation: A guide to practice* (pp. 221–254). Thorofare, NJ: Slack.

CHAPTER 43

Managing Change and Barriers to Evidence-Based Practice

Annie McCluskey

Previous chapters in this section have described the rationale for, and the process of, evidence-based practice. This chapter examines how occupational therapists manage change and barriers to evidence-based practice. Although the profession produces good research, findings are not always used in practice to improve client outcomes. Furthermore, therapists often have difficulty discriminating between "good" research, and research that is of poor methodological quality. Although the process of change can be slow, individuals and organizations need to overcome the research–practice gap, and make the change to evidence-based practice.

First, the nature of change and typical responses to change are described in relation to evidence-based practice. Next, common barriers to using research are examined. Finally, findings from a study are used to illustrate how occupational therapists managed these barriers, what factors helped, and how these therapists started to engage more in the process of evidence-based practice over an 18-month period.

The Change from "Experience-Based" to "Evidence-Based" Practice

Until the mid-1990s, it was reasonable for practice to be based primarily on experience, hence the term "experience-based" practice (Redmond, 1997). When guidelines for clinical reasoning and standards for the education of practitioners were developed, research was not typically the primary source of information. Research references were an optional "extra" in such standards and guidelines.

Today, health professionals are encouraged to use research evidence explicitly when making clinical decisions. Research is also supposed to guide those who educate future practitioners. Furthermore, professionals are expected to appraise and classify studies according to method-ological quality (Sackett, Straus, Richardson, Rosenberg, & Haynes, 2000; Straus, Richardson, Glasziou, & Haynes, 2005; Taylor, 2000). Nonetheless, research evidence is not intended to be used in isolation. Rather, it is combined with clinical experience, clinical reasoning, knowledge from formal education, and information about client needs and values (Pollock & Rochon, 2002). Healthy debate continues about the limited relevance of randomized controlled trials for practice. However, on the whole, professions such as occupational therapy now accept the need to base their practice and teaching on sound research, much more so than they did in the past.

This change from experience-based practice to evidence-based practice (and teaching) requires a substantial change in skills, knowledge, attitudes and behavior. Not surprisingly, practitioners and academics often respond with anxiety to these expectations (Dubouloz, Egan, Vallerand, & von Zweck, 1999), and the degree of change required. Therefore, it can be helpful to understand how different individuals respond to change, and the stages a person moves through during this journey. Individual professionals and managers who are better informed about change can plan ahead, and be proactive instead of reactive (McCluskey & Cusick, 2002).

Different Responses to Change

As with the general population, therapists respond differently to change. Different responses to change will affect the way in which a profession deals with innovation, including the new emphasis on evidence-based practice. Rogers (1983) identifies five categories of individuals, according to how each person responds to innovative ideas:

- Innovators,
- Early adopters,
- The early majority,
- The late majority, and
- Laggards.

Innovators are ahead of the majority and make up the smallest group. They may be isolated and distrusted, perhaps even envied by colleagues, because of their uptake of a new idea such as evidence-based practice. Early adopters are the respected opinion leaders in a group who typically express interest in a new idea ahead of others. This group of opinion leaders may be useful for "marketing" evidence-based practice to others in the workplace or profession (Effective Health Care, 1999; McCluskey & Cusick, 2002).

The early majority refers to people who hold traditional views but will begin to shift their opinions and practice when change becomes inevitable. The early majority can help encourage change in the late majority, or the skeptics within an organization. Typically, the late majority are reluctant to accept new ideas and practices. Finally, the laggards accept change only when this is forced upon them, and may resist even then.

Readiness for Change

In addition to different responses to change, there are also stages that characterize people confronted with change. The staged model of change (Prochaska & DiClemente, 1982; 1983; Prochaska, DiClemente, & Norcross, 1992) is often used to help individuals identify their readiness for change. This model describes five stages:

• Precontemplation,
• Contemplation,
• Preparation,
• Action, and
• Maintenance.

Precontemplation is when an individual has no desire or intention to change, and where there is little reflection on practice. There may be a lack of awareness about the need for change. Some occupational therapists have difficulty moving beyond this stage. They tend to feel anxious or threatened by new developments such as evidence-based practice (Dubouloz et al., 1999). New ways of thinking and working are required. Routines and habits are disturbed by change. Fortunately, many practitioners are interested in acquiring new skills and knowledge, and move on to the stage of contemplation.

> When introducing evidence-based practice, present information about responses to change and the staged model of change. Encourage therapists to reflect on their own response to evidence-based practice, and which stage of change they have reached.

Contemplation is when individuals begin to think about changing their practice. For example, a colleague's enthusiasm about a workshop may lead an occupational therapist to think about change. Evidence-based practice will require significant effort such as regular visits to the library, the acquisition of new skills such as learning to use electronic databases, and a commitment to continuing professional development. At this stage of change, therapists within an organization may find it helpful to identify the pros and cons of evidence-based practice.

The stage of preparation follows, during which individuals start to learn new skills and knowledge in order to support the proposed change. For example, therapists will need search and appraisal skills. They will also need to identify strategies for implementing research findings. Therapists at this stage might, for example, show an interest in organizing or attending an in-service on critical appraisal of research articles.

The stage of action is when a person begins to implement new ideas. Therapists who proceed to this stage will implement research findings by beginning to change their work practices. This stage usually requires significant behavior change. For instance, adoption of evidence-based practice can require discontinuation of treatments that have been accepted practice for decades, and exchanging these for new treatment techniques.

Maintenance is the final stage wherein a permanent change in behavior occurs. Maintenance activities relevant to evidence-based practice might include regular searches of electronic databases such as OTseeker (http://www.otseeker.com). Activities might also include participation in a monthly journal club (Dingle & Hooper, 2000; Phillips & Glasziou, 2004; Taylor, 2000).

The two final stages, action and maintenance, present the biggest challenge to therapists who are trying to be "evidence-based," because it is easy to slip back into old habits. Given typical workloads, most therapists will need encouragement to spend time searching, reading, and appraising research. Working in pairs or small groups or with a mentor may help to maintain motivation (Conroy, 1997). Presenting the findings of a search to other staff members may also act as an incentive.

One of the most important aspects of being an evidence-based practitioner is anticipating and planning for new challenges. For example, in a recent research project (McCluskey, 2004; McCluskey & Lovarini, 2005), occupational therapists were recruited with the primary aim of increasing their skills and knowledge for evidence-

> Most occupational therapists will need support and encouragement to spend time searching, reading, and appraising research. To help maintain motivation, work in pairs or small groups, or with a mentor. Presenting findings to other staff can help to consolidate skills and provides an opportunity for feedback.

based practice. They were asked to identify their stage of readiness for change and to discuss their attitudes to evidence-based practice. Next, they found a "buddy" or peer to work with, in order to promote action and maintenance. They also learned about common barriers to implementing evidence-based practice, and developed a plan of action to address their personal barriers. By explicitly thinking about the change process, they planned ahead, anticipated problems, and put strategies in place to manage these barriers.

Barriers to Evidence-Based Practice

The two primary barriers or reasons reported by health professionals for not using research in practice are a perceived lack of time for reading and interpreting research (Closs & Lewin, 1998) and lack of skills and knowledge when searching for and appraising research literature (Dubouloz et al.,

1999). Therapists typically report that they do not know how to identify a "good" study from a poorly conducted one, nor do they know how to interpret statistics in the results section of a paper (Metcalfe et al., 2001; Pollock, Legg, Langhorne, & Sellars, 2000). Results of two surveys focusing on these barriers are presented in Tables 43.1 and 43.2. These surveys were conducted between 2000 and 2003 with occupational therapists in Australia (McCluskey, 2003, 2004).

Survey 1, 2000

The first survey was conducted with a convenience sample of occupational therapists. All had attended a half-day workshop on evidence-based practice at an occupational therapy conference in Sydney, Australia. They completed the survey before participating in the workshop. Of the 85 therapists in attendance, 64 provided complete data on perceived barriers. In terms of readiness for change, they were mostly in the preparation stage. They were the early majority. Table 43.1 lists the top 10 barriers they identified. Most respondents identified lack of time and a large workload or caseload as the major barriers to adopting EBP, followed by limited searching skills and limited critical appraisal skills.

Survey 2, 2002

The second survey was conducted 2 years later, with a different group of Australian occupational

Table 43.1 Perceived Barriers to Adopting Evidence-Based Practice as Reported by Australian Occupational Therapists in May 2000 ($n = 64$)

Top 10 Barriers Reported	n	%
Lack of time	56	(87.5)
Large caseload	43	(67.2)
Limited searching skills	32	(50.0)
Limited critical appraisal skills	28	(43.7)
Difficulty accessing journals	28	(43.7)
Lack of evidence to support what occupational therapists do	26	(40.6)
Professional isolation	22	(34.4)
Limited resources and funding to support change to EBP	20	(31.2)
Difficulty accessing computer	18	(28.1)
The large volume of published research	16	(25.0)

Note: Participants were asked to choose as many barriers as they wished from the list; therefore the numbers do not add up to 100%.

Adapted from McCluskey, A. (2003). Occupational therapists report a low level of knowledge, skill and involvement in evidence-based practice. *Australian Occupational Therapy Journal, 50*(8) [Table 3]. With permission.

Table 43.2 Perceived Barriers to Adopting Evidence-Based Practice as Reported by Australian Occupational Therapists in 2002 (n = 114)

Top 10 Barriers Reported	Pre-workshop Jan 2002 n = 114	Post-workshop Feb 2002 n = 106	Follow-up October 2002 n = 51
	n (%)	n (%)	n (%)
Lack of time	86 (75%)	100 (94%)	45 (88%)
Large workload/caseload	76 (67%)	79 (75%)	31 (61%)
Limited searching skills	69 (61%)	56 (53%)	12 (24%)
Limited critical appraisal skills	68 (60%)	69 (65%)	21 (41%)
Difficulty accessing journals	51 (45%)	45 (43%)	18 (35%)
The large volume of published research	33 (29%)	34 (32%)	7 (14%)
Lack of evidence to support what occupational therapists do	31 (27%)	34 (32%)	18 (35%)
Professional isolation	24 (21%)	28 (26%)	7 (14%)
Limited resources and funding to support change to EBP	23 (20%)	13 (12%)	4 (8%)
Difficulty accessing a computer	19 (17%)	15 (14%)	6 (12%)

Note: Participants were asked to choose as many barriers as they wished from the list, therefore the numbers do not add up to 100%.

Adapted from McCluskey, A. (2004). *Increasing the use of research evidence by occupational therapists* [Final report]. Penrith South, Australia: School of Exercise and Health Sciences, University of Western Sydney, Table 4.1, p. 15. Full copy available in PDF format from http://www.otcats.com [under 'Project Summary']. With permission.

therapists. The sample was specially recruited for their interest in EBP and willingness to attend a 2-day workshop and to complete a critically appraised topic (CAT) as an assignment. Therefore, they were a self-selected and motivated group. Most were in the preparation or action stages of the change process. Once again, before attending the workshop most of this sample identified key barriers as (See Table 43.2, left column): lack of time, a large caseload, limited searching skills, and limited critical appraisal skills.

Immediately after the 2-day workshop, these therapists were surveyed again (see Table 43.2, middle column). More listed lack of time as a barrier than pre-workshop. By that time, therapists were more aware of the work involved in being an evidence-based practitioner, particularly the work required to complete a critically appraised topic. Similarly, more respondents identified limited critical appraisal skills as a barrier than preworkshop. While therapists had learned about and practiced critical appraisal during the workshop, they had become even more aware of skills they still had to learn. For example, they would need to learn about different research designs and statistical analyses,

to make sense of research articles. Searching skills were seen as less of a barrier than before the workshop, with respondents feeling more confident about searching databases on their own.

Table 43.2 (right column) also indicates that over time and with practice, a greater percentage of therapists improved their skills. Ten months later, fewer therapists felt their searching and appraisal skills were a barrier to being an evidence-based practitioner. Interestingly, the majority still identified lack of time as the primary barrier. Nonetheless, many of these therapists had completed a critically appraised topic and developed their skills. As discussed later in this chapter, it was the way in which these therapists managed and reprioritized their time that was critical to adopting evidence-based practice.

In summary, the barriers to adopting evidence-based practice are remarkably consistent across groups of occupational therapists, across professions (Humphris, Littlejohns, Victor, O'Halloran, & Peacock, 2000; Metcalfe et al., 2001) and countries. Lack of time, a large workload, and limited search and appraisal skills are perceived to be the main problems. Yet little has been done to date to address these barriers or problems. Furthermore, some barriers, such as a perceived lack of time, are unlikely to disappear. Therapists are unlikely to be given, or to find, more time in their day. Instead, they need to reprioritize their time.

Managing Barriers to Evidence-Based Practice

As already noted, some of the occupational therapists in the Australian study successfully managed the barriers and began to adopt evidence-based practice. During the 8 months post-workshop, their use of research evidence was monitored. For example, they were asked how often they conducted a search or engaged in appraisal. Further, their level of knowledge about evidence-based practice and their skills were measured objectively. These data were used to select a purposive sample. After 18 months, 10 of the most proactive, knowledgeable, and skilled therapists were interviewed to ascertain what factors accounted for their success (McCluskey, 2004).

Strategies for Adopting Evidence-Based Practice

The occupational therapists interviewed were more successful than others at managing the primary barriers, lack of time and lack of skills. Three main strategies, presented in Table 43.3, were used to overcome barriers and adopt evidence-based practice:

• Finding time for evidence-based practice,
• Developing skills and knowledge, and
• Staying focused.

First, participants proactively made time by prioritizing use of research ahead of other tasks for part of their week, and by planning ahead. Second, they proactively developed their skills and knowledge upon return to work, by teaching others what they had learned, and getting help when this was needed. Third, they stayed focused and committed to evidence-based practice, and found ways to maintain their motivation.

These therapists reported, and quantitative data confirmed, that new skills and knowledge were acquired relatively quickly as a result of attending the workshop. However, finding time to further develop their skills, and changisng policy and practice in line with new research was much more difficult. Implementation took longer—more than 12 months—and not all of the

Table 43.3 Strategies for Adopting Evidence-Based Practice

Strategies	Subcategories
Finding time for evidence-based practice	• Prioritizing activities • Planning ahead
Developing skills and knowledge	• Using evidence • Teaching EBP to others • Seeking help
Staying focused	• Making a commitment • Being persistent • Being motivated

Adapted from McCluskey, A. (2004). *Increasing the use of research evidence by occupational therapists* [Final report]. Penrith South, Australia: School of Exercise and Health Sciences, University of Western Sydney. Table 5.2, page 33. Full copy available in PDF format from http://www.otcats.com [under 'Project Summary']. With permission.

therapists interviewed had yet reached this stage. Their strategies for success are now described in more detail.

Finding Time for Evidence-Based Practice

The first strategy involved prioritizing activities and planning ahead. Time was the major barrier to engaging in evidence-based practice for all participants, as indicated by one of the therapists:

I'm sure everyone finds time a big issue. It is very difficult. Clinically, with just seeing the clients here, it's very busy. And then there are always loads of additional projects that we're working on, meetings and supervision. So, definitely it is very difficult to find the time.

To find time, successful therapists had to make research utilization a priority. They set time aside, both at work and after hours, for these activities. Less successful therapists complained about lack of time and did not prioritize work and personal time for evidence-based practice. Some were not persistent in maintaining their commitment, partly because they and their organization did not place a high value on activities such as searching, reading, and appraisal. For instance, one therapist observed:

Here, if it doesn't get...a little old lady out the door and back home, well then [it is not considered important].

Searching, reading, and critical appraisal were not always considered an essential part of the occupational therapist's work in some organizations. When these activities were less valued than clinical "hands-on" work, therapists felt guilty engaging in them at work, as one therapist noted:

I found that every month I either had to book over that time for clinical appointments to meet the caseload demands...so that was interesting in itself, my own attitude ...rather then protecting that time and doing evidence-based work, I kept putting it off.

In some cases, therapists had to spend time outside work hours engaged in searching and appraisal. Private practitioners prioritized billable work hours ahead of searching and appraisal, since these activities affected their income. They typically completed their activities outside of work hours. Several participants felt that evidence-based practice had to become part of their routine work for it to be sustainable, with a certain number of hours being allocated per week or month; as one therapist noted,

We've got to change our culture and job descriptions...to include the time...rather than it being something you can tack on when you've got a free moment.

Supportive policies were already in place for some participants. Successful therapists planned ahead by booking blocks of time in their schedule. For instance, one therapist noted:

I have autonomy over my work practices and was able to book in ...big chunks of time...I just booked ahead...I just planned and booked out my [work] diary [i.e., schedule].

In summary, finding time for evidence-based practice was difficult for all participants. Lack of time was the major barrier to adopting evidence-based practice. Most struggled to prioritize and plan. Successful therapists managed their time by prioritizing research-related work ahead of other tasks at certain times, by scheduling time in advance in their diary/schedule, and by devoting some time outside work hours. Effective time management was a characteristic of therapists in this study who started to use research in practice.

Developing Skills and Knowledge

Successful therapists developed skills and knowledge by proactively:

• Using evidence,
• Teaching evidence-based practice to others, and
• Seeking help when faced with difficulties.

Lack of skills and knowledge was a barrier to using evidence for 9 of the 10 participants. They all struggled with critical appraisal and understanding statistics in research articles. However, successful therapists overcame these difficulties by persisting, practicing, and seeking help. The following is one participant's report of the importance of practice and using newly acquired skills:

Makes sense doesn't it? If you allow yourself time to do something, you'll get better at it....The penny eventually dropped...[that] with more practice [my skills and knowledge had increased].

Five of the 10 therapists were actively involved in journal clubs or similar research-focused activities at work, requiring them to regularly use their skills and knowledge. One therapist noted that:

[We] started the new journal club about a year ago...everyone has a group that [they're] in. We meet once a month and pick a topic, and then everyone has a certain task to do in terms of doing the searches, or reading the articles or writing the summary.

Those who were successful were more likely to be involved in a journal club, partly because of organizational expectations, and partly because of routine questioning at their work. These therapists were keen to find and use research, in order to provide best practice to their clients. Although most therapists hoped to change their practice in response to research evidence, none were yet using this routinely in practice.

Teaching evidence-based practice to others helped therapists to consolidate and practice their new skills, and develop confidence in their ability to use evidence. As one therapist noted: "It was good doing the in-service...you often learn something better and

> Effective time management was a characteristic of therapists who started to use research in practice.

practice it more than if you're just reading it." The more successful and active therapists were expected to educate others in the organization about searching and appraisal; as one therapist observed: "It was ...pushed that we had the responsibility to educate [others]." Other therapists who were less active did not encounter the same expectations, and were less likely to feel they had the skills to educate others.

The role of local opinion leader was one that successful therapists adopted upon their return to work. For instance, one therapist commented that she had been "dobbed-in [i.e. nominated] to be the evidence-based champion." These therapists provided in-services at work for other staff, and established journal clubs.

The third way in which successful therapists developed their skills and knowledge was by actively seeking help from others, in person or by phone and e-mail. This help sometimes involved a demonstration of searching techniques, or seeking expert advice about statistics. Librarians were a common source of help and support. Work could be delegated to a librarian in some organizations, as one therapist explained:

To save a bit of time in the process...I develop the clinical question and mail it down to the librarian. She'll do the search for me and send up the result.

Therapists found it helpful to have a buddy. A buddy was someone who worked with participants on their critically appraised topic, the project assignment. A buddy helped maintain motivation, shared the work, and sometimes supplied journal articles; this was underscored by one therapist who observed:

I think the buddy system ...worked really well, with everyone being motivated ... to share out the jobs a little bit, bounce ideas off each other and motivate each other. To also remind each other when deadlines were coming up and that sort of thing. I think that's a great system and it helps you to network a little bit too.

Successful therapists, with and without buddies, located and used experts such as librarians, or the project outreach support person, who conducted support visits, answered e-mail questions, and helped with searching over the telephone. In summary, successful therapists in this study developed skills and knowledge by using evidence in practice regularly, by teaching evidence-based practice to others, and by seeking help during times of difficulty.

Staying Focused

The more successful occupational therapists in the study used the strategy of staying focused. This strategy involved:

- Making a commitment to evidence-based practice,
- Being persistent when barriers were encountered, and
- Being motivated about evidence-based practice.

They changed their work habits and maintained the changes in spite of many distractions. Their activities were not constant. Instead, successful therapists had periods of intense activity, followed by periods of inactivity. However, despite periods of inactivity, and barriers encountered along the way, they did not lose sight of their goals. The first step was making a commitment.

Making a commitment meant holding oneself accountable for completing activities, such as searching and appraisal. One factor that cemented commitment was personal or organizational expectations that a critically appraised topic would be completed. Making a commitment also implied that using evidence was valued, as noted by one therapist:

I suppose I had...this obligation, having been part of the project...[You] signed up, and you knew what you were in for. So we needed to finish it. But that was probably a self-imposed obligation, because all along, we were aware we could drop out.

Being persistent involved hard work, and continuing despite failures and obstacles. It was easier for therapists to persist if they were motivated, committed to using evidence, and had organizational support. Being motivated meant having the desire and drive to finish the critically appraised topic. All had been motivated initially to participate in the study and the workshop: "I did the 2-day workshop and came back very motivated and very keen ... and did quite a lot of work into my question." However, as time progressed and deadlines advanced, motivation diminished for some of the participants interviewed. Lack of motivation was characterized by long periods of inactivity and limited time spent searching or appraising evidence, and therefore, limited time spent developing or practicing skills.

The more successful therapists interviewed were motivated to continue using evidence because of comments made by work colleagues, friends, and managers, and e-mails sent by the outreach support person. They were also motivated by meeting deadlines for the project, such as completing and then presenting their critically appraised topic to others. One therapist stayed focused because her manager showed interest, and asked for e-mail updates on her critically appraised topic. In summary, successful therapists stayed focused on becoming an evidence-based practitioner by making a commitment, being persistent, and being motivated.

Factors and Conditions that Helped Occupational Therapists to Change

In this Australian study, qualitative analysis identified four factors or conditions that helped therapists to change and adopt evidence-based practice, or conversely, that limited their progress and presented additional barriers. These four factors or conditions (Table 43.4) were:

• A personal readiness for change,
• Personal and organizational expectations that they would apply the skills learned and teach others,
• Self-determined deadlines that pushed them along, and
• Support within the organization, such as computers and journals, as well as encouragement from colleagues and managers.

If these conditions were present and positive, participants were more likely to progress. If these conditions were absent or negative, they acted as additional barriers to change, and progress was slower.

Discussion

This chapter has discussed barriers that limit the use of research by occupational therapists, and interfere with the change from "experience-based" practice to "evidence-based" practice. The chapter also focused on factors that allowed therapists to overcome some of these barriers. Research presented found that occupational therapists who successfully engaged in evidence-based practice reprioritized their time, proactively developed their skills and knowledge, and stayed focused on answering one or more clinical questions (McCluskey, 2004). They were in control of the change process. They stopped talking about barriers, and changed how they worked. They acknowledged that they were intellectually ready to change work habits, acquire new skills and knowledge, and prioritize their time differently. Further research is needed to investigate whether these experiences and strategies are similar for other cohorts of occupational therapists.

Changing how time is spent at work is more likely to occur if a person is ready to change, able to persist, and committed (Davis, 2003). Strategies

Table 43.4 Conditions that Promoted Change to Evidence-Based Practice

Conditions	Definition
Readiness for change	Time ready, intellectually ready, resource ready, or skill ready. Readiness to change work habits and allocate time to activities such as searching and appraisal.
Personal and organizational expectations	Personal expectations of achievement. Use of evidence encouraged and expected by individuals and their organization. Managers and supervisors were inquiring and interested, and expected new knowledge to be applied and shared with others in the organization.
Presence of deadlines	Intrinsic or extrinsic, negotiable or nonnegotiable, urgent or nonurgent. The presence of deadlines helped initiate and stimulate further activity levels; provided direction and focus for participants.
Availability of support	Encouragement, physical resources (internet, journals, computer, databases) financial assistance and work concessions. Support from managers, organizations, buddies and peers.

Adapted from McCluskey, A. (2004). *Increasing the use of research* evidence *by occupational therapists* [Final report]. Penrith South, Australia: School of Exercise and Health Sciences, University of Western Sydney. Table 5.3, page 37. Full copy available in PDF format from http://www.otcats.com [under 'Project Summary']. With permission.

Strategies for managing time so that evidence-based practice can be implemented include:

• Using efficient search techniques,
• Completing tasks in small manageable segments,
• Setting and negotiating short-term goals, ideally in conjunction with a manager or supervisor,
• Recognizing the time and skills required to prepare a critically appraised topic, and
• Avoiding procrastination and extended searching (both of which can be ways of avoiding the critical appraisal stage).

for better time use include prioritizing daily tasks (Rogak, 1999), making plans (Dobbins & Pettman, 1998), delegating tasks to allow time for more important activities (Mancini, 1994), setting aside blocks of time (Dobbins & Pettman, 1998), and dividing large overwhelming tasks into smaller sections so they appear more manageable (Kroehnert, 1999). Other strategies include not postponing tasks (Mackenzie, 1997).

It is also important to manage behaviors that waste time. Time wasting activities include procrastination (McGuire, 2003), lack of self-discipline and inadequate planning (Mackenzie, 1997), being reactive rather than proactive, not setting priorities, and poor delegation (Dobbins & Pettman, 1998). Based on prior literature and the recent qualitative study, strategies for managing time so that evidence-based practice can implemented include:

• Using efficient search techniques,
• Completing tasks in small manageable segments,
• Setting and negotiating short-term goals, ideally in conjunction with a manager or supervisor,
• Recognizing the time and skills required to prepare a critically appraised topic, and
• Avoiding procrastination and extended searching (both of which can be ways of avoiding the critical appraisal stage).

> Anyone learning about evidence-based practice should seek opportunities to teach, as well as seek help from, others.

> Searching, reading, and critical appraisal should no longer be considered activities that therapists are expected to "fit in" when there is "spare time."

Developing skills and knowledge for evidence-based practice is an ongoing process (Rosenberg et al., 1998). The skills and knowledge required include learning about the process of evidence-based practice, as discussed previously. Initially therapists need to write a clinical question, a skill that most therapists learn quickly. Following this first step, database search skills need to be developed, which can be more of a challenge. This second step is more of a challenge, demanding focus and avoidance of "busy" work (i.e., searching for and collecting more articles than needed).

Critical appraisal is the third step in the process of evidence-based practice, a skill that many practitioners find difficult to master (Bryar et al., 2003; McCluskey, 2003; Oswald & Bateman, 2000). Appraisal skills are more challenging to learn than searching, and therefore need to be thoroughly addressed during the professional education of occupational therapists. Introducing assignments early in a student's education which demand critical appraisal of published research may help in this regard. Completion of critically appraised topics as a final year assignment can showcase the skills of university graduates (see http://www.otcats.com for examples). However, graduates need to be able to interpret efficacy studies (particularly randomized controlled trials and systematic reviews), as well as qualitative research and studies that compare tests and outcome measures.

Managers also need to address the development of critical appraisal skills, by supporting graduate therapists to attend journal clubs and interactive workshops on evidence-based practice (McCluskey & Cusick, 2002). Local opinion leaders need to be supported and encouraged to act as role models. Experts might be called in to facilitate positive first-time experiences of a journal club (Phillips & Glasziou, 2004).

Previous studies have suggested that once skills and knowledge have been acquired, the time required to complete specialized activities such as searching databases will decrease, as practitioners become more efficient (Bennett et al., 2003). However, skill development and progression requires practice. Outreach support appears to have some effect on skills and knowledge, but regular practice is essential to develop and maintain skills.

Teaching colleagues about evidence-based practice can also help therapists to advance their skills and knowledge. Teaching others can facilitate self-learning, and is recognized as an effective way of improving performance. Teaching occupational therapy students was recently proposed as a strategy for promoting use of research evidence (Craik & Rappolt, 2003). These researchers found that when experienced occupational therapists taught students in clinical practice or on campus, this teaching role consolidated their skills and knowledge. Anyone learning about evidence-based practice should seek opportunities to teach, as well as seek help from, others.

The number of hours in a work day and the size of workloads is unlikely to change. Instead, it is the allocation and prioritization of time, work values, and routines that need to change. Only then will time spent reading, appraising, thinking, and changing what is actually done in practice be considered equally important to direct care and writing reports. In most organizations, a change in the way that time is valued and spent will depend largely on forward thinking managers.

The last two stages of evidence-based practice involve implementing findings in practice, and evaluating the outcome with clients locally. As noted earlier, these appear to be the most difficult stages to implement, and may require the most support. Few studies to date have focused on implementation, particularly the effect of evidence-based practice on client outcomes.

If health professionals are expected to routinely use evidence in practice, it seems reasonable to expect that time will be allocated during work time for searching and appraisal activities. Searching, reading, and critical appraisal should no longer be considered activities that therapists are expected to "fit in" when there is "spare time."

Therefore, evidence-based practice needs to be mentioned in business plans, annual reports, orientation program documentation, and performance appraisals (McCluskey & Cusick, 2002). Evidence-based practice needs to be visible, and should be considered an important criteria for accreditation of healthcare organizations. In the end, organizational culture, and how attitudes and values are espoused by others, particularly managers, appear to enhance or inhibit the adoption of evidence-based practice.

ACKNOWLEDGMENT

Sally Home and Lauren Thompson contributed to qualitative data collection and analysis as part of their occupational therapy undergraduate honours projects in 2003, at the University of Western Sydney, Australia. Categories (stategies and conditions) have been further developed and refined for this chapter.

REFERENCES

Bennett, S., Tooth, L., McKenna. K., Rodger, S., Strong, J., Ziviani, J., Mickan, S., & Gibson, L. (2003). Perceptions of evidence based practice: A survey of occupational therapists. *Australian Occupational Therapy Journal, 50*(1), 13–22.

Bryar, R. M., Closs, S. J., Baum, G., Cooke, J., Griffiths, J., Hostick, T., Kelly, S., Knight, S., Marshall, K., & Thompson, D. R. (2003). The Yorkshire barriers project: Diagnostic analysis of barriers to research utilisation. *International Journal of Nursing Studies, 40*, 73–84.

Closs, S. J., & Lewin, B. J. P. (1998). Perceived barriers to research utilization: A survey of four therapies. *British Journal of Therapy and Rehabilitation, 5*(3), 151–155.

Conroy, M. (1997). 'Why are you doing that?' A project to look for evidence of efficacy within occupational therapy. *British Journal of Occupational Therapy, 60*, 487–490.

Craik, J., & Rappolt, S. (2003). Theory of research utilization enhancement: A model for occupational therapy. *Canadian Journal of Occupational Therapy, 70*, 266–275.

Davis, N. (2003). Stealing time: Time management techniques add hours to each day. *Journal of the American Health Information Management Association, 74*(6), 25–28.

Dingle, J., & Hooper, L. (2000). Establishing a journal club in an occupational therapy service: One service's experience. *British Journal of Occupational Therapy, 63*, 554–556.

Dobbins, R., & Pettman, B. O. (1998). Creating more time. *Equal Opportunities International, 17*(2), 18–27.

Dubouloz, C., Egan, M., Vallerand, J., & von Zweck, C. (1999). Occupational therapists' perceptions of evidence-based practice. *American Journal of Occupational Therapy, 53*, 445–453.

Effective Health Care. (1999). *Getting evidence into practice* [Report]. York, England: University of York,

A range of Internet resources and educational Web sites are available for anyone engaged in teaching, and include the OTseeker site (Occupational Therapy Systematic Evaluation of Evidence, at http://www.otseeker.com), CASP (the Critical Appraisal Skills Program at http://www.phru.nhs.uk/casp/casp.htm), and Netting the Evidence (http://www.shef.ac.uk/scharr/ir/netting/). These sites contain presentations and handouts that can be downloaded for teaching purposes.

National Health Service Centre for Reviews and Dissemination.

Humphris, D., Littlejohns, P., Victor, C., O'Halloran, P., & Peacock, J. (2000). Implementing evidence-based practice: Factors that influence the use of research evidence by occupational therapists. *British Journal of Occupational Therapy, 63,* 516–522.

Kroehnert, G. (1999). *Taming time and how do you eat an elephant?* Roseville, Australia: McGraw-Hill.

Mackenzie, A. (1997). *The time trap* (3rd ed.). New York: American Management Association.

Mancini, M. (1994). *Time management.* New York: McGraw-Hill.

McCluskey, A. (2003). Occupational therapists report a low level of knowledge, skill and involvement in evidence-based practice. *Australian Occupational Therapy Journal, 50*(1), 3–12.

McCluskey, A. (2004). *Increasing the use of research evidence by occupational therapists* [Final report]. Penrith South, Australia: School of Exercise and Health Sciences, University of Western Sydney. Full copy available in PDF format from http://www.otcats.com [under 'Project Summary'].

McCluskey, A., & Cusick, A. (2002). Strategies for introducing evidence-based practice and changing clinician behaviour: A manager's toolbox. *Australian Occupational Therapy Journal, 49,* 63–70.

McCluskey, A., & Lovarini, M. (2005). Providing education on evidence-based practice improved knowledge but did not change behaviour: A before and after study. *BMC Medical Education, 5,* 40.

McGuire, R. (2003). Successful time management. *British Medical Journal, 327,* 117.

Metcalfe, C., Lewin, R., Wisher, S., Perry, S., Bannigan, K., & Moffett, J. (2001). Barriers to implementing the evidence base in four NHS therapies. *Physiotherapy, 87,* 433–441.

Oswald, N., & Bateman, H. (2000). Treating individuals according to evidence: Why do primary care practitioners do what they do? *Journal of Evaluation in Clinical Practice, 6*(2), 139–148.

Phillips, R. S., & Glasziou, P. (2004). What makes evidence-based journal clubs succeed? *Evidence-Based Medicine, 9,* 36–37.

Pollock, A. S., Legg, L., Langhorne, P., & Sellars, C. (2000). Barriers to achieving evidence-based stroke rehabilitation. *Clinical Rehabilitation, 14,* 611–617.

Pollock, N., & Rochon, S. (2002). Becoming an evidence-based practitioner. In M. Law (Ed.), *Evidence-based rehabilitation: A guide to practice* (pp. 31–46). Thorofare, NJ: Slack.

Prochaska, J. O., & DiClemente, C. C. (1982). Transtheoretical therapy: Toward a more integrative model of change. *Psychotherapy: Theory, Research and Practice, 19*(3), 276–288.

Prochaska, J., & Diclemente, C. (1983). Stages and processes of self-change in smoking: Toward an integrative model of change. *Journal of Consulting and Clinical Psychology, 51,* 390–395.

Prochaska, J. O., DiClemente, C. C., & Norcross, J. C. (1992). In search of how people change: Applications to addictive behaviours. *American Psychologist, 47*(9), 1102–1114.

Redmond, A. (1997). Evidence-based medicine: A blueprint for effective practice or the emperor's new clothes? *Podiatry Management, 11,* 123–126.

Rogak, L. (1999). *Smart guide to managing your time.* New York: John Wiley & Sons.

Rogers, E. M. (1983). *Diffusion of innovations.* New York: Free Press.

Rosenberg, W. M., Deeks, J., Lusher, A., Snowball, R., Dooley, G., & Sackett, D. (1998). Improving searching skills and evidence retrieval. *Journal of the Royal College of Physicians of London, 32*(6), 557–563.

Sackett, D. L., Straus, S. E., Richardson, W. S., Rosenberg, W., & Haynes, R. B. (2000). *Evidence-based medicine: How to practice and teach EBP* (2nd ed.). Edinburgh: Churchill Livingstone.

Strauss, S.E., Richardson, W.S., Glasziou, P., & Haynes, R.B. (2005). *Evidence-based medicine: How to practice and teach evidence-based medicine* (3rd ed.). Edinburgh: Elsevier Churchill Livingstone.

Taylor, M. C. (2000). *Evidence-based practice for occupational therapists.* Oxford: Blackwell Science.

RESOURCES

The OTseeker Evidence Database (http://www.otseeker.com)

OTseeker (Occupational Therapy Systematic Evaluation of Evidence) is a free Web-based database that supports evidence-based occupational therapy. Currently, the database contains details of more than 3,000 randomized controlled trials and systematic reviews relevant to occupational therapy. These studies are preappraised and intended to help occupational therapists evaluate the validity and interpretability of current research.

The database has been available since March 2003, and at the time of writing, had received more than 260,000 visits. There is no subscription fee. Funds for development were provided by the Motor Accidents Authority of New South Wales, Australia, and OT-Australia. Funds are now being sought internationally to support ongoing maintenance, and to enable new studies to be added to the database.

When visiting the site, explore diagnoses and interventions relevant to your area of practice. At the time of writing (May 2005), there were 470 articles listed under the category "gerontology," 308 under "pediatrics," 35 under "intellectual disabilities," 477 under "mental health," and 449 under "neurology and neuromuscular disorders." Entries are also categorized by intervention. At the time of writing there were 47 studies catalogued in OTseeker relevant to "case management"; 1051 studies relevant to "consumer education," 92 studies on "assistive technology/adaptive equipment," and 342 studies on "relaxation/stress management."

The site developers, all from Australia, are Drs. Kryss McKenna, Sally Bennett, Tammy Hoffmann, Leigh Tooth and Professor Jenny Strong from the University of Queensland, and Dr. Annie McCluskey from the University of Western Sydney.

Additional links are provided to other databases, which contain "best evidence" on physiotherapy intervention (PEDro or the Physiotherapy Evidence Database, available at http://www.pedro.fhs.usyd.edu.au/) and rehabilitation following acquired brain impairment (PsycBITE, available at http://www.psycbite.com).

Occupational Therapy Critically Appraised Topics (CATs)

A critically appraised topic or CAT is a short summary of evidence on a topic of interest, usually focused around a clinical question. A CAT is like a less rigorous version of a systematic review, summarizing and appraising the best research on a topic. Usually more than one study is appraised in a CAT. When a single study is appraised as the "best" available evidence, the outcome is a critically appraised paper (a CAP). CATs and CAPs are a method of collating and disseminating appraisals to colleagues. CATs are increasingly being used as university assignments to assess students skills in searching and appraisal.

A free CATs Web site for occupational therapists was developed in 2003 and is located at http://www.otcats.com. At the time of writing (May 2005), the site contained more than 30 CATs and CAPs related to occupational therapy interventions. The documents can be printed out and/or saved in PDF format. Students and therapists are invited to submit their own CAT or CAP, and a template is provided on the site for this purpose. The CATs and CAPs are not independently peer reviewed, which is one of their limitations. Nonetheless, the site allows therapists and students to share their completed appraisals, which may have taken several weeks or months to complete. Gradually, a body of critical appraisals is being collected.

For more information, contact Annie McCluskey, the site author (a.mccluskey@uws.edu.au).

Occupational Therapy Critically Appraised Papers (CAPs)

The term *critically appraised paper* (or CAP) refers to the critical appraisal of an original research study, which may be qualitative or quantitative in design, or appraisal of a systematic review. The aim is to help professionals keep up to date with recent advances by appraising and summarizing the results of key research.

The *Australian Occupational Therapy Journal* was the first journal to publish CAPs relevant to occupational therapy practice, commencing a CAPs Department in June 2003. Other journals that contain CAPs include *Evidence-Based Medicine*, *Evidence-Based Nursing*, and the *Australian Journal of Physiotherapy*.

Typically a CAP includes a structured abstract, meaning that the original abstract is rewritten to include details of the study methods, outcome measures, results, and statistics. Sometimes original authors of a study are contacted for missing information or data. Comments on the methodological quality of the study and implications for practice are written as a text summary. The conclusions reached by the appraisers may be the same or different from those reached by the original authors.

CHAPTER 44

Creating Outcome Research Relevant for Evidence-Based Practice

Pimjai Sudsawad

Research Utilization in Evidence-Based Practice

Evidence-based practice (EBP) is frequently defined as the conscientious, explicit, and judicious use of current best evidence in making decisions about the care of individual patients (Sackett, Rosenberg, Gray, Haynes, & Richardson, 1996). Despite the general consensus on the importance of using EBP as a practice approach, there has been a slow uptake of EBP in occupational therapy (Bennett et al., 2003; Curtin & Jaramazovic, 2001; Humphris, Littlejohn, Victor, O'Halloran, & Peacock, 2000; Upton & Lewis, 1998). A number of barriers make it difficult to implement EBP in real practice situations. Difficulty implementing EBP is certainly not unique to occupational therapy. Other rehabilitation professionals such as physical therapy and speech–language pathology also faced the same issue (Meline & Paradiso, 2003; Metcalfe et al., 2001; Turner & Whitfield, 1997).

EBP involves using research evidence, when available, as a basis for practice decisions. However, a number of studies with occupational therapy practitioners indicate that practitioners prefer and continue to use other sources of information more often than research evidence when making practice decisions (Bennett et al, 2003; Dubouloz, Egan, Vallerand, & von Zweck, 1999; Sudsawad, 2004; Sweetland & Craik, 2001). To execute EBP effectively, research evidence has to be used by practitioners. Research articles in professional and interdisciplinary journals have been the main sources of the most current evidence for occupational therapy practitioners, particularly studies of intervention effectiveness. Research evidence that relates to the needs of the practice community and is understandable to the practitioners is conceivably more likely to be used that those who do not have those characteristics.

Practitioners often report difficulties when attempting to use information from research articles for practice. Several difficulties have been identified both in nursing and in rehabilitation such as:

- The lack of someone to help translate findings into practice (Champion & Leach, 1989),
- Failure to make clear the implications for practice in the research presentation (Funk, Champagne, Tornquist, & Wiese, 1995),
- Difficulties with how research is communicated in publications (Kajermo, Nordström, Krusebrant, & Björvell, 2000),
- Practitioners' lack of skills in interpreting research evidence (Law & Baum, 1998),
- Difficulty understanding statistical analyses as presented (Lynn & Moore, 1997; Parahoo, 2000), and
- Perceived lack of relevance, ease of application, or orientation of the research literature to professional practice (Campbell, 1996; Di Fabio, 1999; Dubouloz et al., 1999).

With such difficulties, it is understandable how practitioners would be reluctant to use research evidence for EBP.

Just because research evidence is generated and disseminated does not mean that it will be used or that it is usable. Snell (2003) observed that researchers tend to define the problems and test the solutions apart from practitioners, typically speak a different language, and have a discrepancy in perspectives and goals. Nonetheless, most discussions of EBP focus on practitioners who are expected to learn the skills essential to using research information in its current form. Little emphasis has been placed on researchers and their role in the research application and utilization process (Lynn & Moore, 1997).

Researchers certainly share responsibility for bridging the gap between research and practice. Researchers need to:

- Examine how research is being created,
- Consider its applicability and usability for practice,

- Be open to a different paradigm of creating research evidence, and
- Produce outcome research that can be used for EBP.

Ottenbacher, Barris, and Van Deusen (1986) first raised the issues of research characteristics that could create impediments to occupational therapy practitioners' use of research for practice. They pointed out the problems with using group statistics to determine treatment effectiveness because even if statistically significant differences are found, clinically relevant information cannot be inferred. They also pointed out the difficulties in duplicating the intervention strategies reported in research articles within a clinical environment. They called for both researchers and practitioners to be concerned with the effectiveness with which information generated through research is disseminated and incorporated into practice. Their observations and suggestions are certainly still timely today.

In the following sections, the Diffusion of Innovations theory is introduced as the framework to help identify desirable characteristics of research evidence that could facilitate its use for EBP. The concepts of social validity, ecological validity, and clinical significance are presented as vehicles that can help to create those desirable characteristics when applied to the design and implementation of outcome research in occupational therapy. The discussion in this chapter specifically pertains to the creation of clinical outcome research that is intended to guide practice decisions regarding treatment interventions.

Identifying Desirable Characteristics of Research Evidence

Diffusion of Innovations

The Diffusion of Innovations (Rogers, 2003) is a framework that identifies the process and influencing factors in communicating an innovation (defined as an idea, practice, or object that is perceived as new). This framework has been used widely in fields such as business, marketing, and public health. There are four main elements in a diffusion of an innovation:

- The innovation,
- The communication channels,
- Time, and
- The social systems.

The most influential of these elements for the diffusion of an innovation is the characteristics of the innovation itself, which accounts for 49% to 87% of the variance in predicting its adoption rate (Rogers, 1995).

As identified by Rogers (2003), there are five characteristics of an innovation that could either facilitate or hinder the adoption of an innovation as delineated below:

- Relative advantage: The degree to which an innovation is perceived as better than the idea it supersedes. The degree of relative advantage may be measured in many terms (economic, prestige, convenience, satisfaction, etc.), and the greater the perceived relative advantage of an innovation, the more rapid its rate of adoption will be.
- Compatibility: The degree to which an innovation is perceived as being consistent with the existing values, past experiences, and the needs of the potential adopter. An idea that is incompatible with the values and norms of the social system will not be adopted as rapidly as an innovation that is compatible.
- Complexity: The degree to which an innovation is perceived as difficult to understand and use. The innovations that are readily comprehended by most potential adopters will be adopted more rapidly while the others that are perceived as more complicated will be adopted more slowly.
- Trialability: The degree to which an innovation may be experimented with on a limited basis. If new ideas can be tried on a small scale, it would generally be adopted more quickly.
- Observability: The degree to which the results of an innovation are visible to others. The easier it is for individuals to see the results of an innovation, the more likely they are to adopt.

As shown in Figure 44.1, these characteristics are factors that influence the extent to which the innovation will be adopted and used.

Application of Desirable Characteristics of an Innovation to Research Evidence

Research evidence fits the definition of an innovation because it represents new ideas and/or practice. Therefore, the Diffusion of Innovations framework can be used to examine characteristics that, if present, would likely make research evidence be received more favorably by its potential users. In this case, the potential users of interest are occupational therapy practitioners who would like to use research evidence as a basis for decision-making in practice. The Diffusion of Innovations

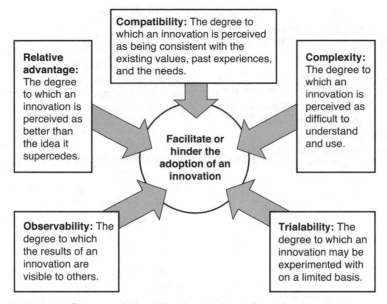

Figure 44.1 Characteristics of an innovation influencing its adoption.

framework can be applied to research characteristics as indicated below.

- First, research must be perceived as containing stronger evidence than other sources so that it is viewed as having a relative advantage over other kinds of evidence.
- Second, the design and conduct of research must be consistent with the existing values, past experiences, and the needs of practitioners and/or occupational therapy consumers to increase compatibility.
- Third, research must be presented in ways that make it easy to understand and use in order to reduce complexity.
- Fourth, the intervention investigated must be easily implemented in the clinical setting to increase the level of trialability.

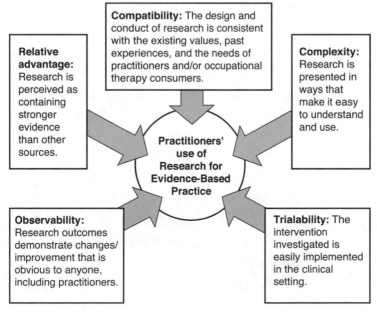

Figure 44.2 Characteristics of outcome research influencing practitioner's use of research for evidence-based practice.

• Last, the research outcomes must demonstrate changes/improvement with a magnitude that is obvious to anyone, including the practitioners, to increase the observability.

Based on the Diffusion of Innovations framework, these characteristics can be conceptualized as factors that influence the extent to which practitioners will use research findings for EBP, as shown in Figure 44.2.

Initial findings suggest that practitioners accept research evidence as stronger than other kinds of evidence (Sudsawad, 2004). It appears that occupational therapy researchers should place an immediate focus on other characteristics to ensure that occupational therapy outcome research is produced such that it is most relevant to practice. Considering the scarcity of the resources available for occupational therapy research, it seems unwise to use those resources to create outcome research that does not lend itself to be used in practice. Creating outcome research that is usable for practice is one of the most important contributions occupational therapy researchers can make toward evidence-based practice.

Concepts and Methods to Fulfill the Desirable Characteristics of Research Evidence

In the following sections, the concepts of social validity, ecological validity, and clinical significance are introduced and their methods discussed in relation to the five desirable characteristics of research information as delineated earlier. Researchers can use these concepts as guides to creating research that is likely to be used in EBP.

These concepts should be used as a supplement to the usual consideration of rigor in the design and conduct of outcome research because scientific rigor in and of itself is not sufficient to make research evidence usable in practice. It is essential that occupational therapy investigators also consider other characteristics to make outcome research maximally relevant for its use in EBP.

> Creating outcome research that is usable for practice is one of the most important contributions occupational therapy researchers can make toward evidence-based practice.

Social Validity

Wolf (1978), who first proposed the concept of social validity, referred to it as something of social importance. According to Wolf (1978) researchers should ask three questions to assess the social validity of outcome research concerning goals, procedures, and outcomes:

• Goals: Are the goals of the intervention being investigated really what society wants?
• Procedures: Are the intervention techniques used acceptable to the consumers, or do they cost too much (e.g., in terms of effort, time, discomfort, ethics, or the like)?
• Outcomes: Are the consumers satisfied with the intervention outcome, both with predicted change and with unpredicted side effects?

The terms "society" and "consumers" include anyone who may be involved with and affected by the intervention process and outcome including the occupational therapy clients, their caregivers, their parents and teachers (in the case of children), community members, disability groups, and others.

There are a variety of methods for operationalizing the social validity concept (e.g., Foster & Mash, 1999; Hawkins, 1991; Kazdin & Matson, 1981; Kendall & Grove, 1988; Schwartz & Baer, 1991). However, this discussion focuses on verification with consumers as a method for establishing social validity.

Schwartz and Baer (1991) identified four different types of consumers who can be approached to determine social validity:

• Direct consumers,
• Indirect consumers,
• Members of the immediate community, and
• Members of the extended community.

Direct consumers are the primary recipients of the intervention. Indirect consumers are those who purchase the intervention for someone else or are strongly affected by the behaviors change targeted in the intervention, but they are not its recipients. Members of the immediate community are those who interact with the direct and indirect consumers on a regular basis, usually through close proximity during work, school, or social situations. The members of the extended community include those who probably do not know or

Verifying the Relevance of Research Questions/Treatment Goals

The following is an example of verifying the relevance of research questions/treatment goals. O'Brien et al. (2000) conducted a study to investigate the effectiveness of an occupational therapy intervention designed to improve playfulness in children. In this study, information obtained from initial home visits and parents' interview were used to determine the area of concern for each child and set up the treatment goal (rather than determining the goal based on the researchers' own opinion).

interact with the direct and indirect consumers but who live in the same community. The point of this delineation is that a few different groups of consumers are available to socially validate the goals, procedures, and outcomes. To strengthen the social validity, more than one consumer group's opinion and perspective may be sought at the same time.

Social validity can be implemented from the initial conception of the research to the conclusion of the study. Occupational therapy researchers can seek the appropriate study topic/research questions (*goals*) by seeking to learn about the topics of interest to practitioners and/or what type of evidence is needed in practice situations. In addition, researchers can include occupational therapy clients to help identify appropriate treatment goals (Feature Box 44.1).

A study's intervention (*procedures*) can be developed such that the reality of practice is taken into consideration. Then, if the intervention studied is found to be effective, practitioners can use it. The acceptability of the intervention can also be verified with service consumers because if consumers found the intervention unacceptable, they may choose not to receive or cooperate with the intervention.

Before the intervention, researchers can verify with the clients that the intervention outcomes (*outcomes*) chosen are important outcomes from their perspective. The social validity of outcomes can also be verified after the intervention by asking clients whether they are satisfied with the outcomes obtained. Practitioners can also help to identify the types of outcomes that may be relevant to their clients.

Relationship Between Social Validity and Desirable Characteristics of Research Evidence

Involving both the consumers and the practitioners in the process of determining research questions/

Verifying Social Appropriateness of Intervention Procedures

The following is an example of verifying the social appropriateness of the intervention procedures and social importance of the outcomes. Schilling, Washington, Billingsley, and Deitz (2003) conducted a study to investigate the effects of using therapy balls as seating on in-seat behaviors and legible word productivity of students with attention deficit hyperactivity disorder (ADHD). They used the social validity methods to verify both the appropriateness of the intervention and the importance of the outcome. The researchers asked teachers, students in the class who were classmates of the study's participants (and also using therapy balls as seating in the classroom at the same time as the study's participants), and the participants themselves to complete a questionnaire to determine whether they observed improvement in performance in the actual classroom setting. The teacher answered questions concerning whether she saw the improvement in students' performance. The students answered questions about whether they saw improvement of their own performance. To verify the acceptability of the intervention, students were also asked whether they preferred using therapy balls than sitting on chairs, and were given an opportunity to put in writing their opinion of sitting on balls in the classroom.

treatment goals, intervention procedures, and intervention outcomes when conducting research studies should increase compatibility—the degree to which research information is perceived as being consistent with the existing values, past experiences, and the needs of the occupational therapy practitioners—either through addressing the consumers' needs (which is the matter of interest to practitioners) or taking into consideration the practitioners' input based on actual practice situations, or both. In addition, investigating intervention methods that are realistic for implementation in practice settings and acceptable by consumers should increase trialability—the degree to which information obtained from research studies can be implemented in practice settings.

Ecological Validity

Ecological validity is related to the social importance of research outcomes; it is the degree to which results obtained in controlled experimental conditions are related to those obtained in naturalistic environments (Tupper & Cicerone, 1990). What a person can do in the artificial experimental environment is not necessarily what the person

Assessing Ecological Validity

Moseley and colleagues (2004) assessed the ecological validity of walking speed measurement
after a traumatic brain injury (TBI) of three clinical gait tests in predicting walking performance
in three natural environments (a corridor in a
brain injury rehabilitation unit, a car park of a
metropolitan shopping center, inside a metropolitan shopping center). They found that for participants with TBI, the agreements between the
speed used in the clinical gait tests and the natural environments was poor. Sudsawad, Trombly,
Henderson, and Tickle-Degnen (2001) assessed
the ecological validity of a standardized handwriting assessment and found that the level of
handwriting performance of children with various
degrees of handwriting illegibility bore almost no
relationship with the children's performance in
the classroom setting as rated by teachers.

does or can do in his or her everyday environment.
Similarly, the interaction between persons' abilities (or disability) and unique environmental demands will yield different performances
(Sbordone, 1996).

Choosing an ecologically valid outcome also
partly relates to the social validity aspect of the
outcome. Not only should the outcome measure
represent performance in real-life environment, it
should also reflect the performance that the clients,
their significant others, or their peers consider to
be important, and with which they are satisfied
(Feature Box 44.3).

Another aspect of ecological validity relates to
the standardized test instruments used for assessment of outcomes. Franzen and Wilhelm (1996)
indicated two general aspects of ecological validity in assessment:

• Verisimilitude, which is the similarity of the data
collection methods in the test to tasks and skills
required in the free and open environment, and
• Veridicality, which is the extent to which test
results reflect or can predict phenomena in the
open environment or "real world."

Verisimilitude will be important in the design
of assessment instruments, but once an instrument
is designed, veridicality becomes more important
(Franzen & Wilhelm, 1996). To achieve ecological
validity, a test must provide information that is relevant to the person's functioning in daily life, not
simply be representative of a hypothetical construct or even a neurological syndrome (Silver,
2000). If a standardized test is to be used as a
measurement instrument in outcome research, it

should have some evidence of ecological validity.
Better yet, real-life performance should be used as
a basis to demonstrate the intervention effectiveness in natural settings whenever possible because
there is no guarantee that a test (or a number of
tests) will predict performance in a natural setting.

Relationship of Ecological Validity to the Desirable Characteristics of Research Evidence

Choosing study outcomes that represent actual
performance in real-life settings can positively
contribute to the use of research evidence for practice. Demonstrating the effect of intervention
in terms of ability or performance in a natural context will help to increase compatibility of research
information for occupational therapy practitioners

Incorporating Real-Life Performance into Outcome Studies

The following studies are examples of how real-
life performance can be incorporated into outcome studies. In a study of the dose–response
effects of a medication for ADHD, Evans et al.
(2001) used everyday tasks in normal classroom
activities as dependent measures including
notetaking quality, quiz and worksheet performance, written language usage and productivity,
teacher ratings on task and disruptive behavior,
and homework completion. The researchers
believed that the measures of behavior and academic performance are needed to assess medication response, rather than using laboratory tasks
as proxy measures of academic functioning, as
past research had showed little correspondence
between performance on such tasks and classroom academic performance.

In the study comparing the effectiveness of
three interventions for stuttering plus a control
group, Craig et al. (1996) measured the participants' stuttering frequency and speech rate not
only during conversations in the clinic with the
clinician, but also in two other relevant contexts
including performance during a telephone conversation with a family member or friend, and in
face-to-face conversation with a family member
or friend in the home environment.

In another study investigating the effectiveness of oral–motor sensory treatment Gisel,
Applegate-Ferrante, Benson, and Bosma (1996)
measured oral–motor skills through the administration of a standardized feeding assessment during observations at lunch/snack time in the
children's accustomed room with the person who
was the child's regular feeder.

because such outcomes reflect the profession's philosophy of enabling clients to be able to engage in an occupation. Presenting the outcome in everyday terms should also reduce the perceived complexity of the information drawn from research evidence because such outcomes can be easily related and understood. Finally, the results of an intervention are more likely to be perceived as easily observed since outcomes were something that can be readily seen by normal observation as opposed to the abstraction of test scores; hence, increase observability of research evidence.

Clinical Significance

Clinical significance refers to the practical value or the importance of the effect of an intervention, that is, whether it makes a real difference in everyday life to the clients, or to others with whom the clients interact (Kazdin, 1999). Statistical significance, while necessary to verify that any changes observed in a study are not likely due to chance, does not ensure that such changes are meaningful for clients' real-life performance. Therefore, statistical significance is an insufficient index for the usefulness of an intervention to improve everyday function. The fact that a treatment effect was probabilistically not "due to chance" is not adequately informative to the practice community (Saunders, Howard, & Newman, 1988). Not surprisingly, agencies and policymakers increasingly demand evidence about real-world effects of interventions in order to invest resources in them (Czaja & Schulz, 2003). Nonetheless, the concept of clinical significance has not been implemented consistently in rehabilitation outcome research (Sudsawad, 2004) or in medical research (Chan, Man-Son-Hing, Molnar, & Laupacis, 2001).

Authors have presented different ways to demonstrate the clinical significance of treatment outcomes including both statistical and nonstatistical methods. The more suitable method that researchers can use to demonstrate clinical significance for their study will depend on many factors such as:

- The study area,
- The study sample,
- The nature of the treated condition, and
- The nature of the expected treatment outcomes.

Some of the methods to demonstrate clinical significance include:

- The use of effect sizes to demonstrate the magnitude of change,
- Using measures of risk potency such as a odds ratio, risk ratio, relative risk reduction, risk difference, and number needed to treat (NNT),
- Comparing both group and individual performance to normative data (Jacobson & Traux, 1991; Kazdin, 1977; Kendall & Grove, 1988),
- Using meta-analysis for a pooled effect size from several studies that is compared with normative data (Nietzel & Trull, 1998),
- Showing that the studied intervention eliminates symptoms/impairments that the intervention is intended to eliminate,
- Demonstrating that the researched intervention enables clients to meet role demands, increases the level of functioning in everyday life, and/or achieves change in quality of life,
- Incorporating subjective judgments of change by the clients, their significant others, or by people who interact with the clients in their natural environments, and
- Documenting satisfaction with the treatment results, including input obtained from the client, his or her significant others or even professionals who are not part of the research team (e.g. a child's regular occupational therapist, teacher, classroom assistant).

Using statistical methods to determine clinical significance (the first four bullet points above) is important to improve the quality of evidence. These methods, however, do not provide information on the impact of the intervention on the client's everyday life and they generate information at a level of abstraction that does not correspond to the everyday world of practice. Focusing on elimination of symptoms/impairments or normative comparison, while useful in some contexts, may not be applicable to many areas of occupational therapy services. Often, the goal of occupational therapy intervention is not to eliminate symptoms or to promote the client's performance to that of the norms, but rather to maximize the client's ability to participate in everyday living as much as possible.

> Statistical significance, while necessary to verify that any changes observed in a study are not likely due to chance, does not ensure that such changes are meaningful for clients' real-life performance.

Making use of client (and others with whom the client is associated) input on the client's performance in natural contexts is a comprehensive approach. For example, assessing a client's satisfaction with change of his or her performance in everyday activities meets the criteria for social validity, ecological validity, and clinical significance. This strategy includes the consumer's perspective and opinion, measures real-life everyday function, and ensures that the change achieved is substantial such that it is satisfactory to the client. On the other hand, if the increased functioning in everyday life is based only on the researcher's observation, it may meet the criteria of ecological validity and clinical significance, but may not have equally strong social validity.

Relationship of Clinical Significance to Desirable Characteristics of Research Evidence

Applying the concept of clinical significance to demonstrate a meaningful change in everyday function can increase the compatibility of research information with the ultimate goal of occupational therapy intervention, which is to positively impact clients' everyday lives. Demonstrating change in ways that are related to everyday functions can also help to decrease the complexity of research information from practitioners' perspectives. They can relate to this type of outcome as evidence of treatment effectiveness more readily than to statistical significance. Clinical significance of treatment outcomes that demonstrate an impact on the study participants' everyday life functioning also increases the observability of findings.

Application of the Diffusion of Innovations Framework in Occupational Therapy

Occupational therapy researchers can use the Diffusion of Innovations framework as a guide, and the social validity, ecological validity, and clinical significance as tools, to create outcome research that is appealing to practitioners. This approach has potential to bridge the gap between research and practice because it emphasizes designing, conducting, and reporting research with the ultimate goal of creating information that is actually related to and usable in real-life practice. The following questions can be used to guide the design and implementation of outcome studies:

- Is the topic of the study what the practitioners/service consumers are interested in or need to know about?
- Is the intervention investigated in the study practical enough to be implemented in practice settings if found to be effective?
- Is the intervention procedure acceptable to the practitioners/service consumers?
- Is the treatment outcome to be measured in the study what practitioners and/or consumers consider to be an important outcome?
- Does the intervention outcome represent performance of daily activities in natural contexts?
- Does the method chosen to measure change/improvement demonstrate an impact on or make a difference in the client's everyday life function?

The use of social validity, ecological validity, and clinical significance concepts simultaneously to design and conduct outcome research, aimed to increase its usability for practice, was termed the Social Validation Model in a recent investigation (Sudsawad, 2004). Based on responses received from more than 900 practitioners in occupational therapy, physical therapy, and speech–language pathology, there was a strong support for the use of the Social Validation Model in rehabilitation outcome research. The majority of practitioners indicated that it was either important or very important that research evidence possesses the key elements included in the questions above. They also indicated that doing so would either likely or very likely increase their use of research information for practice.

Conclusion

It is imperative that occupational therapy researchers create research evidence that not only meets the standards of scientific rigor but also has utility in everyday practice. Moreover, in the current climate of limited available resources, occupational therapy researchers are well advised to produce outcome research that is relevant and applicable to occupational therapy practice. By doing so, researchers will make an important contribution to the progression of evidence-based practice.

REFERENCES

Bennett, S., Tooth, L., McKenna, K., Rodger, S., Strong, J., Ziviani, J., Mickan, S., & Gibson, L. (2003). Perceptions of evidence based practice: A survey of Australian occupational therapists. *Australian Occupational Therapy Journal, 50,* 13–22.

Campbell, T. W. (1996). Systemic therapy practice and basic research. *Journal of Systemic Therapy Practice, 15*(3), 15–39.

Champion, V. L., & Leach, A. (1989). Variables related to research utilization in nursing: An empirical investigation. *Journal of Advanced Nursing, 14,* 705–710.

Chan, K. B. Y., Man-Son-Hing, M., Molnar, F. J., & Laupacis, A. (2001). How well is the clinical importance of study results reported? An assessment of randomized controlled trials. *Canadian Medical Association Journal, 165*(9), 1197–1202.

Craig, A., Hancock, K., Chang, E., McCready, C., Shepley, A., McCaul, A., Costello, D., Harding, S., Kehren, R., Masel, C, & Reilly, K. (1996). A controlled clinical trial for stuttering in persons aged 9 to 14 years. *Journal of Speech and Hearing Research, 39,* 808–826.

Curtin, M., & Jaramazovic, E. (2001). Occupational therapists' views and perceptions of evidence-based practice. *British Journal of Occupational Therapy, 64,* 214–222.

Czaja, S. J., & Schulz, R. (2003). Does the treatment make a real difference? The measurement of clinical significance. (Translating psychosocial research into practice: Methodological issues). *Alzheimer's Care Quarterly, 4*(3), 229–240.

Di Fabio, R. P. (1999). Myth of evidence-based practice. *Journal of Orthopaedic & Sports Physical Therapy, 29,* 632–634.

Dubouloz, C-J., Egan, M., Vallerand, J., & von Zweck, C. (1999). Occupational therapists' perceptions of evidence-based practice, *American Journal of Occupational Therapy, 53,* 445–453.

Evans, S. W., Pelham, W. E., Smith, B. H., Bukstein, O., Gnagy, E. M., Greiner, A. R., Altenderfer, L., & Baron-Myak, C. (2001). Dose-response effects of Methylphenidate on ecologically valid measures of academic performance and classroom behavior in adolescence with ADHD. *Experimental and Clinical Psychopharmacology, 9,* 163–175.

Foster, S. L., & Mash, E. J. (1999). Assessing social validity in clinical treatment research: Issues and procedures. *Journal of Consulting and Clinical Psychology, 67,* 308–319.

Franzen, M. D., & Wilhelm, K. L. (1996). Conceptual foundations of ecological validity in neuropsychological assessment. In R. J. Sbordone & C. J. Long (Eds.), *Ecological validity of neuropsychological testing.* Delray Beach, FL: GR Press/St. Lucie Press.

Funk, S. G., Champagne, M. T., Tornquist, E. M. & Wiese, R. A. (1995). Administrators' views on barriers to research utilization. *Applied Nursing Research, 8,* 44–49.

Gisel, E. G., Applegate-Ferrante, T., Benson, J., & Bosma, J. F. (1996). Oral-motor skills follow a sensory motor therapy in two groups of moderately dysphagic children with cerebral palsy. *Dysphagia, 11,* 59–71.

Hawkins, R. P. (1991). Is social validity what we are interested in? Argument for a functional approach. *Journal of Applied Behavior Analysis, 24,* 205–213.

Humphris, D., Littlejohn, P., Victor, C, O'Halloran, P., & Peacock, J. (2000). Implementing evidence-based practice: Factors that influence the use of research evidence by occupational therapists. *British Journal of Occupational Therapy, 63,* 516–522.

Jacobson, N. S., & Traux, P. (1991). Clinical Significance: A statistical approach to defining meaningful change in psychotherapy research. *Journal of Consulting and Clinical Psychology, 59,* 12–19.

Kajermo, K. N., Nordström, G., Krusebrant, Å., &

Björvell, H. (2000). Perceptions of research utilization: Comparisons between healthcare professionals, nursing students and a reference group of nurse clinicians. *Journal of Advanced Nursing, 31,* 99–109.

Kazdin, A. E. (1977). Assessing the clinical or applied importance of behavior change to social validation. *Behavior Modification, 1,* 427–452.

Kazdin, A. E. (1999). The meanings and measurement of clinical significance. *Journal of Consulting and Clinical Psychology, 67,* 332–339.

Kazdin, A. E., & Matson, J. L. (1981). Social validation in mental retardation. *Applied Research in Mental Retardation, 2,* 39–53.

Kendall, P. C., & Grove, W. M. (1988). Normative comparisons in therapy outcome. *Behavioral Assessment, 10,* 147–158.

Law, M., & Baum, C. (1998). Evidence-based practice occupational therapy. *Canadian Journal of Occupational Therapy, 65,* 131–135.

Lynn, M. R., & Moore, K. (1997). Research utilization by nurse managers: Current practices and future directions. *Seminars for Nurse Managers, 5*(4), 217–223.

Meline, T., & Paradiso, T. (2003). Evidence-based practice in schools: Evaluating research and reducing barriers. *Language, Speech & Hearing Services in Schools, 34,* 273–283.

Metcalfe, C., Lewin, R., Wisher, S., Perry, S., Bannigan, K., & Moffett, J. K. (2001). Barriers to implementing the evidence based in for NHS therapies. *Physiotherapy, 11,* 433–441.

Moseley, A. M., Lanzarone, S., Bosman, J. M., van Loo, M. A., de Bie, R. A., & Hassett, L. (2004). Ecological validity of walking speed assessment after traumatic brain injury: A pilot study. *Journal of Head Trauma Rehabilitation, 19,* 341–348.

Nietzel, M. T., & Trull, T. J. (1998). Meta-analytic approaches to social comparisons: A method for measuring clinical significance. *Behavioral Assessment, 10,* 159–169.

O'Brien, J., Coker, P., Lynn, R., Suppinger, R., Paerigen, T., Rabon, S., St. Aubin, M., & Ward, A. T. (2000). The impact of occupational therapy on a child's playfulness. *Occupational Therapy in Health Care, 12*(2/3), 39–51.

Ottenbacher, K. J., Barris, R., & Van Deusen, J. (1986). Issues related to research utilization in occupational therapy. *The American Journal of Occupational Therapy, 40,* 111–116.

Parahoo, K. (2000). Barriers to, and facilitators of, research utilization among nurses in Northern Ireland. *Journal of Advanced Nursing, 31,* 89–98.

Rogers, E. M. (1995). *Diffusion of innovations* (4th ed.). New York: The Free Press.

Rogers, E. M. (2003). *Diffusion of innovations* (5th ed.). New York: The Free Press.

Sackett, D. L., Rosenberg, W. M. C., Gray, J. A. M., Haynes, R., & Richardson, W. S. (1996). Evidence based medicine: What it is and what it isn't? *British Medical Journal, 312,* 71–72.

Saunders, S. M., Howard, K. I., & Newman, F. L. (1988). Evaluating the clinical significance of treatment effects: Norms and normality. *Behavioral Assessment, 10,* 207–218.

Sbordone, R. J. (1996). Ecological validity: Critical Issues for the neuropsychologist. In R. J. Sbordone & C. J. Long (Eds.), *Ecological validity of neuropsychological testing.* Delray Beach, FL: GR Press/St. Lucie Press.

Schilling, D. L., Washington, K., Billingsley, F. F., & Deitz, J. (2003). Classroom seating for children with attention deficit hyperactivity disorder: Therapy balls versus chairs. *The American Journal of Occupational Therapy, 57,* 534–541.

Schwartz, I. S., & Baer, D. M. (1991). Social validity assessments: Is current practice state of the art? *Journal of Applied Behavior Analysis, 24,* 189–204.

Silver, C. H. (2000). Ecological validity of neuropsychological assessment in childhood traumatic brain injury. *Journal of Head Trauma Rehabilitation, 15,* 973–988.

Snell, M. E. (2003). Applying research to practice: The more pervasive problem? *Research & Practice for Persons with Severe Disabilities, 28*(3), 143–147.

Sudsawad, P. (2004). *Developing a social validation model for effective utilization of disability and rehabilitation research. Project summary.* Submitted to the National Institute of Disability and Rehabilitation Research, US Department of Education, Grant # H133F020023.

Sudsawad, P., Trombly, C. A., Henderson, A., & Tickle-Degnen, L. (2001). The relationship between the Evaluation of Children's Handwriting (ETCH) and teachers' perception of handwriting legibility. *The American Journal of Occupational Therapy, 55,* 518–523.

Sweetland, J., & Craik, C. (2001). The use of evidence-based practice by occupational therapists who treat adult stroke patients. *British Journal of Occupational Therapy, 64,* 256–261.

Tupper, D., & Cicerone, K. (1990). Introduction to the neuropsychology of everyday life. In D. Tupper & K.

Cicerone, *The neuropsychology of everyday life: Assessment and basic competencies.* Boston: Kluwer Academic.

Turner, P., & Whitfield, T. W. A. (1997). Physiotherapists' use of evidence based practice: A cross-national study. *Physiotherapy Research International, 2,* 17–29.

Upton, D., & Lewis, B. (1998). Clinical effectiveness and EBP: Design of a questionnaire. *British Journal of Therapy and Rehabilitation, 5,* 647–650.

Wolf, M. M. (1978). Social validity: The case for subjective measurement or how applied behavior analysis is finding its heart. *Journal of Applied Behavior Analysis, 11,* 203–214.

RESOURCES

Kazdin, A. E. (1999). The meanings and measurement of clinical significance. *Journal of Consulting and Clinical Psychology, 67,* 332–339.

Rogers, E. M. (2003). *Diffusion of Innovations* (5th ed.). New York: The Free Press.

Sbordone, R. J. (1996). Ecological validity: Critical issues for the neuropsychologist. In R. J. Sbordone & C. J. Long (Eds.), *Ecological validity of neuropsychological testing.* Delray Beach, FL: GR Press/St. Lucie Press.

Wolf, M. M. (1978). Social validity: The case for subjective measurement or how applied behavior analysis is finding its heart. *Journal of Applied Behavior Analysis, 11,* 203–214.

Index

Note: Page numbers followed by the letter f refer to figures; those followed by the letter t refer to tables.